149.10

PRINCIPLES and PRACTICE of MOVEMENT DISORDERS

Commissioning Editor: *Lotta Kryhl*
Development Editor: *Louise Cook*
Editorial Assistant: *Kirsten Lowson*
Project Manager: *Joannah Duncan*
Design: *Kirsteen Wright*
Illustration Manager: *Karen Giacomucci*
Illustrator: *Dartmouth Publishing*
Marketing Manager (USA)/(UK): *Helena Mutak/Gaynor Jones*

Video 1.60   Asterixis (negative myoclonus).
Video 1.61   Action and intention myoclonus.
Video 1.62   Palatal myoclonus.
Video 1.63   Palatal myoclonus.
Video 1.64   Ocular myoclonus.
Video 1.65   Opsoclonus (dancing eyes) and mini-polymyoclonus.
Video 1.66   Spinal segmental myoclonus.
Video 1.67   Bouncing gait.
Video 1.68   Myokymia.
Video 1.69   Ocular myorhythmia.
Video 1.70   Faciomasticatory myorhythmia.
Video 1.71   Paroxysmal kinesigenic dyskinesia.
Video 1.72   Paroxysmal nonkinesigenic dyskinesia.
Video 1.73   Tardive dyskinesia (TD).
Video 1.74   Stereotypic hand movements in Rett syndrome.
Video 1.75   Stereotypy.
Video 1.76   Abnormal movements in Kluver–Bucy syndrome.
Video 1.77   Abnormal movements in a boy with normal intelligence.
Video 1.78   Ocular tics.
Video 1.79   Tics in Tourette syndrome.
Video 1.80   Describing the urge to move and produce tics in Tourette syndrome.
Video 1.81   Dystonic tics.
Video 1.82   Tremor at rest.
Video 1.83   Postural and action tremor.
Video 1.84   Intention tremor.
Video 1.85   Orthostatic tremor.
Video 1.86   Dystonic tremor.
Video 1.87   Midbrain tremor.
Video 1.88   Unusual tremor due to Wilson disease.
Video 1.89   Worsening of Wilson disease tremor after initiating penicillamine treatment and improvement with BAL treatment.

CHAPTER 4

Video 4.1   Reemergent tremor.
Video 4.2   Camptocormia.
Video 4.3   Camptocormia.
Video 4.4   Camptocormia.
Video 4.5   Freezing.
Video 4.6   Freezing.

CHAPTER 7

Video 7.1   Deep brain stimulation (DBS) for essential tremor (ET).
Video 7.2   DBS for ET.
Video 7.3   DBS for multiple sclerosis related tremor.
Video 7.4   DBS for PD.
Video 7.5   DBS for PD.
Video 7.6   DBS-induced hemiballism.

CHAPTER 9

Video 9.1   Progressive supranuclear palsy (PSP).
Video 9.2   PSP.
Video 9.3   PSP.
Video 9.4   PSP.
Video 9.5   PSP.
Video 9.6   PSP.
Video 9.7   PSP.
Video 9.8   Multiple system atrophy (MSA).
Video 9.9   MSA.
Video 9.10   Corticobasal degeneration (CBD).
Video 9.11   CBD.
Video 9.12   Lytico-bodig.

CHAPTER 10

Video 10.1   Hemiplegic gait secondary to a stroke.
Video 10.2   Paraplegic gait secondary to hereditary spastic paraplegia.
Video 10.3   Two examples of gait in stiff-person syndrome.
Video 10.4   Ataxic gait in a patient with degenerative ataxia.
Video 10.5   Two examples of gait in patients with dystonia.
Video 10.6   Gait in a patient with Huntington disease.
Video 10.7   Myoclonic gait.
Video 10.8   Three examples of frontal gait.
Video 10.9   Two examples of psychogenic gait.

CHAPTER 11

Video 11.1   Stiff-person syndrome.
Video 11.2   Progressive encephalomyelitis with rigidity.

CHAPTER 12

Video 12.1   Blepharospasm.
Video 12.2   Cervical dystonia.
Video 12.3   Dystonia of leg, with active voluntary movement.
Video 12.4   Writer's cramp.
Video 12.5   Musician's cramp.
Video 12.6   Action focal dystonia of the jaw when chewing.
Video 12.7   Truncal dystonia relieved by dancing or running.
Video 12.8   Truncal dystonia relieved temporarily by placing a hand on the back of the head.
Video 12.9   Retrocollis dystonia relieved by touching the back of the head.
Video 12.10 Postural tremor of the arms associated with dystonia of the arms.
Video 12.11 Generalized torsion dystonia.
Video 12.12 Generalized dystonia.
Video 12.13 Generalized dystonia.
Video 12.14 Generalized dystonia that evolved into a fixed posture.
Video 12.15 Generalized dystonia with inability to walk or crawl.
Video 12.16 Aromatic amino acid decarboxylase deficiency.
Video 12.17 Onset of Oppenheim dystonia involving a leg.
Video 12.18 Worsening of dystonia over time.
Video 12.19 A patient with dopa-responsive dystonia (DRD) in the morning.
Video 12.20 Same patient with DRD, now at night.
Video 12.21 A patient after treatment with levodopa.
Video 12.22 DRD manifesting in infancy.
Video 12.23 Same patient after treatment with levodopa.
Video 12.24 Mother of a patient with DRD who presents with parkinsonism.
Video 12.25 Untreated DRD with onset in childhood, now an adult.
Video 12.26 Myoclonus–dystonia in a boy.
Video 12.27 Myoclonus–dystonia in the father of the previous boy.
Video 12.28 Lubag causing severe oromandibular dystonia.
Video 12.29 Lubag with parkinsonism and lingual dystonia.

CHAPTER 13

Video 13.1   Botulinum toxin (BTX) in cranial dystonia.
Video 13.2   BTX in cervical dystonia.
Video 13.3   BTX in anterocollis.
Video 13.4   Bilateral pallidotomy for generalized dystonia.
Video 13.5   Bilateral DBS for generalized dystonia.
Video 13.6   Bilateral pallidotomy for generalized dystonia.

CHAPTER 14

Video 14.1   Huntington disease (HD).
Video 14.2   HD.
Video 14.3   HD.

Video 14.4   HD.
Video 14.5   HD.
Video 14.6   HD.
Video 14.7   HD.
Video 14.8   HD.
Video 14.9   HD.
Video 14.10   HD.
Video 14.11   HD.
Video 14.12   HD.
Video 14.13   HD.

CHAPTER 15

Video 15.1   Dentatorubral-pallidoluysian atrophy (DRPLA).
Video 15.2   Neuroacanthocytosis.
Video 15.3   Sydenham disease.
Video 15.4   Sydenham disease.
Video 15.5   Levodopa-induced dyskinesia.
Video 15.6   Post-pump chorea.
Video 15.7   Post-pump chorea.
Video 15.8   Hepatic chorea.
Video 15.9   Ballism.
Video 15.10   Ballism.
Video 15.11   Cerebral palsy.

CHAPTER 16

Video 16.1   Facial tics.
Video 16.2   Cervical tics.
Video 16.3   Shoulder tics.
Video 16.4   Limb tics.
Video 16.5   Truncal-abdominal tics.
Video 16.6   Complex tics.
Video 16.7   Simple phonic tics.
Video 16.8   Complex phonic tics.
Video 16.9   Shoulder tics.
Video 16.10   Tonic (isometric) tics.
Video 16.11   Blocking tics.
Video 16.12   Complex motor tics.
Video 16.13   Complex motor tics.
Video 16.14   Peripherally induced tics.
Video 16.15   Coprolalia.
Video 16.16   Self-injurious behavior.
Video 16.17   Self-injurious behavior.
Video 16.18   Tics and tardive dystonia.
Video 16.19   Treatment with botulinum toxin.

CHAPTER 17

Video 17.1   Animal stereotypies.
Video 17.2   Self-gratifying behavior.
Video 17.3   Lesch–Nyhan syndrome.
Video 17.4   Lesch–Nyhan syndrome.
Video 17.5   Rett syndrome.
Video 17.6   Rett syndrome.
Video 17.7   Williams syndrome.
Video 17.8   Subacute sclerosing panencephalitis.
Video 17.9   Tardive akathisia.

CHAPTER 18

Video 18.1   Reemergent tremor.
Video 18.2   Task-specific tremor.
Video 18.3   Task-specific tremor.
Video 18.4   Cerebellar outflow tremor.
Video 18.5   Orthostatic tremor.
Video 18.6   Dystonic tremor.
Video 18.7   Dystonic tremor.
Video 18.8   Psychogenic tremor.
Video 18.9   Hereditary chin tremor.

CHAPTER 19

Video 19.1   Withdrawal emergent syndrome.
Video 19.2   Withdrawal emergent syndrome.
Video 19.3   Oral-buccal-lingual dyskinesia.
Video 19.4   Oral-buccal-lingual dyskinesia with tongue popping.
Video 19.5   Rhythmic rocking movements of the trunk and marching in place.
Video 19.6   Segmental jaw, neck, and arm dystonia, along with classic oral-buccal-lingual dyskinesia.
Video 19.7   Retrocollis as the feature of tardive dystonia.
Video 19.8   Retrocollis, opisthotonus, internal rotation of the arms, extension of the elbows, and flexion of the wrists.
Video 19.9   A combination of dystonia with myoclonic or ballistic movements.
Video 19.10   Moaning as a manifestation of tardive akathisia.
Video 19.11   A combination of tardive dyskinesia and tardive akathisia.
Video 19.12   A combination of tardive dyskinesia, tardive dystonia, and tardive akathisia.

CHAPTER 20

Video 20.1   Examples of different types of myoclonus.
Video 20.2   Examples of negative myoclonus.
Video 20.3   Spinal myoclonus.
Video 20.4   Different types of palatal myoclonus (palatal tremor).
Video 20.5   Cortical tremor.
Video 20.6   Examples of propriospinal myoclonus.
Video 20.7   Hereditary hyperekplexia.
Video 20.8   Latah.
Video 20.9   Posthypoxic myoclonus.
Video 20.10   Negative myoclonus and bouncy gait from posthypoxic myoclonus.
Video 20.11   Subacute sclerosing panencephalitis.
Video 20.12   Opsoclonus–myoclonus syndrome.
Video 20.13   Dystonic myoclonus.
Video 20.14   Psychogenic myoclonus.

CHAPTER 22

Video 22.1   Paroxysmal torticollis in infancy.
Video 22.2   Paroxysmal dystonia in infancy.
Video 22.3   Primary paroxysmal kinesigenic dyskinesia.
Video 22.4   Secondary paroxysmal kinesigenic dyskinesia.
Video 22.5   Primary paroxysmal nonkinesigenic dyskinesia (PNKD).
Video 22.6   Psychogenic PNKD.
Video 22.7   Secondary PNKD.
Video 22.8   Paroxysmal exertional dyskinesia.
Video 22.9   A burst of stereotypic arm and hand wiggling.
Video 22.10   Paroxysmal self-stimulatory behavior.

CHAPTER 23

Video 23.1   Periodic limb movements.
Video 23.2   Hemifacial spasm.
Video 23.3   Jumpy stumps.
Video 23.4   Belly dancer's dyskinesia.
Video 23.5   Painful feet and moving toes.
Video 23.6   Painful arm and moving fingers.
Video 23.7   Peripheral dystonia.

CHAPTER 24

Video 24.1   Examples of Wilson disease.

CHAPTER 25

Video 25.1   Task-specific jaw tremor.
Video 25.2   Head shaking.
Video 25.3   Shaking movements and abnormal postures.
Video 25.4   Paroxysmal tremor.
Video 25.5   Delayed startle, utterances of gibberish.
Video 25.6   Bent gait, episodes of shaking, startle reaction with gibberish.
Video 25.7   Jumping Frenchman syndrome.
Video 25.8   Dystonic postures that persist in sleep.
Video 25.9   Dystonia with fixed contractures.
Video 25.10   Tremors of the hands.
Video 25.11   Deliberate slowness, psychogenic parkinsonism.

PRINCIPLES and PRACTICE of MOVEMENT DISORDERS | SECOND EDITION

Stanley Fahn

MD

H. Houston Merritt Professor of Neurology and Director, Center for Parkinson's Disease and Other Movement Disorders, Department of Neurology, Columbia University Medical Center, The Neurological Institute, New York, New York

Joseph Jankovic

MD

Professor of Neurology, Distinguished Chair in Movement Disorders, Director, Parkinson's Disease Center, and Movement Disorders Clinic, Department of Neurology, Baylor College of Medicine, Houston, Texas

Mark Hallett

MD

Editor in Chief, World Neurology, World Federation of Neurology, Bethesda, Maryland

ELSEVIER
SAUNDERS   Edinburgh   London   New York   Oxford   Philadelphia   St Louis   Sydney   Toronto

ELSEVIER
SAUNDERS

SAUNDERS is an imprint of Elsevier Inc.

© 2011, Stanley Fahn, Joseph Jankovic and Mark Hallett.
Published by Saunders, an imprint of Elsevier Inc. All rights reserved.

First edition 2007

Notices

Knowledge and best practice in this field are constantly changing. As new research and experience broaden our understanding, changes in research methods, professional practices, or medical treatment may become necessary.

Practitioners and researchers must always rely on their own experience and knowledge in evaluating and using any information, methods, compounds, or experiments described herein. In using such information or methods they should be mindful of their own safety and the safety of others, including parties for whom they have a professional responsibility.

With respect to any drug or pharmaceutical products identified, readers are advised to check the most current information provided (i) on procedures featured or (ii) by the manufacturer of each product to be administered, to verify the recommended dose or formula, the method and duration of administration, and contraindications. It is the responsibility of practitioners, relying on their own experience and knowledge of their patients, to make diagnoses, to determine dosages and the best treatment for each individual patient, and to take all appropriate safety precautions.

To the fullest extent of the law, neither the Publisher nor the authors, contributors, or editors, assume any liability for any injury and/or damage to persons or property as a matter of products liability, negligence or otherwise, or from any use or operation of any methods, products, instructions, or ideas contained in the material herein.

British Library Cataloguing in Publication Data
Fahn, Stanley, 1933–
Principles and practice of movement disorders. – 2nd ed.
1. Movement disorders.
I. Title   II. Jankovic, Joseph.   III. Hallett, Mark, 1943–
616.7 – dc22

ISBN-13: 9781437723694
Printed in China
Last digit is the print number: 9   8   7   6   5   4   3   2   1

ELSEVIER your source for books, journals and multimedia in the health sciences
www.elsevierhealth.com

Working together to grow
libraries in developing countries

www.elsevier.com | www.bookaid.org | www.sabre.org

ELSEVIER   BOOK AID International   Sabre Foundation

The publisher's policy is to use **paper manufactured from sustainable forests**

Dedication

We dedicate this book to our loving wives and families in acknowledgment of their understanding and support. We also hope that the book will honor the memory of our close friend and colleague David Marsden.

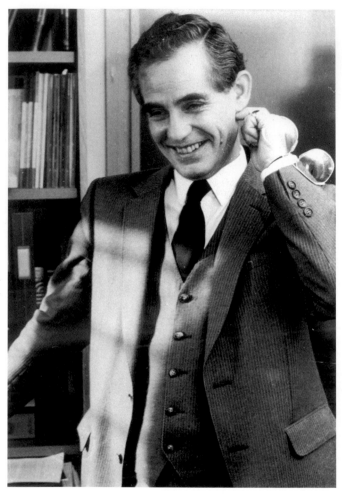

C. David Marsden (1938–1998)

The impetus for this monograph comes directly from the success of "Movement Disorders for the Clinical Practitioner," a continuing medical education course that has been held in Aspen, Colorado, each summer since 1990. The trio of Fahn, Marsden, and Jankovic originated and lectured in the course until Marsden's untimely death. C. David Marsden, DSc, MB, FRCP was professor and head of the Department of Clinical Neurology at the Institute of Neurology in Queen Square, London. Dividing the lectures equally, the three covered the entire field of movement disorders in four half-day sessions that included a large sampling of videos to demonstrate the variety of movement disorders that a neurologist in practice may encounter.

As the course continued to grow in popularity, the three decided to produce a textbook of movement disorders, using as a starting point the annually updated course syllabus. They determined that the book would be not a collection of overlapping chapters by different authors but an integrated work in which the tasks of writing and editing were shared among the three as co-authors. The project began, but it came to a halt on September 29, 1998, with the untimely death of Professor Marsden.

To continue the Aspen course, Fahn and Jankovic invited Mark Hallett, MD, chief of the Human Motor Control Section at the National Institute of Neurological Diseases and Stroke in Bethesda, Maryland (who had trained in the clinical physiology of movement disorders with Professor Marsden), and neuropharmacologist Peter Jenner, PhD (Professor Marsden's longtime colleague and collaborator), to join the faculty and share in delivering the majority of the lectures that Professor Marsden had given. In subsequent years, through 2008, Drs Hallett and Jenner continually updated the portion of the course syllabus that was originally written by Dr Marsden and also incorporated additional topics.

When the book project was resumed, Fahn and Jankovic determined to retain the principle of an integrated work, taking on the responsibility of editing the chapters written by all four authors by incorporating the contributions from Drs Hallett and Jenner. This resulted in the first edition of this book, published in 2007.

Beginning in 2009, the faculty of the Aspen course resumed the three-person format for teaching the course, with Dr Hallett joining Fahn and Jankovic as an equal partner. All three of us have been responsible for lecturing, annually updating the syllabus, and now writing specific sections of the second edition of this book, and each has edited and contributed to all the chapters so that the final product remains an integrated whole.

The three of us greatly miss the intellectual and personal interaction that we enjoyed with our close friend and collaborator David Marsden for so many years and we, therefore, dedicate this book to his memory. We believe that he would be gratified with the extraordinary success of the first edition. This second edition of the book provides a comprehensive update of our current understanding of Parkinson disease and other movement disorders. The main stimulus for preparing this second edition has come from our desire to highlight the rapidly expanding knowledge in the field of movement disorders with clinical, scientific, and therapeutic advances taking place at breath-taking speed. In presenting treatment options, the second edition continues to emphasize evidence based on randomized, controlled trials while also sharing the authors' personal experiences when such data are lacking. We believe this combination of evidence-based medicine and practical "know-how" will greatly aid clinical practitioners in caring for their patients.

The text is divided into three sections – overview, hypokinetic disorders, and hyperkinetic disorders – following the organization of the Aspen course. It is accompanied by an expanded collection of videos – videos from the Aspen course supplemented by new videos that illustrate the rich phenomenology and etiology of movement disorders and provide a visual guide to this most therapeutically oriented specialty of neurology. We hope that readers find the volume comprehensive, current, and enjoyable.

Stanley Fahn MD
Joseph Jankovic MD
Mark Hallett MD
July 2011

Contents

SECTION I: Overview

   1. Clinical overview and phenomenology of movement disorders   1
   2. Motor control: Physiology of voluntary and involuntary movements   36
   3. Functional neuroanatomy of the basal ganglia   55

SECTION II: Hypokinetic disorders

   4. Parkinsonism: Clinical features and differential diagnosis   66
   5. Current concepts on the etiology and pathogenesis of Parkinson disease   93
   6. Medical treatment of Parkinson disease   119
   7. Surgical treatment of Parkinson disease and other movement disorders   157
   8. Nonmotor problems in Parkinson disease   183
   9. Atypical parkinsonism, parkinsonism-plus syndromes, and secondary parkinsonian disorders   197
  10. Gait disorders: Pathophysiology and clinical syndromes   241
  11. Stiffness syndromes   250

SECTION III: Hyperkinetic disorders

  12. Dystonia: Phenomenology, classification, etiology, pathology, biochemistry, and genetics   259
  13. Treatment of dystonia   293
  14. Huntington disease   311
  15. Chorea, ballism, and athetosis   335
  16. Tics and Tourette syndrome   350
  17. Stereotypies   380
  18. Tremors   389
  19. The tardive syndromes: Phenomenology, concepts on pathophysiology and treatment, and other neuroleptic-induced syndromes   415
  20. Myoclonus: Phenomenology, etiology, physiology, and treatment   447
  21. Ataxia: Pathophysiology and clinical syndromes   465
  22. The paroxysmal dyskinesias   476
  23. Restless legs and peripheral movement disorders   496
  24. Wilson disease   507
  25. Psychogenic movement disorders: Phenomenology, diagnosis, and treatment   513

   Index   528

CHAPTER **1**

Clinical overview and phenomenology of movement disorders

Chapter contents

Fundamentals	1	Differential diagnosis of dyskinesias	25
Differential diagnosis of hypokinesias	18	The clinical approach to differentiate the dyskinesias	32
Evaluation of a dyskinesia	24	Conclusions	34

To study the phenomenon of disease without books is to sail an uncharted sea, while to study books without patients is not to go to sea at all.

Sir William Osler

Fundamentals

The quotation from William Osler is an apt introduction to this chapter, which offers a description of the various phenomenologies of movement disorders. Movement disorders can be defined as neurologic syndromes in which there is either an excess of movement or a paucity of voluntary and automatic movements, unrelated to weakness or spasticity (Table 1.1). The former are commonly referred to as *hyperkinesias* (excessive movements), *dyskinesias* (unnatural movements), and *abnormal involuntary movements*. In this text, the term *dyskinesias* is used most often, but all are interchangeable. The five major categories of dyskinesias in alphabetical order are chorea, dystonia, myoclonus, tics, and tremor. Table 1.1 presents the complete list.

The paucity of movement group can be referred to as *hypokinesia* (decreased amplitude of movement), but *bradykinesia* (slowness of movement), and *akinesia* (loss of movement) could be reasonable alternative names. The parkinsonian syndromes are the most common cause of such paucity of movement; other hypokinetic disorders represent only a small group of patients. Basically, movement disorders can be conveniently divided into parkinsonism and all other types; each of these two groups has about an equal number of patients.

Distinguishing between organic and psychogenic causation requires expertise in recognizing the various phenomenologies. Psychogenic movement disorders are covered in Chapter 25.

Those who are interested in keeping up-to-date in the field of movement disorders should refer to the journal *Movement Disorders*, published 12 times per year by The Movement Disorder Society, Inc. (www.movementdisorders.org). The journal, which is accompanied by two DVDs per year, comes with Movement Disorder Society membership, which is open to all interested medical professionals.

Categories of movements

It is important to note that not all of the hyperkinesias in Table 1.1 are technically classified as abnormal involuntary movements, commonly called AIMS. Movements can be categorized into one of four classes: *automatic*, *voluntary*, *semivoluntary* (also called *unvoluntary*) (Lang, 1991; Tourette Syndrome Classification Study Group, 1993; Fahn, 2005), and *involuntary* (Jankovic, 1992). *Automatic* movements are learned motor behaviors that are performed without conscious effort, e.g., walking an accustomed route, and tapping of the fingers when thinking about something else. *Voluntary* movements are intentional (planned or self-initiated) or externally triggered (in response to some external stimulus; e.g., turning the head toward a loud noise or withdrawing a hand from a hot plate). Intentional voluntary movements are preceded by the Bereitschaftspotential (or readiness potential), a slow negative potential recorded over the supplementary motor area and contralateral premotor and motor cortex appearing 1–1.5 seconds prior to the movement. The Bereitschaftspotential does not appear with other movements, including the externally triggered voluntary movements (Papa et al., 1991). In some cases, learned voluntary motor skills are incorporated within the repertoire of the movement disorder, such as camouflaging choreic movements or tics by immediately following them with voluntarily executed movements, so-called parakinesias. *Semivoluntary* (or *unvoluntary*) movements are induced by an inner sensory

DOI: 10.1016/B978-1-4377-2369-4.00001-9

Table 1.1 Movement disorders

Hypokinesias

Akinesia/bradykinesia (parkinsonism)

Apraxia

Blocking (holding) tics

Cataplexy and drop attacks

Catatonia, psychomotor depression, and obsessional slowness

Freezing phenomenon

Hesitant gaits

Hypothyroid slowness

Rigidity

Stiff muscles

Hyperkinesias

Abdominal dyskinesias

Akathitic movements

Ataxia/asynergia/dysmetria

Athetosis

Ballism

Chorea

Dystonia

Hemifacial spasm

Hyperekplexia

Hypnogenic dyskinesias

Jumping disorders

Jumpy stumps

Moving toes and fingers

Myoclonus

Myokymia and synkinesis

Myorhythmia

Paroxysmal dyskinesias

Periodic movements in sleep

REM sleep behavior disorder

Restless legs

Stereotypy

Tics

Tremor

within the cerebral hemispheres (caudate, putamen, and pallidum), the diencephalon (subthalamic nucleus), the mesencephalon (substantia nigra), and the mesencephalic-pontine junction (pedunculopontine nucleus) (see Chapter 3). There are some exceptions to this general rule. Pathology of the cerebellum or its pathways typically results in impairment of coordination (asynergy, ataxia), misjudgment of distance (dysmetria), and intention tremor. Myoclonus and many forms of tremors do not appear to be related primarily to basal ganglia pathology, and often arise elsewhere in the central nervous system, including cerebral cortex (cortical reflex myoclonus), brainstem (cerebellar outflow tremor, reticular reflex myoclonus, hyperekplexia, and rhythmical brainstem myoclonus such as palatal myoclonus and ocular myoclonus), and spinal cord (rhythmical segmental myoclonus and non-rhythmic propriospinal myoclonus). Moreover, many myoclonic disorders are associated with diseases in which the cerebellum is involved, such as those causing the Ramsay Hunt syndrome of progressive myoclonic ataxia (see Chapter 20). The peripheral nervous system can give rise to abnormal movements also, such as the painful legs–moving toes syndrome (Marsden, 1994). It is not known for certain which part of the brain is associated with tics, although the basal ganglia and the limbic structures have been implicated. Certain localizations within the basal ganglia are classically associated with specific movement disorders: substantia nigra with bradykinesia and rest tremor; subthalamic nucleus with ballism; caudate nucleus with chorea; and putamen with dystonia.

Historical perspective

The neurologic literature contains a number of seminal papers, reviews and books that emphasized and established movement disorders as associated with the basal ganglia pathology (Alzheimer, 1911; Fischer, 1911; Wilson, 1912; Hunt, 1917; Vogt and Vogt, 1920; Jakob, 1923; Putnam et al., 1940; Denny-Brown, 1962; Martin, 1967).

An historical perspective of movement disorders can be gained by listing the dates when the various clinical entities were first introduced (Table 1.2).

Epidemiology

Movement disorders are common neurologic problems, and epidemiological studies are available for some of them (Table 1.3). There have been several studies for Parkinson disease (PD), and these have been carried out in several countries (Tanner, 1994; de Lau and Breteler, 2006). Table 1.3 lists the prevalence rates of some movement disorders based on studies in the United States. The frequency of different types of movement disorders seen in the two specialty clinics at Columbia University and Baylor College of Medicine are presented in Table 1.4. More detailed information is provided in the relevant chapters for specific diseases.

stimulus (e.g., need to "stretch" a body part or need to scratch an itch) or by an unwanted feeling or compulsion (e.g., compulsive touching or smelling). Many of the movements occurring as tics or as a response to various sensations (e.g., akathisia and the restless legs syndrome) can be considered unvoluntary because the movements are usually the result of an action to nullify an unwanted, unpleasant sensation. Unvoluntary movements usually are suppressible. *Involuntary* movements are often non-suppressible (e.g., most tremors and myoclonus), but some can be partially suppressible (e.g., some tremors, chorea, dystonia, stereotypies and some tics) (Koller and Biary, 1989).

The origins of abnormal movements

Many movement disorders are associated with pathologic alterations in the basal ganglia or their connections. The basal ganglia are that group of gray matter nuclei lying deep

Genetics

A large number of movement disorders are genetic in etiology, and many of the diseases have now been mapped to specific regions of the genome, and some have even been

Table 1.2 Some notable historical descriptions of movement disorders

Year	Source	Entity	Year	Source	Entity
	Bible	Reference to tremor in the aged	1916	Henneberg	Cataplexy
		Trembling associated with fear and strong emotion	1917	Hunt	Progressive pallidal atrophy
1567	Paracelsus	Mercury-induced tremor	1920	Creutzfeldt	Creutzfeldt–Jakob disease
1652	Tulpius	Spasmodic torticollis	1921	Jakob	Creutzfeldt–Jakob disease
1685	Willis	Restless legs syndrome	1921	Hunt	Dyssynergia cerebellaris myoclonica (Ramsay Hunt syndrome)
1686	Sydenham	Sydenham chorea			
1817	Parkinson	Parkinson disease	1922	Hallervorden/Spatz	Pantothenate kinase deficiency (neurodegenerative disorder with brain iron deposition-1)
1825	Itard	Tourette syndrome			
1830	Bell	Writer's cramp			
1837	Couper	Manganese-induced parkinsonism	1923	Sicard	Akathisia
1848	Grisolle	Primary writing tremor	1924	Fleischhacker	Striatonigral degeneration
1871	Hammond	Athetosis	1926	Davidenkow	Myoclonic dystonia
1871	Traube	Spastic dysphonia	1927	Goldsmith	Hereditary chin quivering
1871	Steinthal	Apraxia	1927	Orzechowski	Opsoclonus
1872	Huntington	Huntington disease	1931	Herz	Myorhythmia
1872	Mitchell	Jumpy stumps	1931	Guillain/Mollaret	Palato-pharyngo-laryngo-oculo-diaphragmatic myoclonus
1874	Kahlbaum	Catatonia			
1878	Beard	Jumpers	1932	De Lisi	Hypnic jerks
1881	Friedreich	Myoclonus	1933	Spiller	Fear of falling
1885	Gilles de la Tourette	Tourette syndrome	1933	Scherer	Striatonigral degeneration
1885	Gowers	Paroxysmal kinesigenic choreoathetosis	1940	Mount/Reback	Paroxysmal nonkinesigenic dyskinesia (paroxysmal dystonic choreoathetosis)
1886	Spencer	Palatal myoclonus			
1887	Dana	Hereditary tremor	1941	Louis-Bar	Ataxia-telangiectasia
1887	Wood	Cranial dystonia	1943	Kanner	Autism
1889	Benedikt	Benedikt syndrome	1944	Asperger	Autism
1891	Unverricht	Progressive myoclonus epilepsy (Unverricht–Lundborg disease)	1946	Titeca/van Bogaert	Dentatorubral-pallidoluysian degeneration
1895	Schultze	Myokymia	1949	Alexander	Alexander disease
1900	Dejerine/Thomas	Olivopontocerebellar atrophy	1953	Adams/Foley	Asterixis
1900	Liepmann	Apraxia	1953	Symonds	Nocturnal myoclonus (periodic movements in sleep)
1901	Haskovec	Akathisia			
1903	Batten	Neuronal ceroid lipofuscinosis	1954	Davison	Pallido-pyramidal syndrome (PARK15)
1904	Holmes	Midbrain ("rubral") tremor			
1908	Schwalbe	Familial dystonia	1956	Moersch/Woltman	Stiff-person syndrome
1910	Meige	Oromandibular dystonia	1957	Schonecker	Tardive dyskinesia
1911	Oppenheim	Dystonia musculorum deformans	1958	Kirstein/Silfverskiold	Startle disease (hyperekplexia)
1911	Lafora	Lafora disease	1958	Smith et al.	Dentatorubral-pallidoluysian degeneration
1912	Wilson	Wilson disease	1958	Monrad-Krohn/Refsum	Myorhythmia
1914	Lewy	Lewy bodies in Parkinson disease	1959	Paulson	Acute dystonic reaction
			1960	Ekbom	Restless legs

Continued

Table 1.2 Continued

Year	Source	Entity	Year	Source	Entity
1960	Shy/Drager	Dysautonomia with parkinsonism (multiple system atrophy)	1977	Hallett et al.	Reticular myoclonus
			1978	Satoyoshi	Satoyoshi syndrome
1961	Hirano et al.	Parkinsonism-dementia complex of Guam	1978	Fahn	Tardive akathisia
1961	Andermann et al.	Facial myokymia	1979	Hallett et al.	Cortical myoclonus
1961	Isaacs	Neuromyotonia, Isaacs syndrome	1979	Rothwell et al.	Primary writing tremor
1962	Kinsbourne	Opsoclonus-myoclonus	1980	Fukuhara et al.	Myoclonus epilepsy associated with ragged red fibers (MERFF)
1963	Lance/Adams	Posthypoxic action myoclonus			
1964	Adams et al.	Striatonigral degeneration	1980	Coleman et al.	Periodic movements in sleep
1964	Steele et al.	Progressive supranuclear palsy	1981	Fahn/Singh	Oscillatory myoclonus
1964	Levine	Neuroacanthocytosis	1981	Lugaresi/Cirignotta	Hypnogenic paroxysmal dystonia
1964	Kinsbourne	Sandifer syndrome	1982	Burke et al.	Tardive dystonia
1964	Lesch/Nyhan	Lesch–Nyhan syndrome	1983	Langston et al.	MPTP-induced parkinsonism
1965	Hakim/Adams	Normal pressure hydrocephalus	1984	Heilman	Orthostatic tremor
1965	Goldstein/Cogan	Apraxia of lid opening	1985	Aronson	Breathy dysphonia
1966	Suhren et al.	Hyperekplexia	1986	Bressman et al.	Biotin-responsive myoclonus
1966	Rett	Rett syndrome	1986	Schenck et al.	REM sleep behavior disorder
1967	Haerer et al.	Hereditary nonprogressive chorea	1986	Schwartz et al.	Oculomasticatory myorhythmia
1968	Rebeiz et al.	Cortical-basal ganglionic degeneration	1987	Tominaga et al.	Tardive myoclonus
			1987	Little/Jankovic	Tardive myoclonus
1968	Delay/Denniker	Neuroleptic malignant syndrome	1990	Iliceto et al.	Abdominal dyskinesias
1969	Horner/Jackson	Hypnogenic paroxysmal dyskinesias	1990	Ikeda et al.	Cortical tremor/myoclonus
1969	Graham/Oppenheimer	Multiple system atrophy	1991c	Brown et al.	Propriospinal myoclonus
			1991	Hymas et al.	Obsessional slowness
1970	Spiro	Minipolymyoclonus	1991	De Vivo et al.	GLUT1 deficiency syndrome
1970	Ritchie	Jumpy stumps	1992	Stacy/Jankovic	Tardive tremor
1971	Spillane et al.	Painful legs and moving toes	1993	Bhatia et al.	Causalgia-dystonia
1975	Perry et al.	Familial parkinsonism with hypoventilation and mental depression	1993	Atchison et al.	Primary freezing gait
			1993	Achiron et al.	Primary freezing gait
1976	Segawa et al.	Dopa-responsive dystonia	2002	Namekawa et al.	Adult-onset Alexander disease
1976	Allen/Knopp	Dopa-responsive dystonia	2002	Okamoto et al.	Adult-onset Alexander disease

Other important dates in the history of movement disorders are 1912, the coining of the term "extrapyramidal" by Wilson; 1985, the founding of the Movement Disorder Society, and 1986, the publication of the first issue of the journal, *Movement Disorders*.

localized to a specific gene (Table 1.5). For example, ten genetic loci have so far been identified with Parkinson disease (PD) or variants of classic PD (PARK4 is a triplication of the normal α-synuclein gene, for which mutations are listed as PARK1). Several genetic loci of movement disorders have been identified with a specific gene and protein. A comprehensive list of movement disorders whose genes have been mapped or identified are listed in Table 1.5. A detailed

chapter (Harris and Fahn, 2003) and an entire book (Pulst, 2003) have been published specifically related to movement disorder genetics. Several inherited movement disorders are due to expanded repeats of the trinucleotide cytosine-adenosine-guanosine (CAG), and Friedreich ataxia is due to the expanded trinucleotide repeat of guanosine-adenosine-adenosine (GAA). Normal individuals contain an acceptable number of these trinucleotide repeats in their genes, but

Table 1.3 Prevalence of movement disorders

Disorder	Rate per 100 000	Reference
Restless legs	9800*	Rothdach et al. (2000)
Essential tremor	415	Haerer et al. (1982)
Parkinson disease	187[†]	Kurland (1958)
Tourette syndrome	29–1052	Caine et al. (1988), Comings et al. (1990)
	2990	Mason et al. (1998)
Primary torsion dystonia	33	Nutt et al. (1988)
Hemifacial spasm	7.4–14.5	Auger and Whisnant (1990)
Blepharospasm	13.3	Defazio et al. (2001)
Hereditary ataxia	6	Schoenberg (1978)
Huntington disease	2–12	Harper (1992), Kokmen et al. (1994)
Wilson disease	3	Reilly et al. (1993)
Progressive supranuclear palsy	2	Golbe (1994)
	2.4	Nath et al. (2001)
	6.4	Schrag et al. (1999)
Multiple system atrophy	4.4	Schrag et al. (1999)

Rates are given per 100 000 population. *For restless legs, the rate cited is in a population 65–83 years of age. [†]For Parkinson disease, the rate is 347 per 100 000 for ages over 39 years (Schoenberg et al., 1985).

Table 1.4 The prevalence of movement disorders encountered in two large movement disorder clinics

Movement disorder	Number of patients	Percent	Movement disorder	Number of patients	Percent
Parkinsonism	**15 107**	**35.3**	Cerebellar	205	
Parkinson disease	10 182		Midbrain ("rubral")	88	
Progressive supranuclear palsy	750		Primary writing	114	
Multiple system atrophy	841		Orthostatic	82	
Cortical-basal ganglionic degeneration	297		Other	1035	
Vascular	867		**Tics (Tourette syndrome)**	**2753**	**6.4**
Drug-induced	327		**Chorea**	**1225**	**2.9**
Hemiparkinsonism–hemiatrophy	116		Huntington disease	690	
Gait disorder	329		Hemiballism	123	
Other	1308		Other	412	
Dystonia	**10 394**	**24.3**	**Tardive syndromes**	**1253**	**2.9**
Primary dystonia	7784		**Myoclonus**	**1020**	**2.4**
Focal		(59%)	**Hemifacial spasm**	**693**	**1.6**
Segmental		(29%)	**Ataxia**	**764**	**1.9**
Generalized		(12%)	**Paroxysmal dyskinesias**	**474**	**1.1**
Secondary dystonia	6610		**Stereotypies (other than TD)**	**246**	**0.6**
Hemidystonia	279		**Restless legs syndrome**	**807**	**1.9**
Tardive	595		**Stiff-person syndrome**	**70**	**0.2**
Other	1737		**Psychogenic movement disorder**	**1268**	**3.0**
Tremor	**6754**	**15.8**	**Grand total**	**42 826**	**100**
Essential tremor	2818				

The above data were obtained from the combined databases of the Movement Disorder Clinics at Columbia University Medical Center (New York City) and Baylor College of Medicine (Houston) for patients encountered through April 2009. Because some patients might have more than one type of movement disorder (such as a combination of essential tremor and Parkinson disease), they would be listed more than once. Therefore, the figures in the table represent the types of movement disorder phenomenology encountered in two large clinics, rather than the exact number of patients.

Table 1.5 Gene localization of movement disorders

Disease	Pattern of inheritance	Chromosome region	Name of gene	Gene identified	Triplet repeat	Name of protein	Function of protein
Parkinson disease							
(1) Familial Parkinson disease	Autosomal dominant	4q21.3	SNCA (PARK1)	Yes	No	α-Synuclein	Synaptic protein
(2) Young-onset Parkinson disease	Autosomal recessive/ dominant	6q25.2–q27	PARKIN (PARK2)	Yes	No	Parkin	Ubiquitin-protein ligase
(3) Susceptibility locus	Autosomal dominant	2p13	PARK3	No	N/I	N/I	N/I
(4) Familial Parkinson disease	Autosomal dominant	4q21	SNCA (PARK4)	Yes	No	Duplication or triplication of α-synuclein region of chromosome	Excess amount of normal α-synuclein
(5) Familial Parkinson disease	Autosomal recessive	4p14	UCHL1 (PARK5)	Yes	No	Ubiquitin carboxy-terminal hydrolase L1	Splits conjugated ubiquitin into monomers
(6) Young-onset Parkinson disease	Autosomal recessive	1p36	PINK1 (PARK6)	Yes	No	PTEN-induced putative kinase 1 (PINK1)	Mitochondrial, anti-stress-induced degeneration
(7) Young-onset Parkinson disease	Autosomal recessive	1p36	DJ-1 (PARK7)	Yes	No	DJ-1	Oxidative stress sensor; supports anti-oxidation
(8) Familial Parkinson disease	Autosomal dominant	12q12	LRRK2 (PARK8)	Yes	No	LRRK2, dardarin	Phosphorylates proteins
(9) Kufor-Rakeb syndrome	Autosomal recessive	1p36	ATP13A2 (PARK9)	Yes	No	ATP13A2	Maintains acid pH in lysosome
(10) Familial Parkinson disease	Autosomal recessive	1p32	PARK10 (Iceland)	No	No	N/I	N/I
(11) Familial Parkinson disease	Autosomal dominant	2q21.2	PARK11 (GIGYF2 in doubt)	Yes (in doubt)	No	GRB10-Interacting GYF protein 2 (in doubt)	N/I
(12) Familial Parkinson disease	X-linked recessive	Xq21–q25	PARK12	No	No	N/I	N/I
(13) Familial Parkinson disease	Autosomal dominant	2p12	HTRA2 (PARK13)	Yes	No	High temperature requirement protein A2 (HTRA2)	Serome protease in endoplasmic reticulum and mitochondria
(14) Familial parkinsonism–dystonia (infantile neuroaxonal dystrophy) (NBIA-2) (also known as adult-onset dystonia–parkinsonism without iron)	Autosomal recessive	22q13.1	PLA2G6 (PARK14)	Yes	No	Phospholipase A2	Releases fatty acids from phospholipids
(15) Early-onset pallido (parkinsonian)–pyramidal syndrome	Autosomal recessive	22q12–q13	FBXO7 (PARK15)	Yes	No	Component of modular E3 ubiquitin protein ligases	Functions in phosphorylation-dependent ubiquitination
(16) Familial Parkinson disease	unknown	1q32	PARK16	?	?	?	?

Table 1.5 Continued

Disease	Pattern of inheritance	Chromosome region	Name of gene	Gene identified	Triplet repeat	Name of protein	Function of protein
(17) Familial Parkinson disease	?	3q26–27	EIF4G1	Yes	?	Eukaryotic initiation factor	Facilitates the recruitment of mRNA to the ribosome
(18) Familial Parkinson disease	Autosomal dominant (homozygous → Gaucher disease)	1q21	GBA	Yes	No	β-glucocerebrosidase	Metabolizes membrane lipid glucosyl ceramide to ceramide and glucose
(19) Familial Parkinson disease	Autosomal dominant	2q22–q23	NR4A2	Yes	No	Nurr1	DA cell development; transcription activator
(20) Perry syndrome (familial parkinsonism with hypoventilation and depression)	Autosomal dominant	2p13	DCTN1	Yes	No	Dynactin 1	Cellular transport functions, including axonal transport
(21) Infantile/ Childhood Parkinson disease	Autosomal recessive	11p15.5	TH	Yes	No	Tyrosine hydroxylase	Converts tyrosine to levodopa
Dopa-responsive dystonia (DRD) – see (109) in Dystonia section							
SCA2 – see (66) in Ataxia section							
SCA17 (susceptibility factor) – see (80) in Ataxia section (Kim et al., 2009)							
(22) Infantile parkinsonism-dystonia	Autosomal dominant	5p15.3	SLC6A3	Yes	No	Dopamine transporter	Reuptake dopamine from synapse
(23) Familial Parkinson disease	Mitochondrial	Mitochondria	N/I	No	No	N/I	Complex I
(24) Familial Parkinson disease	Mitochondrial gene	Mitochondria	MTND4	Yes	No	N/I	Complex I
(25) Familial Parkinson disease	Susceptibility gene	17q21	MAPT	Yes	No	Tau	Fibrils
(26) Familial Parkinson disease	Autosomal recessive	15q25	POLG1	Yes	No	Mt DNA Polymerase gamma	Synthesis, replication and repair of mtDNA
(27) Familial Parkinson disease	Autosomal recessive	21q22.3	PDXK	Yes	No	Pyridoxal kinase	Converts vitamin B6 to pyridoxal-5-phosphate
Parkinson-plus syndromes							
(28) Parkinsonism with ophthalmoplegia	Autosomal dominant	10q24	PEO1	Yes	No	Twinkle	Essential for mtDNA maintenance and regulates mtDNA copy number

Continued

Table 1.5 Continued

Disease	Pattern of inheritance	Chromosome region	Name of gene	Gene identified	Triplet repeat	Name of protein	Function of protein
(29) DLBD	Autosomal dominant	2q35–q36	N/I	No	N/I	N/I	N/I
(30) Frontotemporal dementia	Autosomal dominant	17q21–q23	MAPT	Yes	No	Tau	Microtubules
(31) Frontotemporal dementia	Autosomal dominant	17q21.32	PGRN	Yes	No	Progranulin	Precursor to granulin
(32) Frontotemporal dementia	Autosomal dominant	Chromosome 3	FTD-3	No	No	N/I	N/I
(33) Frontotemporal dementia	Autosomal dominant	16p11.2	FUS	Yes	No	Fusion gene	Translocation of protein to nucleus
(34) Pick disease	Autosomal dominant	17q21–q23	MAPT	Yes	No	Tau	Microtubules
(35) PSP and CBGD	Susceptibility locus	17q21–q23	MAPT	Yes	No	Tau	Microtubules
(36) MSA	?	3p21	ZNF231	Yes	No	Zinc finger protein	Nuclear protein
(37) Parkinson-MELAS syndrome	Mitochondrial gene	Mitochondria	Cytochrome b	Yes	No	Cytochrome b	Complex III
(38) Guamanian PD-ALS-dementia	Autosomal dominant	15q21	TRPM2	Yes	No	Transient receptor potential melastatin 2	Calcium-permeable cation channel
(39) Familial ALS	Autosomal dominant	21q	SOD1	Yes	No	Cu/Zn superoxide dismutase	Convert Superoxide to H_2O_2
(40) Familial ALS	Autosomal dominant	1p36.2	TDP-43	Yes	No	TAR DNA-binding protein 43	TAR DNA-binding protein
Ataxia syndromes							
(41) Friedreich ataxia	Autosomal recessive	9q13–q21.1	X25	Yes	GAA	Frataxin	Phosphoinositide/Fe homeostasis in mitochondria
(42) Friedreich ataxia 2	Autosomal recessive	9p23–p11	FRDA2	No	N/I	N/I	N/I
(43) Early-onset cerebellar ataxia	Autosomal recessive	13q11–q12	No	No	N/I	N/I	N/I
(44) X-linked congenital ataxia	X-linked recessive	X	No	No	N/I	N/I	N/I
(45) Ataxic cerebral palsy	Autosomal recessive	9p12–q12	No	No	N/I	N/I	N/I
(46) Posterior column ataxia with retinitis pigmentosa	Autosomal recessive	1q31–q32	AXPC1	No	No	N/I	N/I
(47) Adult-onset ataxia with tocopherol deficiency	Autosomal recessive	8q13.1–q13.3	α-TTP	Yes	No	α-Tocopherol-transfer protein	Transfers α-tocopherol to mitochondria
(48) Ataxia-telangiectasia	Autosomal recessive	11q22–q23	ATM	Yes	No	PI-3 kinase	DNA repair
(49) Early-onset cerebellar ataxia with oculomotor apraxia (AOA1)	Autosomal recessive	9p13.3	APTX	Yes	No	Aprataxin	N/I

Table 1.5 Continued

Disease	Pattern of inheritance	Chromosome region	Name of gene	Gene identified	Triplet repeat	Name of protein	Function of protein
(50) SCAR1 (AOA2)	Autosomal recessive	9q34	*SETX* (SCAR1)	Yes	No	Senataxin	N/I
(51) SCAR2	Autosomal recessive	9q34–qter	No	No	N/I	N/I	N/I
(52) SCAR3	Autosomal recessive	6p23–p21	No	No	N/I	N/I	N/I
(53) SCAR4 ataxia with saccadic intrusions	Autosomal recessive	1p36	*SCAR4*	No	N/I	N/I	N/I
(54) SCAR5	Autosomal recessive	15q24–q26	No	No	N/I	N/I	N/I
(55) SCAR6 non-progressive infantile ataxia	Autosomal recessive	20q11–q13	No	No	N/I	N/I	N/I
(56) SCAR7	Autosomal recessive	11p15	No	No	N/I	N/I	N/I
(57) SCAR8 (ARCA1)	Autosomal recessive	6q25	*SYNE1* (SCAR8; ARCA1)	Yes	No	Synaptic nuclear envelope protein 1	Nuclear envelope
(58) SCAR9 (ARCA2)	Autosomal recessive	1q41	No	No	N/I	N/I	N/I
(59) SPAX1 hereditary spastic ataxia	Autosomal dominant	12p13	*SPAX1*	No	No	N/I	N/I
(60) SPAX2 hereditary spastic ataxia	Autosomal recessive	17p13	*SPAX2*	No	No	N/I	N/I
(61) SPAX3 hereditary spastic ataxia	Autosomal recessive	2q33–q34	*SPAX3*	No	No	N/I	N/I
(62) Recessive ataxia with epilepsy	Autosomal recessive	16q21–q23	N/I	N/I	N/I	N/I	N/I
(63) Recessive ataxia with intellectual disability (disequilibrium syndrome)	Autosomal recessive	9p24	*VLDLR*	No	N/I	Very low density lipoprotein receptor	Role in triglyceride metabolism
(64) Epilepsy, ataxia, sensorineural deafness, tubulopathy (EAST syndrome)	Autosomal recessive	1q23.2	*KCNJ10*	No	N/I	Inwardly rectifying potassium channel	Recycle potassium for the Na-K-ATPase
(65) SCA1	Autosomal dominant	6p23	*ATXN1*(SCA1)	Yes	CAG40-83	Ataxin-1	N/I
(66) SCA2	Autosomal dominant	12q24	*ATXN2*(SCA2)	Yes	CAG34-59	Ataxin-2	Located in Golgi apparatus
(67) SCA3 (Machado–Joseph disease) MJD	Autosomal dominant	14q24.3–q31	*ATXN3*(SCA3)	Yes	CAG56-86	Ataxin-3	N/I
(68) SCA4	Autosomal dominant	16q22.1	SCA4	No	N/I	N/I	N/I
(69) SCA5	Autosomal dominant	11q13	SCA5	No	N/I	N/I	N/I
(70) SCA6	Autosomal dominant	19p13	*CACNA1A*	Yes	CAG21-31	Alpha-1A calcium channel protein	Ca^{2+} channel

Continued

Table 1.5 Continued

Disease	Pattern of inheritance	Chromosome region	Name of gene	Gene identified	Triplet repeat	Name of protein	Function of protein
(71) SCA7	Autosomal dominant	3p21.1–p12	ATXN7 (SCA7)	Yes	CAG38-200	Ataxin-7	Transcription factor
(72) SCA8	Autosomal dominant	13q21	ATXN8OS (SCA8)	Yes	CTG100-155	N/I	N/I
(73) SCA10	Autosomal dominant	22q13	ATXN10 (SCA10)	No	ATTC800-3800	N/I	N/I
(74) SCA11	Autosomal dominant	15q15.2	TTBK2 (SCA11)	No	No	Tau tubulin kinase-2	Phosphorylates tau and tubulin
(75) SCA12	Autosomal dominant	5q31–q33	PPP2R2B (SCA11)	Yes	CAG66-93	Protein phosphatase PP2A	Regulatory processes
(76) SCA13	Autosomal dominant	19q13.3–q13.4	KCNC3 (SCA13)	Yes	No	Potassium channel subfamily	Voltage-gated potassium channel
(77) SCA14	Autosomal dominant	19q13.4	PRKCG (SCA14)	Yes	No	Protein kinase C gamma	Zinc binding
(78) SCA15	Autosomal dominant	3p26.1–p25.3	ITPR1 (SCA15)	Yes	No	Type 1 inositol 1,4,5-triphosphate receptor	Release calcium ions from intracellular stores
(79) SCA16	Now recognized as identical to SCA15						
(80) SCA17 (also called HDL4)	Autosomal dominant	6q27	TBP (SCA17)	Yes	CAG45-63	TATA-binding protein (TBP)	Transcription initiation factor
(81) SCA18 with sensorimotor neuropathy	Autosomal dominant	7q22–q32	SCA18	N/I	N/I	N/I	N/I
(82) SCA19	Autosomal dominant	1p21–q21	SCA19	N/I	N/I	N/I	N/I
(83) SCA20	Autosomal dominant	11p13–11q11	SCA20	N/I	N/I	N/I	N/I
(84) SCA21	Autosomal dominant	7p21.3–p15.1	SCA21	N/I	N/I	N/I	N/I
(85) SCA22 (same as SCA19)	Autosomal dominant	1p21–q23	SCA22	N/I	N/I	N/I	N/I
(86) SCA23	Autosomal dominant	20p13–p12.3	SCA23	N/I	N/I	N/I	N/I
(87) SCA24	Now called SCAR4; see (53)						
(88) SCA25 ataxia with sensory neuropathy	Autosomal dominant	2p21–p13	SCA25	N/I	N/I	N/I	N/I
(89) SCA26	Autosomal dominant	19p13.3	SCA26	N/I	N/I	N/I	N/I
(90) SCA27	Autosomal dominant	13q34	FGF14 (SCA27)	Yes	No	Fibroblast growth factor 14	Neuronal signaling and axonal trafficking

Table 1.5 Continued

Disease	Pattern of inheritance	Chromosome region	Name of gene	Gene identified	Triplet repeat	Name of protein	Function of protein
(91) SCA28	Autosomal dominant	18p11.22–q11.2	SCA28	N/I	N/I	N/I	N/I
(92) SCA29; congenital, non-progressive	Autosomal dominant	3p26	SCA29	N/I	N/I	N/I	N/I
(93) SCA30	Autosomal dominant	4q34.3–q35.1	SCA30	N/I	N/I	N/I	N/I
(94) Adult-onset Alexander disease	Autosomal dominant	17q21	GFAP	Yes	No	Glial fibrillary acidic protein	Astrocytic protein
Choreic syndromes							
(95) Huntington disease	Autosomal dominant	4p16.3	IT15	Yes	CAG	Huntingtin	N/I
(96) Huntington-like disease-1 (HDL1)	Autosomal dominant	20pter–p12	PRPN	Yes	Octapeptide repeats	Prion protein	N/I
(97) Huntington-like disease-2 (HDL2)	Autosomal dominant	16q24.3	JPH3	Yes	CTG and CAG	Juncto-philin-3	Links the plasma membrane and the endoplasmic reticulum
(98) Huntington-like disease-3 (HDL3)	Autosomal recessive	4p15.3	N/I	No	No	N/I	N/I
(99) Huntington-like disease-4 (HDL4) (same as SCA17; see (80))	Autosomal dominant	6q27	TBP (SCA17)	Yes	CAG45-63	TATA-binding protein (TBP)	Transcription initiation factor
(100) Neuroacanthocytosis	Autosomal recessive	9q21	VPS13A	Yes	No	Chorein	Protein sorting
(101) McLeod syndrome	X-linked recessive	Xp21.2–p21.1	XK	Yes	No	XK	Kell blood group precursor
(102) Benign hereditary chorea	Autosomal dominant	14q13	NKX2-1	Yes	No	Thyroid transcription factor-1 (TITF-1)	Thyroid function
(103) Neonatal brain–thyroid–lung syndrome, a more severe manifestation of above mutation	Autosomal dominant	14q13	NKX2-1	Yes	No	Thyroid transcription factor-1 (TITF-1)	Thyroid function
(104) Benign hereditary chorea	Autosomal dominant	8q21.3–q23.3	N/I	N/I	N/I	N/I	N/I
(105) Dentatorubral-pallidoluysian atrophy (DRPLA)	Autosomal dominant	12p13.31	DRPLA	Yes	CAG	Atrophin-1	N/I
Choreoathetosis							
(106) Choreoathetosis and intellectual disability	X-linked recessive	Xp11	N/I	N/I	N/I	N/I	N/I
Dystonia							
(107) Oppenheim torsion dystonia	Autosomal dominant	9q34	TOR1 DYT1	Yes	No, GAG deletion	TorsinA	Chaperone, ATP binding
(108) Lubag (X-linked dystonia–parkinsonism)	X-linked recessive	Xq13.1	TAF1 DYT3	Yes	No	Multiple transcript system; TAF1	N/I

Continued

Table 1.5 Continued

Disease	Pattern of inheritance	Chromosome region	Name of gene	Gene identified	Triplet repeat	Name of protein	Function of protein
(109) Dopa-responsive dystonia	Autosomal dominant	14q22.1–q22.2	GCH1 DYT5	Yes	No	GTP cyclo-hydrolase 1	Synthesis of BH4
(110) Mixed type dystonia	Autosomal dominant	8p11.21	THAP1 DYT6	Yes	No	THAP1	Regulates endothelial cell proliferation
(111) Familial torticollis	Autosomal dominant	18p?	DYT7	N/I	N/I	N/I	N/I
(112) Myoclonus–dystonia	Autosomal dominant	7q21–q31	SGCE DYT11	Yes	No	Epsilon-sarcoglycan	N/I
(113) Myoclonus–dystonia	Autosomal dominant	18p11	DYT15	N/I	N/I	N/I	N/I
(114) Young-onset dystonia–parkinsonism	Autosomal recessive	2q31.2	DYT16	PRKRA	No	Protein kinase	Stress response
(115) Rapid-onset dystonia–parkinsonism	Autosomal dominant	19q13	DYT12	Yes	No	Na(+)/K(+)-ATPase alpha3 subunit (ATP1A3)	Sodium pump
(116) Alternating hemiplegia of childhood	Autosomal dominant	1q23	ATP1A2	Yes	No	Na(+)/K(+)-ATPase alpha2 subunit (ATP1A2)	Sodium pump
(117) Cervical-cranial-brachial dystonia	Autosomal dominant	1p36.13–p36.32	DYT13	No	N/I	N/I	N/I
(118) Familial dystonia	Autosomal recessive	20p11.2–q13.12	DYT17	No	N/I	N/I	N/I
(119) Aromatic amino acid decarboxylase deficiency	Autosomal recessive	7p11	Aromatic amino acid decarboxylase	Yes	No	Aromatic amino acid decarboxylase	Converts dopa to dopamine
(120) Torticollis	Susceptibility gene	4p16.1–p15.3	Dopamine D5 receptor	Yes	No	Dopamine D5 receptor	Dopamine D5 receptor
(121) Blepharospasm	Susceptibility gene	4p16.1–p15.3	Dopamine D5 receptor	Yes	No	Dopamine D5 receptor	Dopamine D5 receptor
(122) Deafness-dystonia–optic atrophy	X-linked recessive	Xq22	DDP	Yes	No	DDP	Intermembrane protein transport in mitochondria
(123) Dystonic lipidosis (Niemann–Pick type C)	Autosomal recessive	18q11–q12	NPC1	Yes	No	–	Esterification of LDL-derived cholesterol
(124) Neurodegeneration with brain iron accumulation 1 (NBIA-1)	Autosomal recessive	20p12.3–p13	PANK2	N/I	N/I	Pantothenate kinase 2 (PANK2)	Co-enzyme A biosynthesis
(125) Neuroferritinopathy	Autosomal dominant	19q13.3	FTL	Yes	No	Ferritin light polypeptide	Iron binding

Table 1.5 Continued

Disease	Pattern of inheritance	Chromosome region	Name of gene	Gene identified	Triplet repeat	Name of protein	Function of protein
Infantile neuroaxonal dystrophy with parkinsonism dystonia and ataxia (also known as adult-onset dystonia–parkinsonism without iron): see (14)							
(126) Aceruloplasminemia	Autosomal recessive	3q23–q24	CP	No	No	Ceruloplasmin	Oxidizes ferrous ion
(127) Striatal necrosis	Mitochondrial	Mitochondrial	ND6	Yes	No	–	Decreases complex I activity
(128) Striatal necrosis	Autosomal recessive	2q36.3	SLC19A3	Yes	No	Folate (micronutrient) transporter	Biotin-responsive
(129) Striopallido-dentate calcinosis	Autosomal dominant	14q	IBGC1	N/I	N/I	N/I	N/I
(130) Lesch–Nyhan syndrome	X-linked recessive	Xq26–q27.2	HPRT	Yes	No	Hypoxanthine-guanine-phosphoribosyl transferase	
(131) Woodhouse–Sakati syndrome	Autosomal recessive	2q22.3–q35	C2orf37	Yes	N/I	N/I	Nucleolar protein
(132) Spastic paraplegia with dystonia	Autosomal dominant	2q24–q31	N/I	N/I	N/I	N/I	N/I
Hyperekplexia							
(133) Hereditary hyperekplexia	Autosomal dominant	5q32–q31.3	STHE	Yes	No	GLRA1	Glycine receptor
(134) Hereditary hyperekplexia	Autosomal recessive	11p15.2–p15.1	SLC6A5	Yes	No	SLC6A5	Presynaptic glycine transporter
(135) Hereditary hyperekplexia	Autosomal recessive	14q24	GPHN	Yes	No	Gephyrin	Glycine receptor
Myoclonus							
(136) Unverricht–Lundborg disease	Autosomal recessive	21q22.3	EPM1	Yes	Dodecamer repeat expansion	Cystatin B	Cysteine protease inhibitor
(137) Lafora body disease	Autosomal recessive	6q24	EPM2A	Yes	No	Laforin	Tyrosine phosphatase
(138) Lafora body disease	Autosomal recessive	6p22	EPM2B	Yes	No	Malin	E3 ubiquitin ligase
(139) Progressive myoclonus epilepsy	Mitochondrial gene	Mitochondria	tRNA (serine 1 (UCN))	Yes	No	N/I	N/I
(140) Progressive myoclonus epilepsy	Autosomal recessive	7q11.2	KCTD7	Yes	No	Potassium channel	Potassium transport
(141) Progressive myoclonus epilepsy	Autosomal dominant	3q26	SERPINI1	Yes	No	Neuroserpin	Serine proteinase inhibitor

Continued

Table 1.5 Continued

Disease	Pattern of inheritance	Chromosome region	Name of gene	Gene identified	Triplet repeat	Name of protein	Function of protein
(142) Progressive myoclonus epilepsy with or without renal failure	Autosomal recessive	4q13–q21	SCARB2	Yes	No	Scavenger receptor	Lysosomal integral membrane protein
(143) Familial adult myoclonus epilepsy	Autosomal dominant	8q23.3–q24.1	FAME	No	No	N/I	N/I
(144) Familial Creutzfeldt–Jakob disease	Autosomal dominant	20pter–p12	PRNP	Yes	No	Prion protein	N/I
(145) Infantile spasms	X-linked recessive	Xp22.13	ARX	Yes	N/I	N/I	N/I
Paroxysmal dyskinesias							
(146) Episodic ataxia-1/myokymia	Autosomal dominant	12p13	Kv1.1	Yes	No	KCNA1	K+ channel
(147) Episodic ataxia-2/vestibular	Autosomal dominant	19p13	CACNL1A4	Yes	No	CACNL1A4	Ca2+ channel
(148) Episodic ataxia-3/vertigo and tinnitus	Autosomal dominant	1q42	EA-3	N/I	N/I	N/I	N/I
(149) Episodic ataxia-4/diplopia	Autosomal dominant	?	EA-4	N/I	N/I	N/I	N/I
(150) Episodic ataxia-5/vertigo	Autosomal dominant	2q22–q23	CACNB4 (EA-5)	Yes	No	Calcium-channel beta4-subunit	Ca2+ channel
(151) Episodic ataxia-6	Autosomal dominant	5p13	SLC1A3 (EA-6)	Yes	No	Excitatory amino acid transporter 1 (EAAT1)	Glial glutamate transporter
(152) Episodic ataxia-7	Autosomal dominant	19p13	EA-7	N/I	N/I	N/I	N/I
(153) Late-onset episodic ataxia	Autosomal dominant	?	EA-8	N/I	N/I	N/I	N/I
(154) Paroxysmal kinesigenic dyskinesia (PKD)	Autosomal dominant	16p11.2–q11.2	–	No	N/I	N/I	N/I
(155) Paroxysmal kinesigenic dyskinesia (PKD)	Autosomal dominant	16q13–q22.1	EKD2 (DYT19)	No	N/I	N/I	N/I
(156) Paroxysmal nonkinesigenic dyskinesia (PNKD) (Mount–Reback syndrome)	Autosomal dominant	2q34	MR1 (DYT8)	Yes	No	Myofibrillogenesis regulator 1	Detoxify compounds
(157) PNKD2	Autosomal dominant	2q31	–	No	N/I	N/I	N/I
(158) Paroxysmal dyskinesia and spasticity	Autosomal dominant	1p21	Probably SLC2A1	No	No	Probably GLUT1	Glucose transporter
(158a) Paroxysmal dyskinesia and epilepsy	Autosomal dominant	10q22	KCNMA1	No	No	BK channel	Ca-sensitive potassium channel

Table 1.5 Continued

Disease	Pattern of inheritance	Chromosome region	Name of gene	Gene identified	Triplet repeat	Name of protein	Function of protein
(159) Rolandic epilepsy with childhood exercise-induced dyskinesia and writer's cramp	Autosomal recessive	16p12–q11.2	Sodium/glucose cotransporter gene (KST1)	Yes	No	N/I	Cotransport of sodium and glucose
(160) Paroxysmal exertional dyskinesia (PED)	Autosomal dominant	1p35–p31.3	SLC2A1 (DYT18)	Yes	No	Glucose transporter 1 (GLUT1)	Transport of glucose into red blood cells and brain
(161) Familial hypnogenic seizures/dystonia	Autosomal dominant	20q12.2-13.3	CHRNA4	Yes	No	CHRNA4	Nicotinic ACh receptor
(162) Familial hypnogenic seizures/dystonia	Autosomal dominant	15q24	CHRNB2	Yes	No	CHRNB2	Nicotinic ACh receptor
(163) Familial hypnogenic seizures/dystonia	Autosomal dominant	Chromosome 1	N/I	N/I	N/I	N/I	Nicotinic ACh receptor
(164) Allan–Herndon–Dudley syndrome with paroxysmal dyskinesia, spasticity, and intellectual disability	X-linked recessive	Xq13.2	MCT8	Yes	No	Monocarboxylate transporter 8	Active transporter of thyroid hormones
(165) Benign paroxysmal tonic upgaze and torticollis	Autosomal dominant	19p13	CACNL1A4	Yes	No	CACNL 1A4	Ca^{2+} channel
Restless legs syndrome							
(166) Restless legs syndrome (RLS1)	Autosomal recessive	12q12–q21	RLS1	N/I	N/I	N/I	N/I
(167) Restless legs syndrome (RLS2)	Autosomal dominant	14q13–q21	RLS2	N/I	N/I	N/I	N/I
(168) Restless legs syndrome (RLS3)	Autosomal dominant	9p23-24	PTPRD (RLS3)	Yes	No	Protein tyrosine phosphatase receptor type delta	Axonal guidance during development
(169) Restless legs syndrome (RLS4)	Autosomal dominant	2q33	RLS4	N/I	N/I	N/I	N/I
(170) Restless legs syndrome (RLS5)	Autosomal dominant	20p13	RLS5	N/I	N/I	N/I	N/I
(171) Restless legs syndrome	Risk factor	6p21.2	N/I	N/I	N/I	N/I	N/I
Stereotypies							
(172) Rett syndrome	X-linked dominant	Xq28	MECP2	Yes	No	Methyl-CpG-binding protein	Binds CpG proteins
(173) Autism	X-gene duplication	Xq28	MECP2	Yes	No	Methyl-CpG-binding protein	As above; autism and intellectual disability in boys
(174) Autism	Genetic instability	16q11.2	Region of duplications and deletions	No	No	N/I	N/I

Continued

Table 1.5 Continued

Disease	Pattern of inheritance	Chromosome region	Name of gene	Gene identified	Triplet repeat	Name of protein	Function of protein
(175) Head bobbing	Autosomal recessive	6p22	ALDH5A1	Yes	No	Succinic semialdehyde dehydrogenase	Catabolism of GABA
Tics							
(176) Tourette syndrome	Autosomal dominant	15q21–q22	HDC	Yes	No	L-histidine decarboxylase	Rate-limiting enzyme in histamine biosynthesis
(177) Tourette syndrome	Autosomal dominant	11q23	–	No	N/I	N/I	N/I
(178) Tourette syndrome	Susceptibility loci	7q31; 2p11; 8q22	–	No	N/I	N/I	N/I
(179) Tourette syndrome, OCD, chronic tics	Candidate gene	18q22	–	No	N/I	N/I	N/I
(180) Tourette syndrome	Candidate gene	13q31.1	–	N/I	N/I	N/I	N/I
Tremor							
(181) Familial essential tremor	Autosomal dominant	3q13	ETM1	N/I	N/I	N/I	N/I
(182) Familial essential tremor	Autosomal dominant	2p22–p25	ETM2	N/I	N/I	N/I	N/I
(183) Familial essential tremor	Autosomal dominant	6p23	ETM3	N/I	N/I	N/I	N/I
(184) Familial essential tremor	Autosomal dominant (risk factor)	15q24.3	LINGO1	Yes	No	Leucine-rich repeat neuronal protein 1	Axon regeneration and oligodendrocyte maturation
(185) Hereditary geniospasm	Autosomal dominant	9q13–q21	–	N/I	N/I	N/I	N/I
(186) Roussy–Lévy syndrome	Autosomal dominant	17p11.2	CMT-1B	Yes	No	Peripheral myelin protein	Myelin
(187) Fragile X tremor-ataxia syndrome (FXTAS)	X-linked recessive	Xq27.3	FMR1	Yes	CGG repeat 50–200	FMRP	Synaptic structure development
A variety of movements							
Wilson disease							
(188) Wilson disease	Autosomal recessive	13q14.3	ATB7B	Yes	No	Cu-ATPase	Copper transport
Neuronal ceroid lipofuscinoses (Batten disease)							
(189) Infantile	Autosomal recessive	1p32	CLN1	Yes	No	Palmitoyl protein thioesterase	Lysosomal proteolysis
(190) Variant late infantile	Autosomal recessive	1p32	CLN1	Yes	N/I	Palmitoyl protein thioesterase	Lysosomal proteolysis
(191) Late-infantile-classical	Autosomal recessive	9q13–q21	CLN2	Yes	No	Pepstatin-insensitive protease	Lysosomal proteolysis

Table 1.5 Continued

Disease	Pattern of inheritance	Chromosome region	Name of gene	Gene identified	Triplet repeat	Name of protein	Function of protein
(192) Juvenile (Batten)	Autosomal recessive	16p12.1	CLN3	Yes	No	Battenin	Fatty acid desaturase
(193) Adult (Kufs)	Autosomal recessive	N/I	CLN4	No	N/I	N/I	N/I
(194) Finnish late infantile	Autosomal recessive	13q22	CLN5	Yes	No	Unnamed membrane protein	Lysosomal proteolysis
(195) Variant late infantile	Autosomal recessive	15q21-23	CLN6	No	N/I	N/I	N/I
(196) Variant late infantile	Autosomal recessive	4q28.1–q28.2	MFSD8 (CLN7)	No	No	Major facilitator superfamily domain-containing protein-8	Lysosomal

N/I, not yet identified. CAG, cytosine-adenosine-guanosine trinucleotide. GAA, guanosine-adenosine adenosine. GAG, guanosine-adenosine-guanosine. BH4, tetrahydrobiopterin. References for the above listings, in order, are: (1) Polymeropoulos et al., 1996, 1997; Kruger et al., 1998; Zarranz et al., 2004; Ibanez et al., 2004; (2) Matsumine et al., 1997, 1998; Kitada et al., 1998; Abbas et al., 1999; Shimura et al., 2000; Farrer et al., 2001; (3) Gasser et al., 1998; Pankratz et al., 2004; (4) Singleton et al., 2003; (5) Leroy et al., 1998; (6) Valente et al., 2001b; Bentivoglio et al., 2001; Valente et al., 2002; Valente et al., 2004a, 2004b; (7) van Duijn et al., 2001; Bonifati et al., 2003; Healy et al., 2004b; (8) Funayama et al., 2002; Paisan-Ruiz et al., 2004; Zimprich et al., 2004; Clark et al., 2006; (9) Hampshire et al., 2001; Ramirez et al., 2006; (10) Hicks et al., 2002; (11) Pankratz et al., 2003a; Lautier et al., 2008; Nichols et al., 2009; Vilariño-Güell et al., 2009; Zimprich et al., 2009; Di Fonzo et al., 2009a; (12) Pankratz et al., 2003b; (13) Strauss et al., 2005; Bogaerts et al., 2008; (14) Morgan et al., 2006; Kurian et al., 2008; Paisan-Ruiz et al., 2009; (15) Di Fonzo et al., 2009b; (16) Satake et al., 2009; Simón-Sánchez et al., 2009; (17) Chartier-Harlin et al. 2009; (18) Aharon-Peretz et al., 2004; Goker-Alpan et al., 2004, 2006; Clark et al., 2005; (19) Le et al., 2002; Xu et al., 2002; Zheng et al., 2003; (20) Farrer et al., 2009; (21) Knappskog et al., 1995; Lüdecke et al., 1995; Lüdecke et al., 1996; (22) Kurian et al., 2009; (23) Swerdlow et al., 1998; (24) Simon et al., 1999; (25) Healy et al., 2004a; (26) Davidzon et al., 2006; Luoma et al., 2007; (27) Elstner et al., 2009; (28) Baloh et al., 2007; Vandenberghe et al., 2009; (29) Bogaerts et al., 2007; (30) Lynch et al., 1994; Foster et al., 1997; Hutton et al., 1998; Pittman et al., 2004; Pastor et al. 2004; Skipper et al., 2004; (31) Baker et al., 2006; (32) Gydesen et al., 2002; (33) Van Langenhove et al., 2010; (34) Pickering-Brown et al., 2000; (35) Baker et al., 1999; Bugiani et al., 1999; Delisle et al., 1999; Higgins et al., 1999a; Morris et al., 1999; Spillantini et al., 2000; Stanford et al., 2000; Wszolek et al., 2001; (36) Hashida et al., 1998; (37) De Coo et al., 1999; (38) Hermosura et al., 2008; (39) Rosen et al., 1993; (40) Gitcho et al., 2008; Yokoseki et al., 2008; (41) Pandolfo et al., 1993; (42) Christodoulou et al., 2001; (43) Mrissa et al., 2000; (44) Bertini et al., 2000; (45) McHale et al., 2000; (46) Higgins et al., 1999b; (47) Gotoda et al., 1995; (48) Ambrose et al., 1994; Savitsky et al., 1995; (49) Date et al., 2001; Moreira et al., 2001; (50) Duquette et al., 2005; (51) Delague et al., 2001; (52) Bomont et al., 2000; (53) Swartz et al., 2003; (54) Mégarbané et al., 2001; Delague et al., 2002; (55) Tranebjaerg et al., 2003; (56) Breedveld et al., 2004; (57) Gros-Louis et al., 2007; Dupré et al., 2007; (58) Lamperti et al., 2003; Lagier-Tourenne et al., 2008; (59) Meijer et al., 2002; (60) Bouslam et al., 2007; (61) Thiffault et al., 2006; (62). Gribaa et al., 2007; (63) Boycott et al., 2009; (64) Scholl et al., 2009; Bockenhauer et al., 2009; (65) Banfi et al., 1994; (66) Lopes-Cendes et al., 1994a; (67) Kawaguchi et al., 1994; (68) Lopes-Cendes et al., 1994b; Flanigan et al., 1996; Li et al., 2003; (69) Ranum et al., 1994; Burk et al., 2004; (70) Riess et al., 1997; Zhuchenko et al., 1997; (71) David et al., 1996, 1997; Lindblad et al., 1996; La Spada et al., 2001; (72) Koob et al., 1999; (73) Matsuura et al., 1999; Zu et al., 1999; (74) Worth et al., 1999; (75) Fujigasaki et al., 2001a; Holmes et al., 2001b; O'Hearn et al., 2001; (76) Herman-Bert et al., 2000; (77) Yamashita et al., 2000; Brkanac et al., 2002a; Chen et al., 2003; Yabe et al., 2003; (78) Storey et al., 2001; Knight et al., 2003; van de Leemput et al., 2007; Hara et al., 2008; (79) Miyoshi et al., 2001; Miura et al., 2006; (80) Nakamura et al., 2001; Fujigasaki et al., 2001b; Toyoshima et al., 2004; (81) Brkanac et al., 2002b; (82) Verbeek et al., 2002; (83) Knight et al., 2004, 2008; (84) Vuillaume et al., 2002; (85) Chung et al., 2003; (86) Verbeek et al., 2004; (87) see reference (53); (88) Stevanin et al., 2004; (89) Yu et al., 2005; (90) van Swieten et al., 2003; Dalski et al., 2005; (91) Cagnoli et al., 2006; Mariotti et al., 2008; (92) Dudding et al., 2004; (93). Storey et al., 2009; (94) Namekawa et al., 2002; Okamoto et al., 2002; Pareyson et al., 2008; (95) Huntington's Disease Collaborative Research Group, 1993; (96) Xiang et al., 1998; Moore et al., 2001; (97) Margolis et al., 2001; Holmes et al., 2001a; Stevanin et al., 2003; (98) Kambouris et al., 2000; (99) see (80); (100) Rubio et al., 1997, 1999; Rampoldi et al., 2001; Ueno et al., 2001; Dobson-Stone et al., 2002, 2004; (101) Danek et al., 2001; (102) de Vries et al., 2000; Fernandez et al., 2002; Breedveld et al., 2002; Kleiner-Fisman et al., 2003; Devos et al., 2006; (103) Krude et al., 2002; Doyle et al., 2004; (104) Shimohata et al., 2007; (105) Koide et al., 1994; Nagafuchi et al., 1994; Yamada et al., 2001; Okamura-Oho et al., 2003; (106) Reyniers et al., 1999; (107) Kramer et al., 1994; Ozelius et al., 1997; (108) Wilhelmsen et al., 1991; Müller et al., 1994; Nolte et al., 2003; Fabbrini et al., 2005; Makino et al., 2007; (109) Nygaard et al., 1993; Ichinose et al., 1994; (110) Almasy et al., 1997; Saunders-Pullman et al., 2007; T. Fuchs et al., 2009; (111) Leube et al., 1996; (112) Nygaard et al., 1999; Klein et al., 2000; Zimprich et al., 2001; (113) Grimes et al., 2002; (114) Camargos et al., 2008; Seibler et al., 2008; (115) Kramer et al., 1999; Pittock et al., 2000; De Carvalho Aguiar et al., 2004; (116) Bassi et al., 2004; (117) Valente et al., 2001a; (118) Chouery et al., 2008; (119) Hyland et al., 1992; Chang et al., 2004; (120) Placzek et al., 2001; (121) Misbahuddin et al., 2002; (122) Koehler et al., 1999; Jin et al., 1999; Tranebjaerg et al., 2000; Rothbauer et al., 2001; Swerdlow and Wooten, 2001; Ujike et al., 2001; (123) Carstea et al., 1993; Lossos et al., 1997; (124) Taylor et al., 1996; Zhou et al., 2001; Hayflick et al., 2003; (125) Curtis et al., 2001; Mir et al., 2005; (126) Fasano et al., 2008; (127) Solano et al., 2003; (128) Zeng et al., 2005; Debs et al., 2010; (129) Geschwind et al., 1999; (130) Sege-Peterson et al., 1993; Jinnah et al., 2006; (131) Schneider and Bhatia, 2008; Alazami et al., 2008; (132) Gilbert et al., 2009; (133) Shiang et al., 1993; (134) Rees et al., 2006; (135) Rees et al., 2003; (136) Lehesjoki et al., 1993, 1998; (137) Maddox et al., 1997; Minassian et al., 1998; Serratosa et al., 1999; Minassian et al., 2001; (138) Chan et al., 2003a, 2003b; (139) Jaksch et al., 1998; (140) Van Bogaert et al., 2007; (141) Gourfinkel-An et al., 2007; (142) Andermann et al., 1986; Badhwar et al. 2004; Dibbens et al., 2009; (143) Mikami et al., 1999; Plaster et al., 1999; (144) Prusiner, 1993; (145) Stromme et al., 2002; Turner et al., 2002; (146) Browne et al., 1994; Litt et al., 1994; (147) Vahedi et al., 1995; von Brederlow et al., 1995; (148) Steckley et al., 2001; Cader et al., 2005; (149) Damji et al., 1996; (150) Escayg et al., 2000; (151) Jen et al., 2005; de Vries et al., 2009; (152) Kerber et al., 2007; (153) Damak et al., 2009; (154) Tomita et al., 1999; Bennett et al., 2000; (155) Valente et al., 2000; (156) Fouad et al., 1996; Fink et al., 1996, 1997; Hofele et al., 1997; Jarman et al., 1997a; Raskind et al., 1998; Lee et al., 2004; (157) Spacey et al., 2006; (158) Auburger et al., 1996; (158a) Du et al., 2005; (159) Szepetowski et al., 1997; Lee et al., 1998; Carelli et al., 1999; Guerrini et al., 1999; Roll et al., 2002; (160) Weber et al., 2008; Suls et al., 2008; Schneider et al., 2009; Pons et al., 2010; (161) Oldani et al., 1998; Nakken et al., 1999; (162) Phillips et al., 1998, 2001; (163) Gambardella et al., 2000; (164) O. Fuchs et al., 2009; (165) Roubertie et al., 2008; (166) Desautels et al., 2001; Winkelmann et al., 2006; (167) Bonati et al., 2003; Levchenko et al., 2004; (168) Liebetanz et al., 2006; Lohmann-Hedrich et al., 2008; Schormair et al., 2008; (169) Pichler et al., 2006; (170) Levchenko et al., 2006; (171) Stefansson et al., 2007; (172) Sirianni et al., 1998; Amir et al., 1999; Auranen et al., 2001; Ben-Zeev et al., 2002; (173) Ramocki et al. 2009; (174) Weiss et al., 2008; (175) O'Rourke et al., 2010; (176) Ercan-Sencicek et al., 2010; (177) Merette et al., 2000; (178) Petek et al., 2001; Simonic et al., 2001; (179) Cuker et al., 2004; (180) Abelson et al., 2005; (181) Gulcher et al., 1997; (182) Higgins et al., 1997; (183) Deng et al., 2007; (184) Stefansson et al., 2009; (185) Jarman et al., 1997b; (186) Planté-Bordeneuve et al., 1999; (187) Jacquemont et al., 2003, 2004; Hagerman et al., 2004; (188) Bull et al., 1993; Tanzi et al., 1993; (189) Jarvela et al., 1991; Vesa et al., 1995; (190) Das et al., 1998; (191) Sharp et al., 1997; (192) Jarvela et al., 1997; Michalewski et al., 1998; Mole, 1998; Narayan et al., 2006; (193) Berkovic et al., 1988; (194) Savukoski et al., 1998; (195) Sharp et al., 1997; (196) Mole, 1998; Kousi et al., 2009.

Table 1.6 Size of trinucleotide repeats

Disease	Type of nucleotide	In normal individuals	In disease
Huntington	CAG	11–34	37–121
HDL2	CAG	<50	50–60
SCA1	CAG	19–36	42–81
SCA2	CAG	15–29	35–59
SCA3 (Machado–Joseph)	CAG	12–40	66–>200
SCA6	CAG	4–16	21–28
SCA7	CAG		Estimated 64
SCA12	CAG	9–28	55–78
SCA17	CAG	29–42	47–55
DRPLA	CAG	7–34	49–83
Friedreich ataxia	GAA	7–22	120–1700

SCA, spinocerebellar degeneration; DRPLA, dentatorubral-pallidoluysian atrophy. Data in part from Brooks BP, Fischbeck KH. Spinal and bulbar muscular atrophy: a trinucleotide-repeat expansion neurodegenerative disease. Trends Neurosci 1995;18:459–461; Riess O, Schols L, Bottger H, et al. SCA6 is caused by moderate CAG expansion in the alpha(1A)-voltage-dependent calcium channel gene. Hum Mol Genet 1997;6:1289–1293.

these triplicate repeats are unstable, and when expanded, lead to disease (Table 1.6). Neurogenetics is one of the fastest moving research areas in neurology, so the list in Table 1.5 keeps expanding rapidly.

Quantitative assessments

The assessment of severity of disease is a process that is carried out by all clinicians when evaluating a patient. Quantifying the severity provides the means of determining the progression of the disorder and the effect of intervention by pharmacologic or surgical approaches. Many mechanical and electronic devices, including accelerometers, can quantitate specific signs, such as tremor, rigidity, and bradykinesia. These have been developed by physicians and engineers over at least 80 years (Lewy, 1923; Carmichael and Green, 1928), and newer computerized devices continue to be conceived and developed (Larsen et al., 1983; Tryon, 1984; Potvin and Tourtelotte, 1985; Cohen et al., 2003). The advantages of mechanical and electronic measurements are objectivity, consistency, uniformity among different investigators, and rapidity of database storage and analysis. However, these measurements might not be as sensitive as more subjective clinical measurements. In one study comparing objective measurements of reaction and movement times with clinical evaluations, Ward and his colleagues (1983) found the latter to be more sensitive.

The mechanical and electronic methods of measurement have other disadvantages. Instrumentation can usually measure only a single sign, at a single point in time, and in

a single part of the body. Disorders such as parkinsonism encompass a wide range of motor abnormalities, as well as behavioral features. Clinical measurements can cover a wider range of the parkinsonian spectrum of impairments, and have the advantage of being carried out at the bedside or in the office or clinic at the time the patient is being examined by the physician. Equally important, clinical assessment can evaluate disability in terms of activities of daily living (ADL), and the one developed by England and Schwab (1956) and modified slightly (Fahn and Elton, 1987) has proven highly useful.

A number of clinical rating scales have been proposed (e.g., see Marsden and Schachter, 1981). Several that are now considered standards and are in wide use can be recommended: the Unified Parkinson's Disease Rating Scale (UPDRS) (Fahn and Elton, 1987) is the standard scale for rating severity of signs and symptoms; a videotaped demonstration of the assigned ratings has been published (Goetz et al., 1995). A modification of the UPDRS by the Movement Disorder Society is underway (Goetz et al., 2007) and will be known as the MDS-UPDRS. Other standard scales for PD and its complications are the Schwab and England Activities of Daily Living scale for parkinsonism (Schwab and England, 1969) as modified (Fahn and Elton, 1987); the Hoehn and Yahr Parkinson Disease Staging Scale (Hoehn and Yahr, 1967) as modified (Fahn and Elton, 1987); the Goetz dopa dyskinesia severity scale (Goetz et al., 1994); the Lang–Fahn dopa dyskinesia ADL scale (Parkinson Study Group, 2001); the Parkinson psychosis scale (Friedberg et al., 1998); the daily diary to record fluctuations and dyskinesias (Hauser et al., 2004); the core assessment program for intracerebral transplantation (Langston et al., 1992); the PSP Rating Scale (Golbe and Ohman-Strickland, 2007); the Fahn–Marsden Dystonia Rating Scale (Burke et al., 1985); the Unified Dystonia Rating Scale (Comella et al., 2003); the Fahn–Tolosa clinical rating scale for tremor (Fahn et al., 1993); the Bain tremor scale (Bain et al., 1993); and the Unified Huntington's Disease Rating Scale, which also has a published videotaped demonstration of assigned ratings (Huntington Study Group, 1996).

Differential diagnosis of hypokinesias

For a list of hypokinesias, refer to Table 1.1.

Akinesia/Bradykinesia

Akinesia, bradykinesia, and hypokinesia literally mean "absence," "slowness," and "decreased amplitude" of movement, respectively. The three terms are commonly grouped together for convenience and usually referred to under the term of *bradykinesia*. These phenomena are a prominent and most important feature of parkinsonism, and are often considered a *sine qua non* for parkinsonism. Although akinesia means "lack of movement," the label is often used to indicate a very severe form of bradykinesia (Video 1.1). Bradykinesia is mild in early PD, and becomes more severe as the disease worsens; similarly in other forms of parkinsonism. A discussion of the phenomenology of akinesia/bradykinesia requires a brief description of the clinical features of parkinsonism. A fuller discussion is presented in Chapter 4.

Table 1.7 Cardinal features of parkinsonism

Tremor-at-rest
Bradykinesia/hypokinesia/akinesia
Rigidity
Flexed posture of neck, trunk, and limbs
Freezing
Loss of postural reflexes

Table 1.8 Four categories of parkinsonism

1. Primary
2. Secondary
3. Parkinsonism-plus syndromes
4. Heredodegenerative disorders

Parkinsonism is a neurologic syndrome manifested by any combination of six independent, non-overlapping cardinal motor features: tremor-at-rest, bradykinesia, rigidity, flexed posture, freezing, and loss of postural reflexes (Table 1.7). At least two of these six cardinal features should be present before the diagnosis of parkinsonism is made, one of them being tremor-at-rest or bradykinesia. There are many causes of parkinsonism; they can be divided into four major categories: primary, secondary, parkinsonism-plus syndromes, and heredodegenerative disorders (Table 1.8). Primary parkinsonism (Parkinson disease) is a progressive disorder of unknown etiology or of a known gene defect, and the diagnosis is usually made by excluding other known causes of parkinsonism (Fahn, 1992). The complete classification of parkinsonian disorders is presented in Chapter 4. The specific diagnosis of the type of parkinsonism depends on details of the clinical history, the neurologic examination, and laboratory tests.

The primary parkinsonism disorder known as Parkinson disease (PD), also referred to as idiopathic parkinsonism, is the most common type of parkinsonism encountered by the neurologist. But drug-induced parkinsonism is probably the most common form of parkinsonism since neuroleptic drugs (dopamine receptor blocking agents), which cause drug-induced parkinsonism, are widely prescribed for treating psychosis (see Chapter 19). Here, some of the motor phenomenology of parkinsonism is discussed as part of the overview of the differential diagnosis of movement disorders based on phenomenology.

PD begins insidiously. Tremor is usually the first symptom recognized by the patient. However, the disorder can begin with slowness of movement, shuffling gait, painful stiffness of a shoulder, micrographia, or even depression. In the early stages, the symptoms and signs tend to remain on one side of the body (Video 1.2), but with time, the other side slowly becomes involved as well.

Tremor is present in the distal parts of the extremities and the lips while the involved body part is "at rest." "Pill-rolling" tremor of the fingers and flexion–extension or pronation–supination tremor of the hands are the most typical (Video 1.2). The tremor ceases upon active movement of the limb, but re-emerges when the limb remains in a posture against gravity. Resting tremor must be differentiated from postural and kinetic tremors, in which tremor appears only when the limb is being used. These tremors are typically caused by other disorders, namely essential tremor and cerebellar disorders. An occasional patient with PD will have an action tremor of the hand instead of or in addition to tremor-at-rest (Video 1.3). In the cranial structures, the lips, chin, and tongue are the predominant sites for tremor (Video 1.4), whereas head (neck) tremor – although it can occur in PD – is more typical of essential tremor, cerebellar tremor, and dystonic tremor.

Akinesia/bradykinesia/hypokinesia is manifested cranially by masked facies (hypomimia), decreased frequency of blinking, impaired upgaze, impaired ocular convergence, soft speech (hypophonia), loss of inflection (aprosody), and drooling of saliva due to decreased spontaneous swallowing (Video 1.5). When examining cranial structures, one should look for other signs of PD or parkinsonism-plus syndromes. Repetitive tapping of the glabella often reveals non-suppression of blinking (Myerson sign) in patients with PD (Brodsky et al., 2004) (Video 1.6), whereas blinking is normally suppressed after two or three blinks (Brodsky et al., 2004). Eyelid opening after the eyelids were forcefully closed is usually normal in PD, but may be markedly impaired in progressive supranuclear palsy; this has been called "apraxia of eyelid opening" (Video 1.7) even though apraxia is a misnomer. The eyes looking straight ahead are typically quiet in PD, but in some parkinsonism-plus syndromes, square wave jerks may be seen, especially in progressive supranuclear palsy (Video 1.8). Ocular movements are usually normal in PD, except for impaired upgaze and convergence. When saccadic eye movements are impaired, and especially when downgaze is impaired, a parkinsonism-plus syndrome such as progressive supranuclear palsy or cortical-basal ganglionic degeneration is usually indicated (Video 1.9).

In the arms, bradykinesia is manifested by slowness in shrugging or relaxing the shoulder (Video 1.10); slowness in raising the arm; loss of spontaneous movement such as gesturing; smallness and slowness of handwriting (micrographia); slowness and decrementing amplitude of repetitively opening and closing the hands, tapping a finger and twisting the hand back and forth; difficulty with hand dexterity for shaving, brushing teeth, and putting on makeup; and decreased armswing when walking. In the legs, bradykinesia is manifested by slowness and decrementing amplitude in repetitively stomping the foot or tapping the toes; by slowness in making the number 8 with the foot; and by a slow, short-strided, shuffling gait with reduced heel strike when stepping forward. In the trunk, bradykinesia is manifested by difficulty rising from a chair, getting out of automobiles, and turning in bed.

Bradykinesia encompasses a loss of automatic movements as well as slowness in initiating movement on command and reduction in amplitude of the voluntary movement. An early feature of reduction of amplitude is the decrementing of the amplitude with repetitive finger tapping or foot tapping (Video 1.10), which is also manifested by impaired rhythm of the tapping. Decreased rapid successive movements both in amplitude and speed are characteristic of bradykinesia regardless of the etiology of parkinsonism (Video 1.11).

Carrying out two activities simultaneously is impaired (Schwab et al., 1954), and this difficulty may be a manifestation of bradykinesia (Fahn, 1990). With the stimulation of a sufficient sensory input, bradykinesia, hypokinesia, and akinesia can be temporarily overcome (kinesia paradoxica) (Video 1.12). 🎥

Rigidity (described later in this chapter under "Rigidity") is another cardinal feature of parkinsonism. Rigidity is usually manifested in the distal limbs by a ratchety "give" when a joint is passively moved throughout its range of motion, so-called "cogwheel rigidity." Rigidity of proximal joints is easily appreciated by the examiner's swinging the shoulders (Wartenberg sign) (Video 1.13) or rotating the hips. The patient often complains of stiffness of the neck, which is due to rigidity. 🎥

As the disease advances, the patient begins to assume a *flexed posture*, particularly of the neck, thorax, elbows, hips, and knees. The patient begins to walk with the arms flexed at the elbows and the forearms placed in front of the body, and with decreased armswing. With the knees slightly flexed, the patient tends to shuffle the feet, which stay close to the ground and are not lifted up as high as they would be in normal motion; with time there is loss of heel strike, which would normally occur when the foot moving forward is placed onto the ground. Eventually the flexion can become extreme (Video 1.14), leading to camptocormia (Azher and Jankovic, 2005) or pronounced kyphoscoliosis with truncal tilting. 🎥

Loss of postural reflexes occurs later in the disease. The patient has difficulty righting himself or herself after being pulled off balance. A simple test (the "pull test") for the righting reflex is for the examiner to stand behind the patient and give a firm tug on the patient's shoulders towards the examiner, explaining the procedure in advance and directing that the patient should try to maintain his balance by taking a step backwards (Munhoz et al., 2004; Hunt and Sethi, 2006). Typically, after a practice pull, a normal person can recover within two steps (Video 1.15). A mild loss of postural reflexes can be detected if the patient requires several steps to recover balance. A moderate loss is manifested by a greater degree of retropulsion. With a more severe loss the patient would fall if not caught by the examiner (Video 1.16), who must always be prepared for such a possibility. With a marked loss of postural reflexes a patient cannot withstand a gentle tug on the shoulders or cannot stand unassisted without falling. To avoid having the patient fall to the ground, it is wise to have a wall behind the examiner, particularly if the patient is a large or bulky individual. 🎥

A combination of loss of postural reflexes and stooped posture can lead to *festination*, whereby the patient walks faster and faster, trying to catch up with his or her center of gravity to prevent falling (Video 1.17). 🎥

Akinesia needs to be distinguished from the freezing phenomenon, both of which are features of parkinsonism. The *freezing phenomenon* predominantly affects a patient's gait and begins either with start-hesitation – that is, the feet take short, sticking, shuffling steps when the patient initiates walking, or turning-hesitation while walking (Video 1.18). With progression, the feet become "glued to the ground" when the patient walks through a crowded space (e.g., a revolving door) or is trying to move a distance in a short period of time (e.g., crossing the street at the green light or entering an elevator before the door closes). Often, patients develop destination-freezing – that is, stopping before reaching the final destination. For example, the patient might stop too soon when reaching a chair in which he or she intends to sit down. With further progression, sudden transient freezing can occur when the patient is walking in an open space or when the patient perceives an obstacle in the walking path. The freezing phenomenon can also affect arms and speech and is discussed in more detail under "Freezing" later in this chapter. 🎥

In addition to these motor signs, most patients with PD have behavioral signs. *Bradyphrenia* is mental slowness, analogous to the motor slowness of bradykinesia. Bradyphrenia is manifested by slowness in thinking or in responding to questions. It occurs even at a young age in PD and is more common than dementia. The "tip-of-the-tongue" phenomenon (Matison et al., 1982), in which a patient cannot immediately come up with the correct answer but knows what it is, may be a feature of bradyphrenia. With time the parkinsonian patient gradually becomes more passive, indecisive, dependent, and fearful. The spouse gradually makes more of the decisions and becomes the dominant voice. Eventually, the patient would sit much of the day unless encouraged to do activities. Passivity and lack of motivation also express themselves by the patient's not desiring to attend social events. The term *abulia* is used to describe such apathy, loss of mental and motor drive, and blunting of emotional, social, and motor expression. Abulia encompasses loss of spontaneous and responsive motor activity and loss of spontaneous affective expression, thought, and initiative.

Depression is a frequent feature in patients with PD, being obvious in around 30% of cases. The prevalence of *dementia* in PD is about 40%, but the proportion increases with age. Below the age of 60 years, the proportion with dementia is about 8%; older than 80 years, it is 69% (Mayeux et al., 1992). Following PD patients over time, about 80% develop dementia (Aarsland et al., 2003; Buter et al., 2008). The risk of death is markedly increased when a PD patient becomes demented (Marder et al., 1991).

The age at onset of PD is usually above the age of 40, but younger patients can be affected. Onset between ages 20 and 40 is called young-onset Parkinson disease; onset before age 20 is called juvenile parkinsonism. Juvenile parkinsonism does not preclude a diagnosis of Parkinson disease, but it raises questions of other etiologies, such as Wilson disease (Video 1.5) and the Westphal variant of Huntington disease (Video 1.11). Also familial and sporadic primary juvenile parkinsonism might not show the typical pathologic hallmark of Lewy bodies (Dwork et al., 1993). One needs to be aware when reading the literature that in Japan, onset before age 40 is called juvenile parkinsonism and that some research studies have called onset by age 50 young-onset.

PD is more common in men, with a male:female ratio of 3:2. The incidence in the United States is 20 new cases per 100,000 population per year (Schoenberg, 1987), with a prevalence of 187 cases per 100 000 population (Kurland, 1958). For the population over 40 years of age, the prevalence rate is 347 per 100 000 (Schoenberg et al., 1985). With the introduction of levodopa the mortality rate dropped from 3-fold to 1.5-fold above normal. But after the first wave of impaired patients becoming improved with this new and effective treatment, the mortality rate for PD gradually climbed back to the pre-levodopa rate (Clarke, 1995).

Apraxia

Apraxia is a cerebral cortex, not a basal ganglia, dysfunction. Apraxia is traditionally defined as a disorder of voluntary movement that cannot be explained by weakness, spasticity, rigidity, akinesia, sensory loss, or cognitive impairment. It can exist and be tested for in the presence of a movement disorder provided that akinesia, rigidity, or dystonia is not so severe that voluntary movement cannot be executed. The classic work of Liepmann (1920) defined three categories of apraxia.

1. In *ideational apraxia* the concept or plan of movement cannot be formulated by the patient. Some examiners test for ideational apraxia by asking the patient to perform a series of sequential movements such as filling a pipe, lighting it, and then smoking, or putting a letter into an envelope, sealing it, and then affixing a stamp. Ideational apraxia is due to parietal lesions, most often diffuse and degenerative.
2. In *ideomotor apraxia* the concept or plan of movement is intact, but the individual motor engrams or programs are defective. Ideomotor apraxia is commonly tested for by asking patients to undertake specific motor acts to verbal or written commands, such as waving goodbye, saluting like a soldier, combing their hair, or using a hammer to fix a nail, etc. The patients with ideomotor apraxia often improve their performance if asked to mimic the action when the examiner shows them what to do or when given the object or tool to use. Ideomotor apraxia usually does not interfere with normal spontaneous motor actions but requires specific testing for its demonstration. It usually, but not always, is associated with aphasia and is due mainly to lesions in the dominant hemisphere, particularly in the parietotemporal regions, the arcuate fasciculus, or the frontal lobe; such ideomotor apraxia is bilateral, provided that there is not a hemiplegia. Lesions of the corpus callosum can cause apraxia of the nondominant hand.
3. *Limb-kinetic apraxia* is the least understood type. It refers to a higher-order motor deficit in executing motor acts that cannot be explained by simple motor impairments. It has been attributed to lesions of premotor regions in the frontal lobe, such as the supplementary motor area.

The concepts of apraxia are being refined into more discrete identifiable syndromes as knowledge of the functions of the cortical systems controlling voluntary movement advances (for reviews, see Pramstaller and Marsden, 1996; Zadikoff and Lang, 2005). A quick, convenient method for testing for apraxia at the bedside is to ask the patients to copy a series of hand postures shown to them by the examiner.

Ideomotor and limb-kinetic apraxias are found in a number of movement disorders – for example, cortical-basal ganglionic degeneration (CBGD) (Video 1.19) and progressive supranuclear palsy (see Chapter 9). A number of other phenomena reflecting cerebral cortex dysfunction may be seen in such patients. Patients with CBGD frequently have signs of cortical myoclonus (Video 1.20) or cortical sensory deficit. The alien limb phenomenon, also seen in CBGD, consists of involuntary, spontaneous movements of an arm or leg (Video 1.21), which curiously and spontaneously moves to adopt odd postures quite beyond the control or understanding of the patient. Intermanual conflict is another such phenomenon; one hand irresistibly and uncontrollably begins to interfere with voluntary action of the other. The abnormally behaving limb may also show forced grasping of objects, such as blankets or clothing. Such patients often exhibit other frontal lobe signs, such as a grasp reflex or utilization behavior, in which they compulsively pick up objects presented to them and begin to use them. For example, if a pen is presented with no instructions, they pick it up and write. If a pair of glasses is proffered, they place the glasses on the nose; if further pairs of glasses are then shown, the patient may end up with three or more spectacles on the nose!

Blocking (holding) tics

Blocking (or holding) is a motor phenomenon that is seen occasionally in patients with tics and is characterized as a brief interference of social discourse and contact. There is no loss of consciousness and although the patient does not speak during these episodes, he or she is fully aware of what has been spoken. These *blocking tics* appear in two situations: (1) as an accompanying feature of some prolonged tics, such as during a protracted dystonic tic (Video 1.22) or during tic status, and (2) as a specific tic phenomenon in the absence of an accompanying obvious motor or vocal tic. The latter occurrences have the abruptness and duration of a dystonic tic or a series of clonic tics, but they do not occur during an episode of an obvious motor tic.

Although both types can be called blocking tics, the first type can be considered "intrusions" because the interruption of activity is due to a positive motor phenomenon (i.e., severe, somewhat prolonged, motor tics) that interferes with other motor activities. An example would be a burst of tics that is severe enough to interrupt ongoing motor acts, including speech, as seen in Video 1.22.

The second type (i.e., inhibition of ongoing motor activity without an obvious "active" tic) can be considered a negative motor phenomenon, i.e., a "negative" tic. The negative type of *blocking tics* should be differentiated from absence seizures or other paroxysmal episodes of loss of awareness. There is never loss of awareness with blocking tics. Individuals with intrusions and negative blocking recognize that they have these interruptions of normal activity and are fully aware of the environment during them, even if they are unable to speak at that time.

Cataplexy and drop attacks

Drop attacks can be defined as sudden falls with or without loss of consciousness, due either to collapse of postural muscle tone or to abnormal muscle contractions in the legs. About two-thirds of cases are of unknown etiology (Meissner et al., 1986). Symptomatic drop attacks have many neurologic and non-neurologic causes. Neurologic disorders include leg weakness, sudden falls in parkinsonian syndromes including those due to freezing, transient ischemic attacks, epilepsy, myoclonus, startle reactions (hyperekplexia), paroxysmal dyskinesias, structural central nervous system lesions, and hydrocephalus. In some of these, there is loss of muscle tone in the legs, in others there is excessive muscle stiffness with immobility, such as in hyperekplexia. Syncope and cardiovascular disease account for non-neurologic causes. Idiopathic drop attacks usually appear between the ages of 40 and 59 years, the prevalence increasing with advancing age (Stevens and Matthews, 1973), and are a common cause of falls and fractures in elderly people (Sheldon, 1960; Nickens, 1985). A review of drop attacks has been provided by Lee and Marsden (1995).

Cataplexy is another cause of symptomatic drop attacks that does not fit the categories listed previously. Patients with cataplexy fall suddenly without loss of consciousness but with inability to speak during an attack. There is a precipitating trigger, usually laughter or a sudden emotional stimulus. The patient's muscle tone is flaccid and remains this way for many seconds. Cataplexy is usually just one feature of the narcolepsy syndrome; other features include sleep paralysis and hypnagogic hallucinations, in addition to the characteristic feature of sudden, uncontrollable falling asleep. A review of cataplexy has been provided by Guilleminault and Gelb (1995).

Catatonia, psychomotor depression, and obsessional slowness

In 1874, Karl Ludwig Kahlbaum wrote the following description: "the patient remains entirely motionless, without speaking, and with a rigid, mask like facies, the eyes focused at a distance; he seems devoid of any will to move or react to any stimuli; there may be fully developed 'waxen' flexibility, as in cataleptic states, or only indications, distinct, nevertheless, of this striking phenomenon. The general impression conveyed by such patients is one of profound mental anguish" (Bush et al., 1996).

Gelenberg (1976) defined *catatonia* as a syndrome characterized by catalepsy (abnormal maintenance of posture or physical attitudes), waxy flexibility (retention of the limbs for an indefinite period of time in the positions in which they are placed), negativism, mutism, and bizarre mannerisms. Patients with catatonia can remain in one position for hours and move exceedingly slowly to commands, usually requiring the examiner to push them along (Video 1.23). But, when moving spontaneously, they move quickly, such as when scratching themselves. In contrast to patients with parkinsonism, there is no concomitant cogwheel rigidity, freezing, or loss of postural reflexes. Classically, catatonia is a feature of schizophrenia, but it can also occur with severe depression. Gelenberg also stated that catatonia can appear with conversion hysteria, dissociative states, and organic brain disease. However, we believe that his organic syndromes of akinetic mutism, abulia, encephalitis, and so forth should be distinguished from catatonia, and catatonia should preferably be considered a psychiatric disorder.

Depression is commonly associated with a general slowness of movement, as well as of thought, so-called psychomotor retardation, and catatonia can be considered an extreme case of this problem. Although depressed patients are widely recognized to manifest slowness in movement, some – particularly children – might not have the more classic symptoms of low mood, dysphoria, anorexia, insomnia, somatizations, and tearfulness. In this situation, slowness due to depression can be difficult to distinguish from the bradykinesia of parkinsonism. As in catatonia, lack of rigidity and preservation of postural reflexes may help to differentiate psychomotor slowness from parkinsonism. However, there can be loss of facial expression and decreased blinking in both catatonia and depression. Lack of Myerson sign, snout reflex, and palmomental reflexes are the rule, all of which are usually present in parkinsonism. In children with psychomotor depression and motor slowness (Video 1.24), the differential diagnosis is that of juvenile parkinsonism, including Wilson disease and the akinetic form of Huntington disease.

Some patients with obsessive-compulsive disorder (OCD) may present with extreme slowness of movement, so-called *obsessional slowness*. Hymas and colleagues (1991) evaluated 17 such patients out of 59 admitted to hospital with OCD. These patients had difficulty initiating goal-directed action and had many suppressive interruptions and perseverative behaviors. Besides slowness, some patients had cogwheel rigidity, decreased armswing when walking, decreased spontaneous movement, hypomimia, and flexed posture. However, there was no decrementing of either amplitude or speed with repetitive movements, no tremor, and no micrographia. Also there was no freezing or loss of postural reflexes. Like other cases of OCD, this is a chronic illness. Fluorodopa positron emission tomography scans revealed no abnormality of dopa uptake, thereby clearly distinguishing this disorder from PD (Sawle et al., 1991). However, there is hypermetabolism in orbital, frontal, premotor, and midfrontal cortex, suggesting excessive neural activity in these regions.

Freezing

Freezing refers to transient periods, usually lasting several seconds, in which the motor act is halted, being stuck in place. It commonly develops in parkinsonism (see Chapter 4), both primary and atypical parkinsonism (Giladi et al., 1997), and it is one of its six cardinal signs. The freezing phenomenon has also been called motor blocks (Giladi et al., 1992). The terms *pure akinesia* (Narabayashi et al., 1976, 1986; Imai et al., 1986), and *gait ignition failure* (Atchison et al., 1993; Nutt et al., 1993) refer to syndromes in which freezing is the predominant clinical feature with only a few other features of parkinsonism.

In freezing there can be several different phenomena. One is no apparent attempt to move. Another is that the voluntary motor activity being attempted is halted because agonist and antagonist muscles are simultaneously and isometrically contracting (Andrews, 1973), preventing normal execution of voluntary movement. The motor blockage in this circumstance, therefore, is not one of lack of muscle activity, but rather is analogous to being glued to a position so that the patient exerts increased effort to overcome being "stuck." The stuck body part attempts to move to overcome the block, and muscle force (isometric) is being exerted. So, with freezing of gait, by far the most common form of

Table 1.9 Types of freezing phenomena

Start-hesitation (freezing when gait is initiated)
Turning-hesitation (freezing when turning)
Destination-hesitation (freezing when approaching the target)
Freezing when a physical or a temporal "obstacle" is encountered
Spontaneous sudden transient freezing
Palilalia or freezing of speech
"Apraxia" of eyelid opening or levator inhibition
Freezing of limbs

the freezing phenomenon, as the patient attempts to move the feet, short, incomplete steps are attempted, but the feet tend to remain in the same place ("glued to the ground"). After a few seconds, the freezing clears spontaneously, and the patient is able to move at his or her normal pace again until the next freezing episode develops. Often, the patient has learned some trick maneuver to terminate the freezing episode sooner (Videos 1.25 and 1.26). Stepping over an inverted cane when the legs begin to freeze is one method by which patients can manage to ambulate (Video 1.27).

Although freezing most often affects walking, it can manifest in other ways (Table 1.9). Speech can be arrested with the patient repeating a sound until it finally becomes unstuck, and speech then continues (Video 1.28). This can be considered a severe form of parkinsonian palilalia, which usually refers to a repetition of the first syllable of the word the patient is trying to verbally express. Parkinsonian palilalia differs from the palilalia seen in patients with Gilles de la Tourette syndrome, in which there is repetition of entire words or a string of words (see Video 1.22).

Freezing of the arms, such as during handwriting or teeth-brushing, has also been reported (Narabayashi et al., 1976). Difficulty opening the eyes can be another example of freezing (see Video 1.7). This eyelid freezing was originally called *apraxia of eyelid opening*, which is a misnomer because the problem is not an apraxia. Eyelid freezing has also been called "levator palpebrae inhibition" (Lepore and Duvoisin, 1985) and even a form of dystonia. Although previously unrecognized as a freezing phenomenon and usually considered a form of body bradykinesia, difficulty in rising from a chair may be due to freezing in some patients (see Video 1.25). Patients use many tricks to overcome freezing, but these might not always be successful. A discourse on the freezing phenomenon is provided in a review by Fahn (1995).

As was discussed previously, the freezing phenomenon occurs in parkinsonism, whether it be primary (PD) (Giladi et al., 1992), secondary (such as vascular parkinsonism), or parkinsonism-plus syndromes, such as progressive supranuclear palsy and multiple system atrophy. It can also appear as an idiopathic freezing gait without other features of parkinsonism, except for loss of postural reflexes and mild bradykinesia (Achiron et al., 1993; Atchison et al., 1993) (Video 1.29). In some patients, it may be an early sign of impending progressive supranuclear palsy (Riley et al., 1994) or due to nigropallidal degeneration (Katayama et al., 1998).

Hesitant gaits

Hesitant gaits or uncertain gaits are seen in a number of syndromes (see Chapter 10). The *cautious gait* that is seen in some elderly people is slow on a wide base with short steps and superficially may resemble that of parkinsonism except that there are no other parkinsonian features. *Fear of falling*, because of either perceived instability or realistic loss of postural righting reflexes, produces an inability to walk independently without holding onto people or objects. Because this abnormal gait disappears when the person walks holding onto someone, it is often considered to be a psychiatric disorder, a phobia of open spaces (i.e., agoraphobia). But because previous falls usually play a role in patients developing this disorder, it appears to be a true fear of falling that is distinguishable from agoraphobia, which is a separate syndrome. Fear of falling (a psychiatric gait disorder) should be differentiated from psychogenic gait disorders (see Chapter 25). A *cautious gait*, such as in fear of falling, may be superimposed on any other gait disorder.

The *senile gait disorder* (or *gait disorder of the elderly*) is a poorly understood condition that comprises a number of different syndromes (Nutt et al., 1993). In *gait ignition failure* (Atchison et al., 1993), also called *primary freezing gait* (Achiron et al., 1993), the problem is one of getting started. Once underway, such patients walk fairly briskly (see Video 1.29), and equilibrium is preserved. In *frontal gait disorders*, there is also start-hesitation, and walking is with slow, small, shuffling steps, similar to that in PD. However, there are few other signs of parkinsonism, and equilibrium is preserved. Such a gait can occur with frontal lobe tumors, cerebrovascular disease, and hydrocephalus, all causing frontal lobe damage. This pattern has been incorrectly called frontal ataxia or gait apraxia in the older literature.

Other hesitant gaits are those due to *severe disequilibrium*. These types of gait have been associated with frontal cortex and deep white matter lesions (*frontal disequilibrium*) or thalamic and midbrain lesions (*subcortical disequilibrium*) (Nutt et al., 1993). Hesitant gait syndromes are covered in more depth in Chapter 10.

Hypothyroid slowness

Along with decreased metabolic rate, cool temperature, bradycardia, myxedema, loss of hair, hoarseness, and myotonia, severe hypothyroidism can feature motor slowness, weakness, and lethargy. These signs could be mistaken for the bradykinesia of parkinsonism, but the combination of the other signs of hypothyroidism, along with lack of rigidity and loss of postural reflexes, should aid the correct diagnosis.

Rigidity

Rigidity is characterized as increased muscle tone to passive motion. It is distinguished from spasticity in that it is present equally in all directions of the passive movement, equally in flexors and extensors, and throughout the range of motion, and it does not exhibit the clasp-knife phenomenon, nor increased tendon reflexes. Rigidity can be smooth (lead-pipe) or jerky (cogwheel). Cogwheeling occurs in the same range of frequencies as action and resting tremor

(Lance et al., 1963) and appears to be due to superimposition of a tremor rhythm (Denny-Brown, 1962). Cogwheel rigidity is more common than the lead-pipe variety in parkinsonism (nigral lesion), and lead-pipe rigidity can be caused by a number of other central nervous system lesions (Fahn, 1987), including those involving the corpus striatum (hypoxia, vascular, neuroleptic malignant syndrome), cortical-basal (ganglionic degeneration) (Video 1.30), midbrain (decorticate rigidity), medulla (decerebrate rigidity), and spinal cord (tetanus). When a patient does not thoroughly relax to allow passive manipulation of his/her joints, but tends to actively resist, the result is increased muscle tone, so-called Gegenhalten. Gegenhalten is commonly seen in patients with impaired cognition. Often, with Gegenhalten, more force applied by the examiner is met with more resistance by the patient. 🎥

An increase in passive muscle tone can sometimes lead to impaired motor performance or even immobility. Before there was a clear understanding of bradykinesia, rigidity was considered to be responsible for the paucity of movement in parkinsonism. But rigidity is clearly distinct from bradykinesia; the former is more easily treated by levodopa therapy or by stereotactic thalamotomy or stimulation of the subthalamic nucleus, and can be relieved while bradykinesia with residual paucity of movement persists. When rigidity is extremely severe, such that the examiner can barely move the limbs, as in patients with neuroleptic malignant syndrome, the patient is virtually unable to move. The extended neck that is occasionally seen in progressive supranuclear palsy (Steele–Richardson–Olszewski syndrome) may be due to rigidity (versus dystonia); the neck can be immobile in this disorder, and other axial muscles are also rigid.

Rigidity is one part of the neuroleptic malignant syndrome (NMS) (see Chapter 19), which is an idiosyncratic adverse effect of dopamine receptor blocking agents, usually antipsychotic drugs (Smego and Durack, 1982; Kurlan et al., 1984), but it has also been reported to occur on sudden discontinuation of levodopa therapy (Friedman et al., 1985; Keyser and Rodnitzky, 1991). The clinical features of the syndrome are the abrupt onset of a combination of rigidity/dystonia, fever with other autonomic dysfunctions such as diaphoresis and dyspnea, and an altered mental state including confusion, stupor, or coma. The level of serum creatine kinase activity is usually elevated. The dopamine receptor blocking agents may have been administered at therapeutic, not toxic, dosages. There does not seem to be any relationship with the duration of therapy. It can develop soon after the first dose or anytime after prolonged treatment. This is a potentially lethal disorder unless treated; up to 25% of patients die (Henderson and Wooten, 1981). NMS is sometimes called malignant catatonia (Boeve et al., 1994), and needs to be distinguished from malignant hyperthermia.

Stiff muscles

Stiff muscles are defined as being due to continuous muscle firing without muscle disease, and not to rigidity or spasticity. Stiffness syndromes are reviewed in detail in Chapter 11. Briefly, there are four major clinical categories of stiff-muscle syndromes: continuous muscle fiber activity or neuromyotonia, encephalomyelitis with rigidity, the stiff-limb syndrome, and the stiff-person syndrome (Thompson, 1994), with the last three being variations of the same disorder. *Neuromyotonia* is a syndrome of myotonic failure of muscle relaxation plus myokymia and fasciculations. Clinically it manifests as continuous muscle activity causing stiffness and cramps. The best-known neuromyotonic disorder is Isaacs syndrome (Isaacs, 1961).

Encephalomyelitis with rigidity (Whiteley et al., 1976), initially called spinal interneuronitis, manifests with marked rigidity and muscle irritability, with increased response to tapping the muscles, along with myoclonus (Video 1.31). It is now recognized as a severe manifestation of stiff-person syndrome and may respond to steroid therapy. 🎥

Stiff-person syndrome refers to a rare disorder (Spehlmann and Norcross, 1979) in which many somatic muscles are continuously contracting isometrically, resembling "chronic tetanus," in contrast to dystonic movements which produce abnormal twisting and patterned movements and postures. The contractions of stiff-person syndrome are usually forceful and painful and most frequently involve the trunk and neck musculature (Video 1.32). The proximal limb muscles can also be involved, but rarely does the disorder first affect the distal limbs. Benzodiazepines and valproate are usually somewhat effective. Withdrawal of these agents results in an increase of painful spasms. This disorder has now been recognized to be an autoimmune disease, with circulating antibodies against the GABA-synthesizing enzyme, glutamic acid decarboxylase, and also other type of antibodies, including antibodies against insulin (Solimena et al., 1988, 1990; Blum and Jankovic, 1991). Diabetes is a common accompanying disorder. The diagnosis can now be aided by laboratory testing for these antibodies. The syndrome of interstitial neuronitis, also called encephalomyelitis with rigidity and myoclonus, is a more acute variant of the stiff-person syndrome. The so-called stiff-baby syndrome (Video 1.33) is actually due to infantile hyperekplexia, in which the muscles continue to fire repeatedly and so frequently that the muscles appear to contract continuously. 🎥

Evaluation of a dyskinesia

The traditional approach in neurology when evaluating a patient is to ask first where is the lesion, then what is the lesion and finally how do we treat this problem. Essentially, the first question, then, is about localization within the nervous system. This traditional approach is not ordinarily followed when confronting a patient with a movement disorder. Our first question is what is the phenomenology, i.e., what is the type of dyskinesia we are witnessing. The next question is what is the cause, and the third question is how do we treat it. In other words, localization, although important in many situations, is not as important as in recognizing the phenomenology. We can expand upon the three questions with a prior one, namely is the excess movement a dyskinesia or is it a variation of normal motor control.

Thus, the first question to be answered in seeing a person with extraneous movements is whether or not abnormal involuntary movements are actually present. One must consider whether the suspected movements might be purposeful voluntary movements, such as exaggerated gestures, mannerisms or compulsive movements, or whether sustained contracted muscles might be physiologic reflex muscle tightness to reduce pain, so-called guarding. It should also be noted that as a general rule, abnormal involuntary movements are exaggerated with anxiety, and most diminish or disappear during sleep. They may or may not lessen with amobarbital or with hypnosis.

Once it has been decided that abnormal movements are present, the next question is to determine the category of the involuntary movement, such as chorea, dystonia, myoclonus, tics, or tremor. In other words, determine the nature of the involuntary movements. To do so, one evaluates features such as rhythmicity, speed, duration, pattern (e.g., repetitive, flowing, continual, paroxysmal, diurnal), induction (i.e., stimuli-induced, action-induced, exercise-induced), complexity of the movements (complex versus simple), suppressibility by volitional attention or by sensory tricks, and whether the movements are accompanied by sensations such as restlessness or the urge to make a movement that can release a built-up tension. In addition, the examiner must determine which body parts are involved. The evaluation for the type of dyskinesia is the major subject of the next section in this chapter.

The third question is to determine the etiology of the abnormal involuntary movements. Is the disorder hereditary, sporadic, or secondary to some known neurologic disorder? The etiology and workup for the various dyskinesias are discussed in each chapter dealing with specific types of movement disorders in this chapter. As a general rule, the etiology can be ascertained on the basis of the history and judiciously selected laboratory tests.

The final question is how best to treat the movement disorder. Treatments of the various movement disorders are covered in the appropriate chapters of this book.

Differential diagnosis of dyskinesias

The differential diagnosis of movement disorders depends primarily on their clinical features. It is important to observe and describe the nature of the involuntary movements as mentioned previously. In addition, one examines for postural changes, for alteration of muscle tone, for loss of postural reflexes, for motor impersistence, and for any other neurological abnormalities on the general neurological examination.

A list of abnormal involuntary movements is presented alphabetically in Table 1.1 under "Hyperkinesias." A brief description of each of these is now presented along with its major recognizable and differentiating features. Tables 1.10–1.18 list the ordinary process of distinguishing one type of dyskinesia from another by the major stepwise deciphering based on a practical approach.

Abdominal dyskinesias

Abdominal dyskinesias are continuous movements of the abdominal wall or sometimes the diaphragm. The movements persist, and their sinuous, rhythmic nature has led to their being called belly dancer's dyskinesia (Iliceto et al., 1990). They may be associated with abdominal trauma in some cases, and a common result is segmental abdominal myoclonus (Kono et al., 1994) (Video 1.34). Another common cause is tardive dyskinesia. *Hiccups*, which are regularly recurring diaphragmatic myoclonus, do not move the abdomen and umbilicus in a sinewy fashion but with sharp jerks and typically with noises as air is expelled by the contractions, so they should not present a diagnostic problem. Abdominal dyskinesias are discussed in Chapter 23.

Akathitic movements

Akathisia (from the Greek, meaning unable to sit still) refers to a feeling of inner, general restlessness that is reduced or relieved by moving about. The typical akathitic patient, when seated, may caress his or her scalp, cross and uncross the legs, rock the trunk, squirm, get out of the chair often to pace back and forth (Video 1.35), and even make noises such as moaning (Video 1.36). Carrying out these motor acts brings relief from the sensations of akathisia. Akathitic movements are complex and usually stereotyped; the same type of movements are employed over and over. Other movement disorders that show complex movements are tics, compulsions, mannerisms, and the stereotypies associated with intellectual disability, autism, or psychosis.

Akathisia does not necessarily affect the whole body; an isolated body part can be affected. Focal akathisia often produces a sensation of burning or pain, again relieved by moving that body part. Common sites for focal akathisia/pain are the mouth and vagina (Ford et al., 1994).

Akathisia may be expressed by vocalizations, such as continual moaning, groaning, or humming. Other movement disorders associated with moaning sounds or humming are tics, oromandibular dystonia, Huntington disease, parkinsonian disorders (Micheli et al., 1991; Friedman, 1993), and those induced by levodopa (Fahn et al., 1996).

The patient can transiently suppress akathitic movements and vocalizations if he or she is asked to do so.

The most common cause of akathisia is iatrogenic. It is a frequent complication of antidopaminergic drugs, including those that block dopamine receptors (such as antipsychotic drugs and certain antiemetics) and those that deplete dopamine (such as reserpine and tetrabenazine). Akathisia can occur when drug therapy is initiated (acute akathisia), subsequently with the emergence of drug-induced parkinsonism, or after chronic treatment (tardive akathisia). Acute akathisia is eliminated on withdrawal of the medication. Tardive akathisia usually is associated with the syndrome of tardive dyskinesia (see Chapter 19). Like tardive dyskinesia, tardive akathisia is aggravated by discontinuing the neuroleptic, and it is usually relieved by increasing the dose of the offending drug which masks the movement disorder. When associated with tardive dyskinesia, the akathitic movements can be rhythmic, such as body rocking or marching in place. In this situation, it is difficult to be certain whether such rhythmic movements are due to akathisia or to tardive dyskinesia.

The exact mechanism of akathisia is not known, but it seems that the dopamine systems are involved, possibly in the limbic system or frontal cortex. It is of interest that akathisia, both generalized and regional, can be present in patients with PD.

Ataxia/Asynergia/Dysmetria

Ataxia, *asynergia*, and *dyssynergia* are interchangeable terms that refer to decomposition of movement due to breakdown of normal coordinated execution of a voluntary movement. Ataxia is one of the cardinal clinical features of cerebellar disease or of lesions involving the pathways to or from the cerebellum (Video 1.37). Instead of a smooth, continuous movement, the limb wanders off its trajectory attempting to a reach a target, with corrective maneuvers that resemble oscillations of the limb. The limb usually misses the target (*dysmetria*); the ataxia worsens when the limb approaches the target. Common tests for ataxia and dysmetria are the finger-to-nose-to-finger maneuver and the maneuver of heel-to-knee and then the heel sliding down the shin. Limb ataxia is also manifested by *dysdiadochokinesia*, which refers to the breakup and irregularity that occurs when the limb is attempting to carry out rapid alternating movements. The dysmetria with cerebellar dysfunction is due to overshooting (hypermetria) and undershooting (hypometria) of the target. There may be an associated intention (or terminal) tremor (see under "Tremor" later in this chapter). Ataxia is usually associated with hypotonia, loss of check (when a fast voluntary movement is unable to stop precisely on target when the limb reaches its destination), and rebound (when sudden displacement of a limb results in excessive over-correction to return to the baseline position). Ataxia is seen only during voluntary movement and is not a feature of a limb at rest. *Ataxia* of gait is typified by unsteadiness on walking with a wide base, the body swaying, and an inability to tandem walk (heel-to-toe).

Athetosis

Athetosis has been used in two senses: to describe a class of slow, writhing, continuous, involuntary movements, and to describe the syndrome of athetoid cerebral palsy. The latter commonly occurs as a result of injury to the basal ganglia in the prenatal or perinatal period or during infancy. Athetotic movements affect the limbs, especially distally, but can also involve axial musculature, including neck, face, and tongue. When not present in certain body parts at rest, it can often be brought out by having the patient carry out voluntary motor activity elsewhere in the body; this phenomenon is known as *overflow*. For example, speaking can induce increased athetosis in the limbs, neck, trunk, face, and tongue (Video 1.38). Athetosis often is associated with sustained contractions producing abnormal posturing. In this regard, athetosis blends with dystonia. However, the speed of these involuntary movements can sometimes be faster and blend with those of chorea, and the term *choreoathetosis* is used. Athetosis resembles "slow" chorea in that the direction of movement changes randomly and in a flowing pattern (see Chapter 15).

Pseudoathetosis refers to distal athetoid movements of the fingers and toes due to loss of proprioception, which can be due to sensory deafferentation (sensory athetosis) or to central loss of proprioception (Sharp et al., 1994).

Ballism

Ballism refers to very large-amplitude choreic movements of the proximal parts of the limbs, causing flinging and flailing limb movements (see Chapter 15). Ballism is most frequently unilateral, in which case it is referred to as *hemiballism* (Video 1.39). This is often the result of a lesion in the contralateral subthalamic nucleus or its connections or of multiple small infarcts (lacunes) in the contralateral striatum. In rare instances, ballism occurs bilaterally (*biballism*) and is due to bilateral lacunes in the basal ganglia (Sethi et al., 1987). Like chorea, ballism can sometimes occur as a result of overdosage of levodopa.

Chorea

Chorea refers to involuntary, irregular, purposeless, non-rhythmic, abrupt, rapid, unsustained movements that seem to flow from one body part to another. A characteristic feature of chorea is that the movements are unpredictable in timing, direction, and distribution (i.e., random). Although some neurologists erroneously label almost all nonrhythmic, rapid involuntary movements as choreic, many in fact are not. Nonchoreic rapid movements can be tics, myoclonus, and dystonia (see the chapters for each of these disorders); in these conditions, the movements repeat themselves in a set distribution of the body (i.e., are patterned) and do not have the changing, flowing nature of choreic movements, which travel around the body. In rapid dystonic movements, there is a recognizable repetitive recurrence to the movements in the affected body parts, unlike the random nature of chorea. The prototypical choreic movements are those seen in Huntington disease (Video 1.40), in which the brief and rapid movements are irregular and occur randomly as a function of time. In Sydenham chorea and in the withdrawal emergent syndrome (see Chapter 19), the flowing choreic movements have a restless appearance (Video 1.41).

When choreic movements are infrequent, they appear as isolated, small-amplitude, brief movements, somewhat slower than myoclonus but sometimes difficult to distinguish from it. When chorea is more pronounced, the movements occur almost continually, presenting as involuntary movements flowing from one site of the body to another.

Choreic movements can be partially suppressed, and the patient can often camouflage some of the movements by incorporating them into semipurposeful movements, known as *parakinesia*. Chorea is usually accompanied by *motor impersistence* ("negative chorea"), the inability to maintain a sustained contraction. A common symptom of motor impersistence is the dropping of objects. Motor impersistence is detected by examining for the inability to keep the tongue protruded and by the presence of the "milk-maid" grip due to the inability to keep the fist in a sustained tight grip. For details on choreic disorders, see Chapters 14 and 15.

Dystonia

Dystonia refers to movements that tend to be sustained at the peak of the movement, are usually twisting and frequently repetitive, and often progress to prolonged abnormal postures (see Chapter 12). In contrast to chorea, dystonic movements repeatedly involve the same group of muscles – that is, they are patterned. Agonist and antagonist muscles contract simultaneously (cocontraction) to produce the sustained quality of dystonic movements. The speed of the movement varies widely from slow (athetotic dystonia) to shocklike (myoclonic dystonia). When the contractions are very brief (e.g., less than a second), they are referred to as dystonic spasms. When they are sustained for several seconds, they are called dystonic movements. When they last minutes to hours, they are known as *dystonic postures*. When present for weeks or longer, the postures can lead to permanent fixed contractures.

When dystonia first appears, the movements typically occur when the affected body part is carrying out a voluntary action (*action dystonia*) and are not present when that body part is at rest. With progression of the disorder, dystonic movements can appear at distant sites (*overflow*) when other parts of the body are voluntarily moving, such as occurs also in athetosis and in dopa-induced dyskinesias. With further progression, dystonic movements become present when the body is "at rest." Even at this stage, dystonic movements are usually made more severe with voluntary activity. Whereas primary dystonia often begins as action dystonia and may persist as the kinetic (clonic) form, secondary dystonia often begins as sustained postures (tonic form).

One of the characteristic and almost unique features of dystonic movements is that they can often be diminished by tactile or proprioceptive "sensory tricks" (*geste antagoniste*). Thus, touching the involved body part or an adjacent body part can often reduce the muscle contractions. Inexperienced clinicians might assume that this sign indicates that the abnormal movements are psychogenic, but the opposite conclusion should be reached, namely that the presence of sensory tricks strongly suggests an organic etiology (Fahn and Williams, 1988). If the dystonia becomes more severe, sensory tricks providing relief tend to diminish.

When a single body part is affected, the condition is referred to as *focal dystonia*. Common forms of focal dystonia are spasmodic torticollis (cervical dystonia), blepharospasm (upper facial dystonia), and writer's cramp (hand dystonia). Involvement of two or more contiguous regions of the body is referred to as *segmental dystonia*. *Generalized dystonia* indicates involvement of one or both legs, the trunk, and some other part of the body. *Multifocal dystonia* involves two or more regions, not conforming to segmental or generalized dystonia. *Hemidystonia* refers to involvement of the arm and leg on the same side. A variety of these types of dystonia are shown in Videos 1.42 to 1.49.

One type of focal dystonia requires special mention, namely sustained contractions of ocular muscles, resulting in tonic ocular deviation, usually upward gaze (Video 1.50). This is referred to as *oculogyric crisis*. This sustained ocular deviation was encountered in victims of encephalitis lethargica and later in those survivors who developed postencephalitic parkinsonism. Primary torsion dystonia does *not* involve the ocular muscles, hence oculogyria is not truly a feature of dystonia syndromes. Oculogyria is more common today as a complication of dopamine receptor blocking agents (Paulson, 1960) as in drug-induced parkinsonism or other parkinsonian syndromes such as juvenile parkinsonism and the parkinsonism associated with the degenerative disease known as neuronal intranuclear inclusion disease (Kilroy et al., 1972; Funata et al., 1990), and with the biochemical deficiency of the monoamines in the metabolic disorders of aromatic amino acid decarboxylase deficiency

(Hyland et al., 1992; Chang et al., 2004) and pterin deficiencies (Hyland et al., 1998). There has been a case report of oculogyric crises in a patient with dopa-responsive dystonia (Lamberti et al., 1993) and its phenocopy, tyrosine hydroxylase deficiency. *Paroxysmal tonic upgaze* has also been seen in infants and children and often eventually subsides (Ouvrier and Billson, 1988), but it may be a forerunner of developmental delay, intellectual disability, or language delay, indicating impaired corticomesencephalic control of vertical eye movements (Hayman et al., 1998).

Another specific type of action dystonia should be mentioned, lingual feeding dystonia, because is it virtually pathognomonic of a certain diagnosis. When a person with this type of dystonia is eating, the tongue is uncontrollably pushed out of the mouth, often resulting in biting the tongue and dropping food from the mouth (Video 1.51). This characteristic feeding dystonia is seen in the disorder neuroacanthocytosis.

Although classic torsion dystonia may appear initially only as an action dystonia, it usually progresses to manifest as continual contractions. A rarer presentation is when primary dystonia appears initially at rest, and then clears when the affected body part or some other part of the body is voluntarily active; this type has been called *paradoxical dystonia* (Fahn, 1989) (Video 1.52). In contrast to this continual type of classic torsion dystonia, a variant of dystonia also exists in which the movements occur in attacks, with a sudden onset and limited duration – known as *paroxysmal dyskinesias* (see later in this chapter and also Chapter 22). These are categorized among the paroxysmal disorders. Among the other disorders to be differentiated from dystonia are conditions appearing as sustained contractions; these are tonic tics (also called dystonic tics) (see Chapter 16) and conditions referred to as *pseudodystonia*s (see Chapter 12).

Hemifacial spasm

Hemifacial spasm, as the name indicates, refers to unilateral facial muscle contractions. Generally these are continual rapid, brief, repetitive spasms (clonic form of hemifacial spasm), but they can also be more prolonged sustained tonic spasms (tonic form), mixed with periods of quiescence (Video 1.53). Often the movements can be brought out when the patient voluntarily and forcefully contracts the facial muscles; when the patient then relaxes the face, the involuntary movements appear. Hemifacial spasm usually affects both upper and lower parts of the face, but patients are commonly more concerned about closure of the eyelid than about the contractions of the cheek or at the corner of the mouth. The eyebrow tends to elevate with the facial contractions owing to being pulled upwards by the forehead muscles. The disorder involves the facial nerve, and often it is due to compression of the nerve by an aberrant blood vessel (Jannetta, 1982). Hemifacial spasm is an example of a peripherally induced movement disorder (see Chapter 23).

Hemifacial spasm can be easily distinguished from blepharospasm, since the latter involves the face bilaterally and the dystonic contractions often spread to contiguous structures, such as oromandibular and nuchal muscles. Rarely is blepharospasm due to dystonia unilaterally. In such a circumstance, it can be difficult clinically to distinguish it from hemifacial spasm. In contrast to hemifacial spasm, blepharospasm tends to pull the eyebrow down because of contraction of the procerus muscle in addition to the orbicularis oculi. Another condition that has been confused with hemifacial spasm is repetitive facial myoclonus seen with Whipple disease. In this disorder the myoclonic jerks tend to be fairly rhythmical, the contractions usually involve the other side of the face to some extent, and the movements are not sustained. Electromyography may be of assistance since hemifacial spasm is associated with high-frequency repetitive discharges, and sometimes with ephaptic transmission. The contractions in both hemifacial spasm and blepharospasm are intermittent, but both can be sustained.

Hyperekplexia and jumping disorders

Hyperekplexia ("*startle disease*") is an excessive startle reaction to a sudden, unexpected stimulus (Andermann and Andermann, 1986; Brown et al., 1991b; Matsumoto and Hallett, 1994). The startle response can be either a short "jump" or a more prolonged tonic spasm causing falls (Video 1.54). This condition can be familial or sporadic. If patients have a delayed reaction to sudden noise or threat, a psychogenic problem should be considered (Thompson et al., 1992).

Startle syndromes may encompass *jumping disorders* and other similar conditions, with names like Jumping Frenchmen of Maine, latah, myriachit, and Ragin' Cajun, but all of these appear to be influenced by social and group behavior. The names were coined for the ethnic groups in different parts of the world, although their clinical features are similar. In jumping disorders, after the initial jump to the unexpected stimulus, there is automatic speech or behavior, such as striking out. In some of these, there is automatic obedience to words such as "jump" or "throw" (Matsumoto and Hallett, 1994). Such automatic behaviors are not seen in hyperekplexia. The startle disorders are discussed in more detail in Chapter 20.

Hypnogenic dyskinesias: periodic movements in sleep and REM sleep behavior disorder

Most dyskinesias disappear during deep sleep, although they may emerge during light sleep. The major exception is symptomatic rhythmical *oculopalatal myoclonus*, which persists during sleep, in addition to being present while the patient is awake (Deuschl et al., 1990). There are, however, a few movement disorders that are present only when the patient is asleep. The most common hypnogenic dyskinesia is the condition known as *periodic movements in sleep* (Coleman et al., 1980; Lugaresi et al., 1983, 1986; Hening et al., 1986), formerly referred to as *nocturnal myoclonus* (Symonds, 1953). The latter term is unacceptable because the movements are not shocklike, but, in fact, are rather slow. They appear as flexor contractions of one or both legs, with dorsiflexion of the big toe and the foot, and flexion of the knee and hip (Video 1.55). They occur in intervals, approximately every 20 seconds, and hence have been given its new, more acceptable name (Coleman et al., 1980). Periodic movements in sleep are a frequent component of the restless legs syndrome (see Chapter 23). In addition to periodic movements in sleep, this syndrome also is associated with myoclonic-like and dystonic-like movements during sleep and while the patient is drowsy (Hening et al., 1986).

Sleep with rapid eye movements (REM sleep) is the stage of sleep in which dreaming occurs. Along with the ocular movements, there is atonia of the other somatic muscles in the body; this permits people to remain free of body movements when they dream. *REM sleep behavior disorder* (RBD), described by Schenck and colleagues (1986), is a condition in which there is lack of somatic muscle atonia, thus enabling such individuals to move while they dream (acting out their dreams). The affected individual is unaware of these movements unless awakened by falling out of bed or by the bed partner who might have been struck or kicked by the abnormal movements and then awakens the person to stop the movements. RBD may precede by several years the development of a subsequent synucleinopathy (Parkinson disease or multiple system atrophy) (Tan et al., 1996; Postuma et al., 2006; Claassen et al., 2010). RBD may instead develop after the onset of the synucleinopathy, and not all individuals with RBD will develop a synucleinopathy (Postuma et al., 2009).

Another rare nocturnal dyskinesia is hypnogenic paroxysmal dystonia or other dyskinesias that occur only during sleep (Video 1.56) (see Chapter 22). Hypnogenic dystonia can be complex and with sustained contractions, similar to those occurring in torsion dystonia. As its name suggests, such movements occur as a paroxysm during sleep and last only a few minutes. They might or might not awaken the patient. Some may be frontal lobe seizures (Fish and Marsden, 1994).

Jumpy stumps

Jumpy stumps are uncontrollable and sometimes exhausting chaotic movements of the stump remaining from an amputated limb (Video 1.57). When they occur, it is after a delayed period of time following the amputation (Marion et al., 1989).

Moving toes and fingers

The painful legs, moving toes syndrome (see Chapter 23) refers to a disorder in which the toes of one foot or both feet are in continual flexion–extension with some lateral motion, associated with a deep pain in the ipsilateral leg (Spillane et al., 1971). The constant movement has a sinusoidal quality (Video 1.58). The movements and pain are continuous, and both occur even during sleep, though they may be reduced and the normal sleep pattern may be altered (Montagna et al., 1983). The leg pain is much more troublesome to the patient than are the constant movements. In most patients with this disorder, there is evidence for a lesion in the lumbar roots or in the peripheral nerves (Nathan, 1978; Montagna et al., 1983; Dressler et al., 1994). An analogous disorder, "painful arm, moving fingers," has also been described (Verhagen et al., 1985) (Video 1.59).

Myoclonus

Myoclonic jerks are sudden, brief, shocklike involuntary movements caused by muscular contractions (positive myoclonus) or inhibitions (negative myoclonus) (see Chapter

20). The most common form of negative myoclonus is *asterixis*, which frequently accompanies various metabolic encephalopathies. In asterixis, the brief flapping of the outstretched limbs is due to transient inhibition of the muscles that maintain posture of those extremities (Video 1.60). Unilateral asterixis has been described with focal brain lesions of the contralateral medial frontal cortex, parietal cortex, internal capsule, and ventrolateral thalamus (Obeso et al., 1995).

Myoclonus can appear when the affected body part is at rest or when it is performing a voluntary motor act, so-called action myoclonus (Video 1.61). Myoclonic jerks are usually irregular (arrhythmic) but can be rhythmical, such as in *palatal myoclonus* (Video 1.62 and 1.63) or *ocular myoclonus* (Video 1.64), with a rate of approximately 2 Hz. Rhythmic ocular myoclonus due to a lesion in the dentato-olivary pathway needs to be distinguished from arrhythmic and chaotic *opsoclonus* or dancing eyes (Video 1.65) Rhythmic myoclonus is typically due to a structural lesion of the brainstem or spinal cord (therefore also called segmental myoclonus), but not all cases of segmental myoclonus are rhythmic, and some types of cortical epilepsia partialis continua can be rhythmic. Oscillatory myoclonus is depicted as rhythmic jerks that occur in a burst and then fade (Fahn and Singh, 1981). Spinal myoclonus (Video 1.66), in addition to presenting as segmental and rhythmical, can also present as flexion axial jerks triggered by a distant stimulus that travels via a slow-conducting spinal pathway, a type that is called *propriospinal myoclonus* (Brown et al., 1991c). Respiratory myoclonus can be variable and has been called diaphragmatic flutter and diaphragmatic tremor (Espay et al., 2007).

Myoclonic jerks occurring in different body parts are often synchronized, a feature that may be specific for myoclonus. The jerks can often be triggered by sudden stimuli such as sound, light, visual threat, or movement (reflex myoclonus). Some types of myoclonus have a relationship to seizures in that both seem to be the result of hyperexcitable neurons.

Cortical reflex myoclonus usually presents as a focal myoclonus and is triggered by active or passive muscle movements of the affected body part (see Video 1.20). It is associated with high-amplitude ("giant") somatosensory evoked potentials and with cortical spikes that are observed by computerized back averaging, time-locked to the stimulus (Obeso et al., 1985). Spread of cortical activity within the hemisphere and via the corpus callosum can produce generalized cortical myoclonus or multifocal cortical myoclonus (Brown et al., 1991a). Reticular reflex myoclonus (Hallett et al., 1977) is more often generalized or spreads along the body away from the source in the brainstem in a timed-related sequential fashion.

The fact that rhythmic myoclonus consists of synchronous contractions of agonist muscles rather than alternating agonist-antagonist contractions, and the fact that those in one body part are time-relatedly synchronized with contractions elsewhere, are strong arguments for categorizing rhythmic myoclonus as a myoclonic disorder and not a type of tremor. Furthermore, rhythmical myoclonias tend to persist during sleep, whereas tremors usually disappear during sleep.

Action or intention myoclonus is often encountered after cerebral hypoxia–ischemia (Lance–Adams syndrome) and with certain degenerative disorders such as progressive myoclonus epilepsy (Unverricht–Lundborg disease) and progressive myoclonic ataxia (Ramsay Hunt syndrome). Usually action myoclonus is more disabling than rest myoclonus. Negative myoclonus also occurs in the Lance–Adams syndrome, and when it occurs in the thigh muscles when the patient is standing, it manifests as bouncy legs (Video 1.67). In the *opsoclonus-myoclonus* syndrome, originally described by Kinsbourne (1962) and subsequently called both 'dancing eyes, dancing feet' and 'polymyoclonia' by Dyken and Kolar (1968), the amplitude of the myoclonus is usually very tiny, resembling irregular tremors. Because of the small amplitudes of the continuous, generalized myoclonus, it is preferable to use the term *minipolymyoclonus* (Video 1.65), a term that was first used by Spiro (1970) to describe small-amplitude movements in childhood spinal muscular atrophy and subsequently used by Wilkins and colleagues (1985) for the type of myoclonus that is seen in primary generalized epileptic myoclonus.

Myokymia and synkinesis

Myokymia is a fine persistent quivering or rippling of muscles (sometimes called live flesh by patients). The term has evolved since first used (Schultze, 1895), when it described benign fasciculations. Although some may still refer to the benign fasciculations that frequently occur in orbicularis oculi as *myokymia*, Denny-Brown and Foley (1948) distinguished between myokymia and benign fasciculations on the basis of electromyography (EMG). In myokymia, the EMG reveals regular groups of motor unit discharges, especially doublets and triplets, occurring with a regular rhythmic discharge. Myokymia occurs most commonly in facial muscles. Most facial myokymias are due to pontine lesions, particularly multiple sclerosis (Andermann et al., 1961; Matthews, 1966), and less often due to pontine glioma. When due to multiple sclerosis, facial myokymia tends to abate after weeks or months. When due to a pontine glioma, facial myokymia may persist indefinitely and can be associated with facial contracture (Video 1.68). Myokymia is also a feature of neuromyotonia (see under "Stiff muscles," earlier in this chapter). Myokymia can persist during sleep. Continuous facial myokymia in multiple sclerosis has been found by magnetic resonance imaging to be caused by a pontine tegmental lesion involving the postnuclear, postgenu portion of the facial nerve (Jacobs et al., 1994).

Aberrant reinnervation of the facial nerve following denervation, such as from Bell palsy, is manifested by *synkinesis*, which is the occurrence of involuntary movements in one part of the face accompanying voluntary contraction of another part. For example, moving the mouth in a smile may cause the eyelid to close.

For the sake of completeness, it is important to mention fasciculations, the small-amplitude contractions of muscles innervated by a motor unit. This is seen predominantly with disease of the anterior horn cells and presents as low-amplitude intermittent twitching of muscles, due to motor unit discharges, which are usually not strong enough to move a joint, although this can occur, particularly in children.

Myorhythmia

The term *myorhythmia* has been used in different ways over time. Herz (1931, 1944) used it to refer to the somewhat rhythmic movements that are sometimes seen in patients with torsion dystonia. Today, these are simply called dystonic movements and are not distinguished between the movements that are repetitive and those that are not. Dystonic myorhythmia should not be confused with dystonic tremor, which strongly resembles other tremors but is due to dystonia. Monrad-Krohn and Refsum (1958) used the term *myorhythmia* to label what is today called palatal myoclonus or other rhythmic myoclonias. This meaning of the term *myorhythmia* has also been adopted by Masucci and colleagues (1984). The term could be used to represent a somewhat slow frequency (<3 Hz) and a prolonged, rhythmic or repetitive movement, in which the movement does not have the sharp square wave appearance of a myoclonic jerk. Therefore, it would not be applied to palatal myoclonus. Myorhythmia would also not apply to the sinusoidal cycles of most tremors (parkinsonian, essential, cerebellar) because the frequency of these tremors is faster than that defined for myorhythmia.

The most typical disorder in which the term *myorhythmia* is applied is in Whipple disease, in which there are slow-moving, repetitive, synchronous, rhythmic contractions in ocular, facial, masticatory, and other muscles, so-called *oculofaciomasticatory myorhythmia* (Schwartz et al., 1986; Hausser-Hauw et al., 1988; Tison et al., 1992). There is often also vertical supranuclear ophthalmoplegia. Ocular myorhythmia is manifested as continuous, horizontal, pendular, vergence oscillations of the eyes, usually of small amplitude, occurring about every second (Video 1.69). They may be asymmetric and may continue in sleep. They never diverge beyond the primary position. Divergence and convergence are at the same speed. They are not accompanied by pupillary miosis. The movements in the face, jaw, and skeletal muscles are about at the same frequency but may be somewhat quicker and may be more like rhythmic myoclonus (Video 1.70). The abnormal movements of facial and masticatory muscles can also persist in sleep, as is seen also with palatal myoclonus. 📹

Sometimes the term *myorhythmia* may be applied to slow, undulating, rhythmic movements of muscles, unrelated to Whipple disease. Perhaps some of these types of movements are part of the spectrum of complex tics, while in others, they may represent psychogenic movements. Myorhythmias are discussed in Chapter 18.

Paroxysmal dyskinesias

The paroxysmal dyskinesias represent various types of dyskinetic movements, particularly choreoathetosis and dystonia, that occur out of the blue and then disappear after being present for seconds, minutes, or hours (see Chapter 22). The patient can remain unaffected for months between attacks, or there can be many attacks per day.

Paroxysmal kinesigenic dyskinesia is the best described and easiest to diagnose because it is characteristically triggered by a sudden movement, and the abnormal movements last only seconds to a few minutes. Paroxysmal kinesigenic dyskinesia can be hereditary or symptomatic and usually is successfully treated with anticonvulsants. The abnormal movements easily habituate – that is, they fail to recur if the sudden movement is immediately repeated. These movements can be dystonic, ballistic, and choreic (Video 1.71). There may be many brief paroxysmal bursts of movements each day. 📹

Paroxysmal nonkinesigenic dyskinesia can be hereditary or symptomatic, is triggered by stress, fatigue, caffeine or alcohol, and can last minutes to hours (Video 1.72). It is more difficult to treat than the kinesigenic variety, but it sometimes responds to clonazepam or other benzodiazepines and sometimes to acetazolamide. Paroxysmal nonkinesigenic dyskinesia can be familial or sporadic. Sporadic paroxysmal nonkinesigenic dyskinesia in our experience is more often a psychogenic movement disorder (see Chapter 25), particularly if it is a combination of both paroxysmal and continual dystonias. 📹

Paroxysmal exertional dyskinesia can be due to glucose transporter 1 deficiency or be sporadic. The attacks of dyskinesias occur after about 30 minutes of exercising.

When the paroxysmal dyskinesias consist of ataxia or tremor, they have been called *episodic ataxias and tremors*. They are usually familial, and may include vestibular signs and symptoms. The paroxysmal dyskinesias are covered in their own syllabus.

Restless legs

The term *restless legs syndrome* refers to more than just the phenomenon of restless legs, in which the patient has unpleasant crawling sensations in the legs, particularly when sitting and relaxing in the evening, which then disappear on walking (Ekbom, 1945, 1960). The complete syndrome consists of several parts, in which one or more may be present in any individual. While the unpleasant dysesthesias in the legs are the most common symptom, as was mentioned previously in the discussion on nocturnal dyskinesias, the clinical spectrum may also include periodic movements in sleep (Video 1.55), myoclonic jerks, more sustained dystonic movements, or stereotypic movements that occur while the patient is awake, particularly in the late evening (Walters et al., 1991). Other movement disorders associated with a sensory phenomenon are akathisia (feeling of inner restlessness) and tics (feeling of relief of tension or sensory urges upon producing a tic). The restless legs syndrome is covered in Chapter 23. 📹

Stereotypy

Stereotypy refers to coordinated movements that repeat continually and identically. However, there may be long periods of minutes between movements, or the movements may be very frequent. When they occur at irregular intervals, stereotypies may not always be easily distinguished from motor tics, compulsions, gestures, and mannerisms. They can also appear as paroxysmal movements when a child is excited (Tan et al., 1997). In their classic monograph on tics, Meige and Feindel (1907) distinguished between stereotypies and motor tics by describing the latter as acts that are impelling but not impossible to resist, whereas the former, while illogical, are without an irresistible urge. Tics almost always occur intermittently and not continuously – that is, they occur paroxysmally out of a background of normal motor behavior. Although stereotypies can also be bursts of repetitive movements emerging out of a background of normal motor activity, they often repeat themselves in a uniform repetitive fashion for long periods of time (Lees, 1985). Stereotypies typically occur in patients with tardive dyskinesia (Video 1.73) and with schizophrenia, intellectual disability (especially Rett syndrome) (Video 1.74), and autism (Video 1.75), characteristics that assist in separating these from motor tics (Shapiro et al., 1988). Stereotypies apparently occur in Asperger syndrome, a form of mild autism. They have been seen in patients with the Kluver– Bucy syndrome (Video 1.76). Commonly, they are seen in normal children left alone and when not in contact with other people (Video 1.77). 🎥

Although motor tics are often considered to be stereotypic, when a tic bursts out, it is not necessarily a repetition of the previous tic movement. Thus, tics are usually not repetitive from one burst to the next. However, the same type of tic movement will usually recur after some period of time passes, which provides their stereotypic nature. The diversity of motor tics is one feature that sets their phenomenology apart from stereotypies. Tics are rarely continuously repetitive, and when this occurs, the term *tic status* can be applied. As is pointed out in the next section, tics have many other features that aid in their diagnosis, such as their suppressibility, their accompaniment by an underlying urge or compulsion to make the movement, their variability, their migration from one body part to another part, their abruptness, their brevity, and the repetitiveness, rather than randomness, of the particular body part affected by the movements (Fahn, 2005). Therefore, while tics have an element of stereotypy, this type of stereotypy, which can be considered paroxysmal, intermittent, or at most continual (meaning with interruptions), needs to be distinguished from continuous (uninterrupted) involuntary movements that repeat unceasingly. The latter type of continuous stereotypy is what distinguishes the disorders known as stereotypies and is the hallmark of abnormal movements in patients with classic tardive dyskinesia, which is called tardive stereotypy (Jankovic, 2005), the most common type of stereotypy seen in movement disorder clinics.

Compulsions are repetitive, purposeless, usually complex movements seen in patients with *obsessive-compulsive disorder* (OCD). They are associated with an irresistible urge to make the movement. Patients realize that they are making the movements in response to this "need to do so." In this respect, compulsions resemble tics and not stereotypies, which are not accompanied by any urge. In fact, some patients with Gilles de la Tourette syndrome also have OCD, and in this situation it might be impossible to distinguish between tics and compulsions (Jankovic, 2001). Like stereotypies, compulsions could be carried out in a uniform repetitive fashion for long periods of time but at the expense of all other activities because compulsions may be impossible to stop. In contrast, stereotypies can usually be stopped on command, and the patient will have normal motor behavior until they start up again, usually as soon as the patient is no longer paying attention to the command.

Gestures are culturally developed, expressive, voluntary movements that are calculated to indicate a particular state of mind and that may also be used as a means of adding emphasis to oratory (Lees, 1985). *Mannerisms* are sets of movements that include gestures plus more peculiar and individualistic movements that are not considered as bothersome. Mannerisms can be considered to represent a type of motor signature that individualizes a person. Sometimes mannerisms can be bizarre, and these could be considered tics or on the borderline with tics. Because gestures and mannerisms rarely continually repeat themselves, they would not likely be confused with stereotypies, but there may be problems at times distinguishing them from tics.

From this description, stereotypies can be divided into two phenomenologically distinct groups. One type is that in which the stereotypy, though repetitive for prolonged periods, occurs intermittently, normal motor activity being the general background. It is this type that can be difficult to distinguish from tics and compulsions. The second type is that in which the repetitive movements are virtually always there, with less time spent without them. The most common of this type of continuous stereotypy is that of classic *tardive dyskinesia* (TD). The movements that are seen in classic tardive dyskinesia are rhythmic and continuously repetitive complex chewing movements (oral-buccal-lingual dyskinesia) (Video 1.73). Often, this tardive stereotypy will appear together in the same patient with different motor phenomena that make up the tardive dyskinesia syndromes (see Chapter 19), namely dystonia (tardive dystonia), and akathisia (tardive akathisia). All are secondary to exposure to dopamine receptor blocking drugs. Another disorder with continuous stereotypies is the encephalitis due to NMDA receptor antibodies (Dalmau et al., 2007; Dale et al., 2009; Zandi et al., 2009; Ferioli et al., 2010; Irani et al., 2010). 🎥

Tics

Tics consist of abnormal movements (motor tics) or abnormal sounds (phonic tics). When both types of tics are present, the designation of *Gilles de la Tourette syndrome* or *Tourette syndrome* is commonly applied (see Chapter 16). Tics frequently vary in severity over time and can have remissions and exacerbations.

Motor and phonic tics can be simple or complex and occur abruptly for brief moments from a background of normal motor activity. Thus, they are paroxysmal in occurrence unless they are so severe as to be continual. A single simple motor tic may be impossible to distinguish from a myoclonic or choreic jerk; each of these would be an abrupt, sudden, isolated movement. Examples include a shoulder shrug, head jerk, blink, dart of the eyes, and twitch of the nose. Most of the time, such simple tics are repetitive, such as a run of eye blinking or a sequence of several simple tics in a row. In this more complex pattern, tics can be easily distinguished from the other hyperkinesias. Even when tics are simple jerks, more complex forms of tics may also be present in the same patient, allowing one to establish the diagnosis by "the company it keeps." One type of simple tic is quite distinct, namely, ocular (Video 1.78). A single ocular movement is not a feature of chorea or myoclonus, but is common in tics (Frankel and Cummings, 1984). 🎥

Complex motor tics are very distinct, consisting of coordinated patterns of sequential movements that can appear in different parts of the body (Video 1.79) and are not necessarily identical from occurrence to occurrence in the same body part. Examples of complex tics include such acts as touching the nose, touching other people, head shaking with shoulder shrugging, kicking of legs, and jumping. Obscene gesturing (copropraxia) is another example.

Like akathitic movements, tics are usually preceded by an uncomfortable feeling or sensory urge that is relieved by carrying out the movement, like "scratching an itch." Thus, the movements and sounds can be considered "unvoluntary." Unless very severe, tics can be voluntarily suppressed for various periods of time. But when they are suppressed, inner tension builds up and is relieved only by an increased burst of more tics (Video 1.80).

Tics can vary in speed, from being as rapid as myoclonic jerks to being slow and sustained contractions, resembling dystonic movements (Video 1.81). The complex sequential pattern of muscular contractions in dystonic tics makes the diagnosis obvious in most cases. Moreover, torsion dystonia is a continual hyperkinesia, whereas tics are paroxysmal bursts of varying duration.

Involuntary ocular movements can be an important feature for differentiation of tics from other dyskinesias. Whether a brief jerk of the eyes or more sustained eye deviation, ocular movements can occur as a manifestation of tics (see Video 1.78). Very few other dyskinesias involve ocular movements. The exceptions are opsoclonus (dancing eyes) (see Video 1.65), which is a form of myoclonus; ocular myoclonus (rhythmic vertical oscillations at a rate of 2 Hz) (see Video 1.64) that often accompanies palatal myoclonus; ocular myorhythmia, a slow horizontal oscillation (see Video 1.69); and oculogyric crisis (a sustained deviation of the eyes – Video 1.50, thus a dystonia) associated with dopamine receptor-blocking drugs or as a consequence of encephalitis lethargica or other parkinsonian disorders such as neuronal intranuclear hyaline inclusion disease and aromatic amino acid decarboxylase deficiency. See the discussion of oculogyric crises under "Dystonia," earlier in this chapter.

Phonic tics can range from simple throat-clearing sounds or grunts to complex verbalizations and the utterance of obscenities (coprolalia). Sniffing can also be a phonic tic, involving nasal passages rather than the vocal apparatus. Like motor tics, phonic tics can be divided into simple and complex. Throat-clearing and sniffing represent simple phonic tics, whereas verbalizations are considered complex phonic tics.

Involuntary phonations occur in only a few other neurologic disorders beside tics. These include the moaning in akathisia and in parkinsonism; the brief sounds in oromandibular dystonia and Huntington disease; and the sniffing, spitting, groaning, or singing that is occasionally encountered in Huntington disease and neuroacanthocytosis.

Tremor

Tremor is an oscillatory, typically rhythmic and regular, movement that affects one or more body parts, such as the limbs, neck, tongue, chin, or vocal cords. Jerky, irregular "tremor" is usually a manifestation of myoclonus. Tremor is produced by rhythmic alternating or simultaneous contractions of agonist and antagonist muscles. The rate, location, amplitude, and constancy vary depending on the specific type of tremor and its severity. It is helpful to determine whether the tremor is present at rest (with the patient sitting or lying in repose) (Video 1.82), with posture-holding (with the arms or legs extended in front of the body) (Video 1.83), with action (such as writing or pouring water) (Video 1.83), or with intention maneuvers (such as bringing the finger to touch the nose) (Video 1.84). Tremors can, thus, be classified as tremor-at-rest, postural tremor, action tremor, or intention tremor, respectively. Some tremors may be present only during a specific task (such as writing) or with a specific posture such as standing, as in orthostatic tremor (Video 1.85). These are called task-specific and position-specific tremors, respectively, and may overlap with task-specific and position-specific action dystonias, which may also appear as tremors (dystonic tremor) (Video 1.86). Etiologies and treatment of tremors differ according to the type of tremor phenomenology (see Chapter 18). A combination of rest tremor and a worse action and intention tremor is often a manifestation of a lesion in the midbrain (Video 1.87), commonly mislabeled as "rubral" tremor, but is more appropriately called midbrain tremor due to involvement of both the nigrostriatal and dentato-rubro-thalamic pathways. It is important to realize that any tremor, especially wing beating and other unusual tremors, can be a manifestation of Wilson disease (Videos 1.88 and 1.89).

The clinical approach to differentiate the dyskinesias

The process by which one distinguishes one type of dyskinesia from the others is by characterizing the type of abnormal movements that are present and then determining which dyskinesia definition most appropriately encompasses the overall picture and, at the same time, eliminating the dyskinesias that fail to fit. One performs this process in a hierarchic manner, first considering the immediately obvious clinical features (Level A) and proceeding to the next two lower levels in order, each taking longer periods of observation (see Table 1.10).

Level A has four equal factors, and each has its own table dividing movement disorders into those that fit these factors: rhythmicity (Table 1.11), duration of the contractions (Table 1.12), continuity of the contractions (Table 1.13), and their appearance with sleep or when awake (Table 1.14). The second level (Level B), taking a slightly longer period of observation, has three factors. The first is evaluating whether the movements occur when the affected body part is at rest, in a voluntary action, or both (Table 1.15). This table lists those movement disorders that are present when the affected body part is at rest and disappear with action, appear only with action, or are present both at rest and continue with action. By "action," we refer to the presence of the movements when the affected body part is performing a voluntary movement. In the action category are task-specific and posture-specific dyskinesias. Table 1.16 considers whether the movements keep involving the same set of muscles recurring in a repetitive manner (patterned) rather than randomly to involve different muscle groups. Table 1.17 lists disorders

Table 1.10 The clinical approaches to recognizing the various dyskinesias

Level A: Immediate impressions

1. Rhythmic versus arrhythmic (see Table 1.11)
2. Sustained versus nonsustained (see Table 1.12)
3. Paroxysmal versus continual versus continuous* (see Table 1.13)
4. Sleep versus awake (see Table 1.14)

Level B: More prolonged observations

At rest versus with action (see Table 1.15)

Patterned versus nonpatterned (see Table 1.16)

Combinations of varieties of movements (see Table 1.17)

Level C: Features requiring longer observation (see Table 1.18)

Speed: slow versus fast

Amplitude: ballistic versus. not ballistic

Force: powerful (painful) versus easy-to-overcome

Suppressibility

Vocalizations

Self-mutilation

Complexity of movements

Sensory component

*Continual means over and over again; continuous means without stopping or unbroken.

Table 1.11 Differential diagnosis of rhythmic, irregular, and arrhythmic hyperkinesias

Rhythmic	Irregular	Arrhythmic
Tremor	Cortical myoclonus	Akathitic
resting	Minipolymyoclonus	movements
postural	Dystonic tremor*	Athetosis
action		Ballism
intention		Chorea
Dystonic tremor*		Dystonia*
Dystonic myorhythmia*		Hemifacial spasm
Myoclonus, segmental*		Hyperekplexia
Epilepsia partialis		Arrhythmic
continua		myoclonus
Myoclonus, oscillatory		Stereotypy*
Moving toes/fingers		Tics
Myorhythmia*		
Periodic movements in		
sleep		
Tardive dyskinesia		
(tardive stereotypy)*		

*Any apparent incongruity of some dyskinesias appearing on both columns has been explained in the definitions of the different dyskinesias. Dystonia often, but not always, has repetitive movements, which were coined as myorhythmia by Herz (1931, 1944) and now labeled as dystonic tremor and patterned movements. Today, myorhythmia refers to the slow, rhythmic movements, most classically seen in Whipple disease. Segmental myoclonus is typically rhythmic, whereas other forms of myoclonus are arrhythmic. Stereotypies can occur at irregular intervals, and these are in the right hand column above. In contrast, classic tardive dyskinesia movements are continuous, and these stereotypies are placed in the left hand column.

Table 1.12 Differential diagnosis of sustained hyperkinesias

Sustained contractions or postures	Nonsustained contractions
Rigidity	All others
Dystonia	
Oculogyric crisis	
Paroxysmal dystonia	
Dystonic tics	
Pseudodystonias (e.g., Sandifer syndrome)	
Stiff-person syndrome	
Neuromyotonia	
Congenital torticollis	
Orthopedic torticollis	

Table 1.13 Differential diagnosis of paroxysmal and nonparoxysmal hyperkinesias

Paroxysmal	Continual	Continuous
Tics	Ballism	Abdominal
PKD	Chorea	dyskinesias
PNKD	Dystonic movements	Athetosis
PED	Myoclonus,	Tremors
Paroxysmal ataxia	arrhythmic	Dystonic postures
Paroxysmal tremor	Some stereotypies	Minipolymyoclonus
Hypnogenic	Akathitic moaning	Myoclonus, rhythmic
dystonia		Tardive stereotypy*
Stereotypies		Myokymia
Akathitic		Tic status*
movements		Moving toes/fingers
Jumpy stumps		Myorhythmia

Continual means over and over again; continuous means without stopping or unbroken.

Abbreviations used: PKD, paroxysmal kinesigenic dyskinesia; PNKD, paroxysmal nonkinesigenic dyskinesia; PED, paroxysmal exertional dyskinesia.

*Tic status refers to the rare episodes where tics become so severe that they do not stop. Stereotypy and tardive stereotypy (classic tardive dyskinesia) were distinguished in Table 1.11.

Table 1.14 Differential diagnosis of hyperkinesias that are present while asleep or awake

Appears during sleep and disappears when awakened	Persists during sleep	Diminishes during sleep
Hypnogenic dyskinesias	Secondary palatal myoclonus	All others
Periodic movements in sleep	Ocular myoclonus	
REM sleep behavior disorder	Spinal myoclonus	
	Oculofaciomasticatory myorhythmia	
	Moving toes	
	Myokymia	
	Neuromyotonia (Isaacs syndrome)	
	Severe dystonia	
	Severe tics	

Table 1.15 Differential diagnosis of hyperkinesias that are present at rest or with action

At rest only (disappears with action)

Akathitic movements

Paradoxical dystonia*

Resting tremor, but can reemerge with posture holding

Restless legs

Orthostatic tremor (only on standing)

With action only

Ataxia

Action dystonia

Action myoclonus

Orthostatic tremor*

Tremor: postural, action, intention

Task-specific tremor

Task-specific dystonia

At rest and continues with action

Abdominal dyskinesias

Athetosis

Ballism

Chorea

Dystonia*

Jumpy stumps

Minipolymyoclonus

Moving toes/fingers

Myoclonus*

Myokymia

Pseudodystonias*

Tics

*Paradoxical dystonia refers to dystonia that is present only at rest and disappears with action (Fahn, 1989); orthostatic tremor is tremor of the thighs and legs (spreading to the trunk) that occurs only on prolonged standing and disappears with walking or sitting; most dystonias and myoclonias that are present at rest are also present and often worse with action as well; pseudodystonias refer to neuromyotonia and other causes of stiff muscles or postures that are not due to dystonia (common causes are orthopedic deformities and pain).

Table 1.16 Patterned and nonpatterned movements

Patterned (i.e., same muscle groups)	Nonpatterned
Abdominal dyskinesias	All others
Dystonia	
Hemifacial spasm	
Moving toes/fingers	
Segmental myoclonus	
Myorhythmia	
Myokymia	
Most stereotypies	
Tardive stereotypy	
Tremor	

Table 1.17 Combinations of varieties of movements

Psychogenic movement disorders

Tardive syndromes

Neuroacanthocytosis

Wilson disease

Huntington disease

Dentatorubral-pallidoluysian atrophy (DRPLA)

Dystonia*

*Patients with dystonia can have additional dyskinesias that are part of the spectrum of classic torsion dystonia (see the text discussion of dystonia). These include tremor, myoclonus, and choreic-like movements. Dystonia-plus syndromes can have features of parkinsonism or myoclonus in addition to dystonia.

in which there are commonly combinations of various dyskinesias.

The third level (Level C), taking still longer periods of observation, evaluates many factors: speed, amplitude, force, suppressibility, presence of vocalizations, presence of self-mutilation, complexity of the movements, and whether there are associated sensory symptoms (Table 1.18).

Tables 1.10–1.18 are intended to assist the clinician in establishing the correct dyskinesia or syndrome. Once this has been accomplished, it is then the clinician's task to determine the correct etiology that has produced this dyskinesia. The chapters describing the details of each motor phenomenology also describe our approach for evaluating patients to determine their etiologies and treatments.

Conclusions

Working definitions and clinical characteristics of the movement disorders have been presented. Electrophysiologic recordings are adding to our definitions, but they must be compatible with the clinical definitions that have been in use for decades. There are nine predominant movement disorders: akinesia/bradykinesia; rhythmic tremor; the sustained contractions of dystonia (athetosis); three types of usually fast movements – myoclonus, chorea (ballism), and tics; stereotypies (compulsions); paroxysmal dyskinesias; ataxia (asynergia); and hypnogenic dyskinesias. The others are less common. The pathophysiology of movement disorders is beginning to be understood. Many appear to involve

Table 1.18 Clinical features requiring longer observation time

Speed: fast versus slow*

Fastest	Intermediate	Slowest
Minipolymyoclonus	Chorea	Athetosis
Myoclonus	Ballism	Moving toes/fingers
Hyperekplexia	Jumpy stumps	Myorhythmia
Hemifacial spasm	Tremors	Akathitic
	Tardive stereotypy	movements

Amplitude

Large	Medium	Very small
Ballism	Chorea and all others	Minipolymyoclonus
	Jumpy stumps would be large, but a short stump keeps the amplitude at a medium level	

Force

Powerful	Intermediate	Easy-to-overcome
Stiff-person syndrome	Dystonia	All others
Jumpy stump		

Suppressibility

Stereotypies > tics, akathitic movements > chorea > ballism > dystonia > tremor > moving toes

Not suppressible: hemifacial spasm, minipolymyoclonus, myoclonus, hyperekplexia, myorhythmia, moving toes/fingers

Vocalizations

Vocal tics: simple or complex
Akathisia: moaning
Huntington disease
Neuroacanthocytosis
Cranial dystonia

Self-mutilation

Lesch–Nyhan syndrome
Neuroacanthocytosis
Tourette syndrome
Psychogenic movement disorders

Complex movements[†]

Tics
Akathitic movements
Compulsions
Stereotypies
Psychogenic movements

Sensory component

Akathisia
Moving toes, painful legs
Restless legs
Tics

Ocular movements

Tics
Oculogyric crises
Opsoclonus
Ocular myoclonus
Ocular myorhythmia
Ocular dysmetria
Nystagmus

*Tics and dystonic movements can be of all speeds.
[†]Each of the above can also consist of simple movements.

the dopamine system and the basal ganglia, such as too little dopaminergic activity (parkinsonian rigidity and bradykinesia) or too much (chorea, ballism, and tardive dyskinesia). It is hoped that much more knowledge will be gained to provide a better understanding of these disorders, but the first task of the clinician is to recognize the characteristics of the movement disorder in order to decide on the clinical syndrome that the patient presents. The next task is to unravel the etiologic diagnosis to provide information on genetics, prognosis, and treatment.

References available on Expert Consult: www.expertconsult.com

CHAPTER **2**

Motor control
Physiology of voluntary and involuntary movements

Chapter contents

Segmental inputs onto the alpha motoneuron	36	Ataxia	44
Supraspinal control of the alpha motoneuron	37	Cortical control mechanisms	53
The basal ganglia	38	Apraxia	53
Parkinson disease	38	What is a voluntary movement?	54
Dystonia	42	Disorders of willed movement	54
Dyskinesias	44	Acknowledgment	54
Cerebellum	44		

Movement, whether voluntary or involuntary, is produced by the contraction of muscle. Muscle, in turn, is normally controlled entirely by the anterior horn cells or alpha motoneurons. Some involuntary movement disorders arise from muscle, the alpha motoneuron axon, or the alpha motoneuron itself. While this territory might be considered neuromuscular disease, the border can be fuzzy and patients may well appear in the office of the movement disorder specialist. Examples of involuntary movement arising from neuromuscular disorders that will be discussed in subsequent chapters are listed in Table 2.1.

As the sole controller of muscle, the alpha motoneuron is clearly important in understanding the genesis of movement. The influences upon the alpha motoneuron are many and complex, but have been extensively studied. Here only the basics will be reviewed (Hallett, 2003b). Inputs onto the alpha motoneuron can be divided into the segmental inputs and the supraspinal inputs.

Segmental inputs onto the alpha motoneuron

Figure 2.1 depicts the reflex connections onto the alpha motoneuron.

Renshaw cell. The alpha motoneuron axon has a recurrent collateral in the spinal cord that synapses onto the Renshaw cell. Similarly to the neuromuscular junction, the neurotransmitter onto the Renshaw cell is acetylcholine. The Renshaw cell then directly inhibits the alpha motoneuron using glycine as the neurotransmitter. This is called recurrent inhibition. It provides inhibitory feedback to the pool of alpha motoneurons to prevent excessive output.

Ia afferent. The Ia afferent comes from the muscle spindle and provides a sensitive measure of muscle stretch. It synapses monosynaptically with excitation onto the alpha motoneuron using glutamate as the neurotransmitter, and is the substrate of the tendon reflex. Electrical stimulation of the Ia afferents proximal to the muscle spindle produces the H reflex.

Ib afferent. The Ib afferent comes from the Golgi tendon organ and responds to tension of the muscle tendon. It excites the Ib inhibitory interneuron, which in turn inhibits the alpha motoneuron in a disynaptic chain.

Ia afferent from an antagonist muscle. Ia afferents from antagonist muscles excite interneurons in the spinal cord called the Ia inhibitory interneuron. This interneuron provides direct inhibition of the alpha motoneuron disynaptically. Glycine is the neurotransmitter. This is called reciprocal inhibition.

Flexor reflex afferents. Fibers, largely small myelinated and unmyelinated, carrying nociceptive information provide polysynaptic excitation onto the alpha motoneuron. These are the substrate for the flexor reflex.

Presynaptic inhibition. The inhibitory influences described so far are direct on the alpha motoneuron and are largely mediated by the neurotransmitter glycine. Some inhibitory influences, however, are presynaptic on excitatory synapses, such as the Ia afferent synapse. Presynaptic inhibition is commonly mediated by gamma-aminobutyric acid (GABA). Some presynaptic inhibition of the Ia afferent synapse is produced by oligosynaptic input from the antagonist Ia afferent. This effect will cause a "second phase" of reciprocal inhibition following the disynaptic reciprocal inhibition described earlier.

© 2011 Elsevier Ltd, Inc, BV
DOI: 10.1016/B978-1-4377-2369-4.00002-0

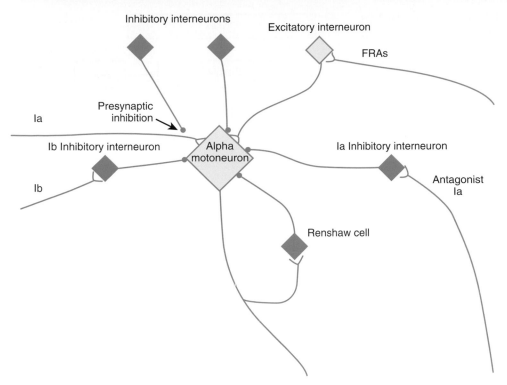

Figure 2.1 Diagram of reflex connections onto the alpha motoneuron. Inhibitory neurons are dark green and excitatory neurons light green. FRAs, flexor reflex afferents.

Table 2.1 Examples of involuntary movements arising from neuromuscular conditions

Muscle

Schwartz–Jampel syndrome

Alpha motoneuron axon

Hemifacial spasm

Peripheral myoclonus

Fasciculation

Neuromyotonia

Anterior horn cell

Fasciculation

Spinal alpha rigidity

Table 2.2 Examples of movement disorders arising from segmental dysfunction

Disorder	Mechanism
Tetanus	Tetanus toxin blocks the release of GABA and glycine at spinal synapses
Stiff-person syndrome	Mainly a disorder of GABA and presynaptic inhibition in the spinal cord
Hereditary hyperekplexia	A disorder of glycine receptors with deficient inhibition at multiple synapses including that from the Ia inhibitory interneuron

All of these mechanisms can be studied in humans, although often limited to only certain muscles. Such studies have illuminated the pathophysiology of both segmental and suprasegmental movement disorders. The reason that suprasegmental movement disorders can be evaluated with these tests is that supraspinal influences can affect segmental function.

Examples of movement disorders arising from segmental dysfunction that will be discussed in subsequent chapters are listed in Table 2.2.

Supraspinal control of the alpha motoneuron

The main supraspinal control comes from the corticospinal tract. Approximately 30% of the corticospinal tract arises from the primary motor cortex, and other significant contributions come from the premotor and sensory cortices. The fibers largely cross in the pyramid, but some remain uncrossed. Some terminate as monosynaptic projections onto alpha motoneurons, and others terminate on interneurons including those in the dorsal horn. Other cortical neurons project to basal ganglia, cerebellum, and brainstem, and these structures can also originate spinal projections. Particularly important is the reticular formation that originates several reticulospinal tracts with different functions (Nathan et al., 1996) The nucleus reticularis gigantocellularis mediates some long loop reflexes and is hyperactive in a form of myoclonus. The nucleus reticularis pontis oralis mediates the startle reflex. The inhibitory dorsal reticulospinal tract may have particular relevance for spasticity (Takakusaki et al., 2001). In thinking about the cortical innervation of the reticular formation, it is possible to speak of a corticoreticulospinal tract. The rubrospinal tract, originating in the magnocellular division of the red nucleus, while important in lower primates, is virtually absent in humans.

Both the basal ganglia circuitry and cerebellar circuitry can be considered as subcortical loops that largely receive information from the cortex and return most of the output back to the cortex via the thalamus. Both also have smaller directly descending projections. Although both loops utilize the thalamus, the relay nuclei are separate, and the loops remain largely separate.

The basal ganglia

The basal ganglia are of critical importance to many movement disorders, and details of their anatomy are presented in Chapter 3.

The basal ganglia loop anatomy is complex with many connections, but a simplification has become popular that has some heuristic value (Bar-Gad et al., 2003; Wichmann and DeLong, 2003a, 2003b; DeLong and Wichmann, 2007) (Fig. 2.2). In this model there are two pathways that go from the cortex and then back to the cortex. The direct pathway is the putamen, internal division of the globus pallidus (GPi), and thalamus (mainly the Vop nucleus). The indirect pathway is the putamen, external division of the globus pallidus (GPe), subthalamic nucleus (STN), GPi, substantia nigra pars reticulata (SNr), and thalamus. The substantia nigra pars compacta (SNc) is the source of the important nigrostriatal dopamine pathway and appears to modulate the loop, although not being in the loop itself. The putaminal neurons of the direct pathway have dopamine D2 receptors and are facilitated by dopamine, while the putaminal neurons of the indirect pathway have dopamine D1 receptors and are inhibited.

Figure 2.2 also has a more complete diagram indicating more connections and some of the complexity. It is now recognized that even this diagram is too simple, and there is also a hyperdirect pathway directly from the cortex to the STN. Additionally, new importance is given to the pedunculopontine nucleus (PPN), an elongated nucleus in the lateral mesencephalon and pons (Aravamuthan et al., 2007; Hamani et al., 2007; Muthusamy et al., 2007; Shimamoto et al., 2010). This nucleus receives output from the STN and GPi and may be important in balance and gait.

What do the basal ganglia contribute to movement? There are likely many contributions, but the topic remains somewhat controversial.

The basal ganglia are anatomically organized to work in a center-surround mechanism. This idea of center-surround organization was one of the possible functions of the basal ganglia circuitry suggested by Alexander and Crutcher (1990). This was followed up nicely by Mink, who detailed the possible anatomy (Fig. 2.3) (Mink, 1996, 2003, 2006). The direct pathway has a focused inhibition in the globus pallidus while the subthalamic nucleus has divergent excitation. The direct pathway (with two inhibitory synapses) is a net excitatory pathway and the indirect pathway (with three inhibitory synapses) is a net inhibitory pathway. Hence, the direct pathway can be the center and the indirect pathway the surround of a center-surround mechanism.

Basal ganglia disorders are characterized by a wide variety of movement signs and symptoms. Often they are divided

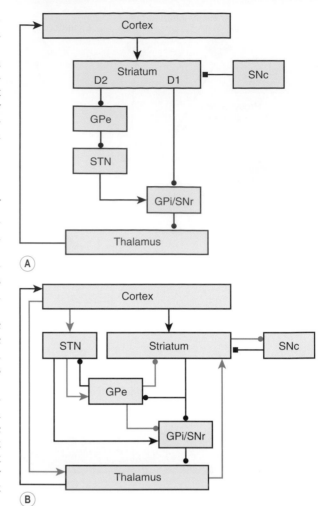

Figure 2.2 The corticobasal ganglia network. The box and arrow network of the different pathways of the basal ganglia. **A** The early network model based on the work of Albin, DeLong, and Crossman. **B** A more up-to-date network. Note that what is missing from these diagrams is that the dopaminergic influence is excitatory on the D1 receptors of the direct pathway and inhibitory on the D2 receptors of the indirect pathway. The early network is in black and later additions are in green. Glutamatergic synapses are denoted by arrows, GABAergic synapses by circles, and dopaminergic synapses by squares. *From Bar-Gad I, Morris G, Bergman H. Information processing, dimensionality reduction and reinforcement learning in the basal ganglia. Prog Neurobiol 2003;71(6):439–73, with permission.*

into hypokinetic and hyperkinetic varieties, implying too little movement on the one hand and too much movement on the other. A full listing of these disorders is in Chapter 1. Here, the pathophysiology of Parkinson disease and dystonia will be emphasized.

Parkinson disease

Parkinson disease (PD) is classically characterized by bradykinesia, rigidity, and tremor-at-rest. All features seem due to the degeneration of the nigrostriatal pathway, but it has not been possible to define a single underlying pathophysiologic mechanism that explains everything. Nevertheless, there are considerable data that give separate understanding to each of the three classic features (Hallett, 2003a; Rodriguez-Oroz et al., 2009).

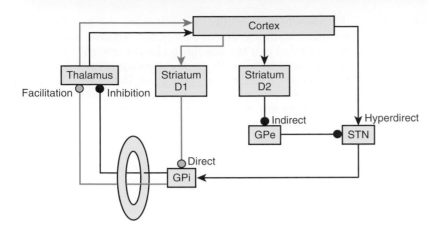

Figure 2.3 The figure illustrates how the organization of the basal ganglia can support a center-surround mechanism of motor control. Excitatory synaptic connections are arrows and inhibitory synaptic connections are circles. The "center" loop (green) including the direct pathway facilitates movement. Note that in the entire loop, there are two inhibitory neurons, so the net action is facilitation. The "surround" loop (black) including both the indirect and hyperdirect pathways inhibits movement. The indirect pathway has three inhibitory neurons and the hyperdirect pathway has one inhibitory neuron, so the net action of both is inhibition. The center loop works by reducing inhibitory influence on the thalamus; the surround loop works by increasing inhibitory influence on the thalamus.

Bradykinesia

The most important functional disturbance in patients with PD is a disorder of voluntary movement prominently characterized by slowness. This phenomenon is generally called bradykinesia, although it has at least two components, which can be designated as bradykinesia and akinesia (Berardelli et al., 2001). Bradykinesia refers to slowness of movement that is ongoing. Akinesia refers to failure of willed movement to occur. There are two possible reasons for the absence of expected movement. One is that the movement is so slow (and small) that it cannot be seen. A second is that the time needed to initiate the movement becomes excessively long.

While self-paced movements can give information about bradykinesia, the study of reaction time movements can yield information about both akinesia and bradykinesia. In the reaction time situation, a stimulus is presented to a subject, and the subject must make a movement as rapidly as possible. The time between the stimulus and the start of movement is the *reaction time*; the time from initiation to completion of movement is the *movement time*. Using this logic, prolongation of reaction time is akinesia, and prolongation of movement time is bradykinesia. Studies of PD patients confirm that both reaction time and movement time are prolonged. However, the extent of abnormality of one does not necessarily correlate with the extent of abnormality of the other (Evarts et al., 1981). This suggests that they may be impaired by separable physiologic mechanisms. In general, prolongation of movement time (bradykinesia) is better correlated with the clinical impression of slowness than is prolongation of reaction time (akinesia).

Some contributing features of bradykinesia are established. One is that there is a failure to energize muscles up to the level necessary to complete a movement in a standard amount of time. This has been demonstrated clearly with attempted rapid, monophasic movements at a single joint (Hallett and Khoshbin, 1980). In this circumstance, movements of different angular distances are accomplished in approximately the same time by making longer movements faster. The electromyographic (EMG) activity underlying the movement begins with a burst of activity in the agonist muscle of 50–100 ms, followed by a burst of activity in the antagonist muscle of 50–100 ms, followed variably

by a third burst of activity in the agonist. This "triphasic" pattern has relatively fixed timing with movements of different distance, correlating with the fact of similar total time for movements of different distance. Different distances are accomplished by altering the magnitude of the EMG within the fixed duration burst. The pattern is correct in patients with PD, but there is insufficient EMG activity in the burst to accomplish the movement. These patients often must go thorough two or more cycles of the triphasic pattern to accomplish the movement. Interestingly, such activity looks virtually identical to the tremor-at-rest seen in these patients. The longer the desired movement, the more likely it is to require additional cycles. These findings were reproduced by Baroni et al. (1984), who also showed that levodopa normalized the pattern and reduced the number of bursts.

Berardelli and colleagues (1986) showed that PD patients could vary the size and duration of the first agonist EMG burst with movement size and added load in the normal way. However, there was a failure to match these parameters appropriately to the size of movement required. This suggests an additional problem in scaling of actual movement to the required movement. A problem in sensory scaling of kinesthesia was demonstrated by Demirci et al. (1997). PD patients used kinesthetic perception to estimate the amplitude of passive angular displacements of the index finger about the metacarpophalangeal joint and to scale them as a percentage of a reference stimulus. The reference stimulus was either a standard kinesthetic stimulus preceding each test stimulus (task K) or a visual representation of the standard kinesthetic stimulus (task V). The PD patients' underestimation of the amplitudes of finger perturbations was significantly greater in task V than in task K. Thus, when kinesthesia is used to match a visual target, distances are perceived to be shorter by the PD patients. Assuming that visual perception is normal, kinesthesia must be "reduced" in PD patients. This reduced kinesthesia, when combined with the well-known reduced motor output and probably reduced corollary discharges, implies that the sensorimotor apparatus is "set" smaller in PD patients than in normal subjects.

In a slower, multijoint movement task, PD patients show a reduced rate of rise of muscle activity that also implies deficient activation (Godaux et al., 1992). On the other hand, Jordan and colleagues (1992) showed that release of force was just as slowed as increase of force, suggesting that slowness to change and not deficient energization was the main problem. If termination of activity is an active process, then this finding really does not argue against deficient energization.

A second physiologic mechanism of bradykinesia is that there is difficulty with simultaneous and sequential movements (Benecke et al., 1987). That PD patients have more difficulty with simultaneous movements than with isolated movements was first pointed out by Schwab and colleagues (1954). Quantitative studies show that slowness in accomplishing simultaneous or sequential movements is more than would be predicted from the slowness of each individual movement. With sequential movements, there is another parameter of interest, the time between the two movements designated the inter-onset latency (IOL) by Benecke and colleagues (1987). The IOL is also prolonged in patients with PD. This problem, similar to the problem with simple movements, can also be interpreted as insufficient motor energy.

Akinesia would seem to be multifactorial, and a number of contributing factors are already known. As noted above, one type of akinesia is the limit of bradykinesia from the point of view of energizing muscles. If the muscle is selected but not energized, then there will be no movement. Such phenomena can be recognized on some occasions with EMG studies where EMG activity will be initiated but will be insufficient to move the body part. Another type of akinesia, again as noted above, is prolongation of reaction time; the patient is preparing to move, but the movement has not yet occurred. Considerable attention has been paid to mechanisms of prolongation of reaction time. One factor is easily demonstrable in patients with rest tremor, who appear to have to wait to initiate the movement together with a beat of tremor in the agonist muscle of the willed movement (Hallett et al., 1977; Staude et al., 1995).

Another mechanism of prolongation of reaction time can be seen in those circumstances where eye movement must be coordinated with limb movement (Warabi et al., 1988). In this situation, there is a visual target that moves into the periphery of the visual field. Normally, there is a coordinated movement of eyes and limb, the eyes beginning slightly earlier. In PD, some patients do not begin to move the limb until the eye movement is completed. This might be due to a problem with simultaneous movements, as noted above. Alternatively, it might be that PD patients need to foveate a target before they are able to move to it.

Many studies have evaluated reaction time quantitatively with neuropsychological methods (Hallett, 1990). The goal of these studies is to determine the abnormalities in the motor processes that must occur before a movement can be initiated. In order to understand reaction time studies, it is useful to consider from a theoretical point of view the tasks that the brain must accomplish. The starting point is the "set" for the movement. This includes the environmental conditions, initial positions of body parts, understanding the nature of the experiment and, in particular, some understanding of the expected movement. In some circumstances, the expected movement is described completely, without ambiguity. This is the "simple reaction time" condition. The movement can be fully planned. It then needs to be held in store until the stimulus comes to initiate the execution of the movement. In other circumstances, the set does not include a complete description of the required movement. It is intended that the description be completed at the time of the stimulus that calls for the movement initiation. This is the "choice reaction time" condition. In this circumstance, the programming of the movement occurs between the stimulus and the response. Choice reaction time is always longer than simple reaction, and the time difference is due to this movement programming.

In most studies, simple reaction time is significantly prolonged in patients compared with normal subjects (Hallett, 1990). On the other hand, patients appear to have normal choice reaction times or the increase of choice reaction time over simple reaction time is the same in patients and normal subjects. Many studies in which cognitive activity was required for a decision on the correct motor response have shown that PD patients do not have apparent slowing of thinking, called bradyphrenia. The study of choice reaction times was extended by considering three different choice reaction time tasks that required the same simple movement, but differed in the difficulty of the decision of which movement to make (Brown et al., 1993). Comparing PD patients to normal subjects, the patients had a longer reaction time in all three conditions, but the difference was largest when the task was the easiest and smallest when the task was the most difficult. Thus, the greater the proportion of time there is in the reaction time devoted to motor program selection, the closer to normal are the PD results. Labutta et al. (1994) have shown that PD patients have no difficulty holding a motor program in store. Hence, the difficulty must be in executing the motor program. Execution of the movement, however, lies at the end of choice reaction time, just as it does for simple reaction time. How then can it be abnormal and choice reaction time be normal? The answer may be that in the choice reaction time situation both motor programming and motor execution can proceed in parallel.

Transcranial magnetic stimulation (TMS) can be used to study the initiation of execution. With low levels of TMS, it is possible to find a level that will not produce any motor evoked potentials (MEPs) at rest, but will produce an MEP when there is voluntary activation. Using such a stimulus in a reaction time situation between the stimulus to move and the response, Starr et al. (1988) showed that stimulation close to movement onset would produce a response even though there was still no voluntary EMG activity. A small response first appeared about 80 ms before EMG onset and grew in magnitude closer to onset. This method divides the reaction time into two periods. In the first period, the motor cortex remains "unexcitable"; in the second, the cortex becomes increasingly "excitable" as it prepares to trigger the movement. Most of the prolongation of the reaction time appeared due to prolongation of the later period of rising excitability (Pascual-Leone et al., 1994a). This result has been confirmed (Chen et al., 2001). The finding of prolonged initiation time in PD patients is supported by studies of motor cortex neuronal activity in reaction time movements in monkeys rendered parkinsonian with 1-methyl-4-phenyl-1,2,3,6-tetrahydropyridine (MPTP) (Watts and Mandir, 1992). In these investigations, there was a prolonged time between initial activation of motor cortex neurons and movement onset.

Thus, an important component of akinesia is the difficulty in initiating a planned movement. This statement would not be a surprise to PD patients, who often say that they know what they want to do, but they just cannot do it. A major problem in bradykinesia is a deficiency in activation of muscles, whereas the problem in akinesia seems to be a deficiency in activation of motor cortex. The dopaminergic system apparently provides energy to many different motor tasks, and the deficiency of this system in PD leads to both bradykinesia and akinesia.

Another factor that should be kept in mind is that patients appear to have much more difficulty initiating internally triggered movements than externally triggered movements. This is clear clinically in that external cues are often helpful in movement initiation. Examples include improving walking by providing an object to step over or playing march music. This can also be demonstrated in the laboratory with a variety of paradigms (Curra et al., 1997; Majsak et al., 1998).

How does bradykinesia arise from dysfunction of the nigrostriatal pathway? Thinking about the simple basal ganglia diagram, dopamine facilitates the direct pathway and inhibits the indirect pathway. Loss of dopamine will lead to lack of facilitation of movement in both pathways. This could certainly be represented by bradykinesia. This has been referred to as a loss of "motor motivation" (Mazzoni et al., 2007).The origin of rigidity and tremor is less understandable, but also less directly linked to dopamine deficiency clinically (Rodriguez-Oroz et al., 2009).

Rigidity

Tone is defined as the resistance to passive stretch. Rigidity is one form of increased tone that is seen in disorders of the basal ganglia ("extrapyramidal disorders"), and is particularly prominent in PD. Increased tone can result from changes in (1) muscle properties or joint characteristics, (2) amount of background contraction of the muscle, and (3) magnitude of stretch reflexes. There is evidence for all three of these aspects contributing to rigidity. For quantitative purposes, responses can be measured to controlled stretches delivered by devices that contain torque motors. The stretch can be produced by altering the torque of the motor or by altering the position of the shaft of the motor. The perturbation can be a single step or more complex, such as a sinusoid. The mechanical response of the limb can be measured: the positional change if the motor alters force or the force change if the motor alters position. Such mechanical measurements can directly mimic and quantify the clinical impression (Hallett et al., 1994; Hallett, 1999).

Patients with PD do not relax well and often have slight contraction at rest. This is a standard clinical as well as electrophysiologic observation, and it is clear that this mechanism plays a significant part in rigidity.

There are increases in long-latency reflexes in PD patients. Generally, this is neurophysiologically distinct from the increases in the short-latency reflexes seen in spasticity, increase in tone of "pyramidal" type. The short-latency reflex is the monosynaptic reflex. Reflexes occurring at a longer latency than this are designated long latency. When a relaxed muscle is stretched, in general only a short-latency reflex is produced. When a muscle is stretched while it is active, one or more distinct long-latency reflexes are produced following the short-latency reflex and prior to the time needed to produce a voluntary response to the stretch. These reflexes are recognized as separate because of brief time gaps between them, giving rise to the appearance of distinct "humps" on a rectified EMG trace. Each component reflex, either short or long in latency, has about the same duration, approximately 20–40 ms. They appear to be true reflexes in that their appearance and magnitude depend primarily on the amount of background force that the muscle was exerting at the time of the stretch and the mechanical parameters of the stretch; they do not vary much with whatever the subject might want to do after experiencing the muscle stretch. By contrast, the voluntary response that occurs after a reaction time from the stretch stimulus is strongly dependent on the will of the subject.

Long-latency reflexes are best brought out with controlled stretches with a device such as a torque motor. While long-latency reflexes are normally absent at rest, they are prominent in PD patients (Rothwell et al., 1983, Tatton et al., 1984; Hallett et al., 1994; Hallett, 1999). Long-latency reflexes are also enhanced in PD with background contraction. Since some long-latency stretch reflexes appear to be mediated by a loop through the sensory and motor cortices, the enhancement of long-latency reflexes has been generally believed to indicate increased excitability of this central loop.

There is some evidence that at least one component of the increased long-latency stretch reflex in PD is a group II mediated reflex. This suggestion was first made by Berardelli et al. (1983) on the basis of physiologic features, including insensitivity to vibration. It was subsequently supported by the observation that an enhanced late stretch reflex response could not be duplicated with a vibration stimulus (Cody et al., 1986). Some studies show a correlation between clinically measured increased tone and the magnitude of long-latency reflexes (Berardelli et al., 1983), while others do not (Bergui et al., 1992; Meara and Cody, 1993). Long-latency reflexes contribute significantly to rigidity, but are apparently not completely responsible for it.

Tremor-at-rest

The so called "tremor-at-rest" is the classic tremor of PD and other parkinsonian states such as those produced by neuroleptics or other dopamine-blocking agents such as prochlorperazine and metoclopramide (Elble and Koller, 1990; Hallett, 1991, 1999; Elble, 1997). It is present at rest, disappears with action, but may resume with static posture. That the tremor may also be present during postural maintenance is a significant point of confusion in regard to naming this tremor "tremor-at-rest." It can involve all parts of the body and can be markedly asymmetrical, but it is most typical with a flexion–extension movement at the elbow, pronation and supination of the forearm, and movements of the thumb across the fingers ("pill-rolling"). Its frequency is 3–7 Hz, but is most commonly 4 or 5 Hz; EMG studies show alternating activity in antagonist muscles.

The anatomical basis of the tremor-at-rest may well differ from the classic neuropathology of PD, that of degeneration of the nigrostriatal pathway. For example, 18F-dopa uptake in the caudate and putamen declines with bradykinesia and rigidity, but is unassociated with degree of tremor (Otsuka et al., 1996). Evidence from a PET study suggests that tremor is associated with a serotonergic deficiency (Doder et al., 2003). Another point in favor of this idea is that the tremor may be successfully treated with a stereotactic lesion or deep brain stimulation of the ventral intermediate (VIM) nucleus of the thalamus, a cerebellar relay nucleus (Jankovic et al., 1995; Benabid et al., 1996).

In parkinsonian tremor-at-rest, there may be some mechanical-reflex component and some 8–12 Hz component, but the most significant component comes from a pathologic central oscillator at 3–5 Hz. This tremor component is unaffected by loading. Evidence for the central oscillator includes the facts that the accelerometric record and the EMG are not affected by weighting, and small mechanical perturbations do not affect it. On the other hand, it can be reset by strong peripheral stimuli such as an electrical stimulus that produces a movement of the body part five times more than the amplitude of the tremor itself (Britton et al., 1993a). Where this strong stimulus acts is not clear, but it does not have to be on the peripheral loop. Additionally, the tremor can be reset by TMS (Britton et al., 1993b; Pascual-Leone et al., 1994b), presumably indicating a role of the motor cortex in the central processes that generate the tremor. In the studies of Pascual-Leone et al. (1994b), using a relatively small stimulus, the tremor was reset with TMS, but not with transcranial electrical stimulation. Since TMS affects the intracortical circuitry more, this seems to be further evidence for a role of the motor cortex.

While cells in the globus pallidus may have oscillatory activity, they are not as well related to the tremor as the cells in the VIM of the thalamus (Hayase et al., 1998; Hurtado et al., 1999). Lenz and colleagues have studied the physiologic properties of cells in the VIM in relation to tremor production (Zirh et al., 1998). They have tried to see if the pattern of spike activity is consistent with specific hypotheses. They examined whether parkinsonian tremor might be produced by the activity of an intrinsic thalamic pacemaker or by the oscillation of an unstable long loop reflex arc. In one study of 42 cells, they found 11 with a sensory feedback pattern, 1 with a pacemaker pattern, 21 with a completely random pattern, and 9 that did not fit any pattern (Zirh et al., 1998). In another study of thalamic neuron activity, some cells with a pacemaker pattern were seen, but these did not participate in the rhythmic activity correlating with tremor (Magnin et al., 2000). These results confirm those of Lenz et al. suggesting that the thalamic cells are not the pacemaker. Using sophisticated analytical techniques, it can be demonstrated that oscillations both in the VIM and in the STN play an efferent role in tremor generation, but that the tremor itself feeds back to these same structures to influence the oscillation (Tass et al., 2010). This does suggest that in some sense the whole loop is responsible for the tremor. The basal ganglia loop may well trigger the cerebellar loop to produce the tremor (Helmich et al., 2011).

Wherever the pacemaker for the tremor, it is important to note that while the tremor is synchronous within a limb, it is not synchronous between limbs (Hurtado et al., 2000). Hence a single pacemaker does not influence the whole body.

There are other types of tremor in PD including an action tremor looking like essential tremor, but these have not been extensively studied.

Dystonia

Dystonia is characterized by abnormal muscle spasms producing distorted motor control and undesired postures (Defazio et al., 2007; Breakefield et al., 2008). Early on, dystonia is produced only by action, but then it can occur spontaneously. There are presently three general lines of work that may indicate the physiologic substrate for dystonia.

Loss of inhibition

A principal finding in focal dystonia is that of loss of inhibition (Hallett, 2004, 2006a, 2006b, 2011). Loss of inhibition is likely responsible for the excessive movement seen in dystonia patients. Excessive movement includes abnormally long bursts of EMG activity, co-contraction of antagonist muscles, and overflow of activity into muscles not intended for the task (Cohen and Hallett, 1988). Loss of inhibition can be demonstrated in spinal and brainstem reflexes. Examples are the loss of reciprocal inhibition in the arm in patients with focal hand dystonia (Nakashima et al., 1989; Panizza et al., 1990) and abnormalities of blink reflex recovery in blepharospasm (Berardelli et al., 1985). Loss of reciprocal inhibition can be partly responsible for the presence of co-contraction of antagonist muscles that characterizes voluntary movement in dystonia.

Loss of inhibition can also be demonstrated for motor cortical function including the transcranial magnetic stimulation techniques of short intracortical inhibition, long intracortical inhibition, and the silent period (Hallett, 2007a, 2011).

Short intracortical inhibition (SICI) is obtained with paired pulse methods and reflects interneuron influences in the cortex (Ziemann et al., 1996). In such studies, an initial conditioning stimulus is given, enough to activate cortical neurons, but small enough that no descending influence on the spinal cord can be detected. A second test stimulus, at suprathreshold level, follows at a short interval. Intracortical influences initiated by the conditioning stimulus modulate the amplitude of the MEP produced by the test stimulus. At short intervals, less than 5 ms, there is inhibition that is likely largely a GABAergic effect, specifically GABA-A (Di Lazzaro et al., 2000). (At intervals between 8 and 30 ms, there is facilitation, called intracortical facilitation, ICF). There is a loss of intracortical inhibition in patients with focal hand dystonia (Ridding et al., 1995). Inhibition was less in both hemispheres of patients with focal hand dystonia, and this indicates that this abnormality is more consistent as a substrate for dystonia.

The silent period (SP) is a pause in ongoing voluntary EMG activity produced by TMS. While the first part of the SP is due in part to spinal cord refractoriness, the latter part is entirely due to cortical inhibition (Fuhr et al., 1991). This type of inhibition is likely mediated by GABA-B receptors (Werhahn et al., 1999). SICI and the SP show different modulation in different circumstances and clearly reflect different aspects of cortical inhibition. The SP is shortened in focal dystonia.

Intracortical inhibition can also be assessed with paired suprathreshold TMS pulses at intervals from 50 to 200 ms

(Valls-Solé et al., 1992). This is called long intracortical inhibition, or LICI, to differentiate it from SICI as noted above. LICI and SICI differ as demonstrated by the facts that with increasing test pulse strength, LICI decreases but SICI tends to increase, and that there is no correlation between the degree of SICI and LICI in different individuals (Sanger et al., 2001). The mechanisms of LICI and the SP may be similar in that both seem to depend on GABA-B receptors. Chen et al. (1997) investigated long intracortical inhibition in patients with writer's cramp and found a deficiency only in the symptomatic hand and only with background contraction. This abnormality is particularly interesting since it is restricted to the symptomatic setting, and therefore might be a correlate of the development of the dystonia.

There is also neuroimaging evidence consistent with a loss of inhibition. Dopamine D2 receptors are deficient in focal dystonias (Perlmutter et al., 1997). There is weak evidence for reduced GABA concentration both in basal ganglia and motor cortex utilizing magnetic resonance spectroscopy (Levy and Hallett, 2002; Herath et al., 2010).

Loss of cortical inhibition in motor cortex can give rise to dystonic-like movements in primates. Matsumura et al. showed that local application of bicuculline, a GABA antagonist, onto the motor cortex led to disordered movement and changed the movement pattern from reciprocal inhibition of antagonist muscles to co-contraction (Matsumura et al., 1991). In a second study, they showed that bicuculline caused cells to lose their crisp directionality, converted unidirectional cells to bidirectional cells, and increased firing rates of most cells including making silent cells into active ones (Matsumura et al., 1992).

There is a valuable animal model for blepharospasm that supports the idea of a combination of genetics and environment, and, specifically, that the background for the development of dystonia could be a loss of inhibition (Schicatano et al., 1997). In this model, rats were lesioned to cause a depletion of dopamine; this reduces inhibition. Then the orbicularis oculi muscle was weakened. This causes an increase in the blink reflex drive in order to produce an adequate blink. Together, but not separately, these two interventions produced spasms of eyelid closure, similar to blepharospasm. Shortly after the animal model was presented, several patients with blepharospasm after a Bell's palsy were reported (Chuke et al., 1996; Baker et al., 1997). This could be a human analog of the animal experiments. The idea is that those patients who developed blepharospasm were in some way predisposed. A gold weight implanted into the weak lid of one patient, aiding lid closure, improved the condition, suggesting that when the abnormal increase in reflex drive was removed, the dystonia could be ameliorated (Chuke et al., 1996).

Loss of surround inhibition, a functional consequence of loss of inhibition

A principle for function of the motor system may be "surround inhibition" (Hallett, 2006a, 2006b; Beck and Hallett, 2011). Surround inhibition is a concept well accepted in sensory physiology (Angelucci et al., 2002). Surround inhibition is poorly known in the motor system, but it is a logical concept. When making a movement, the brain must activate the motor system. It is possible that the brain just activates the specific movement. On the other hand, it is more likely that the one specific movement is generated, and, simultaneously, other possible movements are suppressed. The suppression of unwanted movements would be surround inhibition, and this should produce a more precise movement, just as surround inhibition in sensory systems produces more precise perceptions. For dystonia, a failure of "surround inhibition" may be particularly important since overflow movement is often seen and is a principal abnormality.

There is now good evidence for surround inhibition in human movement. Sohn et al. (2003) have shown that with movement of one finger there is widespread inhibition of muscles in the contralateral limb. Significant suppression of MEP amplitudes was observed when TMS was applied between 35 and 70 ms after EMG onset. Sohn and colleagues have also shown that there is some inhibition of muscles in the ipsilateral limb when those muscles are not involved in any way in the movement (Sohn and Hallett, 2004b). TMS was delivered to the left motor cortex from 3 ms to 1000 ms after EMG onset in the flexor digitorum superficialis muscle. MEPs from abductor digiti minimi were slightly suppressed during the movement of the index finger in the face of increased F-wave amplitude and persistence, indicating that cortical excitability is reduced.

Surround inhibition was studied similarly in patients with focal hand dystonia (Sohn and Hallett, 2004a). The MEPs were enhanced similarly in the flexor digitorum superficialis and abductor digiti minimi indicating a failure of surround inhibition. Using other experimental paradigms, a similar loss of surround inhibition in the hand has been found (Stinear and Byblow, 2004; Beck et al., 2008).

How can the abnormalities of dystonia be related to the basal ganglia? This is not completely clear, but a number of investigators have felt that there is an imbalance in the direct and indirect pathways so that the direct pathway is relatively overactive (or that the indirect pathway is relatively underactive). This should lead to excessive movement and, in particular, a loss of surround inhibition.

Abnormal plasticity

There is abnormal plasticity of the motor cortex in patients with focal hand dystonia (Quartarone et al., 2006; Weise et al., 2006). This has been demonstrated using the technique of paired associative stimulation (PAS) (Stefan et al., 2000). In PAS, a median nerve shock is paired with a TMS pulse to the sensorimotor cortex timed to be immediately after the arrival of the sensory volley. This intervention increases the amplitude of the MEP produced by TMS to the motor cortex. It has been demonstrated that the process of PAS produces motor learning similar to long-term potentiation (LTP). In patients with dystonia, PAS produces a larger increase in the MEP than that seen in normal subjects. There is also an abnormality in homeostatic plasticity. Homeostatic plasticity is the phenomenon whereby plasticity remains within limits; this can be exceeded in dystonia (Quartarone et al., 2006).

Increased plasticity may arise from decreased inhibition so the inhibitory problem may well be more fundamental. This abnormality may be an important link in demonstrating how environmental influences can trigger dystonia.

Abnormal plasticity can arise, at least in part, from abnormal synaptic processes in the basal ganglia (Peterson et al., 2010).

The possibility of increased plasticity in dystonia had been suspected for some time given that repetitive activity over long periods seems to be a trigger for its development. An animal model supported this idea (Byl et al., 1996). Monkeys were trained to hold a vibrating manipulandum for long periods. After some time, they became unable to do so, and this motor control abnormality was interpreted as a possible dystonia. The sensory cortex of these animals was studied, and sensory receptive fields were found to be large. The interpretation of these results was that the synchronous sensory input caused the receptive field enlargement, and that the abnormal sensory function led to abnormal motor function. The results suggested that the same thing might be happening in human focal dystonia: repetitive activity caused sensory receptive field changes and led to the motor disorder.

Abnormal sensory function

Stimulated by the findings of sensory dysfunction in the primate model, investigators began examining sensory function in patients with focal hand dystonia and found it to be abnormal. Although there is no apparent sensory loss on a clinical level, detailed testing of spatial and temporal discrimination revealed subtle impairments (Molloy et al., 2003). The abnormality is present on both hands of patients with unilateral hand dystonia and also on hands of patients with cervical dystonia and blepharospasm. The identification of abnormality of sensation beyond the symptomatic body parts indicated that the sensory abnormality could not be a consequence of abnormal learning, but is more likely a pre-existing physiologic state.

Sensory dysfunction can also be demonstrated with somatosensory evoked potential (SEP) testing (Bara-Jimenez et al., 1998). The dipoles of the N20 from stimulation of individual fingers show disordered representation in the primary sensory cortex (Bara-Jimenez et al., 1998) and these abnormalities are present on both hands of patients with focal hand dystonia (Meunier et al., 2001). The bilateral SEP abnormality was the first indication in the literature that the sensory abnormality was more likely endophenotypic than a consequence of repetitive activity. PET studies show that the sensory cortex is more activated than normal with writing and is more activated when patients are experiencing more dystonia (Lerner et al., 2004). Voxel-based morphometry studies in patients with focal hand dystonia show an increase in gray matter in the primary sensory cortex (Garraux et al., 2004). Such observations indicate that dystonia is a sensory disorder as well as a motor disorder.

There are data from sensory function that are compatible with loss of surround inhibition. Tinazzi and colleagues (2000) studied median and ulnar nerve somatosensory evoked potentials (SEPs) in patients who had dystonia involving at least one upper limb. They compared the amplitude of SEP components obtained by stimulating the median and ulnar nerves simultaneously (MU) with the amplitude value being obtained from the arithmetic sum of the SEPs elicited by stimulating the same nerves separately (M + U). The ratio of MU to (M + U) indicates the interaction between afferent inputs from the two peripheral nerves. No significant difference was found between SEP amplitudes and latencies for individually stimulated median and ulnar nerves in dystonic patients and normal subjects, but recordings in patients yielded a significantly higher percentage ratio for spinal N13, brainstem P14, and cortical N20, P27 and N30 components. The authors state that "these findings suggest that the inhibitory integration of afferent inputs, mainly proprioceptive inputs, coming from adjacent body parts is abnormal in dystonia. This inefficient integration, which is probably due to altered surrounding inhibition, could give rise to an abnormal motor output and might therefore contribute to the motor impairment present in dystonia."

Another demonstration of loss of surround inhibition in sensory function is in the temporal domain. Patients have difficulty recognizing two stimuli when they are close together. This abnormality seems due to a loss of a short latency inhibition, identified using SEP recovery curves (Tamura et al., 2008).

Dyskinesias

The dyskinesias include the choreas such as Huntington disease, hemiballismus, and dopa-induced dyskinesia. These are characterized by involuntary movements that generally appear randomly. These might arise due to a substantial failure of the indirect pathway of the basal ganglia loop. This would be a failure of the inhibitory role of the basal ganglia and involuntary movement would result. Evidence for this in regard to Huntington disease is that the initial degeneration of the putamen is for those neurons bearing dopamine D2 receptors.

Cerebellum

The anatomy of the cerebellar pathways, like the basal ganglia pathways, is complex, but there are simplified models that aid thinking (Schmahmann, 1994; Schmahmann and Pandya, 1997) (Fig. 2.4). The main cortico-cerebellar-cortical loop is frontal lobe, pontine nuclei, cerebellar cortex (via middle cerebellar peduncle), deep cerebellar nuclei, red nucleus and ventral lateral nucleus of thalamus (via superior cerebellar peduncle), and motor cortex. The input fibers to the cerebellar cortex are the mossy fibers that synapse onto granule cells which in turn synapse onto the Purkinje cells. There is also extensive sensory input via spinocerebellar tracts, largely carried in the inferior cerebellar peduncle. A critical modulatory loop involves the inferior olivary nucleus. The inferior olive innervates both the cerebellar cortex and deep nuclei via the inferior cerebellar peduncle and the climbing fibers that synapse directly onto Purkinje cells. Feedback returns to the inferior olive by a dentate-olivary pathway that travels in the superior cerebellar peduncle, goes around the red nucleus, and descends in the central tegmental tract.

Ataxia

The term *ataxia*, literally meaning *without order*, refers to disorganized, poorly coordinated or clumsy movement

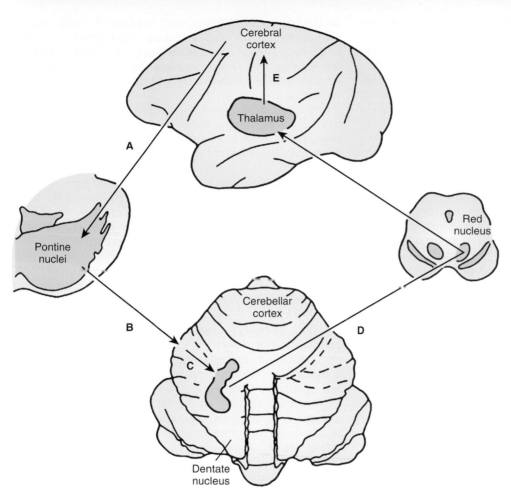

Figure 2.4 Diagram of the cerebrocerebellar circuit. Note that the path from the cortex to cerebellum is crossed (path B) and the return path is also crossed (path D); hence the cortical and cerebellar hemispheres are on opposite sides; while the motor cortex is contralateral to movement, the cerebellar activity is ipsilateral. *From Schmahmann JD. The cerebellum in autism. Clinical and anatomical perspectives. In: Bauman ML, Kemper TL, eds. The Neurobiology of Autism. Baltimore: Johns Hopkins University Press; 1994, pp. 195–226, with permission.*

(Massaquoi and Hallett, 2002). Since the time of Holmes (1939), it has been applied more specifically to clumsiness that is due to lesions of the cerebellum and its immediate connecting pathways, of proprioceptive sensory pathways or sometimes of the vestibular system. In order to identify the presence of ataxia, it should not be explained by any abnormality in (maximal isometric) strength, segmental reflexes, muscular tone, ability to isolate movement of individual body parts, or gross motor sequencing or spatial planning. The clumsiness is also not due to spontaneous involuntary movements. Ataxia may be associated with any voluntary movement and with many reflex movements. It commonly affects upright balance, gait, manual coordination and speech, yielding stagger, clumsy manipulation and slurring dysarthria which appear drunken. Indeed, the motor coordination-impairing effects of ethanol are attributed to its specific interference with cerebellar function.

Tonic force control abnormalities: hypotonia and asthenia

Normal individuals have very low, barely perceptible muscle tone when fully relaxed. Holmes noted, however, that acutely injured soldiers with penetrating wounds to the cerebellum had further reduced resistance to passive movement. He viewed hypotonia as a fundamental abnormality which underlies many cerebellar motor deficits (Holmes, 1939). This hypotonia tended to be characteristic especially of the upper extremities and to normalize gradually over weeks to months depending on the severity of the injury. Gilman et al. (1981) have shown that in primates this change parallels the recovery of muscle spindle sensitivity which was acutely depressed by loss of cerebellar fusimotor facilitation.

Large-scale surgical cerebellar ablation in monkeys is generally reported to produce acute weakness especially of the extensor muscles (Gilman et al., 1981). In humans, Holmes clearly distinguished the weakness that followed acute massive damage to the cerebellar hemispheres, *asthenia*, from that associated with corticospinal tract lesions, *paresis*. The former did not affect specific muscle groups more than others and was not necessarily associated with changes in tendon reflex sensitivity. Interestingly, *asthenia* was noted particularly when strength was tested during movement. Static resistance to the examiner was most often normal. Indeed, weakness per se is a very inconstant complaint in cerebellar patients. Further questioning often reveals the problem to be one of easy fatigability and/or a lack of coordination or stability, not of peak strength. Holmes also drew attention to the inability of some patients to maintain steady force levels (*astasia*, after Luciani). Patients sometimes complain of sudden losses of strength, such as a leg "giving out" or the tendency of an item to drop suddenly from the hand. Holmes attributed these episodes to hypotonia, but their nature remains unclear.

As with hypotonia, true asthenic weakness is most often seen in the context of acute cerebellar injury, especially, Holmes felt, when deep nuclei were involved. This was presumably related to the abrupt withdrawal of cerebellar facilitation from certain spinal, brainstem and perhaps cerebral centers. Recovery usually takes place over the course of weeks to months. Although chronically ataxic patients clearly have difficulty generating force rapidly, their strength, as indicated by peak levels of isometric force that can be achieved, is most often normal. Certainly, though, coincidental weakness superimposed upon cerebellar or sensory dysfunction markedly worsens the patient's disability.

Even in the presence of normal strength and muscular tone, easy fatigability (a second aspect of asthenia) is a prominent complaint of many patients with cerebellar ataxia (Holmes, 1939). The fatigue may affect an individual body part, but may also be sensed more globally. Most patients report that all of the aspects of their ataxia worsen when they are fatigued. A poor night's sleep, or a particularly busy previous day, predisposes to a day of especially poor motor control. Patients frequently take naps during the day which provide considerable benefit. Fatigue in cerebellar patients appears to be central, and not muscular in origin. Electrophysiologic studies of fatigue in non-depressed patients with cerebellar ataxia by Samii et al. (1997) showed decreased post-exercise facilitation of motor potentials evoked from transcranial magnetic stimulation. This is a central activation defect, similar to that seen in patients with depression and chronic fatigue syndrome. As in these disorders, patients sometimes complain of decreased concentration and mild difficulties with thinking. In this regard, the fatigue is also qualitatively similar to that seen in Parkinson disease. Ultimately, the general fatigue in cerebellar disease and other movement disorders may be related to the increased mental concentration needed to compensate for degraded automatic motor control.

Force-rate and movement amplitude scaling deficits: dysmetria, impaired check, and past-pointing

Classic descriptions of cerebellar ataxia include various clinical signs such as dysmetria, dyssynergia (asynergia, decomposition of movement), dysdiadochokinesia, dysrhythmia, and kinetic (intention) and postural tremors (Holmes, 1939; Gilman et al., 1981). Characteristically, ataxic individuals have particular difficulty in properly generating, guiding, and terminating high-speed movements. Movements accelerate somewhat slowly and are relatively late in onset if executed in reaction to a cue. Movements may then either partially arrest prior to reaching their targets or gradually accelerate to excessive speed and overshoot their targets to an abnormal degree. These two types of errors are examples of dysmetria, hypometria and hypermetria, respectively. Two distinct motor control abnormalities appear to underlie dysmetria: force-rate inadequacy and step amplitude mis-scaling. The former causes brief, more consistent velocity-sensitive inaccuracies and the latter, more variable protracted errors.

At a fundamental level, the patient with cerebellar ataxia has difficulty changing voluntary force levels abruptly (Mai et al., 1988). Both acceleration and braking are impaired. In point-to-point movements, for example, this voluntary force-rate deficit is generally corroborated by a slowness in the build-up of agonist EMG and a prolonged agonist action with delayed onset of antagonist EMG (Hallett et al., 1991; Hallett and Massaquoi, 1993). In patients attempting rapid, single-joint movement, the first agonist burst is frequently prolonged regardless of the distance and speed of the movement, and the most striking kinematic abnormality is prolonged acceleration time. The pattern of acceleration time exceeding deceleration time is common in patients but uncommon in normal subjects. Duration of the first agonist burst correlates with, and is largely responsible for, acceleration time. Altered production of appropriate acceleration for rapid voluntary movements may therefore be the primary abnormality in cerebellar dysfunction for attempted rapid voluntary movements. Hypermetria would be the expected resultant movement error unless there is compensation. Hypometria has been attributed to over-compensation, to asthenia in the acute setting, to tremor, or to failure of timely relaxation of the antagonist during movement initiation (Manto et al., 1998). Any of these mechanisms may be contributory in a given movement, and the topography of the lesion might correlate with the type of deficit (Manto et al., 1998).

For point-to-point movements of any given duration, ataxic movements exhibit greater overshoot than normal. In their study of rapid point-to-point elbow flexions, Hore et al. (1991) noted in normal subjects a transient overshoot of about 5–10% of the movement distance. Ataxic patients overshot the target by more than 20% and as much as 35% of the movement distance. On the other hand, whenever there is no observable overshoot, the movements of ataxic individuals are usually abnormally slow or are hypometric. From the point of view of Fitts' speed–accuracy tradeoff, ataxic patients display decreased motor control bandwidth. Generally, therefore, in the assessment of ataxia it is important to note both the degree of overshoot and the movement time. Appropriate abnormality of either may be consistent with ataxia. Because, however, there may be alternative explanations for increased movement time, slowness is a much less specific finding than overshoot. Due to the inherent tradeoff between speed and accuracy, patients often slow down intentionally in order to maintain error levels that are acceptable to them. Therefore, if it is important to observe maximal speed in a motor task, the examiner must explain that large errors are acceptable and may be, in fact, unavoidable. Even with this encouragement, the examiner is sometimes uncertain that the maximum achievable speed has been elicited.

In spinocerebellar atrophy type 6 (SCA6), there is an abnormality of a voltage-sensitive calcium channel. Hyperventilation enhances the defective function of the channel and increases the behavioral dysfunction. In addition to modifying nystagmus, hypermetria in single-joint movements is exaggerated with hyperventilation (Manto, 2001). This may be a useful clinical provocative test.

Patients with cerebellar deficits also have abnormalities in termination of movement. This problem has been explicitly studied in a task where subjects were asked to make a rapid elbow flexion on the background of tonic elbow extension needed to hold a position against a background force (Hallett et al., 1975). In this circumstance, the tonic triceps activity typically stops before the phasic biceps activity occurs (the "Hufschmidt phenomenon"). Patients with cerebellar dysfunction have a delay in terminating the triceps activity so that it overlaps the beginning of the biceps activity. This delay in stopping leads to overlap of the end of one movement with the beginning of the next.

The practical consequence of sluggishness in termination can be seen at the bedside with the sign called *impaired check*. If a patient's elbow which was flexed strongly against the grasp of the examiner is suddenly released, it is difficult for the patient to avoid striking himself/herself with the hand. Impaired check can also be attributed to delay in the triggering of the antagonist muscle (Terzuolo et al., 1973). The distinction between sluggish reduction and delayed changes in force is partially artificial.

In addition to transient overshoot, some patients may show movements that come to rest briefly, or nearly come to rest, at locations that are different from that of the target, most often beyond it (*past-pointing*). Unlike dynamic overshoot which is always speed-dependent, this effective mis-scaling of the overall movement amplitude is less consistently related to the movement velocity, and often improves with repetition. The sign can be elicited using the Barany pointing test, in which the patient is asked to extend an arm forward, holding it parallel to the floor, and to note its position carefully (Gilman et al., 1981). Next, the patient closes the eyes and points the arm toward the ceiling. The arm is then rapidly brought down to a level as close to its original horizontal position as possible. The ataxic patient without demonstrable proprioceptive deficits may return at least briefly to a steady position beyond (lower than) the original, as if there is an error in the calculation of the distance moved or to have been moved. Among ataxic patients, past-pointing is less consistently observed than is dynamic overshoot, and it is not known whether past-pointing is as closely linked to movement acceleration as is dynamic overshoot. If the patient is allowed to practice and view the error a few times, he or she may become able correct the final position using a second movement while maintaining the eyes closed. It is as if a more precise proprioceptive measurement system can be employed after movement completion. Eventually, the patient may learn to produce a normally scaled movement. That the initial mis-scaling is often correctable may be related to residual cerebellar function, to a retained ability to increase dependence on proprioceptive information, or to rescaling movement at extracerebellar sites.

Exaggerated postural reactions: rebound

When the cerebellar patient is asked to maintain a steady outstretched arm position and the examiner applies a gentle downward tap, there typically follows a rapid, excessive upward displacement termed *rebound* (note that the term currently has a meaning slightly different from the original). Rebound often occurs transiently in normal individuals, and is usually quickly attenuated with re-perturbation as the normal subject adapts to the amplitude or force of the disturbance. Due to the excessive rate and magnitude of the response, the patient initially yields less than normal to the perturbation, but overshoots in the opposite direction. Rebound may be partially due to sluggish braking as occurs with *impaired check*. However, an excess force-rate abnormality is at least contributory.

The same phenomenon is seen as persistently excessive postural responses to platform perturbations observed by Horak and Diener (1994) in patients with injury to the anterior lobe of the cerebellum. As with rebound in the upper extremity, the excessive initial component of the platform postural response does not attenuate with repetition. Consistent with a cerebellar mechanism, attenuation of initial platform responses in normal subjects appears to be subconscious. Because of secondary, long-latency stabilizing responses, cerebellar patients were still able to avoid falling during the experiments.

Abnormal control of simple multijoint movements: dyssynergia

In ataxic simple multijoint movements, such as intended straight point-to-point hand movements, there is a breakdown in the normal coordination of joint rotations. This has been termed *dyssynergia* or *asynergia* and is described as a type of *movement decomposition*. This typically causes abnormal movement path deviations. As the movements of normal subjects usually display some natural deviation from perfect linearity, abnormality in path is a matter of degree of curvature and of specific pattern. Evidence is now accumulating that ataxic multijoint movements exhibit characteristic trajectory abnormalities (Massaquoi and Hallett, 1996). Thach et al. (1993) have attributed the pronounced ataxia seen in multijoint movements to a hypothetically preferential role for the cerebellum in the coordination of multijoint movement. While the neuroanatomical organization of the cerebellum makes it particularly well suited for coordinating muscle actions of different body parts, the function of the cerebellum in both single and multijoint control may be fundamentally similar.

Analysis of simple, horizontal planar two-joint arm movements suggests that the deficits in acceleration and braking observed at single joints may account, at least in part, for the dyssynergia observed (Hallett and Massaquoi, 1993; Massaquoi and Hallett, 1996). It appears that the force-rate deficit may be accentuated at the joint having the greatest torque-rate demand, which causes an imbalance in the joint accelerations leading to hand movement curvature. This suspected mechanism is consistent with the marked worsening of dyssynergia with increases in intended acceleration. Massaquoi and Slotine (1996) have proposed a theoretical model of intermediate cerebellar function that relates the force production deficit in both single and multijoint limb movements to a common failure of a long-loop feedback control system. The model accounts for the underdamped quality of ataxic motions and reproduces the characteristic curvature of cerebellar patients' hand trajectories in horizontal planar movements.

As noted by Holmes, ataxia may be especially apparent in multijoint movements because the control problem is more demanding. In addition to the need for forces to launch and stop, there is a requirement for rapid compensation for the disturbing effects of multiple interaction torques between body segments, as well as the need to coordinate more muscles having different individual actions. Because of the additional degrees of force and motion freedom available, failure to compensate for muscular forces and body interaction torques may lead to multidirectional path errors in addition to overall dysmetria. Indeed, several groups have specifically related multijoint trajectory errors in cerebellar ataxia to deficits in interaction torque compensation (Bastian et al., 1996, 2000; Topka et al., 1998). Moreover, Sainburg et al. (1993) have shown deficits in interaction torque control in subjects with sensory ataxia due to peripheral neuropathy. These findings appear to point to similar mechanisms underlying both sensory and cerebellar ataxia.

Several investigators have suggested other mechanisms for asynergia that may be also or alternatively operative. Multijoint movements may be sometimes decomposed into multistep single-joint movement components as a voluntary strategy to simplify programming by minimizing interaction torques between the joints (Bastian et al., 1996). Dyssynergy may be due to the general difficulties cerebellar patients have with timing tasks (Keele and Ivry, 1990). These might yield problems with coordinating the actions of the different joints or muscles within the synergy as suggested by Thach et al. (1992). From this perspective, dysmetria and dyssynergy within simple (single intended velocity peak) single and multijoint movements may have a mechanism similar to that which underlies *dysdiadochokinesia*, a disruption of compound movements involving more than one intended velocity peak (see below). On the other hand, a servo-control model, such as Massaquoi's, predicts that timing derangements within single movements occur as secondary effects of muscular activation (force) rate deficits (Massaquoi and Slotine, 1996). The latter view is supported by the prediction, based on dynamics, of a preferred direction for the interjoint timing abnormality (i.e., lag or lead) for a given intended planar hand movement, and therefore of a certain preferred trajectory pattern, rather than random path aberrations.

Abnormalities in timing and coupling movements and other processes: dysrhythmia, dysdiadochokinesia, delayed reaction time and impaired time interval assessment

Ataxia also includes disruption of the normally smooth concatenation and coordination of compound movement subcomponents. This gives rise to a particular degradation of the rhythm of repetitively alternating single movements (*dysrhythmia*), and of the synchronization of single-joint movement components within repetitively alternating multijoint movements yielding *dysdiadochokinesia* (*adiadochokinesia*), a second type of movement decomposition. Although clinical testing for dysrhythmia and dysdiadochokinesia typically employs rapidly alternating oppositely-directed movements which maximize the sensitivity for detecting errors in the timing of movement onsets and offsets, timing difficulties may be noted in a variety of tasks that involve sequential movements. Bedside testing for dysrhythmia can be done by asking the patient to tap out a rhythm with a single-joint movement. Tests for dysdiadochokinesia include alternately slapping the palmar and dorsal surfaces of the hand on the thigh, or making rapid pincer movements of the index finger tip to the opposing mid-thumb crease. Accurate slapping or tapping requires precise synchronization of rotations of more than one joint (the elbow and radioulnar joints in the first case, the interphalangeal and metacarpophalangeal joints in the latter). In these two tasks, ataxic patients display both an irregular underlying rhythm and inaccurately placed contacts owing to failed multijoint coordination. Dysdiadochokinesia can therefore be seen as a combination of dysrhythmia and dyssynergia.

Thus, in multicomponent movements, considering that each subcomponent movement is subject to imprecise execution due to simple movement control deficits discussed above, it is clear that at least some timing derangement is associated with, if not due to, abnormal acceleration, braking or scaling. That is, it results from serial dysmetria, as well as serial dyssynergia in the multijoint case. If a patient is asked to perform even multicomponent movements very slowly, both temporal and spatial accuracy tend to improve substantially.

In addition to timing aberrations that are associated with, and in fact may result from, clumsy movement execution, there appears to be a separate timing abnormality due to failure of a cerebellum-dependent "central clock" (Keele and Ivry, 1990). Theoretically, this clock assists in the timely launching of movements with respect to preceding movements (Diener et al., 1993; Grill et al., 1997). The same system may generally help to launch movements with respect to other events, both external and internal. In all types of reaction tasks, not only does agonist EMG build up more slowly in cerebellar patients, but the EMG onset itself is significantly delayed with respect to the time of the stimulus, as if a triggering system was defective (Grill et al., 1997).

Much physiologic evidence has been accumulated to suggest that the lateral cerebellar hemispheres and dentate nucleus are preferentially involved in context-dependent triggering of movements, while the intermediate and medial regions of the cerebellum control the evolution of ongoing movement of single or multiple body parts. Supporting the existence of an internal triggering/timing system that is separate from that for movement execution control, is the finding by Wing and Kristofferson that timing errors in a simple rhythmic finger tapping task could be partitioned into "implementation" (executional) mistiming and internal clock mistiming, according to a two-component statistical model (Wing et al., 1984). Subsequently, Ivry and Keele found that in cerebellar patients, increased implementation errors were associated with lesions of the medial cerebellum, while clock errors occurred in those having lesions of the lateral hemispheres (Keele and Ivry, 1990). Moreover, cerebellar patients with lateral hemisphere lesions also had difficulty in accurately assessing the difference in the lengths of time intervals between two pairs of tones, while those with medial cerebellar lesions did not. Also noteworthy is their observation that patients with clumsy movements due to either sensory neuropathy or deafferentation showed only executional mistiming. It is not clear, however, whether their abnormal movements appeared clinically identical to cerebellar ataxia.

Abnormalities in motion assessment and prediction: impairment of tracking and mass estimation

Probably closely related to their problems with assessment of time intervals and movement amplitude scaling is cerebellar patients' basic difficulty in using sensory information to assess and predict motion characteristics. This applies both to body parts, as shown by Grill et al. (1994) and as exhibited in past-pointing tests, and to external objects. Especially in rapid multicomponent movements, a certain amount of motion prediction ability is important for effective performance. Because of the delays in the transmission of neural signals, initiation of movement subcomponents may need to take place well in advance of completion of the preceding subcomponent (Grill et al., 1997). Often, however, details of the plan for the second motion may depend upon the progress of the first motion. For example, in throwing a ball, timing of release must be coordinated with the movement of the arm to produce a properly directed trajectory (e.g., Becker et al., 1990). Similarly, for any control system having nontrivial feedback delays, high-precision tracking of a moving target requires a certain amount of predictive control. This may take the form of additional open-loop (feedforward) predictive signals or the processing of higher derivatives of error information (e.g., velocity error information for position control) which inherently include some predictive information.

The cerebellum appears to be involved in both predictive feedforward and velocity feedback control. Motion prediction deficits can often be identified at the bedside by asking the patient to track, with his or her finger, the examiner's finger as it moves slowly back and forth in a smooth motion. A motion should be used which would be normally easy to predict and at a speed that would not engender overshoot in a simple point-to-point movement. Cerebellar patients will nevertheless frequently lag the examiner during the motion and/or overshoot at the direction reversals, presumably because they fail to assess properly the examiner's rate of acceleration and deceleration or the rhythm of the examiner's overall movement (Morrice et al., 1990). Very slow manual tracking in cerebellar patients also shows breakdown into a sequence of small movements in "staircase" pattern which has been attributed to loss of velocity feedback control (Beppu et al., 1984, 1987).

Holmes (1939) and, more recently Angel (1980), have noted in hemiataxic patients a tendency to overestimate the weight of objects in the affected hand. However, Holmes found no difference between the sides in being able to discriminate accurately between two different weights placed successively in the same hand. Keele and Ivry (1990) also did not find an abnormality in the perception of static force in cerebellar patients. Thus, the cerebellar patient appears compromised in terms of absolute but not relative weight determination. The explanation favored by Holmes and Angel is that individuals tend to assess weight (or mass, as opposed to force per se) by moving an object up and down with their hands, presumably attempting to relate the applied force, or perhaps more accurately, the applied effort, to the rate of acceleration or oscillation frequency. Given patients' difficulties with the kinesthetic assessment of motion characteristics (Grill et al., 1994), and possibly an element of asthenia, it would not be surprising if a patient's ability to relate movement effort to hand acceleration is compromised, thus disturbing the assessment of mass as a secondary effect.

Sensory information acquisition and analysis, and motor control

The critical role of sensory information in successful motor control has been long recognized. Based on the deficits that have been noted in cerebellar patients that were described earlier and on the afferent neuroanatomical connections of the cerebellum, it is evident that it plays an important role in processing sensory information to influence motor performance. However, the nature of this influence has been debated. Although it would appear that improved stability and accuracy of body motion are principal purposes of cerebellar function, Bower has put forward the controversial suggestion that the cerebellum is primarily concerned with fine control of the acquisition of sensory information rather than control of movement per se (Gao et al., 1996; Bower, 1997). In particular, it may be chiefly designed to coordinate the positioning and movement of tactile sensory surfaces to optimize the information received.

However, the question of whether the cerebellum is primarily interested in acquiring sensory information or a motor controller is substantially moot from the point of view of modern feedback control system design, which often incorporates sophisticated afferent signal processing. The job of any motor feedback controller is to assist in minimizing the discrepancy between an intended body state (position and velocity) and the actual state as it is deduced or predicted from available information. If the output is effectively employed for continuous control, the controlled body part will be guided so that its associated sensors register or nearly register measurements of the intended state. In a real sense, feedback-controlled motion is always planned in sensory coordinates. Whether the purpose of the motion is to acquire other sensory information or to transport the body part varies with the task. If the controller output is not applied to the motor command, the controller may be used simply for state estimation or other types of processing of its sensory input (e.g., filtering or prediction) depending on its design. For example, computation of the slide rate along the skin of a contact point is as useful for control of active tactile exploration as it is for monitoring the progress of an object slipping from a stationary hand, or of a passive hand slipping from a support. Because, in practice, the detection of slip may be used to trigger certain behaviors when the slide approaches a critical point, even the distinction between motor control and passive sensory data acquisition is not fundamental. The state of seemingly passive sensory monitoring may in fact be readily employed within a discrete response-type motor control loop.

Increased movement variability

Ataxic motor performance is frequently described as being more variable than normal (Hallett and Massaquoi, 1993; Palliyath et al., 1998). However, aside from the presence of involuntary movements, ataxic variability may arise more as a consequence of enhanced susceptibility to perturbation and of the sequential compounding of errors, than of an inherent noise as might result from the presence of an unstable autonomous generator. This is suggested by the fact that when tasks are constrained sufficiently, ataxic movements become much less variable (Massaquoi and Hallett, 1996). Thus, especially for experimentally conducted single- and two-joint movements for which there is a single attempted movement speed and direction, and where head, eyes, and trunk are fixed, and in the absence of external contacts and forces (i.e., not against gravity), ataxic movements though inaccurate, are much more consistent in their inaccuracy. Because of the loosened control over executive action in the cerebellar patient, movements and perhaps certain cognitive processes are more vulnerable to both internal and external environmental disturbances. Most natural tasks involve multijoint movements which inherently have many degrees of movement freedom, as well as ongoing efforts to guide motion. Elemental trajectory errors may therefore interact, propagate, and become compounded; a process that effectively produces motor control noise.

Cerebellar tremors

Two types of action cerebellar tremor are commonly identified: kinetic and postural tremor. Lesions of the dentate, of the interpositus, and of the cerebellar outflow via the brachium conjunctivum appear to be the most frequently associated with action tremors. Both manifest alternating EMG bursting in agonist and antagonist muscles (Hallett, 1987). All types of cerebellar action tremors may be exacerbated near the point of attempted fixation if greater effort is made to maintain position precisely. Tremor frequency may differ between limbs and the oscillations are generally not synchronous in non-adjacent body parts. However, as are most tremors, cerebellar action tremors are worsened by fatigue. Cerebellar action tremors are often improved and sometimes eliminated by eye closure (Sanes et al., 1988). Propranolol has no substantial effect and alcohol tends to worsen cerebellar action tremors.

Basic mechanisms that have been suggested to underlie cerebellar tremor have included (1) serial voluntary corrections for positioning error (serial dysmetria) (Hallett, 1987), (2) abnormality of transcortical and segmental proprioceptive feedback loops (Hore and Flament, 1986), and (3) action of central oscillators (Ito, 1984). Sufficient evidence has accumulated to indicate that each of these mechanisms is likely to be important to some component of body oscillations in ataxic patients under various circumstances. It is apparent clinically from the slowness of cerebellar voluntary reactions and in performance of rapid alternating movements that serial dysmetria is unlikely to be operative at frequencies greater than around 1–2 Hz at proximal joints or perhaps 3 Hz at the fingers. Thus, only the irregular, low-frequency, ataxic movements exhibited by patients' limbs as they approach a target are a manifestation of serial dysmetria. Because of the voluntary nature and gross irregularity of these movements, however, serial dysmetria is not really tremor.

Holmes (1939) also drew attention to the intermittent recoveries of posture that patients exhibit when fatigued. These movements consist of slow drifting *downward* from the intended posture followed by faster upward corrections that appeared voluntary. While these movements can be viewed as a coarse, asymmetric tremor, their nystagmoid character distinguishes them from the more regular, higher-frequency, involuntary oscillations *around* the intended posture or trajectory that would be characteristic of "true" cerebellar tremors.

The modification of cerebellar tremor by external perturbations and mechanical state (Sanes et al., 1988) indicates at least a partial dependence on peripheral factors, while the persistence of these cerebellar tremors during deafferentation indicates the presence of some central neural instability (Gilman et al., 1976). Several experimental results and models of cerebellar function include the interaction between central and peripheral feedback loops that could be consistent with these observations (Massaquoi and Slotine, 1996).

Increased postural sway and titubation

Ataxic patients exhibit increased irregular sway when standing and sometimes a more regular tremor (titubation). The characteristics of these involuntary movements vary according to the site of the cerebellar system lesion. Diener and Dichgans have performed extensive studies of postural balance in patients with cerebellar system disease (Diener and Dichgans, 1992; Diener et al., 1984). Common to all ataxic patients, except those with lesions restricted to the hemispheres, is the tendency to have abnormally large amplitude sway when the eyes are closed. Patients with anterior lobe atrophy due to chronic alcohol intake and malnutrition and patients with Friedreich ataxia have a high "Romberg quotient," meaning that they sway considerably more with eyes closed. In general, the eyes-closed instability is greater in Friedreich ataxia patients, who typically have significant proprioceptive loss and may fall without vision. By contrast, the anterior lobe lesion patients tend to oscillate markedly without falling when their eyes are closed. Patients with anterior lobe damage also tend to move much more in an anteroposterior direction while those with Friedreich ataxia have an abnormal degree of lateral sway.

Patients with vestibulocerebellar lesions display increased, omnidirectional, low-frequency (~1 Hz) sway and may fall with eyes both open and closed, and therefore have a normal Romberg quotient. Patients who have hemispheric lesions may exhibit slightly increased sway relative to normal subjects, but balance instability is not prominent. Those with diffuse cerebellar damage exhibit a mixture of characteristics. They may be differentiated from normal subjects, but not from each other on the basis of posturography.

In addition to low-frequency (~1 Hz) sway, a characteristic 2–3 Hz body tremor is seen exclusively in patients with anterior lobe dysfunction when the eyes are closed. Unlike the irregular head and trunk titubation that may be seen with various other cerebellar lesions, the anterior lobe tremor consists of regular anteroposterior oscillation at the head, hip, and ankle. The hip is 180° out of phase with the head so that the center of gravity moves little and balance is maintained despite marked titubation. This tremor has been attributed to increased duration and amplitude of long-latency stretch responses. These long-latency responses are likely to be the scalable, secondary responses observed by Horak and Diener (1994) following exaggerated postural responses. Although abnormally large, these responses eventually stabilize the body after a few decaying oscillations at about 2–3 Hz when the eyes are open. Presumably, persistent titubation occurs especially with eyes closed because the gain of these scalable responses is increased in an effort to compensate for the loss of visual input. This is consistent with the view of titubation as a postural tremor.

Dysarthria

When ataxia affects speech, it is manifested as a clumsy, slurring, poorly modulated dysarthria. No disruption of language usage, structure, or content is attributable to the cerebellar dysfunction. As noted by Gilman et al. (1981), adjectives commonly used to describe cerebellar speech include scanning, slurring, staccato, explosive, hesitant, slow, altered accent, and garbled. These investigators have identified 10 elemental speech abnormalities which are present to varying degrees in different cerebellar patients: (1) imprecise consonants, a feature basic to all dysarthrias; (2) excess and equal stress, the inappropriate allocation of emphasis and accent; (3) irregular articulatory breakdown, the elision of syllables or phonemes; (4) distorted vowels; (5) harshness; (6) prolonged phonemes; (7) prolonged intervals; (8) monopitch; (9) monoloudness; and (10) slow rate. Cerebellar speech may also be tremulous and may trail off to a whisper. However, it should again be noted that many patients are intentionally slow and perhaps regularize their speech, i.e., voluntarily generate "scanning" speech to increase its intelligibility.

Perhaps analogous to the two types of timing deficits in finger movements described by Keele and Ivry (1990), at least two levels of speech control may be abnormal in cerebellar dysarthria. First, it is evident that on simple repetition of syllables, the peak repetition rate is considerably reduced in cerebellar patients and the sounds are not crisp. This could easily be attributed to a difficulty with rapid production and termination of force in the musculature of the vocal tract and respiration. In addition, however, there seems to be a poor regulation of the normal speech prosody or rhythm that is not simply due to decreased ability to speak quickly. Correspondingly, at least two locations for cerebellar control of speech have been suggested. Holmes described dysarthria in gunshot wound patients with damage to the cerebellar hemispheres that was more pronounced when the vermis was also damaged, suggesting important roles for both the vermis and hemispheres.

Dysarthria has been reported in cases where lesions were apparently confined to the vermis (Kadota et al., 1994) and Chiu et al. (1996) have stressed the importance of the vermis and fastigial nuclei in speech integration. On the other hand, Lechtenberg and Gilman (1978) have identified a paravermal site in the left cerebellar hemisphere that is specifically related to cerebellar dysarthria. They speculate that this cerebellar region functions in association with prosody areas in the right cerebral hemisphere to help regulate the timing of speech. The left hemisphere site is probably the more important of at least two cerebellar regions involved in normal speech production.

Gait ataxia

A deterioration in the stability of ambulation is the chief complaint of the majority of patients afflicted with cerebellar dysfunction. This is apparently due to two factors. First, the vermis of the cerebellum appears to be preferentially or initially affected in many degenerative conditions. This is especially the case for alcoholic/nutritional degeneration, but also for cases of multiple system atrophy. Second, walking, which consists of carefully managing a series of controlled collisions with the environment, is very demanding dynamically. Unlike the vocal tract and the arms, which are mechanically stable and will come to rest upon relaxation, the upright body, virtually an inverted pendulum, is unstable. Thus, the body does not automatically return to a consistent initial condition following each step. Rather, each successive step depends sensitively on the manner in which the preceding step was completed. This aspect of bipedal locomotion probably contributes significantly to the variability of foot placement in ataxic gait.

Despite the variability in ataxic locomotion there are still consistent kinematic patterns (Palliyath et al., 1998). As in upper extremity multijoint movement tasks, lower extremity multijoint coordination is characteristically abnormal. In particular, when walking, patients show a relatively greater delay of plantar flexion at the ankle than in flexion at the knee, as well as a relatively sluggish dorsiflexion of the ankle at the onset of swing. In walking, the largest and fastest required force transients are the forceful ankle plantar flexion at the end of stance and the rapid ankle dorsiflexion that follows immediately at the onset of swing. Therefore, as argued with respect to the shoulder in upper extremity multijoint coordination failure, each of these two lower extremity coordination abnormalities is consistent with a force-rate deficit (or perhaps force-delay) at the joint, in this case the ankle, that has the greatest force-rate demand. The situation is not completely clear, however, because a similar ankle–knee relationship may be seen in elderly subjects without ataxia. Further quantitative studies are needed. In any case, owing at least in part to the sluggishness of dorsiflexion, there is a tendency for ataxic patients to trip as their toes fail to clear the ground during swing. That no significant abnormality was noted in the height of toe lift during swing phase by Palliyath et al. (1998) may well be because trials in which stumbles occurred were excluded from analysis.

Ataxic gait, when under control, tends to be slower than normal and to have shortened strides. As argued by Palliyath et al. (1998), this is at least partially a voluntary compensation for the loss of control that occurs at higher speeds. Because walking involves controlled falling, both forward and laterally onto the next foot placement, walking with too slow a cadence demands prolonged balancing on each leg, which is difficult for the ataxic patient. Therefore, as patients slow down, they will tend to adopt a much shorter stride to maintain their cadence, or a wider base to stabilize themselves laterally. Possibly because of the resulting waddle, patients sometimes report that they walk "better" when they move at a moderate speed rather than very slowly, even though they may become more prone to veer or to trip than when they waddle.

Impaired motor learning

The consideration that ataxic patients should have difficulty with motor learning follows from the apparent logic that if they could learn, then why would they still be clumsy. Motor learning itself is a complex phenomenon with a number of different components (Hallett et al., 1996; Hallett and Grafman, 1997). One aspect can be defined as a change in motor performance with practice. Other aspects would include increasing the repertoire of motor behavior and maintenance of a new behavior over a period of time. Even considering only a change in motor performance, there are likely to be several different phenomena. Adaptation and skill learning can be distinguished. Adaptation is simply a change in the nature of the motor output while skill learning is the development of a new capability.

Adaptation learning clearly involves the cerebellum. Adaptation to lateral displacement of vision as produced by prism glasses is a method for assessing learning of a visual-motor task. When prism glasses are used, there is at first a mismatch between where an object is seen and where the pointing is directed. With experience, normal human subjects adjust to this and begin to point correctly. This correct pointing can be a product of both a true change in the visual-motor coordination or an intellectual decision to point in a different direction than where the object appears to be so that the correct movement is made. When the glasses are removed, typically the subject initially points in the opposite direction to that when the glasses were put on. In the naive subject, this is an excellent measure of true change in the visual-motor task since there is no reason for making any intellectual decision to point other than in the direction that the object appears to be. With additional experience, the subjects return to correct performance again. Patients with cerebellar damage show poor or no adaptation (Weiner et al., 1983; Martin et al., 1996). Another paradigm that can test adaptation learning is a task with a change in the visual-motor gain. An example is making movements of the elbow by matching targets on a computer screen. If the gain of the elbow with respect to the display on the computer screen is changed, then the amount of movement to match the targets will change. In the normal circumstance after a gain change, there would be an error that gradually would be reduced with continued practice. Deuschl et al. (1996) found that ataxic patients showed much slower learning than the normal controls.

Eye blink conditioning is recognized as a form of motor learning and could be argued to fit the definition proposed here for adaptation learning. In nonhuman animal studies, eye blink conditioning seems to require the cerebellum, at least for the expression and timing of the response. A number of groups have studied eye blink conditioning in patients with cerebellar lesions and found them to be markedly deficient (Daum et al., 1993; Topka et al., 1993).

There have been fewer studies of motor skill learning. Topka et al. (1998) evaluated the ability of patients to learn a multijoint two-dimensional trajectory with the upper extremity. While the performance of the patients was clearly impaired, they improved their performance as much as the normal subjects as long as the task was done slowly. With rapid movements, learning did slow down abnormally in the patients. Skill learning has many components including features such as the sequencing of the different components. Other parts of the brain play important roles in these other functions and can be responsible for the learning in the ataxic patients. Functional imaging studies, for example, show increased activation with learning in motor cortex, premotor cortex, and parietal areas (Hallett et al., 1996; Hallett and Grafman, 1997). The cortical network becomes more tightly connected (Wu et al., 2008).

Clinical localization

Virtually any lesion of the cerebellar parenchyma can be associated with ataxia. Presumably due to the considerable redundancy, complex interconnectedness, and plasticity of cerebellar circuits, as well as to inter-individual physiologic differences, attempts at precisely localizing cerebellar function on the basis of experimental and natural lesions have yielded inconsistent results. Similarly, it is usually not possible to predict lesion site within the cerebellum with great accuracy from the clinical examination. The clinicoanatomic correlations described below should therefore be viewed only as predominant patterns. See Timmann et al. (2008) for a review.

The cerebellum is often considered to be functionally divided into four parts on the basis of its output nuclei. Three sagittal zones – midline, intermediate, and lateral – project, respectively, to the fastigius, interpositus (globose and emboliform nuclei in combination), and dentate nuclei, while the vestibulocerebellum (flocculonodular lobe) projects to the lateral vestibular nucleus, which effectively functions as a fourth cerebellar deep nucleus. From a clinical point of view, however, partitioning into simply midline, lateral (or vermis and hemispheres), and vestibular cerebellum is usually sufficient. The vestibulocerebellum, owing to its large involvement in head, eye, and balance control, can be considered part of the midline region. At least for tasks used in bedside examination, the functions of the intermediate and lateral zones of the hemispheres are not readily distinguished. In addition, it is also useful to keep in mind that tremor appears to be seldom due to lesions of the cerebellar cortex alone and that the superior/anterior portion of the vermis, in particular, is affected in relative isolation by vitamin deficiency (often secondary to chronic alcohol intoxication) and tumors (especially in children), which produce a fairly pure ataxia of upright stance and gait with minimal, if any, limb ataxia, dysarthria, or nystagmus.

In general, signs that involve only the limbs unilaterally are most often due to lesions of the ipsilateral cerebellar hemispheres. However, this is not uniformly the case. In a series of 106 patients having unilateral or predominantly unilateral hemispheric injury (most postsurgical cases) studied by Lechtenberg and Gilman (Gilman et al., 1981), predominantly right limb dysmetria was associated with right hemisphere damage in 22 of 26 (85%) cases and left limb dysmetria with left hemispheric damage in 37 of 42 (88%) cases. For dysdiadochokinesia, ipsilateral hemispheric lesions were seen in 11 of 12 (91%) right predominant cases and 25 of 32 (78%) left predominant cases. The mechanism of strictly contralateral hemispheric effects on limb

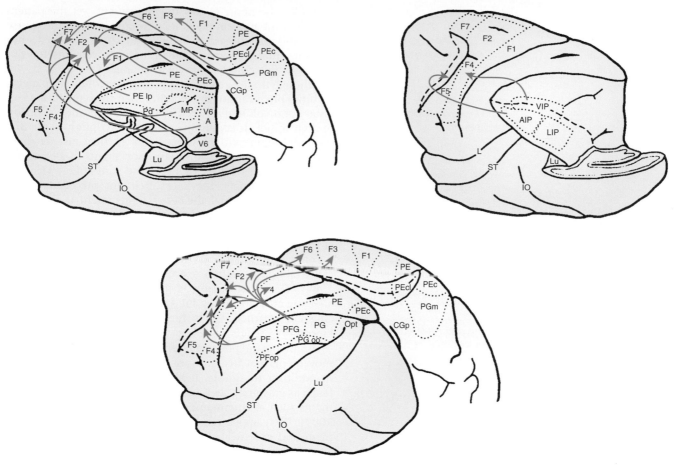

Figure 2.5 Diagram of the multiple parieto-frontal connections as identified in the primate. The critical concept is that there are multiple parietal areas and multiple frontal areas and that there are highly specific parietal-frontal connections between them; each connection has a specific motor function. For abbreviations, see original reference. *From Rizzolatti G, Luppino G, Matelli M. The organization of the cortical motor system: new concepts. Electroencephalogr Clin Neurophysiol 1998;106(4):283–96, with permission.*

movement is not known. The handedness of the subjects was not reported. However, assuming the usual prevalence, the findings for dysdiadochokinesia are consistent with a mild additional impairment of the nondominant hand. This is consistent with the apparent importance of cerebrocerebellar interaction with rapid alternating movements (see above). When vermal lesions affected the limbs, the deficits were usually seen bilaterally and when there was asymmetry of deficit, the left limbs tended to be more severely affected. Overall, tremor was found less often than dysmetria or dysdiadochokinesia, but it occurred with similar rates in vermal and unilateral hemispheric disease.

Deficits involving the head, trunk, balance, and gait in isolation tend to be related preferentially to vermal lesions. However, other sites are possible. As discussed earlier, dysarthria, deficits involving the mouth, though midline, may be due to vermal or hemispheric dysfunction.

Cortical control mechanisms

As noted earlier, the primary motor cortex provides the principal output to the corticospinal tract. Thus, its inputs determine the brain's contribution to movement. The main inputs come from the premotor cortices, including the lateral premotor cortex, the supplementary motor area, and the caudal parts of the cingulate motor area. These areas in turn receive their input from wide areas of brain including the presupplementary motor area, rostral parts of the cingulate motor area, dorsolateral prefrontal cortex, and parietal areas. Considerable attention has been given recently to the parietal-premotor connections, which are highly specific and appear to provide important links between sensory and motor function (Rizzolatti et al., 1998; Rizzolatti and Luppino, 2001) (Fig. 2.5).

Apraxia

The apraxias are disorders of motor control, characterized by a loss of the motor program, not explicable by more elemental motor, sensory, coordination, or language impairments (Haaland et al., 2000; Hanna-Pladdy et al., 2001; Zadikoff and Lang, 2005; Gross and Grossman, 2008). Idiomotor apraxia is present when there is knowledge of the task, but there are temporal and spatial errors in performance (Wheaton and Hallett, 2007). It has long been suspected to be due to a disconnection between parietal and premotor areas. Table 2.3 lists the types of apraxias.

Table 2.3 Types of apraxia

Limb kinetic apraxia	Loss of hand and finger dexterity; significantly affecting manipulative movements
Ideomotor apraxia	Deficit in pantomiming tool use and gestures with temporal and spatial errors. Knowledge of tasks is still present
Ideational apraxia	Failure to carry out a series of tasks using multiple objects for an intended purpose; problem in the sequencing of actions. Tools are identifiable
Conceptual apraxia	Loss of tool knowledge; inappropriate use of tools and objects; inability to solve mechanical problems
(Verbal-motor) Dissociation apraxia	Failure to respond to verbal commands, but use of objects is appropriate
Conduction apraxia	Problems with imitating, but not with responding to verbal commands

Modified from Wheaton LA, Hallett M. Ideomotor apraxia: A review. J Neurol Sci 2007;260:1–10.

What is a voluntary movement?

While clearly much is known about the anatomy and physiology of the motor system, there is still considerable difficulty with the concept of voluntariness. Many movements are triggered by sensory stimuli, and the physiology of this mechanism is relatively clear. However, there are certainly movements that appear to be "internally triggered" and humans have the sense that they have willed the movement. The self-initiation of movement and conscious awareness of movement appear to involve mesial motor structures such as the supplementary motor area and the dorsolateral prefrontal cortex (Deiber et al., 1999). As pointed out by Paus (2001), the mesial motor structures including the anterior cingulate cortex, in particular, is a place of convergence for motor control, homeostatic drive, emotion, and cognition. Looked at critically, the sense of voluntariness is clearly a "perception of consciousness" (what can be called a quale). There is very little understanding of how this evolves.

Disorders of willed movement

In neurology, there are many disorders where the issue of will arises (Hallett, 2006c, 2007b, 2009).

There are patients who have movements that are commonly held as being involuntary. Myoclonus is such an example. The brain makes the movement, yet the patient interprets the movement as involuntary. Early in the course of Huntington disease, patients with chorea often do not recognize that there are any involuntary movements. It is not clear why this happens or why it changes later.

Although tics are generally considered involuntary, patients with tics often cannot say whether their movements are voluntary or involuntary. This may not be a relevant distinction in their minds. It is perhaps a better description to say that they can suppress their movements or they just let them happen. Tics look like voluntary movements in all respects from the point of view of EMG and kinesiology (Hallett, 2000). Interestingly, they are often not preceded by the normal brain potential, the Bereitschaftspotential, and hence the brain mechanisms for their production clearly differs from ordinary voluntary movement (Obeso et al., 1981; Karp et al., 1996).

The symptom of loss of voluntary movement is often called abulia or, in the extreme, akinetic mutism (Fisher, 1983). The classic lesion is in the midline frontal region affecting areas including the supplementary motor area and cingulate motor areas. The bradykinesia and akinesia of Parkinson disease are related.

The alien hand phenomenon is characterized by unwanted movements that arise without any sense of their being willed. In addition to simple, unskilled, quasi-reflex movements (such as grasping), there can also be complex, skilled movements such as intermanual conflict or interference (Fisher, 2000). There appears to be difficulty in self-initiating movement and excessive ease in the production of involuntary and triggered movements. In cases with discrete lesions, this seems to have its anatomical correlation in the territory of the anterior cerebral artery.

Conversion psychogenic movements are movements interpreted by the patient as involuntary. Their etiology is actually obscure since the physiology of conversion is really unknown. EEG investigation of these movements shows a normal looking Bereitschaftspotential preceding them (Toro and Torres, 1986; Terada et al., 1995). The normal brain potential, however, indicates that there must be substantial sharing of brain voluntary movement mechanisms (Hallett, 2010).

Acknowledgment

The ataxia section of the chapter is updated from a syllabus written for the 1999 meeting of the American Academy of Neurology, which itself was extensively modified and updated from a chapter by Massaquoi and Hallett (1998). The Parkinson disease section is modified from an earlier chapter (Hallett, 2003a). The dystonia section is modified from earlier chapters (Hallett, 2004).

References available on Expert Consult: www.expertconsult.com

CHAPTER **3**

Functional neuroanatomy of the basal ganglia

Chapter contents

Introduction	55	Circuitry of the basal ganglia	62
Neurotransmitters	55	Physiology	64
Components of the basal ganglia	60		

Introduction

The basal ganglia comprise a collection of nuclear structures deep in the brain and have been defined anatomically and functionally. Anatomically, the basal ganglia are the deep nuclei in the telencephalon. Functionally, three closely associated structures, the subthalamic nucleus (in the diencephalon), the substantia nigra and pedunculopontine nucleus (both in the mesencephalon), are also included as part of the motor part of the basal ganglia. The definition of which structures are included has varied over the years and depends also in part on a preconceived notion of their function. Most of the time, and for the purposes of the study of movement disorders, the basal ganglia are viewed as having primarily a motor function. Indeed, the early movement disorders included in the concept, such as Parkinson disease (PD) (see Table 3.1 for all abbreviations in this chapter) and Huntington disease (HD), were primarily basal ganglia related, and interested neuroscientists would meet at "basal ganglia clubs." It is now clear, however, that the basal ganglia also play a role in cognitive, behavioral, and emotional functions. For example, the limbic system interacts extensively with the basal ganglia, and some components of the basal ganglia, such as the amygdala (archistriatum), nucleus accumbens, and ventral pallidum, serve these functions (Haber and Knutson, 2010).

The core motor structures of the basal ganglia include the caudate and putamen, collectively called the neostriatum (commonly abbreviated as the striatum), the globus pallidus (GP) (paleostriatum), the subthalamic nucleus (STN), the substantia nigra (SN), and the pedunculopontine nucleus (PPN) (Figs 3.1, 3.2, and 3.3). The putamen and globus pallidus together are sometimes called the lenticular nucleus. The main informational processing loop of the basal ganglia comes from the cortex and goes back to the cortex via the thalamus. The substantia nigra pars compacta (SNc) is largely a modulator of this main loop, with dopamine as its neurotransmitter. Other modulators are the locus coeruleus (LC), with norepinephrine as neurotransmitter, and the median raphe nucleus (MRN), which uses serotonin as neurotransmitter. The notion that the basal ganglia provide an "extrapyramidal" control of movement separate from the cortical-pyramidal control is not correct since the main output of the basal ganglia projects to the cortex. Therefore, the term "extrapyramidal disorders" for disorders arising from dysfunction of the basal ganglia is a misnomer.

In this chapter, we will first consider the neurotransmitters and their receptors that are involved in basal ganglia circuitry. Next, we will consider the main components of the basal ganglia and the way that they interact with each other. At the end, we will review some features of the physiologic activity, and consider what the main functions of the basal ganglia might be.

Neurotransmitters

Dopamine (DA)

It is appropriate to start out the discussion of neurotransmitters with a consideration of dopamine, the most "prominent" neurotransmitter since it is depleted in PD and because we have the means to manipulate this transmitter in therapeutics. The main sources of dopamine are the lateral SNc (A9), the medial ventral tegmental area (VTA, A10), and the retrorubral area (A8) (Fig. 3.2). The SNc innervates the striatum via the nigrostriatal pathway, while the VTA and retrorubal areas give rise to the mesolimbic innervation of the ventral striatum (nucleus accumbens) and the mesocortical innervation of the dorsolateral and ventromedial prefrontal cortex regions (Fig. 3.4) (Van den Heuvel and Pasterkamp, 2008).

© 2011 Elsevier Ltd, Inc, BV
DOI: 10.1016/B978-1-4377-2369-4.00003-2

Table 3.1   **Abbreviations**

AAADC	Aromatic L-amino acid decarboxylase	L-dopa	Levodopa
ACh	Acetylcholine	LFP	Local field potential
AChE	Acetylcholinesterase	M1	Primary motor cortex
ADP	Adenosine diphosphate	MAO	Monoamine oxidase
AMPA	α-Amino-3-hydroxyl-5-methyl-4-isoxazole-propionate	mAChR	Muscarinic acetylcholine receptor
ATP	Adenosine triphosphate	MEA	Midbrain extrapyramidal area
BuChE	Butyrylcholinesterase (pseudocholinesterase)	MPTP	1-Methyl-4-phenyl-1,2,3,6-tetrahydropyridine
cAMP	Cyclic adenosine monophosphate	MRN	Median raphe nucleus
ChAT	Choline acetyltransferase	3-MT	3-Methoxytyramine (3-O-methydopamine)
CM	Centrum medianum nucleus of the thalamus	nAChR	Nicotinic acetylcholine receptor
COMT	Catechol-O-methyltransferase	NE	Norepinephrine
DA	Dopamine	NMDA	N-methyl-D-aspartic acid
DAG	Diacylglycerol	PD	Parkinson disease
DAT	Dopamine transporter	Pf	Parafascicular nucleus of the thalamus
DBH	Dopamine beta-hydroxylase	PMv	Premotor cortex, ventral division
DBS	Deep brain stimulation	PPN	Pedunculopontine nucleus
DOPAC	3,4-Dihydroxyphenylacetic acid	PPNc	Pedunculopontine nucleus, pars compacta
EAAT	Excitatory amino acid transporter	PPNd	Pedunculopontine nucleus, pars dissipatus
GABA	Gamma-amino butyric acid	SERT	Serotonin transporter
GABA-T	GABA-transaminase	SMA	Supplementary motor area
GAD	Glutamic acid decarboxylase	SN	Substantia nigra
GAT	GABA transporter	SNc	Substantia nigra, pars compacta
Glu	Glutamate	SNr	Substantia nigra, pars reticulata
GP	Globus pallidus	STN	Subthalamic nucleus
GPe	Globus pallidus externa	TANs	Tonically active neurons
GPi	Globus pallidus interna	TH	Tyrosine hydroxylase
HD	Huntington disease	VA	Ventral anterior nucleus of thalamus
5-HT	5-Hydroxytryptamine, serotonin	VAChT	Vesicular ACh transporter
5-HTP	5-Hydroxytryptophan	VL	Ventral lateral nucleus of thalamus
HVA	Homovanillic acid	VMAT2	Vesicular monoamine transporter 2
IP3	Inositol triphosphate	VTA	Ventral tegmental area
LC	Locus coeruleus	ZI	Zona incerta

DA is formed from levodopa (L-dopa) by the enzyme aromatic L-amino acid decarboxylase (AAADC), which is commonly called dopa decarboxylase (Fig. 3.5) (Stahl, 2008). Once synthesized, DA is taken up into synaptic vesicles by the vesicular monoamine transporter 2 (VMAT2). In vivo, levodopa is synthesized from L-tyrosine by the enzyme tyrosine hydroxylase (TH). L-tyrosine is an essential amino acid in the brain, because it cannot be synthesized from L-phenylalanine, as it can in the rest of the body. DA can be metabolized by monoamine oxidase (MAO) to 3,4-dihydroxyphenylacetic acid (DOPAC), by catechol-O-methyltransferase (COMT) to 3-methoxytyramine (3-MT)

(also called 3-O-methydopamine), and by both enzymes serially to homovanillic acid (HVA). MAO exists in two forms, MAO-A and MAO-B, both found in the mitochondria of neurons and glia (Bortolato et al., 2008). COMT is a membrane-bound enzyme (Bonifacio et al., 2007). Physiologically, DA action is terminated by reuptake back into the dopaminergic nerve terminal by action of the dopamine transporter (DAT). Once in the cytosol, it can be taken back up into synaptic vesicles by VMAT2. Dopamine neurons have MAO-A (Demarest et al., 1980), but virtually no COMT. DA not taken up into vesicles will therefore be metabolized to DOPAC. If DA remains non-metabolized in the cytosol,

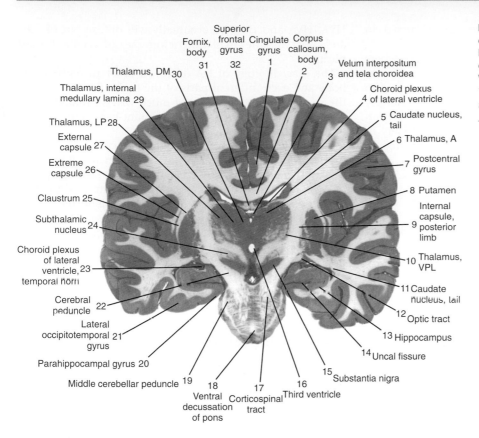

Superior
Fornix, frontal Cingulate Corpus
body gyrus gyrus callosum,
31 32 1 body
Thalamus, DM 30 2
3 Velum interpositum
Thalamus, internal and tela choroidea
medullary lamina 29 Choroid plexus
4 of lateral ventricle
Thalamus, LP 28 5 Caudate nucleus,
External tail
capsule 27 6 Thalamus, A
Extreme 7 Postcentral
capsule 26 gyrus
Claustrum 25 8 Putamen
Subthalamic Internal
nucleus 24 9 capsule,
posterior
Choroid plexus limb
of lateral 10 Thalamus,
ventricle, 23 VPL
temporal horn 11 Caudate
Cerebral nucleus, tail
peduncle 22 12 Optic tract
Lateral 13 Hippocampus
occipitotemporal 21 14 Uncal fissure
gyrus 15 Substantia nigra
Parahippocampal gyrus 20
Middle cerebellar peduncle 19 18 17 16
Ventral Corticospinal Third ventricle
decussation tract
of pons

Figure 3.1 Anatomy of the basal ganglia. A coronal section of the brain showing most of the basal ganglia nuclei. A, anterior nucleus; DM, dorsomedial nucleus; LP, lateral posterior nucleus; VPL, ventral posterior lateral nucleus. *From Woolsey TA, Hanaway J, Gado MH. The Brain Atlas. A Visual Guide to the Human Central Nervous System, 3rd ed. Hoboken, NJ: John Wiley & Sons, Inc.; 2008.*

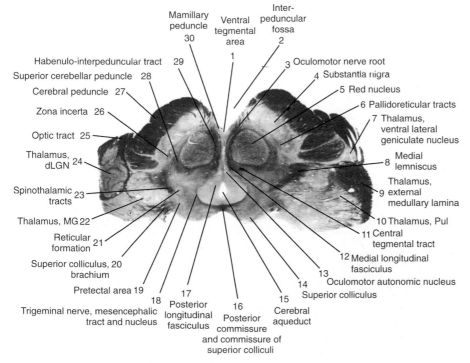

Inter-
Mamillary Ventral peduncular
peduncle tegmental fossa
30 area 2
1
Habenulo-interpeduncular tract 29 3 Oculomotor nerve root
Superior cerebellar peduncle 28 4 Substantia nigra
Cerebral peduncle 27 5 Red nucleus
Zona incerta 26 6 Pallidoreticular tracts
Optic tract 25 7 Thalamus,
Thalamus, ventral lateral
dLGN 24 geniculate nucleus
Spinothalamic 23 8 Medial
tracts lemniscus
Thalamus, MG 22 9 Thalamus,
Reticular external
formation 21 medullary lamina
Superior colliculus, 20 10 Thalamus, Pul
brachium 11 Central
Pretectal area 19 tegmental tract
18 17 16 15 12 Medial longitudinal
Trigeminal nerve, mesencephalic Posterior Posterior Cerebral 13 fasciculus
tract and nucleus longitudinal commissure aqueduct 14 Oculomotor autonomic nucleus
fasciculus and commissure of Superior colliculus
superior colliculi

Figure 3.2 An axial section at the midbrain level showing the principal nuclei for the origin of dopamine projections, the substantia nigra and the ventral tegmental area. Pul, pulvinar; MG, medial geniculate nucleus; dLGN, dorsal lateral geniculate nucleus. *From Woolsey TA, Hanaway J, Gado MH. The Brain Atlas. A Visual Guide to the Human Central Nervous System, 3rd ed. Hoboken, NJ: John Wiley & Sons, Inc.; 2008.*

it might contribute to oxidative stress, as discussed in Chapter 5.

DOPAC can diffuse out of the presynaptic terminal where it might confront COMT on the postsynaptic neuron, endothelial cells or possibly glial cells and be converted to HVA. MAO-B is prominent in the basal ganglia, and is largely in glial cells. Any DA not taken up in the presynaptic terminal might diffuse into glial cells (DAT is not necessary in nondopaminergic cells) where it would be converted to

HVA. HVA and DOPAC eventually will diffuse out of cells and either into the circulation or into the CSF via the choroid plexus.

The exact biology of DA differs in different parts of the body and even different parts of the brain. For example, in the cerebral cortex there is not much DAT so that after DA release, COMT is much more important in terminating DA action (Matsumoto et al., 2003).

There are five subtypes of dopamine receptors, D1–D5, in two families, D1-like and D2-like (Missale et al., 1998; Beaulieu and Gainetdinov, 2011). The D1-like family, composed of D1 and D5, activates adenyl cyclase and causes conversion of adenosine triphosphate (ATP) to cyclic adenosine monophosphate (cAMP). Raising the concentration of cAMP is typically excitatory. The D2-like family, composed of D2, D3, and D4, inhibits adenyl cyclase and reduces the concentration of cAMP. Lowering cAMP is typically inhibitory. Some D2 receptors, called autoreceptors, are on the presynaptic side of dopamine synapses, regulating release by negative feedback.

Acetylcholine (ACh)

Cholinergic neurons have two different types of roles (Pisani et al., 2007). One is as an interneuron, and the "giant aspiny interneuron" of the striatum is cholinergic. A second role is as a projection neuron. There are two prominent cholinergic projection systems in the brain. The best known are the neurons of the basal forebrain, such as the nucleus basalis of Meynert, that innervate wide areas of cortex, are involved with functions such as memory, and are deficient in Alzheimer disease. The other is the set of projections from the meso-pontine tegmental complex, which includes the PPN. These are importantly involved in the basal ganglia motor system.

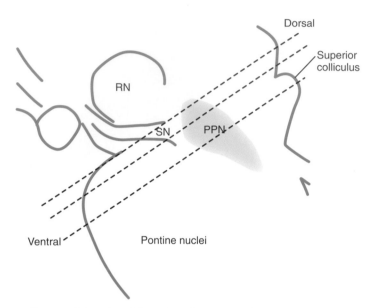

Figure 3.3 Location of the pedunculopontine nucleus (PPN) with respect to the red nucleus (RN) and the substantia nigra (SN). *From Jenkinson N, Nandi D, Muthusamy K, et al. Anatomy, physiology, and pathophysiology of the pedunculopontine nucleus. Mov Disord 2009;24(3):319–28.*

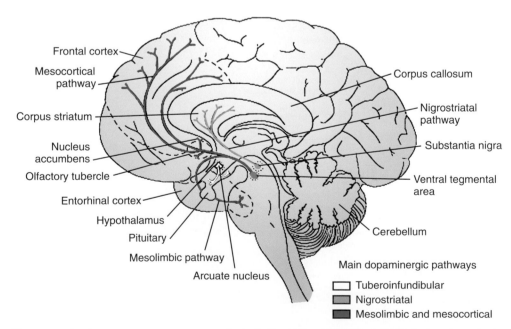

Figure 3.4 The dopamine projection systems in the brain. The nigrostriatal pathway begins in the substantia nigra (light green), the mesolimbic and mesocortical pathways begin in the ventral tegmental area (dark green), and the tuberoinfundibular pathway begins in the arcuate nucleus (white). *From www.australianprescriber.com.*

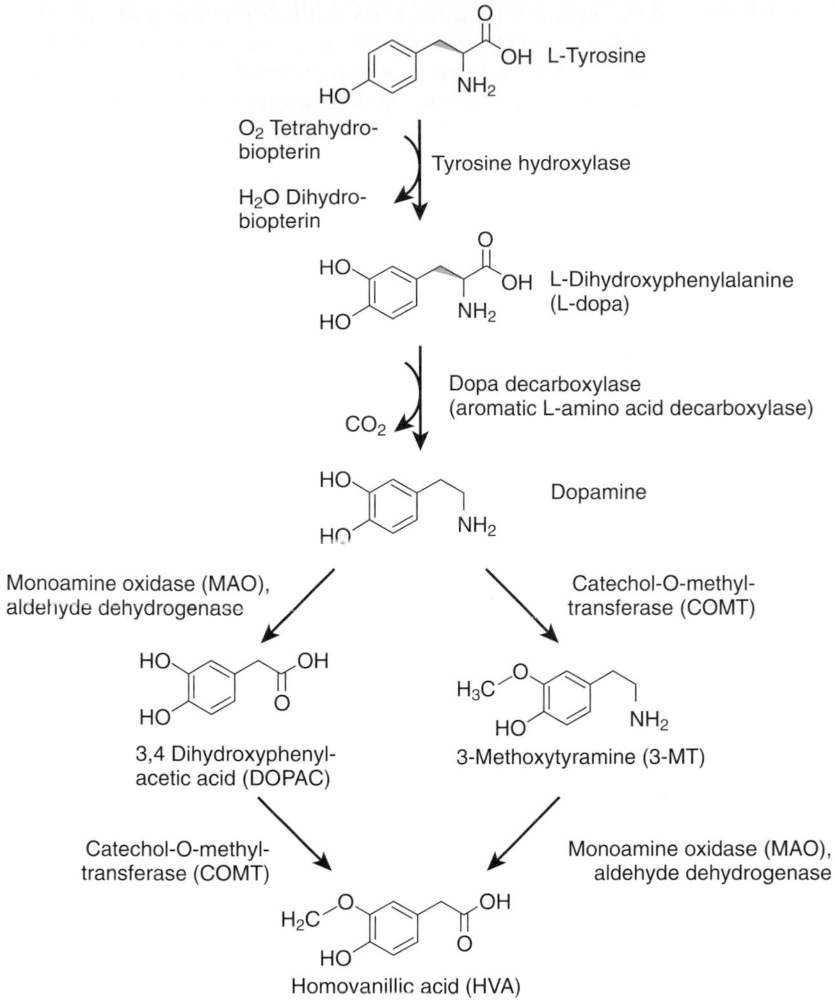

Figure 3.5 Metabolism of dopamine. *From: http://en.wikipedia.org/wiki/Dopamine.*

Acetylcholine is synthesized in neurons from choline and acetyl-CoA by the enzyme choline acetyltransferase (ChAT). After synthesis it is collected into vesicles by the enzyme vesicular ACh transporter (VAChT). Once released from the nerve terminals it is broken down by acetylcholinesterase (AChE), which is both pre- and postsynaptic, and butyrylcholinesterase (BuChE), also called pseudocholinesterase, that resides in glia (Cooper et al., 2003; Siegel et al., 2006). The resultant choline is taken back up into the presynaptic cell by a choline transporter (Stahl, 2008).

There are two broad classes of ACh receptors, nicotinic and muscarinic. Nicotinic receptors (nAChR) are ionotropic and are prominent outside the brain at the neuromuscular junction and autonomic ganglia, but are also in the brain (Albuquerque et al., 2009). Activation at an nAChR will open a nonselective cation channel allowing flow of sodium, potassium, and sometimes calcium. Muscarinic receptors (mAChR) are metabotropic and also found both inside and outside the brain. Activation at an mAChR couples to a variety of types of G proteins (Eglen, 2005, 2006). There are many types of nAChR and these are generally described by their subunit composition. Designations of M_1–M_5 are given to the mAChRs. Both nAChR and mAChR are found in the basal ganglia, and there are both excitatory and inhibitory effects.

Glutamate (Glu)

Glutamate is the primary excitatory neurotransmitter in the brain and as such it has a prominent role in the excitatory cortical-striatal input and in the excitatory projection from the STN to the globus pallidus interna (GPi). Glutamate is a central molecule in many cellular processes, and is also the precursor for the most important inhibitory neurotransmitter in the brain, GABA. Glutamate is made from glutamine in mitochondria by glutaminase. It is then taken up into synaptic vesicles by the vesicular glutamate transporter. Upon release, its action is terminated by its being taken up into glial cells via an excitatory amino acid transporter (EAAT) and then converted to glutamine by glutamine synthetase. Glutamine transporters then move the glutamine from the glial cell into the neuron (Siegel et al., 2006; Stahl, 2008).

Glutamate receptor biology is very complex and the details are well beyond this chapter. There are three groups of metabotropic glutamate receptors, groups I, II, and III, depending on mGluR composition. There are also three classes of ionotropic receptors, α-amino-3-hydroxyl-5-methyl-4-isoxazole-propionate (AMPA), N-methyl-D-aspartic acid (NMDA), and the kainate (KA) receptors. Hence, glutamate not only transmits an excitatory signal by opening calcium channels, but also sets many metabolic processes in action, such as creating short- and long-term changes in synaptic excitability. Such changes are thought to be fundamental in brain plasticity (Lovinger, 2010).

Gamma-amino butyric acid (GABA)

GABA is the main inhibitory neurotransmitter in the brain, and this includes the major inhibitory connections in the basal ganglia. It is synthesized by glutamic acid decarboxylase (GAD) from glutamate. Once synthesized, it is collected into synaptic vesicles by vesicular inhibitory amino acid transporters. After release, its action is terminated by its being taken back into the presynaptic cell by the GABA transporter (GAT). If the nerve ending has too much GABA in it, then it can be broken down by GABA transaminase (GABA-T).

There are three classes of GABA receptors: A, B, and C (Stahl, 2008). GABA-A and GABA-C are ionotropic, and have inhibitory action by opening chloride and potassium channels. There is much known about GABA-A, but only little about GABA-C. GABA-A channels have many subclasses depending on the subunit makeup. An important distinction between subclasses is whether they are sensitive to benzodiazepines or not, depending on whether the benzodiazepines bind to them or not. In the sensitive channels, benzodiazepines can increase the inhibitory action of a GABA-A synapse. GABA-B is a metabotropic receptor (Filip and Frankowska, 2008), and produces a longer duration inhibition than GABA-A by promoting potassium channels and inhibiting calcium channels.

Norepinephrine (NE)

NE influence on the basal ganglia comes from the strong projection to it from the LC. NE is made from DA (in noradrenergic neurons) by the action of dopamine beta-hydroxylase (DBH). After synthesis, it is stored in vesicles by action of VMAT2 (similar to DA). After release, it is taken back up presynaptically by the NE transporter. Like DA, it can be metabolized by MAO-A or MAO-B or COMT, but similar to DA, the main enzyme in the presynaptic terminal is MAO-A.

There are a large number of NE receptors; the different classes are alpha 1A, 1B, 1D, alpha 2A, 2B, 2C, and beta 1, 2 and 3 (Stahl, 2008). All can be postsynaptic, and the alpha 2 receptors can also be presynaptic. Activation of the presynaptic receptors inhibits further NE release. The alpha 1 receptors are G protein coupled, and increase levels of phospholipase C, inositol trisphosphate (IP3), and calcium. The alpha 2 receptors are G protein coupled, with an action to inactivate adenylate cyclase and reduce concentrations of cAMP. The beta receptors couple to G proteins that activate adenylate cyclase and increase cAMP.

Serotonin (5-hydroxytryptamine, 5-HT)

5-HT influence on the basal ganglia comes from the median raphe nuclei (MRN). 5-HT is synthesized from the amino acid tryptophan. Tryptophan is converted to 5-hydroxytryptophan (5-HTP) by tryptophan hydroxylase, and then 5-HTP is converted to 5-HT by aromatic amino acid decarboxylase (AAADC). As with dopamine and NE, after synthesis, 5-HT is taken up into vesicles by the action of VMAT2. After release it is metabolized by MAO-A or taken back up into the serotonergic neuron by the serotonin transporter (SERT). Serotonergic neurons contain both MAO-A and MAO-B.

There are many subtypes of 5-HT receptors, categorized into seven families, 5-HT_1 to 5-HT_7. 5-HT_3 is a ligand-gated Na^+ and K^+ channel that depolarizes membranes. The other family members are G protein coupled. 5-HT_1 and 5-HT_{5A} decrease cAMP; 5-HT_4, 5-HT_6, and 5-HT_7 increase cAMP; 5-HT_2 increases inositol triphosphate (IP3) and diacylglycerol (DAG). 5-HT_{1A} and $5\text{-HT}_{1B/D}$ receptors are presynaptic and act to reduce 5-HT release, a negative feedback influence. Postsynaptic receptors include 5-HT_{1A}, $5\text{-HT}_{1B/D}$, 5-HT_{2A}, 5-HT_{2C}, 5-HT_3, 5-HT_4, 5-HT_5, 5-HT_6, and 5-HT_7. Serotonin actions are complex. Activation of the 5-HT_{1A} receptor is generally inhibitory but also increases dopamine release. Activation of the 5-HT_{2A} receptor is generally excitatory but also inhibits dopamine release (Stahl, 2008). Monoamine interactions in general are very complex; for example, NE can influence 5-HT release, and 5-HT can influence NE release.

Adenosine

Adenosine is a purine nucleoside and is an endogenous molecule in the brain (Benarroch, 2008a). Part of ATP, ADP, and cAMP, adenosine is a critical molecule in cellular energy metabolism, but it also plays a role as a neurotransmitter. Adenosine is found both intra- and extracellularly, and the concentration in the synaptic area is regulated by adenosine transporters (Hasko et al., 2008). There are four subtypes of adenosine receptors, A1, A2A, A2B, and A3, all G protein coupled. Caffeine is an important antagonist at the adenosine receptors. The A1 receptor is generally inhibitory, while the A2 receptors are excitatory, increasing levels of cAMP. Adenosine A2A receptors are colocalized with striatal DA D2 receptors on GABAergic medium spiny neurons which project via the "indirect" striatopallidal pathway to the globus pallidus externa (GPe) (Fuxe et al., 2007). Adenosine at the A2A receptor reduces binding of DA to the D2 receptor, and an antagonist of adenosine, like caffeine, therefore enhances dopamine binding (Simola et al., 2008; Stahl, 2008).

Components of the basal ganglia

Striatum

The striatum is composed of the caudate, putamen, and ventral striatum. As will be discussed below when dealing with circuitry, the different parts of the striatum have different functions related to different patterns of connectivity with the rest of the brain. In general, the putamen is the motor part, the caudate is the associative or cognitive part, and the ventral striatum, which includes the nucleus accumbens, is the limbic part.

A large majority of cells in the striatum (80–95%) are medium spiny neurons (MSN), primarily affected in HD (Martinez-Torres et al., 2008). These are GABAergic cells that

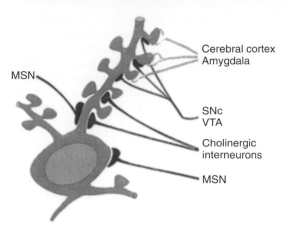

Figure 3.6 Sites of synaptic input onto medium spiny neurons (MSNs) in the striatum. Note in particular that the cortical input is on the head of the spine and the dopaminergic input, from both SNc and VTA, are on the neck of the spine. *From Groenewegen HJ. The basal ganglia and motor control. Neural Plast 2003;10(1–2):107–20.*

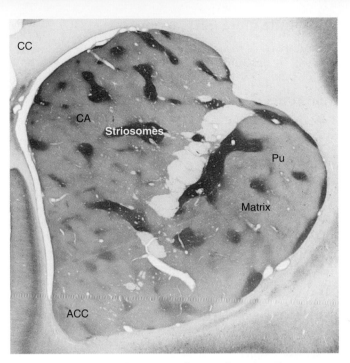

Figure 3.7 Striosomes in the striatum of *Macaca fascicularis*. The striosomes are stained against potassium voltage-gated channel-interacting protein 1. ACC, nucleus accumbens; CA, caudate; CC, corpus callosum; Pu, putamen. *From BrainMaps.org, copyright UC Regents Davis campus.*

project out of the striatum to the GP. They receive glutamatergic input from the cortex and the thalamus. The centrum medianum (CM) nucleus of the thalamus projects to the putamen and the parafascicular (Pf) nucleus to the caudate. These cells also receive important dopaminergic input from the SNc. Additional input from the LC is noradrenergic and from the MRN is serotonergic. The glutamatergic input comes to the dendritic spines on these cells, and the dopaminergic input comes to the neck of these spines (Fig. 3.6). It certainly appears that DA regulates the glutamatergic influence on these cells. There are two types of the MSNs that are differentiated by the DA receptors on their surface. Those that have D1 receptors, in addition to GABA, also contain the polypeptide neurotransmitters substance P and dynorphin. These cells project directly to the GPi. Those that have D2 receptors, in addition to GABA, also contain the polypeptide neurotransmitter enkephalin. These cells project to the GPe, as the first step of the circuit to the GPi known as the indirect pathway.

The striatum also contains interneurons, which are aspiny, and do not project outside the striatum. There are at least four classes of these cells. One of these neurons is the giant aspiny cholinergic cell that has axons with large terminal fields (Pisani et al., 2007). These cells receive their principal input from the cortex (glutamate) and the SNc (dopamine). The cortical input activates the cells and the nigral input inhibits them. The cells have autonomous spontaneous activity and are also known as the tonically active neurons (TANs). This spontaneous action means that there is a tonic release of ACh in the striatum. The extracellular level of ACh will be modulated by AChE and by negative feedback mediated by presynaptic muscarinic receptors. These interneurons are also influenced by adenosine, GABA, NE, and 5-HT (Pisani et al., 2007). The cells play a role in reward processing and modulation of dopamine-dependent neuroplasticity.

There are three classes of GABAergic interneurons in the striatum. These are identified by their containing parvalbumin, calretin, or somatostatin/nitric oxide/neuropeptide Y. All these cells are obviously inhibitory in nature.

Staining of the striatum for AChE revealed an interesting organization of the cells, which had not been anticipated by simple histology. There are regions called patches or striosomes that are AChE-poor, embedded in a matrix that is AChE-rich (Fig. 3.7). This organization presumably comes from segregated influences of the cholinergic interneurons. The matrix appears to receive more sensorimotor and associative input, while the patches receive more limbic input (Eblen and Graybiel, 1995). The output of the two compartments also differs slightly (Fujiyama et al., 2011).

Globus pallidus (GP)

The GP is divided into the dorsal part and the ventral part (ventral striatum) and into the internal and external divisions, GPi and GPe, respectively, which are separated by the medial medullary lamina. There are only a few interneurons as most neurons are large, parvalbumin-positive, GABAergic neurons with large arbors of dendrites. The cells are shaped as flat disks that are parallel to each other (Yelnik et al., 1984). The GP gets input from all parts of the striatum, and the motor part is posterolateral. The pars reticulata of the SN (SNr) is similar in histology and connectivity to the GPi, from which it is separated by the internal capsule.

Subthalamic nucleus (STN)

The main neurons of the STN are glutamatergic with long dendrites (Yelnik and Percheron, 1979; Hamani et al., 2004). There are about 7.5% GABAergic interneurons (Levesque and Parent, 2005). The dorsolateral part of STN is motor, whereas the ventral part is associative and the medial part projects to limbic areas (Benarroch, 2008b).

Substantia nigra (SN)

The two parts of the SN are rather different from each other and will be described separately.

Substantia nigra pars compacta (SNc)

The majority of the neurons of the SNc are dopaminergic and are the cells of origin of the nigrostriatal projection. It is clear that the SNc facilitates movement, and there is good evidence as well for a role of DA in facilitating specific reward behaviors. These cells contain neuromelanin which makes them dark, giving rise to the name of the nucleus ("nigra"). As the death of these cells gives rise to the motor symptoms in Parkinson disease, their cell biology has been studied extensively. Neuromelanin is derived from conjugation of dopamine-quinone, an oxyradical, thereby protecting the dopaminergic neurons from oxidative stress (Sulzer et al., 2000). Neuromelanin can chelate iron and can bind a variety of toxins (Zecca et al., 2001). Some of the dendrites of the dopaminergic cells extend into the SNr, where they have GABAergic receptors. About 15% of cells are interneurons, at least some of which are GABAergic (Hebb and Robertson, 2000).

Substantia nigra pars reticulata (SNr)

The SNr is similar to the GPi in its histology, connectivity, and even pattern of degeneration in neurologic disorders. Hence, it is often considered a part of the GPi that has been separated by anatomical accident. In addition to connectivity similar to the GPi, it has an important output to the superior colliculus, which plays an important role in the control of saccadic eye movements.

Pedunculopontine nucleus (PPN)

The PPN has important reciprocal connections with other parts of the basal ganglia, and it is crucial to understand its role. It appears to be a critical component in the midbrain locomotor area, among other functional activities. The PPN region is rather complex, and is composed of a number of subregions that are not always completely distinct from each other. Many of the details of the subregions, their exact localization in humans, their connectivities, and their neurotransmitters are still being worked out. The PPN itself can be divided into the compacta (PPNc) and dissipatus (PPNd) (Pahapill and Lozano, 2000; Hamani et al., 2007; Zrinzo et al., 2008; Jenkinson et al., 2009). Other nuclei in the vicinity include the midbrain extrapyramidal area (MEA) (Steininger et al., 1992), the peripeduncular nucleus (Zrinzo and Hariz, 2007), and the sub-cuneiform nucleus (Piallat et al., 2009).

The PPNc is composed mainly of cholinergic cells. The PPNd may be mostly glutamatergic cells, but has also cholinergic cells.

Lateral habenula

As we learn more about the basal ganglia, it becomes apparent that there are many structures with important influence on their function. There has been considerable recent interest in the lateral habenula (Hikosaka et al., 2008). The habenula is located above the posterior thalamus near the midline. The cells have a mixture of neurotransmitters. The lateral part of the habenula has a strong inhibitory influence on the SNc as well as the MRN. It appears to exert its inhibition when there is a negative result from action, thus inhibiting a possible favorable effect of dopamine in facilitating rewarded behavior (Bromberg-Martin et al., 2010).

Zona incerta (ZI)

The ZI is a distinct nucleus, which appears to be an extension of the reticular nucleus of the thalamus, sitting ventral to the thalamus and between the fields of Forel, the fiber tracts conveying the pallidal output to the thalamus (Plaha et al., 2008). It receives input from the GPi and SNr, the ascending reticular activating system, the cerebellum, and different regions of the cerebral cortex. Its output cells are GABAergic and go to the CM/Pf and the VA/VL thalamic nuclei, as well as the MEA, medial reticular formation, and reciprocal connections to the cerebellum, GPi/SNr and cerebral cortex. The ZI may act to help synchronize activity across the many regions that it contacts (Plaha et al., 2008).

Other nuclei

The LC is the source of noradrenergic input to the basal ganglia. The MRN is the source of serotonergic input. The thalamus, although not part of the basal ganglia itself, is a main relay station for output from the GPi and SNr to the cortex. There are two important nuclear target regions, the ventral anterior/ventral lateral (VA/VL) nuclei, which are the classic relay nuclei, and the centrum medianum/parafascicular (CM/Pf) nuclei, which are midline thalamic nuclei and serve as internal feedback to the basal ganglia. These thalamic neurons are all glutamatergic.

Circuitry of the basal ganglia

General circuitry

The connectivity of the basal ganglia is clearly crucial in carrying out its functions. The connections are complex, and it is necessary to have some general model for how they are organized. Such a model was proposed about two decades ago independently by three groups of investigators, each using a different technique: Crossman (Crossman, 1987); Albin, Young, and Penney (Albin et al., 1989); and DeLong (DeLong, 1990). This model has been extremely helpful in organizing thinking, planning pharmaceutical strategies for basal ganglia disorders, and even developing surgical approaches to patients. However, there were always difficulties with the model, and in more recent years, it has become apparent that this model is not sufficient to explain what we now know. Hence, a new model is emerging that takes into account many more of the known connections and basal ganglia functions. It is worthwhile to present the older, "classic" model first, since it does form a foundation for the new model and much current thinking is still based on it.

The classic model is shown in Chapter 2, Figure 2.2A, and is a part of the model shown in Figure 3.8. In this model,

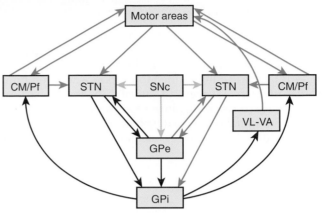

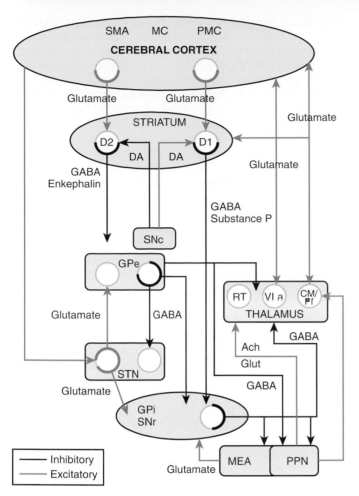

Figure 3.8 Basal ganglia circuitry. Abbreviations are standard for this chapter except for: MC motor cortex, PMC premotor cortex, RT reticular nucleus of thalamus, VLa anterior part of VL nucleus of thalamus. *From Kopell BH, Rezai AR, Chang JW, Vitek JL. Anatomy and physiology of the basal ganglia: implications for deep brain stimulation for Parkinson's disease. Mov Disord 2006;21(Suppl 14):S238–46.*

Figure 3.9 Basal ganglia circuitry. Green arrows are for glutamate, black arrows are for GABA, and the light green arrows (from the SNc) are for dopamine. *From Obeso JA, Marin C, Rodriguez-Oroz C, et al. The basal ganglia in Parkinson's disease: current concepts and unexplained observations. Ann Neurol 2008;64(Suppl 2):S30–46.*

described also in Chapter 2, there are two parallel loops from the cortex through the basal ganglia and back to the cortex, the direct and indirect pathway. The direct pathway starts with cortical glutamatergic input to the striatal cells bearing D1 receptors. These GABAergic neurons project directly to the GPi. The GABAergic neurons of the GPi project to the VA/VL nuclei of the thalamus, and the thalamic cells return glutamatergic input to the cortex. This four-neuron circuit has two inhibitory neurons and would be net excitatory. The indirect pathway starts with cortical glutamatergic input to the striatal cells bearing D2 receptors. These GABAergic cells project to the GPe, which has a GABAergic projection to the STN, which has a glutamatergic projection to the GPi. The final part of the path from GPi through thalamus to cortex is the same as the direct pathway. This is a six-neuron pathway with three inhibitory neurons, and therefore this would be net inhibitory. The SNc is a modulator of both direct and indirect pathways. Via its influence on D1 and D2 receptors, it will facilitate those striatal neurons of the direct pathway and inhibit those striatal neurons of the indirect pathway. Thus the influence of the SNc is to facilitate the facilitatory pathway and inhibit

the inhibitory pathway. While it is not the role of this chapter to discuss pathophysiology, it is immediately apparent why dysfunction of the SNc should give rise to bradykinesia as seen in Parkinson disease. Other movement disorders appear superficially to be similarly easily explained.

There are many connections that are left out of the classic model, and it appears that many of them are rather important. Figure 3.8 (and Chapter 2, Fig. 2.2B) shows the connections of the more complete model, and Figure 3.9 shows the model in a different form to emphasize different connections. This model does not dispute any of the old connections, it adds new, apparently important connections. A missing node in the network is the CM/Pf nucleus of the thalamus. The GPi projects to it as well as to VA/VL, and the CM/Pf in turn projects back both to striatum and STN. CM projects mainly to the putamen, and Pf to caudate and ventral pallidum. CM/Pf also has reciprocal connections to the cortex. There is a strong connection from the cortex directly to the STN; this is called the hyperdirect pathway. Additionally, the SNc projects to STN, and the STN projects back to the GPe, as a reciprocal connection to what was in the classic model. The GPe itself plays a more critical role, now not only getting input from the striatum, but also from STN and SNc. The major new aspects are increased importance of STN and GPe as integrative nodes, and more widespread direct influence of SNc (Obeso et al., 2008).

Even this newer model, discussed in the last paragraph, does not include the brainstem influences. These come from the LC (NE), the MRN (5-HT), the ZI, the lateral habenula, and the PPN. The lateral habenula and the PPN have several different neurotransmitters, but the PPN is the main source of cholinergic input to the basal ganglia. The PPN has reciprocal connections with virtually every part of the basal ganglia circuitry (Fig. 3.10). The most important inputs come from GPi and STN, and the most important outputs go to STN, GPi, SNc, thalamus, and brainstem. The latter output to the brainstem is now thought to be the major directly descending motor influence from the basal ganglia. The PPN is also reciprocally connected directly to the cortex.

Parallel pathways

Another important principle of basal ganglia circuitry is its parallel organization (Alexander et al., 1986). Each part of the cortex has a separate pathway through the whole circuit (Fig. 3.11). In broad brush, the motor loop would run from motor cortex, to putamen, to lateral GPi, to VL, back to cortex. An executive or cognitive loop would run from dorsolateral prefrontal cortex, to dorsolateral caudate, to medial GPi, to medial dorsal and VA nuclei of the thalamus, back to cortex. A limbic loop would run from anterior cingulate cortex, to ventral striatum, to ventral pallidum, to medial dorsal nucleus of thalamus, back to cortex. These loops do not interact with each other, or only in a very limited way. The loops are even more fine-grained, so that, for example, in the motor system, different parts of the motor system have different loops and somatotopy of different body parts is maintained throughout the loop (Middleton and Strick, 2000). For example, the primary motor area (M1), the supplementary motor area (SMA), and the ventral premotor area (PMv) will have separate loops. The cerebellum has similar isolated loops, and generally the cerebellar and basal ganglia loops do not interact either. However, there is at least some connection between cerebellar and basal ganglia loops in the GPe (Hoshi et al., 2005).

Physiology

Cellular activity

Most information about normal cellular activity comes from recordings in animals. There are considerable data from primates. Human information comes largely from recordings when placing electrodes for deep brain stimulation (DBS) surgery, and thus is pathologic rather than normal. By comparing human pathologic data with animal models, such as the MPTP monkey model of Parkinson disease, it has been generally concluded that primate information is likely quite similar to that of humans.

The medium spiny neurons (MSN) in the striatum have a low firing rate, on average 0.5–2 Hz (van Albada and Robinson, 2009). Cells are often in a hyperpolarized, or down state, because of an intrinsic inwardly rectifying K^+ current (Hammond et al., 2007). Cells will fire largely only when there is a convergence of inputs onto the cell. Excitatory inputs come mainly from cortex and thalamus. The excitatory input will be modulated by the striatal interneurons and the nigrostriatal dopamine neurons that have input at the base of the dendritic spine and on the shaft of the dendrite itself (Fig. 3.6). The cholinergic interneurons, the tonically active neurons (TANs), appear to be the most

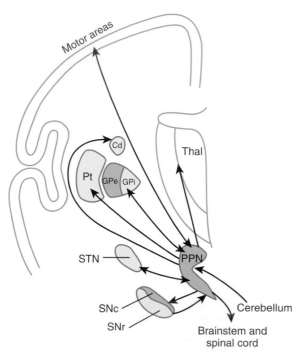

Figure 3.10 Connections of the pedunculopontine nucleus (PPN). Cd caudate nucleus, GPe external division of the globus pallidus, GPi internal division of the globus pallidus, Pt putamen, SNc substantia nigra pars compacta, SNr substantia nigra pars reticulata, STN subthalamic nucleus, Thal thalamus. *From Jenkinson N, Nandi D, Muthusamy K, et al. Anatomy, physiology, and pathophysiology of the pedunculopontine nucleus. Mov Disord 2009;24(3):319–28.*

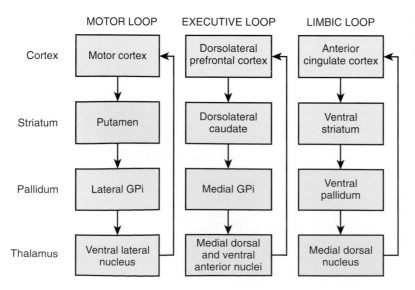

Figure 3.11 Segregated loops through the basal ganglia. *Redrawn from Purves D, Augustine GJ, Fitzpatrick D, et al. Neuroscience, 2nd ed. Sunderland, MA: Sinauer Associates, Inc.; 2001.*

spontaneously active neurons in the striatum. They fire at 2–10 Hz, and are modulated to some extent during learning (Aosaki et al., 1995).

Cellular activity in the GPi is the opposite of the striatum; cells are tonically active at 60–90 Hz (van Albada and Robinson, 2009). Activity in the GPe shows two types of behavior. About 85% of cells have high-frequency bursts together with long intervals of silence for up to several seconds, and an average firing rate of 55 Hz. The other 15% have a slower average rate of about 10 Hz, with occasional bursts (van Albada and Robinson, 2009). Cells in the STN also show spontaneous activity, at about 20–30 Hz, and spikes may be in pairs or triplets (van Albada and Robinson, 2009). Cells in the VA/VL of the thalamus fire at about 18–19 Hz (van Albada and Robinson, 2009).

Circuit physiology

Exactly what the basal ganglia ordinarily contribute to brain processing is not certain. However, the cellular processing should give some insight into this. Inputs from cortex (and thalamus) come to the striatum, and, as noted above, only a strong, convergent input will get neurons active. Activity of MSNs of the direct pathway will then suppress the tonically rapid firing cells in the GPi, which will release a region of the thalamus from tonic inhibition. This should be a net facilitation back to the cortex. At the same time that the GPi is inhibited by the direct pathway, there are a number of sources of excitation (or lessened inhibition). The GPe delivers less inhibition. Other inputs arrive via the STN, which gets less inhibition via the classic indirect pathway and excitation via the hyperdirect pathway. Thus, the output of the STN on the GPi is to excite it. The GPi therefore has to integrate its opposing inputs for a properly balanced output.

The basal ganglia clearly provide important signal processing, but there is strong evidence that they are also involved in motor learning. The basal ganglia show significant plasticity of synaptic connections. DA plays an important role in this plasticity, conveying reward signals that indicate the importance of what should be learned (Schultz, 2010).

Another measure of cellular activity is called a local field potential (LFP). LFPs summate large number of neurons and synaptic activity, similar to the EEG. Like the EEG, LFPs can sometimes show rhythmic behavior in different frequency ranges. Cellular activity in the basal ganglia nuclei is not typically synchronized and LFPs do not show prominent oscillations. In Parkinson disease, there is synchronization and oscillations in both STN and GPi in the 10–30 Hz (beta)

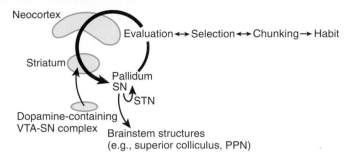

Figure 3.12 Proposed basal ganglia function of making movements automatic and habitual by iterative cycling through the basal ganglia. *From Graybiel AM. Habits, rituals, and the evaluative brain. Annu Rev Neurosci 2008;31:359–87.*

range (Brown, 2007; Galvan and Wichmann, 2008; Israel and Bergman, 2008). The origin of this beta rhythm is not completely clear, but it appears to correlate with bradykinesia and tremor (Chen et al., 2010; Tass et al., 2010). The beta rhythm may also be coupled to even higher-frequency oscillations (Lopez-Azcarate et al., 2010).

There are a number of theories as to what the basal ganglia contribute to movement processing, and by analogy to processing of cognitive and limbic information as well. One such theory is movement selection, which has been discussed in Chapter 2. According to this theory the direct pathway selects a movement to be facilitated, and the inhibitory influences by the indirect and hyperdirect pathways inhibit undesired movements. Other concepts include the automatic running of motor programs (Marsden, 1982), and learning and release of habits (Graybiel, 2008). The latter idea is that certain behaviors that get rewarded and get repeated, eventually become automatic (Fig. 3.12). As is abundantly clear in this book, considering all the hyperkinetic and hypokinetic disorders that derive from basal ganglia dysfunction, the basal ganglia must have something to do with the regulation of amount of motor output. It seems also to be the case that the function of the basal ganglia must to some extent be a parallel pathway of brain function, since a large stroke destroying most of the basal ganglia or an ablative lesion of the GPi, such as done with pallidotomy in Parkinson disease, can allow the patient to perform reasonably well.

References available on Expert Consult: www.expertconsult.com

CHAPTER 4

Parkinsonism: Clinical features and differential diagnosis

Chapter contents

Introduction	66	Sleep disorders	79
Clinical features	66	Sensory abnormalities	80
Bradykinesia	69	Clinical-pathologic correlations	81
Tremor	69	Subtypes and natural history of Parkinson disease	82
Rigidity and flexed posture	70	Differential diagnosis	85
Loss of postural reflexes	71	Clinical rating scales and other assessments	85
Freezing	72	Epidemiology	88
Other motor abnormalities	73	Laboratory tests	89
Nonmotor manifestations	74	Presymptomatic diagnosis and biomarkers	90
Autonomic dysfunction	74	Pathologic findings	92
Cognitive and neurobehavioral abnormalities	75		

Introduction

Parkinsonism is a syndrome manifested by a combination of the following six cardinal features: tremor-at-rest, rigidity, bradykinesia, loss of postural reflexes, flexed posture, and freezing (motor blocks). A combination of these signs is used to clinically define definite, probable, and possible parkinsonism (Table 4.1). The most common form of parkinsonism is the idiopathic variety known as Parkinson disease (PD), first recognized as a unique clinical entity by James Parkinson in 1817, who in his *An Essay on the Shaking Palsy* identified six cases, three of whom he personally examined and the others he observed on the streets of London (Parkinson, 1817). Previously referred to as "paralysis agitans," Charcot later in the nineteenth century gave credit to Parkinson by referring to the disease as "maladie de Parkinson" and pointed out that slowness of movement should be distinguished from weakness; he also recognized non-tremulous forms of PD (Kempster et al., 2007). With the recognition of marked clinical-pathologic heterogeneity of parkinsonism due to a single mutation and some uncertainty whether PD should be defined clinically, pathologically, or genetically, a variety of other names have been proposed for this neurodegenerative disorder, including "Parkinson complex" and "Parkinson Lewy disease" (Langston, 2006), but it is unlikely that these names will replace the traditional name "Parkinson disease." Some have argued that PD is not a single entity, a notion supported by genetic forms of parkinsonism with variable clinical and pathologic features (Weiner, 2008).

It was not until 100 years after Parkinson's landmark paper that the loss of dopamine-containing cells in the substantia nigra (SN) was recognized (Tretiakoff, 1919). In 1960, Ehringer and Hornykiewicz (1960) first noted that the striatum of patients with PD was deficient in dopamine, and the following year, Birkmayer and Hornykiewicz (1961) injected levodopa in 20 patients with PD and postencephalitic parkinsonism and noted marked improvement in akinesia but not in rigidity. Later in the same decade, Cotzias and colleagues (1967, 1969) are credited with making levodopa clinically useful in patients with PD. The recent disclosure of the diagnosis of PD in several public figures has contributed to increased awareness about the disease, which should translate into greater research funding.

Clinical features

There are dozens of symptoms and signs associated with PD, and the clinician must become skilled in eliciting the appropriate history and targeting the neurologic examination in a way that will bring out and document the various neurologic signs (Jankovic and Lang, 2008; Tolosa et al., 2006; Jankovic, 2007, 2008). The manifestation of PD may vary from a barely perceptible tremor to a severe disability during the end-stage of the disease. Rest tremor in the hands or in the

DOI: 10.1016/B978-1-4377-2369-4.00004-4

Table 4.1 Parkinsonism diagnostic criteria

1. Tremor-at-rest
2. Bradykinesia
3. Rigidity
4. Loss of postural reflexes
5. Flexed posture
6. Freezing (motor blocks)

Definite: At least two of these features must be present, one of them being 1 or 2.

Probable: Feature 1 or 2 alone is present.

Possible: At least two of features 3 to 6 must be present

Table 4.2 Frequency of different movement disorders in a referral movement disorders clinic

Primary movement disorder	Total number		Percentage total	
Parkinsonism	10,952	–	31.86%	–
Parkinson's disease	–	6,975	–	20.29%
Dystonia	6,446	–	18.75%	–
Tremor (other than PD)	4,862	–	14.14%	–
Tics (including Tourette's Syndrome)	2,341	–	6.81%	–
Chorea	1,445	–	4.20%	–
Huntington's Disease	617	–	1.79%	–
Ballism	60	–	0.20%	–
Athetosis	13	–	0.04%	–
Myoclonus	676	–	1.97%	–
Other	6,960	–	20.24%	–
Restless Leg Syndrome	–	827	–	2.41%
Stereotypies (including tardive dyskinesia)	–	899	–	2.61%
Akathisia	–	78	–	0.23%
Ataxia	–	414	–	1.20%
Psychogenic	–	1,752	–	5.10%
All Other	–	2,990	–	8.70%
TOTAL	34,380	–	100.00%	–

These figures represent the number of reported disorders in each patient. Patients may have more than one disorder.

Courtesy of Parkinson's Disease Center and Movement Disorders Clinic: Baylor College of Medicine, Houston, Texas.

lips might be not just socially embarrassing but may cause a severe handicap in people whose occupation depends on a normal appearance. Therefore, it is important that the severity of the disease be objectively assessed in the context of the individual's goals and needs. In some cases, unintended movements accompanying voluntary activity in homologous muscles on the opposite side of the body, the so-called mirror movements, may occur even in early, asymmetric PD (Espay et al., 2005; Li et al., 2007), although one study showed that mirror movements actually occur less frequently in PD patients than in healthy controls (29% vs. 71%, $P < 0.0001$) (Ottaviani et al., 2008).

In a retrospective study of patients with PD, early nonspecific symptoms that were reported included generalized stiffness, pain or paresthesias of the limbs, constipation, sleeplessness, and reduction in volume of the voice (Przuntek, 1992). More specific complaints that were elicited on a detailed history as the disease progressed included problems with fine motor skills, decreased sense of smell, loss of appetite, and a tremor occurring with anxiety. Family members retrospectively reported decreased arm swing on the affected side, decreased emotional expression, and personality changes, including more introversion and inflexibility. Using strict criteria for asymmetry, 46% of patients with PD had characteristic asymmetric presentation that correlated with handedness (Uitti et al., 2005). Handedness, however, did not predict the onset of PD motor symptoms in another study (Stochl et al., 2009). The mechanisms of the observed asymmetry of PD symptoms and signs are not well understood, but the side of predominant involvement may be stochastically determined, similar to other complex diseases such as cancer (Djaldetti et al., 2006). The notion that the side of predominant involvement is merely coincidental and determined by chance alone is supported by seemingly random right and left distribution without correlation to hand dominance, lack of concordance for the affected side within family members of genetically determined PD, and the frequent presence of asymmetric involvement in drug-induced parkinsonism. In some cases, parkinsonism may remain confined to one side and may be associated with hemiatrophy. In one study, the mean age at onset of the 30 patients who satisfied the criteria for hemiparkinsonism–hemiatrophy was 44.2 (15–63) years with a mean duration of symptoms of 9.7 (2–20) years (Wijemanne and Jankovic, 2007) (Table 4.2). Half of all patients had dystonia at onset and dystonia was present in 21 (70%) of all patients during

the course of the syndrome. The majority of patients were responsive to levodopa, and perinatal and early childhood cerebral injury appeared to play an important role in about half of the cases. This syndrome of hemiparkinsonism–hemiatrophy also suggests that some cases of PD may start prenatally, and as a result of the low number of dopaminergic neurons from birth and subsequent age-related attrition, develop PD symptoms in middle age (Le et al., 2009) (Fig. 4.1). The asymmetrical lateral ventricular enlargement that is associated with PD motor asymmetry (Lewis et al., 2009) may represent a nonspecific marker of underlying neurodegeneration or may suggest an early insult, similar to what has been postulated in hemiparkinsonism–hemiatrophy (Wijemanne and Jankovic, 2007).

Clinical heterogeneity of PD and the rich phenomenology associated with the disease are well recognized. In a survey of 181 treated PD patients, Bulpitt and colleagues (1985) found at least 45 different symptoms that were attributable to the disease, nine of which were reported by the patients with more than fivefold excess compared with a control population of patients randomly selected from a general

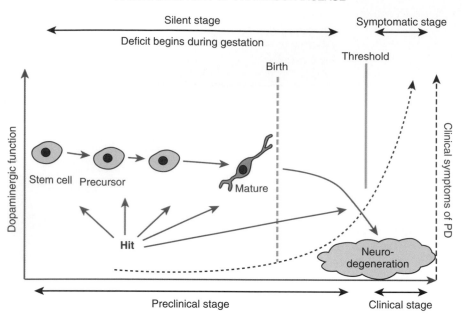

NATURAL HISTORY OF PARKINSON DISEASE

Figure 4.1 Developmental progression of neurodegeneration.

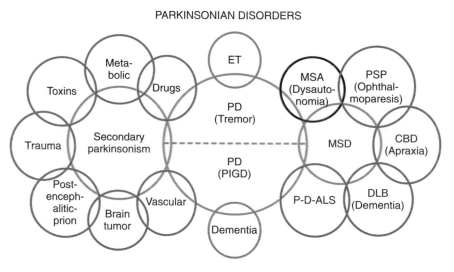

PARKINSONIAN DISORDERS

Figure 4.2 Differential diagnosis of PD. CBD, corticobasal degeneration; DLB, dementia with Lewy bodies; ET, essential tremor; MSA, multiple system atrophy; MSD, multiple system degeneration; P-D-ALS, parkinsonism–dementia–amyotrophic lateral sclerosis difficulty; PIGD, postural instability-gait; PSP, progressive supranuclear palsy.

practice. These common symptoms included being frozen or rooted to a spot, grimacing, jerking of the arms and legs, shaking hands, clumsy hands, salivation, poor concentration, severe apprehension, and hallucinations. Hallucinations, although usually attributed to dopaminergic therapy, may be part of PD, particularly when there is a coexistent dementia and depression (Fenelon et al., 2006; Marsh et al., 2006). However, even these frequent symptoms are relatively nonspecific and do not clearly differentiate PD patients from diseased controls. Gonera and colleagues (1997) found that 4–6 years prior to the onset of classic PD symptoms, patients experience a prodromal phase characterized by more frequent visits to general practitioners and specialists in comparison to normal controls. During this period, PD patients, compared to normal controls, had a higher frequency of mood disorder, fibromyalgia, and various pains (Defazio et al., 2008), particularly shoulder pain (Stamey et al., 2008; Madden and Hall, 2010). In one study of 25 PD patients and 25 controls, PD patients had 21 times the odds of having

shoulder pain compared with those without PD (Madden and Hall, 2010).

Because of the marked heterogeneity of clinical symptoms and natural progression, several studies have attempted to identify clinical subtypes of PD. Using cluster analysis, a systematic review of the literature confirmed the existence of the following disease subtypes: (1) young age at onset and slow disease progression, (2) old age at onset and rapid disease progression, (3) tremor-dominant, and (4) postural instability and gait difficulty (PIGD) (Jankovic et al., 1990) dominated by bradykinesia and rigidity (van Rooden et al., 2009). Patients who manifest predominantly axial symptoms, such as dysarthria (Ho et al., 1999), dysphagia, loss of equilibrium, and freezing of gait, are particularly disabled by their disease in comparison to those who have predominantly limb manifestations (Jankovic et al., 1990; Muslimovic et al., 2008). The poor prognosis of patients in whom axial symptoms predominate, many of whom have either the PIGD form of PD or some atypical parkinsonism (Fig. 4.2), is partly due to a lack of response of these symptoms to dopaminergic drugs (Jankovic et al., 1990; Kompoliti et al., 2000). In this regard, one study suggested that an abnormal tandem gait (the "ten steps" test) is much more common in patients with atypical parkinsonism than in those with typical PD and this test seems to differentiate the two groups with 82% sensitivity and 92% specificity (Abdo et al., 2006). In another classification of PD subtypes, the differences are largely driven by the severity of "nondopaminergic" features and levodopa-related motor complications (van Rooden et al., 2011).

Bradykinesia

Bradykinesia, the most characteristic clinical hallmark of PD, may be initially manifested by slowness in activities of daily living and slow movement and reaction times (Cooper et al., 1994; Touge et al., 1995; Giovannoni et al., 1999; Jankovic et al., 1999a; Rodriguez-Oroz et al., 2009). In addition to whole-body slowness, bradykinesia is often manifested by impairment of fine motor movement, demonstrated on examination by slowness in rapid alternating movements. Although speed and amplitude are usually assessed together on the Unified Parkinson's Disease Rating Scale (UPDRS) Part III, there is some evidence that amplitude is disproportionately more affected than speed in patients with PD and may be due to different motor mechanisms and should probably be assessed separately (Espay et al., 2009). Other manifestations of bradykinesia include drooling due to failure to swallow saliva (Bagheri et al., 1999; Lal and Hotaling, 2006), monotonic and hypophonic dysarthria, loss of facial expression (hypomimia), and reduced arm swing when walking (loss of automatic movement). Micrographia has been postulated to result from an abnormal response due to reduced motor output or weakness of agonist force coupled with distortions in visual feedback (Teulings et al., 2002). Bradyphrenia refers to slowness of thought. Bradykinesia, like other parkinsonian symptoms, is dependent on the emotional state of the patient. With a sudden surge of emotional energy, the immobile patient may catch a ball or make other fast movements. This curious phenomenon, called kinesia paradoxica, demonstrates that the motor programs are intact in PD but that patients have difficulty utilizing or accessing the programs without the help of an external trigger. Therefore, parkinsonian patients are able to make use of prior information to perform an automatic or preprogrammed movement, but they cannot use this information to initiate or select a movement. Although PD represents the most common form of parkinsonism, there are many other causes of bradykinesia, the parkinsonian clinical hallmark (Table 4.2).

The pathophysiology of bradykinesia is not well understood, but it is thought to result from failure of basal ganglia output to reinforce the cortical mechanisms that prepare and execute the commands to move (Jankovic, 2007). This is manifested by slowness of self-paced movements and prolongation of reaction and movement time. Evarts and colleagues (1981) first showed that both reaction (RT) and movement (MT) times are independently impaired in PD. The RT is influenced not only by the degree of motor impairment but also by the interaction between the cognitive processing and the motor response. This is particularly evident when choice RT is used and compared to simple RT. Bradykinetic patients with PD have more specific impairment in choice RT, which involves a stimulus categorization and a response selection and reflects disturbance at more complex levels of cognitive processing. Ward and colleagues (1983b) found that of the various objective assessments of bradykinesia, the MT correlates best with the total clinical score, but it is not as sensitive an indicator of the overall motor deficit as the clinical rating.

Reduced dopaminergic function has been hypothesized to disrupt normal motor cortex activity, leading to bradykinesia. In recordings from single cortical neurons in free-moving rats, a decrease in firing rate correlated with haloperidol-induced bradykinesia, demonstrating that reduced dopamine action impairs the ability to generate movement and causes bradykinesia (Parr-Brownlie and Hyland, 2005). The premovement EEG potential (Bereitschaftspotential) is reduced in PD, probably reflecting inadequate basal ganglia activation of the supplementary motor area (Dick et al., 1989). On the basis of electromyographic (EMG) recordings in the antagonistic muscles of parkinsonian patients during a brief ballistic elbow flexion, Hallett and Khoshbin (1980) concluded that the most characteristic feature of bradykinesia was the inability to energize the appropriate muscles to provide a sufficient rate of force required for the initiation and maintenance of a large, fast (ballistic) movement. Therefore, PD patients need a series of multiple agonist bursts to accomplish a larger movement. Thus, the amount of EMG activity in PD is underscaled (Berardelli et al., 2001). Although many patients with PD complain of "weakness," this subjective symptom is probably due to a large number of factors including bradykinesia, rigidity, fatigue, and also reduced power due to muscle weakness, particularly when lifting heavy objects (Allen et al., 2009).

Of the various parkinsonian signs, bradykinesia correlates best with a reduction in the striatal fluorodopa uptake measured by positron emission tomography (PET) scans and in turn with nigral damage (Vingerhoets et al., 1997). This is consistent with the finding that decreased density of SN neurons correlates with parkinsonism in the elderly, even without PD (Ross et al., 2004). PET scans in PD patients have demonstrated decreased ^{18}F-fluorodeoxyglucose uptake in the striatum and accumbens-caudate complex roughly proportional to the degree of bradykinesia (Playford and Brooks, 1992). Studies performed initially in monkeys made parkinsonian with the toxin 1-methyl-4-phenyl-1,2,3,6-tetrahydropyridine (MPTP) (Bergman et al., 1990) and later in patients with PD provide evidence that bradykinesia results from excessive activity in the subthalamic nucleus (STN) and the internal segment of globus pallidus (GPi) (Dostrovsky et al., 2002). Thus, there is both functional and biochemical evidence of increased activity in the outflow nuclei, particularly subthalamic nucleus and GPi, in patients with PD.

Tremor

By using the term *shaking palsy*, James Parkinson in his *An Essay on the Shaking Palsy* (1817) drew attention to tremor as a characteristic feature of PD. Indeed, some parkinsonolo-gists regard rest tremor as the most typical sign of PD, and its absence should raise the possibility that the patient's parkinsonism is caused by a disorder other than PD. The typical rest tremor has a frequency between 4 and 6 Hz, and the tremor is almost always most prominent in the distal part of an extremity. In the hand, the tremor has been called a "pill-rolling tremor." In the head region, tremor occurs most commonly in the lips, chin and jaw, but while a common manifestation of essential tremor, head tremor is rare in PD (Roze et al., 2006; Gan et al., 2009). Some patients with PD complain of an internal, not visible, tremor, called "inner tremor." Rest tremor of PD is often exacerbated during potential provocations, such as walking and counting back-wards (Raethjen et al., 2008).

As pointed out below, presentation with tremor as the initial symptom often confers a favorable prognosis with slower progression of the disease and some have suggested the term "benign tremulous parkinsonism" for a subset of patients with minimal progression, frequent family history of tremor, and poor response to levodopa (Josephs et al., 2006; O'Suilleabhain et al., 2006). Rajput and colleagues (1991) noted that 100% of 30 patients with pathologically proven PD experienced some degree of rest tremor at some time during the course of their disease. However, in another clinical-pathologic study, only 76% of pathologically proven cases of PD had tremor (Hughes, et al., 1992b). In an expanded series of 100 pathologically proven cases of PD, tremor was present at onset in 69%; 75% had tremor during the course of the illness, and 9% lost their tremor late in the disease (Hughes et al., 1993).

Although rest tremor is a well-recognized cardinal feature of PD, many PD patients have a postural tremor that is more prominent and disabling than the classic rest tremor. Postural tremor without parkinsonian features and without any other known etiology is often diagnosed as essential tremor (ET), but isolated postural tremor may be the initial presentation of PD, and it may be found with higher-than-expected frequency in relatives of patients with PD (Brooks et al., 1992b; Jankovic et al., 1995; Jankovic, 2002; Louis et al., 2003). Jankovic and colleagues (1995) and others (Louis et al., 2003) have shown that relatives of patients with tremor-dominant PD have a significantly higher risk of having action tremor than relatives of patients with the PIGD form of PD, but it is not yet clear whether the iso-lated tremor in the relatives is ET or whether it represents an isolated manifestation of PD. The two forms of postural tremor, ET and PD, can be differentiated by a delay in the onset of tremor when arms assume an outstretched posi-tion. Most patients with PD tremor have a latency of a few seconds (up to a minute) before the tremor reemerges during postural holding, hence the term *reemergent tremor* (Jankovic et al., 1999b) (Video 4.1). In contrast, postural tremor of ET usually appears immediately after arms assume a horizontal posture. Since the reemergent tremor has a frequency similar to that of rest tremor and both tremors generally respond to dopaminergic drugs, reemer-gent tremor most likely represents a variant of the more typical rest tremor. In addition to the rest and postural tremors, a kinetic tremor, possibly related to enhanced physiologic tremor, may also impair normal reach-to-grasp movement (Wenzelburger et al., 2000).

While bradykinesia and rigidity are most likely associated with nigrostriatal dopaminergic deficit, the pathophysiology of PD rest tremor is probably more complicated and most likely results from dysfunction of both the striato-pallidal-thalamocortical and the cerebello-dentato-thalamo-cortical circuits (Boecker and Brooks, 2011). The pallidum, in particular, appears to play a fundamental role in genera-tion of tremor as suggested by a 4-8 Hz GPi neuronal firing in primate models of parkinsonism, correlation of tremor severity with pallidal (but not striatal) dopamine depletion, and complete abolition or a marked improvement of tremor with GPi ablation or DBS (Helmich et al., 2011).

As a result of the abnormal neuronal activity at the level of the GPi, the muscle discharge in patients with PD changes from the normal high (40 Hz) to pulsatile (10 Hz) contrac-tions. These muscle discharges, which may be viewed as another form of PD-associated tremor, can be auscultated with a stethoscope (Brown, 1997).

Rigidity and flexed posture

Rigidity, tested by passively flexing, extending, and rotating the body part, is manifested by increased resistance through-out the range of movement. Cogwheeling is often encoun-tered, particularly if there is associated tremor or an underlying, not yet visible, tremor. In 1926 Froment and Gardere published a series of papers based on their studies of parkinsonian rigidity, including the observation of enhanced resistance to passive movement of a limb about a joint detected during voluntary movement of a contralateral limb ("Froment's maneuver") (Broussolle et al., 2007). Rigidity may occur proximally (e.g., neck, shoulders, and hips) and distally (e.g., wrists and ankles). At times, it can cause discomfort and actual pain. Painful shoulder, possibly due to rigidity but frequently misdiagnosed as arthritis, bur-sitis, or rotator cuff, is one of the most frequent initial mani-festations of PD (Riley et al., 1989; Stamey et al., 2008). In a prospective, longitudinal study of 6038 individuals, mean age 68.5 years, who participated in the Rotterdam study and had no dementia or parkinsonian signs at baseline, subjec-tive complaints of stiffness, tremor, and imbalance were associated with increased risk of PD with hazard ratios of 2.11, 2.09, and 3.47, respectively (de Lau et al., 2006). During the mean 5.8 years of follow-up, 56 new cases of PD were identified.

Rigidity is often associated with postural deformity result-ing in flexed neck and trunk posture and flexed elbows and knees. But rigidity is a common sign in early PD, whereas flexed posture occurs later in the disease. Some patients develop "striatal hand" deformity, characterized by ulnar deviation of hands, flexion of the metacarpophalangeal joints, and extension of the interphalangeal joints (Fig. 4.3), and there may be extension of the big toe ("striatal toe") or flexion of the other toes, which can be confused with arthri-tis (Jankovic and Tintner, 2001; Ashour et al., 2005; Ashour and Jankovic, 2006; Jankovic, 2007). Striatal toe was found to be present in 13 of 62 (21%) of patients with clinically diagnosed PD (Winkler et al., 2002).

Other skeletal abnormalities include extreme neck flexion ("dropped head" or "bent spine") (Oerlemans and de Visser, 1998; Askmark et al., 2001; Ashour and Jankovic, 2006;

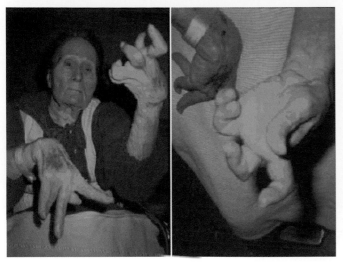

Figure 4.3 Striatal hand deformity associated with PD.

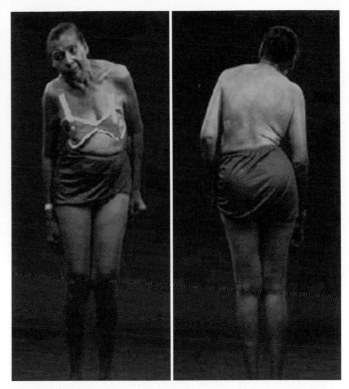

Figure 4.4 Scoliosis associated with PD.

Kashihara et al., 2006; Gdynia et al., 2009; Oyama et al., 2009) and truncal flexion (camptocormia) (Djaldetti et al., 1999; Umapathi et al., 2002; Azher and Jankovic, 2005; Tiple et al., 2009; Sako et al., 2009). Askmark and colleagues (2001) found 7 patients out of 459 with parkinsonism who had a head drop attributed to neck extensor weakness. Myopathic changes on EMG were noted in all seven, and five patients who consented had abnormal muscle biopsy, with mitochondrial abnormalities in two. Isolated neck extensor myopathy was reported in other patients with anterocollis associated with parkinsonism (Lava and Factor, 2001; van de Warrenburg et al., 2007; Gdynia et al., 2009), although its true frequency in patients with PD, multiple system atrophy (MSA), and other parkinsonian disorders is unknown. The following etiologies have also been identified in various series of patients with head drop (head ptosis or anterocollis), bent spine, or camptocormia: dystonia, disproportionately increased tone in the anterior neck muscles resulting in fibrotic and myopathic changes, amyotrophic lateral sclerosis, focal myopathy, inclusion body myositis, polymyositis, nemaline myopathy, facioscapulohumeral dystrophy, myasthenia gravis, encephalitis, dopamine agonists (Uzawa et al., 2009), and valproate toxicity (Umapathi et al., 2002; Gourie-Devi et al., 2003; Schabitz et al., 2003; Azher and Jankovic, 2005; van de Warrenburg et al., 2007).

Camptocormia is characterized by extreme flexion of the thoracolumbar spine that increases during walking and resolves in supine position (Videos 4.2, 4.3, 4.4). It appears to be more common in patients with more severe PD and if they had prior vertebral surgery (Tiple et al., 2009). The term was coined during World War I when young soldiers who were apparently attempting to escape the stress of battle developed this peculiar posture, perhaps promoted by a stooped posture when walking in the trenches. There appear to be two possible mechanisms of camptocormia: (1) dystonia due to a central disorder and (2) extensor trunkal muscle myopathy (Bloch et al., 2006; Lepoutre et al., 2006; Melamed and Djaldetti, 2006; Gdynia et al., 2009).

Other truncal deformities include scoliosis and tilting of the trunk, referred to as the Pisa syndrome (Villarejo et al., 2003) (Fig. 4.4). The axial dystonias resulting in scoliosis

and camptocormia may improve with botulinum toxin injections into the paraspinal or rectus abdominis muscles (Azher and Jankovic, 2005; Bonanni et al., 2007). In some cases, dystonia may be the presenting symptom of PD, particularly the early-onset Parkinson disease (EOPD) variety such as is seen in patients with the *parkin* mutation (Lücking et al., 2000; Jankovic and Tintner, 2001; Hedrich et al., 2002). In addition, several autosomal recessive disorders, including PANK2, PLA2G6, ATP13A2, FBX07, TAF1, and PRKRA-associated neurodegeneration, are manifested by the dystonia–parkinsonism combination (Schneider et al., 2009). Another form of dystonia associated with PD is paroxysmal exercise-induced foot dystonia, which may be the presenting feature of young-onset PD (YOPD) (Bozi and Bhatia, 2003).

Loss of postural reflexes

Loss of postural reflexes is a characteristic feature in PD patients who exhibit the PIGD phenotype and usually occurs in more advanced stages of the disease along with freezing of gait and other symptoms that often lead to falling. One of the distinguishing features of PD fallers is their tendency to overestimate balance performance on functional reach testing compared to controls, and this overestimation worsens with worsening disease severity and when concurrently performing complex motor (e.g., carrying a tray) and cognitive tasks (e.g., performing mental arithmetic). In contrast to controls, PD patients are willing to sacrifice motor performance to complete competing tasks and make significantly more motor errors when performing a complex motor-cognitive task, whereas controls were more likely to preserve motor performance while sacrificing cognitive accuracy (Bloem et al., 2006). The loss of protective reactions further contributes to fall-related injuries. In one study, a fall in the past year, abnormal axial posture, cognitive impairment, and freezing of gait were independent risk factors for falls and predicted 38/51 fallers (75%) and 45/62 non-fallers (73%) (Latt et al., 2009). Additional measures contributing to falls include frontal impairment, poor leaning balance, and leg weakness. In another study, female gender, symmetrical onset, postural and autonomic instability appear to be the most reliable predictors of falls in PD (Williams et al., 2006). Using a battery of neurologic and functional tests in 101 patients with early PD and in an optimally medicated state, 48% reported a fall and 24% more than one fall in a prospective follow-up over 6 months (Kerr et al., 2010). The following measures provided the best sensitivity (78%) and specificity (84%) for predicting falls: UPDRS total score, total freezing of gait score, occurrence of symptomatic postural orthostasis, Tinetti total score, and extent of postural sway in the anterior-posterior direction.

The average period from onset of symptoms to the first fall in progressive supranuclear palsy (PSP) is 16.8 months, as compared to 108 months in PD, 42 months in MSA, 54 months in dementia with Lewy bodies, and 40.8 months in vascular parkinsonism. Many patients with postural instability, particularly when associated with flexed truncal posture (camptocormia), have festination, manifested by faster and faster walking as if chasing their center of gravity to prevent falling. When combined with axial rigidity and bradykinesia, loss of postural reflexes causes the patient to collapse into the chair when attempting to sit down. The pull test (pulling the patient by the shoulders) is commonly used to determine the patient's degree of retropulsion or propulsion (see above) (Visser et al., 2003; Hunt and Sethi, 2006; Valkovic et al., 2008). Alterations in cholinergic rather than dopaminergic neurotransmission have been implicated in disturbed balance and falls associated with PD, partly because of evidence that gait control depends on cholinergic system-mediated higher-level cortical and subcortical processing, including pedunculopontine nucleus (PPN) function. This is supported by a cross-sectional study of 44 patients with PD without dementia and 15 control subjects who underwent a clinical assessment and [^{11}C] methyl-4-piperidinyl propionate (PMP) acetylcholinesterase (AChE) and [^{11}C]dihydrotetrabenazine (DTBZ) vesicular monoamine transporter type 2 (VMAT2) brain PET imaging (Bohnen et al., 2009). The study found reduced cortical AChE hydrolysis rates demonstrated in the PD fallers (−12.3%) compared to PD nonfallers (−6.6%) and control subjects ($P = 0.0004$). In another study, involving 22 normal controls, 12 patients with PD, 13 with MSA-P, and 4 with PSP, PET with [^{11}C]PMP showed a significant decrease in AChE activity in most cerebral cortical regions in PD and MSA-P, and a nonsignificant decrease in PSP. On the other hand, subcortical cholinergic activity was significantly more decreased in MSA-P and PSP than in PD. The authors suggested that the more substantial decrease in subcortical AChE in MSA-P and PSP reflects greater impairment in the pontine cholinergic group (PPN) and may account for the greater gait disturbances in the early stages of these two disorders compared to PD (Gilman et al., 2010). Thus cholinergic hypofunction, possibly related to PPN degener-

ation, may be contributing to falls in patients with PD (Thevathasan and Aziz, 2010).

Freezing

One of the most disabling symptoms of PD is freezing, also referred as *motor blocks*, considered by some as a form of akinesia (loss of movement) (Giladi et al., 1997, 2001; Giladi and Nieuwboer, 2008; Morris et al., 2008) (Videos 4.5, 4.6). Although it most often affects the legs when walking, it can also involve upper limbs and the eyelids (apraxia of eyelid opening or eyelid closure) (Boghen, 1997). Freezing consists of sudden, transient (a few seconds) inability to move. It typically causes start hesitation when initiating walking and the sudden inability to move feet (as if glued to the ground) when turning or walking through narrow passages (such as the door or the elevator) (Almeida and Lebold, 2010), when crossing streets with heavy traffic, or when approaching a destination (target hesitation). Freezing is the most common cause of falls in patients with PD that can result in injuries, including hip fractures. Patients often adopt a variety of cues or tricks to overcome the freezing attacks: marching to command ("left, right, left, right"), stepping over objects (the end of a walking stick, a pavement stone, cracks in the floor, etc.), walking to music or a metronome, shifting body weight, rocking movements, and others (Dietz et al., 1990; Fahn, 1995; Marchese et al., 2001; Rubinstein et al., 2002; Suteerawattananon et al., 2004; Nieuwboer, 2008). "Off" gait freezing was found to correlate with dopa-responsive abnormal discriminatory processing as determined by abnormally increased temporal discrimination threshold (Lee et al., 2005). Freezing may be a manifestation of the "off" phenomenon in PD patients who fluctuate but may also occur during "on" time ("on freezing"), independent of bradykinesia and tremor (Bartels et al., 2003). Based on responses by 6620 patients to a questionnaire sent to 12 000 members of the German Parkinson Association, 47% of patients reported freezing, and it was present more frequently in men than women and less frequently in patients who considered tremor as their main symptom (Macht et al., 2007). When freezing occurs early in the course of the disease or is the predominant symptom, a diagnosis other than PD should be considered. Disorders associated with prominent freezing include progressive supranuclear palsy (PSP), MSA, and vascular (lower body) parkinsonism (FitzGerald and Jankovic, 1989; Elble et al., 1996; Winikates and Jankovic, 1999; Jankovic et al., 2001). Freezing has been thought to be related to noradrenergic deficiency as a result of degeneration of the locus coeruleus (Zarow et al., 2003), as suggested by possible response to noradrenergic agents such as L-threo-dihydroxy-phenylserine, or DOPS (Narabayashi, 1999). Neurophysiologic studies in monkeys treated with MPTP found that dopamine depletion is associated with impaired selection of proprioceptive inputs in the supplementary motor area, which could interfere with motor planning and may be related to motor freezing (Escola et al., 2002). Integrating EMG signals over real time while recording EMG activity from lower extremities before and during freezing, Nieuwboer and colleagues (2004) showed significantly abnormal timing in the tibialis anterior and gastrocnemius muscles, although reciprocity is preserved. Thus, before freezing, the tibialis anterior and gastrocnemius contract prematurely, and the duration of contraction is shortened in the tibialis anterior, but the amplitude of the EMG burst is increased (probably a compensatory strategy pulling the leg into swing), whereas the contraction is prolonged in the gastrocnemius during the actual swing phase. Isolated freezing usually suggests a diagnosis other than PD and may be present in atypical forms of parkinsonism or brainstem strokes (Kuo et al., 2008). The pathologic involvement of brainstem in patients with pure akinesia and gait freezing is suggested by decreased glucose metabolism on PET scans in the midbrain of such patients, similar to the findings in patients with PSP (Park et al., 2009). Neither medical (Giladi, 2008) nor surgical (Ferraye et al., 2008; Nashatizadeh and Jankovic, 2008) treatments generally provide satisfactory control of freezing. 📹

Other motor abnormalities

Some patients exhibit the reemergence of primitive reflexes attributed to a breakdown of the frontal lobe inhibitory mechanisms that are normally present in infancy and early childhood, hence the term *release signs* (Vreeling et al., 1993; Thomas, 1994; Rao et al., 2003). The glabellar tap reflex, also known as Meyerson sign, has often been associated with PD. However, its diagnostic accuracy has not been subjected to rigorous studies. The glabellar tap reflex is elicited through repeated stimuli to the glabellar region of the forehead, inducing concomitant blinking with each tap. In the normal subject, the reflex blinking habituates or the subject stops blinking with each stimulus tap after the second to fifth tap. Brodsky and colleagues (2004) examined the glabellar reflex and the palmomental reflex in 100 subjects, which included patients with PD ($n = 41$), patients with PSP ($n = 12$), patients with MSA ($n = 7$), and healthy, age-matched controls ($n = 40$). Using a standardized protocol and a "blinded" review of videotapes, we found that (1) both reflexes were present significantly more frequently in patients with PD as compared to normal controls; (2) glabellar, but not palmomental, reflex was more frequently present in patients with PSP than in controls; (3) there was no difference in the frequency of these reflexes between normal controls and patients with MSA; (4) the two reflexes occurred with similar frequency among the three parkinsonian disorders; (5) glabellar, but not palmomental, reflex correlated with parkinsonian motor deficit; and (6) the primitive reflexes correlated with mental deficit. While relatively sensitive signs of parkinsonian disorders, particularly PD, these primitive reflexes lack specificity, as they do not differentiate among the three most common parkinsonian disorders (Brodsky et al., 2004). Abnormal spontaneous blinking, particularly the longer pauses between closing and opening phase, compared to normal controls suggests that the decreased blinking in PD reflects underlying bradykinesia (Agostino et al., 2008). In addition to these primitive reflexes, there are other "frontal" and "cortical disinhibition" signs, such as the applause sign (Wu et al., 2008), but none of them are specific for PD.

Besides the classic cardinal signs, there are many other motor abnormalities that may be equally or even more disabling. One of the most prominent features of motor impairment in PD is the inability to perform multiple tasks simultaneously. Using functional magnetic resonance imaging (fMRI), Wu and Hallett (2008) found that during dual task execution, greater activity was recorded in the precuneus region, cerebellum, premotor area, and parietal and prefrontal cortex. They concluded that difficulties in dual task performance in PD were associated with limited attentiveness and defective central executive function, and that training may improve the performance. The bulbar symptoms (dysarthria, hypophonia, dysphagia, and sialorrhea) are thought to result from orofacial-laryngeal bradykinesia and rigidity (Hunker et al., 1982). PD-associated speech and voice impairment, often referred to as hypokinetic dysarthria, is characterized by low volume (hypophonia), uniform (monotonous) loudness and pitch (aprosody), imprecise consonants, hesitation, and short rushes of speech (tachyphemia). Other speech characteristics include a variable (abnormally slow or increased) speech rate, palilalia, and stuttering. PD patients have been found to have higher speech acceleration than controls and a significant reduction in the number of pauses, indicating abnormal speech rate and rhythm (Skodda and Schlegel, 2008). A history of childhood stuttering that had remitted can subsequently recur with onset of PD, suggesting an involvement of the dopaminergic system in this speech disorder (Shahed and Jankovic, 2001). When speech therapy designed to stimulate increased vocal fold adduction with instructions to "think loud, think shout," the Lee Silverman Voice Treatment (Ramig et al., 2001), was compared with "speak loud and low," the Pitch Limiting Voice Treatment (de Swart et al., 2003), the two methods produced the same increase in loudness, but the latter method was found to prevent strained voicing. Other treatment strategies for PD-related dysarthria include the use of various verbal cues to regulate speech volume (Ho et al., 1999), but deep brain stimulation has a variable effect (Pinto et al., 2004). The low-volume voice in PD has been attributed in part to vocal fold bowing due to loss of muscle mass and control (Schulz et al., 1999), and augmentation of vocal folds with collagen injections provides improvement in voice quality and has a significantly beneficial impact on quality of life (Hill et al., 2003). Respiratory difficulties result from a variety of mechanisms, including a restrictive component due to rigid respiratory muscles and levodopa-induced respiratory dyskinesias (Rice et al., 2002).

In addition to categorization of patients into clinical subtypes, there is a growing appreciation for differences in clinical presentation depending on genetic background. Thus patients with *parkin* mutations (PARK2), who account for nearly a third of patients with early-onset PD, tend to develop levodopa-induced dyskinesias and hallucinations relatively early in the course of the disease. They also may present with dystonic gait, cervical dystonia, dopa-responsive dystonia, hemiparkinsonism–hemiatrophy, freezing, festination, retropulsion, leg tremor at rest and on standing, marked sleep benefit, hyperreflexia, ataxia, peripheral neuropathy, and dysautonomia (Klein and Lohmann, 2009). Carriers of *LRRK2* G2019S mutation are more likely to manifest the PIGD subtype of PD rather than the tremor-dominant phenotype, although in contrast to the PIGD in patients with sporadic PD, *LRRK2* patients tend to have a much slower, less aggressive course (Alcalay et al., 2009; Dächsel and Farrer, 2010). Other studies have confirmed that in comparison with genetically undefined patients, *LRRK2* mutation carriers had more severe motor symptoms, a higher rate of dyskinesia, and less postural tremor, whereas *PINK1* mutation carriers have younger age at onset and slower progression, but similar to *LRRK2* PD patients have an increased rate of drug-induced dyskinesia and a lower rate of postural tremor (Nishioka et al., 2010).

Nonmotor manifestations

Although James Parkinson in his original description focused on the motor symptoms, he also drew attention to several nonmotor features, including problems associated with sleep and gastrointestinal function (Parkinson, 1817). Traditionally viewed as primarily a motor disorder, there is growing recognition that nonmotor symptoms of PD, which occur in 88% of all patients, are as troublesome if not more so than the classic motor features (Simuni and Sethi, 2008). The nonmotor manifestations and fluctuations in nonmotor symptoms have been found to be more disabling than the motor symptoms in 28% of PD patients (Witjas et al., 2002). These nonmotor, nondopaminergic symptoms have been largely ignored, but several recent studies have highlighted their frequency and their serious impact on quality of life, particularly in more advanced stages of the disease (Lang and Obeso, 2004; Chaudhuri et al., 2006a, 2006b, 2007; Ahlskog, 2007; Martinez-Martin et al., 2007; Pfeiffer, 2007; Lim et al., 2009). The Sydney Multicenter Study showed that PD patients treated with "modern" initial therapy continue to die at a rate in excess of their peers, with only one-third of original study subjects remaining alive at 15 years after diagnosis, and most were disabled more by their nonmotor than motor symptoms: 84% experienced cognitive decline with 48% meeting diagnostic criteria for dementia, 58% were unable to live alone, and 40% were in long-term care facilities (Hely et al., 2005). After 20 years' follow-up, only 36 (26%) survived and the standardized mortality ratio reached 3.1 (Hely et al., 2008). Of the 30 included in this longitudinal study, 100% had levodopa-induced dyskinesia and end of dose failure, dementia was present in 83%, and 48% were in nursing homes. Other problems included excessive daytime sleepiness in 70%, falls in 87%, freezing in 81%, fractures in 35%, symptomatic postural hypotension in 48%, urinary incontinence in 71%, moderate dysarthria in 81%, choking in 48%, and hallucinations in 74%. Of the 87 patients followed prospectively in the Sydney study whose brain was examined at autopsy, the final diagnosis was PD in 29, PD with dementia in 52, and dementia with Lewy bodies (DLB) in 6 (Halliday et al., 2008). The clinical-pathologic correlations suggested that there were three groups of patients: (1) younger-onset patients with a typical PD clinical course; brainstem Lewy bodies predominate in those surviving to 5 years, and by 13 years, 50% of cases have a limbic distribution of Lewy bodies; (2) older-onset PD cases with shorter survival and with higher Lewy body loads and additional plaque pathology; and (3) early malignant, dementia-dominant syndrome and severe neocortical disease, consistent with DLB. In a multicenter study of 1072 consecutive patients with PD in 55 Italian centers, the so-called Priamo study, 98.6% of patients reported a mean of 7.8 (range 0–32) nonmotor symptoms, such as fatigue (58%), anxiety (56%), leg pain (38%), insomnia (37%),

urinary urgency and nocturia (35%), drooling of saliva (31%) and difficulties in maintaining concentration (31%) (Barone et al., 2009). Apathy was the symptom associated with worse PDQ-39 score but presence of fatigue, attention/memory, and psychiatric symptoms also had a negative impact on quality of life. The nonmotor features associated with PD are presumably related to involvement of the non-dopaminergic systems and even pathology outside the central nervous system (Djaldetti et al., 2009).

Autonomic dysfunction

Autonomic failure is typically associated with MSA and may be the presenting feature of that disease, but it may also herald the onset of PD (Kaufmann et al., 2004; Mostile and Jankovic, 2009). In contrast to PD associated with dys-autonomia, due to predominantly peripheral (ganglionic and postganglionic) involvement, in MSA the primary lesion is preganglionic; also dysautonomic symptoms are more severe at baseline and become more global in MSA as compared to PD (Lipp et al., 2009). Rating scales for dysautonomia associated with PD have been developed (Evatt et al., 2009). Dysautonomia, such as orthostatic hypotension, sweating dysfunction, sphincter dysfunction, and sexual impotence occur frequently in patients with PD (Senard et al., 1997; Swinn et al., 2003). In one study, 7 of 51 (14%) patients with early, untreated PD had a decrease of more than 20 mmHg in systolic blood pressure (Bonuccelli et al., 2003). Another community-based study of a cohort of PD patients showed that 42 of 89 (47%) met the diagnostic criteria for orthostatic hypotension (Allcock et al., 2004). Orthostatic hypotension, however, is not often detected in the clinic. Although the symptom of orthostatic lightheadedness has a relatively high specificity, it seems to have low sensitivity in predicting orthostatic hypotension, partly because it is more likely to occur after tilting than on standing, and is often delayed by longer than the recommended 3 minutes (Jamnadas-Khoda et al., 2009). Autonomic symptoms, particularly orthostatic hypotension, seem to be more common in the PIGD form of PD (Allcock and et al., 2006). Autonomic symptom severity was associated with more motor dysfunction, depressive symptoms, cognitive dysfunction, psychiatric complications, nighttime sleep disturbances, and excessive daytime sleepiness ($P < 0.01$) (Verbaan et al., 2007a). While dysautonomia is typically associated with MSA, it may also be prominent in PD, although autonomic testing might not always differentiate between PD and MSA (Riley and Chelimsky, 2003).

Orthostatic hypotension in patients with PD has been traditionally attributed to dopaminergic therapy, but recent studies have provided evidence that orthostatic hypotension in PD is due to failure of reflexive sympathetically mediated cardiovascular stimulation from sympathetic denervation, as demonstrated by markedly decreased 6-[^{18}F]-fluorodopamine-derived radioactivity in septal and ventricular myocardium (Goldstein et al., 2002). This sympathetic nervous system deficit involved postganglionic catecholaminergic, not cholinergic, nerves (Sharabi et al., 2003).

Sweating dysfunction, hyperhidrosis, and to a lesser extent hypohidrosis, were reported by 64% of patients with PD as compared to 12.5% of controls ($P < 0.005$) (Swinn et al.,

2003). These symptoms did not correlate with the severity of the disease but occurred most frequently during the "off" periods and during "on with dyskinesia" periods. Because sudomotor skin response was reduced in the palms, the axial hyperhidrosis has been suggested to be a compensatory phenomenon for reduced sympathetic function in the extremities (Schestatsky et al., 2006). Sweating may be a particularly troublesome symptom during wearing off (Pursiainen et al., 2007). The presence of α-synuclein deposits in the dermis of a patient with pure autonomic failure provides evidence that this disorder as well as other disorders associated with autonomic failure (e.g., PD, DLB, and MSA) should be viewed as variant synucleinopathies (Kaufmann and Goldstein, 2010; Shishido et al., 2010).

Bladder and other urologic symptoms are frequent in PD and are among the most common complaints requiring medical attention (Blackett et al., 2009; Sakakibara et al., 2010). One survey found that over one-fourth of men with PD had urinary difficulty, most often causing urinary urgency (Araki and Kuno, 2000). In one study, urge episodes and urge incontinence were observed in 53% and 27% of the patients with PD, respectively, and detrusor overactivity in 46% of the patients with PD, which was less prevalent than in patients with dementia with Lewy bodies and Alzheimer disease, while mean voided volume, free flow, cystometric bladder capacity, and detrusor pressor were similar in the groups (Ransmayr et al., 2008).

Despite the possibility of hypersexuality, usually related to dopaminergic drugs, many patients with PD have sexual dysfunction (Celikel et al., 2008; Meco et al., 2008; Hand et al., 2010). In a review of sexual functioning of 32 women and 43 men with PD, women reported difficulties with arousal (87.5%), reaching orgasm (75.0%), and sexual dissatisfaction (37.5%) (Bronner et al., 2004). Men reported erectile dysfunction (68.4%), sexual dissatisfaction (65.1%), premature ejaculation (40.6%), and difficulties reaching orgasm (39.5%). Reduced sexual drive and dissatisfaction with orgasm was particularly common in female PD patients (Celikel et al., 2008). Among 90 patients with PD, loss of libido was reported by 65.6%, and 42.6% of men also complained of erectile dysfunction (Kummer et al., 2009). Aging, female gender, lower education, and depression were significantly associated with decreased sexual desire. Premorbid sexual dysfunction may contribute to cessation of sexual activity during the course of the disease (among 23.3% of men and 21.9% of women). Associated illnesses, use of medications, motor difficulties, depression, anxiety, and advanced stage of PD contributed to sexual dysfunction.

Drooling (sialorrhea) is one of the most embarrassing symptoms of PD (Chou et al., 2007). While some studies have shown that PD patients actually have less saliva production (Proulx et al., 2005) than normal controls, others have suggested that the excessive drooling is due to a difficulty with swallowing (Bagheri et al., 1999). Salivary sympathetic denervation, however, could not be demonstrated by 6-[^{18}F]-fluorodopamine scanning (Goldstein et al., 2002). Dysphagia (Hunter et al., 1997) along with delayed gastric emptying (Hardoff et al., 2001) and constipation (Ashraf et al., 1997; Bassotti et al., 2000; Winge et al., 2003; Cersosimo and Benarroch, 2008) represent the most frequent gastrointestinal manifestations of PD. In addition to constipation, PD patients often experience pharyngeal and esophageal dysphagia and 60% have evidence of delayed gastric emptying (Krygowska-Wajs et al., 2009).

When PD patients were compared to healthy controls, those with PD were found to swallow significantly more often during inhalation, at low tidal volumes, and exhibited significantly more post-swallow inhalation (Gross et al., 2008). Impaired coordination of breathing and swallowing may contribute to the high frequency of aspiration pneumonia in PD.

Gastrointestinal dysfunction in PD has been attributed to many mechanisms such as involvement, including neurodegeneration and the presence of Lewy bodies, of the dorsal motor nucleus of the vagus, paravertebral sympathetic ganglia, and intrinsic neurons of the enteric nervous system (Cersosimo and Benarroch, 2008). On the basis of information on the frequency of bowel movements in 6790 men in the Honolulu Heart Program, Abbott and colleagues (2001) concluded that infrequent bowel movements are associated with increased risk for future PD. Based on the observation from the Honolulu-Asia Aging Study that bowel frequency was lower in subjects who were found to have incidental Lewy bodies in their brains at postmortem examination than in controls, the investigators suggested that constipation was one of the earliest symptoms of PD (Abbott et al., 2007). Also, constipation was associated with low SN neuron density (Petrovitch et al., 2009). Based on a review of Mayo Clinic medical records of 196 case-control pairs ($N = 392$), constipation preceding PD was more common in cases than in controls (odds ratio 2.48; $P = 0.0005$) (Savica et al., 2009). Constipation in patients with PD is associated with slow colonic transit, weak abdominal strain, decreased phasic rectal contraction, and paradoxical sphincter contraction on defecation (Sakakibara et al., 2003). Dermatologic changes such as seborrhea, hair loss, and leg edema may represent evidence of peripheral involvement in PD, although some of these changes may be exacerbated by anti-PD drugs (Tabamo and Di Rocco, 2002; Tan and Ondo, 2000).

Autonomic complications, coupled with motor and mental decline, contribute to a higher risk of hospitalization and nursing home placement. Examination of hospital records of 15 304 cases of parkinsonism and 30 608 age- and sex-matched controls showed that PD patients are six times more likely to be admitted to hospital with aspiration pneumonia than are nonparkinsonian controls (Guttman et al., 2004). Other comorbid medical conditions significantly more common in patients with PD include fractures of the femur, urinary tract disorders, septicemia, and fluid/electrolyte disorders. But similarly to other reports (Jansson and Jankovic, 1985; Gorell et al., 1994; Vanacore et al., 1999; Inzelberg and Jankovic, 2007), this study showed that cancer might be less common in patients with PD, with the major exception being malignant melanoma with an almost twofold increased risk (Olsen et al., 2005) and a higher risk of family history of melanoma (Gao et al., 2009).

Cognitive and neurobehavioral abnormalities

Cognitive and neuropsychiatric disturbances have as much impact on the quality of life of a patient with PD as the motor symptoms (Aarsland et al., 2009). Cognitive deficits have been found in 30% of patients with early PD (Elgh et al., 2009). The Sydney Multicenter Study showed that after 15 years of follow-up, 84% have cognitive decline and 48% meet diagnostic criteria for dementia, 58% were unable to live alone, and 40% were in long-term care facilities (Hely et al., 2005). A long-term follow-up study of 233 subjects in Norway found that 60.1% of subjects by 12 years into the course of the disease had evidence of dementia (Buter et al., 2008). Based on this study, a 70-year-old man with PD but without dementia has a life expectancy of 8 years, 3 of which will be marked by coexistent dementia. In 537 patients with dementia associated with PD (PDD), 58% had associated depression, 54% apathy, 49% anxiety, and 44% hallucinations (Aarsland et al., 2007). A structured interview of 50 patients with PD found that anxiety (66%), drenching sweats (64%), slowness of thinking (58%), fatigue (56%), and akathisia (54%) were the most frequent nonmotor fluctuations. Many patients, for example, exhibit neurobehavioral disturbances, such as depression, dementia, tip-of-the-tongue phenomenon and other word-finding difficulties (Matison et al., 1982), various psychiatric symptoms, and sleep disorders (van Hilten et al., 1994; Aarsland et al., 1999; Pal et al., 1999; Tandberg et al., 1999; Olanow et al., 2000; Wetter et al., 2000; Ondo et al., 2001; Emre, 2003; Grandas and Iranzo, 2004; Adler and Thorpy, 2005; Goetz et al., 2008a). Although neurobehavioral abnormalities are often considered late features of PD, cognitive impairment affecting attention, psychomotor function, episodic memory, executive function, and category fluency (Elgh et al., 2009) may be detected even in early stages of the disease, and depression (Alonso et al., 2009) may be one of the earliest symptoms of PD.

A variety of instruments have been developed, designed to assess behavioral and cognitive impairments associated with PD (Goetz et al., 2008a). On the basis of the most frequently affected cognitive domains in PD, Marinus and colleagues (2003) proposed the SCOPA-COG (Scales for Outcomes of Parkinson's disease – cognition). Using this scale and the search of the literature, they concluded that the cognitive functions that are most frequently affected in PD include attention, active memory, executive, and visuospatial functions, whereas verbal functions, thinking, and reasoning are relatively spared. PD patients may have a limited perception of large spatial configurations (seeing trees but not the forest) (Barrett et al., 2001). Aarsland and colleagues (2001) found in a community-based, prospective study that patients with PD have an almost six-fold increased risk of dementia. In an 8-year prospective study of 224 patients with PD, they found that 78.2% fulfilled the DSM-III criteria for dementia (Aarsland et al., 2003). The mean annual decline on Mini-Mental State Examination (MMSE) in patients with PD is 1 point, in patients with PD and dementia, it is 2.3 points (Aarsland et al., 2004). While the MMSE has been used traditionally to screen for cognitive deficits, it often fails to detect early cognitive decline because of its ceiling effect, and, therefore, the Montreal Cognitive Assessment (MoCA) has been developed to detect mild cognitive impairment in PD (Gill et al., 2008). In a study designed to compare the two scales in 88 patients with PD, the percentage of subjects scoring below a cutoff of 26/30 (used by others to detect mild cognitive impairment) was higher on the MoCA (32%) than on the MMSE (11%) ($P < 0.000002$), suggesting that the MoCA is a more sensitive tool to identify early

cognitive impairment in PD (Zadikoff et al., 2007). Of the various scales specifically designed to assess cognitive impairment in PD the SCOPA-COG, which mainly assesses "frontal-subcortical" cognitive defects, and the PD-CRS (Parkinson's Disease – Cognitive Rating Scale), which assesses "instrumental-cortical" functions, have been most rigorously validated (Kulisevksy and Pagonabarraga, 2009). The MMP (Mini-Mental Parkinson) and PANDA (Parkinson Neuropsychiatric Dementia Assessment) are brief screening tests that still require more extensive clinimetric evaluations.

A variety of measures have been investigated for their predictability of cognitive impairment. In the DATATOP study of patients with early PD, cumulative incidence of cognitive impairment, defined as scoring 2 standard deviations below age- and education-adjusted MMSE norms, was 2.4% (95% confidence interval 1.2–3.5%) at 2 years and 5.8% (3.7–7.7%) at 5 years (Uc et al., 2009a). Risk factors for cognitive impairment in this group of 740 patients was older age, hallucinations, male gender, increased symmetry of parkinsonism, increased severity of motor impairment (except for tremor), speech and swallowing impairments, dexterity loss, and presence of gastroenterologic/urologic disorders at baseline.

Functional imaging has been also used to study risk factors for cognitive decline in PD. Temporoparietal cortical hypometabolism is present in patients with PD and may be a useful predictor of future cognitive impairment (Hu et al., 2000). Another predictor of cognitive dysfunction appears to be reduced ^{18}F-fluorodopa uptake in the caudate nucleus and frontal cortex (Rinne et al., 2000) as well as in the mesolimbic pathways (Ito et al., 2002). Using event-related fMRI to compare groups of cognitively impaired and unimpaired patients, Lewis and colleagues (2003) showed a significant signal intensity reduction during a working-memory paradigm in specific striatal and frontal lobe sites in PD patients with cognitive impairment. These studies indicate that cognitive impairments in early PD are related to reductions in activity of frontostriatal neural circuitry. In a PET study of brain activation during frontal tasks, such as trial-and-error learning, Mentis and colleagues (2003) found that even in early PD when learning is still relatively preserved, PD patients had to activate four times as much neural tissue as the controls in order to achieve learning performance equal to controls. Although the sequence learning is impaired even in early PD, this learning deficit does not appear to reflect impairments in motor execution or bradykinesia and may be related to reduced attention (Ghilardi et al., 2003).

Patients with PD have nearly twice the risk for developing dementia as controls, and siblings of demented PD patients have an increased risk for Alzheimer disease (Marder et al., 1999). In addition to the MMSE, other tests (e.g., the Frontal Assessment Battery) have been developed and validated to assess the cognitive and frontal lobe function (Dubois et al., 2000) in patients with dementia with or without parkinsonism. In agreement with basal forebrain cholinergic denervation even in early PD, prominent and widespread reduction in cortical, particularly the medial occipital secondary visual cortex (Brodmann area 18), acetylcholinesterase can be demonstrated using N-[^{11}C]methyl-4-piperidyl acetate PET (Shimada et al., 2009). These changes were more pronounced but similar in patients with PDD and DLB.

There are several reasons why patients with PD have an associated dementia. Pathologically, dementia correlates with cortical pathology, including Lewy bodies (Hughes et al., 1993; Hurtig et al., 2000), especially in the cingulate and entorhinal cortex (Kovari et al., 2003). But the significance of cortical Lewy bodies is not clear, since most patients with PD have some detectable Lewy bodies in the cerebral cortex, and patients with PD with no dementia during life have been found to have neuropathologic findings diagnostic of Lewy body dementia (Colosimo et al., 2003). In contrast to earlier studies showing relatively low frequency of dementia in PD, more recent studies suggest that the cumulative prevalence may be as high as 78%, correlating best with cortical and limbic Lewy bodies (Emre, 2004).

Depression is a common comorbid condition in patients with PD, with clinically significant depression present in about a third of all PD patients (Reijnders et al., 2008; Stella et al., 2008; Pankratz et al., 2008) and it may precede other symptoms or signs of PD (Alonso et al., 2009). Death or suicide ideation has been reported in 28% and 11% respectively, and 4% of PD patients have a lifetime suicide attempt, correlated with severity of depression, impulse control disorder, and psychosis (Nazem et al., 2008; Weintraub, 2008). The severity and impact of depression in PD may be assessed by several instruments, but the Hamilton Depression Scale (HAM-D), Beck Depression Inventory (BDI), Hospital Anxiety and Depression Scale (HADS), Montgomery-Asperg Depression Rating Scale (MADRS), and Geriatric Depression Scale (GDS) have been found particularly useful for screening purposes and HAM-D, MADRS, BDI, and the Zung Self-Rating Depression Scale (SDS) have been recommended for assessment of severity (Schrag et al., 2007a). While the HADS and the GDS may be particularly useful in measuring severity of depression, these scales are not apparently sensitive enough to detect a change in patients with severe depression. In addition to instruments used to assess depression, scales for apathy and anhedonia (Leentjens et al., 2008a) and for anxiety (Leentjens et al., 2008b) associated with PD have been developed and validated. Even without these tools, using DSM-IV-TR and a diagnostic examination by psychiatrists, a 49% lifetime prevalence of anxiety was found in a physician-based sample of 127 patients with PD (Pontone et al., 2009).

A community-based study showed that 7.7% of PD patients met the criteria for major depression, 5.1% met those for moderate to severe depression, and another 45.5% had mild depressive symptoms (Tandberg et al., 1996). Depression in PD, clearly a multifactorial disorder, has a major impact on the quality of life (Schrag, 2006). In 139 patients with PD, Aarsland and colleagues (1999) found at least one psychiatric symptom in 61% of the patients. These included depression (38%), hallucinations (27%), and a variety of other behavioral and cognitive changes. In a study of 114 PD patients, 27.6% screened positive for depression during the average 14.6 months of follow-up; 40% were neither treated with antidepressants nor referred for further psychiatric evaluation (Ravina et al., 2007a). Furthermore, depression, as assessed by the GDS-15, correlated with impairment in activities of daily living (ADLs) ($P < 0.0001$). Subsequent analysis showed that increasing severity of depressive symptoms, older age, and longer PD duration predicted a lower likelihood of symptom resolution (Ravina

et al., 2009). Patients with depression may be three times more likely to later develop PD (Schuurman et al., 2002). In one study, depression was found in 15% of patients with PD, and it had more impact on the ADLs than on the motor subscale of UPDRS (Holroyd et al., 2005). Anhedonia is another frequent symptom of PD, which is independent from depression or motor deficits (Isella et al., 2003). Despite the high frequency of depression, patients with PD appear to have higher levels of anger control, consistent with the recognized stoic personality trait (Macías et al., 2008). Stage of illness, motor impairment, and functional disability clearly correlate with depressive symptoms (Pankratz et al., 2008).

Using [^{11}C]RTI-32 PET as a marker of both dopamine and norepinephrine transporter binding in 8 PD patients with and 12 without depression, Remy and colleagues (2005) showed significantly lower binding of this ligand in the locus coeruleus and various limbic regions in depressed and anxious patients compared to those without these psychiatric symptoms. In a group of 94 patients with primary depression, Starkstein and colleagues (2001) found that 20% of patients had parkinsonism that was reversible on treatment of the depression. Blunted reactivity to aversive (pleasant and unpleasant) stimuli has been found in a group of nondemented PD patients (Bowers et al., 2006). Some investigators have attributed the various nonmotor symptoms associated with PD, such as depression, anxiety, lack of energy, and sexual dysfunction, to comorbid testosterone deficiency (found in 35% of PD patients) and suggested that testosterone treatment may be the appropriate therapy for these patients (Okun et al., 2002) and may also improve apathy associated with PD (Ready et al., 2004; Kirsch-Darrow et al., 2006). However, in a subsequent control clinical trial, testosterone was not found to be beneficial in men with PD (Okun et al., 2006).

Psychosis has been long recognized to complicate the course of PD and several scales have been developed to assess this symptom (Fernandez et al., 2008). Diagnostic criteria for psychosis in PD emphasize primarily the presence of paranoid delusions, visual hallucination, illusions, and false sense of presence in contrast to auditory hallucinations and thought disorder typically seen in patients with schizophrenia (Ravina et al., 2007b). Several studies have shown that the occurrence of psychosis is frequently associated with other psychiatric comorbidities, especially depression, anxiety, and apathy (Marsh et al., 2004), and with dementia (Factor et al., 2003). One study concluded that the presence of hallucinations is the strongest predictor of nursing home placement and death (Aarsland et al., 2000). The prognosis of PD-associated psychosis, however, has improved with the advent of atypical neuroleptics in that the incidence of death within 2 years of nursing home placement decreased from 100% to 28%. Minor hallucinations may occur in as many as 40% of patients with PD, illusions in 25%, formed visual hallucinations in 22%, and auditory hallucinations in 10% (Fénelon et al., 2000). Risk factors for hallucinations include older age, duration of illness, depression, cognitive disorder, daytime somnolence, poor visual acuity, family history of dementia (Paleacu et al., 2005), and dopaminergic drugs (Barnes and David, 2001; Goetz et al., 2001; Holroyd et al., 2001). Hallucinations seem to correlate with daytime episodes of rapid eye movement (REM) sleep as well as daytime non-REM and nocturnal REM sleep, suggesting that hallucinations and psychosis may represent a variant of narcolepsy-like REM sleep disorder (Arnulf et al., 2000) and that dream imagery plays an important role in visual hallucinations (Manni et al., 2002). Other studies, however, have found no correlation between hallucinations and abnormal sleep patterns (Goetz et al., 2005). The sleep abnormalities observed in patients with PD may possibly be related to a 50% loss of hypocretin (orexin) neurons (Fronczek et al., 2007; Thannickal et al., 2007).

Besides the cardinal motor signs, there are many behavioral and cognitive symptoms associated with PD, such as depression, sleep disorders, and fatigability, that can adversely influence the overall quality of life in patients with PD (Karlsen et al., 1999). In one study, 50% of patients with PD had significant fatigue that had a major impact on health-related quality of life (Herlofson and Larsen, 2003). PD-related fatigue contributes to poor functional capacity and physical function (Garber and Friedman, 2003; Chaudhuri and Behan, 2004; Friedman et al., 2007). A 16-item self-report instrument designed to measure fatigue associated with PD has been developed (Brown et al., 2005). One study showed that depression, postural instability, and cognitive impairment have the greatest influence on quality of life (Schrag et al., 2000). In a prospective longitudinal study of 111 patients followed for 4 years, Karlsen and colleagues (2000) showed significantly increased distress, based on health-related quality of life, not only due to motor symptoms but also because of pain, social isolation, and emotional reactions.

Variants of bradyphrenia (slowness of thought), such as abulia (severe apathy and lack of initiative and spontaneity) as well as akinetic mutism and catatonia (immobility, mutism, refusal to eat or drink, staring, rigidity, posturing, grimacing, negativism, waxy flexibility, echophenomenon, and stereotypy), have been recognized in patients with parkinsonism. Apathy in PD appears to be related to the underlying disease process rather than being a psychologic reaction to disability or to depression (Kirsch-Darrow et al., 2006) and is closely associated with cognitive impairment (Pluck and Brown, 2002). Various studies have reported that 32–54% exhibit apathy (Aarsland et al., 2007; Dujardin et al., 2007; Aarsland et al., 2009). Although depression and dementia are the most frequent comorbidities associated with apathy, about 13% of patients with PD exhibit apathy alone (Starkstein et al., 2009). Whether these symptoms represent a continuum of bradykinesia–bradyphrenia or different disorders is not easy to answer with the current rudimentary knowledge of these disorders (Muqit et al., 2001).

There have been several studies attempting to address the question of "premorbid parkinsonian personality." Twin and other studies have suggested that since childhood, PD patients tend to be more introverted, cautious, socially alert, tense, nervous, and rigid compared to controls (Ishihara and Brayne, 2006). Some have found PD patients, even before onset of motor symptoms, to often avoid risk-seeking behavior, such as smoking (Ward et al., 1983a), and to exhibit lower impulsive and less novelty-seeking behavior (Menza et al., 1993; Fujii et al., 2000; Evans et al., 2004). Since dopamine is involved in the reward system, presymptomatic dopamine deficiency may predispose some individuals to exhibit a "non-smoking personality," thus accounting for the lower frequency of smokers among PD patients (Wirdefeldt et al., 2005). Many studies have demonstrated that even before they first develop any motor symptoms, PD patients tend to have relatively characteristic personality traits, such as industriousness, seriousness, inflexibility, and a tendency to be "honest" (Przuntek, 1992; Macías et al., 2008; Abe et al., 2009). One study of 32 patients, using F-fluorodeoxyglucose PET scans, showed that PD patients are indeed "honest" and have difficulties making deceptive responses, and that this personality trait might be derived from dysfunction of the prefrontal cortex (Abe et al., 2009). Many patients with PD also develop obsessive-compulsive behavior, addictive personality, and impulse control disorder, particularly exemplified by compulsive gambling and shopping, hypersexuality, hoarding and other compulsive behaviors (Molina et al., 2000; Alegret et al., 2001; Geschwandtner et al., 2001; Driver-Dunckley et al., 2003; Ondo and Lai, 2008; Stamey and Jankovic, 2008; Mamikonyan et al., 2008; Ferrara and Stacy, 2008; Robert et al., 2009; O'Sullivan et al., 2010). In one study at Baylor College of Medicine, 300 consecutive patients taking dopamine agonists for PD ($n = 207$), restless legs syndrome ($n = 89$), or both ($n = 4$), 19.7% reported increased impulsivity: 30 gambling, 26 spending, 11 sexual activity, and 1 wanton traveling, but only 11/59 (18.6%) felt the change was deleterious (Ondo and Lai, 2008). Increased impulsivity correlated with a younger age ($P = 0.01$) and larger doses of dopamine agonist. Using perfusion TC99m single-photon emission computed tomography (SPECT) to study brain activity, PD patients with pathologic gambling have been found to have resting state dysfunction of the mesocorticolimbic network involved in addictive behavior (Cilia et al., 2008). Thus it is postulated that in such patients there is lack of the usual reduction in cortical perfusion typically associated with the neurodegenerative process and that pathologic gambling results from abnormal drug-induced overstimulation of the relatively spared mesocorticolimbic dopamine system. Increased striatal dopamine release has been postulated in PD patients with pathologic gambling, based on findings from raclopride PET scans (Steeves et al., 2009).

Various intrusive cognitive events with associated repetitive behaviors, representing the spectrum of obsessive-compulsive disorder in PD, include the following domains: (1) checking, religious, and sexual obsessions; (2) symmetry and ordering; (3) washing and cleaning; and (4) punding. Punding is characterized by intense fascination with repetitive handling, examining, sorting, and arranging of objects, inordinate writing, doodling, painting, collecting things, shuffling through personal papers, journaling/blogging, internet play, excessive cleaning or gardening or sorting household objects, humming or singing, and reciting long, meaningless soliloquies without an audience (Evans et al., 2004; Voon, 2004; Silveira-Moriyama et al., 2006). The behavior may be based on one's past experiences and hobbies or may be more related to obsessive-compulsive disorder features such as gambling, which in turn may be exacerbated by dopaminergic drugs (Kurlan, 2004). In a survey of 373 consecutive patients with PD, only 1.4% exhibited punding behavior (Miyasaki et al., 2007). Compulsive singing may be another variant of punding (Bonvin et al., 2007). Pathologic gambling has been attributed most frequently to the use of dopamine agonists (Kurlan, 2004; Dodd et al., 2005; Stamey and Jankovic, 2008), but levodopa and even subthalamic nucleus deep brain stimulation have been also reported to cause pathologic gambling. The obsessive-compulsive disorder that is associated with PD has been reported to improve with high-frequency stimulation of the subthalamic nucleus (Mallet et al., 2002).

Another behavioral abnormality, possibly related to underlying obsessive-compulsive disorder, is "hedonistic homeostatic dysregulation." This behavior is seen particularly in males with young-onset or early-onset PD (YOPD) who misuse and abuse dopaminergic drugs and develop cyclic mood disorder with hypomania or manic psychosis (Giovannoni et al., 2000; Pezzella et al., 2005). Other behavioral symptoms associated with dopamine dysregulation syndrome include compulsive dopaminergic replacement (Lawrence et al., 2003), craving, binge eating, compulsive foraging, euphoria, dysphoria, hypersexuality, pathologic gambling, compulsive shopping, aggression, insulting gestures, paranoia, jealousy, phobias, impulsivity, and other behaviors (Evans and Lees, 2004; Isaias et al., 2008; Mamikonyan et al., 2008; Stamey and Jankovic, 2008; Weintraub, 2008). Dopaminergic drugs, particularly dopamine agonists, have been demonstrated to precipitate or exacerbate behavioral symptoms of impulse control disorder and the symptoms usually improve with reduction of dosage or cessation of the offending drug (Mamikonyan et al., 2008).

Sleep disorders

Sleep disorders are being increasingly recognized as a feature of PD. An instrument consisting of 15 questions for assessing sleep and nocturnal disability has been described (Chaudhuri et al., 2002). While most studies have attributed the excessive daytime drowsiness and irresistible sleep episodes (sleep attacks) to anti-PD medications (Ondo et al., 2001), some authors believe that these sleep disturbances are an integral part of PD and are age-related (Gjerstad et al., 2006). Increasing the nighttime sleep with antidepressants or benzodiazepines may not necessarily alleviate daytime drowsiness (Arnulf et al., 2002). In a study of 303 PD patients, 63 (21%) had symptoms of restless legs syndrome, possibly associated with low ferritin levels, but there was no evidence that restless legs syndrome leads to PD (Ondo et al., 2002). These results are nearly identical to another study that found restless legs syndrome in 22% of 114 patients with PD (Gomez-Esteban et al., 2007). In another study, 10 of 126 (7.9%) patients with PD and 1 of 129 (0.8%) controls had symptoms of restless legs syndrome (Krishnan et al., 2003). Tan and colleagues (2002) found motor restlessness in 15.2% of their patients with PD, but the prevalence of restless legs syndrome, based on diagnostic criteria proposed by the International Restless Legs Syndrome Study Group, in the PD population was the same as that in the general or clinic population. Degeneration of the diencephalospinal dopaminergic pathway has been postulated to be the mechanism of restless legs syndrome in patients with PD (Nomura et al., 2006).

Several studies have provided evidence that up to 50% of patients presenting with idiopathic rapid eye movement (REM) sleep behavior disorder (RBD) eventually developed parkinsonism and idiopathic RBD is now considered to represent a pre-parkinsonian state (Schenk et al., 1996; Plazzi et al., 1997; Comella et al., 1998; Wetter et al., 2000; Ferini-Strambi and Zucconi, 2000; Matheson and Saper, 2003; Gagnon et al., 2006; Iranzo et al., 2006; Postuma et al., 2006; Boeve et al., 2007; Britton and Chaudhuri, 2009; Postuma et al., 2009a; Postuma et al., 2010). RBD seems to be predictive of PD-associated dysautonomia, particularly orthostatic hypotension (Postuma et al., 2009b). The RBD Screening Questionnaire (RBDSQ) seems to be a sensitive instrument that captures most of the characteristics of RBD and may be useful as a screening tool (Stiasny-Kolster et al., 2007). In one study, 86% of patients with RBD had associated parkinsonism (PD: 47%; MSA: 26%; PSP: 2%) (Olson et al., 2000). RBD was found in 11 of 33 (33%) patients with PD, and 19 of 33 (58%) had REM sleep without atonia (Gagnon et al., 2002). In another study, RBD preceded the onset of parkinsonism in 52% of patients with PD (Olson et al., 2000). The strong male preponderance that is seen in patients with RBD is much less evident in patients who eventually develop MSA. Although considered a parkinsonian symptom, RBD is often exacerbated by dopaminergic therapy (Gjerstad et al., 2008). [^{11}C]-dihydrotetrabenazine PET (Albin et al., 2000) and [^{123}I]-iodobenzamide SPECT (Eisensehr et al., 2000) found evidence of significantly reduced dopaminergic terminals and striatal D2 receptor density, respectively, in patients with RBD, though not to the same degree as in patients with PD. Patients with RBD are significantly less likely to have the tremor-dominant form of PD, have higher frequency of falls, and are less responsive to medications than PD patients without RBD (Postuma et al., 2008). Furthermore, patients with RBD have been found to have a high incidence of mild cognitive impairment (Gagnon et al., 2009), impaired color discrimination, olfactory dysfunction, and dysautonomia, in addition to motor impairment (Postuma et al., 2006). RBD has been also found to predict cognitive impairment in PD patients without dementia (Vendette et al., 2007). Sleep walking has been also demonstrated in PD patients with RBD (Poryazova et al., 2007). Only two cases with RBD have been examined at autopsy, showing evidence of Lewy body disease associated with degenerative changes in the SN and locus coeruleus in one case, but not in the other case (Boeve et al., 2007). Thus individuals with symptoms of RBD have a significantly increased risk of developing parkinsonism, particularly if functional imaging shows decreased nigrostriatal dopaminergic activity, over the next decade, but progression to neurodegenerative disease is not inevitable (Britton and Chaudhuri, 2009; Postuma et al., 2009a).

There is a growing body of evidence supporting the notion that dopamine activity is normally influenced by circadian factors (Rye and Jankovic, 2002). For example, tyrosine hydroxylase falls several hours before the person wakes, and its increase correlates with motor activity. It has been postulated that low doses of dopaminomimetic drugs stimulate D2 inhibitory autoreceptors located on cell bodies of neurons in the ventral tegmental area resulting in sedation. This is consistent with the findings that local (ventral tegmental area) application of D2 antagonists causes sedation while administration of amphetamines initiates and maintains wakefulness. Although the cerebrospinal fluid levels of hypocretin (Sutcliffe and de Lecea, 2002) have been reported to be normal in three PD patients with excessive daytime drowsiness, further studies are needed to explore the relationship between hypocretin and sleep disorders associated with PD (Overeem et al., 2002). Since the loss of dopamine in PD generally progresses from putamen to the caudate and eventually to the limbic areas, it has been postulated that it is loss of dopamine in these latter circuits, most characteristic of advanced disease, that is a potential factor in the expression of excessive daytime drowsiness and sleep-onset REM in PD (Rye and Jankovic, 2002).

Sensory abnormalities

In addition to motor and behavioral symptoms, PD patients often exhibit a variety of sensory deficits. Sensory complaints, such as paresthesias, akathisia, and oral and genital pain (Comella and Goetz, 1994; Ford et al., 1996; Djaldetti et al., 2004; Tinazzi et al., 2006; Defazio et al., 2008) are frequently not recognized as parkinsonian symptoms and result in an inappropriate and exhaustive diagnostic evaluation.

Olfactory function is typically impaired in 90% of PD cases, but hyposmia may be present in 25% of controls due to head trauma, rhinitis, and other causes. Several studies have demonstrated that hyposmia may be present even in very early stages of PD (Stern et al., 1994; Katzenschlager and Lees, 2004; Lee et al., 2006; Silveira-Moriyama et al., 2009b), and may predate other clinical symptoms of PD by at least 4 years (Ross et al., 2008). One study showed that idiopathic olfactory dysfunction (hyposmia) may be associated with a 10% increased risk of developing PD (Ponsen et al., 2004). Camicioli and colleagues (2001) found that a combination of finger tapping, olfaction ability (assessed by the University of Pennsylvania Smell Identification Test, or UPSIT), and visual contrast sensitivity, or Paired Associates Learning, discriminated between PD patients and controls with 90% accuracy. A color-coded probability scale has been developed to interpret UPSIT in patients with suspected parkinsonism (Silveira-Moriyama et al., 2009a). In one study, after 5 years of prospective follow-up 5/40 (12.5%) hyposmic first-degree relatives of patients with PD fulfilled clinical diagnostic criteria for PD; none of the other 349 relatives available for follow-up developed PD (Ponsen et al., 2010). All hyposmic individuals developing PD had an abnormal baseline 2beta-carboxymethoxy-3-beta-(4[^{123}I]iodophenyl) tropane (β-CIT) SPECT scan. Thus a two-step approach using olfactory testing followed by dopamine transporter (DAT) SPECT scanning in hyposmic individuals appears to have a high sensitivity and specificity in detecting PD. The mechanism of olfactory loss in PD is not well understood, but it does not appear to be due to damage to the olfactory epithelium, but rather results from abnormalities in central regions involved in odor perception (Witt et al., 2009). In fact, recent studies indicate that cholinergic denervation of the limbic archicortex is a more important determinant of hyposmia than nigrostriatal dopaminergic denervation in patients with PD and that deficits in odor identification are associated with greater cognitive impairment (Bohnen et al., 2010). These findings are based on a study of 58 patients with PD who underwent PET scans using [^{11}C]PMP acetylcholinesterase as a cholinergic ligand. The investigators found that odor identification test scores correlated

positively with acetylcholinesterase activity in the hippocampal formation ($r = 0.56$, $P < 0.0001$), amygdala ($r = 0.50$, $P < 0.0001$) and neocortex ($r = 0.46$, $P = 0.0003$) and with cognitive measures such as episodic verbal learning ($r = 0.30$, $P < 0.05$).

To determine which signs in very early, presymptomatic or prodromal phase of the disease predict the subsequent development of PD, Montgomery and colleagues (1999) studied 80 first-degree relatives of patients with PD and 100 normal controls using a battery of tests of motor function, mood, and olfaction (Tissingh et al., 2001; Double et al., 2003). They found that 22.5% of the relatives and only 9% of the normal controls had abnormal scores. It is, of course, not known how many of the relatives with abnormal scores will develop PD; therefore, the specificity and sensitivity of the test battery in predicting PD cannot be determined. UPSIT administered to 62 twin pairs who were discordant for PD showed that smell identification was reduced in the twins affected with PD in comparison to those without symptoms (Marras et al., 2005a). After a mean interval of 7.3 years, 19 of the twins were retested. Neither of two twins who developed new PD had had impaired smell identification at baseline, although their UPSIT scores declined more than those of the other 17 twins. The authors concluded that "smell identification ability may not be a sensitive indicator of future PD 7 or more years before the development of motor signs." In another study of 295 PD patients and 150 controls, olfactory impairment was found to be an independent feature of PD, unrelated to other PD symptoms (Verbaan et al., 2008). Furthermore, *parkin* and *DJ-1* mutation carriers had normal olfaction. Impaired olfaction correlates well with decreased β-CIT uptake and may precede the onset of motor symptoms of PD (Berendse et al., 2002; Siderowf et al., 2005) and with decreased ^{123}I-metaiodobenzylguanidine (MIBG) cardiac uptake (Lee et al., 2006). Reduced olfaction in PD may be related to a neuronal loss in the corticomedial amygdala (Harding et al., 2002) or to an increase of dopaminergic neurons in the olfactory bulb (dopamine inhibits olfactory transmission), as determined by increased tyrosine hydroxylase-reactive neurons (Huisman et al., 2004). It is important to point out, however, that olfaction is impaired in the elderly population. Using the San Diego Odor Identification Test and self-report, Murphy and colleagues (2002) found that 24.5% of people between the ages of 53 and 97 have impaired olfaction, and the incidence is 62.5% in people over age 80. Loss of smell is characteristic of PD and Alzheimer disease but is usually not present in ET, PSP, corticobasal degeneration, vascular parkinsonism (Katzenschlager et al., 2004), or parkinsonism due to *parkin* mutation (Khan et al., 2004). Within PD, patients with the tremor-dominant form with family history were found to have less olfaction loss than those without family history, suggesting that the familial tremor-dominant form of PD might be a different disease from sporadic PD (Ondo and Lai, 2005). In 19 patients with PARK8 (*LRRK2* G2019S mutations), the mean UPSIT scores were significantly lower than in healthy controls ($P < 0.001$) and similar to that of patients with PD, but the score was normal in two asymptomatic carriers (Silveira-Moriyama et al., 2008). α-Synuclein pathology, including Lewy bodies, was found in the rhinencephalon of four brains of the *LRRK2* patients who had hyposmia. Biopsy of olfactory nasal neurons does not aid in differentiating PD and Alzheimer disease from the other neurodegenerative disorders (Hawkes, 2003). Some investigators think that olfactory testing is comparable to other diagnostic tests, such as MRI, SPECT, and neuropsychologic testing, in differentiating PD from other parkinsonian disorders and in early detection of PD (Katzenschlager and Lees, 2004). Olfactory impairment early in the course of PD has led to the hypothesis for the pathogenesis of PD suggesting that some infectious, prion-like process, or environmental agent enters the brain via the olfactory route (Doty, 2008; Lerner and Bagic, 2008). The prodromal phase, often associated with olfactory deficit, dysautonomia, and sleep disorder, lasts months or years before the onset of typical motor features of PD (Hawkes, 2008).

There are other sensory abnormalities in patients with PD. One study showed that patients with PD who experience pain have increased sensitivity to painful stimuli (Djaldetti et al., 2004). Using quantitative sensory testing with thermal probes, laser-evoked potentials (LEPs), and laser-induced sudomotor skin responses (1-SSRs) in "off" and "on" conditions, Schestatsky et al. (2007) found lower heat pain and laser pinprick thresholds, higher LEP amplitudes, and less habituation of sympathetic sudomotor responses to repetitive pain stimuli in patients with PD who complained of primary central pain as compared with PD patients without pain and control subjects, suggesting an abnormal control of the effects of pain inputs on autonomic centers. Joint position has been found to be impaired in some patients with PD (Zia et al., 2000).

There is some evidence that while the visual acuity in PD is usually spared, some patients experience progressive impairment of color discrimination, contrast sensitivity (especially in the blue-green axis), visual speed, visual construction, and visual memory (Bodis-Wollner, 2002; Diederich et al., 2002; Uc et al., 2005). A review of 81 PD patients found nonmotor tasks were affected by visual or visuospatial impairment (Davidsdottir et al., 2005). Motor disturbances were directly attributed to visual hallucinations, double vision, and estimating spatial relations, and most often produced freezing of gait. Although color visual discrimination, as measured by the Farnsworth Munsell 100 Hue Test, has been found to be abnormal in some patients with PD, this does not appear to be an early marker for PD (Veselá et al., 2001). It is not known whether this visual dysfunction is due to retinal or postretinal abnormality. In their review of ophthalmologic features of PD, Biousse and colleagues (2004) noted that any of the following may contribute to the ocular and visual complaints in patients with PD: decreased blink rate, ocular surface irritation, altered tear film, visual hallucinations, blepharospasm, decreased blink rate, and decreased convergence. Electrophysiologic testing has revealed prolonged visual evoked potential latencies and abnormal electroretinographic patterns, suggesting retinal ganglion cell impairment playing a role in the loss of acuity in PD subjects (Sartucci et al., 2003). Disturbances in visual pathway from the retina to the occipital cortex have been demonstrated and may account for a large variety of visual disturbances experienced by patients with PD (Archibald et al., 2009). In one study, levodopa was found to significantly increase response time for reflexive (stimulus driven) prosaccades and reduced error rate for voluntary (internally guided) antisaccades, suggesting that medicated patients are better able to plan and execute voluntary eye movements, mediated by the frontostriatal system (Hood et al., 2007).

Motor fluctuations related to levodopa therapy are well recognized, but what is not readily appreciated is that many patients also experience nonmotor fluctuations, such as sensory symptoms, dyspnea, facial flushing, hunger (and sweet cravings), and other symptoms (Hillen and Sage, 1996). Weight loss is another, though poorly understood, typical manifestation of PD (Jankovic et al., 1992; Ondo et al., 2000; Chen et al., 2003; Lorefalt et al., 2004; Bachmann and Trenkwalder, 2006; Uc et al., 2006b; Barichella et al., 2009). In one study, PD patients lost 7.7% ± 1.5% of body weight over a mean of 7.2 years of follow-up, as compared to only 0.2% ± 0.7% over a mean of 10 years (55.6% of PD patients vs. 20.5% of controls lost >5% of weight, $P < 0.001$) (Uc et al., 2006b). The weight loss correlated with worsening of parkinsonism, age at diagnosis, visual hallucinations, and possibly dementia. In Huntington disease, weight loss has been attributed to higher sedentary energy expenditure (Pratley et al., 2000), but the mechanism of weight loss in PD is not well understood, though it is not thought to be due to reduced energy intake (Chen et al., 2003). It is important to note that these nonmotor symptoms may be as disabling as the classic motor symptoms or even more so (Lang and Obeso, 2004).

While most animal models of PD have focused on the motor symptoms, there is growing interest in developing models with both motor and nonmotor features to better simulate the human condition. Mice genetically engineered to have vesicular monoamine 2 (VMAT2) deficiency, in addition to progressive loss of striatal dopamine, levodopa-responsive motor deficits, α-synuclein accumulation, and nigral dopaminergic cell loss, also display progressive deficits in olfactory discrimination, delayed gastric emptying, altered sleep latency, anxiety-like behavior, and age-dependent depressive behavior (Taylor et al., 2009). Restoring monoamine function in these animals (and patients with PD) may be beneficial in treating the disease.

Clinical-pathologic correlations

The clinical heterogeneity in parkinsonian patients suggests that there is variable involvement of the dopaminergic and other neurotransmitter systems. Alternatively, the subgroups might represent different clinical-pathologic entities, thus indicating that PD is not a uniform disease but a syndrome. By using statistical cluster analysis of 120 patients with early PD, four main subgroups were identified: (1) young-onset, (2) tremor-dominant, (3) non-tremor-dominant with cognitive impairment and mild depression, and (4) rapid disease progression but no cognitive impairment (Lewis et al., 2005). A systematic review of 242 pathologically verified cases of PD showed that the cases were segregated into earlier disease onset (25%), tremor-dominant (31%), non-tremor-dominant (36%), and rapid disease progression without dementia (8%) subgroups (Selikhova et al., 2009). As noted before, the non-tremor cases were more likely to have cognitive disability, the earlier disease onset group had the longest duration to death and greatest delay to the onset of falls and cognitive decline, and rapid disease progression was associated with older age, early depression, and early midline motor symptoms. Furthermore, the non-tremor dominant subgroup had significantly more cortical Lewy bodies, amyloid-beta plaque load, and cerebral amyloid angiopathy than early disease onset and tremor-dominant groups.

Highly predictive diagnostic criteria are essential to select an appropriate patient population for genetic studies and clinical trials (Gelb et al., 1999; Dickson et al., 2009). In support of the notion that the PIGD subgroup represents a distinct disorder, separate from PD, is the finding that only 27% of patients with the PIGD form of idiopathic parkinsonism have Lewy bodies at autopsy (Rajput et al., 1993). In the London brain bank series, only 11% of the 100 pathologically proven cases of PD had tremor-dominant disease, and 23% had "akinetic/rigid" disease; the rest (64%) were diagnosed as having a "mixed pattern" (Hughes et al., 1993). In contrast to the 76–100% occurrence of tremor in PD, only 31% of those with atypical parkinsonism (progressive supranuclear palsy, or PSP; striatonigral degeneration, or SND; Shy–Drager syndrome, or SDS; and the combination of SND and olivopontocerebellar atrophy, or OPCA) had rest tremor (Rajput et al., 1991), and 50% of the 24 cases with non-PD parkinsonism in the London series had tremor, type not specified (Hughes et al., 1992b). Women tend to have the tremor-dominant form of PD, which has a slower progression than the non-tremor forms.

In a clinical-pathologic study, Hirsch and colleagues (1992) have demonstrated that patients with PD and prominent tremor have degeneration of a subgroup of midbrain (A8) neurons, whereas this area is spared in PD patients without tremor. Other clinical-pathologic studies have confirmed that the tremor-dominant type of PD shows more damage to the retrorubral field A8, containing mainly calretinin-staining cells but only a few tyrosine hydroxylase and dopamine transporter immunoreactive neurons (Jellinger, 1999). Also the tremor-dominant PD seems to be associated with more severe neuron loss in medial than in lateral zona compacta of SN. The ventral (rostral and caudal) GPi seems to be relatively spared in tremor-dominant PD as the dopamine levels in this area are essentially normal, but are markedly decreased in the other pallidal regions (Rajput et al., 2008). In contrast, A8 is rather preserved in the PIGD, rigid-akinetic PD, possibly owing to the protective role of calcium-binding protein. Using voxel-based morphometry of 3 teslas, T1-weighted MR images in 14 patients with tremor-dominant PD and 10 PD patients without rest tremor, decreased gray matter volume in the cerebellum was associated with parkinsonian rest tremor (Benninger et al., 2009). These findings support the hypothesis that differential damage of subpopulations of neuronal systems is responsible for the diversity of phenotypes seen in PD and other parkinsonian disorders. Detailed clinical-pathologic-biochemical studies will be required to prove or disprove this hypothesis.

Using ^{18}F-6-fluorodopa, Vingerhoets and colleagues (1997) demonstrated that bradykinesia is the parkinsonian sign that correlates best with nigrostriatal deficiency. In contrast, patients with the tremor-dominant PD have increased metabolic activity in the pons, thalamus, and motor association cortices (Antonini et al., 1998). The presence of tremor in PD also seems to correlate with serotonergic dysfunction as suggested by a 27% reduction in the midbrain raphe 5-HT$_{1A}$ binding demonstrated by ^{11}C-WAY 100635 PET scans

(Doder et al., 2003). In contrast to dopamine, which is reduced by >80% in the caudate and >98% in the putamen of brains of patients with PD, serotonin markers are reduced by 30–66% (Kish et al., 2008). While the reduction of serotonin in the caudate nucleus has been suggested to be associated with "associative-cognitive problems," the clinical significance of relative serotonin preservation in the putamen is not known. The role of serotonin in motor dysfunction, levodopa-induced dyskinesias, mood, and psychosis associated with PD has been recently reviewed, but because of lack of data no definite conclusions can be made (Fox et al., 2009).

There is a growing appreciation not only for the clinical heterogeneity of PD, but also for genetic heterogeneity (Tan and Jankovic, 2006). As a result, the notion of PD is evolving from the traditional view of a single clinical-pathologic entity to "Parkinson diseases" with different etiologies and clinical presentations. For example, the autosomal recessive juvenile parkinsonism (AR-JP) due to mutation in the *parkin* gene on chromosome 6q25.2–27 (PARK2) may present with a dystonic gait or camptocormia during adolescence or early adulthood (or even in the sixth or seventh decade) and with levodopa-responsive dystonia and may be characterized by symmetric onset, marked sleep benefit, early levodopa-induced dyskinesias, hemiparkinsonism–hemiatrophy, hyperreflexia, and "slow" orthostatic tremor. Patients with *parkin* mutation seem to have a slower disease course (Lücking et al., 2000; Rawal et al., 2003; Schrag and Schott, 2006). Furthermore, similar to EOPD, patients with *parkin* mutations show marked decrease in striatal ^{18}F-FDOPA PET, but in contrast to PD, *parkin* patients show additional reductions in caudate and midbrain as well as significantly decreased raclopride binding in striatal, thalamic, and cortical areas (Scherfler et al., 2004). PARK2 (due to *parkin* mutations) is the most common cause of parkinsonism (EOPD), followed by *DJ-1*, and *PINK1* mutations, although these genetic causes accounted for only 9% of all cases of EOPD (Macedo et al., 2009). Other causes of levodopa-responsive juvenile parkinsonism or EOPD include dopa-responsive dystonia, spinocerebellar atrophy type 2 (SCA2), SCA3, and other causes (Paviour et al., 2004).

Subtypes and natural history of Parkinson disease

The rich and variable clinical expression of PD has encouraged a search for distinct patterns of neurologic deficits that may define parkinsonian subtypes and predict the future course (Jankovic, 2005; Le et al., 2009). On the basis of an analysis of a cohort of 800 PD patients, two major subtypes were identified: one characterized by tremor as the dominant parkinsonian feature and the other dominated by PIGD (Zetusky et al., 1985; Jankovic et al., 1990; McDermott et al., 1995). The mean tremor score was defined as the mean of the sum of the baseline tremor (UPDRS Part II) and tremor scores (UPDRS Part III) for face, right and left hand, right and left foot, and right and left hand action tremor. The mean PIGD score was defined as the sum of an individual's baseline falling, freezing, walking, gait, and postural stability UPDRS scores divided by five. Patients were categorized as having tremor-dominant PD if the ratio of the mean tremor score to the mean PIGD score was ≥1.50 and as PIGD dominant if the ratio was ≤1.00 (Jankovic et al., 1990). The tremor-dominant form of PD seems to be associated with a relatively preserved mental status, earlier age at onset, and a slower progression of the disease than the PIGD subtype, which is characterized by more severe bradykinesia and a more rapidly progressive course (Post et al., 2007). Furthermore, several studies have demonstrated that patients with the PIGD form of PD have more cognitive impairment than those with the tremor-dominant form of PD (Verbaan et al., 2007b). A presentation with bradykinesia and the PIGD type of PD seems to be associated with a relatively malignant course, whereas PD patients who are young and have tremor at the onset of their disease seem to have a slower progression and a more favorable prognosis. In a meta-analysis of 1535 titles and abstracts, of which 27 fulfilled a set of predetermined criteria, higher age at onset and higher PIGD score provided the strongest evidence of poor prognosis (Post et al., 2007). In one study, the relative risk of death in patients with the tremor-dominant form of PD was significantly lower than in PD patients without rest tremor (1.52 vs. 2.04, $P < 0.01$) (Elbaz et al., 2003). Using the SPES/SCOPA rating scale (Marinus et al., 2004) in 399 PD patients, four distinct motor patterns were identified: tremor-dominant, bradykinetic-rigid, and two types of axial patterns: (a) rise, gait, postural instability (similar to PIGD) and (b) freezing, speech, and swallowing, the latter related to complications of dopaminergic therapy (van Rooden et al., 2009). In a random sample of 173 patients, four different subtypes were identified: rapid disease progression subtype, young-onset subtype, non-tremor-dominant subtype (associated with hypokinesia, rigidity, postural instability and gait disorder, cognitive deterioration, depressive and apathetic symptoms, and hallucinations), and a tremor-dominant subtype (Reijnders et al., 2009). The AAN Practice Parameter on diagnosis and prognosis of new-onset PD made the following conclusions: (1) Early falls, poor response to levodopa, symmetry of motor manifestations, lack of tremor, and early autonomic dysfunction are probably useful in distinguishing other parkinsonian syndromes from PD. (2) Levodopa or apomorphine challenge and olfactory testing are probably useful in distinguishing PD from other parkinsonian syndromes. (3) Predictive factors for more rapid motor progression, nursing home placement, and shorter survival time include older age at onset of PD, associated comorbidities, presentation with rigidity and bradykinesia, and decreased dopamine responsiveness (Suchowersky et al., 2006).

The more favorable course of the tremor-dominant form of PD is also supported by the finding that the reduction in FDOPA uptake, as measured by PET and expressed as K_i, was 12.8% over a 2-year period in PD patients with severe tremor compared with a 19.4% reduction in the mild or no tremor group ($P = 0.04$) (Whone et al., 2002). Furthermore, Hilker and colleagues (2005) provided evidence for a variable progression of the disease based on the clinical phenotype. Similar to other studies (Jankovic and Kapadia, 2001), they showed that patients with the tremor-dominant form of PD progressed at a slower rate than patients with the other PD subtypes (Figs 4.5 and 4.6). A clinicopathologic study of 166 patients with PD followed for over 39 years (1968–2006) showed that the age at onset was significantly younger,

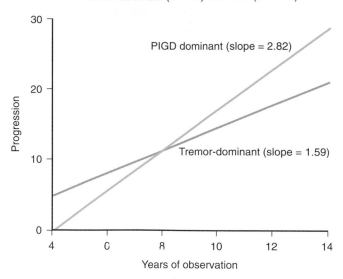

Figure 4.5 More rapid progression of PIGD versus tremor-dominant form of PD. *Data from Jankovic J, Kapadia AS. Functional decline in Parkinson's disease. Arch Neurol 2001;58:1611–1615.*

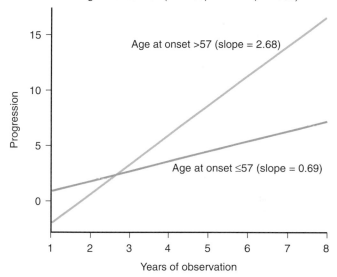

Figure 4.6 Young-onset PD progresses at a slower rate than late-onset PD. *Data from Jankovic J, Kapadia AS. Functional decline in Parkinson's disease. Arch Neurol 2001;58:1611–1615.*

progression to Hoehn and Yahr stage 4 was slower, and dementia was least common in the tremor-dominant cases (Rajput et al., 2009). In addition, the tremor-dominant form of PD is associated with a more frequent family history of tremor, and it is more likely to have coexistent ET (Jankovic et al., 1995; Shahed and Jankovic, 2007). In 22 patients with PD with family history of ET, 90% (20 of 22) had the tremor-predominant subtype of PD (Hedera et al., 2009). Axial impairment, probably mediated predominantly by non-dopaminergic systems, is associated with incident dementia (Levy et al., 2000). While executive function was found to be impaired in both familial and sporadic PD, explicit memory recall is more impaired in the sporadic form of PD (Dujardin et al., 2001).

To determine whether age at onset is a predictor of the future course and response to levodopa, 48 patients with YOPD (onset between 20 and 40 years of age) were compared to 123 late-onset PD (LOPD) patients (onset at 60 years of age or older) (Jankovic et al., 1997). YOPD patients presented more frequently with rigidity, while LOPD presented more frequently with PIGD; there was no difference in the occurrence of tremor at onset. YOPD patients generally respond to levodopa better but are more likely to develop dyskinesias and "wearing-off" (Quinn et al., 1987; Jankovic et al., 1997; Schrag et al., 1998; Kumar et al., 2005; Schrag and Schott, 2006; Wickremaratchi et al., 2009). Furthermore, the YOPD subtype is characterized by slower progression of disease, increased rate of dystonia and levodopa-induced dyskinesia, and less motor and cognitive disability (Graham and Sagar, 1999; Diederich et al., 2003; Wickremaratchi et al., 2009). Many, if not most, YOPD patients have been found to have *parkin* mutations (PARK2) or other mutations in other gene loci (PARK6 and PARK7), but their clinical characteristics and ^{18}F-FDOPA uptake are similar to those in other YOPD patients without mutations (Thobois et al., 2003). PD seems to have a much greater psychosocial impact on YOPD patients in terms of loss of employment, disruption of family life, perceived stigmatization, and depression than on LOPD patients (Schrag et al., 2003).

There is growing evidence that the progression of PD is not linear and that the rate of deterioration is much more rapid in the early phase of the disease (Jankovic, 2005; Schapira and Obeso, 2006; Lang, 2007; Maetzler et al., 2009). This is also supported by functional imaging (FDOPA PET) (Brück et al., 2009) and postmortem pathologic studies (Fearnley and Lees, 1991) (see below). To study the overall rate of functional decline and to assess the progression of different signs of PD, 297 patients (181 males) with clinically diagnosed PD for at least 3 years were prospectively followed (Jankovic and Kapadia, 2001) (Figs 4.5 and 4.6). Data from 1731 visits over a period of an average of 6.36 years (range: 3–17) were analyzed. The annual rate of decline in the total UPDRS scores was 1.34 units when assessed during "on" and 1.58 when assessed during "off." Patients with older age at onset had a more rapid progression of disease than those with younger age at onset. Furthermore, the older-onset group had significantly more progression in mentation, freezing, and Parts I and II UPDRS subscores. Handwriting was the only component of UPDRS that did not significantly deteriorate during the observation period. Regression analysis of 108 patients, whose symptoms were rated during their "off" state, showed a faster rate of cognitive decline as the age at onset increased. The slopes of progression in UPDRS scores, when adjusted for age at initial visit, were steeper for the PIGD group of patients than in the tremor-dominant group. In a study of 573 patients with newly diagnosed PD, PIGD, cognitive impairment, and hallucinations were among the most reliable predictors of high mortality (Lo et al., 2009).

These results are similar to the 1.5-point annual decline, based on longitudinal assessments using the motor function (Part III) portion of the UPDRS, reported by Louis and colleagues (1999) in a community-based study of 237 patients with PD who were followed up prospectively for a mean of 3.30 years. Another prospective study, involving 232 patients with PD, showed annual decline in UPDRS motor score of 3.3 points (range 0–108; 3.1%) and 0.16 points in Hoehn–Yahr stage (range 0–5; 3.2%), with slower and more restricted decline in YOPD cases (Alves et al., 2005). In a prospective study of 145 clinic-based patients followed for 1 year and 124 community-based patients followed for 4 years, the annual mean rate of deterioration in motor and disability scores ranged between 2.4% and 7.4% (Schrag et al., 2007b). These findings, based on longitudinal follow-up data, provide evidence for a variable course of progression of the different PD symptoms, thus implying different biochemical or degenerative mechanisms for the various clinical features associated with PD. Although the deterioration in motor scores seems to flatten in more advanced stages of the disease, disability scores continued to progress, probably because of emergence of nonmotor symptoms. The study by Greffard and colleagues (2006) has also suggested that the rate of progression might not be linear and that the disease might progress more rapidly initially (about 8–10 UPDRS points in the first year) and the rate of deterioration slows in more advanced stages of the disease. This is supported by the findings in moderately advanced cases of PD requiring levodopa treatment compared with patients in early stages of the disease such as those enrolled in the DATATOP study (Parkinson Study Group, 1998). In that study of early, previously untreated patients, the rate of annual decline in the total UPDRS score was 14.02 ± 12.32 (mean ± SD) in the placebo-treated group. This is nearly identical to the 1 UPDRS unit of decline per month in the ELLDOPA study (Fahn et al., 2004). In contrast, in a group of 238 patients treated with levodopa, bromocriptine, or both in whom progression was estimated on the basis of a retrospectively determined duration of the symptoms, the annual rate of decline in bradykinesia score was 3.5% during the first year but was estimated to be only 1.5% in the tenth year (Lee et al., 1994). More rapid progression in the early stages than in more advanced stages of the disease is also suggested by the finding of mean of 0.5 annual decline in FDOPA influx constant in the contralateral putamen in the first 2 years and only 0.2 during the subsequent 3 years (Brück et al., 2009).

Interestingly, in a study of 787 older (mean age at baseline: 75.4 years) Catholic clergy without clinically diagnosed PD who were prospectively followed for up to 7 years, the average decline in UPDRS units was 0.69 per year (Wilson et al., 2002). In those subjects who had some worsening of their global UPDRS score (79% of all subjects), the risk of death was 2.93 times the rate in those without progression (21%). The risk of death was associated with worsening of gait and posture but not with rigidity or postural reflex impairment, even though the latter two signs (but not bradykinesia or tremor) also worsened. The average reported rate of decline in total UPDRS is about 8 units per year. A systematic review of 13 studies investigating predictors of prognosis concluded that greater baseline impairment, early cognitive disturbance, older age, and lack of tremor at onset are relatively predictive of a poor prognosis (Marras et al., 2002). The aging process has been found to contribute particularly to the axial (gait and postural) impairment in PD (Levy et al., 2005) and advancing age, rather than duration of the disease, seems to be the most important determinant of clinical progression (Levy, 2007).

The natural history of PD appears to be influenced not only by the age at onset and the clinical presentation, but also by a number of other factors, such as stress (Tanner and Goldman, 1996), pregnancy (Shulman et al., 2000), intercurrent illness (Onofrj and Thomas, 2005), and therapy. Infection, gastrointestinal disorder, and surgery are among the most common causes of the syndrome of acute akinesia, a sudden deterioration in motor performance that usually last 4–26 days and represents a life-threatening complication of PD, usually requiring hospitalization (Onofrj and Thomas, 2005). Although therapeutic advances have had a positive impact on the quality of life, epidemiologic studies have not been able to demonstrate that levodopa significantly prolongs life (Clarke, 1995). Several studies, however, have concluded that PD patients have a nearly normal life expectancy (Lilienfeld et al., 1990; Clarke, 1995; Parkinson Study Group, 1998). In a prospective study of 800 patients who were followed longitudinally from the early stages of their disease for an average of 8.2 years, the overall death rate was 2.1% per year, which was similar to that of an age- and gender-matched US population without PD (Parkinson Study Group, 1998). In a 10-year Sydney multicenter follow-up of 149 patients with PD initially enrolled in a double-blind study of levodopa-carbidopa versus bromocriptine, the standardized mortality ratio (SMR) was 1.58, which was significantly higher than that of the Australian population ($P < 0.001$) (Hely et al., 1999). In a subsequent report, based on a population-based study, Morgante and colleagues (2000) showed a relative risk of death in patients with PD of 2.3 (95% confidence interval 1.60–3.39). In another study of 170 elderly patients with PD, with a mean age at death of 82 years, who were followed for a median of 9.4 years, the relative risk of death compared to referent subjects was 1.60 (95% confidence interval 1.30–1.8), and the mean duration of illness was 12.8 years (Fall et al., 2003). Pneumonia was the most frequent cause of death in both studies. The SMR was reported to be 1.52 in a community-based study of a Norwegian population (Herlofson et al., 2004). The hazard ratio for mortality was 1.64 for patients with PD compared to controls, but the mortality increased if there was associated dementia, depression, or both (Hughes et al., 2004). In a 15-year follow-up of patients who were originally enrolled in the Sydney Multicenter Study of PD comparing levodopa with low-dose bromocriptine, the SMR was 1.86 (Hely et al., 2005). In a comprehensive review of the literature, SMR has been reported to range between 1 and 3.4 (Ishihara et al., 2007). On the basis of 296 deaths in a cohort of patients who were originally enrolled in the DATATOP study and followed for 13 years, survival was found to be strongly related to response to levodopa (Marras et al., 2005b). SMR based on a cohort analysis of 22 071 participants in the Physicians' Health Study, with 560 incident cases of PD, was found to be 2.32 (95% CI 1.85–2.92) (Driver et al., 2008). Age-specific life expectancy was found to be reduced in patients with PD, particularly those with young-onset PD (Ishihara et al., 2007). In a 20-year follow-up study of 238 consecutive patients with PD, the SMR was 0.9 by 10 years and 1.3 by 20–30 years (Diem-Zangerl et al., 2009). The authors concluded that when PD patients are "Under regular specialist care using all currently available therapies, life expectancy in PD does not appear seriously compromised, but male gender, gait disorder, and absent rest tremor at presentation are associated with poorer long-term survival."

Differential diagnosis

Causes of parkinsonism other than PD can be classified as secondary, multiple system degeneration, or the parkinsonism-plus syndromes and heredodegenerative disorders (Stacy and Jankovic, 1992) (Table 4.3). Features that are found to be particularly useful in differentiating PD from other parkinsonian disorders include absence or paucity of tremor, early gait abnormality (such as freezing), postural instability, pyramidal tract findings, and poor response to levodopa (Tables 4.1 and 4.4). Although good response to levodopa is often used as an index of well-preserved postsynaptic receptors, supporting the diagnosis of PD, only 77% of pathologically proven cases had "good" or "excellent" initial levodopa response in the London series (Hughes et al., 1993). Furthermore, two patients with pathologically proven Lewy body parkinsonism but without response to levodopa have been reported (Mark et al., 1992). Therefore, while improvement with levodopa supports the diagnosis of PD, response to levodopa cannot be used to reliably differentiate PD from other parkinsonian disorders (Parati et al., 1993). Subcutaneous injection of apomorphine, a rapidly active dopamine agonist, has been used to predict response to levodopa and thus to differentiate between PD and other parkinsonian disorders (Hughes et al., 1990; D'Costa et al., 1991; Bonuccelli et al., 1993). Although PD patients are much more likely to improve with apomorphine, this test is cumbersome, and it does not reliably differentiate PD from the atypical parkinsonian disorders. Furthermore, response to apomorphine test is not superior to chronic levodopa therapy in diagnosis of PD; therefore, this test adds little or nothing to the diagnostic evaluation (Clarke and Davies, 2000). The differences in response to dopaminergic drugs may be partly explained by differences in the density of postsynaptic dopamine receptors. These receptors are preserved in PD, in which the brunt of the pathology is in the SN, whereas they are usually decreased in other parkinsonian disorders in which the striatum is additionally affected.

Perhaps expression analysis of genes in brains of patients with various neurodegenerative disorders, and recognizing disease-specific patterns will in the future assist in differentiating PD from other parkinsonian disorders. For example, using microarray technology in SN samples from six patients with PD, two with PSP, one with frontotemporal dementia–parkinsonism (FTDP), and five controls, Hauser and colleagues (2005) found 142 genes that were differentially expressed in PD cases and controls, 96 in the combination of PSP-FTDP, and 12 that were common to all three disorders. Further studies are needed to confirm this intriguing finding.

Clinical rating scales and other assessments

Although a variety of neurophysiologic and computer-based methods have been proposed to quantitate the severity of the various parkinsonian symptoms and signs, most studies rely on clinical rating scales, particularly the Unified

Table 4.3 Classification of parkinsonism (see also Table 9.1 for a more complete list)

I. Primary (idiopathic) parkinsonism

- Parkinson disease
- Juvenile parkinsonism

II. Multisystem degenerations (parkinsonism-plus)

- Progressive supranuclear palsy (PSP), Steele–Richardson–Olszewski disease (SRO)
- Multiple system atrophy (MSA)
- Striatonigral degeneration (SND or MSA-P)
- Olivopontocerebellar atrophy (OPCA or MSA-C)
- Dementia with Lewy Bodies (DLBD)
- Lytico-bodig or parkinsonism–dementia–ALS complex of Guam (PDACG)
- Cortical-basal ganglionic degeneration (CBGD)
- Progressive pallidal atrophy
- Pallidopyramidal disease (PARK15)

III. Heredodegenerative parkinsonism

- Hereditary juvenile dystonia–parkinsonism
- Autosomal dominant Lewy body disease
- Huntington disease
- Wilson disease
- Hereditary ceruloplasmin deficiency
- Neurodegeneration with brain iron accumulation
- Aceruloplasminemia
- Neuroferritinopathy
- Pantothenate kinase associated neurodegeneration (PKAN)
- PLA2G6 associated neurodegeneration (PLAN)
- Fatty acid hydroxylase associated neurodegeneration (FAHN)
- ATP13A2 mutation (Kufor–Rakeb disease) and lysosomal disorders
- Woodhouse–Sakati syndrome (WSS)

- Olivopontocerebellar and spinocerebellar degenerations
- Spinocerebellar ataxia (SCA) type 2, 3, 6, 12, 21
- Frontotemporal dementia
- Gerstmann–Sträussler–Scheinker disease
- Familial progressive subcortical gliosis
- Lubag (X-linked dystonia–parkinsonism)
- Familial basal ganglia calcification
- Mitochondrial cytopathies with striatal necrosis
- Ceroid lipofuscinosis
- Familial parkinsonism with peripheral neuropathy
- Parkinsonian-pyramidal syndrome
- Neuroacanthocytosis
- Hereditary hemochromatosis

IV. Secondary (acquired, symptomatic) parkinsonism

- Infectious: postencephalitic, AIDS, subacute sclerosing panencephalitis, Creuzfeldt–Jakob disease, prion diseases
- Drugs: dopamine receptor blocking drugs (antipsychotic, antiemetic drugs), reserpine, tetrabenazine, alpha-methyl-dopa, lithium, flunarizine, cinnarizine
- Toxins: 1-methyl-4-phenyl-1,2,3,6-tetrahydropyridine, CO, Mn, Hg, CS_2, cyanide, methanol, ethanol
- Vascular: multi-infarct, Binswanger disease
- Trauma: pugilistic encephalopathy
- Other: parathyroid abnormalities, hypothyroidism, hepatocerebral degeneration, brain tumor, paraneoplastic, normal pressure hydrocephalus, noncommunicating hydrocephalus, syringomesencephalia, hemiatrophy-hemiparkinsonism, peripherally induced tremor and parkinsonism, and psychogenic

Reprinted with permission from Jankovic J, Lang AE: Classification of movement disorders. In Germano IM (ed): Surgical Treatment of Movement Disorders. Lebanon, NH, American Association of Neurological Surgeons, 1998, pp. 3–18.

Table 4.4 Motor and nonmotor symptoms associated with PD

Motor	Nonmotor
Tremor, bradykinesia, rigidity, postural instability	Behavioral: depression, apathy, anhedonia, pseudobulbar effect, cautious personality, fatigue
Hypomimia, dysarthria, dysphagia, sialorrhea	Cognitive: bradyphrenia, tip-of-the-tongue, dementia
Microphagia, difficulties cutting food, feeding, dressing, hygiene; slow ADL	Sensory: anosmia, ageusia, impaired visual acuity, contrast, and color sensitivity, paresthesias, pain (shoulder)
Decreased arm swing, shuffling gait, freezing, festination, difficulty rising from chair, turning in bed	Dysautonomia: orthostatic hypotension, constipation, urinary and sexual dysfunction, abnormal swelling, seborrhea, rhinorrhea, weight loss
Glabellar reflex, blepharospasm, dystonia, skeletal deformities, striatal hand/foot	Sleep disorders: RBD, vivid dreams, daytime drowsiness, sleep fragmentation, restless legs syndrome?

Parkinson's Disease Rating Scale (UPDRS), Hoehn–Yahr Staging Scale (Goetz et al., 2004), and Schwab–England Scale of activities of daily living (Fahn et al., 1987; Goetz et al., 1994, 1995; Bennett et al., 1997; Stebbins et al., 1999; Ramaker et al., 2002). The historical section of the UPDRS can be self-administered and reliably completed by nondemented patients (Louis et al., 1996).The Short (0 to 3) Parkinson's Evaluation Scale (SPES) and the Scale for Outcomes in Parkinson's Disease (SCOPA) are both short, reliable scales that can be used in both research and practice (Marinus et al., 2004). Although the UPDRS has a number of limitations (Movement Disorder Society Task Force on Rating Scales for Parkinson's Disease, 2003) such as ambiguities in the written text, inadequate instructions for raters, some metric flaws, and inadequate screening questions for nonmotor symptoms, the scale is the most frequently used instrument in numerous clinical trials. In order to address some of the limitations of the original UPDRS scale, a revised scale, MDS-UPDRS, has been developed (Goetz et al., 2007, 2008b). This new MDS-UPDRS retains the original UPDRS structure of four parts with a total summed score, but the parts have been modified to provide a section that integrates nonmotor elements of PD: I: Nonmotor

Experiences of Daily Living; II: Motor Experiences of Daily Living; III: Motor Examination; IV: Motor Complications. All items have five response options with uniform anchors of 0 = normal, 1 = slight, 2 = mild, 3 = moderate, 4 = severe. In some studies, the UPDRS is supplemented by more objective timed tests, such as the Purdue Pegboard test and movement and reaction times (Jankovic and Lang, 2008; Jankovic, 2007). When a particular aspect of parkinsonism requires more detailed study, separate scales should be employed, such as certain tremor scales or the Gait and Balance Scale (GABS) (Thomas et al., 2004). Also, it is important that in performing the UPDRS, the instructions are followed exactly. For example, one study of a pull test, a measure of postural instability (Hunt and Sethi, 2006), in 66 subjects, performed by 25 examiners showed marked variability in the technique among the examiners, and only 9% of the examinations were rated as error-free (Munhoz et al., 2004). Another study showed that the "push and release test" predicts which PD patients will be fallers better than the pull test (Valkovic et al., 2008). The standard pull test consists of a sudden, firm, and quick shoulder pull without prior warning, but with prior explanation, and executed only once (Visser et al., 2003). If the patient takes more than two steps backward, this is considered abnormal. When performing the push and release test, patients are instructed to stand in a comfortable stance with their eyes open while the examiner stands behind them. The patient is then instructed to push backward against the palms of the examiner's hands placed on the patient's scapulae while the examiner flexes his elbows to allow slight backward movement of the trunk. The examiner then suddenly removes his hands, requiring the patient to take a backward step to regain balance.

There are also many scales, such as the Parkinson disease questionnaire-39 (PDQ-39) (Hagell and Nygren, 2007) and the Parkinson disease quality-of-life questionnaire (PDQL) (de Boer et al., 1996), that attempt to assess the overall health-related or preference-based quality of life (Marinus et al., 2002; Siderowf et al., 2002; Den Oudsten et al., 2007) and the impact of the disease on the performance of activities of daily living (Lindeboom et al., 2003). The Parkinson's Disease Quality of Life Scale (PDQUALIF), developed by the Parkinson Study Group, is being used in clinical trials designed to assess the impact of PD on quality of life (Welsh et al., 2003). The briefer version of PDQ-39, the PDQ-8, has been found to be a longitudinally reliable and responsive measure of health-related quality of life (HRQoL) and to estimate the minimally important difference (MID) or minimal clinically important change (MCIC) in response to therapeutic intervention (Schrag et al., 2006; Luo et al., 2009). In addition to these quantitative measures of PD-related disability, screening tools have been developed and validated to enhance early recognition of parkinsonism. One such instrument has used nine questions that were found to reliably differentiate patients with early PD from those without parkinsonism (Hoglinger et al., 2004). The generic 15D instrument has been found to be valid for measuring HRQoL in PD (Haapaniemi et al., 2004). In a study of 227 patients, 82 of whom were followed for up to 8 years, Forsaa et al., (2008) measured changes in HRQoL over time using the Nottingham Health Profile; they found that the steepest progression was in physical mobility,

followed by social isolation and emotional reactions. Several instruments have been developed utilizing questionnaires, such as questions about the nonmotor symptoms of PD, including the nonmotor questionnaire or NMS Quest (Barone et al., 2009) and the nonmotor scale or the NMS Scale (Chaudhuri et al., 2006b), or on life satisfaction: "general life satisfaction" (QLSM-A) and "satisfaction with health" (QLSM-G), in which each item is weighted according to its relative importance to the individual. In one study these instruments were validated against the 36-item short form health survey (SF-36) and the EuroQol (EQ-5D) (Kuehler et al., 2003). When the initial questionnaires were reduced to 12 items for a "movement disorder module" (QLSM-MD), and 5 items for a "deep brain stimulation module" (QLSM-DBS), psychometric analysis revealed Cronbach's α values of 0.87 and 0.73, and satisfactory correlation coefficients for convergent validity with SF-36 and EQ-5D. Other quality-of-life instruments have been used in assessing the response to therapies, particularly surgery as this treatment intervention is especially susceptible to a placebo effect (Martinez-Martin and Deuschl, 2007; Diamond and Jankovic, 2008).

One of the most important factors contributing to quality of life is the ability to drive. Using a standardized open-route method of assigning driving abilities and safety, Wood and colleagues (2005) found that patients with PD are significantly less safe than are controls and, more important, that the driver's perception of his or her ability to drive correlated poorly with the examiner's assessment. Distractibility and impaired cognition, visual perception, and motor function, associated with sleepiness, are among the major factors in driving safety errors committed by PD patients (Newman, 2006; Uc et al., 2006a; Singh et al., 2007; Uc et al., 2009c). One study found the following commonest errors committed by PD patients while driving: indecisiveness at T-junctions and reduced usage of rear view and side mirrors (Cordell et al., 2008). Driving simulation under low-contrast visibility conditions, such as fog or twilight, showed that a larger proportion of drivers with PD crashed (76.1% vs. 37.3%, $P < 0.0001$) and the time to first reaction in response to incursion was longer (median 2.5 vs. 2.0 seconds, $P < 0.0001$) compared with controls (Uc et al., 2009b). The strongest predictors of poor driving outcomes among the PD cases were worse scores on measures of visual processing speed and attention, motion perception, contrast sensitivity, visuospatial construction, motor speed, and activities of daily living score.

To assess the impact of the various nonmotor symptoms in patients with PD on their quality of life, a 30-item nonmotor symptom screening questionnaire (NMSQuest) was developed, containing nine dimensions: cardiovascular, sleep/fatigue, mood/cognition, perceptual problems, attention/memory, gastrointestinal, urinary, sexual function, and miscellany (Chaudhuri et al., 2007). In 242 patients, mean age 67.2 years and mean duration of symptoms of 6.4 years, the mean score was 56.5 ± 40.7 (range: 0–243); symptoms that were "flagged" by the NMSQuest included: nocturia (61.9%), urinary urgency (55.8%), constipation (52.5%), sad/blues (50.1%), insomnia (45.7%), concentrating (45.7%), anxiety (45.3%), forgetfulness (44.8%), dribbling (41.5%), and restless legs (41.7%) (Martinez-Martin et al., 2007).

Epidemiology

The frequency of PD varies depending on the diagnostic criteria, study population, and epidemiologic methods used, although the prevalence is generally thought to be about 0.3% in the general population and 1% in people over the age of 60 years; the reported incidence figures have ranged from 8 to 18 per 100 000 person-years (de Lau and Breteler, 2006). In a study of 364 incident cases of parkinsonism among residents of Olmsted County, MN, for the period from 1976 through 1990, 154 with PD (42%), 72 with drug-induced parkinsonism (20%), 61 unspecified (17%), 51 with parkinsonism in dementia (14%), and 26 with other causes (7%) were identified (Bower et al., 1999). The average annual incidence rate of parkinsonism (per 100 000 person-years) in the age group 50–99 years was 114.7 and the incidence increased exponentially with age from 0.8 in the age group 0–29 years to 304.8 in the age group 80–99 years. The cumulative incidence of parkinsonism was 7.5% to age 90 years. Men had higher incidence than women at all ages for all types of parkinsonism except drug-induced. In the US studies, African-Americans have been found to be half as likely to be diagnosed with PD as white Americans; these differences could not be explained by differences in age, sex, income, insurance, or access to health care (Dahodwala et al., 2009). Based on a meta-analysis of 29 studies reporting familial aggregation, the relative risk of PD is 2.9 in a first-degree relative, 4.4 in siblings, and 2.7 for a child–parent pair (Thacker and Ascherio, 2008).

Validated screening instruments, designed to detect symptoms of PD with high sensitivity and specificity, are currently lacking. Rest tremor, difficulty walking, difficulty rising from a chair, and walking slowly have been found to be highly specific (93.8–95.9%), but less sensitive (35.9–49.1%) for detecting parkinsonian motor symptoms, while other parkinsonian features such as micrographia and olfactory dysfunction are less specific, but more sensitive (Ishihara et al., 2005). A self-administered, 16-item Baylor Health Screening Questionnaire (BHSQ) is being developed for a web-based use as a potential tool to detect early symptoms of parkinsonism with 91% sensitivity and 92% specificity based on pilot data (Hunter et al., 2008). The instrument used in this study is easy to administer and may be used in mass screenings to identify individuals with undiagnosed PD. If high sensitivity and specificity are confirmed by large prospective studies, this instrument may be used for epidemiologic studies as well as for referrals to appropriate health care or research facilities.

Several diagnostic criteria have been developed for PD, including the UK Parkinson's Disease Society Brain Bank criteria used in various clinical-pathologic studies (Hughes et al., 1992a, 1992b) (Table 4.5). During a workshop sponsored by the National Institute of Neurological Disorders and Stroke (NINDS), a set of diagnostic criteria for PD was proposed, based on a review of the literature regarding the sensitivity and specificity of the characteristic clinical features (Gelb et al., 1999; Jankovic, 2008). The reliability of the different diagnostic criteria, however, has not been vigorously tested by an autopsy examination, which is commonly considered the gold standard (de Rijk et al., 1997). Early clinical-pathologic series concluded that only 76% of patients with

Table 4.5 UK Parkinson's Disease Society Brain Bank's clinical criteria for the diagnosis of probable Parkinson disease

Step 1
1. Bradykinesia
2. At least one of the following criteria:
   A. Rigidity
   B. 4–6 Hz rest tremor
   C. Postural instability not caused by primary visual, vestibular, cerebellar, or proprioceptive dysfunction

Step 2: Exclude other causes of parkinsonism

Step 3: At least three of the following supportive (prospective) criteria:
1. Unilateral onset
2. Rest tremor present
3. Progressive disorder
4. Persistent asymmetry affecting side of onset most
5. Excellent response (70–100%) to levodopa
6. Severe levodopa-induced chorea (dyskinesia)
7. Levodopa response for 5 years or more
8. Clinical course of 10 years or more

Data from Hughes AJ, Daniel SE, Kilford L, Lees AJ. Accuracy of clinical diagnosis of idiopathic Parkinson's disease: A clinico-pathological study of 100 cases. J Neurol Neurosurg Psychiatry 1992;55:181–184; and Hughes AJ, Ben-Shlomo Y, Daniel SE, Lees AJ: What features improve the accuracy of clinical diagnosis in Parkinson's disease: A clinical pathological study. Neurology 1992;42:1142–1146.

a clinical diagnosis of PD actually met the pathologic criteria; the remaining 24% had evidence of other causes of parkinsonism (Hughes et al., 1992a, 1992b). This study was based on autopsied brains collected from 100 patients who had been clinically diagnosed with PD by the UK Parkinson's Disease Society Brain Bank (Hughes, et al., 1992a, 1992b). Similar findings were reported in another study, which was based on autopsy examinations of brains from 41 patients who were followed prospectively by the same neurologist over a 22-year period (Rajput et al., 1991). When Hughes et al. (2001) examined the brains of patients diagnosed with PD by neurologists, the diagnostic accuracy increased to 90%; 6% had MSA, 2% had PSP, 1% had neurofibrillary tangles, and 1% had evidence of vascular parkinsonism. In a study of 143 cases of parkinsonism that came to autopsy and had a clinical diagnosis made by neurologists, the positive predictive value of the clinical diagnosis was 98.6% for PD and 71.4% for the other parkinsonian syndromes (Hughes et al., 2002). In the DATATOP study, 800 patients were prospectively followed by trained parkinsonologists from early, untreated stages of clinically diagnosed PD for a mean of 7.6 years (Jankovic et al., 2000). An analysis of autopsy data, imaging studies, response to levodopa, and atypical clinical features indicated an 8.1% inaccuracy of initial diagnosis of PD by Parkinson experts, but the final diagnosis was not based on pathologic confirmation in all cases. In a study of 89 incident patients initially diagnosed with parkinsonism by experienced clinicians, the diagnosis was subsequently changed in 22 (33%) during the median follow-up of 29 months (Caslake et al., 2008). In this cohort, 38% of those initially diagnosed with PD had their diagnosis changed to DLB; other common misdiagnosis was ET in patients initially thought to have PD and vice versa. This and other studies underscore the need for valid diagnostic criteria to be used in assessing patients with initial manifestations of parkinsonism. In a community-based study of 402 patients taking antiparkinsonian medications, parkinsonism was confirmed in 74% and clinically probable PD in 53%. The commonest causes of misdiagnosis were essential tremor (ET), Alzheimer disease, and vascular parkinsonism. Over one-quarter of subjects did not benefit from antiparkinsonian medication (Meara et al., 1999). Parkinsonian signs, including rigidity, gait disturbance, and bradykinesia, may also occur as a consequence of normal aging, although comorbid medical conditions, such as diabetes, may significantly increase the risk of these motor signs (Arvanitakis et al., 2004). There is considerable debate whether levodopa responsiveness should be included among diagnostic criteria for PD. Although nearly all patients with PD do respond, a small minority with "documented" PD have a poor or no response, although levodopa responsiveness has not been well defined in the literature (Constantinescu et al., 2007).

Nearly all epidemiologic studies of PD show that both incidence and prevalence of PD are 1.5–2 times higher in men than in women (Haaxma et al., 2007). While there is no obvious explanation for this observed male preponderance, exposure to toxins, head trauma, neuroprotection by estrogen in women, mitochondrial dysfunction, or X-linked genetic factors have been suggested (Wooten et al., 2004; Haaxma et al., 2007). The most plausible explanation is that symptoms of PD may be delayed in women by higher striatal dopamine levels, possibly due to the effects of estrogen (Haaxma et al., 2007; Taylor et al., 2007), but this would not explain the lack of female preponderance in Asian, particularly Chinese populations (de Lau and Breteler, 2006).

Laboratory tests

Neuroimaging

Although there is no blood or cerebrospinal fluid test that can diagnose PD, certain neuroimaging techniques may be helpful in differentiating PD from other parkinsonian disorders. MRI in patients with typical PD is usually normal; but a high-field-strength (1.5 T) heavily T2-weighted MRI may show a wider area of lucency in the SN that is probably indicative of increased accumulation of iron (Olanow, 1992). Diffusion-weighted imaging (DWI) provides information on neuronal integrity by quantitating motion of water molecules, which is impaired in axonal cell membranes damaged by a neurodegenerative disease, such as PD. Applying this technique to 17 patients with PD, 16 (94%) were correctly discriminated with a sensitivity of 100% and a specificity of 88% (Scherfler et al., 2006). These patients showed significant increases of diffusivity in the region of both olfactory tracts. Using the Spin-Lattice Distribution Index (SI), a measure of MRI signal in the substantia nigra pars compacta (SNc), provides a "highly sensitive" marker for PD (Hutchinson and Raff, 2008). In a study of 14 patients with early, untreated, PD and 14 age- and gender-matched controls using a 3-tesla MRI and high-resolution diffusion tensor imaging (DTI) protocol, fractional anisotropy (FA) was reduced in the SN of subjects with PD compared with controls ($P < 0.001$), particularly in the caudal SN compared with the rostral region of interest, with 100% sensitivity and

specificity for distinguishing patients with PD from healthy subjects (Vaillancourt et al., 2009). The method used apparently corrected for eddy currents-induced distortion but it is not clear that this is the essential element that accounted for the high sensitivity and specificity of this imaging technique or whether the reported decreased FA was a result of impaired water diffusion through iron-induced field gradients in the SN. Although there is a high correlation between DTI findings and number of SNc dopaminergic neurons lost with MPTP intoxication in a murine model of PD, there is no apparent correlation between the FA values and UPDRS motor scores.

By using [18F]-fluorodopa PET scans to assess the integrity of the striatal dopaminergic terminals, characteristic reduction of the [18F]-fluorodopa uptake, particularly in the putamen, can be demonstrated in virtually all patients with PD, even in the early stages (Brooks, 1991). Using [11C]-raclopride to image dopamine D2 receptors, Brooks and colleagues (1992a) showed that in patients with untreated PD, the striatal D2 receptors are well preserved, whereas patients with atypical parkinsonism have a decrease in the density of dopamine receptors. Involvement of the postsynaptic, striatal dopamine receptor-containing neurons in the atypical parkinsonian syndromes is also suggested by decreased binding of iodobenzamide, a dopamine receptor ligand, as demonstrated by SPECT scans (Schwarz et al., 1992). In addition to reduced density of the dopamine receptors, patients with atypical parkinsonism have decreased striatal metabolism as demonstrated by PET scans (Eidelberg et al., 1993). Besides imaging of postsynaptic D2 receptors, SPECT imaging of the striatal dopamine reuptake sites with I-123 labeled β-CIT and of presynaptic vesicles with [11C]-dihydrotetrabenazine may be also helpful in differentiating PD from atypical parkinsonism (Gilman et al., 1996; Marek et al., 1996; Booij et al., 1997). Dopamine transporter (DAT) imaging using DAT SPECT has been found to be a useful tool in reliably differentiating between PD, essential tremor, dystonic tremor, drug-induced, psychogenic, and vascular parkinsonism (Kägi et al., 2010). Although the imaging tests cannot yet be used to reliably differentiate PD from other parkinsonian disorders, future advances in this technology will undoubtedly improve their diagnostic potential.

Besides clinical rating, neuroimaging techniques have been used to assess progression of PD and other neurodegenerative disorders (Antonini and DeNotaris, 2004; Jankovic, 2005; Brooks, 2007; Nandhagopal et al., 2008a; Martin et al., 2008). Abnormal proton transverse relaxation rate (R2*) measured by 3-tesla MRI, consistent with iron deposition in the lateral SNc, seems to correlate with progression of motor symptoms and as such may have potential utility as a biomarker for disease progression (Martin et al., 2008). Neuroimaging techniques can be used not only in diagnosis but also in following the progression of the disease (Wu et al., 2011). Several studies have shown that the annualized rate of reduction in striatal dopaminergic markers, such as uptake of 18F-FDOPA or DAT binding, to range from 4% to 13% for patients with PD and 0% to 2.5% in healthy controls. Jennings and colleagues (2000) found, on the basis of sequential β-CIT and SPECT imaging at intervals ranging from 9 to 24 months, the annual rate of loss of striatal β-CIT uptake to be 7.1% in subjects having a diagnosis of PD for fewer than 2 years compared with a 3.7% rate in those having a diagnosis of PD for longer than 4.5 years. In another study using ^{18}F-FDOPA PET, Nurmi and colleagues (2001) showed a $10.3 \pm 4.8\%$ decline in the uptake in the putamen over a 5-year period. Using serial FDOPA PET in a prospective, longitudinal study of 31 patients with PD followed for more than 5 years (mean follow-up: 64.5 ± 22.6 months), Hilker and colleagues (2005) found an annual decline in striatal FDOPA ranging from 4.4% (caudate) to 6.3% (putamen), consistent with most other similar studies (Morrish et al., 1998). They concluded that "the neurodegenerative process in PD follows a negative exponential course," and in contrast to the long-latency hypothesis, they estimated that the preclinical disease period is relatively short: only about 6 years. Morrish and colleagues (1998), using a similar design, but with an interscan interval of only 18 months, came to the same conclusion. This is similar to the results of other longitudinal studies of PD progression, using imaging ligands either measuring dopamine metabolism (FDOPA PET) or targeting dopamine transporter (β-CIT SPECT), demonstrating an annualized rate of reduction in these striatal markers of about 4–13% in PD patients compared with a 0–2.5% change in healthy controls (Parkinson Study Group, 2002). In a PET follow-up brain graft study of patients with advanced PD, Nakamura and colleagues (2001) found a 4.4% annual decline in the sham operated patients. Thus, longitudinal studies of PD progression, imaging ligands targeting dopamine metabolism ([18F]-dopa) and dopamine transporter density (β-CIT) using PET and SPECT, respectively, have demonstrated an annualized rate of reduction in striatal [18F]-dopa or [123I]β-CIT uptake of about 11.2% (6–13%) in PD patients compared with 0.8% (0–2.5%) change in healthy controls (Marek et al., 2001).

With improved methodology of β-CIT SPECT scans, the annualized rate of decline is now estimated to be 4–8% (Parkinson Study Group, 2002). These imaging studies are consistent with pathologic studies showing that the rate of nigral degeneration in PD patients is eightfold to tenfold higher than that of healthy age-matched controls. The several studies, including the one by Hilker and colleagues (2005), that suggest that the rate of progression of PD is not linear over time, being more rapid initially and slowing in more advanced stages of the disease, argue against the long-latency hypothesis for presymptomatic period in PD (Jankovic, 2005). Finally, on the basis of clinical-pathologic correlation, Fearnley and Lees (1991) suggested that there is a 30% age-related nigral cell loss at disease onset, again indicating rapid decline in nigral dopaminergic cells in the early stages of the disease. Genetic studies have found that the age at onset of PD (and Alzheimer disease) is strongly influenced by a gene on chromosome 10q (Li et al., 2002).

Increased echogenicity on brain parenchyma transcranial sonography (TCS) is an ultrasound sign that has been found to be relatively specific for PD and that has been used to differentiate PD from atypical parkinsonism, mostly MSA (Walter et al., 2003; Berg et al., 2008). The investigators found that 24 of 25 (96%) patients with PD exhibited hyperechogenicity, whereas only 2 of 23 (9%) patients with atypical parkinsonism showed a similar pattern. They concluded that brain parenchyma sonography may be highly specific in differentiating between PD and atypical parkinsonism. In another study the sensitivity of TCS was 90.7% and the specificity was 82.4%; the positive predictive value was 92.9%

(Gaenslen et al., 2008). In this study, however, tremor-dominant PD patients were excluded. Furthermore, in about 10% of patients SN cannot be imaged because of inadequate temporal bone window. Since the hyperechogenicity seems to be constant over time, TCS possibly may be used to detect this sign as a marker for PD before the onset of neurologic symptoms.

Presymptomatic diagnosis and biomarkers

One of the most important challenges in PD research is to identify individuals who are at risk for PD and to diagnose the disease even before the initial appearance of symptoms. Searching for sensitive biomarkers, such as clinical, motor, physiologic, and olfactory testing, cerebrospinal fluid proteomics, genetic testing, sleep and autonomic studies, and neuroimaging, that detect evidence of PD even before clinical symptoms first appear, has been the primary focus in many research centers around the world (Michell et al., 2004; Hawkes, 2008; Marek et al., 2008; Halperin et al., 2009; Mollenhauer and Trenkwalder, 2009; Wu et al., 2011) (Fig. 4.7). These biomarkers, if found to be useful, should reliably predict: (1) risk (clinical, genetic, blood/CSF test, imaging), (2) diagnosis, (3) progression (prognosis), and (4) response to treatment. As was noted previously, impaired olfaction is one of the earliest signs of PD, present even before the onset of motor symptoms.

Neuroimaging of the presynaptic nigrostriatal terminals has been suggested as a potential biomarker for diagnosis of early PD and for early differentiation between PD and other parkinsonian disorders. Presymptomatic carriers of the *LRRK2* mutation have been shown to have decreased dopaminergic activity and a greater rate of decline in dopaminergic imaging markers, particularly dopamine transporter binding, compared to healthy controls, suggesting that functional neuroimaging may provide a sensitive signal for subclinical dopaminergic deficiency (Nandhagopal et al., 2008b). To evaluate the diagnostic accuracy of dopamine transporter imaging using ([123I]β-CIT, Jennings

PARKINSON DISEASE

Symptomatic

Presymptomatic
- Gene mutations
- Essential tremor
- Anosmia
- Constipation
- REM behavioral disorder
- Shoulder pain
- Red or blond hair color
- Slow reaction time
- Lower impulsiveness
- Low uric acid
- Low LDL
- Nurr1 in lymphocytes
- Blood/CSF proteomics
- Imaging: MRI-DTI, PET, SPECT, sonography

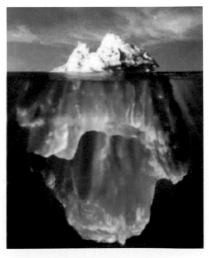

Figure 4.7 Premotor markers of PD.

et al. (2004) evaluated 35 patients referred by community neurologists with suspected early PD. The clinical diagnosis was "confirmed" by two movement disorder experts, which represented the diagnostic "gold standard." A disagreement between the "gold standard" diagnosis and imaging diagnosis occurred in only 8.6% of cases, giving the imaging sensitivity of 0.92 and specificity of 1.00. They concluded that (^{123}I)β-CIT and SPECT imaging is a useful diagnostic tool to differentiate between patients with early PD and other parkinsonian disorders.

Many studies provide evidence suggesting that the latency between the onset of neuronal degeneration (or onset of the disease process) and clinical symptoms might not be as long as was initially postulated (Morrish et al., 1996). On the basis of a study of 36 control and 20 PD brains, Fearnley and Lees (1991) suggested that the presymptomatic phase of PD from the onset of neuronal loss to the onset of symptoms might be only 5 years, thus arguing against aging as an important cause of PD. With advancing age, there is 4.7% per decade rate of loss of pigmented neurons from the SNc, whereas in PD, there is 45% loss in the first decade. Since the rate of progression is so highly variable, it is perhaps not surprising that the estimates of the presymptomatic period vary between 40 years and 3.1 years, depending on the method used (Morrish et al., 1996). The shorter presymptomatic period has been suggested by longitudinal ^{18}F-FDOPA PET studies (Morrish et al., 1996). Although UPDRS has been used in these longitudinal studies as a measure of clinical progression, the instrument is currently being revised to include additional items, including nonmotor experiences of daily living, to capture symptoms that reflect nondopaminergic involvement in PD. Whether the progression as measured with the current or revised UPDRS correlates with nigral and extranigral pathology associated with PD awaits future clinical-pathologic validation.

One of the benefits of longitudinal imaging studies, such as the one by Hilker and colleagues (2005; see also Jankovic, 2005), is that they can be used to estimate duration of the presymptomatic period. Assuming that the threshold at which symptoms are first manifested is at 69% of the normal putaminal FDOPA uptake, Hilker and colleagues (2005) concluded that the preclinical disease period must be relatively short: only about 6 years. This is consistent with other imaging and with autopsy data (Fearnley and Lees, 1991). The 31% loss of striatal dopaminergic terminals needed before onset of symptoms, demonstrated by Hilker and colleagues (2005), is substantially lower than the 60–80% loss of dopaminergic neurons in the SN that is traditionally cited as being required before symptoms of PD first become evident. The difference may be explained by compensatory changes in response to presynaptic dopaminergic loss, such as enhanced synthesis of dopamine in surviving dopaminergic neurons, upregulation of striatal dopa-decarboxylase activity, and increased dopaminergic innervation of the striatum (Jankovic, 2005). Furthermore, there may be functional compensatory changes, as suggested by the finding of increased FDOPA uptake in the globus pallidus interna, in early PD. This enhanced function of the nigropallidal dopaminergic projection maintains a more normal pattern of pallidal output in early stages of the disease, but these compensatory mechanisms eventually fail, and the disease starts to progress. Thus, because of the compensatory changes,

FDOPA PET more accurately reflects dopaminergic function at the striatal terminal rather than a cell loss in the SN. These compensatory mechanisms may also explain why despite age-related loss of nigral neurons, there is little or no change in FDOPA uptake with normal aging (Sawle et al., 1990) and why up to 15% of patients with signs of PD, as determined by experienced parkinsonologists, have normal FDOPA or β-CIT scans without evidence of dopaminergic deficit (SWEDD) (Marek et al., 2003; Whone et al., 2003; Clarke, 2004; Fahn et al., 2004; Jankovic, 2005; Scherfler et al., 2007). These SWEDDs might represent patients with PD and compensatory striatal changes or with other disorders. They might also represent false-negative results and therefore highlight the relative lack of sensitivity of these functional neuroimaging studies as potential biomarkers for detection of PD, particularly at early stages of the disease (Michell et al., 2004). Since individuals with SWEDDs fail to develop dopaminergic deficit and fail to show clinical worsening, it is likely that these individuals were incorrectly diagnosed. This is supported by normal olfaction in SWEDD individuals (Silveira-Moriyama et al., 2009b). One possible condition misdiagnosed as PD, but with SWEDD, is adult-onset dystonic tremor, which may present as unilateral or asymmetric rest tremor and decreased arm swing (Schneider et al., 2007).

To the extent that future protective therapies may prevent or even halt the neurodegenerative process, it is essential that they be implemented early in the course of the disease. Therefore, recent clinical and basic studies have focused on a search for presymptomatic biomarkers of PD (Michell et al., 2004). An identification of a disease-specific diagnostic test would be immensely helpful not only in defining the various PD subtypes and in differentiating PD from atypical parkinsonian syndromes, but also, more importantly, in identifying populations that are at increased risk for developing PD. Such potentially vulnerable populations could then be targeted for protective therapy. Novel imaging techniques are being developed not only to monitor the progression of the disease, but also as diagnostic tools in clinically uncertain cases. Using the dopamine transporter ligand [I-123] (N)-(3-iodopropene-2-yl)-2beta-carbomethoxy-3beta-(4-chlorophenyl) tropane (IPT), and SPECT, Schwarz and colleagues (2000) showed a reduction of dopamine transporter binding in patients with early PD, suggesting that this technique has potential in detection of preclinical disease. Comparing inversion recovery MRI and ^{18}F-FDOPA PET in 10 patients with Hoehn and Yahr stage 3 and 4 PD and 8 normal controls, Hu and colleagues (2001) found that discriminant function analysis of the quantified MRI nigral signal correctly classified the combined PD patient/control group, but three patients with PD were incorrectly classified as "normal," whereas with PET, 100% of PD patients and controls were correctly classified. In a study of 118 patients with clinically uncertain parkinsonian syndromes, all patients with presynaptic parkinsonism had abnormal ^{123}I-ioflupane SPECT (DaTSCAN, Amersham Health), whereas 94% with "non-presynaptic" parkinsonism had a normal scan (Catafau and Tolosa, 2004). Abnormal echogenicity on transcranial sonography may be detected in early, and possibly even in presymptomatic PD (Weise et al., 2009). Decreased cardiac MIBG uptake was found even in de novo patients with PD, suggesting that this test could be used to detect early or even presymptomatic PD (Oka et al., 2006; Lee et al., 2006).

Reduction in myocardial MIBG uptake seems to correlate with presynaptic nigrostriatal dopaminergic deficit as measured by putaminal [^{123}I]FP-CIT SPECT, suggesting that brain and extracranial neurodegeneration in PD are coupled (Spiegel et al., 2007). Cardiac sympathetic degeneration and Lewy body pathology, even in the presymptomatic phase of PD, is likely responsible for these abnormalities, although PD-related clinically evident heart disease has not been demonstrated (Fujishiro et al., 2008).

Besides loss of olfaction, constipation, shoulder pain, RBD, and imaging studies, there are other tests that are being explored as potential biomarkers for early detection of PD. For example, mRNA expression of nuclear receptor related 1 protein (Nurr1) on peripheral lymphocytes has been found to be decreased in patients with PD as compared to other dopaminergic disorders (Pan et al., 2004). Furthermore, mRNA expression of co-chaperone ST13 in peripheral blood, which stabilizes heat-shock protein 70, a modifier of α-synuclein misfolding, has been found to be lower in patients with PD than in controls ($P = 0.002$) in two independent populations (Scherzer et al., 2007).

Pathologic findings

In the absence of a specific biologic marker or a diagnostic test, the diagnosis of PD can be made with certainty only at autopsy. PD is pathologically defined as a neurodegenerative disorder characterized chiefly by (1) depigmentation of the SN associated with degeneration of melanin- and dopamine-containing neurons, particularly in the SNc and in the norepinephrine-containing neurons in the locus coeruleus, and (2) the presence of Lewy bodies (eosinophilic cytoplasmic inclusions) in the SNc and other brain regions, including the locus coeruleus and some cortical areas. In fact, some studies have found that, despite the universally accepted notion that SN is the site of the brunt of the pathology in PD, neuronal loss in the locus coeruleus is more severe (Zarow et al., 2003). These criteria are open to question, however, since typical cases of levodopa-responsive parkinsonism have been reported without Lewy bodies and with or without neurofibrillary tangles in the SN (Rajput et al., 1991). In contrast, the pathologically typical form of Lewy body parkinsonism has been described with atypical clinical features such as poor response to levodopa (Mark et al., 1992). Both the Canadian (Rajput et al., 1991) and the London Parkinson's Disease Society Brain Bank study (Hughes et al., 1992b) showed that 24% of patients in each series had a pathologic diagnosis other than PD. Furthermore, in patients with pathologically documented PD, other disorders may be present that can cloud the clinical picture. For example, in 100 cases of pathologically proven PD, Hughes and colleagues (1993) found 34 with coexistent pathology in the striatum and 28 outside the nigrostriatal system; vascular changes involving the striatum were found in 24 patients, Alzheimer changes in 20 (3 had striatal plaques confined to the striatum), and diffuse Lewy body disease or dementia with Lewy bodies in 4. As was noted previously, in a subsequent study, the diagnostic accuracy had improved markedly (Hughes et al., 2002). Until parkinsonian disorders can be differentiated by either disease-specific biologic or etiologic markers, neuroimaging, or other laboratory tests, the separation of the different parkinsonian disorders still depends largely on clinical-pathologic correlations.

While the emphasis in PD research has been on dopaminergic deficiency underlying motor dysfunction, there is a growing body of evidence that the caudal brainstem nuclei (e.g., dorsal motor nucleus of the glossopharyngeal and vagal nerves), anterior olfactory nucleus, and other non-dopaminergic neurons might be affected long before the classic loss of dopaminergic neurons in the SN, based on accumulation of Lewy neurites detected by staining for α-synuclein (Braak et al., 2003, 2004; Braak and Del Tredici, 2008). According to the Braak staging, in presymptomatic stage 1, the Lewy neurite pathology remains confined to the medulla oblongata and olfactory bulb. In stage 2, it has spread to involve the pons. In stages 3 and 4, the SN and other nuclear grays of the midbrain and basal forebrain are the focus of initially subtle and then more pronounced changes, at which time the illness reaches its symptomatic phase. In end-stages 5 and 6, the pathologic process encroaches on the telencephalic cortex. A clinical-pathologic study of 129 brains in the UK Brain Bank, focusing on the late phase of PD, indicates that while it takes longer for young-onset patients to reach the end-stage of the disease, marked by more rapid physical and cognitive decline, this terminal stage is rather similar irrespective of age at onset (Kempster et al., 2010). This, according to the authors, supports "a staging system based on the rostral extent and severity of Lewy body pathology, although other pathologies may play a synergistic role in causing cognitive disability", consistent with the Braak hypothesis.

The Braak staging, however, has been challenged for several reasons, including lack of cell counts to correlate with the described synuclein pathology and no observed asymmetry in the pathologic findings that would correlate with the well-recognized asymmetry of clinical findings. In addition, there is controversy as to the classification of dementia with Lewy bodies; Braak viewed it as part of stage 6, but others suggest that it is a separate entity, since these patients often have behavioral and psychiatric problems before the onset of motor or other signs of PD. This staging proposal, however, has been challenged as there are no cell counts to correlate with the described synuclein pathology, no immunohistochemistry to identify neuronal types, no observed asymmetry in the pathologic findings that would correlate with the well-recognized asymmetry of clinical findings, bulbar symptoms are late not early features of PD despite the suggested early involvement of the dorsal motor nucleus of the vagal nerve, exclusion of cases of dementia with Lewy bodies, the idiopathic Lewy body cases were preselected for the presence of α-synuclein deposition, cases with well-documented α-synuclein inclusions at higher levels in the neuraxis without involvement of caudal brainstem have been reported, the pathologic examination did not include the spinal cord and peripheral autonomic nervous system, and brain synucleinopathy consistent with Braak stages 4 and 6 has been found in individuals without any neurologic signs (Burke et al., 2008).

References available on Expert Consult: www.expertconsult.com

CHAPTER 5

Current concepts on the etiology and pathogenesis of Parkinson disease

Chapter contents

Anatomical and biochemical pathology of PD	93
Interconnected pathogenic mechanisms of PD	99
Genetics as an etiologic factor of PD	100
Environmental factors contributing to etiology of or protection against PD	104
Endogenous factors that contribute to the etiology of PD	107
Where does PD pathology begin? How does it progress? Braak's staging system	110
Clues on pathogenesis from monogenic PD	114
Lewy bodies in fetal dopaminergic neurons; infectious protein hypothesis	116
Multiple hit hypothesis with a central role of α-synuclein	117
Animal models	118

Anatomical and biochemical pathology of PD

Historical introduction

Parkinson disease (PD) was first described in 1817 with the publication by James Parkinson of a book entitled *An Essay on the Shaking Palsy* (Parkinson, 1817). In it, he described six individuals with the clinical features that have come to be recognized as a disease entity. One of the people was followed in detail over a long period of time; the other five consisted of brief descriptions, including two of whom he had met walking in the street, and another whom he had observed at a distance. Such distant observations without a medical examination demonstrate how easily distinguishable the condition is. The physical appearance of flexed posture, resting tremor, and shuffling gait are readily recognizable. Parkinson's opening description has his key essentials: "Involuntary tremulous motion, with lessened muscular power, in parts not in action and even when supported; with a propensity to bend the trunk forward, and to pass from a walking to a running pace: the senses and intellects being uninjured." In the small monograph, Parkinson provided a detailed description of the symptoms and also discussed the progressive worsening of the disorder, which he called "the shaking palsy" and also its Latin term "paralysis agitans."

After the publication of Parkinson's Essay, the disease was widely accepted in the medical community. It took 70 years for the name of the disorder to be referred to as "Parkinson's disease," as recommended by the French neurologist Charcot (1879) who argued against the term "paralysis agitans" (see Goetz, 1987, for English translation) and recommended the disorder be named after James Parkinson. Charcot argued that there is no true paralysis, but rather the "lessened muscular power" is what is today called akinesia, hypokinesia, or bradykinesia; all three terms often being used interchangeably by clinicians, although these three terms specifically refer to lack of movement, small movement, and slow movement, respectively. These terms represent a paucity of movement not due to weakness or paralysis. Similarly, Charcot emphasized that tremor need not be present in the disorder, so "agitans" and "shaking" are not appropriate as part of the name of the disorder.

The clinical features of PD and its differential diagnosis are presented in Chapter 4.

Incidence, prevalence, and mortality

Although PD can develop at any age, it begins most commonly in older adults, with a peak age at onset around 60 years. The likelihood of developing PD increases with age, with a lifetime risk of about 2% (Elbaz et al., 2002). A positive family history doubles the risk of developing PD to about 4%. A summation from seven population-based studies in various European countries found the overall prevalence of PD in people aged over 65 to be 1.8%, with an increase from 0.6% for persons aged 65–69 years to 2.6% for people aged 85–89 years (de Rijk et al., 2000). Twin studies indicate that PD with an onset under the age of 50 years is more likely to have a genetic relationship than for patients with an older age at onset (Tanner et al., 1999). Males have higher prevalence (male-to-female ratio of 3:2) and incidence rates than females (Fig. 5.1) (Bower et al., 2000), but the age-specific incidence rates have not varied over the past 70 years (Fig. 5.2) (Rocca et al., 2001). The

DOI: 10.1016/B978-1-4377-2369-4.00005-6

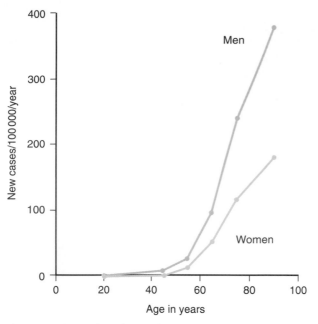

Figure 5.1 Age- and gender-specific incidence rates (new cases per 100 000 person-years) of PD in Olmsted County, MN, 1996–1990. *From Bower JH, Maraganore DM, McDonnell SK, Rocca WA. Influence of strict, intermediate, and broad diagnostic criteria on the age- and sex-specific incidence of Parkinson's disease. Mov Disord 2000;15(5):819–825.*

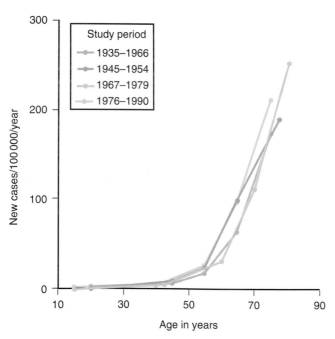

Figure 5.2 Comparison of age-specific incidence rates of parkinsonism in Olmsted County, MN, over seven decades. *From Rocca WA, Bower JH, McDonnell SK, Peterson BJ, Maraganore DM. Time trends in the incidence of parkinsonism in Olmsted County, Minnesota. Neurology 2001;57(3):462–467.*

incidence rates vary among studies, but average between 11.0 and 13.9/100 000 population per year (Van Den Eeden et al., 2003). In a northern California study, the incidence rates varied among ethnic groups, being highest in Hispanics, then non-Hispanic whites, then Asians, and lowest in African-Americans (Van Den Eeden et al., 2003).

The prevalence rates of PD have varied in different studies and in different countries. The figure of 187 per 100 000 population given by Kurland (1958) is a reasonable estimate in the US. But if the population is restricted to adults older than 39 years of age, the prevalence rate is 347 per 100 000 (Schoenberg et al., 1985) since both prevalence and incidence rates increase with age. At age 70, the prevalence is approximately 550 per 100 000, and the incidence is 120 per 100 000/year. At the present time, approximately 850 000 individuals in the US have PD, although one recent estimate is less than this (Hirtz et al., 2007). The number is expected to grow as the population ages (Dorsey et al., 2007). Advancing age is the single greatest risk factor for developing sporadic PD. Approximately 2% of the population will have PD by the time they reach the age of 80 years.

In the pre-levodopa era, mortality was reported to be three-fold greater in patients with PD (Hoehn and Yahr, 1967). The mortality rate was reduced to 1.6-fold greater than age-matched non-PD individuals after the introduction of levodopa (Yahr, 1976; Elbaz et al., 2003). Today, patients with PD can live 20 or more years, depending on the age at onset (Kempster et al., 2007). Death in PD is usually due to some concurrent unrelated illness or due to the effects of decreased mobility, aspiration, or increased falling with subsequent physical injury. The Parkinson-plus syndromes typically progress at a faster rate and often cause death within 9 years. Thus, the diagnosis of PD versus other forms of parkinsonism is of prognostic importance, as well as of therapeutic significance because it almost always responds to at least a moderate degree with levodopa therapy, whereas the Parkinson-plus disorders usually do not.

Anatomical pathology of PD

It was many years after Parkinson's original description before the basal ganglia were recognized by Meynert in 1871 as being involved in disorders of abnormal movements. And it was not until 1895 that the substantia nigra (SN) was suggested to be affected in PD. Brissaud (1895) suggested this on the basis of a report by Blocq and Marinesco (1893) of a tuberculoma in that site that was associated with a contralateral hemiparkinsonian tremor. These authors were careful to point out that the pyramidal tract and the brachium conjunctivum above and below the level of the lesion contained no degenerating fibers. The importance of the SN was emphasized by Tretiakoff in 1919. He studied the SN in nine cases of PD, one case of hemiparkinsonism, and three cases of postencephalitic parkinsonism, finding neuronal loss in this nucleus in all cases. With the hemiparkinsonian case, Tretiakoff found a lesion in the nigra on the opposite side, concluding that the nucleus served the motor activity on the contralateral side of the body. The SN, so named because of its normal content of neuromelanin pigment, was noted to show depigmentation, loss of nerve cells, and gliosis. These findings remain the principal and essential histopathologic features of the disease. In his study, Tretiakoff also found Lewy bodies in the SN, expanding the earlier observation of Lewy (1912, 1914), who had discovered the presence of these cytoplasmic inclusions in the substantia innominata and the dorsal vagus nucleus in PD. Lewy bodies (Fig. 5.3) are now widely recognized as the major pathologic hallmark of the disorder. Lewy bodies have since been seen in autonomic

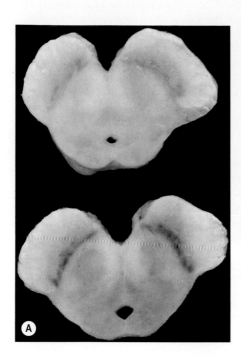

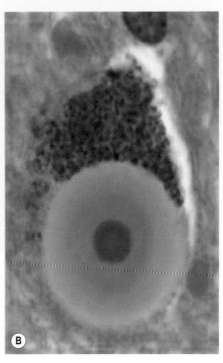

Figure 5.3 Pathology of PD. **A** Cross-section of a midbrain from a patient with PD (upper) and from an individual without PD (lower). This demonstrates the depigmentation of the substantia nigra in PD. **B** A high-powered view of a pigmented nigral neuron containing an intracytoplasmic eosinophilic inclusion, the Lewy body. *Courtesy of Jean-Paul Vonsattel, MD.*

ganglia, the peripheral nervous system and in other regions of the central nervous system, including the cerebral cortex (Jellinger, 2009a).

Foix and Nicolesco (1925) made a detailed study of the pathology of PD in 1925 and found that the most constant and severe lesions are in the substantia nigra. Since then many workers, including Hassler (1938) and Greenfield and Bosanquet (1953), have confirmed these findings and added other observations, including involvement of other brainstem nuclei such as the locus coeruleus and the raphe nuclei. The pigmented cells of the locus coeruleus contain neuromelanin; these cells are also lost in PD, with many of those remaining containing Lewy bodies. The asymmetry of clinical signs in PD is reflected by the asymmetrical and more severe contralateral loss of substantia nigra pars compacta (SNc) neurons. Neuronal loss extends beyond loss in SNc, locus coeruleus, and raphe, with loss of neurons in the dorsal motor vagal nucleus, hypothalamus, the nucleus basalis of Meynert, and sympathetic ganglia (Forno, 1982; Jellinger, 1987). There are also losses of glutamatergic projection neurons from thalamus to the basal ganglia (Henderson et al., 2000) and glutamatergic projection neurons from the presupplementary motor cortex to the premotor cortices (Halliday et al., 2005).

PD and the Parkinson-plus syndromes have in common a degeneration of SNc dopaminergic neurons, with a resulting deficiency of striatal dopamine due to loss of these nigrostriatal neurons. Accompanying this neuronal loss is an increase in glial cells in the nigra and a loss of the neuromelanin normally contained in the dopaminergic neurons. There is a reduction of nigral neurons and striatal dopamine with aging also (Carlsson and Winblad, 1976; McGeer et al., 1977; Fearnley and Lees, 1991) (Fig. 5.4), and although PD is associated with increasing age, the greater rate (Fig. 5.5) and the pattern of cell loss in the SN differs between that in

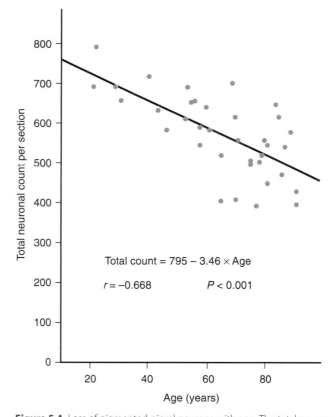

Total count = 795 − 3.46 × Age

$r = -0.668$ $P < 0.001$

Figure 5.4 Loss of pigmented nigral neurons with age. The total neuronal count equals the number of pigmented cell bodies in one section of the caudal substantia nigra. *From Fearnley JM, Lees AJ. Ageing and Parkinson's disease: substantia nigra regional selectivity. Brain 1991;114:2283–2301.*

aging and that in PD (Figs 5.6, 5.7) (Fearnley and Lees, 1991). Clinical features begin to emerge when approximately 80% of striatal dopamine content (or 60% of nigral dopaminergic neurons) are lost (Bernheimer et al., 1973). The course of clinical decline is associated with the progressive reduction of striatal dopamine (Riederer and Wuketich, 1976).

Pathologically, almost all patients with PD have Lewy bodies in the SN and locus coeruleus. Juvenile PD (Dwork et al., 1993; Hattori et al., 2000), now recognized as being due mainly to homozygous *parkin* mutations, is a major exception. Another exception is with PD due to the R1441G mutation in the *LRRK2* gene (Martí-Massó et al., 2009). The pathology has not yet been described in juvenile PD patients due to homozygous mutations in *DJ-1* genes, but in one case of young-onset PD with *PINK1* mutation, the autopsy showed the presence of Lewy bodies (Samaranch et al., 2010). There are no Lewy bodies in the Parkinson-plus syndromes or in postencephalitic parkinsonism (Jellinger, 2009b).

The presence of Lewy bodies in the SNc and the locus coeruleus plus the clinical features of PD (without the characteristic clinical features of some other form of parkinsonism) are usually used to make the pathologic diagnosis of PD, but there is no complete agreement among neuropathologists about the pathologic criteria for the diagnosis of PD (Forno, 1982, 1996). Some patients with clinical PD die with nigral degeneration without Lewy bodies (Rajput et al., 1991; Hughes et al., 1992, 2002). In fact, as mentioned

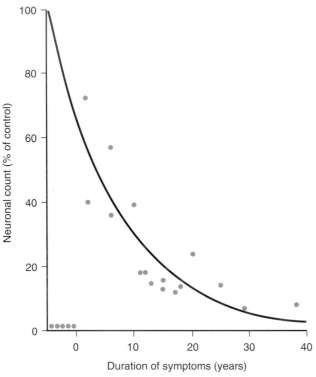

Figure 5.5 Total pigmented nigral neurons with disease duration. *From Fearnley JM, Lees AJ. Ageing and Parkinson's disease: substantia nigra regional selectivity. Brain 1991;114:2283–2301.*

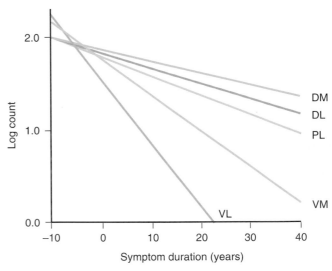

Figure 5.7 Logarithm of regional age-adjusted neurons with PD duration. DM, Dorsal tier medial. DL, Dorsal tier lateral. PL, Dorsal tier pars lateralis. VM, Ventral tier medial. VL, Ventral tier lateral. *From Fearnley JM, Lees AJ. Ageing and Parkinson's disease: substantia nigra regional selectivity. Brain 1991;114:2283–2301.*

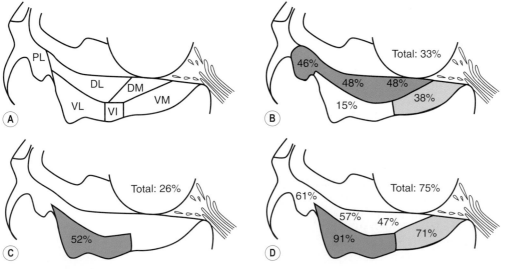

Figure 5.6 Regional pigmented neuronal loss in aging and in Parkinson disease. **A** Normal anatomy. **B** Aging. Numbers indicate percentage of neurons lost between ages 20 and 90. **C** Incidental Lewy body disease. **D** Parkinson disease. In **C** and **D**, numbers indicate average percentage loss compared to normal individuals. Dorsal tier: PL, pars lateralis; DL, lateral; DM, medial. Ventral tier: VL, lateral; VI, intermediate; VM, medial. *From Fearnley JM, Lees AJ. Ageing and Parkinson's disease: substantia nigra regional selectivity. Brain 1991;114:2283–2301.*

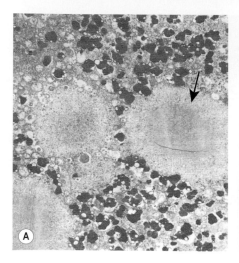
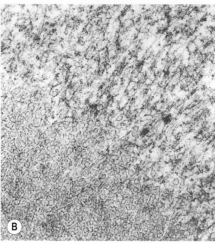

Figure 5.8 Electron microscopic appearance of the Lewy body. There is a dense central core surrounded by radiating filamentous material. **A** A lower resolution of two Lewy bodies. The arrow points to the radiating filamentous material. **B** A higher power resolution of a Lewy body at the junction of the dense core and the surrounding radiating filamentous material. *From Fahn S, Duffy P. Parkinson's disease. In Goldensohn ES, Appel SH, eds: Scientific Approaches to Clinical Neurology, Philadelphia: Lea & Febiger; 1977, pp. 1119–1158.*

Table 5.1 Age-specific prevalence of incidental Lewy bodies

Age	No.	Percent
<20	0/2	
20–29	0/6	
30–39	0/6	
40–49	1/7	3.7
50–59	0/20	
60–69	2/51	3.9
70–79	3/56	5.4
80–89	6/49	12.2
90–99	1/8	12.5

Data from Fearnley JM, Lees AJ. Ageing and Parkinson's disease: substantia nigra regional selectivity. Brain 1991,114:2283–2301.

above, patients with juvenile PD usually do not have Lewy bodies, especially those with homozygous *parkin* mutations (Dwork et al., 1993; Hattori et al., 2000). Thus, Lewy bodies confirm the diagnosis and are a critical pathologic marker to confirm the diagnosis, but they are not necessary and their presence is not pathognomonic for PD (Forno 1982). They are found in 4–6% of routine autopsies (Forno, 1982), the incidence rate increases with age as in PD (Fearnley and Lees, 1991) (Table 5.1), and people dying with such incidental Lewy bodies are considered to have a presymptomatic state of PD. The site of regional nigral neuronal loss in incidental Lewy body disease is the lateral region in the ventral tier, the same as for PD (Fig. 5.6) (Fearnley and Lees, 1991). These brains show a reduction in striatal dopaminergic markers (e.g., tyrosine hydroxylase and vesicular monoamine transporter 2), but not as severe as those with clinical PD (Delle-Donne et al., 2008; Dickson et al., 2008). Cortical Lewy bodies in patients with dementia and no parkinsonism could be a separate disease or a variant in the presentation of the same disorder that causes PD. Lewy bodies consist of a dense inner core surrounded by a radiating filamentous

outer zone (Fig. 5.8) (Duffy and Tennyson, 1965; Forno and Norville, 1976).

Biochemical pathology of PD

The pigmented neurons of both the SNc and the ventral tegmental area (medial to the SN in the midbrain) contain dopamine. The former neurons project to the neostriatum, the latter to the limbic system and the neocortex. In PD, the mesolimbic and mesocortical neurons are relatively spared, whereas the nigrostriatal neurons are progressively lost. As a result, there is a corresponding decrease of dopamine content in both the nigra and the striatum, with the innervation of the posterior putamen affected first and most severely, as can be detected in FDOPA PET scans (Fig. 5.9). Whereas dopamine is reduced initially in the posterior striatum in PD, over time, as the disease progresses, all striatal subregions are affected to a similar degree (Nandhagopal et al., 2009).

The pigmented neurons of the locus coeruleus contain norepinephrine, and these neurons project widely in the CNS. A third set of monoaminergic neurons are those containing serotonin (5-HT), located in the raphe of the pons and medulla. In PD there is a progressive loss of all three types of monoaminergic cells, particularly the dopaminergic cells. So, in addition to a depletion of striatal dopamine, there is also a reduction in brain norepinephrine and 5-HT (Ehringer and Hornykiewicz, 1960; Hornykiewicz, 1966) (Table 5.2). There is also a reduction in other neurotransmitters (Agid et al., 1987) as well as enzyme activities for the synthesis of other neurotransmitters (Table 5.2), indicating that the biochemical changes in PD extend beyond the loss of only the monoamines.

In addition to the motor features of PD, the symptoms that define the clinical diagnosis, there are also a host of nonmotor symptoms, some occurring before the motor symptoms and some occurring after (see Chapter 8). The early motor symptoms of bradykinesia and rigidity and tremor are associated with monoaminergic cell and chemical loss. The later motor symptoms of flexed posture, loss of postural reflexes, and the freezing phenomenon appear to correlate poorly with dopaminergic deficit. The nonmotor symptoms probably are the result of loss of neuronal

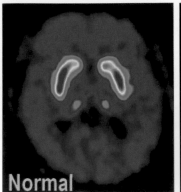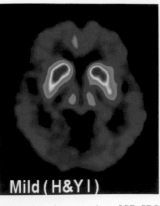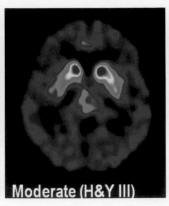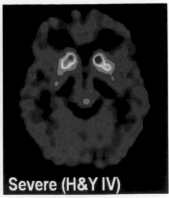

Figure 5.9 Examples of FDOPA PET scans with clinical progression of PD. FDOPA uptake is lost in a progressive pattern, first and most severely in the posterior putamen, then the anterior putamen, and finally the caudate nucleus. In the most severe state shown here, there is still FDOPA uptake in the caudate nucleus. H&Y, Hoehn and Yahr stage. *Courtesy of David Eidelberg, MD.*

Table 5.2   Concentration of neurotransmitters, their metabolites, and synthesizing enzymes in selected regions of brain of controls and PD

Brain region	DA	HVA	NE	5-HT	GAD	CAT
Putamen						
Controls	5.06	4.92	0.10	0.32	622	1656
PD	0.14	0.54	0.05	0.14	292	780
Caudate						
Controls	4.06	2.92	0.09	0.33	659	1460
PD	0.20	1.19	0.04	0.12	321	694
Globus pallidus						
Controls	0.5	2.92	0.06	0.23	553	231
PD	0.2	0.72	0.05	0.13	388	39
Substantia nigra						
Controls	0.46	2.32	0.23	0.55	637	63
PD	0.07	0.41	0.11	0.26	263	12
Nucleus accumbens						
Controls	3.79	4.38	1.29	–	–	–
PD	1.61	3.13	0.52	–	–	–

DA, dopamine; HVA, homovanillic acid, a metabolite of DA; NE, norepinephrine; 5-HT, serotonin; GAD, glutamic acid decarboxylase; CAT, choline acetyltransferase. All results are mean values. Results of the monoamines and HVA are means expressed as µg/g wet tissue. Results of GAD activity are expressed as nmol/CO_2/h/mg protein. Results of CAT activity are expressed as pmol/min/mg protein.
Data from Hornykiewicz O. Brain neurotransmitter changes in Parkinson's disease. In Marsden CD, Fahn S, eds. Movement Disorders. London, Butterworth Scientific, 1982;41–58.

function other than dopamine. Catecholamine reduction in PD is seen in the autonomic nervous system and accounts for the reduction in MIBG SPECT scan labeling in the heart in PD due to loss of postganglionic myocardial sympathetic nerve fibers (Rascol and Schelosky, 2009).

Among the neurotransmitter changes is the reduction of brain acetylcholine (Bohnen and Albin, 2010). Acetylcholinesterase (AChE), which serves as a marker for cholinergic neurons, can be measured by PET scanning (Shimada et al., 2009). A reduction of AChE begins early in PD (Bohnen and Albin, 2009). Reduced thalamic AChE activity correlates with falling in PD (Bohnen et al., 2009), and in part represents decreased cholinergic output of the pedunculopontine nucleus (PPN), which appears to be important for gait. Cortical loss of acetylcholine probably contributes to the dementia seen in PD (Shimada et al., 2009; Bohnen and Albin, 2010). Overall, reduced AChE is more widespread and

profound both in PD with dementia and in dementia with Lewy bodies (Shimada et al., 2009).

There are compensatory changes, such as supersensitivity of dopamine receptors, so that symptoms of PD are first encountered only when there is about an 80% reduction of dopamine concentration in the putamen (or a loss of 60% of nigral dopaminergic neurons) (Bernheimer et al., 1973). Another compensatory mechanism is an increase in neurotransmitter turnover, as detected by an increased HVA/DA ratio. In a major review, Hornykiewicz (1966) correlated loss of dopamine concentration in the striatum with severity of bradykinesia and rigidity in PD. With further loss of dopamine concentration, parkinsonian bradykinesia becomes more severe. The progressive loss of the dopaminergic nigrostriatal pathway can be detected during life using PET and SPECT scanning (Fig. 5.9); these show a continuing reduction of FDOPA and dopamine transporter ligand binding in the striatum that correlates with the bradykinesia score in the Unified Parkinson's Disease Rating Scale (Brooks et al., 1990; Snow et al., 1994; Seibyl et al., 1995; Morrish et al., 1996; Vingerhoets et al., 1997; Broussolle et al., 1999; Benamer et al., 2000). Using special statistical techniques, FDG PET also shows a correlation between worsening brady-kinesia and increase of lentiform metabolism (Eidelberg et al., 1995). In fact, using FDG PET demonstrates a meta-bolic network characteristic of PD compared to other forms of parkinsonism (Hirano et al., 2009; Tang et al., 2010). While postsynaptic dopamine receptors have been thought to be preserved in PD, a recent study suggested a downregu-lation of the D3 receptors in drug-naive PD patients (Boileau et al., 2009).

Interconnected pathogenic mechanisms of PD

The best correlation of symptoms with progressive loss of striatal dopamine are those of bradykinesia and rigidity, which relate to striatal dopamine deficiency and loss of SNc dopaminergic neurons and can be correlated with a progres-sive decrease of dopaminergic imaging by PET or SPECT (see above). Since these symptoms are two of the cardinal fea-tures of the disease, research efforts have concentrated on the pathogenic mechanisms that cause loss of the nigrostriatal dopamine system, and this will be reflected in this review. Similar mechanisms might involve the other monoaminer-gic systems (noradrenergic and serotonergic). But there is little knowledge of the pathogenesis of neuronal loss for nonaminergic neurons. It seems likely that loss of these other monoamines might be instrumental in the high rate of depression (Mayeux et al., 1984) and anxiety in patients with PD. Little is known about the anatomical or biochemi-cal associations for the other clinical features of the disease, including motoric features of tremor, freezing, flexed posture and loss of postural reflexes, and the multitude of nonmotor features.

A variety of pathogenic mechanisms have been uncovered for the loss of dopamine neurons, and probably more will be uncovered. The reader is referred to reviews on this topic for details (Dauer and Przedborski, 2003; Jenner and Olanow, 2006; Gupta et al., 2008). With the development of genetic causes of PD, a multiple hit hypothesis was pro-posed by Sulzer (2007), discussed later in this chapter. Evi-dence has accumulated over decades from pathologic and biochemical findings that implicate oxidative stress, mito-chondrial dysfunction, excitotoxicity, inflammation, and apoptosis as taking place in the SNc (Fig. 5.10). More recently protein aggregation in the form of Lewy bodies and Lewy neurites has placed a major emphasis on the accumulation of toxic protein as perhaps the most important pathogenic factor. Each of these factors cross-interact with the others to add to the pathogenesis of cell death. Toxic proteins accu-mulate because of insufficient degradation or an excess syn-thesis that the normal degradation process cannot handle.

Oxidative stress

A key source of oxidative stress in monoaminergic neurons is via monoamine metabolism and auto-oxidation (dis-cussed in more detail below). Since most research in PD

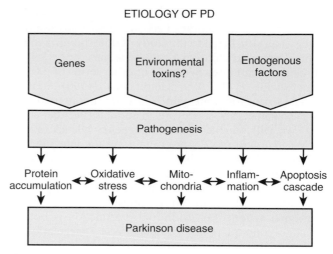

ETIOLOGY OF PD

Figure 5.10 Pattern of etiologic and pathogenic factors leading to dopamine neuron loss and the clinical motor features of PD.

neurodegeneration has been applied to dopaminergic neurons, we will focus on dopamine. Antioxidant defenses protect cells, and one of the leading antioxidants is reduced glutathione (GSH), and this is reduced in the SNc of PD patients at postmortem (Perry et al., 1982; Sian et al., 1994). This reduction of GSH is specific to PD brains, and is not seen in atypical parkinsonisms with nigral degenera-tion. The reduction of GSH likely reflects an excess utiliza-tion of this reducing agent, implying a high degree of oxidative stress taking place there. The decrease in GSH in the SNc occurs in incidental Lewy bodies as well as in PD, suggesting that oxidative stress has occurred prior to nerve cell loss. Some evidence suggests that GSH depletion itself may play an active role in PD pathogenesis (Martin and Teismann, 2009). Iron accumulation in the nigra also con-tributes to oxidative stress (Dexter et al., 1989a). Oxidized products of lipids, DNA, and protein are also seen in the PD nigra (Dexter et al.,1989b; Sanchez-Ramos et al., 1994), providing postmortem evidence of oxidative stress. The for-mation of neuromelanin in dopamine neurons is derived from the condensation of oxidized dopamine products, and thus represents a protective mechanism by the cell to defend itself against oxidative stress (Sulzer et al., 2000). One of the mutant genes that can cause PD, *DJ-1*, functions normally to protect against oxidative stress and is discussed below.

It is of interest that an endogenous substance, uric acid, which has antioxidant properties, has been correlated with a reduction in developing PD (Weisskopf et al., 2007). Sub-sequent studies evaluating urate levels in plasma in the PRECEPT (Schwarzschild et al., 2008) and CSF in the DATATOP (Ascherio et al., 2009) clinical trials found that higher urate levels in men were associated with a slower rate of progression of PD.

Mitochondrial dysfunction

Mitochondria appear to play an important role in the pathogenesis of PD (Banerjee et al., 2009). The finding that 1-methyl-4-phenyl-1,2,3,6-tetrahydropyridine (MPTP) intoxication causes parkinsonism (Langston et al., 1983), and the discovery that MPTP selectively destroys dopamine neurons and impairs complex I activity in the mitochondria (Nicklas et al., 1987) led to the study of mitochondria in PD patients. Decreased complex I activity is seen in the SNc of PD brains and not elsewhere, nor in other forms of parkinsonism (Mizuno et al., 1989; Schapira et al., 1990). Another complex I toxin, rotenone, which is a commonly used pesticide, also damages SNc neurons in animals (Betarbet et al., 2000). We will see below that two genes related to PD, namely *parkin* and *PINK1*, help maintain the integrity and function of the mitochondria, and loss of function of these genes results in PD. Mitochondrial dysfunction impairs ATP production, which hinders energy-dependent mechanisms of degradation of misfolded proteins by the ubiquitin-proteasomal system. Mitochondrial dysfunction is both a cause and a consequence of oxidative stress. Deregulation of mitochondrial respiration leads to generation of reactive oxygen species, contributing to oxidative stress, while oxidative and nitrosative stress deteriorates mitochondrial function. An early event in MPTP toxicity is oxidative stress, which is the consequence of an inability to transport electrons due to the inhibition of mitochondrial complex I. The accumulating electrons are a source of oxidative stress (Zhou et al., 2008). Besides their role in electron transport and oxidative phosphorylation, mitochondria are a major cellular source of free radicals, affect calcium homeostasis, and instigate cell-death pathways via apoptosis (Henchcliffe and Beal, 2008; Schapira, 2008).

Other mechanisms

Excitotoxicity from excessive glutamatergic activity results in an increase in calcium and can damage mitochondria; this has been implicated in PD (Beal, 1998). Nitrosative stress is induced by nitric oxide forming peroxynitrite, leading to protein nitration, and has also been suggested as a pathogenic factor (Tsang and Chung, 2009). Inflammation is seen in PD SN (McGeer et al., 1988a, 1988b), but is not considered an early event (Zhou et al., 2008). Rather, inflammation appears to augment the continuing degeneration (Tansey et al., 2007; Hirsch and Hunot, 2009; Saijo et al., 2009; Przedborski, 2010). Apoptosis is thought to represent the cellular death mechanism in PD (Mochizuki et al., 1996; Hirsch et al., 1999).

Accumulation of toxic proteins

The accumulation of too much protein in the cell has invoked the concept that these proteins are toxic and can lead to cell death. The concept of accumulated unwanted protein derived from genetic studies with the discovery that the protein α-synuclein is present in Lewy bodies (discussed below). Proteins are commonly damaged by misfolding or some other alteration, so that they are not functioning normally, and the cell attempts to repair them or eliminate them through degradation by either the ubiquitin-proteasomal system or by autophagy via the lysosome. Thus, misfolded, damaged, or altered proteins are either repaired or else removed from the cell, otherwise they would accumulate and act as toxins that would damage the cell. The first step to eliminate such proteins is to try to repair them through chaperone-mediated mechanisms. If this fails,

the ubiquitin-proteasomal system attempts to remove the unwanted protein. If this is not capable of removing the protein, then autophagy via the lysosome takes place (Kopito, 2000; Pan et al., 2008). Autophagy appears to play a major role in removing α-synuclein and other unwanted proteins. This mechanism is described later in this chapter.

A host of etiologic factors trigger the various pathogenic mechanisms discussed above, with genetic, environmental, and endogenous factors being suspected as major players. An interaction between genes and the other two seem important, e.g., certain gene mutations act to increase susceptibility to neuronal damage.

Genetics as an etiologic factor of PD

Familial PD

Families with PD occurring in several members have been recognized over the years, with approximately 10% of newly diagnosed patients reporting someone else in the family having PD. One of the earliest to describe a family with multiple affected members was Allen (1937). Perhaps the largest pedigree of PD described to date and with many generations affected was that reported by Mjönes (1949) of a Swedish and Swedish-American family. He found an autosomal dominant inheritance pattern in this family with 60% penetrance. But generally, since most PD patients are sporadic without a positive family history, the disease was not thought to have a genetic etiology.

Twin studies

To study the possibility of a genetic cause of PD though, Duvoisin, Eldridge and their colleagues (1981) evaluated twins with PD. They found zero concordance in 12 monozygotic twin pairs and concluded that "genetic factors appear not to play a major role in the etiology of PD." This group (Ward et al., 1983) continued to analyze twin pairs and now in 43 monozygotic (MZ) and 19 dizygotic (DZ) pairs with the index case having definite PD, the frequency of PD in MZ twins was similar to that expected in an unrelated control group matched for age and sex. The authors again concluded that "the major factors in the etiology of PD are nongenetic." A Finnish twin study 5 years later (Martilla et al., 1988) also found low concordance in MZ twin pairs and also concluded that PD appears to be "an acquired disease not caused by a hereditary process." However, Bill Johnson, then at Columbia University, began to question the conclusions of the twin studies (Johnson et al., 1990), saying they were too small to be statistically conclusive and recommended that linkage studies be conducted.

The momentum toward a genetic etiology of PD

In 1990 Golbe and Duvoisin and their colleagues described a large kindred with autosomal dominant PD originating in Contoursi, Italy, with some of the family having emigrated to the US. This led Duvoisin to rethink his previous conclusions that PD is largely nongenetic (Duvoisin and Johnson, 1992).

At this time there were also reports that FDOPA PET scans can detect decreased FDOPA uptake in some nonaffected relatives, including twins with an affected co-twin (Brooks, 1991). A large PET study in twins indicated that the concordance for decreased striatal FDOPA uptake in PD twins is greater than previously realized (Burn et al., 1992). With the availability of the Contoursi kindred and with the tools of linkage analysis, the stage was set for finding a gene mutation in familial PD.

Finding the first gene mutation in PD

Linkage analysis was carried out on the Contoursi kindred, and after several years of searching, linkage to chromosome 4q21–q23 was found (Polymeropoulos et al., 1996). By the next year, Polymeropoulos and colleagues (1997) identified the mutated gene, SNCA, for the protein α-synuclein. The Contoursi family actually originated in Greece and immigrated to Italy. The mutation (Ala53Thr) was also found in three small, unrelated Greek families. Subsequently, two other mutations were found in SNCA, which also caused autosomal dominant PD, namely Ala30Pro in a German family (Krüger et al., 1998) and Glu46Lys in a Spanish family (Zarranz et al., 2004). Families with SNCA mutations have a younger age at onset (usually in their forties) and a more rapidly worsening course of PD, and also with some early cognitive impairment. So, the gene mutation, on average, causes a more severe form of the disease than the typical adult-onset sporadic case. The SNCA gene was originally labeled PARK1.

Although all these SNCA mutations are rare in causing all worldwide cases of both familial and sporadic PD, the protein α-synuclein has taken on a premier and most important role as being highly likely involved in the disease's pathogenesis, including the sporadic cases. Immediately after the gene mutation was discovered (Polymeropoulos et al., 1997), Spillantini and colleagues (1997) found that fibrillary α-synuclein is a major component of the Lewy body, a finding confirmed the following year (Mezey et al., 1998). In fact, staining microscopic brain slices with the antibody for α-synuclein has become the pathologist's tool to detect Lewy bodies, and probably accounts for the recognition that diffuse Lewy body disease (DLBD), also known as dementia with Lewy bodies (DLB), is the second most common cause of dementia after Alzheimer disease. Prior to staining for α-synuclein, ubiquitin antibodies were used because ubiquitin is another protein found within the Lewy body. Ubiquitin is located in the central core and α-synuclein in the surrounding halo (Fig. 5.11). Autopsies on patients with mutated or excess amounts of α-synuclein show an abundance of Lewy bodies (Seidel et al., 2010).

Other gene mutations in PD

After the SNCA gene mutation was found, other investigators began collecting families with PD and conducting linkage analyses on them and then cloning the gene when linkage was obtained. Japanese investigators discovered the second gene to cause PD, which they called parkin and designated as PARK2, with the protein also called parkin (Kitada et al., 1998). The gene mutation was initially reported in a family with autosomal recessive juvenile parkinsonism without

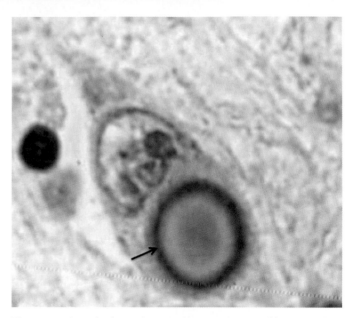

Figure 5.11 Lewy body in substantia nigra immunostained for α-synuclein. The arrow depicts the deposition of α-synuclein in the halo area of the Lewy body. *From Hishikawa N, Hashizume Y, Yoshida M, Sobue G. Clinical and neuropathological correlates of Lewy body disease. Acta Neuropathol 2003;105(4):341–350.*

Lewy bodies that had been linked to chromosome 6q25.2–q27 (Matsumine et al., 1998). Discovery was aided because many patients had deletions of large sections of chromosome 6, where the gene resides. Parkin mutations have now been identified pan-ethnically and are thought to be the cause of approximately 50% of familial young-onset PD and 15–20% of sporadic young-onset PD (<50 years). Over 70 mutations, including exon rearrangements, point mutations, and deletions, have been identified, many of them recurrent in different populations. The identification of parkin mutations is inversely correlated with age of onset, with the earliest age of onset having the greatest association. However, PARK2 does not appear to be restricted to young-onset PD, and parkin mutations have been identified in individuals over 50 (Lücking et al., 2000). Juvenile parkin-related PD is associated with mutations in both parkin alleles (homozygotes or compound heterozygotes). Some heterozygotes have now been recognized as having adult-onset PD with Lewy bodies (Farrer et al., 2001; Pramstaller et al., 2005). A single parkin mutation (heterozygote) may be responsible for instances of later onset PD (Foroud et al., 2003), and numerous heterozygote cases have now been found (Pramstaller et al., 2005). This is a crucial finding in the search for the cause of idiopathic PD, and it is clear that parkin plays an important role. The frequency and penetrance of parkin mutations have yet to be determined. PARK2, especially in juvenile cases, has been characterized by slow clinical progression, sustained response to levodopa, high likelihood of levodopa-induced dyskinesias, dystonia, sleep benefit, and hyperreflexia. The rate of loss of FDOPA striatal uptake is much slower in symptomatic and asymptomatic parkin carriers, compatible with the slow clinical worsening in this form of PD (Pavese et al., 2009).

The locus for PARK3 has been localized by linkage to chromosome 2p13 in a small group of European families with autosomal dominant PD with incomplete penetrance

(Gasser et al., 1998). Affected individuals have clinical and pathologic findings similar to sporadic late-onset PD, including age of onset. The sepiapterin reductase gene is a likely candidate for PARK3 (Karamohamed et al., 2003; Sharma et al., 2006). Sepiapterin reductase is an enzyme in the pathway for tetrahydrobiopterin synthesis, a cofactor for tyrosine hydroxylase. At present PARK3 is considered a susceptibility gene.

The evolution of the gene identification for PARK4 is a fascinating story. Waters and Miller (1994) described a kindred with autosomal dominant Lewy body parkinsonism in four generations, with an early age at onset (PARK4). The kindred was extended (Muenter et al., 1998; Farrer et al., 1999; Gwinn-Hardy et al., 2000), and action tremor similar to essential tremor and dementia were prominent within the family, and widespread Lewy bodies were seen in the cerebral cortex. Linkage was reported to chromosome 4p, but this haplotype also occurred in individuals in the pedigree who did not have clinical Lewy body parkinsonism but rather suffered from postural tremor only (Farrer et al., 1999). A second genome-wide search in this family found linkage on chromosome 4q and the mutation to be a triplication of a region of the chromosome that includes the *SNCA* gene (Singleton et al., 2003), the same gene that is mutated in PARK1. Instead of a mutation, though, this triplication produces a doubling of the normal, wild-type α-synuclein protein. A second PD family (this one being Swedish-American) with PD dementia with triplication of *SNCA* has also been reported (Farrer et al., 2004). The large Swedish family reported originally by Mjönes (1949) has been genetically analyzed and found to consist of duplications and triplications of normal *SNCA* (Fuchs et al., 2007). The remarkable thing about it is that the family has an α-synuclein duplication in one branch, and a triplication in the other, with a correspondingly different clinical picture (late versus early onset, respectively).

PARK5, an autosomal dominant mutation of the gene for ubiquitin-carboxy-terminal-hydrolase L1 (*UCHL1*), was found in a single family and was mapped to chromosome 4p14 (Leroy et al., 1998). Additional families with this mutation are necessary before concluding that *UCHL1* is a definite causative gene. But since this enzyme is part of the ubiquitin-proteasomal system, it implicates this degradative pathway as being important in the pathogenesis of PD (see below). Another potential pathogenic mechanism is the association of UCH-L1 with cellular membranes, including the endoplasmic reticulum (Liu et al., 2009). The membrane-associated form of UCH-L1 has been correlated with the intracellular level of α-synuclein.

Families with autosomal recessive, young-onset PD in southern Europe were mapped to chromosome 1p35–p36, labeled as PARK6 (Valente et al., 2002), and Valente and her colleagues (2004) identified two homozygous mutations in the PTEN-induced putative kinase 1 (*PINK1*) gene. Novel homozygous mutations in this gene were subsequently found in six unrelated Asian families (Hatano et al., 2004). Other families around the globe have been reported, and heterozygosity appears to increase susceptibility to developing PD (Hedrich et al., 2006). PINK1 is a mitochondrial serine/threonine kinase, and appears important in combating oxidative stress. The patients with *PINK1* mutations resemble those with *parkin* mutations. Excessive parkin can

rescue the PINK1 mutant phenotype, indicating that parkin works downstream from PINK1 in a common pathway. One autopsy of a young-onset patient with PD due to *PINK1* mutations showed the presence of Lewy bodies (Samaranch et al., 2010).

PARK7, the *DJ-1* gene mutation, is another cause of early-onset, autosomal recessive PD and is due to mutations on chromosome 1p36 (Bonifati et al., 2003). The mutations and gene identification were found in a consanguineous Dutch family and families in Italy and Uruguay. PARK7, like *parkin* and *PINK1*, is characterized by slow progression and a good response to levodopa. No autopsies have been reported for individuals with *DJ-1*. The crystal structure of DJ-1 reveals a redox-reactive center. DJ-1 may be activated in the presence of reactive oxygen species under conditions of oxidative stress. DJ-1, therefore, is an important redox-reactive signaling intermediate controlling oxidative stress (Kahle et al., 2009). *DJ-1* and *PINK1* are both important for mitochondrial function (Cookson, 2010). Knock-out mutants of DJ-1 enhance mitochondrial oxidative stress produced by pacemaking of SNc neurons (Guzman et al., 2010).

The most common PD gene mutation found so far has been PARK8, the gene located on chromosome 12p11.2–q13.1 for the protein leucine-rich repeat kinase 2 (LRRK2) (Zimprich et al., 2004), which is also called dardarin (Paisan-Ruiz et al., 2004). Initially, linkage to chromosome 12 was reported in a large Japanese autosomal dominant family without Lewy bodies (Funayama et al., 2002). But the Zimprich and Paisan-Ruiz families included subjects with Lewy body pathology, tangle pathology, and without Lewy bodies. One *LRRK2* mutation, G2019S, is the most common and is seen in more than 2% in sporadic North American and English PD patients (Gilks et al., 2005; Nichols et al., 2005). The highest frequencies are in the Portuguese (Bras et al., 2005), Ashkenazi Jewish (Clark et al., 2006; Ozelius et al., 2006), and North African Arab (Lesage et al., 2006) patients, even in the absence of a family history of PD. The clinical, pathologic, and genetic epidemiology of *LRRK2* were reviewed by Haugarvoll and Wszolek (2006) and mixed pathology resembling typical PD, tauopathies (tangles), and multiple system atrophy (MSA) were seen. However, patients with typical MSA were not found to have the *LRRK2* G2019S mutation (Ozelius et al., 2007). In the Chinese population the G2019S mutation is rare, but about 9% of PD patients have a heterozygous G2385R mutation (Fung et al., 2006; Farrer et al., 2007). *LRRK2* mutations show the typical age at onset and are not prone to be young onset (Clark et al., 2006). Penetrance is not complete and variable rates have been reported. Penetrance increases with age. In one report, it increases from 28% at age 59 years, to 51% at 69 years, and 74% at 79 years (Healy et al., 2008), and in another report the penetrance rate was 24% at the age of 80 (Clark et al., 2006).

How mutations in *LRRK2* cause PD is not clear. Increased kinase activity appears to be involved. Enhanced kinase activity (approximately three-fold) has been consistently reported for G2019S; but four disease mutants, R1441C, R1441G, Y1699C, and I2020T, have kinase activity less than two-fold of the wild-type protein (Dauer and Ho, 2010). Inhibitors of LRRK2 kinase have been found to be protective in both in vitro and in vivo models of LRRK2-induced neurodegeneration. These results establish that LRRK2-induced degeneration of neurons in vivo is kinase-dependent (Lee et al., 2010).

PARK9 is actually a Parkinson-plus disorder rather than PD. The autosomal recessive disorder has a mutation for the A form of parkinsonism-plus seen with a mutation of lysosomal type 5 ATPase, *ATP13A2*, on chromosome 1q36, known as PARK9. There is juvenile onset, and the disorder was originally known as the Kufor-Rakeb syndrome, after the village in Jordan where the affected families reside (Najim al-Din et al., 1994). This syndrome had features of Parkinson-plus with pyramidal signs, dystonia, and supranuclear gaze palsy. The disorder is levodopa-responsive, and some cases show putaminal and caudate iron accumulation, making it another neurodegeneration with brain iron accumulation (NBIA) (Schneider et al., 2010).

A genome-wide screen on 117 Icelandic patients with classic late-onset Parkinson disease and 168 of their unaffected relatives from 51 families resulted in linkage to chromosome 1p32 (Hicks et al., 2002). This susceptibility gene for PD was designated as PARK10.

A genome-wide screen on 150 families with PD resulted in finding linkage for a susceptibility gene on chromosome 2q36–q37, designated as PARK11 (Pankratz et al., 2003a). Mutations in the gene coding for GRB10-interacting GYF protein 2 (GIGYF2) was reported (Lautier et al., 2008), but this has been questioned by other investigators (Guo et al., 2009; Nichols et al., 2009).

A genome-wide search also found a positive LOD score for a locus on chromosome Xq21–q25 (Pankratz et al., 2003b), which has been designated as PARK12.

Using a candidate gene approach based on the phenotype of motor neuron degeneration in mice, a genome search on German PD patients found a novel mutation of a mitochondrial serine protease HTRA2 (high temperature requirement protein A2) in four patients (Strauss et al., 2005; Plun-Favreau et al., 2008). This mutation has been listed as PARK13.

Homozygosity for a missense mutation in the *PLA2G6* gene was discovered in a large consanguineous Pakistani family with neurodegeneration with brain iron accumulation (NBIA2), a condition known as infantile neuroaxonal dystrophy (Morgan et al., 2006). Spasticity, cerebellar ataxia, and optic atrophy are common in these infants (Kurian et al., 2008). But the phenotypic spectrum has been found to be much broader. It can cause autosomal recessive dystonia–parkinsonism at all ages, including adults, and without evidence of brain iron accumulation (Paisan-Ruiz et al., 2009). It has been labeled PARK14.

Parkinsonism with spasticity occurring in the first decade of life has been called pallido-pyramidal syndrome (Davison, 1954). It is a recessive disorder that responds well to levodopa therapy (Horowitz and Greenberg, 1975; Bronstein and Vickrey, 1996). It has also been called parkinsonism-pyramidal syndrome, and the mutation was found in the *FBXO7* gene coding for the F-box only protein 7 (Di Fonzo et al., 2009). It has been labeled PARK15.

PARK16 was discovered by a large genome-wide association study in the Japanese population on chromosome 1q32 (Satake et al., 2009). This finding was replicated in a large genome-wide association study in the European population (Simón-Sánchez et al., 2009) as did another replication study, which showed an association in ethnic Chinese but no association in caucasians of European ancestry

(Vilariño-Güell et al., 2010). The nature of the abnormal gene is unknown.

A mutation in the *EIF4G1* gene on chromosome 3q27 was recently found in European and American families, all with the same ancestral haplotype (Chartier-Harlin et al., 2009).

Although not designated with a PARK label, heterozygotic mutations of the lysosomal enzyme, β-glucocerebrosidase (*GBA*) gene on chromosome 1q21 (homozygotes are the cause of Gaucher disease) have been associated with PD (Goker-Alpan et al., 2004; Aharon-Peretz et al., 2004, 2005; Clark et al., 2005) and in other Lewy body disorders (Goker-Alpan et al., 2006). Mutations of GBA are most common in the Ashkenazi Jewish population. Between 17–30% of the Ashkenazi sporadic PD patients are heterozygotes for the *GBA* mutation (Aharon-Peretz et al., 2005; Clark et al., 2007). The *GBA* mutation is associated with onset younger than 50 years compared to the older age onset in sporadic PD (Clark et al., 2007). Heterozygous mutations have been found in patients with PD in all ethnic groups, and has been designated a risk factor for PD. Being a lysosomal enzyme, it implies a link between autophagy malfunction and PD.

Evaluating eight mutations of *GBA* among 420 patients with PD and 4138 controls of Israeli Ashkenazi origin, the relative frequency of mutation carriers was 18% versus 4% and severe mutations were associated with 13-fold increased risk of PD compared to two-fold risk increase in subjects with mild mutations (Gan-Or et al., 2008). In addition, 14% of the studied patients had the G2019S *LRRK2* mutation. Thus more than a third of all PD Ashkenazi Jewish patients carried the *GBA* or the *LRRK2* mutation. In one study involving a Japanese population of 534 patients with PD and 544 controls, 55 patients with PD (9.4%) and only 2 controls (0.37%), odds ratio (OR) 28.0, had at least one of 11 pathogenic heterozygous variants in the *GBA* gene (Mitsui et al., 2009). In another study, involving 790 British (non-Jewish) PD patients and 257 controls, *GBA* mutations were found in 33 (4.18%) of patients and 3 (1.17%) of controls (OR 3.7) (Neumann et al., 2009). The *GBA* positive patients were younger at onset and 45% had visual hallucinations and 48% had cognitive decline or dementia. Diffuse neocortical Lewy body pathology occurred more frequently in the 17 *GBA*-positive patients examined at autopsy, than in controls. A large worldwide 16-center collaborative project involving 5691 patients with PD and 4898 controls revealed an OR of 5.43 for any *GBA* mutation in patients versus controls (Sidransky et al., 2009).

Compared to the general population, parkinsonism in patients with Gaucher disease is more frequent, occurs at an earlier age, responds less well to levodopa, and is more frequently associated with cortical dysfunction (Kraoua et al., 2009). Enzyme replacement therapy and substrate reduction therapy were ineffective. The independently increased risk of *GBA* mutations in patients with PD, together with the identification of mutations in a lysosomal type 5 P-type ATPase gene responsible for the PARK9 locus, suggests the link between neurodegeneration producing the PD phenotype and impaired autophagic lysosomal mechanisms (Pan et al., 2008). For those with Gaucher disease 5–7% develop PD by age 70, and 9–12% before age 80 years (Rosenbloom et al., 2011).

Families with compound heterozygosity in the DNA polymerase gamma 1 (POLG1) were discovered to have early onset PD in addition to a polyneuropathy (Davidson et al., 2006; Orsucci et al., 2011). This enzyme is involved in the replication of mitochondrial DNA, indicating that impaired mitochondrial function can lead to PD.

Perry syndrome is a rapidly progressive disease with familial parkinsonism, hypoventilation, depression, and weight loss (Perry et al., 1975; Wider and Wszolek, 2008). In addition to severe neuronal loss in the substantia nigra and locus coeruleus, there is also loss of putative respiratory neurons in the ventrolateral medulla and raphe nucleus (Tsuboi et al., 2008). There are neuronal and glial inclusions that stain positive for TAR DNA-binding protein-43 (TDP-43) (Wider et al., 2009), as seen in ALS and frontotemporal dementia. Mutations in the *DCTN1* gene, which codes for dynactin 1, has been found (Farrer et al., 2009). The dynactin complex is important for many cellular transport functions including axonal transport of vesicles.

An *infantile dystonia–parkinsonism* disorder due to homozygous loss-of-function mutations in the *SLC6A3* gene encoding the dopamine transporter has been reported (Kurian et al., 2009). Such mutations have been associated with attention deficit hyperactivity disorder. One would expect increased synaptic dopamine, and therefore a hyperkinetic disorder rather than a parkinsonian-dystonia disorder, which is usually associated with a deficiency of striatal dopamine and thus decreased synaptic dopamine reaching the dopamine receptor. The CSF contained an elevated level of homovanillic acid (HVA), the final metabolite of dopamine, indicating a high turnover of dopamine. It would appear that the synaptic dopamine is being rapidly metabolized by monoamine oxidase (MAO) and catechol-O-methyltransferase. Perhaps the dopamine receptor was downregulated. There was a poor response to levodopa therapy.

Other familial or childhood-onset *dystonia–parkinsonisms* are those due to homozygous mutations of the gene for tyrosine hydroxylase and the heterozygous mutations of the gene for the tyrosine hydroxylase cofactor, GTPCH1. Both of these disorders are discussed in Chapter 12.

There is emerging evidence that some patients with parkinsonism are born with fewer than normal dopaminergic neurons as a result of some in utero or perinatal event or as a result of mutations in genes that code for various transcription factors, such as nuclear receptor-related 1 (*NURR1*) (Bensinger and Tontonoz, 2009), human achaete-scute homolog 1 (*HASH1*), and paired-like homeodomain transcription factor 3 (*PITX3*), and other genes necessary for the development and maintenance of the dopaminergic system (Le et al., 2009).

A summary of the genetic alterations described above is presented in Table 5.3.

Environmental factors contributing to etiology of or protection against PD

Environmental toxic factors

A gene–environment interaction is a common theme in the etiology of PD. With the discovery of MPTP as a toxin causing parkinsonism due to dopamine neuron degeneration (Langston et al., 1983), an environmental etiology seemed likely. MPTP is the protoxin; it is oxidized by MAO-B to MPP+, which can be taken up into dopamine nerve terminals via the dopamine transporter. Once there, it inhibits complex I in the mitochondrial respiratory chain, thereby reducing ATP synthesis and increasing superoxide radicals (for review, see Dauer and Przedborski, 2003). But MPTP-induced parkinsonism is not PD; moreover inhibition of MAO-B with selegiline (Parkinson Study Group, 1993) or rasagiline (Parkinson Study Group, 2004) does not halt progression of PD. Rotenone is used to poison unwanted fish in lakes, and like MPP+ inhibits complex I and can cause experimental parkinsonism (Betarbet et al., 2000). Whether it is an important environmental factor is questionable, although the association of PD in men with pesticide exposure is positive whereas exposure to other chemicals is not (Frigerio et al., 2006). Two pesticides in particular, maneb and paraquat, show a high risk for PD, and the risk is even greater if a person is exposed to both (Costello et al., 2009).

There are other pesticides known to cause dopaminergic damage, including ziram, which has been shown to inhibit the ubiquitin/proteasome system in primary ventral mesencephalic cultures (Chou et al., 2008). In an analysis of serum samples of 50 PD patients and 43 controls, beta-hexachlorocyclohexane (β-HCH) was more often detectable in patients with PD (76%) than controls (40%) (Richardson et al., 2009). One study showed the world's highest prevalence of PD may be among the Amish in the northeast United States. The prevalence of PD was 5703/100 000 (nearly 6%) of people 60 years old or older, more than three times the prevalence for the rest of the United States (Racette et al., 2009). Since normal subjects were more related to each other than were subjects with clinically definite PD, this suggests that environmental factors, such as high use of pesticides, may contribute to the high prevalence of PD in this community. To investigate occupation, specific job tasks or exposures, and risk of parkinsonism and clinical subtypes, a multicenter case-control study comparing lifelong occupation and job-task histories was created to determine associations with parkinsonism. In the study, referred to as SEARCH (Study of Environmental Association and Risk of Parkinsonism using Case-Control Historical Interviews), 519 patients and 511 controls were analyzed. Increased risk of parkinsonism was found with pesticide use (OR 1.9, 95% CI 1.12–3.21), whereas tobacco and greater caffeine intake were inversely associated with PD risk (Tanner et al., 2009).

Other than pesticides, there is little consistent evidence for environmental factors. Other putative risk factors are head trauma, certain occupations, and milk consumption (Tanner, 2010). Against a strong, new environmental factor is the lack of clusters of PD and an unchanging incidence rate over decades (Rocca et al., 2001). With the discovery of individual genes causing PD, a major genetic contribution to the etiology of PD has become predominant. It is likely that there are specific genes that can cause familial PD and susceptibility genes that make the individual with those genes sensitive to triggers to pathogenesis from environmental or endogenous factors, such as oxidative stress. Endogenous factors, such as dopamine in nigral neurons and autonomous cell firing through calcium channels with the aging process, are discussed below under pathogenesis.

Infectious agents remain a possible etiologic factor. For example, the highly pathogenic H5N1 avian influenza

Table 5.3 Gene alterations causing parkinsonism

Gene	Locus	Protein	Mode of inheritance	Mean age at onset (years)	Progression; clinical features	Protein function
SCNA (PARK1)	4q21.3	α-Synuclein; A53T, A30P, and E46K mutations	AD	45 (20–85)	Rapid; dementia, hypoventilation, myoclonus, abnormal extraocular movements, incontinence	Possibly synaptic vesicle trafficking; elevated in bird song learning
PRKN (PARK2)	6q25.2–q27	Parkin	AR in juvenile onset; AD in older onset	Young (3–64); usually below 20	Very slow; dystonia at onset; sleep benefit; no Lewy bodies in AR juvenile form	Ubiquitin E3 ligase, attaches short ubiquitin peptide chains to proteins for degradation
PARK3	2p13	Unknown	AD	59 (37–89)	Slow; indistinguishable from idiopathic PD	–
SCNA (formerly PARK4)	4q21 region duplication and triplication	Excess wild-type α-synuclein	AD	33	Rapid; wide range of symptoms from idiopathic PD to dementia with Lewy bodies	Same as PARK1
UCHL1 (PARK5)	4p14	Ubiquitin-C-terminal hydrolase L1	AD	~50	Indistinguishable from idiopathic PD	Removes polyubiquitin in ubiquitin-proteasomal cycle
PINK1 (PARK6)	1p35–p36	PTEN-induced putative kinase 1	AR	40 (30–68)	Slow	Mitochondrial serine-threonine kinase; modulates mitochondrial dynamics
DJ-1 (PARK7)	1p36	DJ-1	AR	33 (27–40)	Slow; as in parkin, but with behavioral problems and focal dystonia	Possible atypical peroxiredoxin; protects against oxidative stress
LRRK2 (PARK8)	12p11.2–q13.1	Leucine rich repeat kinase 2 (dardarin)	AD	~60	Indistinguishable from idiopathic PD; ↓ penetrance	Probably a cytoplasmic kinase
ATP13A2 (PARK9)	1p36	Lysosomal ATPase	AR	12–16	Kufor-Rakeb syndrome, similar to PD and to pallidopyramidal syndrome (PARK15)	Maintain acid pH in lysosome
PARK10	1p32	Unknown	AR	Typical late onset	Standard PD; families in Iceland	–
(*GIGYF2* in doubt) (PARK11)	2q21.2	GRB10-Interacting GYF protein 2 (in doubt)	AD	Typical late onset	Indistinguishable from idiopathic PD	Gene identification is in doubt
PARK12	Xq21–q25	Unknown	X-linked recessive	Typical late onset	Indistinguishable from idiopathic PD	–
HTRA2 (PARK13)	2p12	High temperature requirement protein A2 (HTRA2)	AD	Typical late onset	Indistinguishable from idiopathic PD	Serine protease primarily localized in the endoplasmic reticulum and mitochondria

Continued

Table 5.3 Continued

Gene	Locus	Protein	Mode of inheritance	Mean age at onset (years)	Progression; clinical features	Protein function
PLA2G6 (PARK14)	22q13.1	Phospholipase A2	AR	Infants, children, and adults	(1) Infantile neuroaxonal dystrophy with spasticity, ataxia and iron accumulation (NBIA2); (2) dystonia–parkinsonism in adults without iron	Phospholipase A2, releases fatty acids from phospholipids
FBXO7 (PARK15)	22q12–q13	F-box only protein 7	AR	Childhood onset	Pallidopyramidal disease; parkinsonian-pyramidal syndrome	Component of modular E3 ubiquitin protein ligases; functions in phosphorylation-dependent ubiquitination
PARK16	1q32	Unknown	Unknown	Typical late onset	Discovered by genome-wide association studies in Japan and Europe	–
EIF4G1	3q26–q27	Eukaryotic translation initiation factor 4-gamma, 1	AD	Typical late onset	Families from France, Ireland, Italy, and the US and all affected carriers appear to have the same ancestral haplotype	Eukaryotic initiation factor: facilitates the recruitment of mRNA to the ribosome
GBA	1q21	β-glucocerebrosidase	AD	Slightly younger than average	Indistinguishable from idiopathic PD; all ethnic groups; most common in Ashkenazi Jews; homozygotes → Gaucher disease	Lysosomal enzyme; metabolizes membrane lipid glucosyl ceramide to ceramide and glucose
DCTN1	2p13	Dynactin 1	AD	Early onset	Perry syndrome; familial parkinsonism with hypoventilation, depression, and weight loss; neuronal and glial inclusions that stain positive for TAR DNA-binding protein-43 (TDP-43)	Cellular transport functions, including axonal transport
POLG1	15q25	Polymerase gamma 1	AD	Early onset	Families with PD and peripheral neuropathy	DNA polymerase gamma 1, replication of mitochondrial DNA
GCH1 Dopa-responsive dystonia (DYT5)	14q22.1–q22.2	GTP cyclo-hydrolase 1	AD	Childhood onset with gait disorder; adult onset with parkinsonism	Dopa-responsive dystonia; penetrance is higher in females	Cofactor for tyrosine hydroxylase
TH	11p15.5	Tyrosine hydroxylase	AR	Infantile parkinsonism and dystonia	Dopa-responsive dystonia	Converts tyrosine to levodopa
SLC6A3 (DAT1)	5p15.3	Solute carrier family 6; dopamine transporter	AD	Infantile parkinsonism and dystonia	Elevated CSF HVA; poor response to levodopa	Reuptake dopamine from synapse
ATXN2 (SCA2)	12q24	Ataxin-2	AD	Young and late onsets	Ataxia, but can have a parkinsonian phenotype	Ataxin-2 is predominantly located in the Golgi apparatus

AD, Autosomal dominant; AR, autosomal recessive.

viruses enter the CNS and cause activation of microglia and α-synuclein phosphorylation and aggregation; in the SN there is loss of dopaminergic neurons (Jang et al., 2009a). Viruses known to induce parkinsonism include Coxsackie, Japanese encephalitis B, St Louis, West Nile, and HIV viruses (Jang et al., 2009b).

Environmental protective factors

There are a couple of environmental factors that are consistently associated with a *reduced* risk for developing PD, namely smoking (Ritz et al., 2007) and caffeine consumption. In the huge study (more than 140 000 men and women) in the Cancer Prevention Study II Nutrition Cohort, there was a lower risk of developing PD that correlated with (a) more years smoked, (b) smoking more cigarettes per day, (c) older age at quitting smoking, and (4) fewer years since quitting smoking (Thacker et al., 2007). It was concluded that the dependence of this association on the timing of smoking during life is consistent with a biologic effect.

Coffee consumption was also found to be associated with a lower risk of developing PD. First discovered by Ross and colleagues (2000) in Japanese-American men in Hawaii, this association has held up in subsequent epidemiologic studies. Ascherio and colleagues (2001) evaluated this association in two other large cohorts being followed, and found a similar association with coffee consumption and a mild lowered risk of developing PD in men (the authors speculated that estrogen use in women eliminated the caffeine benefit). Focus centered on caffeine and then speculation about the adenosine A2A receptor since this is affected by caffeine (Checkoway et al., 2002; Hernan et al., 2002; Schwarzschild et al., 2002; Ascherio et al., 2003, 2004).

A higher serum urate level is correlated with a reduction in developing PD (Weisskopf et al., 2007). Subsequent studies evaluating urate levels in plasma in the PRECEPT (Schwarzschild et al., 2008) and CSF in the DATATOP (Ascherio et al., 2009) clinical trials found that higher urate levels in men were associated with a slower rate of progression of PD. Urate has antioxidant properties. Use of anti-inflammatory drugs is another putative protective factor (Gagne and Power, 2010).

Endogenous factors that contribute to the etiology of PD

Gene mutations described above are not restricted to the cells that succumb in PD. Therefore, there must be some other factors that make these cells, in particular, more vulnerable. There are some unique features of dopamine neurons, and it is plausible that one or more contribute to the selective vulnerability of these cells. Three of them have gained prominence: (1) the presence of dopamine; (2) the interaction between dopamine and α-synuclein; (3) the autonomous firing of the SNc dopaminergic neurons using influx of calcium ions to trigger the action potential.

Dopamine induces oxidative stress

The SNc neurons are dopaminergic, and this monoamine provides a steady source of oxidative stress (Fahn and Cohen,

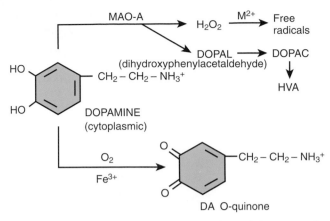

Figure 5.12 Auto-oxidation and enzymatic oxidation of dopamine to form oxyradicals and dihydroxyphenylacetaldehyde (DOPAL).

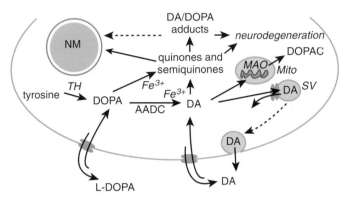

Figure 5.13 Metabolic pathways for levodopa and dopamine forming neuromelanin in dopaminergic nerve cells. NM, neuromelanin; TH, tyrosine hydroxylase; SV, synaptic vesicle; AADC, amino acid decarboxylase; DOPAC, dihydroxyphenylacetic acid; DA, dopamine; MAO, monoamine oxidase; Mito, mitochondria. *From Sulzer D, Bogulavsky J, Larsen KE, Behr G, Karatekin E, Kleinman MH, et al. Neuromelanin biosynthesis is driven by excess cytosolic catecholamines not accumulated by synaptic vesicles. Proc Natl Acad Sci USA 2000;97.11869–11874.*

1992). Levodopa and dopamine can be auto-oxidized to oxyradicals (semiquinones and quinones) and dopamine can be enzymatically oxidized by MAO-A (located in the dopamine nerve terminals) to form the intermediate dihydroxyphenylacetaldehyde (DOPAL) and final metabolite, homovanillic acid (HVA) (Fig. 5.12). For every molecule of dopamine metabolized by MAO, a molecule of hydrogen peroxide is formed, which can be a precursor of more oxyradicals. DOPAL has been found to enhance aggregation of α-synuclein (W.J. Burke et al., 2008). This may be an important mechanism of nigral neuron cell death because injection of DOPAL into rat nigra results in dopamine neuron loss (W.J. Burke et al., 2008).

The cell's defense is to condense the oxidized products and turn them into insoluble neuromelanin (Sulzer et al., 2000) (Fig. 5.13). This could explain why the most susceptible cells are those with the most neuromelanin (Hirsch et al., 1988, 1989); not because neuromelanin itself is toxic, but rather because its presence indicates these are the cells with the most oxidative stress. Cytosolic dopamine quinone can also

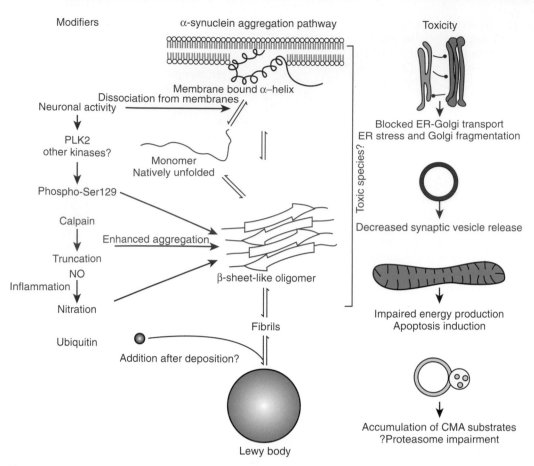

Figure 5.14 Schematic showing the different forms of α-synuclein and the pathway to fibrillogenesis. Natively unfolded or disordered α-synuclein monomers can also be in an alpha-helical form when within a membrane. It can form β-sheet-rich oligomers that comprise a transient population of protofibrils of heterogeneous structure that may include spheres, chains, or rings. The protofibrils may give rise to more stable amyloid-like fibrils. α-Synuclein fibrils eventually aggregate and precipitate to form LBs in vivo. CMA, chaperone-mediated autophagy; ER, endoplasmic reticulum. *From Cookson MR. alpha-Synuclein and neuronal cell death. Mol Neurodegener 2009;4:9.*

form adducts with other compounds, including cysteine to make a toxic compound.

Interaction between dopamine and α-synuclein

In the dopamine neuron, a special situation occurs for wild-type α-synuclein. α-Synuclein is a soluble protein in cytoplasm that is natively unfolded. By virtue of its containing an A2 alpha helix domain, it can associate with vesicle membranes (Clayton and George, 1998). A potential role for binding to synaptic vesicles is suggested by an enhanced synaptic recovery for evoked DA release in the knock-out animal (Maroteaux et al., 1988) and alterations in the distal synaptic vesicle pool in mutants (Abeliovich et al., 2000; Cabin et al., 2002). α-Synuclein can form into oligomers (also called protofibrils), which are beta-sheets that consist of spheres, chains, and rings. These protofibrils permeabilize the synaptic vesicles that store dopamine by forming pore-like assemblies on their surface (Mosharov et al., 2006). This allows leakage of vesicular dopamine into the cytosol, thus enriching cytosolic dopamine to enhance oxidative stress. A vicious cycle is at play because cytosolic dopamine reacts with α-synuclein to form a covalent adduct that slows the conversion of protofibrils to fibrils, thus sustaining the

presence of the protofibrils (oligomers) (Conway et al., 2000; Rochet et al., 2004). The presence of the oligomers then leads to more permeabilization of the synaptic vesicles and more cytosolic dopamine (Sulzer, 2010). A diagram of normal soluble α-synuclein forming oligomers, fibrils, aggregates and their deposition in Lewy bodies is seen in Figure 5.14.

Another critical peculiarity of α-synuclein-dopamine adducts is that they block chaperone-mediated autophagy (CMA) by binding and blocking the receptors on the lysosome from accepting other proteins and from being broken down by the CMA mechanism (Martinez-Vicente et al., 2008). This would lead to accumulation of toxic proteins in the cell, which would lead to the cell's dysfunction and death. A more complete discussion about the role of autophagy in removing damaged proteins is presented below.

Calcium influx into SNc dopaminergic neurons

A remarkable feature in the pathology of PD is that while SN dopamine neurons, particularly those located in the ventral tier of the SNc, undergo selective death, the neighboring dopamine neurons of the ventral tegmental area (VTA) are generally unaffected. The reason for this selective pattern of dopaminergic neuronal death remains unclear and should

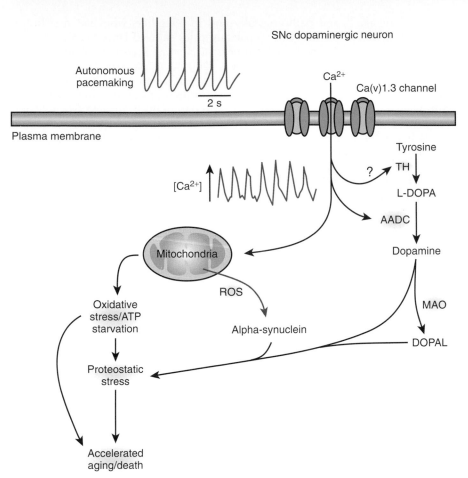

Figure 5.15 Calcium enhancement of dopamine synthesis leads to increased stress in substantia nigra dopaminergic neurons. *From Surmeier DJ. alpha-Synuclein at the synaptic gate. Neuron 2010;65(1):3–4.*

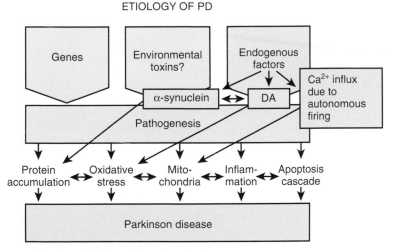

Figure 5.16 Endogenous factors contributing to the pathogenesis of dopamine neuron loss in PD.

be an important clue to pathogenesis. There are differences between the dopaminergic neurons in the SN and the VTA. There is less neuromelanin (apparently indicating less long-term oxidative stress from cytosolic dopamine) and there is more of the calcium-binding protein, calbindin (Iacopino et al., 1992). The expression of the vesicular monoamine transporter (VMAT2) that delivers cytosolic dopamine into the synaptic vesicles may also be somewhat higher in the VTA (Peter et al., 1995). Adult SNc dopaminergic neurons fire autonomously due to calcium ion influx, but VTA dopaminergic neurons use sodium ions (Surmeier, 2007).

A physiologic explanation has been suggested by Surmeier (2007). Unlike most neurons in the brain, SNc dopamine neurons are autonomously active; that is, they generate action potentials at a clock-like 2–4 Hz in the absence of synaptic input. In this respect, they are much like cardiac pacemakers. Juvenile dopamine-containing neurons in the substantia nigra pars compacta use sodium ion influx as the pacemaking mechanism. But these mechanisms remain latent in adulthood (Chan et al., 2007). Instead their adult autonomous activity is generated by Ca^{2+} ions whereas most neurons use channels that allow Na^+ ions across the membrane. The SNc dopamine neurons rely on L-type Ca(v)1.3 Ca^{2+} channels. With increased intracellular calcium, mitochondrial function can be affected with increased demand on oxidative phosphorylation, leading to increased production of reactive oxygen species and eventually cellular damage. As the cells undergo more stress over time, they thus "age faster." This would be a link with the risk factor of age (Surmeier, 2007). Blocking Ca(v)1.3 Ca^{2+} channels in adult neurons induces a reversion to the juvenile form of pacemaking (Chan et al., 2007). Such blocking ("rejuvenation") protects these neurons in both in-vitro and in-vivo models of PD, pointing to a new strategy that could slow or stop the progression of the disease (Chan et al., 2007; Surmeier, 2007). An intriguing finding is that a case-control analysis within the UK-based General Practice Research Database revealed that calcium-channel blockers when used to treat hypertension are associated with a lower prevalence of PD in those individuals compared to other antihypertensive therapies (Becker et al., 2008). This finding has been substantiated by a similar epidemiologic analysis of the Danish medical database. Subjects prescribed centrally-acting dihydropyridines (calcium channel blockers) prior to 2 years before the index date (onset of PD in affected subjects) were less likely to develop PD (OR 0.73, 95% CI 0.54–0.97) (Ritz et al., 2010). In contrast, risk estimates were close to null for the peripherally-acting dihydropyridine amlodipine and for other antihypertensive medications.

Mosharov and colleagues (2009) found that an interaction between Ca^{2+}, cytosolic dopamine, and α-synuclein appears to underlie the susceptibility of SN neurons in PD. α-Synuclein is critical, for without it, dopaminergic neurons are resistant to levodopa toxicity, and Ca^{2+} influx through L-type channels elevates dopamine synthesis to potentially toxic levels (Mosharov et al., 2009). Figure 5.15 illustrates how Ca^{2+} influx influences mitochondria and oxidative stress and may lead to cell death. Figure 5.16 illustrates how all the above endogenous factors influence the pathogenesis of PD.

Where does PD pathology begin? How does it progress? Braak's staging system

Following the development of Lewy neurites

Braak and his colleagues, using staining techniques to identify α-synuclein in neurons (Lewy neurites), studied 30 autopsied brains that were observed to have incidental Lewy body pathology (Del Tredici et al., 2002). Instead of finding α-synuclein staining fibers in the substantia nigra, they found them in non-catecholaminergic neurons of the dorsal glossopharyngeus–vagus complex, in projection neurons of the intermediate reticular zone, and in specific nerve cell types of the gain-setting system (coeruleus–subcoeruleus complex, caudal raphe nuclei, gigantocellular reticular nucleus), olfactory bulb, olfactory tract, and/or anterior olfactory nucleus, all in the absence of nigral involvement (Fig. 5.17). None of the melanized areas were affected, and the first of these to show Lewy changes was the locus coeruleus. Based on these findings of the location of Lewy neurites, these investigators proposed that PD begins in the lower brainstem and the olfactory apparatus.

Braak followed this study with one investigating Lewy neurites in 41 autopsies that were characteristic of PD clinically

and pathologically and in 69 others who had no clinical features but whose autopsies showed Lewy neurites so that he could determine if there was a pattern of progression (Braak et al., 2003, 2004). A pattern of α-synuclein-immunopositive Lewy neurites and Lewy bodies was discerned, in which these features began in the anterior olfactory nucleus and in the lowest part of the brainstem (stage 1) and then progressed rostrally up the brainstem. The raphe and locus coeruleus were the next to be involved (in stage 2). The substantia nigra became involved in stage 3, the mesocortex and thalamus in stage 4, the neocortex association areas and prefrontal cortex in stage 5, and the entire neocortex, but only mildly so in primary motor and sensory areas, in stage 6 (Fig. 5.18). As the stages develop, the sites involved in the earlier stages become more severely affected.

In a subsequent titled lecture, Braak and colleagues (2006) reinforced his staging system and cited support from other neuropathologic reports. They state that their samples did not include cases of diffuse Lewy body disease, which has its Lewy bodies starting in the cerebral cortex. All 110 cases they examined fell into one of six different subgroups based on the location of the brain regions involved (Fig. 5.19). Each of the subgroups displayed newly affected regions and those previously involved were worse. They pointed out that long unmyelinated axons, which the nigrostriatal pathway has, are the susceptible sites for Lewy neurites.

Although α-synuclein accumulation may not start in the nigra, unless the nigra becomes involved, the symptoms of PD do not develop. On the other hand, it is possible that symptoms of decreased sense of smell, depression, decreased assertiveness, impaired spatial sense, and even constipation may be preclinical symptoms of PD (Fig. 5.20) (Langston, 2006). Such a concept is leading researchers to seek clinical and laboratory biomarkers to detect PD before it becomes manifest with motor symptoms.

Are Lewy bodies and Lewy neurites toxic or protective?

Since they were first discovered, most neurologists and neuropathologists assumed that Lewy bodies somehow contribute to the cause or pathogenesis of the disease. Only recently has this assumption come under serious doubt. In fact, there is a large school of scientists who consider the formation of Lewy bodies as a means for the neuron to protect itself. Initiated by Lansbury and colleagues (2002, 2006), the concept has evolved that oligomers (protofibrils) of α-synuclein are toxic, in part because they permeabilize synaptic vesicle membranes. The protofibrils can be fibrillated (aggregated) into amyloid, thereby removing them, and thus protecting the neuron (Figs 5.21, 5.22). These aggregates thus represent a protective mechanism by the cell against oligomers' toxicity. This view is not universally accepted, and some neuroscientists believe that the fibrils are the toxic element. This remains a controversial point.

Is the Braak staging system for PD established as denoting the progression of pathology in PD?

A comprehensive appraisal of the Braak hypothesis was conducted by R.E. Burke and colleagues (2008). From their

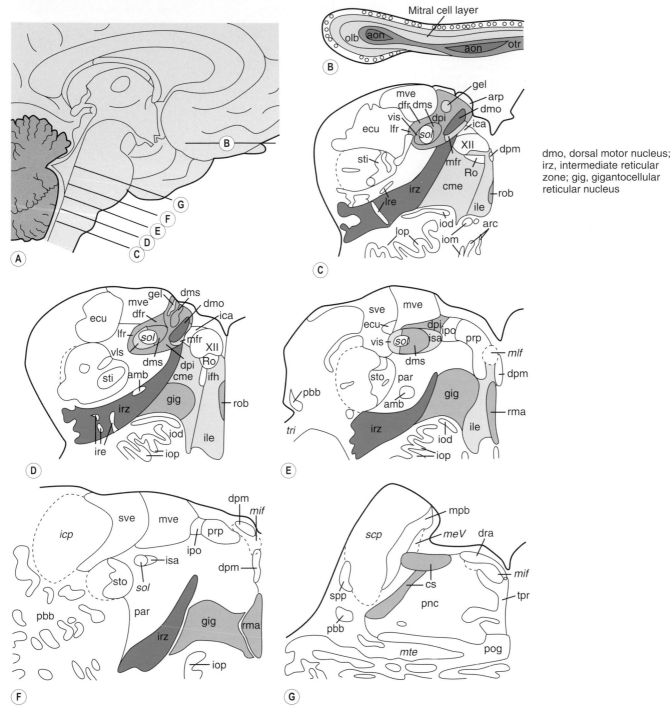

dmo, dorsal motor nucleus; irz, intermediate reticular zone; gig, gigantocellular reticular nucleus

Figure 5.17 Location of Lewy neurites in people with incidental Lewy bodies, and without clinical PD or DLBD. The more intense the color, the greater amount of Lewy neurites are present. *From Del Tredici K, Rub U, De Vos RA, et al. Where does Parkinson disease pathology begin in the brain? J Neuropathol Exp Neurol 2002;61(5):413–426.*

analysis, it is clear that the caudal-to-rostral spread of Lewy neurites is not entirely universal. Here, we summarize the arguments they made in concluding that this pattern of abnormal synucleinopathy – from caudal brainstem toward rostral structures over time – is not completely established for PD, but augmented with more recent findings, suggesting that the majority of PD patients might follow this pattern.

1. Unlikely that PD is universally preceded by caudal synucleinopathy. Many brains with incidental Lewy bodies with reduced numbers of nigral dopamine neurons do not show lower brainstem synucleinopathy. In a study by Parkkinen and her colleagues (2005), 16% of subjects with incidental Lewy bodies in the nigra did not have synuclein pathology in the lower brainstem. In another study looking at distribution of incidental Lewy bodies (iLBD), 34 of 235 brains studied had iLBD (14.5%) and all but one could be assigned a Braak PD stage (Frigerio et al., 2009). There were three patterns of distribution of α-synuclein pathology: (1) diffuse

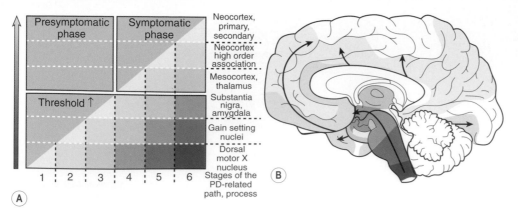

Figure 5.18 Braak staging of PD based on development of Lewy neurites. *From Braak H, Ghebremedhin E, Rub U, et al. Stages in the development of Parkinson's disease-related pathology. Cell Tissue Res 2004;318(1):121–134.*

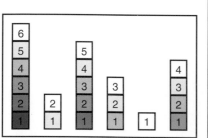

6: Neocortex, primary, secondary
5: Neocortex high order association
4: Mesocortex, thalamus
3: Substantia nigra, amygdala
2: Gain setting nuclei
1: Dorsal motor X nucleus

Figure 5.19 All 110 cases of Braak et al. (2006) fall into just one of six categories of locations of Lewy neurites. *From Braak H, Ghebremedhin E, Rub U, Bratzke H, Del Tredici K. Stages in the development of Parkinson's disease-related pathology. Cell Tissue Res 2004;318(1):121–134.*

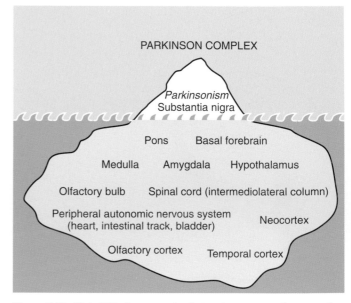

Figure 5.20 Clinical PD diagrammed as being the overt manifestation of a more complex disorder, in which several nonmotor features are considered part of PD. *From Langston JW. The Parkinson's complex: parkinsonism is just the tip of the iceberg. Ann Neurol 2006;59(4):591–596.*

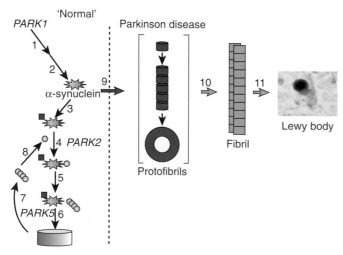

Figure 5.21 Excess or altered α-synuclein that is unable to be removed by the cell can form oligomers (protofibrils) and ultimately fibrils, which are deposited in Lewy bodies. *From Lansbury PT Jr, Brice A. Genetics of Parkinson's disease and biochemical studies of implicated gene products. Curr Opin Genet Develop 2002;12:299–306.*

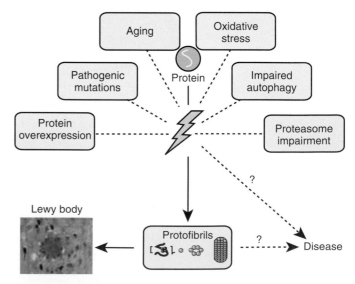

Figure 5.22 Factors that lead to the formation of α-synuclein protofibrils that could result in neurodegeneration. *From Lansbury PT, Lashuel HA. A century-old debate on protein aggregation and neurodegeneration enters the clinic. Nature 2006;443(7113):774–779.*

cortical and subcortical; (2) no cortical, but a caudal-to-rostral ascending pattern, primarily involving brainstem; and (3) intermediate between these two categories. Also, 6/33 cases failed to follow the pattern of contiguous spread proposed by Braak. These findings suggest dichotomy in the distribution of iLBD: some cases fit the Braak ascending scheme, conceptually consistent with preclinical PD, whereas others displayed prominent cortical involvement that might represent preclinical DLB.

2. **Dementia with Lewy bodies (DLB) in the cerebral cortex often does not have brainstem synucleinopathy.** Braak and colleagues (2003) excluded DLB in their series; yet many DLB cases have features of PD. In the autopsy series by Parkkinen and colleagues (2008), there were 226 cases of Lewy bodies in either the dorsal motor nucleus of vagus, substantia nigra or basal forebrain; 55% in Braak stage 5 or 6 lacked clinical features of dementia or parkinsonism. Moreover, of cases with dementia, 28% did not fit the Braak scheme of brainstem Lewy neurites being present.

3. **Many elderly people have Braak pathology from stages 1 through 6 and die without developing PD.** R.E. Burke and colleagues (2008) analyzed cases from the literature and plotted the Braak stages and the age at death, which showed no correlation between these two. Therefore, there is no certainty that those with early Braak stages will develop PD, and not everyone with advanced Braak stages has PD.

4. **No correlation between Braak stages and the clinical severity of PD.** R.E. Burke and colleagues (2008) plotted the Hoehn and Yahr (H&Y) scores published by Braak and colleagues (2003) and reported that individuals either had no clinical PD or had H&Y scores of 3–5 without a relationship to the Braak stage.

5. **REM sleep behavior disorder (RBD) usually does not necessarily precede PD and not everyone with RBD develops PD.** RBD is suspected of arising in the pons-medulla area, and therefore the Braak scheme would have RBD occurring before PD, if RBD is a component of PD. In the survey of their PD patients, Scaglione and colleagues (2005) found that only 33% had RBD. Of these, PD preceded RBD in 73%, an average of 8 years after onset of PD. In another study, RBD preceded PD in only 22% (De Cock et al., 2007). Postuma and colleagues (2009) followed patients with idiopathic RBD and found the risk for developing any neurodegenerative disease (PD, DLB, MSA, or Alzheimer disease) is 17.7% by 5 years, 40.6% by 10 years, and 52.4% by 12 years. Only 14 out of 93 developed PD. Subsequent studies reveal that approximately 50% of individuals with idiopathic RBD will develop PD and that the more severe the loss of atonia on baseline polysomnograms, the better the prediction of the development of PD (Postuma et al., 2010).

6. **PD due to *LRRK2* mutations does not always have Lewy body pathology.** In patients with *LRRK2* mutations who have PD, nigral degeneration is seen, but many do not have Lewy bodies, even though they may have the identical molecular mutation as those who do have Lewy bodies (Haugarvoll and Wszolek, 2006). Some patients have tau pathology. This is another example, like those described above, that Lewy bodies are not essential to have PD. Because the genetics are the same in these *LRRK2* families, one can question the role of α-synuclein in the pathogenesis of all cases of PD.

In addition to the above arguments, there are many other concerns about the Braak hypothesis (Attems and Jellinger, 2008; Halliday et al., 2008; Parkkinen et al., 2008; Kalaitzakis et al., 2009). For example, the progression outlined by Braak is not consistent with the natural history of PD (Lees et al., 2009). A study evaluating 71 PD cases showed that caudorostral spread did not occur in 47% of the cases and that extensive synucleinopathy can occur without overt neurological signs (Kalaitzakis et al., 2008). Some pathologists have, therefore, proposed of a "multicentric" origin of PD (Dickson et al., 2008).

7. **Results of neuroimaging do not completely match the pattern of the Braak pattern of progression.** Brooks (2010) has analyzed alterations in PET to see if they correlated with the Braak staging. Microglial activation as detected by PET has been seen in the cerebral cortex prior to dementia in early PD, suggesting a Braak level 5 or 6 at that early stage. Braak staging suggests that the serotonergic and noradrenergic systems could become dysfunctional ahead of the dopaminergic system in PD. But PET studies with serotonergic markers show less midbrain pathology than the dopaminergic nigrostriatal system. FDOPA uptake in the locus coeruleus appears to be preserved until late disease, indicating that the loss of noradrenergic function is a late phenomenon in PD, despite the presence of Lewy body pathology in Braak stage 2. Assessment of cholinergic function reveals a significant reduction in parietal and occipital cortex in early PD, although this would represent Braak stage 4 disease. In the heart, MIBG and ^{18}F-dopamine studies suggest early involvement of the sympathetic ganglia in PD, which is in keeping with Braak staging. Even so, in Hoehn and Yahr stage 1 PD, 50% of patients have normal MIBG uptake.

8. **Some nonmotor features of PD appear before the motor signs as predicted by the Braak staging hypothesis.** Autonomic involvement accounts for constipation seen in PD. A case-control study at the Mayo Clinic matched each incident case of PD ($n = 196$) by age and gender to the general control population (Savica et al., 2009). Constipation preceding PD was more common in cases than in controls ($P = 0.0005$). This association of constipation was found to have occurred for 20 or more years before the onset of motor symptoms of PD.

Bowel movement frequency was monitored and compared with postmortem SN neuronal loss in the Honolulu-Asia Aging Study (Petrovitch et al., 2009). There were evaluations in 414 men aged 71–93 years who later had postmortem evaluations. Men with 1 or more bowel movements daily had a significantly higher density of neurons in the SN compared to those with <1 daily. Constipation was associated with low SN neuron density independent of the presence of Lewy bodies. Incidental Lewy bodies were evaluated in these men. For men with <1, 1, and >1 bowel movement/day, corresponding percentages of incidental Lewy bodies were 24.1%, 13.5%, and 6.5% (Abbott et al., 2007), reflecting that fewer bowel movements were associated with more Lewy bodies.

Olfaction dysfunction (hyposmia) also precedes the motor signs of PD. Olfaction was assessed in 2267 men in the Honolulu-Asia Aging Study and followed for up to 8 years (Ross et al., 2008). The odds ratio for developing PD in the lowest quartile of smell sensitivity was 5.2 compared with

PARKINSON DISEASE TIMELINE

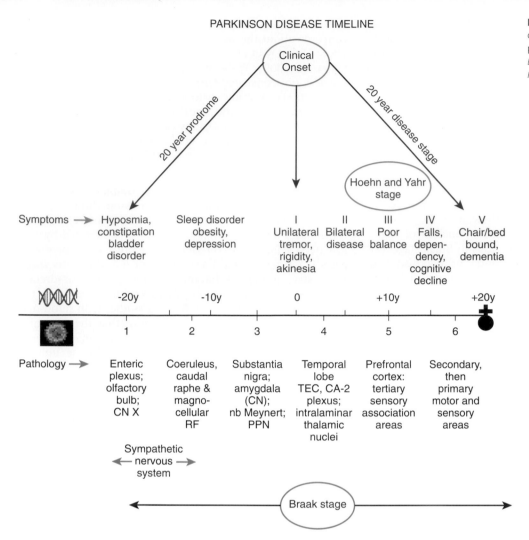

Figure 5.23 Diagram of a 40-year duration of PD, with 20 years being premotor. *From Hawkes CH, Del Tredici K, Braak H. A timeline for Parkinson's disease. Parkinsonism Relat Disord 2010;16(2):79–84.*

the top two quartiles. In another prospective study, involving nonaffected relatives of PD patients, 40 hyposmic and 38 normosmic individuals were studied at baseline and 2 years later with clinical evaluation and a dopamine transporter (DAT) scan (Ponsen et al., 2004). By 2 years, 10% of the individuals with hyposmia, who also had strongly reduced DAT binding at baseline, had developed clinical PD as opposed to none of the other relatives in the cohort. In the remaining nonparkinsonian hyposmic relatives, the average rate of decline in DAT binding was significantly higher than in the normosmic relatives. These results indicate that idiopathic olfactory dysfunction is associated with an increased risk of developing PD of at least 10%.

Supporting evidence that peripheral nervous system is affected before CNS Lewy neurites was the finding that cardiac sympathetic denervation – as measured by MIBG scintigraphy – precedes nigrostriatal loss (Tijero et al., 2010).

9. Human autopsy study to determine validity of Braak staging scheme. Dickson and colleagues (2010) studied the density and distribution of Lewy bodies (LBs) in several conditions. They found that the proportion of cases that fitted the PD staging scheme was 67% for incidental LBs (*n* = 12); 86% for progressive supranuclear palsy (PSP) with incidental LBs (*n* = 18); 86% for pure Lewy body disease

(LBD) with minimal or no Alzheimer type pathology (*n* = 52); 84% for LBD with concomitant Alzheimer disease (AD) (*n* = 84); and only 6% for AD with amygdala predominant LBs (*n* = 64). They conclude that the PD staging scheme of Braak is valid, except in the setting of advanced AD.

Braak and his colleagues are now estimating that the disease (pathology of Lewy neurites) begins in the olfactory and autonomic system by approximately 20 years before the onset of the motor symptoms of PD, and they have tried to correlate the Braak staging with the Hoehn and Yahr staging of clinical PD (Hawkes et al., 2010) (Fig. 5.23).

Clues on pathogenesis from monogenic PD

PARK1 (*SNCA*) and PARK4 (*SNCA*) and α-synuclein accumulation as Lewy neurites and Lewy bodies

Based on the presence of α-synuclein in Lewy bodies and on the pattern of progressive Lewy neurite formation from the caudal to rostral areas of the brain, it is clear that α-synuclein has a special place in the pathogenesis of PD. The normal function of α-synuclein, however, may have little or nothing to do with its role in pathogenesis. Its ability to self-aggregate, its presence in Lewy bodies, the apparent ability of pathogenic mutations or nitrated or DA-reacted proteins to be more prone to aggregation, the ability of protofibrils to disrupt membrane, and the identification of PARK4 as a triplication of the chromosomal region that contains the α-synuclein gene, all seem to point to a toxic function of α-synuclein itself. This notion is also supported by the finding that mice that lack α-synuclein expression are resistant to MPTP toxicity, although neuronal and synaptic vesicle uptake appear unaltered (Dauer et al., 2002). Expression of mutant α-synuclein also causes an apparent increase in cytosolic DA levels, suggesting a link between genetic and oxidative stress pathways (Lotharius et al., 2002). Thus, it may be that the disease stems from inappropriate or dysregulated degradation of this protein. The accumulated, insoluble, aggregated α-synuclein appears to play a vital role in the pathogenesis, leading to the suggestion that impaired protein degradation may be a key problem.

An approach to treating the toxicity from the accumulation of α-synuclein may be by the use of inhibitors of sirtuin 2. Sirtuins are members of the histone deacetylase family of proteins that participate in a variety of cellular functions and play a role in aging. Inhibition of SIRT2 rescued α-synuclein toxicity and modified inclusion morphology in a cellular model of PD and in a *Drosophila* model of the disease (Outeiro et al., 2007). The results suggest a link between neurodegeneration and aging.

PARK2 (*PRKN*) and PARK5 (*UCHL1*) and the ubiquitin-proteasomal system (UBS)

The key mechanisms through which misfolded or toxic proteins are degraded are the ubiquitin-proteasomal system (UBS) and autophagy via the lysosome. The cell initially attempts to restore such proteins using specific chaperones (heat-shock proteins) (Kopito, 2000), but if that is unsuccessful, the cell degrades the protein. The first attempt by the cell to remove these unwanted proteins is via the ubiquitin-proteasomal system. If that is unsuccessful, the process of autophagy is employed, using the lysosomes (Martinez-Vicente and Cuervo, 2007; Pan et al., 2008). Attention was initially directed to UBS because of the normal function of the proteins of PARK 2 (parkin) and PARK5 (UCHL1). The former is an E3 ligase and the latter separates the polyubiquitin chain into its separate components, both of which are active processes in the UBS. More recently, studies indicate that parkin is also related to mitochondria integrity and function (Mortiboys et al., 2008). PINK1 regulates parkin to its localization in the mitochondria by phosphorylating parkin (Kim et al., 2008). Both mutant *parkin* and *PINK1* result in swollen mitochondria. Parkin also stabilizes PINK1 (Shiba et al., 2009) to maintain the mitochondria. When expressed in a *Drosophila* model of PD, wild-type parkin protects against LRRK2 G2019S mutant-induced dopaminergic neurodegeneration (Ng et al., 2009). Parkin also promotes macroautophagy of damaged mitochondria (Narendra et al., 2008). This is another example of the important role of the autophagy by the lysosome in PD. Parkin may play a role in sporadic PD because it is inactivated by nitrosative, oxidative, and dopaminergic stress (Dawson and Dawson, 2010).

Protein degradation by autophagy – its importance in PD discovered by studying degradation of mutated α-synuclein

The lysosome degrades cell products by three different mechanisms – macroautophagy, microautophagy, and chaperone-mediated autophagy (Martinez-Vicente and Cuervo, 2007; Pan et al., 2008).

1. *Macroautophagy* involves the "in bulk" degradation of complete regions of the cytosol. Initially, these regions are sequestered by a limiting membrane, which seals to form a double membrane compartment known as an autophagosome. Because this vesicle lacks any enzymes, the trapped contents are not degraded until the autophagosome fuses with a lysosome, which provides all the hydrolases required for degradation of the contents. Macroautophagy occurs under stress conditions and has two major purposes: as a source to generate essential macromolecules and energy in conditions of nutritional scarcity or as a mechanism for the removal of altered intracellular components.

2. *Microautophagy* involves sequestering cytosolic regions directly into the lysosome through invaginations into the lysosomal lumen where they are rapidly degraded. Microautophagy participates in the continuous turnover of cellular components in normal cellular conditions.

3. *Chaperone-mediated autophagy (CMA)* is a mechanism to remove selective proteins, which are recognized by chaperones that deliver them to the surface of the lysosome. The substrate proteins interact with a receptor protein at the lysosomal membrane, and, assisted by a chaperone located inside lysosomes, the substrate proteins cross the membrane to be degraded in the lysosomal lumen. With impairment of the ubiquitin-proteasomal system and CMA, the misfolded protein could form fibers or oligomers and would need to be handled by macroautophagy. In conditions in which not even macroautophagy can remove the altered proteins, these aggregates usually trap other still-functional proteins inside aggregates. This is a serious event and can lead to cell death.

Wild-type α-synuclein is degraded by the ubiquitin-proteasomal system and chaperone-mediated autophagy (Cuervo et al., 2004, 2010). Mutated α-synuclein is unable to enter the lysosome; it becomes trapped at the lysosomal surface and that blocks other material from entering the lysosome and being degraded. Thus, mutated α-synuclein itself is not degraded, and "gums" up the process for other substrates. In addition to mutated α-synuclein being unable to penetrate the lysosome, the same problem exists for altered α-synuclein (phosphorylated, nitrated, or oxidized α-synuclein); these compounds bind to lysosomal membrane with high affinity and are not translocated into the lysosome (Fig. 5.24) (Martinez-Vicente and Cuervo, 2007). As mentioned above in the discussion about endogenous factors leading to selective vulnerability of dopamine neurons, the same problem develops with adducts of α-synuclein and dopamine; these adducts block the translocation of other CMA-attached proteins into the lysosome.

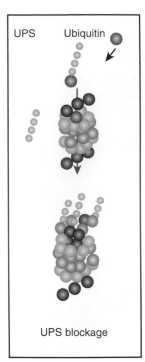

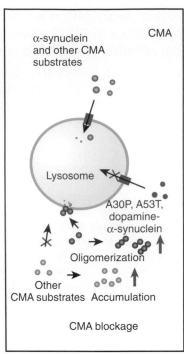

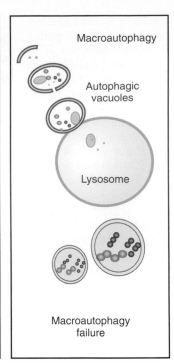

Figure 5.24 Altered α-synuclein degradation in Parkinson disease. Normal α-synuclein can be selectively degraded by the ubiquitin/proteasome system (UPS) (left) or in lysosomes by chaperone-mediated autophagy (CMA; middle). Pathogenic mutations and certain posttranslational modifications in α-synuclein promote its organization into complex structures no longer amenable to degradation via the proteasome or CMA (left and middle bottom). Furthermore, α-synuclein oligomers and preaggregates can block those two proteolytic systems. Macroautophagy undertakes the removal of organized abnormal α-synuclein and delivers it to lysosomes in sealed double membrane vesicles (autophagosomes; right). Changes in the lysosomal system due to the increasing amount of toxic α-synuclein complexes or indirectly through the action of aggravating factors, such as aging or oxidative stress, could result in macroautophagy failure and the consequent cellular compromise (right bottom). *From Cuervo AM, Wong ES, Martinez-Vicente M. Protein degradation, aggregation, and misfolding. Mov Disord 2010;25(Suppl 1):S49–54.*

PARK6 (*PINK1*), PARK7 (*DJ-1*), and PARK8 (*LRRK2*)

The PARK8 mutation is the one with the highest prevalence for PD of all the known gene mutations. The protein dardarin (also known as leucine rich repeat kinase 2 (LRRK2) has GTPase and kinase enzymatic domains plus at least two protein–protein interaction domains (Hardy et al., 2006). The common G2019S mutation and an adjacent mutation are located at the N-terminal portion in the kinase domain. This site contains the Mg^{2+} ion required for kinase function. Mutated *LRRK2* is disinhibited and has increased kinase activity and induces a progressive reduction in neurite length and branching both in primary neuronal cultures and in the intact rodent CNS (MacLeod et al., 2006). In contrast, *LRRK2* deficiency leads to increased neurite length and branching (MacLeod et al., 2006). Because most patients with PARK8 have Lewy bodies, the biochemical defect appears to be upstream of α-synuclein, but because some patients do not have Lewy bodies and may have other inclusions, such as tau tangles, the exact pathogenesis of PARK8's effect is still not clear.

PINK1 harbors a mitochondrial targeting motif and a serine/threonine kinase domain (Valente et al., 2004). PINK1 protein appears to accumulate within the intermembrane space of mitochondria (Silvestri et al., 2005). There is genetic interaction between *PINK1* and *parkin*; *Drosophila* deficient in *PINK1* can be restored to health with overexpression of *parkin*, but not vice versa (Abeliovich and Beal,

2006). This suggests a genetic pathway, with *parkin* functioning downstream of *PINK1*.

DJ-1 appears to play a role in protecting against oxidative stress, including that produced by dopamine (Lev et al., 2009). *DJ-1* deficiency sensitizes dopamine neurons to oxidative stressors in vitro and in the intact CNS (Abeliovich and Beal, 2006). Over-expression appears to protect against oxidative insults.

Lewy bodies in fetal dopaminergic neurons; infectious protein hypothesis

In the May 2008 issue of *Nature Medicine* three papers were published about postmortem findings of Lewy bodies in a few of the many surviving fetal dopaminergic neurons that were implanted into subjects with PD more than 11 years earlier. In two of the papers three of the subjects – implanted 11, 14 and 16 years earlier – had rare α-synuclein-containing inclusions resembling Lewy bodies (Li et al., 2008; Kordower et al., 2008). In the third paper, these α-synuclein-containing inclusions were sought out but not found in the brains of five subjects who were implanted 9–14 years earlier (Mendez et al., 2008). A fourth patient with PD who died 14 years posttransplantation also was found to have Lewy bodies in some of the otherwise numerous healthy grafted cells (Kordower et al., 2008).

Clearly, the differences between the studies need to be sorted out. The Lewy body findings, however, suggest a factor in the host striatum that can lead to α-synuclein accumulation and Lewy body formation. It also suggests that some factor(s) in the striatum may play a role in PD pathogenesis. This would imply that dopamine nerve terminals – and not the cell bodies – may be the initial site of pathology for the demise of the dopaminergic nigrostriatal neuron. The findings support the concept that the pathogenic process is chronically active in the PD brain, as McGeer and colleagues (1988a) have pointed out by their observations of continuing inflammation in the striatum. One speculation is that a prion-like mechanism might explain how PD pathology can transfer from the host to the graft (Kordower and Brundin; 2009).

Desplats and colleagues (2009) explored that possibility of neuron-to-neuron transfer of labeled α-synuclein from neuronal cells to neural stem cells in both in-vitro and in-vivo systems. α-Synuclein was transmitted via endocytosis to neighboring neurons and neuronal precursor cells, forming Lewy-like inclusions. With impaired autophagy, there was accumulation of transmitted α-synuclein and inclusion formation. The authors suggest that this mechanism may explain the topographical progression of Lewy pathology in PD suggested by Braak et al. (2003). Olanow and Prusiner (2009) proposed that the topographical spread of α-synuclein would be analogous to the spread of prion protein in prion diseases. Supporting this concept, Hansen and colleagues (2011) showed that exogenous dopaminergic cells can take up α-synuclein grafted into mice with overexpressed α-synuclein.

Multiple hit hypothesis with a central role of α-synuclein

Sulzer (2007) divides the genetic mutations resulting in PD into several categories as follows.

- Proteins affecting mitochondria (e.g., PINK1, DJ-1, Omi/HtrA2 and POLG).
- Proteins that might be involved in organelle trafficking and vesicular fusion (e.g., α-synuclein and tau).
- Proteins of macromolecular degradation pathways, such as ubiquitination or ubiquitination-like degradation pathways (e.g., parkin and DJ-1) and lysosomal function (e.g., β-glucocerebrosidase).
- Proteins that modify oxidative stress or antioxidant function (e.g., sepiapterin, DJ-1 and fibroblast growth factor-20 (FGF-20)).

With so many etiologic and pathogenic factors all resulting in the common denominator of loss of dopaminergic SNc cells, it is difficult to grasp a single unifying concept. Sulzer (2007) attempts to do just that with his multiple hit hypothesis. He suggests that "multiple hits" that combine toxic stress, for example, from dopamine oxidation or mitochondrial dysfunction, with an inhibition of a neuroprotective response, such as loss of function of parkin or stress-induced autophagic degradation, underlie selective neuronal death.

Despite the multiple hits that may be necessary for sporadic PD, α-synuclein appears to play a central role. This concept is supported by (1) its presence in Lewy bodies, which are found in all cases except those caused by *parkin*, some cases of *LRRK2*, and possibly *DJ-1*; (2) awareness that excess of wild-type α-synuclein can cause PD, and (3) indications that it may have prion-like properties. This would imply that preventing the accumulation of α-synuclein or finding means to eliminate it could be an effective approach to arrest and even reverse the disease process. A diagram illustrating how some of the genetic and pathogenic factors cause dopaminergic neuronal death is presented in Figure 5.25.

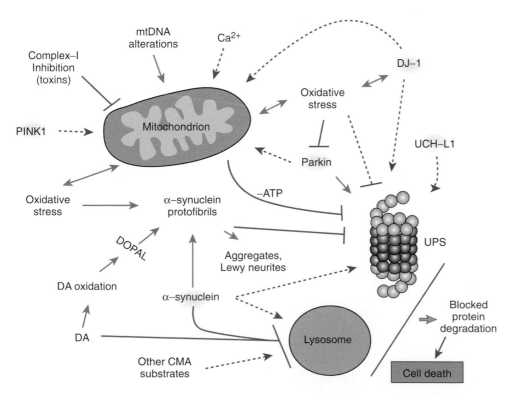

Figure 5.25 Diagram linking some of the genetic and pathogenic factors leading to impaired protein degradation in dopaminergic neurons via the lysosome and the ubiquitin-proteasomal system (UPS). Multiple hits may be involved before cell death can develop. *Design of diagram modified from Moore DJ, West AB, Dawson VL, Dawson TM. Molecular pathophysiology of Parkinson's disease. Annu Rev Neurosci 2005;28:57–87.*

Animal models

A reliable animal model that produces excess α-synuclein and manifests the PD phenotype could prove invaluable. A number of animal models manifesting features of PD have been developed. Perhaps the first was the reserpinized animal. Reserpine, discovered in India as rauwolfia, was known to produce a state of akinesia, i.e., drug-induced parkinsonism. One of the pioneering discoveries was that L-dopa is able to reverse this akinesia (Carlsson et al., 1957). Over the years, other agents were used to damage the dopamine neurons. These include 6-hydroxydopamine, MPTP (Halliday et al., 2009), and rotenone (Pan et al., 2009a). Systemically administered proteasome inhibitors have not been found to consistently produce dopaminergic. When lactacystin, a proteasome inhibitor, is injected in the region of the SN, it does produce pathologic, biochemical, and behavioral changes, suggestive of parkinsonism (Pan et al., 2009b).

The disappointment with the above animal models is that they are good for finding symptomatic therapies, but they have not been successful in helping to find neuroprotective therapies. Drugs that are effective by providing protection in some animal models have not been found to be protective in patients (Rascol et al., 2003; Lang et al., 2006; Olanow et al., 2006; Parkinson Study Group PRECEPT Investigators, 2007). Thus, these models, which are toxin models such as MPTP, have not been proven helpful in finding neuroprotective agents. Perhaps a genetic model would prove useful. Until recently knock-in, knock-out, and transgenic models have resulted in loss of dopaminergic SNc neurons but without the clinical phenotype of PD. More recently Li and colleagues (2009) developed a transgenic mouse model with an altered missense mutation on the *LRRK2* gene that produced some aspects of the parkinsonian phenotype, including older age at onset of symptoms and response to levodopa therapy. There was axonal pathology of the nigrostriatal neurons, but no loss of dopaminergic SNc cells. It will be interesting to use this animal model for neuroprotective studies and then see if successful agents will prove beneficial in patients with PD.

References available on Expert Consult: www.expertconsult.com

CHAPTER **6**

Medical treatment of Parkinson disease

Chapter contents

Introduction	119	Treatment of early-stage Parkinson disease	127
Therapeutic principles	119	Treatment of mild-stage Parkinson disease	134
Therapeutic choices available for Parkinson disease	121	Treatment of moderate-stage Parkinson disease	139
Medications available for Parkinson disease	121	Treatment of advanced-stage Parkinson disease	141

Introduction

If treatment of Parkinson disease (PD) with levodopa, the most efficacious drug available for this disorder, were uniformly successful and free of complications, there would be no controversies or complexities, and treatment of this disease would be easy. Moreover, treatment with levodopa would begin when the diagnosis of PD was made. But because of levodopa's propensity to cause motor complications (wearing-off and dyskinesia), which can impair a patient's quality of life, strategies have been developed to avoid or delay these motor complications. Also, strategies have been developed to overcome these complications once they have appeared. Thus, treatment strategies have evolved to deal with the different phases of the natural history of PD and also the presence of the motor complications. The natural history of PD is one of gradual worsening, not only of the cardinal motor symptoms, but also increasing prominence of nonmotor features; these are discussed in Chapter 8, which covers nonmotor symptoms due to the illness as well as those due to the medication. The natural history of the prototypical person who develops PD is someone who develops the first symptoms around age 60 and lives approximately 20 years, and has clinical problems as illustrated in Figure 6.1. The early stages, including problems of motor complications from medications, are largely treatable. It is the later stages with intractable motor symptoms and dementia that are virtually untreatable at present.

Therapeutic principles

Before discussing the phases of the disease and the treatment choices for each phase, we will discuss general principles of therapy for the patient with PD.

Give priority to any therapies, such as drugs or surgery, that have been established as protective

If any drug could slow the progression of the disease process, it would make sense to use it as soon as the disease is diagnosed. As of this writing, no proven protective or restorative effect of a drug has been demonstrated with certainty. But studies are in progress looking at various agents to determine if they have such an effect. Drugs that have been specifically evaluated in controlled clinical trials for slowing disease progression have been selegiline and tocopherol (Parkinson Study Group, 1989b, 1993a), selegiline alone (Myllyla et al., 1992; Parkinson Study Group, 1996a; Palhagen et al., 1998, 2006), riluzole (Rascol et al., 2003), neuroimmunophilin (NINDS NET-PD Investigators, 2007), coenzyme Q10 (Shults et al., 2002; NINDS NET-PD Investigators, 2007), glial-derived neurotrophic factor (GDNF) (Lang et al., 2006), and rasagiline (Parkinson Study Group, 2004a; Olanow et al., 2009). Two antiapoptic drugs that that were studied in controlled trials were a propargyline that inhibits glyceraldehyde 3-phosphate dehydrogenase (Waldmeier et al., 2000) and an inhibitor of the mixed lineage kinase-3 family that lies upstream of the c-Jun N-terminal kinase signal transduction pathway to apoptotic cell death (Xia et al., 2001). Both studies failed to show benefit (Olanow et al., 2006; Parkinson Study Group PRECEPT Investigators, 2007). Controlled trials with an antibiotic, minocycline, and an energy enhancer, creatine, using a futility design (Tilley et al., 2006), failed to show these drugs to be superior to their comparison placebo group (NINDS NET-PD Investigators, 2006, 2008). The same results were obtained for coenzyme Q10 and neuroimmunophylin (NINDS NET-PD Investigators, 2007). The MAO-B inhibitors, selegiline and rasagiline, have been studied in

DOI: 10.1016/B978-1-4377-2369-4.00006-8

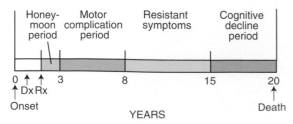

Figure 6.1 Natural history of PD in a prototypical patient with onset at age 60 and death 20 years later. Despite best available therapies, the clinical features of the disease progress through these phases.

clinical trials, with positive results suggesting they may modify disease progression, and many neurologists utilize one of these agents at the time of diagnosis, but whether either would delay the long-term, dopa-nonresponsive features is unknown. A discussion of the results of these completed studies is presented in the section "Treatment of early-stage PD."

Encourage patients to remain active and mobile

PD leads to decreased motivation and increased passivity. An active exercise program, even early in the disease, can often avoid this. Furthermore, such a program involves patients in their own care, allows muscle stretching and full range of joint mobility, and enhances a better mental attitude towards fighting the disease. By being encouraged to take responsibility in fighting the devastations of the disease, the patient becomes an active participant. Physical therapy, which can be implemented in the form of a well-constructed exercise program, is useful in all stages of disease. In early stages, a physical therapy program can instruct the patient in the proper exercises, and the regimen forces the patient to exercise if he or she lacks the motivation to exercise on his or her own. In advanced stages of PD, physical therapy may be even more valuable by keeping joints from becoming frozen, and providing guidance on how best to remain independent in mobility. Therefore, exercise is beneficial in both the early and later stages. It has been shown that PD patients who exercise intensively and regularly have better motor performance (Reuter et al., 1999; Behrman et al., 2000; Craig et al., 2006) and quality of life (Rodrigues de Paula et al., 2006). If exercise is not maintained, the benefit is lost (Lokk, 2000).

A number of basic science studies have discovered that exercise, particularly enriched exercise, can reduce the loss of dopaminergic neurons after 1-methyl-4-phenyl-1,2,3,6-tetrahydropyridine (MPTP) exposure. When such exercise is initiated shortly after rodents were given experimental lesions of the nigrostriatal dopamine pathway, the result was a significantly less amount of damage to the dopamine pathway (Tillerson et al., 2001, 2002, 2003; Cohen et al., 2003; Bezard et al., 2003; Fisher et al., 2004; Mabandla et al., 2004). The mechanism appears to be the induction of increased trophic factors, such as GDNF (Smith and Zigmond, 2003) and brain-derived neurotrophic factor (BDNF) (Bezard et al., 2003).

Table 6.1 Five major responses to >5 years of levodopa therapy (n = 330 patients)

	No.	%
1. Smooth, good response	83	25
2. Troublesome fluctuations	142	43
3. Troublesome dyskinesias	67	20
4. Toxicity at therapeutic or subtherapeutic dosages	14	4
5. Total or substantial loss of efficacy	27	8

Thirty-six patients had troublesome fluctuations and troublesome dyskinesias. Data from Fahn S. Adverse effects of levodopa. In Olanow CW, Lieberman AN, eds: *The Scientific Basis for the Treatment of Parkinson's Disease.* Carnforth, England: Parthenon Publishing Group, 1992; pp. 89–112.

Keep the patient functioning independently as long as possible

There are a number of drugs that have a favorable impact on the clinical features of the disease by reducing its symptoms, but to date none have been shown to stop the progression of the disease. Since PD is a progressive disease and since no medication prevents ultimate worsening, the long-term goal in treating PD is to keep the patient functioning independently for as long as possible. Clearly, if medications that provide symptomatic relief can continue to be effective and without producing adverse effects, this would be excellent. For example, if levodopa therapy could persistently reverse parkinsonian signs and symptoms, we would not have a problem with therapeutic strategy. The difficulty is that 75% of patients have serious complications after 5 years of levodopa therapy (Table 6.1) (Fahn, 1992a), and younger patients (less than 60 years of age) are particularly prone to develop the motor complications of fluctuations and dyskinesias (Quinn et al., 1987; Kostic et al., 1991; Gershanik, 1993; Wagner et al., 1996). Some physicians therefore recommend utilizing dopamine agonists in younger patients, rather than levodopa, when beginning therapy, in an attempt to delay the onset of these problems (Quinn, 1994b; Fahn and Przedborski, 2010). Controlled clinical trials comparing dopamine agonists and levodopa as the initial therapeutic agent have proven that motor complications are less likely to occur with dopamine agonists (Parkinson Study Group, 2000; Rascol et al., 2000; Oertel et al., 2006). But each of these studies also showed that levodopa was more effective in improving parkinsonian symptoms and signs as measured quantitatively by the Unified Parkinson's Disease Rating Scale (UPDRS) (Fahn and Elton, 1987). But ultimately symptoms develop that are not responsive to levodopa or other dopaminergic agents (Hely et al., 2005, 2008).

Individualize therapy

The treatment of PD needs to be individualized, i.e., each patient presents with a unique set of symptoms, signs, response to medications, and a host of social, occupational, and emotional problems that need to be addressed.

Table 6.2 Individualizing treatment according to disease severity

Early stage of PD: mild symptoms, no threat to activities, not in need of symptomatic treatment

Mild stage: when PD symptoms and signs begin to interfere with activities, in need of symptomatic treatment

Moderate stage: inadequate response to nondopa medications or low dose levodopa, no complications

Advanced disease: complications from medications or presence of freezing or falling or abnormal posture or dementia or psychosis

End stage: poor response despite all available treatments; patient disabled

Table 6.3 Dopaminergic agents

Dopamine precursor: levodopa (combined with carbidopa in immediate-release, extended-release, and dissolvable-in-mouth formulations) (also combined with carbidopa and entacapone)

Decarboxylase inhibitor: carbidopa, benserazide

Dopamine agonists: bromocriptine, pergolide, pramipexole (immediate and extended release), ropinirole (immediate and extended release), rotigotine dermal patch, apomorphine, cabergoline, lisuride, piribedil

Catechol-O-methyltransferase inhibitors: entacapone, tolcapone

Dopamine releaser: amantadine

Dopamine receptor blocker: domperidone

Type B MAO inhibitor: selegiline, Zydis selegiline, selegiline dermal patch, rasagiline, lazabemide

Type A and B MAO inhibitor: tranylcypromine, phenelzine

Dopamine synthesizer: zonisamide

Table 6.4 Dopamine agonists and dopamine receptors

Agonist	D1	D2	D3	D4	D5
Bromocriptine	−	++	++	+	+
Lisuride	+	++	?	?	?
Pergolide	+	++	+++	?	+
Cabergoline	−	+++	?	?	?
Ropinirole	−	++	++++	+	−
Pramipexole	−	++	++++	++	?

Table 6.5 Nondopaminergic agents for motor symptoms

Antimuscarinics: trihexyphenidyl, benztropine, ethopropazine

Antihistaminics: diphenhydramine, orphenadrine

Antiglutamatergics: amantadine, dextromethorphan, riluzole

Muscle relaxants: cyclobenzaprine, diazepam, baclofen

Antioxidant vitamins: ascorbate, tocopherol

Mitochondrial enhancer: coenzyme Q10

Adenosine A_{2A} receptor antagonists (in clinical trials): istradefylline, preladenant and others

Neurotrophins: neuroimmunophilins, GDNF (neither were successful in clinical trials), neurturin (currently in a clinical trial)

As mentioned above, a major goal is to keep the patient functioning independently as long as possible. Practical guides for how to direct the treatment are to consider the patient's symptoms, the degree of functional impairment, and the expected benefits and risks of available therapeutic agents. Determine what the issues are for the individual patient by asking the patient to list the specific symptoms that trouble him/her the most. Attempt to treat the most troublesome symptoms, which is the way to maximize quality of life.

Also, keep in mind that younger patients are more likely to develop motor fluctuations and dyskinesias; older patients are more likely to develop confusion, sleep–wake alterations, and psychosis from medications. We have divided the severity of PD into five stages and describe treatment for each of them except end stage, which is resistant to treatment: early, mild, moderate, advanced, and end stage (Table 6.2).

Therapeutic choices available for Parkinson disease

Treatment of patients with PD can be divided into three major categories: physical (and mental health) therapy, medications, and surgery. Physical exercise and physiotherapy were discussed in a previous paragraph. Speech therapy plays a similar role in those with problems of communication. Dysarthria, palilalia, and tachyphemia are difficult to treat, but hypophonia can be overcome by training the patient to shout, known as the Lee Silverman Voice Treatment (Ramig et al., 2001). Psychiatric assistance may be required to handle depression and the social and familial problems that can develop with this chronic, disabling illness. Electroconvulsive therapy (ECT) may have a role in patients with severe, intractable depression; some psychiatrists have been promoting it to help overcome the motor symptoms of PD, but at best ECT provides only short-term motor benefit, and it may not be replicated on repeat treatments. The current practice parameters on treatment of depression, psychosis, and dementia in patients with PD have been summarized in the 2006 report by the American Academy of Neurology Quality Standards Subcommittee (Miyasaki et al., 2006); this topic is covered in Chapter 8.

Neurosurgery for PD is becoming increasingly available as the technique of deep brain stimulation has been developed. This major topic is covered in Chapter 7, and is only mentioned here to be complete in understanding the choices available.

Medications available for Parkinson disease

A great many drugs have been developed for PD. Tables 6.3 through 6.6 classify them according to their mechanisms of action. Selection of the most suitable drugs for the individual patient and deciding when to utilize them in the course of the disease are challenges to the treating clinician. In many of the parkinsonism-plus disorders, the response to treatment is not satisfactory, but the principles for treating PD are the basis for treating these disorders as well. Because

Table 6.6 Nondopaminergic agents for nonmotor symptoms

Behavioral

Dementia: donepezil (Aricept), rivastigmine (Exelon), galantamine (Razadyne)

Depression: selective serotonin reuptake inhibitors, tricyclics, ECT

Psychosis: clozapine, quetiapine, donepezil, rivastigmine

Stress/anxiety: benzodiazepines: diazepam, lorazepam, alprazolam

Apathy: methylphenidate

Fatigue: modafinil

Sleep-related

Daytime sleepiness: modafinil

Insomnia: quetiapine, zolpidem, benzodiazepine, mirtazapine, amitriptyline, trazodone

REM-sleep behavior disorder: clonazepam

Restless legs: dopamine agonists, opioids (e.g., propoxyphene, tramadol, oxycodone)

Autonomic

Orthostasis: fludrocortisone, midodrine (ProAmatine), pyridostigmine

Urinary urgency: trospium (Sanctura), oxybutynin (Ditropan), tolterodine (Detrol)

Impotence: sildenafil (Viagra) and related drugs

Gastrointestinal

Constipation: fiber, "rancho recipe," polyethylene glycol (MiraLax), pyridostigmine

Nausea: trimethobenzamide (Tigan), domperidone

Sialorrhea: propantheline, glycopyrrolate, trospium (Sanctura), botulinum toxin injections

Table 6.7 Major symptoms after 15 years of PD

Living in aged care facility – 40%	Employed – 0%
Motor symptoms	**Nonmotor symptoms**
Choking – 50%	Symptomatic orthostasis – 35%
Falls – 84%	Urinary incontinence – 41%
Fractures – 24%	Depression – 50%
Motor complications – 95%	Hallucinations – 50%
	Cognitive decline – 84%
	Dementia – 48%

Data from Hely et al. (2005) on following subjects enrolled in a study comparing bromocriptine and levodopa therapies. Although approximately 95% of subjects have experienced dopa-induced dyskinesia/dystonia and wearing-off, in the majority these symptoms were not disabling. Dyskinesia and dystonia were delayed by early use of bromocriptine, but wearing-off appeared at a similar time once levodopa was added. The most disabling long-term problems of PD relate to the emergence of symptoms that are not improved by levodopa.

Table 6.8 Major symptoms after 20 years of PD

Living in aged care facility – 48%	Living independently – 1/36
Motor symptoms	**Nonmotor symptoms**
Choking – 48%	Symptomatic orthostasis – 48%
Falls – 87%	Urinary incontinence – 71%
Fractures – 35%	Depression – 70%
Freezing – 81%	Hallucinations – 74%
Moderate dysarthria – 81%	Dementia – 83%
	Excessive daytime sleepiness – 70%

Data from Hely et al. (2008) on following subjects enrolled in a study comparing bromocriptine and levodopa therapies. The most disabling long-term problems of PD relate to the emergence of symptoms that are not improved by levodopa, particularly dementia.

PD is a chronic progressive disease, patients require lifelong treatment. Medications and their doses will change over time as adverse effects and new symptoms are encountered. Tactical strategy is based on the severity of the disease.

Almost all drug trials evaluate a drug's short-term symptomatic benefit, but the leading unmet need is to stop or slow progression. Dopaminergic medications usually are effective in controlling the early motor symptoms of PD, but ultimately many patients develop new symptoms that do not respond to dopaminergic medication. The Sydney Multicenter Study of Parkinson disease has reported the problems experienced by people who survived 15 years (Table 6.7) (Hely et al., 2005) and 20 years (Table 6.8) (Hely et al., 2008) from diagnosis. The major problems are the development of symptoms that are not responsive to dopaminergic therapy (Tables 6.7 and 6.8), with dementia reaching 81% in 20-year survivors. Only 26% survived 20 years. The standardized mortality ratio, although less than in the pre-levodopa era of 3.0 (Hoehn and Yahr, 1967), was still significantly elevated at 1.86 at 15 years, but was 3.1 between 15 and 20 years. None were employed. Nonmotor symptoms were prevalent.

Dopaminergic agents

Because most of the major motoric symptoms of PD are related to striatal dopamine deficiency (Hornykiewicz, 1966), dopamine replacement therapy is the major medical approach to treating these features of the disease. Table 6.3 lists these dopaminergic drugs. The most powerful drug is levodopa. It is usually administered with a peripheral decarboxylase inhibitor. In Table 6.3, both carbidopa and benserazide are listed as peripheral dopa decarboxylase inhibitors, although in the United States only carbidopa is available. In many other countries, benserazide is also available. Carbidopa/levodopa is marketed as Sinemet or as a generic drug; the combination is available in immediate-release (e.g., Sinemet standard) and extended-release (e.g., Sinemet CR) formulations. The former allows a more rapid "on" and shorter half-life, and the latter allows for a delayed "on" and a slightly longer plasma half-life. Benserazide/levodopa is marketed as standard Madopar and Madopar HBS (for slow release). The peripheral decarboxylase inhibitors potentiate levodopa, allowing about a four-fold reduction of levodopa dosage to obtain the same benefit. Moreover, by preventing the formation of peripheral dopamine, which can act at the area postrema (vomiting center with a lack of a blood–brain barrier), they block the development of nausea and vomiting. If additional carbidopa is needed for patients in whom nausea persists, it can be prescribed, and patients can obtain it from their pharmacy; the additional peripheral decarboxylase inhibitor may overcome the nausea. Keep in mind that levodopa is absorbed only in the proximal small intestine. The slow release of levodopa from the extended-release versions is such that only about two-thirds to three-quarters of levodopa is absorbed per tablet compared to standard Sinemet. This is because some of the levodopa in the slow-dissolving tablet has not been released before the tablet reaches the large intestine. Levodopa is not absorbed from the rectum, so suppository administration is not useful. There is also an immediate-release formulation of carbidopa/levodopa that dissolves in the mouth and is swallowed with saliva, with the trade name of Parcopa. It can be taken without water, which may be an advantage for some patients, e.g., those who have trouble swallowing or who need to be without food or water pre- and postsurgery.

Levodopa is universally accepted as the most effective drug available for symptomatic relief of many of the motor features of PD. If it were uniformly and persistently successful and also free of complications, new strategies utilizing other treatments would not be needed. Unfortunately, 75% of patients have serious complications after 5 years of levodopa therapy (Table 6.1). Fahn (2008) has reviewed the discovery of levodopa as a useful drug and the history of dopamine's role in PD.

The absorption of levodopa may be increased by eradicating gastric Helicobacter pylori with omeprazole, amoxicillin, and clarithromycin in PD patients documented to be infected with this bacterium (Pierantozzi et al., 2006; Lee et al., 2008). About 50% of the general population is infected with the bacterium.

The question of whether to use levodopa in a patient who has a history of malignant melanoma needs to be considered. Levodopa is an intermediary metabolite in the synthesis of skin melanin, so the concern is whether lurking melanoma cells can be activated by the use of levodopa therapy. A review of the literature does not provide evidence of a definite relationship between treatment with levodopa and the development or reemergence of malignant melanoma (Pfutzner and Przybilla, 1997; Zanetti et al., 2006; Olsen et al., 2007). Epidemiologic studies have shown that people with PD have an increased prevalence of malignant melanoma (Olsen et al., 2006). A clinical trial in which the development of melanoma was a secondary outcome measure showed that patients with PD on the placebo arm of the trial had a much higher rate of developing malignant melanoma than would have been predicted; no association between levodopa therapy and the incidence of melanoma was found (Constantinescu et al., 2007). Yet, it is would seem prudent not to treat with levodopa in a patient with a history of a malignant melanoma if other antiparkinson agents remain effective. Once it becomes necessary to use levodopa to improve quality of life, the patient needs to be informed that he should be observed carefully for changes in or development of new pigmented lesions.

Besides being metabolized by aromatic amino acid decarboxylase (also called dopa decarboxylase), levodopa is also metabolized by catechol-O-methyltransferase (COMT) to form 3-O-methyldopa. Two COMT inhibitors are currently available – tolcapone and entacapone. These agents extend the plasma half-life of levodopa without increasing its peak plasma concentration, and can thereby prolong the duration of action of each dose of levodopa. These drugs are used in conjunction with levodopa to reduce the wearing-off effect, a common motor fluctuation adverse effect of levodopa therapy. The net effect with multiple dosings a day, though, is to elevate the average plasma concentration but smooth out the variations in the concentration. Tolcapone has two potential adverse effects that need to be explained to the

patient. The most serious is that a small percentage of patients will develop elevated liver transaminases, and patients need to have baseline and follow-up liver function tests. Death from hepatic necrosis has occurred in three patients who had no liver function surveillance (Watkins, 2000). Entacapone has not shown these hepatic changes. With tolcapone, a small percentage of patients will develop diarrhea, which does not appear until about 6 weeks after starting the drug. The diarrhea can be explosive, so the patient might not have any warning. Entacapone appears not to have these adverse effects. Many clinicians believe that tolcapone is more effective than entacapone in reducing motor fluctuations, but one should not prescribe the former unless the latter has not been effective in relieving wearing-off. Patients on entacapone can be easily switched to tolcapone if the former had less than the desired effect, and a double-blind comparison showed tolcapone to be slightly more effective in reducing the amount of "off" time (Entacapone to Tolcapone Switch Study Investigators, 2007). We advise starting tolcapone at a low dose of 100 mg/day and increasing gradually to 100 mg three times daily.

Elevated total plasma homocysteine, a risk factor for strokes, heart attacks, and dementia, has been found in PD patients using levodopa. The increase of plasma homocysteine with levodopa therapy is thought to be due to the utilization of the methyl group from methionine in the COMT reaction, converting levodopa to 3-O-methyldopa, while converting methionine to homocysteine. A study evaluating the immediate effects of initiating levodopa therapy found a modest elevation of homocysteine and a modest lowering of vitamin B12 levels (O'Suilleabhain et al., 2004). These investigators did not see a reversal with levodopa reduction, agonist treatment, or entacapone treatment. In another study, entacapone also did not reduce homocysteine levels (Nevrly et al., 2010). Another study reported that levodopa treatment does not affect B12 levels, but does reduce folate levels (Lamberti et al. 2005). These investigators found that the addition of COMT inhibitors could reduce the amount of homocysteine, but other investigators did not. Whether the increase in plasma homocysteine with levodopa therapy puts the patient at a greater risk for other medical problems is unknown (Postuma and Lang, 2004).

Adding entacapone to levodopa for patients who are not experiencing motor fluctuations did not add any improvement to motor performance in one study (Olanow et al., 2004), but improved the activities of daily living (ADL) score in another (Brooks and Sagar, 2003). In the FIRST-STEP study, levodopa/carbidopa/entacapone (LCE) 100/25/200 mg three times daily was compared with levodopa/carbidopa (LC) 100/25 mg three times daily in patients with early PD for 39 weeks (Hauser et al., 2009). LCE treatment resulted in slightly better UPDRS Part II activities of daily living (ADL) scores ($P = 0.025$), but not Part III motor scores.

The concept that intermittent brain levels of levodopa and dopamine contribute to the development of motor complications (see below in discussion of advanced PD) has led to the concept that continuous dopaminergic stimulation may avoid these complications from levodopa. So far, one study (STRIDE-PD) testing this hypothesis has yielded the opposite effect, i.e., an earlier onset of dyskinesias (Stocchi et al., 2010). A total of 747 patients with early PD were randomized to LCE 100/25/200 mg or LC 100/25 mg with flexible dosing to reach 400 mg/day, with a dose 3.5 h apart. The results showed that time to dyskinesia was statistically significantly shorter in LCE-treated patients compared to LC-treated patients. The incidence of dyskinesia during the study period was higher in LCE-treated patients in comparison to the LC group.

The next most powerful drugs, after levodopa, in treating PD symptoms are the dopamine agonists. Of those listed in Table 6.3, bromocriptine, pramipexole, ropinirole, and apomorphine are available in the United States, and these are discussed below. Lisuride, pergolide, cabergoline, rotigotine and piribedil are marketed in some countries. Lisuride is water soluble and can be infused subcutaneously; it has considerable 5-HT agonist activity. Cabergoline is the longest acting and could be taken just once a day (Ahlskog et al., 1996; Hutton et al., 1996); it might prove to be the most important in terms of preventing or reducing the "wearing-off" effect. Piribedil is relatively weak, but has been touted as having an anti-tremor effect. Rotigotine is a dopamine agonist that is utilized as a transdermally applied skin patch (Parkinson Study Group, 2003; Poewe and Luessi, 2005; LeWitt et al., 2007; Poewe et al., 2007; Watts et al., 2007) and was marketed in summer 2007. After the discovery that crystals of rotigotine appear on the patch, the drug was withdrawn from the USA.

Other than apomorphine and rotigotine, the other dopamine agonists in Table 6.3 are effective orally. Apomorphine needs to be injected subcutaneously or sprayed intranasally. Bromocriptine is the weakest clinically in comparison to the others. Pergolide, pramipexole, and ropinirole appear to be comparable in clinical practice, but some patients will respond better to one than the others. There are some differences between these agonists in their affinity for the dopamine receptor subtypes, as depicted in Tables 6.4 and 6.9. Only apomorphine (strong) and pergolide and lisuride (modest) have agonist activity at the D1 receptor. The activation of the D2 receptor is known to be important in obtaining an anti-PD response, whereas it is unknown how important D3 receptor activation is for improving the anti-PD response. Bromocriptine, pergolide, pramipexole, and ropinirole activate the dopamine D3 as well as the D2 receptor, but their ratios of affinities for these two receptors are different (Table 6.9) (Perachon et al., 1999). All dopamine agonists are less likely to induce dyskinesias compared to levodopa (Schrag et al., 1998). The agonists can be used as adjuncts to levodopa therapy (e.g., Lieberman et al., 1998;

Pinter et al., 1999) or as monotherapy (e.g., Kieburtz et al., 1997b; Brooks et al., 1998; Kulisevsky et al., 1998; Rinne et al., 1998a; Sethi et al., 1998). Adverse effects that are more common with dopamine agonists than with levodopa are drowsiness, sleep attacks, confusion, orthostatic hypotension, nausea, and ankle/leg edema associated commonly with erythema (Parkinson Study Group, 2000; Rascol et al., 2000). Edema can spread to involve other areas of the body including the arms and face.

Apomorphine, being water soluble and injectable, is usually employed as a rapidly acting dopaminergic to overcome "off" states, i.e., provide a rescue. It is either injected subcutaneously or applied intranasally. Because of its emesis-producing propensity, the patient must be pretreated with an antinauseant, such as domperidone or trimethobenzamide. Apomorphine and lisuride (also water soluble) are also being used by continuous subcutaneous infusion to provide a smooth response for patients who fluctuate between dyskinetic and "off" states. Apomorphine may be the most powerful dopamine agonist and activates both the dopamine D1 and D2 receptors.

Having several dopamine agonists to choose from allows the opportunity to find one that is better tolerated as well as one that might have more effect. Adverse effects may be the deciding factor as to which drug a patient will do best on. Unfortunately, all these drugs can induce confusion and hallucinations in elderly patients. Leg edema occurs in some patients, usually after a few years. Pramipexole and ropinirole, and other dopaminergics as well, though with probably less frequency, can cause sleepiness and sleep attacks. This could be dangerous for the patient who drives an automobile, and motor vehicle accidents have occurred when patients fell asleep at the wheel (Frucht et al., 1999; Ferreira et al., 2000; Hoehn, 2000; Schapira, 2000). So when deciding to place a patient on pramipexole or ropinirole, the physician should determine the extent of the driving to be done by the patient, and warn the patient about this potential hazard. Short trips, e.g., 10 minutes or so, should be without risk. Should sudden falling asleep occur in any non-driving activity, this event can serve as a warning against driving or else it would be best to taper and even discontinue these medications if driving is necessary. Dopamine agonists also are more likely to induce impulse control problems, such as gambling, hypersexuality, shopping, and binge eating (see Chapter 8) (Weintraub et al., 2010).

Amantadine has several actions. It activates release of dopamine from nerve terminals, blocks dopamine uptake into the nerve terminals, has antimuscarinic effects, and blocks glutamate receptors. Its dopaminergic actions make it a useful drug to reduce symptoms in about two-thirds of patients, and it has a quick onset of action (within 2 days). But it can induce livedo reticularis, ankle edema, visual hallucinations, and confusion, the latter two mainly in older individuals. Its antiglutamatergic action is discussed later in this section.

Domperidone is a peripherally active dopamine receptor blocker and is useful in preventing gastrointestinal upset from levodopa and the dopamine agonists. Although it does not enter the central nervous system (CNS), it can still block the dopamine receptors in the area postrema, thereby preventing nausea and vomiting. By not penetrating the CNS, it does not block the dopamine receptors in the striatum,

Table 6.9 Dopamine agonists and affinities for the dopamine D1, D2, and D3 receptors

Agonist	D1	D2	D3	D2/D3 ratio
Bromocriptine	0	+++	++	10:1
Pergolide	+	+++	+++	1:1
Ropinirole	0	++	+++	1:10
Pramipexole	0	++	+++	1:10

Data extracted from Perachon S, Schwartz JC, Sokoloff P. Functional potencies of new antiparkinsonian drugs at recombinant human dopamine D-1, D-2 and D-3 receptors. Eur J Pharmacol 1999;366:293–300.

thus not interfering with the action of dopamine or dopamine agonists. Domperidone is not marketed in the United States, but US patients can obtain it from Canada.

Monoamine oxidase (MAO) inhibitors offer mildly effective symptomatic benefit. Type B MAO inhibitors eliminate concern about the "cheese effect" that can occur with type A inhibitors and a high tyramine meal. Although there is debate about possible protective benefit with selegiline, it does have mild symptomatic effects when used alone (Parkinson Study Group, 1993a, 1996a, 1996b) and also potentiates levodopa when used in combination with it (Lees, 1995). A more thorough discussion of selegiline's possible protective effect is presented below in the section entitled "Selegiline, rasagiline, and antioxidants." Selegiline has a mild ameliorating effect for mild "wearing-off" from levodopa (Golbe et al., 1988). Zydis selegiline is a form of selegiline that dissolves in the mouth and is absorbed through the oral mucosa, avoiding first pass metabolism in the liver (Waters et al., 2004). This preparation of selegiline, formulated in a freeze-dried tablet that contains a fast dissolving selegiline (Zelapar), has been approved by the Food and Drug Administration in 2006 for clinical use (Clarke and Jankovic, 2006).

Like selegiline, rasagiline is another irreversible type B MAO inhibitor with mild symptomatic benefit (Rabey et al., 2000; Parkinson Study Group, 2002a, 2004a) and with a similar chemical structure; both are propargylamine compounds. Rasagiline is available for use in both early and advanced stages of PD and has a good safety record (Goetz et al., 2006). Both the TEMPO trial and the subsequent larger ADAGIO trial using a delayed-start design showed that starting earlier with rasagiline allows a better clinical outcome than starting later (Parkinson Study Group, 2004a; Olanow et al., 2009). A more thorough discussion of rasagiline's possible protective effect is presented below in the section entitled "Selegiline, rasagiline, and antioxidants."

Lazabemide is another type B MAO inhibitor, but is a reversible inhibitor. It shows the same symptomatic effect in PD (Parkinson Study Group, 1993b) as does selegiline and rasagiline. It is not known whether it has a neuronal rescue effect. Lazabemide is not commercially available in the United States. In contrast to selegiline, neither lazabemide nor rasagiline is metabolized to methamphetamine. Type B MAO inhibitors should not require a tyramine-restricted diet, provided that the dose remains no higher than the FDA-authorized dose. Higher doses will begin to inhibit MAO type A, and could cause severe hypertension (the so-called "cheese effect") if the diet contained too much tyramine. A controlled tyramine challenge showed that rasagiline up to 2 mg/day did not induce a significant blood pressure or pulse change when tyramine was added (deMarcaida et al., 2006). Inhibitors of both type A and type B MAO would offer greater inhibition of dopamine oxidation in the brain and thus the combination would theoretically be more capable of reducing oxidative stress as well as providing more symptomatic effect (Fahn and Chouinard, 1998). But tranylcypromine and phenelzine (both nonselective inhibitors of types A and B MAO) cannot be taken in the presence of levodopa therapy because of the "cheese effect," and even in the absence of levodopa, patients on these drugs need to adhere to a reduced tyramine diet (Gardner et al., 1996).

We will return to discuss MAOIs and antioxidants below in their possible role in treating early-stage PD. Next, we will review the nondopaminergic drugs that are useful in treating PD, both the motor problems (Table 6.5) and the nonmotor problems (Table 6.6).

Nondopaminergic agents for motor symptoms

Nondopaminergic agents (Table 6.5) are also useful to treat motoric PD symptoms, particularly antimuscarinic drugs (commonly referred to as anticholinergics), which have been widely used since the 1950s, but these are much less effective than the dopaminergic agents, including amantadine. Antimuscarinic drugs have been thought to be somewhat helpful in reducing all symptoms of PD, but they have found special favor in reducing the severity of tremor. But because of sensitivity to memory impairment and hallucinations in the elderly population, antimuscarinic drugs should usually be avoided in patients over the age of 70 years. The antihistaminics, tricyclics, and cyclobenzaprine (Flexeril) have milder anticholinergic properties that make them useful in PD, particularly in older patients who should not take the stronger anticholinergics.

Amantadine, listed in Table 6.3 as a dopaminergic agent, is listed also in Table 6.5 because it has antiglutamatergic effects; this property might account for its usefulness in reducing choreic dyskinesias induced by levodopa (Rajput et al., 1997; Metman et al., 1998a). Dextromethorphan is another antiglutamatergic agent, and it has been found effective in reducing the severity of dyskinesias by 50% (Metman et al., 1998b). Another useful class of drugs is the benzodiazepines to reduce anxiety, and thereby decrease parkinsonian tremor that is exacerbated by stress. Diazepam is usually well tolerated and does not exacerbate parkinsonian symptoms, whereas chlordiazepoxide can (Schwarz and Fahn, 1970). Lorazepam and alprazolam are other useful benzodiazepine agents; the latter has the added benefits of being short-acting and having antidepressant effects. The muscle relaxants listed in Table 6.5 might help in treating "off" and peak-dose dystonias. Because oxidative stress appears to play a role in the pathogenesis of PD, high doses of antioxidant vitamins have been tried for patients with PD. The DATATOP study showed that tocopherol by itself has no effect, but the combination of ascorbate and tocopherol may be more effective than either of these two vitamins alone (Fahn, 1992b; Yoshikawa, 1993). Ascorbate has proven effective in blocking degeneration of nerve cells in vitro induced by levodopa (Mena et al., 1993; Mytilineou et al., 1993; Pardo et al., 1993, 1995; Lai and Yu, 1997). Adenosine A2A receptors are located on GABA neurons in the striatum and antagonize the effect of dopamine on these neurons (Benarroch, 2008). Antagonizing adenosine A2A receptors has a behavioral effect similar to enhancing dopaminergic transmission. One of these receptor antagonists, istradefylline, has undergone clinical trials for patients with motor fluctuations (Bara-Jimenez et al., 2003; Hauser et al., 2003, LeWitt et al., 2008; Stacy et al., 2008), but the results were mixed, with insufficient relief of fluctuations while enhancing dyskinesias. Another adenosine A2A receptor antagonist, preladenant, is currently undergoing clinical trials.

Nondopaminergic agents for nonmotor symptoms

Many nonmotor problems are commonly present in patients with PD; these are discussed in more detail in Chapter 8. But a list of the common drugs used for these nonmotor symptoms is provided in Table 6.6, and a brief explanation of some of the drugs used is provided here. Drugs that are available to improve memory in Alzheimer disease may be tried in patients with Parkinson disease who have dementia, whether from diffuse Lewy body disease or from concomitant Alzheimer disease. These drugs are the centrally active cholinesterase inhibitors, donepezil, rivastigmine, and galantamine. Initial concern that they might worsen tremor and bradykinesia have not been borne out, perhaps because dopaminergic agents are also being given in these patients. These drugs have also been reported to be useful in treating levodopa-induced psychosis.

Because depression is common in patients with PD, this symptom needs to be vigorously attacked if present; otherwise it is difficult to reduce parkinsonian symptoms. The tricyclics and selective serotonin reuptake inhibitors are useful antidepressants in PD. It is not certain whether one type of antidepressant class of compounds is superior to the other in treating the depression accompanying PD. The selective serotonin uptake inhibitors may aggravate parkinsonism if antiparkinsonian drugs are not being utilized concurrently. If insomnia is a problem for the patient, using an antidepressant at bedtime that is also a soporific, such as amitriptyline, can be doubly advantageous. Amitriptyline has considerable somnolence-inducing effect. The type B MAO inhibitor selegiline is not effective as an antidepressant, unless used in a transdermal form to achieve both types A and B inhibition. The oral inhibitors of both types A and B MAO are very effective, but they cannot be given in the presence of levodopa because of swings in blood pressure, and they must also be accompanied by a tyramine-restrictive diet at all times.

Psychosis induced by levodopa and the dopamine agonists can often be controlled by clozapine and quetiapine without worsening the parkinsonism. Both agents are dibenzodiazepine antipsychotic drugs. They are called atypical antipsychotics because they rarely cause drug-induced parkinsonism. They are relatively selective D4 receptor antagonists, although they have some D2 blocking action, particularly at high doses, because akathisia (Safferman et al., 1993; Friedman, 1993), acute dystonic reaction (Kastrup et al., 1994; Thomas et al., 1994), and tardive dyskinesia (Dave, 1994) have been associated with them. Clozapine is the most effective agent in treating levodopa-induced psychosis in patients with PD without aggravating the PD (Friedman and Lannon, 1990; Pfeiffer et al., 1990; Kahn et al., 1991; Factor and Brown, 1992; Greene et al., 1993; Pinter and Helscher, 1993; Factor et al., 1994; Diederich et al., 1995; Rabey et al., 1995; Factor and Friedman, 1997; Ruggieri et al., 1997; Friedman et al., 1999; Pollak et al., 2004). But weekly monitoring of white blood cells is necessary with clozapine to prevent irreversible agranulocytosis that can occur rarely with clozapine; this allow a timely discontinuation of this drug when a drop of leukocytes is observed. Because of this need for weekly blood counts, quetiapine is a useful, although somewhat less effective

substitute for clozapine, and it is now the drug of first choice. Both clozapine and quetiapine are given at bedtime because of their soporific effect. Olanzapine is an effective antipsychotic, but the dose needs to be kept small because it can worsen PD (Jimenez-Jimenez et al., 1998). There is a window of dosing with olanzapine by which psychosis can be reduced without increasing parkinsonism.

Stress, excitement, and anxiety make parkinsonian symptoms worse, especially tremor. In fact, tremor that is otherwise well controlled can reemerge under stress. The benzodiazepines, by reducing anxiety, can partially offset this worsening of tremor. Apathy and fatigue are common in PD, and no medication as yet has been found satisfactory.

Various sleep problems are encountered in PD. Excessive drowsiness can occur after a dose of levodopa or dopamine agonist. Modafinil can sometimes help to overcome this problem. Insomnia needs to be treated, otherwise quality of life suffers and daytime sleepiness is enhanced. Hypnotics, such as zolpidem and benzodiazepines, can be safely used in PD. Quetiapine and clozapine often allow a good night's sleep, and can be utilized even in the absence of psychosis. Acting out dreams, so-called REM-sleep behavior disorder, is not uncommon and is usually treated with clonazepam at bedtime. Restless legs syndrome (RLS) and periodic movements in sleep are quite common in patients with PD. If the dopaminergic agent they are taking is ineffective, then an opioid such as propoxyphene, tramadol or oxycodone can be effective. These should be administered an hour or so before the usual onset of these symptoms. Because dopaminergic medication can augment an existing restless legs syndrome, it is reasonable to consider that these agents might also induce it to develop, when previously it did not exist. Thus, restless legs could be considered a complication of dopaminergic medications in PD patients who develop RLS after starting these medications. In a survey of 447 consecutive Korean patients with PD, 16.3% had RLS (Lee et al., 2009). Multivariate logistic regression analysis revealed that the duration of antiparkinson therapy was the most significant factor contributing to the development of RLS in patients with PD, and this supports the notion that medications are likely a causative factor. RLS and its treatment is covered more thoroughly in Chapters 8 and 23.

Although common in multiple system atrophy, orthostatic hypotension also can occur in PD, often as a complication of dopaminergic or other medications. Fludrocortisone to increase salt retention and midodrine as an α_1-adrenergic receptor agonist can be effective in overcoming syncope. Dyssynergia of bladder sphincters can sometimes be a problem, and relief can be obtained with peripheral antimuscarinics. Oxybutynin (Ditropan) and tolterodine (Detrol) are commonly used for this condition. Difficulty obtaining erections can occur in patients with PD, and these men have reported benefit with sildenafil and related drugs.

One of the most common complaints by patients with PD is constipation. This symptom can be a factor of both the disease and the medications used to treat PD. A high fiber diet, including dried fruits, is often sufficient to relieve constipation. The "rancho recipe" is given in Chapter 8. If that is not effective, one can try the standard laxatives or polyethylene glycol (MiraLax). Nausea can be a complication of dopamine agonists and levodopa. Domperidone, a peripheral dopamine receptor blocker, is effective. Because domperidone is not available in the United States, trimethobenzamide (Tigan) can be tried. Sialorrhea is due to infrequent and inadequate spontaneous swallowing of saliva. Peripherally active peripheral antimuscarinics such as propantheline and glycopyrrolate can be quite effective. Injecting botulinum toxin into the parotid glands may benefit some patients (Racette et al., 2003).

Treatment of early-stage Parkinson disease

The earliest stage of PD begins when the symptoms are first noticed and the diagnosis is made. At this stage, symptoms are mild, and there is no threat to the patient's activities. The designation of "early stage" lasts until the symptoms begin to become troublesome to the patient, and intervention with symptomatic medications is needed. All symptomatic drugs can induce side effects, and if a patient is not troubled by mild symptoms socially or occupationally, the introduction of these drugs can be delayed until symptoms become more pronounced. The clinician needs to discuss this choice with the patient and his/her family. Most neurologists do not use levodopa or other potent antiparkinson agents when the diagnosis is first established and the disease presents with no threat to physical, social, or occupational activities (Fahn, 1991, 1999; Fahn et al., 1996).

Because symptomatically beneficial medications are not needed and because there is no proven neuroprotective treatment, patients in the early, recently diagnosed stage of PD are excellent candidates for participating in a clinical trial in which a placebo is one of the treatment arms. A literature review of clinical trials related to neuroprotection in PD has been conducted by Fahn and Sulzer (2004) and by the Quality Standards Subcommittee of the American Academy of Neurology (Suchowersky et al., 2006). Another elective option is to use one of the drugs described in this section for which hints of neuroprotection have been demonstrated in controlled clinical trials.

One should keep in mind that the generic label *neuroprotection* can be divided into at least three different classes of action: slowing the pathogenetic cascade that leads to cell death so that the natural history of the disease is less progressive (neuroprotection), restoring injured dysfunctional neurons (neurorescue, neurorestoration), and replacing dead neurons (neuroregeneration) (Fig. 6.2). In this section we discuss the rationale and results of clinical trials for neuroprotection of PD.

Selegiline, rasagiline, and antioxidants

The first controlled clinical trial for the purpose of evaluating medications as neuroprotective agents for PD was the DATATOP (Deprenyl and Tocopherol Antioxidative Therapy of Parkinsonism) study (Parkinson Study Group, 1989a, 1989b). Deprenyl (selegiline) is an irreversible noncompetitive inhibitor of type B MAO with a long duration of action (MAO-B inhibition half-life of 40 days (Fowler et al., 1994)). Selegiline was tested along with the antioxidant alpha-tocopherol (vitamin E), in a 2×2 design. Patients were enrolled in the study early in the course of the illness, and did not require symptomatic therapy. They were placed on

SLOWING THE DISEASE PROGRESSION

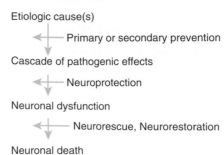

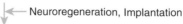

Figure 6.2 Neuroprotection – terminology.

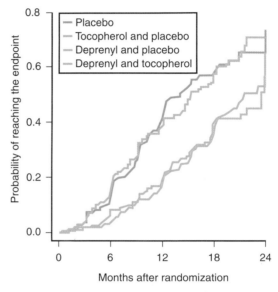

Figure 6.3 DATATOP endpoints. Kaplan–Meier curves of the cumulative probability of reaching the endpoint (need for dopaminergic therapy) in DATATOP. *From Parkinson Study Group. Effects of tocopherol and deprenyl on the progression of disability in early Parkinson's disease. N Engl J Med 1993;328:176–183.*

selegiline (5 mg twice daily), alpha-tocopherol (1000 IU twice daily), the combination, or double placebo, with approximately 200 subjects in each of the four treatment arms. The primary endpoint was the need for dopaminergic therapy. The study showed that tocopherol had no effect in delaying parkinsonian disability, but selegiline delayed symptomatic treatment by 9 months (Fig. 6.3) (Parkinson Study Group, 1993a). It also reduced the rate of worsening of the UPDRS by half (Table 6.10). Other investigators conducted other studies testing selegiline, showing similar results (Myllyla et al., 1992; Palhagen et al., 1998).

Because selegiline has a mild symptomatic effect that is long lasting (Parkinson Study Group, 1993a), one could explain its ability to delay progression of disability entirely on this symptomatic effect. In favor of some neuroprotective effect is that after 2 months of washout of the drug, patients had slightly milder PD than did those on placebo (Parkinson Study Group, 1993a). But because of selegiline's very long

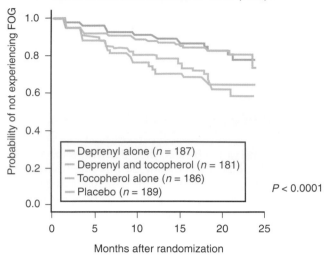

KAPLAN-MEIER SURVIVAL CURVES OF NOT EXPERIENCING FREEZING OF GAIT (FOG)

— Deprenyl alone ($n = 187$)
— Deprenyl and tocopherol ($n = 181$)
— Tocopherol alone ($n = 186$)
— Placebo ($n = 189$)

$P < 0.0001$

Figure 6.4 Freezing in DATATOP. Kaplan–Meier curves showing probability of not experiencing freezing of gait (FOG) in the absence of levodopa in the DATATOP study. *From Giladi N, McDermott MP, Fahn S, Przedborski S, Jankovic J, Stern M, Tanner C. Freezing of gait in PD: Prospective assessment in the DATATOP cohort. Neurology 2001;56:1712–1721.*

duration of action as an inhibitor of MAO-B (Parkinson Study Group, 1995), this observation could represent an insufficient washout period. Furthermore, selegiline's benefit in delaying the introduction of levodopa gradually diminishes over time (Parkinson Study Group, 1993a), with the best results occurring in the first year of treatment. The odds ratio increased from 0.35 for the first 6 months, to 0.38 in the second 6 months, to 0.77 in the third 6 months, and to 0.86 after 18 months. Follow-up of DATATOP subjects showed that placebo-treated subjects fared better than selegiline-treated subjects when the drug was reintroduced after a 2-month washout period and that the two groups were identical in developing levodopa complications (Parkinson Study Group, 1996a, 1996b). The net understanding by the year 2000 was that there is no convincing evidence that selegiline delayed the need for levodopa because of any protective effect; all results could be those of a drug with a continuing mild symptomatic benefit.

On the other hand, basic scientific research was finding that in animal models, tiny doses of selegiline have a neuronal rescue effect (Tatton, 1993). This effect is not via its MAO inhibitor mechanism of action, but is believed to be due to enhanced protein synthesis of a neurotrophic agent, which is antagonized by amphetamine. Ultimately this finding led to investigation of other agents for their rescue effect, resulting in the discovery of a propargyline drug that was tested in a clinical trial (Waldmeier et al., 2000, 2006).

When the DATATOP study was evaluated to better understand the development of freezing of gait, it was discovered that the group that was treated with selegiline had a statistically significantly decreased risk for developing freezing (Fig. 6.4) (Giladi et al., 2001b). It could not be discerned whether this benefit was because of selegiline's mild symptomatic benefit or because of some unknown neuroprotection effect. Whichever it was, the authors concluded that one should consider using selegiline in patients who are likely to develop freezing of gait (absence of tremor, gait involvement as the initial symptom).

Based on the BLIND-DATE study, it now appears that the decreased risk of freezing of gait with selegiline is not simply from its symptomatic effect as an enhancer of dopamine. The investigators of the DATATOP study, while continuing to follow their subjects, carried out a re-randomization in a controlled trial (called the BLIND-DATE study). A total of 368 subjects who were now on both selegiline and levodopa

Table 6.11 Change in total UPDRS after second randomization to either selegiline or placebo while taking levodopa

Duration after randomization	Placebo	Selegiline	Difference
1 month	0.50 ± 7.73	−1.52 ± 7.54	2.02
3 months	1.57 ± 9.41	−0.85 ± 9.42	2.42
9 months	4.18 ± 10.12	1.63 ± 10.61	2.55
15 months	5.63 ± 10.73	0.46 ± 10.88	5.17
21 months	7.06 ± 12.70	1.51 ± 10.36	5.55
↑Levodopa mg/day	181 ± 246	106 ± 205	$P = 0.003$

therapy agreed to be randomized to either selegiline or placebo, while remaining on levodopa. The results were dramatic. The subjects on selegiline required a lower dosage of levodopa, had a slower rate of worsening of symptoms and signs of PD (Table 6.11), and had less freezing of gait (Fig. 6.5) (Shoulson et al., 2002). These results support the view that selegiline does provide some neuroprotective effect or else it has a symptomatic effect separate from dopamine. The possibility that this benefit is derived from an anti-apoptotic effect rather than its antioxidative effect is discussed below.

A similar study was carried out by Palhagen and colleagues (2006), who followed patients for at least 7 years after they entered a controlled clinical trial evaluating selegiline versus placebo in those with early, untreated PD. Then, when any subject required symptomatic therapy, open-label levodopa was added, while maintaining the blind on selegiline versus

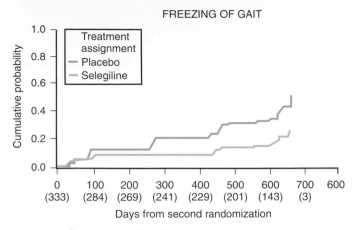

FREEZING OF GAIT

Figure 6.5 Freezing in BLIND-DATE. Kaplan–Meier curves showing probability of experiencing freezing of gait in the presence of levodopa in the BLIND-DATE study. *From Shoulson I, Oakes D, Fahn S, et al. Impact of sustained deprenyl (selegiline) in levodopa-treated Parkinson's disease: A randomized placebo-controlled extension of the deprenyl and tocopherol antioxidative therapy of parkinsonism trial. Ann Neurol 2002;51:604–612.*

placebo. During the 7 years of follow-up from the start of the study, the selegiline-treated group had a statistically significantly slower rate of worsening of clinical signs and symptoms as measured by UPDRS scores. Like the Shoulson and colleagues (2002) study mentioned above, this also shows the added benefit that selegiline provides in slowing clinical symptoms. Whether this can be attributed to a neuroprotective effect or to a symptomatic effect that does not appear to be through dopamine is undetermined by the two studies.

The safety of selegiline was raised, though, in an open-label clinical trial in the United Kingdom (Lees, 1995). The use of selegiline when combined with levodopa was reported to be associated with a higher mortality rate than was seen in the patients assigned to levodopa treatment alone. Analysis of this result by others found a number of flaws in the study to refute this conclusion (Olanow et al., 1996). The UK investigators followed up their report with a more detailed analysis of the cause of death (Ben-Shlomo et al., 1998). The excess mortality in the selegiline + levodopa group was greatest in the third and fourth year of treatment. The cause of the increase in deaths showed the excess to be from PD only, and to occur particularly in patients with dementia and a history of falls. No significant differences in mortality were found for revised diagnosis, disability rating scores, autonomic or cardiovascular events, other clinical features, or drug interactions. Other studies with selegiline have failed to find any excess mortality from the combination treatment with levodopa (Myllyla et al., 1997; Aaltonen et al., 1998; Olanow et al., 1998). After being followed by the Parkinson Study Group for an average of 8.2 years, the subjects in the DATATOP study showed no difference in mortality between the groups assigned to treatment with selegiline, tocopherol, or placebo; the death rate averaged 2.1% per year (Parkinson Study Group, 1998), much lower than in the UK study.

A meta-analysis of 17 controlled clinical trials involving type B MAO inhibitors found that no significant difference in mortality existed between patients on type B MAO inhibitors and control patients (Ives et al., 2004). The

analysis also found that subjects randomized to type B MAO inhibitors had significantly better total scores, motor scores, and ADL scores on the UPDRS at 3 months compared with patients taking placebo; they were also less likely to need additional levodopa or to develop motor fluctuations. No difference existed between the two groups in the incidence of side effects or withdrawal of patients.

High-dosage vitamin E has also been suggested to increase mortality, but analysis of the DATATOP cohort followed for up to 13 years failed to find any difference in mortality between the groups on vitamin E and the group on placebo (Marras et al., 2005).

In a more recent analysis of retrospective observational data from Scotland (Donnan et al., 2000) comparing PD patients with a comparable control population, the patients with PD had a higher rate of mortality than those without PD (rate ratio (RR) 1.76; 95% confidence interval (CI) 1.11–2.81). There was significantly greater mortality in monotherapy (RR = 2.45, 95% CI 1.42–4.23) relative to the comparators, adjusting for previous cardiovascular drug use and diabetes. However, there was no significant difference in mortality in patients with PD who received combination therapy of selegiline with levodopa and other drugs in relation to the comparators (RR = 0.92, 95% CI 0.37–2.31). Thus, from this study, selegiline did not increase the mortality rate, whether used as monotherapy or in combination with levodopa. In fact, levodopa monotherapy had the highest mortality rate.

Mortality in PD patients was also determined in a multicenter European study (Berger et al., 2000). As in the Scotland study (Donnan et al., 2000), the mortality rate was twice that of a controlled population (RR 2.3; 95% CI 1.8–3.0). The risk for death in men with PD (RR 3.1; 95% CI 2.1–4.4) was higher than that in women with PD (RR 1.8; 95% CI 1.2–5.1). Women with PD had a fivefold higher risk of living in a care facility than men with PD.

Rasagiline, based on the delayed-start studies, TEMPO (Parkinson Study Group, 2004a), and ADAGIO (Olanow et al., 2009), also can reduce the rate of clinical worsening in patients with early PD. But there were inconsistent outcomes between these two studies. In TEMPO, the 2 mg dose of rasagiline had a superior result compared to the 1 mg dose. In ADAGIO, only the 1 mg dose was superior to placebo; the 2 mg dose was no better than placebo (Fig. 6.6). Starting a symptomatically effective drug early does not automatically lead to a reduced rate of clinical worsening as tested by the delayed-start design. For example, pramipexole, an effective dopaminergic agent, does not give a superior clinical result if started early compared to starting it later (Schapira et al., 2009). Thus, there would appear to be a special property of the MAO inhibitors to be able to delay clinical worsening in a delayed-start study.

As mentioned above, the dose of selegiline and rasagiline should not exceed their specificity as selective type B inhibitors of MAO. Selegiline greater than 10 mg/day and rasagiline greater than 2 mg/day will also inhibit type A MAO. A woman given rasagiline at 4 mg/day in the presence of levodopa therapy developed the serotonin syndrome of hyperpyrexia, confusion, agitation and episodic periods of unconsciousness (Fernandes et al., 2011). Because selegiline is metabolized to amphetamine and methamphetamine, insomnia could develop, and one should avoid taking it late

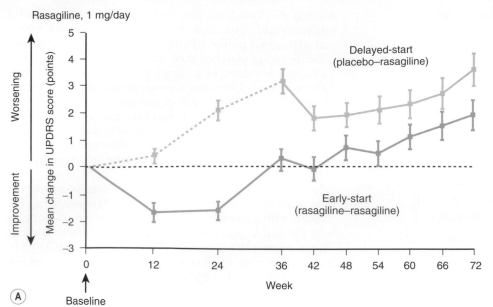

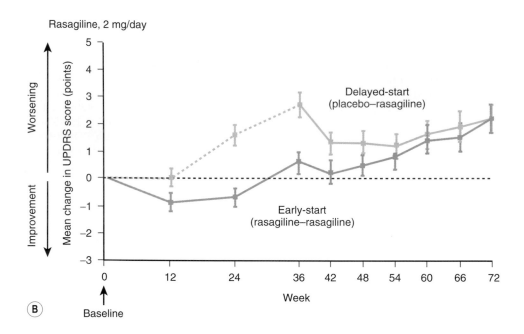

Figure 6.6 ADAGIO trial showed that 1 mg/day (**A**) of rasagiline resulted in a lower UPDRS score at 18 months if started earlier rather than 9 months later, but the 2 mg/day dose (**B**) showed no difference whether started earlier or later. *From Olanow CW, Rascol O, Hauser R, et al.; ADAGIO Study Investigators. A double-blind, delayed-start trial of rasagiline in Parkinson's disease. N Engl J Med. 2009;361(13):1268–1278. © 2009 Massachusetts Medical Society. All rights reserved.*

in the day. It may be necessary to limit selegiline to 5 or 10 mg in the morning only if insomnia is a problem. Male impotence is not common with MAO inhibitors. In the presence of levodopa, MAO inhibitors potentiate levodopa's effect, and lower doses of levodopa can usually be achieved (Lees, 1995; Shoulson et al., 2002). Selegiline does not prevent the development of levodopa-induced complications of fluctuations and dyskinesias (Parkinson Study Group, 1996b). Selegiline decreases the risk of patients developing freezing of gait (Giladi et al., 2001b; Shoulson et al., 2002). It is not clear if rasagiline has this ability. Interestingly, type A MAO inhibitors, but not type B MAO inhibitors, have been shown to reduce stress-induced freezing behavior in rats (Maki et al., 2000).

The DATATOP study showed that selegiline inhibits MAO activity by about 20% in the CNS (Parkinson Study Group, 1995). Because the original premise for the DATATOP study was that selegiline might be neuroprotective by inhibiting MAO (reducing formation of hydrogen peroxide and thereby decreasing oxidant stress), the CSF analysis of homovanillic acid indicates that selegiline is a poor inhibitor of CNS MAO. This finding could explain the lack of success of selegiline as a powerful neuroprotective agent. Whether a more potent inhibitor of MAO could be more successful remains to be determined. In the meantime, it is reasonable for patients to consider an inhibitor of both types A and B, as possibly augmenting inhibition of MAO in the brain. Such MAO inhibitors can induce the "cheese effect," so the MAO inhibitor diet, avoiding dietary tyramine, needs to be utilized. Such MAO inhibitors can be used only in the absence of levodopa because the combination will create marked blood pressure fluctuations.

Because the oxidant stress hypothesis is widely held as one of the pathogenic mechanisms in PD (Graham et al., 1978; Cohen, 1983, 1986; Fahn, 1989; Fornstedt et al., 1990; Olanow, 1990, 1992; Jenner, 1991; Fahn and Cohen, 1992; Jenner et al., 1992a, 1992b; Zigmond et al., 1992; Spencer et al., 1995; Alam et al., 1997), the use of a combination of antioxidants seems a reasonable approach.

Fahn has used tranylcypromine (Parnate), an irreversible inhibitor of both types A and B MAO, along with high dosages of antioxidants (Fahn and Chouinard, 1998). As measured by cerebrospinal fluid concentration of the metabolite of dopamine, selegiline just partially inhibits dopamine oxidation, reducing hydrogen peroxide formation by only 20% (Parkinson Study Group, 1995), whereas tranylcypromine inhibits by 75% (Fahn et al., 1998). Using tranylcypromine requires the patient to be placed on an MAO inhibitor diet, which is not onerous (Gardner et al., 1996), and if adhered to, avoids the "cheese effect." In the presence of an irreversible type A MAO inhibitor, tyramine cannot be deaminated in the gut. The absorption of tyramine results in the release of norepinephrine from sympathetic nerve terminals, thereby raising blood pressure, and potentially creating a hypertensive crisis ("cheese effect"). Some patients can develop intracerebral hemorrhage during an episode of such a crisis. The usual dose of tranylcypromine is 10 mg three times daily, but doses up to 60 mg per day can be used. Insomnia and male impotence are fairly common adverse effects that would require shifting the times of the dosages from the evening hours or reducing or discontinuing the drug. A side benefit is the lifting of any existing depression. Levodopa cannot be given in the presence of an inhibitor of type A MAO because the combination produces a volatile blood pressure. Meperidine (Demerol) and antidepressants such as tricyclics and selective serotonin uptake inhibitors are also to be avoided because of the potential for psychiatric and autonomic reactions ("serotonin syndrome") that could be fatal.

The antioxidants ascorbate (vitamin C) and tocopherol (vitamin E) are recommended solely on the basis of the oxidant stress hypothesis of the pathogenesis of PD. Although the DATATOP trial showed that tocopherol by itself is ineffective in slowing down the progression of PD, a combination of ascorbate and tocopherol potentiates the antioxidant efficacy of both (Yoshikawa, 1993; Hamilton et al., 2000). This combination of antioxidants in early PD patients has been used since 1979 and has not produced any harmful effects (Fahn, 1992b). The dosages gradually reached in four divided doses are 3000 mg per day of ascorbate and 3200 IU per day of d-alpha-tocopherol. Coenzyme Q10 and vitamin E need each other as antioxidants (Kagan et al., 2000). There is evidence that the natural form of tocopherol (d-alpha) achieves higher blood levels than the synthetic racemic (d,l-alpha) tocopherol (Acuff et al., 1994).

Riluzole

Glutamate is the major excitatory neurotransmitter in the CNS and can induce excitotoxicity. A slow excitotoxic process has been proposed by Beal (1998) to be a possible mechanism of cell death in PD. Riluzole impairs glutamatergic neurotransmission by blocking voltage-dependent sodium channel currents. In experimental animal models of PD, riluzole was found to have neuroprotective effects (Benazzouz et al., 1995; Barneoud et al., 1996; Boireau et al., 2000; Obinu et al., 2002). However, in controlled clinical trials in patients with early PD, riluzole was not found to be effective as a neuroprotective agent (Jankovic and Hunter, 2002; Rascol et al., 2003).

Providing trophic factors

Glial-derived neurotrophic factor (GDNF) promotes the survival of DA neurons (Burke et al., 1998), DA neuron neurite outgrowth, and quantal size (the amount of DA released per synaptic vesicle exocytic event) (Pothos et al., 1998). When GDNF was injected into the midbrain of primates rendered parkinsonian by MPTP, there was improvement of the parkinsonian features (Gash et al., 1996). Moreover, DA concentration in the substantia nigra (SN) was increased on the injected side and the nigral DA neurons were 20% larger with an increased fiber density. In a subsequent study, primates received infusions of GDNF into a lateral ventricle (Grondin et al., 2002). This approach also showed restoration of the nigrostriatal dopaminergic system and improved the motor function in rhesus monkeys. The functional improvements were associated with pronounced upregulation and regeneration of nigral DA neurons and their processes innervating the striatum. However, in a randomized, double-blind, placebo-controlled trial of infusing GDNF into the lateral ventricle of patients with PD, there was no clinical improvement (Nutt et al., 2003). Nausea, anorexia, and vomiting were common, hours to several days after injections of GDNF. Weight loss occurred in the majority of subjects receiving 75 μg or larger doses. Paresthesias, often described as electric shocks (Lhermitte sign), were common in GDNF-treated subjects.

One subsequent open-label study in five patients with PD showed that infusing GDNF directly into the putamen improved motor performance, and that there was increased FDOPA uptake on PET scans in some of the patients (Gill et al., 2003). However, a subsequent larger placebo-controlled trial failed to show clinical improvement although FDOPA uptake did increase (Lang et al., 2006).

Another approach of delivering GDNF directly into the brain was successfully achieved in primates using lentoviral vectors containing the gene for producing GDNF (Kordower et al., 2000). Lenti-GDNF was injected into the striatum and SN of rhesus monkeys that had been treated 1 week previously with MPTP. Lenti-GDNF reversed functional deficits and completely prevented nigrostriatal degeneration. Long-term gene expression (8 months) was seen in intact monkeys that were given this treatment.

A novel nonimmunosuppressive immunophilin ligand, GPI-1046 (henceforth called neuroimmunophilin), was found to have trophic activity, including regenerative sprouting from spared nigrostriatal dopaminergic neurons following MPTP toxicity in mice or 6-hydroxydopamine toxicity in rats (Steiner et al., 1997). Since then, there have been reports supporting a regenerative effect by neuroimmunophilins (Guo et al., 2001) and with a proposed mechanism of increasing glutathione in the brain (Tanaka et al., 2001,

2002). On the other hand, there have been many reports that failed to find such benefits in various animal models of PD, including primates (Harper et al., 1999; Bocquet et al., 2001; Emborg et al., 2001; Eberling et al., 2002). One controlled clinical trial testing neuroimmunophilin in patients was unsuccessful, and a subsequent larger and longer one also failed to show benefit.

Enhancing mitochondria and energy function

Coenzyme Q10 is the electron acceptor for mitochondrial complexes I and II and is also a potent antioxidant. Complex I activity was found to be affected by MPTP, and subsequently found to be selectively decreased postmortem in SN in patients with PD (Schapira et al., 1990). Coenzyme Q10 is reduced in the mitochondria (Shults et al., 1997) and in sera of patients with PD (Matsubara et al., 1991). Oral supplementation of coenzyme Q10 in rats resulted in increases of coenzyme Q10 in cerebral cortex mitochondria (Matthews et al., 1998). A controlled clinical pilot trial of coenzyme Q10 was undertaken in 80 patients with early PD. They were randomized into four equal arms and were assigned 300 mg/day, 600 mg/day, 1200 mg/day, or placebo and followed up to 16 months (Shults et al., 2002). There was a positive trend ($P = 0.09$) for a linear relationship between the dosage and the mean change in the total UPDRS score. The highest dose group (total UPDRS change of +6.69) was statistically less than the UPDRS change of +11.99 for the placebo group (Fig. 6.7). The change in UPDRS for the lower doses showed no significant difference from the placebo group. There was a slower decline in the change of all three components of the UPDRS scores in the 1200 mg/day group, with the greatest effect in Part II (the subjective ADL component) (Fig. 6.8). This raises the question of whether patients on 1200 mg/day of coenzyme Q10 might simply feel better rather than having an objective improvement of their motoric features of PD. After 1 month of treatment, there was improvement of the Part II UPDRS (ADL) score in the 1200 mg/day group of −0.66, compared to worsening in the placebo group of

+0.52. This wash-in effect supports the concern that there might be a "feel good" response from coenzyme Q10 rather than a neuroprotective effect. Also, it should be noted that those who were treated with the 1200 mg/day failed to show a delay in the need for dopaminergic therapy. Of course, the study was not powered for a modest effect, and the study investigators urged caution in interpretation of the results until a larger study could be conducted and evaluated. A futility trial showed little difference over time between coenzyme Q10 and placebo in the clinical progression of PD (NINDS NET-PD Investigators, 2007). Also, coenzyme Q10 showed no symptomatic benefit (Storch et al., 2007).

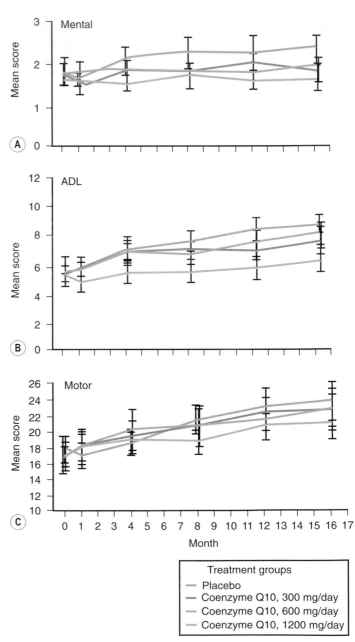

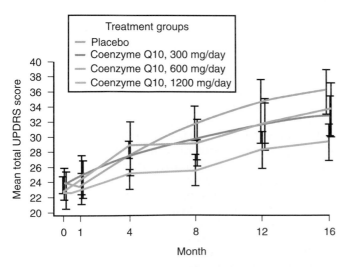

Figure 6.7 Change in total UPDRS with different dosages of coenzyme Q10. *From Shults CW, Oakes D, Kieburtz K, et al. Effects of coenzyme Q(10) in early Parkinson disease – evidence of slowing of the functional decline. Arch Neurol 2002;59(10):1541–1550.* © American Medical Association. All rights reserved.

Figure 6.8 Change in the different components of the UPDRS with coenzyme Q10. *From Shults CW, Oakes D, Kieburtz K, et al. Effects of coenzyme Q(10) in early Parkinson disease – evidence of slowing of the functional decline. Arch Neurol 2002;59(10):1541–1550.* © American Medical Association. All rights reserved.

Creatine is a guanidine-derived compound that is generated in the body. The creatine/phosphocreatine system functions as an energy buffer between the cytosol and mitochondria (Beal, 2003). Creatine has been proposed to serve as a neuroprotectant in neurodegeneration, and has been tested in a controlled clinical futility trial in early PD. Creatine was found not to be futile and is deserving of a phase III trial (NINDS NET-PD Investigators, 2006, 2008).

Counteracting inflammation

Gliosis and reactive microglia are seen in the substantia nigra of patients with PD, indicating an ongoing inflammatory process. Such changes have also been seen following MPTP (Vila et al., 2001) and rotenone (Betarbet et al., 2000) neurotoxicity. Inflammation is considered to be a secondary effect, but may play an important role in enhancing neurodegeneration by the production of cytokines and prostaglandins. Experimental animal models have shown that treatment with the antibiotic minocycline can reduce the level of degeneration by MPTP (Du et al., 2001; Wu et al., 2002). As a result of these reports, a controlled clinical futility trial testing minocycline was conducted, showing minocycline not to be futile (NINDS NET-PD Investigators, 2006).

Inhibiting apoptosis

Studies on selegiline, in an effort to explain its effectiveness in the DATATOP study, have shown it to have a neuronal rescue effect that is independent of its MAO inhibition (Tatton, 1993). This finding led to the investigation of other agents for their neuronal rescue effect, resulting in the discovery that propargylamines have an anti-apoptotic action. A search for similar compounds but without inhibiting MAO resulted in the discovery of one agent (TCH346) that is anti-apoptotic and that may act by stabilizing glyceraldehyde-3-phosphate dehydrogenase (Waldmeier et al., 2000). This drug was tested in a controlled clinical trial, but was found not to be effective in slowing progression of PD (Waldmeier et al., 2006; Olanow et al., 2006). The propargylamine rasagiline is also anti-apoptotic in laboratory and animal models. It was studied in a delayed-start neuroprotective trial, and the press release in June 2008 stated that the study was successful. The results have not yet been reported in a scientific meeting or publication. Another anti-apoptotic drug, CEP1347, which inhibits mitogen linear kinases was shown to be an effective neuroprotectant in animal models of PD. This drug was tested in a large controlled clinical trial that was stopped early because of lack of effectiveness of the drug (Parkinson Study Group PRECEPT Investigators, 2007).

Dopamine agonists

There are four published trials comparing a dopamine agonist and levodopa in patients with PD who were in need of symptomatic therapy. These compared cabergoline and levodopa (Rinne et al., 1998a) ropinirole and levodopa (Rascol et al., 2000), pramipexole and levodopa (the so-called CALM-PD trial) (Parkinson Study Group, 2000), and pergolide and levodopa (Oertel et al., 2006). The clinical outcomes of these studies are discussed below in

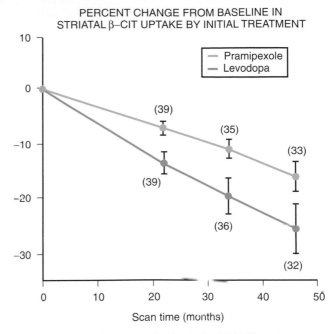

PERCENT CHANGE FROM BASELINE IN STRIATAL β–CIT UPTAKE BY INITIAL TREATMENT

Figure 6.9 Striatal β-CIT SPECT binding in the CALM-PD study. *From Parkinson Study Group. Dopamine transporter brain imaging to assess the effects of pramipexole vs levodopa on Parkinson disease progression. JAMA 2002;287:1653–1661.*

"Treatment of mild-stage Parkinson disease." In this section regarding neuroprotection, the results of the neuroimaging component of these trials are discussed. In the CALM-PD (pramipexole vs. levodopa) trial, the 4-year imaging results show a statistically significant lesser rate of decay of dopamine transporter binding (β-CIT SPECT) (a marker of integrity of nerve terminals of the dopaminergic nigrostriatal fibers) in the striatum in the group originally assigned to pramipexole treatment (Fig. 6.9) (Parkinson Study Group, 2002b). A separate study evaluating FDOPA PET scans, a marker of dopa uptake and dopa decarboxylase activity, showed a similar statistically significant lesser rate of decay of labeling in the striatum in a controlled trial in the group assigned to ropinirole compared to the group assigned to levodopa therapy (Whone et al., 2003).

Because there was no placebo comparator in either study, interpretation is difficult. Whether dopamine agonists slow the rate of progression of PD, whether levodopa hastens it, and whether both explanations are playing a role, are possibilities. Another possibility would be a pharmacodynamic effect on the dopamine transporter and dopa decarboxylase by either the agonists or levodopa. For example, if levodopa downregulated the dopamine transporter, β-CIT SPECT binding would be reduced. If levodopa downregulated dopa decarboxylase, FDOPA PET binding would be reduced. Short trials of levodopa showed no change in these imaging markers, so there is no evidence that levodopa affects either type of imaging study in such a pharmacologic manner. But a consensus conference concluded that there is insufficient information about the effect of medications on dopaminergic imaging to recommend neuroimaging as a biomarker for disease progression in the presence of medication (Ravina et al., 2005). Without knowing whether the agonists actually slow the rate of progression, it is not possible to recommend the starting treatment on the basis of these results alone.

Pramipexole was tested in a delayed-start trial and failed to show any slowing of PD (Schapira et al., 2009).

Inhibiting calcium entry

Substantia nigra pars compacta (SNc) dopamine neurons are autonomously active; that is, they generate action potentials at a clock-like 2–4 Hz in the absence of synaptic input (Surmeier et al., 2005). In this respect, they are much like cardiac pacemakers. Juvenile dopamine-containing neurons in the SNc use sodium influx as the pacemaking mechanisms common to neurons not affected in PD, but the sodium mechanism remains latent in adulthood (C.S. Chan et al., 2007). Instead, the autonomous activity is generated by Ca^{2+} influx (Mercuri et al., 1994; C.S. Chan et al., 2007; Surmeier, 2007). The SNc dopamine neurons rely on L-type $Ca(v)1.3$ Ca^{2+} channels. With increased intracellular calcium, mitochondrial function can be affected with increased demand on oxidative phosphorylation, leading to increased production of reactive oxygen species and eventually cellular damage. As the cells undergo more stress over time, they thus "age faster." This would be a link with the risk factor of age (Surmeier, 2007). Blocking $Ca(v)1.3$ Ca^{2+} channels in adult neurons induces a reversion to the juvenile form of pacemaking. Such blocking ("rejuvenation") protects these neurons in both in-vitro and in-vivo models of Parkinson disease, pointing to a new strategy that could slow or stop the progression of the disease (C.S. Chan et al., 2007; Surmeier, 2007).

As it turns out, use of calcium channel blockers for treating hypertension has been shown to be associated with less risk for developing PD in two database-mining studies (Becker et al., 2008a; Ritz et al., 2010), but not in a third (Simon et al., 2011). A clinical trial to evaluate the dihydropyridine isradipine, a calcium channel blocker, is currently underway and has been shown to be well tolerated (Simuni et al., 2010).

Statins and NSAIDs

One epidemiologic study in California surveying use of statins in patients with PD and a control population found that statin use was more common in the controls (Wahner et al., 2008), but another study surveying statin use in the UK, did not find any difference between patients with PD and controls (Becker et al., 2008b). One data-mining epidemiologic study reported that ibuprofen, but not other nonsteroidal anti-inflammatory drugs (NSAIDs), was associated with a lower risk of developing PD (Gao et al., 2011).

Treatment of mild-stage Parkinson disease

Strategy

The mild stage of PD occurs when the signs and symptoms of the illness are beginning to interfere with daily activities or with quality of life. The judgment to initiate symptomatic drug therapy is made in discussions between the patient and the treating physician. According to a survey (Parkinson Study Group, 1989a) the most common problems that clinicians consider important for the decision to initiate symptomatic agents are (1) threat to employability, (2) threat to ability to handle domestic, financial, or social affairs, (3) threat to ability to handle activities of daily living, and (4) appreciable worsening of gait or balance. According to a Norwegian quality of life study (Karlsen et al., 1999), the factors that produce the highest distress for PD patients compared to healthy elderly people are depressive symptoms, self-reported insomnia, and a low degree of independence, measured by the Schwab and England scale. Severity of parkinsonian motor symptoms contributed, but to a lesser extent. A sense of lack of energy was seen in half of the PD patients compared to a fifth of controls, and this could be only partially accounted for by depressive symptoms and the UPDRS motor scores.

The choice of drugs (Tables 6.3 and 6.5) is wide, but the degree of disability and the age (or mental acuity) of the patient are two critical factors. If the delay in initiating symptomatic treatment was so prolonged that the symptoms now threaten employment or endanger falling, one needs to begin levodopa to get a quick response. The advantages of using levodopa when the symptoms are this pronounced, in preference to a dopamine agonist or other medications, are that a therapeutic response is both rapid and virtually guaranteed, because nearly all patients with PD will respond to levodopa and relatively quickly. In contrast, only a minority of patients with severe symptoms will benefit sufficiently from a dopamine agonist given alone, and it takes more time (often months) to build up the dose to adequate levels to discover this. If levodopa is to be utilized, inhibitors of type A MAO must be discontinued. If selegiline (or another selective type B MAO inhibitor) was the MAO inhibitor that was utilized, this drug can be continued. A type A MAO inhibitor can be used safely with dopamine agonists.

If the symptoms are not severe enough to require levodopa and the patient is younger than 60 (younger than 70 if the patient is mentally young), we prefer to employ a dopasparing strategy to avoid as long as possible the development of levodopa-induced dyskinesias and motor fluctuations (mainly the wearing-off effect). These complications are more likely to occur in younger patients (Quinn et al., 1987; Kostic et al., 1991; Gershanik, 1993; Wagner et al., 1996). The choices are dopamine agonists, amantadine, and anticholinergics. Tranylcypromine can be continued in the presence of any of these drugs. Dopamine agonists are the most potent antiparkinsonian agents among this group of drugs. Four-year results of the pramipexole versus levodopa trial reveal that levodopa is clinically more potent, but is also much more likely to induce dyskinesias and clinical fluctuations (Holloway and Parkinson Study Group, 2004). For patients older than 70 years or those with any cognitive decline, employ levodopa as the initial therapy. Not only is there less need for a dopa-sparing strategy in these elderly patients, they are more susceptible to confusion, psychosis, or drowsiness from other antiparkinson drugs, including dopamine agonists. Levodopa provides the greatest benefit for the lowest risk of these adverse effects compared to the other drugs.

Rationale for dopa-sparing strategy in young patients

As was mentioned earlier, younger patients (less than 60 years of age) are particularly prone to develop the motor complications of fluctuations and dyskinesias (Quinn et al., 1987; Kostic et al., 1991; Gershanik, 1993; Wagner et al., 1996). Some physicians therefore recommend utilizing dopamine agonists, rather than levodopa, in younger patients when beginning therapy, in an attempt to delay the onset of these problems (Quinn, 1994b; Fahn and Przedborski, 2010; Montastruc et al., 1999). But others prefer starting with levodopa (Weiner, 1999). A conference on this topic failed to produce a consensus (Agid et al., 1999).

Choice of drug when employing a dopa-sparing strategy

Dopamine agonists

The dopamine agonists are the group of agents that is next most powerful in reducing the symptoms of PD after levodopa therapy. Thus, they are a good choice. Based on a clinical trial, there is no evidence that they provide neuroprotection (Schapira et al., 2009a). Perhaps the main reason many patients are started with this class of drugs, is that they are less likely to induce dyskinesias and motor fluctuations (Rinne et al., 1998a; Parkinson Study Group, 2000; Rascol et al., 2000; Holloway and Parkinson Study Group, 2004).

Rinne (1989a, 1989b) first proposed that early use of the dopamine agonists would reduce the likelihood of developing complications from chronic levodopa therapy. However, the Rinne reports were on retrospective analyses, using historical rather than contemporary controls. In one double-blind study, Weiner and colleagues (1993) could not confirm Rinne's findings. However, in another controlled trial, Montastruc and colleagues (1994) reported that there were fewer motor complications in patients who started on bromocriptine, to which levodopa was later added. Studies of dopamine agonists as primary monotherapy in early PD have shown that, even with sustained treatment, drug-induced dyskinesias rarely develop, but that monotherapy is successful for more than 3 years in only about 30% of all PD patients (Poewe, 1998). In addition to this benefit, the dopamine agonists are the most powerful antiparkinson medications after levodopa. Therefore, if one wants to use dopa-sparing strategies, one should choose among the dopamine agonists.

The first double-blind study comparing an agonist with levodopa was with cabergoline. A smaller percentage of patients in the cabergoline group developed motor fluctuations (22%) versus 34% on levodopa ($P < 0.02$) (Rinne et al., 1998a). Controlled clinical trials comparing ropinirole (Rascol et al., 2000), pramipexole (Parkinson Study Group, 2000), and pergolide (Oertel et al., 2006) have shown that starting treatment with a dopamine agonist is less likely than treatment with levodopa to induce dyskinesias. On the other hand, these studies all showed that levodopa is more potent and improves UPDRS scores more than the agonists did. Moreover, the agonists are more likely to produce hallucinations and sedation than levodopa.

Post hoc analysis revealed that starting treatment with ropinirole (Rascol et al., 2006) or pramipexole (Kieburtz et al., 2006) delays levodopa-induced dyskinesias by delaying the start of levodopa therapy. A 10-year follow-up of the ropinirole trial showed that motor complications remained fewer in those subjects who started on ropinirole, but there was no difference in UPDRS. (Hauser et al., 2007). Of course, all subjects were taking levodopa at that time. A similar finding was found in the 6-year follow-up of the CALM-PD subjects (initiating levodopa or pramipexole) (Parkinson Study Group CALM Cohort Investigators, 2009).

The dopamine agonists that are currently available are the ergots pergolide (Permax) in some countries (not the United States) and bromocriptine (Parlodel), and the non-ergots pramipexole (Mirapex) and ropinirole (Requip). The longer-duration ergot cabergoline is available in some countries. Rotigotine (Neupro) is absorbed transdermally, and was available on the global market until crystals of the drug were found on the dermal patch; the dermal patch of rotigotine was withdrawn from the US market, and the company is currently attempting to remedy the problem.

Ergots rarely can induce red, inflamed skin (St Anthony's fire), which is reversible on discontinuing the drug. They also have the potential (although rare) with long-term use to induce fibrosis: retroperitoneal, pleuropulmonary, and pericardial (Pfitzenmeyer et al., 1996; Ling et al., 1999; Shaunak et al., 1999). Pergolide has also been seen in association with fibroproliferative changes in heart valves, initially reported in three patients (Pritchett et al., 2002). Since then there have been other reports (Baseman et al., 2004; Horvath et al., 2004; Van Camp et al., 2004). The frequency of this complication is still being resolved. The reports of this complication raised new concerns, and questions as to whether pergolide should be used as a drug for PD unless other dopamine agonists have been unsatisfactory in terms of benefits or adverse effects (Agarwal et al., 2004). Now echocardiograms performed on patients taking pergolide have revealed a much higher prevalence, about 33%, of restrictive valvulopathies (Van Camp et al., 2004). This indicates that all patients on pergolide need to undergo echocardiography. Fortunately, the valvulopathy is reversible in some patients if pergolide is discontinued. If this ergoline can cause this problem, then it is possible that the other ergoline agonists can do likewise. It seems prudent to utilize non-ergot dopamine agonists rather than starting pergolide on other patients. With the publication of larger studies (Peralta et al., 2006; Zanettini et al., 2007; Dewey et al., 2007) and the analysis of the United Kingdom General Practice Research Database for cardiac valve regurgitation showing pergolide and cabergoline to increase its incidence rate (Schade et al., 2007), the FDA issued a strong warning, and the pharmaceutical company discontinued manufacturing pergolide in 2007.

Heart valves contain 5-HT$_{2B}$ receptors. Drugs like fenfluramine that activate these receptors can induce thickening of the heart valves. Roth (2007) reviewed the effect on 5-HT receptors by dopamine agonists. The only two dopamine agonists that are also potent 5-HT$_{2B}$ agonists are pergolide and cabergoline, and these are the only ones that were significantly associated with cardiac valve disease (Schade et al., 2007). Lisuride, which is an agonist at 5-HT$_{2A}$ and 5-HT$_{2C}$ receptors, but not at 5-HT$_{2B}$ receptors, was not associated with valve disease. Although regurgitation was reported with bromocriptine, restrictive valvulopathy was not (Tan et al., 2009).

Pramipexole and ropinirole, as was mentioned earlier, appear more readily to produce drowsiness and sleep attacks in which patients fall asleep without warning, including while driving, although there have now been rare incidences of sleep attacks with all dopamine agonists and levodopa (Frucht et al., 1999; Hoehn, 2000; Schapira, 2000; Ferreira et al., 2000). The Epworth Sleepiness Scale is not predictive as to which patient may develop a sleep attack (Hobson et al., 2002). Korner and colleagues (2004) sent a questionnaire to 12 000 patients and received responses from 63%, 42% of whom reported that they had experienced sudden onset of sleep; 10% of these had not experienced sleepiness before their first sleep attack. Predicting factors were nonergoline dopamine agonists, age less than 70 years, and disease duration less than 7 years. Modafinil has successfully been used to prevent sleep attacks (Hauser et al., 2000).

Adverse effects that are more common with agonists than with levodopa are orthostatic hypotension, nausea (because nausea from levodopa is blocked by carbidopa), drowsiness, hallucinations, and leg edema. All agonists have a propensity to produce ankle and leg edema (Tan and Ondo, 2000), which is not an early problem, but tends to occur after a few years of treatment. In a retrospective review of developing pedal edema with pramipexole treatment, there was no relationship between dose of pramipexole and incidence and severity of pedal edema. The risk of development of pedal edema was 7.7% in the first year after initiation of pramipexole therapy, with more rapid development of edema among those with a history of coronary artery disease (Kleiner-Fisman and Fisman, 2007). The edematous skin is often red, and some clinicians, unaware of this adverse effect, assume that there is a deep vein thrombosis. The edema and redness persists unless the drug is stopped. Diuretics are only partially effective in relieving the edema. Whether it is dangerous to continue to allow the edema to persist is not known. But continued use of the agonist can eventually result in discolored, indurated skin in the lower part of the legs where the edema was located. The tight skin prevents edema from accumulating there, so the edema is seen above the induration. Substituting one agonist for another may occasionally allow the edema to dissipate, but more often than not, once the edema has occurred, it persists in the presence of other dopamine agonists as well. The only satisfactory treatment of the edema is to discontinue the agonist, and substitute levodopa, which does not cause this problem. The edema of the legs that is induced by dopamine agonists resembles that induced by amantadine.

A new adverse effect was reported in 2010 by Rabinak and Nirenberg, who described the "dopamine agonist withdrawal syndrome (DAWS)." This was defined as a cluster of physical and psychological symptoms that correlate with dopamine agonist withdrawal, causing clinically significant distress or social/occupational dysfunction, and are refractory to levodopa and other PD medications, and cannot be accounted for by other clinical factors. Symptoms of DAWS resembled those of other drug withdrawal syndromes and included anxiety, panic attacks, agoraphobia, depression, dysphoria, diaphoresis, fatigue, pain, orthostatic hypotension, and drug cravings. Some of those with DAWS needed to be restarted on the dopamine agonist.

An experimental study in MPTP-treated primates showed that treatment with dopamine agonists (ropinirole and bromocriptine in this study) significantly less likely to cause severe dyskinesias than treatment with levodopa (Pearce

et al., 1998). The investigators titrated dosages that produced similarly increased locomotion and improved motor disability. However, these investigators also showed that an agonist will elicit comparable dyskinesia once levodopa priming has occurred, and they therefore recommended early use of dopamine agonists. Controlled clinical trials comparing ropinirole (Rascol et al., 2000), pramipexole (Parkinson Study Group, 2000), and pergolide (Oertel et al., 2006) have shown that starting treatment with a dopamine agonist is less likely than treatment with levodopa to induce dyskinesias.

Each of the dopamine agonists easily induces orthostatic hypotension, particularly when the drug is first introduced (Kujawa et al., 2000). After that period, this complication is much less common. Therefore it is best to start with a tiny dose (bromocriptine 1.25 mg at bedtime; pergolide 0.05 mg at bedtime; pramipexole 0.125 mg at bedtime) for the first 3 days, and then switch from bedtime to daytime dosing for the remainder of the first week. Ropinirole can be started at 0.25 mg three times daily for the first week. The daily dose can be increased gradually (bromocriptine 1.25 mg every week; pergolide 0.125 mg weekly; pramipexole 0.125 mg every 2 days for 10 days, then 0.125 mg per day weekly; ropinirole 0.5 mg/day twice weekly), building the dosage up on a four times a day dosing schedule until benefit or a dose around 40 mg/day (bromocriptine), 4–6 mg/day (pergolide and pramipexole), or 24 mg/day (ropinirole) is reached. Use the lowest dose that provides adequate benefit.

Bromocriptine appears to be the weakest of the four agonists, yet it can induce psychotoxicity just as readily as the other agonists, if not more so. That is why bromocriptine is not used as much and therefore not presented in Table 6.12. The choice between the other three drugs is one of personal preference and experience, and perhaps should be based on adverse effects because the benefits are similar. Some patients may benefit from all three equally; some may get adverse effects from one, but not the others. By having these three drugs available, the clinician has the ability to switch from one to another should one of them not be tolerated. Switching can be done rapidly using a ratio of 1:1:5 for pergolide:pramipexole:ropinirole, without having to build up the dose of the new drug from a much lower level. If the response is less than satisfactory, and it is desired to maintain the dopa-sparing strategy for as long as possible, one can then add amantadine or an anticholinergic (see below). If none of these agents is helpful or tolerated, the patient moves into the next stage of illness, the stage in which levodopa is required. Nausea and vomiting are other potential side effects that would limit the usefulness of the dopamine agonists. These symptoms are usually avoided by increasing the dose slowly. The peripherally-acting dopamine antagonist domperidone will block these gastrointestinal side effects. The usual dose is 10–20 mg thrice daily. Even if a dopamine agonist is effective, many patients require the addition of levodopa within a year or two.

One can quickly switch from one dopamine agonist to another without having to build up the dose slowly for the new one (Canesi et al., 1999). Using a conversion factor, the new agonist can begin at full dosage at the beginning of the day while the current one is suddenly discontinued. A conversion table is provided (Table 6.13), in which pergolide is given at unity (1). Pramipexole is also 1, ropinirole

Table 6.12 Suggested schedule for dopamine agonist therapy

Agonist	Initial dose	Titration phase	Lowest dose likely to be effective	Typical maintenance dose	Typical maximum dose
Pramipexole	0.05 mg at bedtime for 3 nights; then switch to daytime	Increase by 0.25 mg every 2 days for 10 days, using a t.i.d. schedule; then 0.125 mg per day weekly	0.75 mg t.i.d.	1.5 mg t.i.d.	2–3 mg t.i.d.
Ropinirole	0.125 mg t.i.d.	0.5 mg per day twice weekly	2 mg t.i.d.	4–5 mg t.i.d.	7–9 mg t.i.d.
Ropinirole extended release	2 mg once a day	2 mg every 1–2 weeks	6 mg	12–18 mg	24 mg per day
Rotigotine (patch)	2 mg patch once a day	2 mg patch weekly	2 mg	6 mg patch daily	6 mg daily

This is just one schedule; many other related schedules can be used. t.i.d., three times a day.

Table 6.13 Conversion factors for the dopamine agonists

Agonist	Ratio
Pergolide	1
Pramipexole	1
Ropinirole	5
Bromocriptine	10

is 5, and bromocriptine is 10. This means that if the dose of pergolide or pramipexole were 2 mg/day, ropinirole and bromocriptine equivalents would be 10 and 20 mg/day, respectively.

Amantadine

Amantadine is a mild indirect dopaminergic, acting by augmenting dopamine release from storage sites and possibly blocking reuptake of dopamine into the presynaptic terminals. It also appears to have some anticholinergic properties, as well as glutamate receptor blocking activity. In the mild stage of PD it is effective in about two-thirds of patients (Fahn and Isgreen, 1975). A major advantage is that substantial benefit, if it occurs, is seen in a couple of days. Unfortunately, its benefit in more advanced PD is often short-lived, with patients reporting a fall-off effect after several months of treatment in the absence of concomitant levodopa. The mechanism appears to be a depletion of already reduced dopamine stores in the dopaminergic nerve terminals so that the effect of amantadine is exhausted. A common adverse effect is livedo reticularis (a reddish mottling of skin) around the knees; this is not dangerous, although it can be cosmetically a problem for some patients. Occasional adverse effects are ankle edema and visual hallucinosis. Sometimes when the drug is discontinued, there can be a gradual worsening of parkinsonian signs, indicating that the drug has been helpful. The usual dosage is 100 mg twice daily, but sometimes a higher dose (up to 400 mg) may be required.

Amantadine can be useful, not only in the early phases of symptomatic therapy, thereby forestalling the introduction of levodopa or reducing the required dosage of levodopa, but also in the advanced stage of the disease as an adjunctive drug to levodopa and the dopamine agonists. It is also effective in reducing levodopa-induced dyskinesias (Rajput et al., 1997; Metman et al., 1998a; Thomas et al., 2004), probably from its antiglutamatergic activity.

Amantadine is excreted mostly unchanged in the urine, so the dose needs to be reduced in patients with renal impairment. The half-life is long, about 28 hours, so twice daily dosing is adequate. CNS adverse effects of myoclonus, hallucinations, and delirium are associated with very high plasma levels of amantadine, which can be due to overdosage (Fahn et al., 1971) or from impaired renal function (Nishikawa et al., 2009).

Antimuscarinic drugs (anticholinergics)

The anticholinergics are less effective antiparkinson agents than the dopamine agonists. The anticholinergics are estimated to improve parkinsonism by about 20%. Many clinicians find that if tremor is not relieved by an agonist or levodopa, then the addition of an anticholinergic drug is often effective. Sometimes, the anticholinergic can lessen tremor severity even in the absence of levodopa, so clinicians can use such an agent as monotherapy for tremor. If this is not helpful, then continuing to use the drug while a dopamine agonist or levodopa is added can be helpful. Later, if tremor is relieved by the dopaminergic agent, one can try to discontinue the anticholinergic. Commonly used anticholinergics are trihexyphenidyl (Artane) and benztropine mesylate (Cogentin); but there are many others. To minimize adverse effects, start with low doses (trihexyphenidyl 1 mg twice daily; benztropine 0.5 mg twice daily) and increase gradually to 2 mg three times daily for trihexyphenidyl and 1 mg three times daily for benztropine. As would be expected, if anticholinergics lessen parkinsonism, cholinergic agents aggravate parkinsonian symptoms (Duvoisin, 1967), including nicotine (Ebersbach et al., 1999).

Peripheral anticholinergic adverse effects include blurred vision (treated with pilocarpine eye drops, which also must be utilized if glaucoma is present), dry mouth, and urinary retention. Pyridostigmine, up to 60 mg three times daily if necessary, can sometimes be helpful in overcoming dry mouth and urinary difficulties. The predominant central side effects are forgetfulness and decreased short-term memory. Occasionally hallucinations and psychosis can occur, particularly in the elderly. Powerful anticholinergics should be

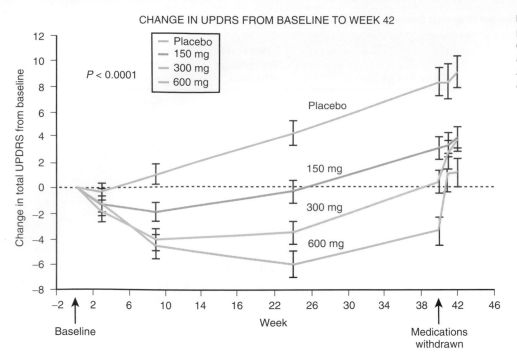

CHANGE IN UPDRS FROM BASELINE TO WEEK 42

Figure 6.10 Levodopa and the progression of PD. *From Parkinson Study Group. Levodopa and the progression of Parkinson's disease. N Engl J Med 2004;351(24):2498–2508.* © 2004 Massachusetts Medical Society. All rights reserved.

avoided in patients older than 70 years of age. If tremor persists in this age range despite the presence of levodopa or dopamine agonists, utilize drugs with a weaker anticholinergic effect, such as diphenhydramine (Benadryl), orphenadrine (Norflex), cyclobenzaprine (Flexeril), and amitriptyline (Elavil). Diphenhydramine and amitriptyline can cause drowsiness; therefore they can also be used as a hypnotic. For tremor control, one needs to increase the dose gradually until at least 50 mg three times daily is reached for diphenhydramine and orphenadrine, 20 mg three times daily for cyclobenzaprine, and 25 mg three times daily for amitriptyline.

There is concern that use of anticholinergic drugs in PD may hasten cognitive decline. In one study, where patients were followed for 8 years, cognitive decline was higher in those who were begun with anticholinergic drugs (Ehrt et al., 2010). Their median decline on the Mini-Mental State Examination (MMSE) was 6.5 points compared with a 1 point decline in those who had not taken such drugs ($P = 0.025$). The duration of using these drugs also correlated with a greater decline in MMSE scores ($P = 0.032$).

Another point of view: utilize levodopa as the first drug

There are a number of neurologists who advocate starting with levodopa when symptomatic therapy is needed (Agid, 1998; Weiner, 1999; Factor, 2000), and for the sake of the reader, this point of view should be made known. The argument is that there is no proof that levodopa itself causes either neurotoxicity or the motor complications of dyskinesias and "off" states. Rather, they suggest that it is the severity of the disease that allows these complications to appear with levodopa. Therefore, they prefer to use the most effective drug first when the symptoms are mild in order to provide the highest quality of life. However, despite the ELLDOPA trial (Parkinson Study Group, 2004b), uncertainty about

neurotoxicity remains, and until there is a follow-up controlled clinical trial to answer the uncertainties from that trial, the justification can be made that unless a dopamine agonist is not tolerated or effective, levodopa can be delayed until needed (Fahn, 1999).

The ELLDOPA study was a controlled clinical trial evaluating the effect of levodopa on the natural history of PD (Parkinson Study Group, 2004b). Unexpectedly, the clinical results showed that subjects treated with levodopa had less clinical progression 2 weeks after stopping the drug than subjects treated with placebo, and this effect was dose-dependent (Fig. 6.10). But concern has been raised that perhaps the 2-week washout of levodopa was insufficient to eliminate all of its symptomatic benefit. Moreover, the ELLDOPA study showed a discordance between the neuroimaging component and the clinical results. The dopamine transporter binding ligand imaging study was compatible with a more rapid decline of dopamine neurons. But that result has now raised the question as to whether levodopa itself interferes with this binding. Therefore, the interpretation of the ELLDOPA study remains uncertain. On the other hand, a computer simulation of the ELLDOPA results, combined with the DATATOP results, supports the conclusion that levodopa slows disease progression (P.L. Chan et al., 2007). It is of interest that in subsequent clinical trials, such as the PRECEPT study, subjects reach endpoint at a lower level of severity of parkinsonism compared to the DATATOP study which was conducted prior to the ELLDOPA study (Marras et al., 2009). Subjects may feel that starting levodopa sooner is not as serious a threat to their well-being, having seen the ELLDOPA results.

Another argument is that levodopa has delayed mortality, and therefore it should be used early. However, the initial improvement of mortality rates occurred when levodopa was first introduced and most likely was from the improvement of mobility, not from the drug itself. Improved or maintained mobility with another antiparkinson agent would probably be just as effective. Actually, mortality rates have gone back to their earlier increased level, now that levodopa has taken care of the backlog of disabled patients (Clarke, 1995). In a more recent analysis of retrospective data from Scotland (Donnan et al., 2000) comparing PD patients with their treatment assignment, levodopa monotherapy had a higher mortality rate than did selegiline monotherapy or selegiline plus levodopa.

From the DATATOP study, the 387 subjects who reached endpoint, i.e., the need for symptomatic therapy, were placed on levodopa, and their UPDRS scores were reduced by approximately 33% (from approximately 43 units to 29 units) (Fig. 1 in Growdon et al., 1998).

Whether levodopa actually provides a better quality of life (Martinez-Martin, 1998; Glozman et al., 1998) for patients with mild-stage PD remains to be determined, particularly as compared to dopamine agonists in patients with early PD. In one study – the levodopa versus pramipexole controlled clinical trial (Holloway and Parkinson Study Group, 2004) – health-related quality of life (HRQOL) was assessed by three different measures. All three measures resulted in similar profiles over time characterized by initial improvement over the first 3–6 months and followed by a gradual decline in years 2, 3, and 4 (Noyes et al., 2006). The difference in HRQOL between the treatment arms widened in favor of pramipexole in years 3 and 4 for all HRQOL measures used. Because levodopa had a superior result in UPDRS scores, the results suggest that pramipexole and levodopa affect HRQOL via improvement on different domains of well-being: nonmotor effect for pramipexole and mobility improvement for levodopa.

Whether the motor complications that are seen with chronic levodopa therapy in patients with PD are actually caused by long-term levodopa therapy or simply reflect the progression of the disease is unknown and widely debated (de Jong et al., 1987; Quinn et al., 1987; Blin et al., 1988; Roos et al., 1990; Caraceni et al., 1991; Cedarbaum et al., 1991). Advanced disease with altered sensitivity of dopamine receptors is a critical factor, but one does not see these motor complications if the patient was never exposed to levodopa and was treated only with the other antiparkinson agents. In untreated, but advanced PD, levodopa-induced dyskinesias occur shortly after levodopa is started (Onofri et al., 1998). In the parkinsonian states of postencephalitic parkinsonism and MPTP-induced parkinsonism there is rapidly severe depletion of nigral neurons (Bernheimer et al., 1973; Davis et al., 1979; Burns et al., 1983; Langston et al., 1984). These patients may develop dyskinesias and fluctuations within weeks to months after starting levodopa (Calne et al., 1969; Sacks et al., 1970; Duvoisin et al., 1972; Sacks, 1974; Langston et al., 1983; Langston and Ballard, 1984; Ballard et al., 1985). But if patients with those diseases had been treated with dopamine agonists instead of levodopa, it is likely that those motor complications would not have occurred.

In deciding the choice of drug therapy, it is important to keep in mind the principles of therapy listed at the beginning of this chapter: individualize therapy to fit the patient and keep the goal in mind of maintaining the patient as independent as possible for as long as possible.

If one chooses to use levodopa in the mild-stage disease, there is evidence to suggest keeping the dose as low as possible (Poewe et al., 1986; Lesser et al., 1979). One strategy is to build the dosage from carbidopa/levodopa 25/100 mg to 50/200 mg three times daily and then add a dopamine agonist if the patient needs more symptomatic relief. (For older patients, stay with levodopa and increase that if more medication is needed – see the next section.)

Treatment of moderate-stage Parkinson disease

Moderate-stage PD is when the disability is beyond the scope of efficacy of dopamine agonists, amantadine, anticholinergics, and a MAO-B inhibitor; treatment with levodopa is necessary to control symptoms. The rule of thumb is to utilize the lowest dosage that brings about adequate symptom reversal, not the highest dosage that the patient can tolerate, in an attempt to avoid response fluctuations and dyskinesias. This recommendation seems contra to the ELLDOPA results (Parkinson Study Group, 2004b), which suggests that higher doses may offer more neuroprotection. But interpretation of that study is difficult because a longer duration of benefit may exceed the 2-week washout period, and the imaging results suggest the opposite interpretation, namely that levodopa may enhance loss of dopamine nerve terminals. Until the uncertainties are clarified, we are left with the reality that levodopa dosage contributes to the development of motor complications, as recorded in the ELLDOPA study.

Levodopa is usually given combined with a peripheral decarboxylase inhibitor (carbidopa (Sinemet and generics) or benserazide (Madopar)) to prevent the formation of dopamine peripherally, thereby usually avoiding the otherwise common peripheral adverse effects of anorexia, nausea, and vomiting. Many patients require at least 50–75 mg of carbidopa a day to have adequate inhibition of peripheral dopa decarboxylase. If the dose of levodopa is less than 300 mg/day, then one should use the 25/100 mg strength tablets and not the 10/100 mg tablets. In some patients even 75 mg per day of carbidopa is inadequate, and nausea, anorexia, or vomiting still occurs. In such patients, one needs to use higher doses of carbidopa; carbidopa tablets (Lodosyn) are available by prescription.

Carbidopa/levodopa is marketed in both immediate release (Sinemet and generics) and extended release (Sinemet CR and generic carbidopa/levodopa ER) tablets; the latter provides a longer plasma half-life and lower peak plasma levels of levodopa compared to standard Sinemet. Unfortunately, Sinemet CR has not been shown to avoid the development of response fluctuations. A 5-year study in 618 dopa-naive patients compared Sinemet CR and standard Sinemet therapy. There was no difference between the two groups in the development of either fluctuations or dyskinesias (Block et al., 1997; Koller et al., 1999). An Italian study found that using small, divided doses during the day is more likely to lead to loss of the long duration response (Zappia et al., 2000).

A pre-bedtime dose of Sinemet CR may allow the patient some mobility during the night. Disadvantages of Sinemet CR are the lack of a rapid response with each dose and a delayed response that can be excessive, resulting in sustained severe dyskinesias that cannot be controlled except by sedating the patient. Moreover, the response to individual doses of Sinemet CR is less predictable than the response to standard Sinemet. It is complicated to use both standard Sinemet and Sinemet CR to smooth out fluctuations, but this is often necessary. Finally, one should keep in mind that not all of the carbidopa/levodopa in Sinemet CR is absorbed because some of the medication may have reached the large intestine before all of it was absorbed in the small intestine. A dose of Sinemet CR is equal to about two-thirds to three-quarters of an identical dose of standard Sinemet.

On the other hand, Sinemet CR is useful as a first line drug in patients older than age 70 years to slow the rate of absorption and lower the peak plasma level of levodopa, making it less likely for the patient to develop peak-dose drowsiness or confusion. For younger patients, in whom cognitive adverse effects are less likely to occur, standard carbidopa/levodopa is preferred in order to observe the response and better monitor the effectiveness of the drug. In these younger patients there may be merit in utilizing a combination of immediate and extended release tablets simultaneously in an effort to provide smoother, stabler plasma and brain concentrations of levodopa, in an attempt to lessen the development of dyskinesias and wearing-off.

Sinemet CR is available in two strengths, carbidopa/levodopa 50/200 mg tablet, which is scored and can be broken in half, and a 25/100 mg unscored tablet. Crushing either tablet loses the slow release property because the matrix is no longer intact. When Sinemet CR is added in a patient taking a dopamine agonist, a dose of 25/100 mg three times daily (built up gradually by 25/100 mg weekly) often suffices. When it is used alone, it often is necessary to use these dosages after meals to reduce initial nausea and vomiting; the dose can later be increased to 50/200 mg three or four times daily. If greater relief is required, a dopamine agonist should then be added.

Immediate release carbidopa/levodopa is available in 10/100, 25/100, and 25/250 mg tablets. Because of the desire to have at least 75 mg per day of carbidopa, one should start with the 25/100 mg tablets when the drug is introduced. An increase by 25/100 mg per day per week until three times daily dosing is achieved is often adequate. A 25/100 mg three times daily dosing is the most common plateau schedule neurologists aim for (Fahn and Mazzoni, 2006). Not every symptom of PD responds equally well. Bradykinesia and rigidity respond best, while tremor can be more resistant. If a response is seen, but with symptoms later returning or worsening, increasing to 50/200 mg three times daily is a reasonable goal before adding a dopamine agonist. If agonists are already being taken, and there is still an inadequate response, the dosage of levodopa should be increased gradually, switching to the 25/250 mg tablets as necessary. A dose of 25/250 mg four times daily may be required. A reasonably high dose before concluding that levodopa is ineffective is 2000 mg of levodopa per day.

A clinical trial was conducted to determine if entacapone should be given with levodopa when the latter is introduced. There was a widespread belief that continuous dopaminergic therapy, which is the method utilized to treat fluctuations and dyskinesias, would also prevent the development of these motor complications to levodopa. (For more detailed discussion on motor complications and continuous dopaminergic stimulation, see the section entitled "Treatment of advanced-stage Parkinson disease.") Subjects requiring dopaminergic treatment were randomized to be on either levodopa with carbidopa (LC group) or with entacapone added to the tablet (LCE group). The opposite outcome than what was expected happened. The LCE group developed dyskinesias earlier, and more subjects in that group developed dyskinesias compared to the LC group (Stocchi et al., 2010). One possible explanation is that when levodopa dosage equivalents were calculated, the LCE group received higher dosages than the LC group. Based on the results of this study, we cannot recommend entacapone be administered at the beginning of levodopa therapy; it should be reserved for the treatment of fluctuations, as described in the section "Treatment of advanced-stage Parkinson disease."

A patient's response or lack of response to levodopa is a very important piece of information to help differentiate PD from parkinsonism-plus syndromes. If the response is nil or minor, it is most likely that the disorder is not PD (Marsden and Fahn, 1982). However, a beneficial response does not ensure that a diagnosis of PD is correct. All cases of presynaptic disorders (e.g., reserpine-induced, MPTP-induced, postencephalitic parkinsonism) will respond to levodopa. Also, patients in the early stages of multiple system atrophy and progressive supranuclear palsy may improve with levodopa; later in these diseases, when dopamine receptors are lost, the response is lost. Some patients with Shy–Drager syndrome and olivopontocerebellar atrophy may continue to have intact dopamine receptors in the striatum and continue to respond to levodopa. The only effective drugs in situations in which levodopa is not effective are the anticholinergics and amantadine, even though only mildly so.

It takes a mean of 9.3 ± 1.8 days to achieve maximum response when beginning treatment with Sinemet CR and 6.8 ± 3.0 days for the parkinsonism severity to return to baseline levels after stopping chronic Sinemet CR treatment (Barbato et al., 1997). This compares to a decay time of 6.2 ± 1.7 days following withdrawal of the dopamine agonist ropinirole (9–21 mg daily). These studies support the concept that the long-duration effect of levodopa and ropinirole might be due to some slowly evolving postsynaptic pharmacodynamic change in the CNS (Barbato et al., 1997).

It is important to avoid sudden withdrawal of levodopa, which is sometimes done for a surgical procedure (Stotz et al., 2004). A "neuroleptic malignant-like" syndrome can ensue, with fever, rigidity, and incoherence (Friedman et al., 1985; Hirschorn and Greenberg, 1988; Gordon and Frucht, 2001; Ueda et al., 2001). Tapering levodopa over 3 days appears to be safe (Parkinson Study Group, 2004b).

As PD worsens, the duration of effectiveness of a dose of levodopa becomes shorter (Contin et al., 1998a). The effective clinical half-life of a dose of levodopa declines in relation to both worsening of symptoms and duration of disease. While the pharmacokinetic half-life remains constant, around 90 minutes, the clinical half-life declines from a mean of 262 minutes in stage I patients, to 142 minutes in stage II, to 54 minutes in stage III. The rate of decline becomes smaller as the disease progresses. The mean annual reduction of the effective half-life slows down as the disease worsens, dropping by 37 minutes/year in stage I patients and by 6.5 minutes/year in stage III, and is about 17% per year of the disease. Contin and colleagues (1998a) determined this "effective" half-life by administering a standard oral fasting dose (100 mg) of levodopa (with a peripheral decarboxylase inhibitor). Motor response was measured by finger tapping speed and walking speed. The decline in effective half-life is equivalent to the loss of the long-duration response from levodopa to only a short-duration response as the disease worsens, and as first reported by Muenter and Tyce (1971).

Treatment of advanced-stage Parkinson disease

Advanced PD is that stage of the disease in which there is at least one of the following conditions: (1) sufficient disability to interfere with independence despite levodopa therapy, (2) sufficient loss of postural reflexes so that one must be cautious when walking, (3) the presence of the freezing phenomenon to make walking difficult, (4) pronounced postural deformity, or (5) the presence of complications (fluctuations, dyskinesias, psychosis) from levodopa that have become the focus of treatment. Because it is only the last group that is somewhat amenable to therapy, the discussion will concentrate on methods to overcome these complications. In advanced PD, because of the severity of the clinical situation, all patients should be receiving levodopa therapy or at least have had a trial of this drug, but have not been able to remain on it because of disabling adverse effects. The Quality Standards Subcommittee of the American Academy of Neurology conducted an evidence-based literature review of clinical trials related to treating dyskinesias and fluctuations (Pahwa et al., 2006).

Description of motor (and sensory) complications

The motor complications can be divided into two categories: fluctuations ("off" states) and dyskinesias; these are subdivided into their temporal relationship with a dose of levodopa and the clinical motor and sensory phenomena seen as features of these levodopa-related complications (Table 6.14). The "off" states usually consist of a return of parkinsonian symptoms and signs, such as bradykinesia, tremor, rigidity, immobility, and freezing (so-called "off freezing"). There are also other features of "off" states in many patients. "Off dystonia" is the presence of sustained contractions and spasms, often painful, and most common early in the morning on arising and in the feet. Because technically "off dystonia" is an abnormal involuntary movement (dyskinesia), this is listed in Table 6.14 in the dyskinesia column, but it should be recognized clinically as an "off" phenomenon. "Off" dystonia shows an abnormal irregular firing of globus pallidus interna neurons similar to that seen in primary dystonia (Hashimoto et al. 2001). So-called "sensory offs," "behavioral offs," and "autonomic offs" are the sensory, behavioral, and autonomic phenomena that may accompany a motor (parkinsonian) "off" or be present as an "off" in the absence of any motoric parkinsonian signs. Sensory/behavioral/autonomic "offs" can consist of any combination of pain, akathisia, depression, anxiety, dysphoria, panic, drenching sweating, abdominal bloating, and dyspnea. Sensory/behavioral "offs" are often unrecognized and, like dystonic "offs," are extremely poorly tolerated. It is often the presence of one of these sensory and behavioral phenomena – more so than motoric parkinsonian or dystonic "offs"

Table 6.14 Major fluctuations and dyskinesias as complications of levodopa

Fluctuations ("offs")

Slow "wearing-off"

Sudden "off"

Random "off"

"Super off"

Yo-yo-ing

Delayed "on"

Episodic failure to respond (dose failure)

Response varies in relationship to meals

Weak response at end of day

Sudden transient freezing

Dyskinesias

Peak-dose chorea, ballism, and dystonia

Diphasic chorea and dystonia

End-of-day dyskinesia

"Off" dystonia

Myoclonus

Simultaneous dyskinesia and parkinsonism

Sensory/Behavioral/Autonomic "offs"

Pain

Akathisia

Depression

Anxiety

Dysphoria

Panic

Drenching sweats

Abdominal bloating

Dyspnea

Sensation of urinary urgency

– that drives the patient to take more and more levodopa, turning the patient into a "levodopa junkie." The sensory/behavioral/autonomic "offs" are covered in Chapter 8.

There is usually a pattern of progressively worsening response fluctuations in patients who are on chronic levodopa therapy. Response fluctuations usually begin as mild wearing-off (end-of-dose failure). Wearing-off can be defined to be present when an adequate dosage of levodopa does not last at least 4 hours. Typically, in the first couple of years of treatment, there is a long-duration response (Muenter and Tyce, 1971). As the disease progresses or as levodopa treatment continues, the long-duration response fades and the short-duration response becomes predominant, leading to the wearing-off effect (Fig. 6.11).

The "offs" tend to be mild at first but, over time, often become deeper with more severe parkinsonism; simultaneously, the duration of the "on" response becomes shorter. Eventually, some patients develop sudden "offs" in which the deep state of parkinsonism develops over minutes rather than tens of minutes, and they are less predictable in terms of timing with the dosings of levodopa, and can be called random "offs" in this situation. A "super off" is where the "off" state is more severe than the untreated parkinsonian state. The "super off" appears either at the end of an "on"

LONG-DURATION BENEFIT

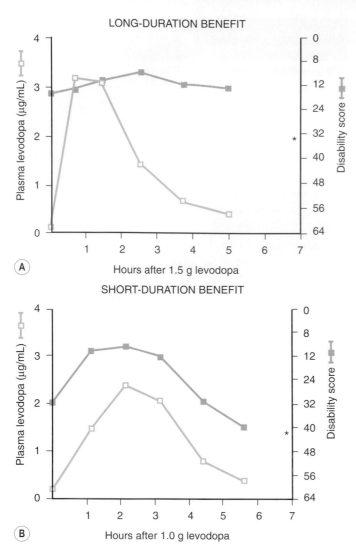

(A) Hours after 1.5 g levodopa

SHORT-DURATION BENEFIT

(B) Hours after 1.0 g levodopa

Figure 6.11 Clinical response to a dose of levodopa. **A** Long-duration response. **B** Short-duration response. The asterisk represents the level of clinical disability before the dose of levodopa. *From Muenter MD, Tyce GM. L-dopa therapy of Parkinson's disease: Plasma L-dopa concentration, therapeutic response, and side effects. Mayo Clin Proc 1971;46:231–239.*

patients respond best to levodopa given as the first dose of the day, and get a weaker response with the later doses, resulting in a weak response at end of day. This may reflect lower plasma levels of levodopa with each succeeding dose. Sudden transient freezing is not technically an "off" state; it is part of the freezing phenomenon, and can occur with "off" or "on" freezing.

Levodopa-induced dyskinesias appear to be related to the degree of dopamine receptor supersensitivity. It is difficult to induce dyskinesias in healthy animals or people, but with a high-enough dose, this has been achieved in monkeys (Sassin et al., 1972; Togasaki et al., 2001; Pearce et al., 2001). With increasing denervation, resulting in increased receptor sensitivity, there is more likelihood of developing choreic dyskinesias at a lower dose of levodopa (Cedarbaum et al., 1991). Dystonic reactions (forceful sustained contractions) may evolve over time in patients who earlier had choreic dyskinesias. However, some patients develop peak-dose dystonia at relatively low dosages; these may be patients with multiple system atrophy (Quinn, 1994a). Dyskinesias tend to first appear and remain more severe on the side of the body that PD presents itself clinically, in keeping with being contralateral to the more supersensitive dopamine receptors. In general, developing dyskinesias in PD can be viewed in a favorable light because the phenomenon indicates that dopamine receptors remain responsive so that motor symptoms of parkinsonism can be reduced by levodopa therapy. Also, the presence of dyskinesias does not have a significant negative effect on quality of life (Marras et al., 2004).

Dyskinesias usually occur at the peak concentration of the levodopa dose reaching the brain. The most common phenomenon is chorea. Rarely, the chorea can be so severe, it takes the form of ballism. More commonly, chorea can evolve into dystonia, and many patients will have a combination of chorea and dystonia. Peak-dose dyskinesias fade as the concentration of levodopa in the brain diminishes. Diphasic chorea and dystonia is when the dyskinesia begins at the beginning or the end of the dose, labeled as D-I-D by Muenter and colleagues (1977) (Fig. 6.12). The dyskinesias are typically present in the legs, whereas peak-dose dyskinesias are most common in the neck and upper body. End-of-day dyskinesia is the last end-of-dose dyskinesia of the day. "Off" dystonia is technically an "off" phenomenon, but instead of being a parkinsonian state, it is a painful dystonic state. Myoclonus can occur as a form of being overdosed from a dopaminergic (including amantadine) usually when there is mental confusion also. Some parts of the patient's body may be more sensitive to levodopa, and then will develop dyskinesias in that body part while the rest of the body may still be in a parkinsonian "off" state, so-called simultaneous dyskinesia and parkinsonism. A more detailed description of dyskinesias is available in a review by Fahn (2000).

The sensory/behavioral/autonomic "offs" resemble the same phenomena if they were to occur unrelated to the levodopa medication. It is likely that the dopamine receptors responsible for these symptoms are not neostriatal, but rather limbic and cortical for the behavioral and sensory symptoms, hypothalamic and possibly peripheral for the autonomic symptoms. All dopamine receptors would be activated by levodopa therapy, and become partially desensitized by such sustained activation. When the dopamine

period or immediately after a dose of levodopa (Merello and Lees, 1992). The latter situation is difficult to explain (Nutt et al., 1988). Many patients who develop response fluctuations also develop abnormal involuntary movements (i.e., dyskinesias). Yo-yo-ing is the state where the patient moves from an "off" to "on" with dyskinesia, and then back to being "off" again, with almost no time spent in-between, i.e., a state of "on" without dyskinesias. A delayed "on" is when the levodopa takes longer than 30 minutes after being swallowed for it to "kick in." This is the result of delayed gastric emptying. Levodopa is absorbed in the upper small intestine, predominantly the duodenum. Levodopa is absorbed utilizing the large neutral amino acid transport system. Dose failures are where the levodopa failed to "kick in" at all. The levodopa remained in the stomach. This often happens after a full meal. The meals can influence the speed of turning "on" after a dose of levodopa in those patients who have lost the long-duration benefit and are now dependent on the short-duration benefit (Muenter and Tyce, 1971). Many

ONSET AND END OF DOSE DYSKINESIA

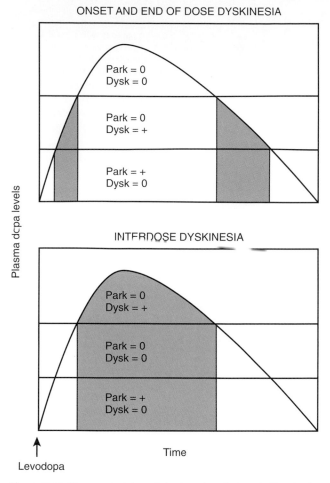

Figure 6.12 Diagram depicting diphasic and peak-dose dyskinesias. *From Agid Y, Bonnet AM, Signoret JL, Lhermitte F. Clinical, pharmalogical, and biochemical approach of "onset-, and end-of-dose" dyskinesias. Adv Neurol 1979;24:401–410.*

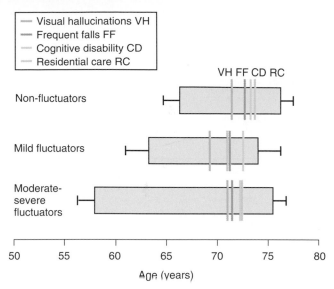

Figure 6.13 Milestones of disease advancement and total disease course in non-fluctuators and fluctuators. Error bars for standard error of the mean. The blue rectangles represent disease duration. *From Kempster PA, Williams DR, Selikhova M, et al. Patterns of levodopa response in Parkinson's disease: a clinicopathological study. Brain 2007;130(Pt 8):2123–2128.*

levels drop when the levodopa levels are low, these receptors are inadequately activated, and as a result produce symptoms as noted.

Clinicopathologic correlation of motor complications

Kempster and colleagues (2007) carried out a clinicopathologic correlation of PD patients with and without motor complications (fluctuations and dyskinesias) (Fig. 6.13). Ninety-seven cases of proven PD brains with good clinical descriptions were available. Clinically, the cases were divided into non-fluctuators ($n = 35$), mild fluctuators ($n = 17$) and moderate-severe fluctuators ($n = 45$). Patients with motor fluctuations had a younger age of onset and longer disease course ($P < 0.001$), although mean age at death was almost the same. Four milestones of advanced disease (frequent falls, visual hallucinations, cognitive disability, and need for residential care) occurred at a similar time from death in each group; this interval was not proportionate to the disease duration. There were no significant differences in the severity or distribution of Lewy body or other pathologies. Irrespective of the pattern of levodopa response, patients reach a common pathologic endpoint at a similar age, and the duration and manifestations of end-stage disease are alike.

Pathogenesis of motor complications

The known major risk factors for peak-dose dyskinesias appear to be severity of the disease (Horstink et al., 1990a; Ahlskog and Muenter, 2001), levodopa dosage (Poewe et al., 1986; Parkinson Study Group, 2004b), age of the patient (Quinn et al., 1987; Kostic et al., 1991; Kempster et al., 2007), and duration of levodopa therapy (Horstink et al., 1990b; Roos et al., 1990, Rajput et al., 2002, Van Gerpen et al., 2006). Although pulsatile administration of levodopa has been proposed as a risk factor (Chase, 1998; Chase et al., 1993), an attempt to smooth out plasma levels in advance of developing dyskinesias has had the opposite effect; it resulted in more and earlier dyskinesias (Stocchi et al., 2010). On the other hand, once wearing-off develops, it can be ameliorated by smoothing out plasma levels by continuous administration (Fig. 6.14) (Shoulson et al., 1975).

Fluctuations ("off" states)

The wearing-off phenomenon (also known as end-of-dose failure) is the gradual return of parkinsonism; it correlates with the falling concentration of levodopa in the plasma (and therefore the brain) (Muenter and Tyce, 1971; Shoulson et al., 1975; Fahn, 1982). The "on-off" phenomenon, as originally defined (Duvoisin, 1974b; Fahn, 1974), is a label for a sudden and random event in which the patient suddenly becomes parkinsonian. That is, the benefit from levodopa suddenly disappears, like turning off a light switch – hence the name. To avoid ambiguity, because the term "on-off" is sometimes used to refer to any type of fluctuation in parkinsonian patients, the phenomenon for sudden "offs" is labeled here as either "sudden off" or "on–off" in contrast to "wearing-off." In addition to worsening of motor performance during "off" states, there is often decreased mood accompanied by anxiety and sometimes pain (Maricle et al.,

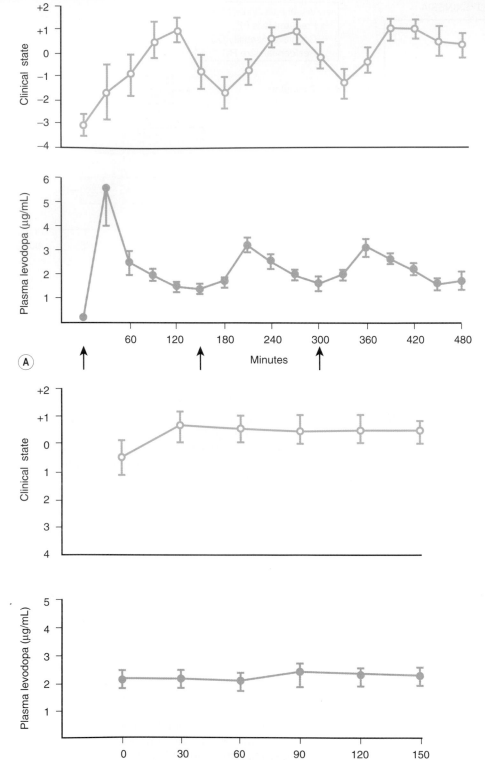

Figure 6.14 Relationship between clinical state and plasma levodopa concentration as mean scores in patients with clinical fluctuations. **A** Graphs are with the subjects taking oral levodopa at the times indicated by the arrows. **B** Graphs are with the subjects receiving intravenous levodopa infusions. *From Shoulson I, Glaubiger GA, Chase TN. "On-off" response: Clinical and biochemical correlations during oral and intravenous levodopa administration. Neurology 1975;25:1144–1148.*

1995; Ford et al., 1996; Hillen and Sage, 1996). These fluctuating mood and pain states can respond to the pharmacologic effects of levodopa.

On–off phenomenon

In "on–off," the patient can improve just as suddenly, even without taking another dose of levodopa. Pharmacologic studies have revealed plasma levels of levodopa to be in the declining phase when the "offs" appear (Fig. 6.15) (Fahn, 1974). It has been speculated that the "sudden off" problem is due to a sudden and transient desensitization of the dopamine receptors that would be compatible with the receptor switching from a high-affinity to a low-affinity state (Fahn, 1974). Response of a "sudden off" state to a new dose

TWO EPISODES OF SUDDEN "OFFS"

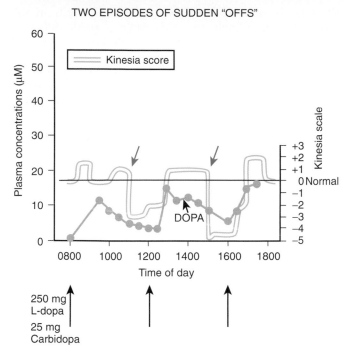

Figure 6.15 Two episodes of sudden "offs" (green arrows) during the declining slope of plasma levodopa concentrations. *From Fahn S. "On-off" phenomenon with levodopa therapy in parkinsonism: Clinical and pharmacologic correlations and the effect of intramuscular pyridoxine. Neurology 1974;24:431–441.*

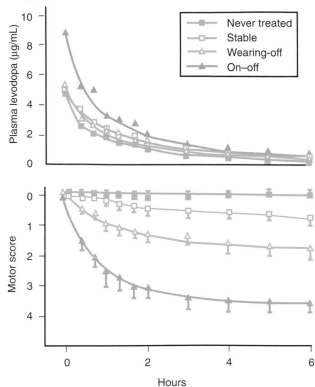

Figure 6.16 Plasma decay curves of levodopa and decay of symptoms. The upper graph shows the falling levodopa plasma levels after stopping the drug. The curves are very similar. The lower graph shows the fading of clinical response after stopping levodopa. The most severe fluctuators have the fastest decay of the clinical benefit. Those patients with no fluctuations have a long-duration benefit with no decay after stopping the drug. *From Fabbrini G, Juncos J, Mouradian MM, et al. Levodopa pharmacokinetic mechanisms and motor fluctuations in Parkinson's disease. Ann Neurol 1987;21:370–376.*

of levodopa or to a subcutaneous injection of apomorphine (Clough et al., 1984; Frankel et al., 1990) is compatible with the stimulation of a desensitized receptor; the receptor being presented with a higher concentration of dopamine (or dopamine agonist) will now respond. This result is not incompatible with the hypothesis that a desensitized receptor might be responsible for the "sudden off."

Wearing-off phenomenon

When patients have wearing-off, the clinical improvement from a dose of levodopa lasts only as long as the plasma concentration of levodopa is high (Muenter and Tyce, 1971). As the plasma level gradually falls, there is a loss of clinical response. In stable patients without clinical fluctuations, they maintain the long-duration response despite a fall in plasma levels of levodopa. Patients with wearing-off and on–off have lost the long-duration response and have only a short-duration response. In the study by Fabbrini et al. (1987) discontinuation of steady intravenous infusion of levodopa was followed by a decay in the plasma concentration of levodopa, identical in all groups of patients, representing an unchanged pharmacokinetic profile. With the falling plasma concentration of levodopa, the stable patients maintain their clinical response with only a gradual decay in the response over time (Fig. 6.16 upper). However, the patients with wearing-off and on–off have a rapid loss of the anti-PD effect, more closely paralleling the falling plasma concentration (Fig. 6.16 lower) (Fabbrini et al., 1987).

If the plasma level can be maintained, the clinical response can also be maintained (Figs 6.14, 6.17) (Shoulson et al., 1975; Hardie et al., 1984; Mouradian et al., 1990). Providing a continuous supply of dopamine or dopamine agonist to the striatum, such as by intravenous (Nutt, 1987) or

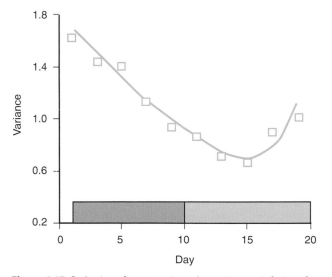

Figure 6.17 Reduction of motor variance by continuous infusion of levodopa. *From Mouradian MM, Heuser IJE, Baronti F, Chase TN. Modification of central dopaminergic mechanisms by continuous levodopa therapy for advanced Parkinson's disease. Ann Neurol 1990;27:18–23.*

intestinal (Sage et al., 1989a, 1989b; Bredberg et al., 1993; Kurth et al., 1993b; Nyholm et al., 2005) infusion of levodopa, or by subcutaneous infusion of dopamine agonist (Obeso et al., 1989b) can overcome this type of fluctuation. Thus, continuous benefit in the unstable patient (advanced PD) depends on a steady supply of levodopa in the plasma reaching the brain in a constant influx. This type of necessary bioavailability of plasma levodopa is not a factor with patients who have a smooth response to levodopa because such individuals have the same type of plasma half-life of levodopa as do those with fluctuations (Fabbrini et al., 1987).

Plasma concentrations of large neutral amino acids (LNAA), which compete with levodopa for transport into the brain, contribute to motor fluctuations, even when levodopa is being steadily infused (Nutt et al., 1997). These LNAAs play an even bigger role when the daily dosage of levodopa is higher. On the other hand, severity of PD did not predict fluctuations during the infusions. In addition to this obvious peripheral pharmacokinetic mechanism, because fluctuations are more prominent in patients who have taken larger daily doses of levodopa, pharmacodynamic factors are also implicated.

Some other factor(s) must be playing a role. It seems that central (such as small dopamine storage capacity and dopamine receptor alterations), as well as peripheral, pharmacokinetic, and pharmacodynamic mechanisms are involved in the pathophysiology of these problems (Mouradian et al., 1988, 1989; Obeso et al., 1989a).

Small dopamine-storage capacity

After 16 hours of infusion of levodopa intravenously in patients, and then suddenly discontinuing the infusion, patients with "on–off" and wearing-off, respectively, show the fastest return of parkinsonian symptoms, compared to those with a stable response to levodopa or those who have never been treated with levodopa (Fig. 6.16 lower) (Fabbrini et al., 1987). The patients with dyskinesias have a faster decay of their dyskinesias than of their anti-PD benefit, suggesting different receptors for the two functions are involved (Fig. 6.18) (Mouradian et al., 1989). The loss of the anti-PD

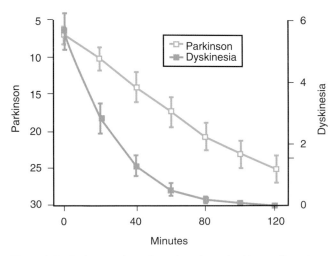

Figure 6.18 Dyskinesias decay faster than the antiparkinson effect when levodopa is withdrawn. *From Mouradian MM, Heuser IJE, Baronti F, et al. Pathogenesis of dyskinesias in Parkinson's disease. Ann Neurol 1989;25:523–526.*

effect as the plasma levodopa concentration falls in the above studies strongly indicates either a small buffering capacity for levodopa storage or a short-duration receptor response in patients with fluctuations.

The synaptic concentration of dopamine as a function of the timing of levodopa dosing was studied indirectly by evaluating D2 receptor ligand PET scans in patients who eventually developed wearing-off and those who remained stable, as non-fluctuators (de la Fuente-Fernandez et al., 2001). The former group showed higher synaptic dopamine 1 hour after a dose, but lower concentrations 3 hours later than the latter group. This result suggests increased dopamine turnover, i.e., decreased storage of dopamine.

Supporting the concept of a small buffering capacity are studies performed in rats with different degrees of 6-hydroxydopamine lesions of the nigrostriatal pathway (Papa et al., 1994). The rats are then treated with twice daily injections of levodopa. Rats with over 95% loss of dopaminergic neurons evidenced a progressive shortening in the duration of levodopa's motor effects (equivalent to wearing-off) as well as a failure of nearly 8% of levodopa injections to elicit any response (equivalent to dose failures) after the first week of treatment. In contrast, response changes resembling those associated with wearing-off fluctuations in parkinsonian patients did not occur in the less severely lesioned rats. These results suggest that the extent of a dopamine neuron loss must exceed a relatively high threshold before intermittent levodopa treatment produces changes favoring the appearance of motor fluctuations.

If the wearing-off phenomenon is due, at least in part, to loss of storage sites of dopamine in the striatum, severity of parkinsonism, regardless of duration of parkinsonism, should be associated with the wearing-off effect. This would explain why fluctuations occurred early in the course of treatment in patients with MPTP-induced parkinsonism (Ballard et al., 1985); these patients had a severe destruction of dopaminergic nigrostriatal pathway. In contrast, those with PD develop the wearing-off problem as a function of duration of treatment (McDowell and Sweet, 1976), which could also be a reflection of duration of illness.

Levodopa may contribute to the development of fluctuations

Dopamine storage capacity alone does not explain why younger patients are more prone to develop fluctuations than older patients (Pederzoli et al., 1983). Nor would it explain why using low doses of levodopa instead of high doses would delay the development of this problem (Poewe et al., 1986; Lesser et al., 1979). Furthermore, treatment with direct-acting agonists does not eliminate the problem, although it does ameliorate it somewhat by making the depths of the "off" state less severe. These three observations would imply that levodopa itself or the peaks and valleys of supplying the brain with levodopa may also be responsible for contributing to this problem. Some investigators have found that the major risk factors for fluctuations appear to be duration (Horstink et al., 1990b; Roos et al., 1990) and dosage (Poewe et al., 1986; Fabbrini et al., 1988) of levodopa therapy.

The CALM-PD clinical trial, comparing levodopa and pramipexole, clearly showed that levodopa was statistically more likely than the dopamine agonist to induce fluctuations (and dyskinesias), after both 2 years (Parkinson Study

Group, 2000) and 4 years of observation (Holloway and Parkinson Study Group, 2004). Whether the effect is inherent to levodopa, the potency of levodopa compared to the agonist, or the short duration of levodopa's half-life is uncertain. A further analysis of the CALM-PD data revealed that motor complications that occur within the first 4 years of treatment of PD do not have a significant negative effect on quality of life (Marras et al., 2004).

Pharmacokinetic mechanisms. Murata and Kanazawa (1993) repeatedly administered levodopa to intact rats and found that this treatment induced (1) acceleration of dopa absorption at the gut and the blood–brain barrier, (2) reduction of dopamine retention in the striatum, and (3) loss of "supersensitive response" of dopamine receptors. These authors concluded that long-term levodopa treatment is the cause of the wearing-off effect. Murata and colleagues (1996) subsequently studied plasma pharmacokinetics in 55 parkinsonian patients. They showed that long-term levodopa therapy markedly increased the peak levodopa concentration (C_{max}) and the area under the time-concentration curve (AUC); whereas it decreased time to the peak concentration (T_{max}) and the elimination half-life ($T_{1/2}$). These results suggest that long-term levodopa therapy accelerates the absorption of levodopa. These changes were seen in patients who were stable as well as in those with the wearing-off effect, although the fluctuators had a higher C_{max} and AUC and a shorter T_{max} and $T_{1/2}$ than the non-fluctuators. In an FDOPA PET study, Torstenson and colleagues (1997) showed that levodopa infusion during the scanning decreased FDOPA influx in mild PD, but upregulated the influx in patients with advanced PD. These findings could help explain the less graded clinical response to levodopa in advanced PD.

Pharmacodynamic mechanisms. Direct alterations of dopamine receptors and storage sites by levodopa, dopamine, or their metabolites is another possibility. D2 receptors were studied by raclopride PET scanning in patients early in the course of treatment with levodopa and then 3–5 years later, when motor fluctuations had appeared (Antonini et al., 1997). Raclopride binding was elevated (supersensitive receptors) after 3–4 months of levodopa therapy and returned to normal (downregulated) after 3–5 years of treatment.

One indication that dopamine receptors play a role in the loss of the anti-PD benefit as the plasma concentration of levodopa falls is the dichotomy of the decay of dyskinesia and the return of the parkinsonism (Fig. 6.18) (Mouradian et al., 1989). The dyskinesia decays faster than the loss of the anti-PD benefit. Dyskinesia half-time (time required to reduce severity score by 50%) was 25.3 minutes; the anti-PD half-time (time required to increase PD severity scores to 50% of their maximum) was 50.4 minutes. The shape of the two curves differs: the decay of dyskinesia is quadratic, the return of PD severity is linear. This suggests that dyskinesia effect and anti-PD effect represent different dopamine receptors (e.g., D1 and D2 receptors, respectively).

Chase and his colleagues (1993, 1998) suggest that intermittent (compared to continuous) administration of levodopa contributes to this problem. Chase proposes that there is an alteration of the striatal dopaminoceptive medium spiny neurons, with a potentiation of glutamate receptors (of the N-methyl-D-aspartate (NMDA) subtype) on these

GABAergic striatal efferents, and that these cells are producing the motor complications. In 6-hydroxydopamine-lesioned rats, an animal model of PD, Chase found increased phosphorylation of striatal NMDA receptor subunits on serine and tyrosine residues. Along with this concept is the finding from his laboratory that an NMDA antagonist can reverse the shortened levodopa response time in these rats (Blanchet et al., 1997). Furthermore, the intrastriatal administration of selective inhibitors of certain serine and tyrosine kinases alleviates the motor complications (Chase et al., 2000). He believes the same mechanism is responsible for both motor fluctuations and dyskinesias.

Although Chase incriminates intermittent administration of levodopa as the primary cause of motor complications, another potential mechanism is that dopamine can lead to the formation of free radicals by auto-oxidation or by enzymatic oxidation, and these oxyradicals could be the culprits attacking dopamine receptors (Fahn and Cohen, 1992; Fahn, 1996).

Once established, motor complications are seemingly irreversible. Substituting dopamine agonists for levodopa therapy diminishes the severity of the complications but does not eliminate them. Dopamine receptors may have irreversible changes, much like the irreversible alteration that is seen with tardive syndromes after exposure to dopamine receptor blocking agents (see Chapter 19). The healing process takes a long time without exposure to the offending agent before the process disappears, which often never happens.

Altered dopamine receptors

The dose–response curve to a bolus of levodopa injected intravenously was studied in patients with "on–off" and wearing-off, as well as those with a stable response to levodopa and those who had never been treated with levodopa (Fig. 6.19) (Mouradian et al., 1988). The antiparkinsonian response showed a linear dose–response curve in the latter

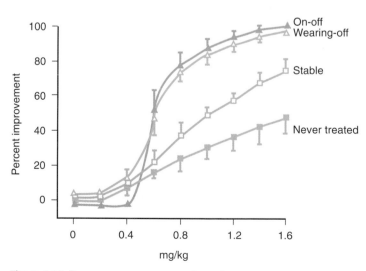

Figure 6.19 Dose–response curves vary depending on presence or absence of motor fluctuations. Fluctuators have more sensitive DA receptors. *From Mouradian MM, Juncos JL, Fabbrini G, et al. Motor fluctuations in Parkinson's disease: Central pathophysiological mechansims, Part II. Ann Neurol 1988;24:372–378.*

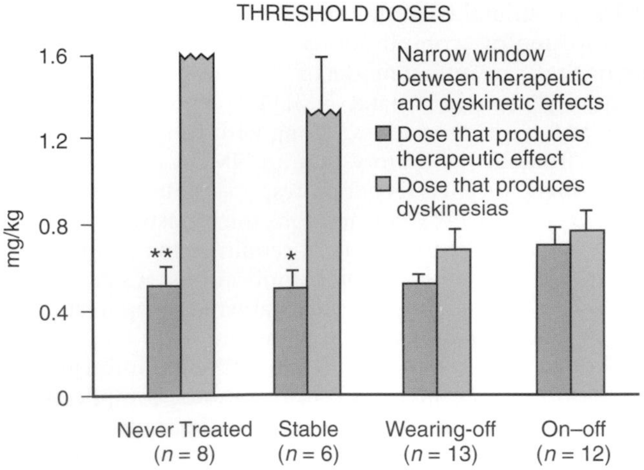

Figure 6.20 Narrow window between antiparkinson and dyskinetic effects in fluctuators compared to non-fluctuators. *$P < 0.006$, **$P < 0.0001$ for difference from dyskinesia threshold. *From Mouradian MM, Juncos JL, Fabbrini G, et al. Motor fluctuations in Parkinson's disease: Central pathophysiological mechansims, Part II. Ann Neurol 1988;24:372–378.*

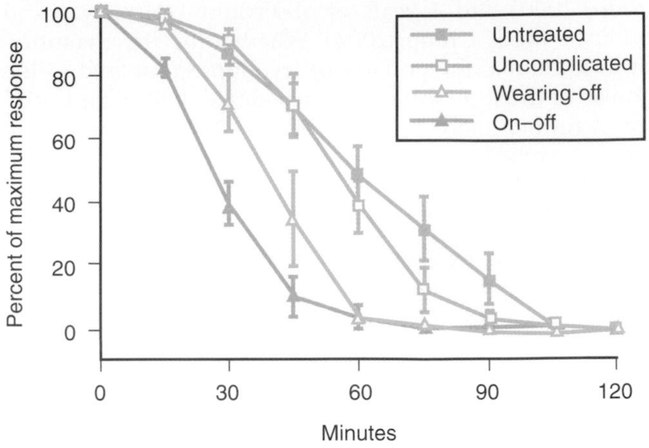

Figure 6.21 Differential decay rates of the antiparkinsonian effect among fluctuators and non-fluctuators after withdrawal of apomorphine. *From Bravi D, Mouradian MM, Roberts JW, Davis TL, Sohn YH, Chase TN. Wearing-off fluctuations in Parkinson's disease: Contribution of postsynaptic mechanisms. Ann Neurol 1994;36:27–31.*

two groups, but an S-shape curve for the first two groups. Thus, patients with fluctuations have a brittle response to levodopa. Because the peripheral pharmacokinetics are the same in all groups, this increased sensitivity to levodopa, despite identical antiparkinsonian threshold, strongly implies an alteration of the dopamine receptor, probably the D2 receptor, in patients with fluctuations. There is also a narrow window between antiparkinson and dyskinetic effects in patients who have fluctuations and dyskinesias (Fig. 6.20) (Mouradian et al. 1988).

Already mentioned was that the dichotomy of the decay rates for dyskinesia and anti-PD benefit when levodopa was withdrawn after a steady intravenous infusion suggested different dopamine receptors may be responsible for dyskinesias and for the anti-PD effect of levodopa (Fig. 6.18) (Mouradian et al., 1989). A more direct evaluation of dopamine receptors is by using a dopaminergic agent that acts only at the postsynaptic dopamine receptors for its effect. After a steady-state optimal-dose infusion of apomorphine, a direct-acting dopamine agonist that is not dependent on storage of dopamine, the apomorphine was withdrawn, and the loss of the anti-PD effect was faster in patients who had fluctuations than in stable patients with a stable response (Fig. 6.21) (Bravi et al., 1994). Because apomorphine's effect is not dependent on presynaptic terminals, postsynaptic mechanisms must play a role in the loss of the long-duration response and hence the wearing-off effect.

Other studies supporting the notion that postsynaptic dopamine receptors play a role in wearing-off are those by Colosimo and colleagues (1996) and Metman and colleagues (1997a). These showed that duration of response to apomorphine is shorter in advanced, complicated parkinsonian patients compared to early, levodopa-naive patients or stable patients. Also, the dose–response slope steepened, and the therapeutic window narrowed. The plasma levels of apomorphine were identical in the stable and fluctuating patients.

This conclusion was supported by another study comparing duration of response between the more and less affected sides in patients with PD to an infusion of levodopa and to subcutaneous apomorphine. Rodriguez and colleagues (1994) showed that the more affected side had a shorter response duration, increased latency, and greater response magnitude than the less affected side. These differences were more pronounced in patients receiving chronic levodopa treatment than in untreated patients. As apomorphine is not dependent on dopamine storage capacity, these findings suggest that postsynaptic mechanisms play an important part in the origin of motor fluctuations in PD. Could these postsynaptic mechanisms develop because of inconstant and pulsating activation of receptors by dopamine related to levodopa therapy or possibly from dopamine-mediated oxyradicals or other toxins related to levodopa therapy?

Implicating the intermittent administration of chronic levodopa therapy

Ten days of continuous, round-the-clock administration of levodopa intravenously producing a stable plasma concentration of levodopa gradually reduced fluctuations of response to levodopa in patients with the "on–off" or wearing-off effects (Fig. 6.17) (Mouradian et al., 1990). Because smoothing out the plasma (and brain) concentrations provided this benefit, the authors suggested that the chronic, routine method of intermittent oral treatment with levodopa may be underlying the development of motor fluctuations. Continuous intravenous treatment increased the threshold to levodopa for both the anti-PD and dyskinesia response (Table 6.15), with an increase in the therapeutic window by about 50% (computed as the difference between the dyskinesia threshold dose and the anti-PD threshold dose).

The S-shape of the dose–response curve for the fluctuators remained, but with a shift of the curve to the right indicating the decreased sensitivity to levodopa. At the increased threshold dosage for dyskinesia, the anti-PD response increased 76% (despite the shift of the curve to the right) with no

Table 6.15 Effect of continuous therapy with levodopa on its dose–response measures

Measure	Pretreatment (mg/kg)	Posttreatment (mg/kg)	*P* value
Antiparkinsonian threshold dose	0.59 ± 0.07	0.9 ± 10.07	<0.0001
Dyskinesia threshold dose	0.66 ± 0.08	1.0 ± 0.09	<0.0001
Therapeutic window	0.061 ± 0.04	0.092 ± 0.04	

The threshold for both the antiparkinsonian and dyskinesia response increased.
Data from Mouradian MM, Heuser IJE, Baronti F, Chase TN. Modification of central dopaminergic mechanisms by continuous levodopa therapy for advanced Parkinson's disease. Ann Neurol 1990;27:18–23.

change in the severity of the dyskinesias. Once the continuous infusions were discontinued, the fluctuations returned. Nutt and colleagues (1993) believe that tolerance actually develops after continuous infusions; when the infusion is stopped, the duration of response is shorter after a long infusion than after a shorter one. It is well recognized that once developed, "on–off" problems are difficult to eliminate.

A 5-year study of 618 dopa-naive patients compared Sinemet CR and standard Sinemet therapy. There was no difference between the two groups in the development of either fluctuations or dyskinesias (Block et al., 1997; Koller et al., 1999). Whether this study adequately tested the intermittent versus continuous levodopa hypothesis for the cause of fluctuations is unlikely. But in terms of therapeutics, it showed no advantage for beginning with either preparation over the other.

Summary of pathogenesis of fluctuations

Chase (1998) and Metman and colleagues (2000) summarized their views on the mechanisms leading to the development of fluctuations from levodopa therapy. They believe that the fluctuations are related to altered dopaminergic mechanisms at both the presynaptic and postsynaptic levels. Wearing-off phenomena initially reflect the loss of dopamine storage capacity of the degenerating nigrostriatal system. Then, with increasing degeneration of the nigrostriatal system, swings in plasma levodopa concentrations associated with standard dosage regimens produce nonphysiologic fluctuations in intrasynaptic dopamine. As a result of long-term discontinuous stimulation, secondary changes occur at sites downstream from the dopamine system and now appear to underlie the progressive worsening of wearing-off phenomena as well as the eventual appearance of other response complications. Chronic intermittent stimulation of normally tonically active dopaminergic receptors activates specific signaling cascades in striatal dopaminoceptive medium spiny neurons, and this evidently results in long-term potentiation of the synaptic efficacy of glutamate receptors of the NMDA subtype on these GABAergic efferents due to increased phosphorylation of the serine and tyrosine moieties in these receptors. As a consequence of their increasing sensitivity to excitation by cortical glutamatergic projections, it would, however, appear that medium spiny neuron function changes to favor the appearance of response fluctuations of the "on–off" type and peak-dose dyskinesias. The inability of standard levodopa treatment to restore striatal dopaminergic function in a more physiologic manner clearly contributes to the appearance of motor complications.

Continuous dopaminergic replacement not only reverses these complications in parkinsonian patients but also prevents their development in animal models of PD. Nutt (2007) presented a scholarly critique of the continuous dopaminergic stimulation hypothesis and argued that an adequate clinical trial needs to rigorously test it.

Another explanation from both primate studies and postmortem human studies is that long-term levodopa therapy leads to glutamate receptor supersensitivity in the putamen, and this plays a role in the development of motor complications (both wearing-off and dyskinesias) following long-term levodopa therapy in PD (Calon et al., 2003).

Dyskinesias

When dyskinesias first appear, their onset coincides with the onset of the antiparkinsonian effect from levodopa (Nutt et al., 2010). The offset of the so-called "peak-dose" dyskinesias also coincides with the offset of the antiparkinsonian response. The latency to the onsets of dyskinesia and the antiparkinsonian response tended to shorten during long-term levodopa therapy, suggesting that both responses were sensitized by long-term levodopa.

A PET study suggests that dopamine reuptake after its release is reduced in patients who have dopa-induced dyskinesias (Troiano et al., 2009). The study utilized two ligands: [^{11}C]-d-threo-methylphenidate (MP) and [^{11}C]-(+/−) dihydrotetrabenazine (DTBZ). The former measures the function of the dopamine transporter, the latter dopamine nerve terminal density. The putaminal MP/DTBZ ratio was significantly reduced in patients with dyskinesias compared to those without.

Another suggestion for a mechanism for the production of dopa-induced dyskinesias is based on postmortem chemical studies performed on primates, ranging from normal, parkinsonian, nondyskinetic dopa-treated and dyskinetic dopa-treated (Aubert et al., 2005). These investigators found that the sensitivity of the D1 receptor is linearly related to dyskinesias. This implies that dopa-induced dyskinesia results from increased dopamine D1 receptor-mediated transmission at the level of the direct pathway.

Risk factors for peak-dose dyskinesias were retrospectively analyzed by using the Kaplan–Meier survival method in 100 consecutive patients treated with levodopa for 1–18 years. Blanchet and colleagues (1996) found that 56% of patients developed dyskinesia after a mean of 2.9 years. Dyskinetic patients were significantly younger at disease onset, but their mean latency to dyskinesia induction after levodopa initiation was not different from that of older dyskinetic individuals. In the study by Kumar and colleagues (2005), the 5-year risk of dyskinesias is 50% for PD onset 40–59 years, and 26% with onset ages 60–69 and 16% age 70 or over. Dosage of levodopa is another factor in causing dyskinesias (Parkinson Study Group, 2004b).

The levodopa dosage threshold for dyskinesia is much lower for patients with fluctuations than for patients with a stable response or for those who have never been treated before. This was determined by bolus injections of levodopa intravenously (Fig. 6.20) (Mouradian et al., 1988). Those who had never been treated and those with a stable response to levodopa had such a high threshold for dyskinesias that dyskinesias never appeared in some of these patients at the highest doses tested. After 16 hours of steady intravenous infusion of levodopa, followed by sudden discontinuation, the loss of dyskinesias is faster than the return of parkinsonism (Mouradian et al., 1989). These studies indicate that dyskinetic effects and antiparkinsonian effects may represent responses to different dopamine receptors. The investigators proposed that these are very likely the D1 and D2 receptors, respectively.

In a study looking at severity of PD after overnight drug withdrawal, Schuh and Bennett (1993) found that continuous intravenous levodopa shifted the dyskinesia dose–response curve to the right and reduced maximum dyskinesia activity, but did not significantly alter dose response for relief of parkinsonism. These results support the hypothesis that relief of parkinsonism and production of dyskinesia by levodopa occur by separate mechanisms.

Possession of a single common allele of the brain-derived neurotrophic factor (BDNF) gene doubles the risk for developing levodopa-induced dyskinesia, and possessing two alleles quadruples the risk (Foltynie et al., 2009). Two alleles of the BDNF gene differ at position 66, encoding either a valine or methionine amino acid. In the general white population the genotype frequencies are 60% val/val, 36% val/met, and 4% met/met. Patients with PD have increased risk for developing levodopa-induced dyskinesia for each additional met allele in their BDNF gene.

Treatment of motor fluctuations associated with levodopa therapy

When levodopa or other antiparkinson medication no longer provides a smooth, adequate, long-duration response, treatment requires skill; it becomes an art form utilizing approaches to control the various complications that have developed in a given patient. At this stage of treatment, the clinician is usually placed in a position analogous to that of a firefighter, being called on to "put out fires." Every time a new problem arises in a response-complicated patient, the clinician uses his or her skill to control the new developments arising from levodopa therapy. The following subsections describe various complications and the approaches that can be taken to control them.

Wearing-off phenomenon in the absence of dyskinesias

There are many choices available to control wearing-off. When mild, it may be ameliorated with the addition of selegiline (Golbe et al., 1988) (introduced as 5 mg daily, and increasing to 5 mg twice daily, as necessary). Selegiline potentiates the action of levodopa, and its introduction can induce confusion and psychosis, particularly in the elderly, and dyskinesias. A lower dose of levodopa might be necessary. Rasagiline, another type B MAO inhibitor, also decreases the amount of daily "off" time – by about 1 hour per day (Parkinson Study Group, 2005) and in a comparative study with entacapone, had the same degree of benefit (Rascol et al., 2005). Sinemet CR can also be effective in patients with mild wearing-off (Bush et al., 1989; Hutton and Morris, 1992; Pahwa et al., 1993), and one can gradually switch from standard carbidopa/levodopa to Sinemet CR, beginning with the last dose of the day and working forward each day. Because it takes over an hour for slow-release medication to become effective, most patients will also require supplemental standard carbidopa/levodopa to obtain an adequate response. Because not all of Sinemet CR is absorbed before the tablet passes through the small intestine (absorption of carbidopa/levodopa is achieved only via the small intestine), the same dosages of Sinemet CR and standard Sinemet are not identical. Only about two-thirds to three-quarters of Sinemet CR is absorbed. Therefore to achieve the equivalent of 100 mg of levodopa in standard Sinemet, a patient would require between 130 and 150 mg of levodopa in Sinemet CR.

COMT inhibitors have an advantage because if effective, they are effective immediately. They increase the amount of "on" time by about an hour per day (Kieburtz et al., 1997a; Adler et al., 1998; Rinne et al., 1998b). Entacapone has a shorter duration of action than tolcapone does and its 200 mg tablet needs to be given simultaneously with carbidopa/levodopa, working with that dose only. Thus, if only one or two doses of levodopa result in wearing-off, then entacapone can be given just with those doses. Entacapone does not require any precautions for assessing liver function, whereas tolcapone does. Tolcapone can produce fulminant hepatitis; this is rare, but has caused death (Assal et al., 1998; Watkins, 2000). Therefore, patients should not be given tolcapone unless the clinical fluctuations are a great problem and other medications have failed to relieve the clinical fluctuations. Patients need a baseline liver transaminase profile which should be followed biweekly. Discontinuing tolcapone if a rise in transaminase activity is seen should be sufficient to reverse the hepatic change. Patients should also be warned that diarrhea, including explosive diarrhea, could develop in 6–8 weeks on tolcapone. Entacapone causes less of a problem with diarrhea, but it turns the urine a yellow-orange. Tolcapone comes in 100 and 200 mg tablets. Start with 100 mg once daily and increase fairly rapidly to three times daily dosing. If not effective, switch to the 200 mg tablets. Although entacapone can reduce the amount of "off" time, it does not appear to improve quality of life (Reichmann et al., 2005).

With any of these additions to the treatment regimen, if dyskinesias develop, the dosage of carbidopa/levodopa needs to be reduced.

Another approach is to utilize standard carbidopa/levodopa alone, giving the doses closer together. But ultimately most patients will develop progressively shorter durations of effectiveness from these doses, so patients would require as many as six or more doses per day. Then, eventually, dose failures often develop. Investigation of this problem of shorter response time with smaller, more frequent doses of levodopa has shown that response time continues to increase when suprathreshold doses of levodopa are given, although increased dyskinesias also are seen (Metman et al., 1997b).

Direct-acting dopamine agonists, which have a longer biological half-life than levodopa, can also be used in combination with standard Sinemet or Sinemet CR (Parkinson Study Group, 1997). As a general rule, dopamine agonists are useful to improve the severity of the "off" state, but can also reduce the amount of "off" time per day. Pergolide, pramipexole, and ropinirole are more effective than bromocriptine and are preferred. These drugs in combination with levodopa can increase dyskinesias while reducing the depths of the "offs." In this situation the levodopa dosage would need to be reduced. Because of its long half-life, cabergoline can be effective even with once-a-day dosage (Geminiani et al., 1996; Inzelberg et al., 1996). Utilizing dopamine agonists and delaying the introduction of levodopa can delay the start of the wearing-off effect and reduce the risk of developing it (Montastruc et al., 1994; Przuntek et al., 1996; Rinne et al., 1998a; Parkinson Study Group, 2000; Rascol et al., 2000; Oertel et al., 2006).

The anti-epileptic drug zonisamide has been shown to be effective to reduce "off" time without worsening dyskinesias (Murata et al., 2007). Adenosine A2A antagonists, still in clinical trials, have been purported to reduce "off" time also. A critical factor in reducing "off" time is not to simultaneously increase dyskinesias. If a drug can accomplish this, it would be a major advance in therapeutics. So far, no drug has accomplished this with corroborative evidence.

Patients with a deep "off" would benefit from a rescue dose of anti-PD medication. Dissolving levodopa in carbonated water and drinking it usually provides a response in about 10–15 minutes. Subcutaneous injections or intranasal sprays of apomorphine provides a similar response (Dewey et al., 1998). Etilevodopa, a dispersible form of levodopa ethylester, was expected to improve these types of delayed "off" responses (Djaldetti and Melamed, 1996), but a study by the Parkinson Study Group (Blindauer et al., 2006) of 327 patients with PD who were taking levodopa and had a latency of ≥90 minutes each day before the onset of drug benefit (measured as time to "on") showed that the mean improvements were similar in the etilevodopa-carbidopa and levodopa-carbidopa groups (reductions of 0.58 and 0.79 hours, respectively).

Sudden "offs"

The "sudden off" phenomenon is a more difficult problem to overcome. It is now clear that direct-acting dopamine agonists, slow-release levodopa, amantadine, and selegiline are ineffective. Subcutaneous injections of the dopamine agonist apomorphine are effective in turning the patient back "on" quickly (Hughes et al., 1993), as is an oral administration of dissolved Sinemet. To block nausea and vomiting by apomorphine, the peripheral dopamine receptor antagonist domperidone or trimethobenzamide needs to be taken in addition. Increasingly severe on-phase dyskinesias and postural instability mar the long-term therapeutic response of apomorphine in many patients.

Our approach is to attempt to utilize dopamine agonists as the major therapeutic agents and reduce the amount of levodopa as much as possible. If even a small amount of Sinemet added to the dopamine agonist causes too much dyskinesia, one should try to substitute plain levodopa without any carbidopa in place of Sinemet. We have not been able to eliminate sudden "offs" if levodopa is the major therapeutic agent.

Random "offs"

Often a sudden "off" appears unrelated to the timing of the last dose of levodopa, leading to the name "random off." With careful plotting of these off periods, a pattern can often be seen, so these "random offs" might not be so random. These "random offs" are usually sudden in onset. The treatment strategy is the same as for "sudden offs."

Dose failures (episodic failure to respond to each dose, no "on")

Failure of the patient to respond to each dose of levodopa is related to poor gastric emptying (Rivera-Calimlin et al., 1970; Fahn, 1977). A radionuclide gastric emptying study showed that PD patients had prolonged gastric emptying compared with the normal control subjects and that this was increased in fluctuating patients with dose failures compared to non-fluctuators (Djaldetti et al., 1996). The problem of dose failures can be overcome by dissolving levodopa in liquid before ingesting it. For this situation, individual doses of Sinemet can be liquefied at the time it is needed. It dissolves readily in carbonated water because of the acidity of the water, and the formation of bubbles that toss the Sinemet tablet around, quickly dissolving it. When a dose failure occurs, the patient can take dissolved Sinemet and will usually respond in 10–15 minutes. Another approach is to use apomorphine injections (Ostergaard et al., 1995).

Response failures are probably more common than is usually recognized. In a survey of their patients Melamed and colleagues (1986) found a number of patients with this difficulty. It is not clear whether the delayed gastric emptying is due to levodopa therapy itself or whether the disorder develops because frequent dosing will statistically result in some tablets not passing through the stomach quickly enough to reach the proximal small intestine where absorption takes place.

Delayed "on"

Melamed and colleagues (1986) reported that patients with fluctuations often also have a problem in getting an "on" with the first dose in the morning. These patients tend to have a longer delay with this dose that the non-fluctuator. The mechanism is not clear, but it might have to do with obtaining adequate plasma levels. We have noticed that many patients need a larger dosage of levodopa as their first dose of the day to "kick-in" a response to the medication. Since the first dose is often accompanied by a higher plasma level of levodopa than later doses (Shoulson et al., 1975; Fahn, 1982), the problem might not be entirely pharmacokinetic. Rather, it is possible that the dopamine receptors are in a low-affinity state and require more dopamine agonism to activate them. To treat the delayed "on" by obtaining a higher plasma level of levodopa sooner, the patient should dissolve Sinemet before swallowing.

"Super offs"

"Super offs" are a more severe "off" state than the standard "wearing-off" or the "practically defined off," which occurs at the beginning of the day before the first dose and about 12 hours after the patient's last dose at bedtime the night before. Patients with pronounced tremor, for example, could have an even more severe tremor during a "super off." The severity of the "super off" is greater than if the patient were withdrawn from her/his levodopa and let the natural parkinsonian state reappear. The "super off" state might represent a desensitized state of the dopamine receptor during that "super off" period.

Weak response at end of day

Most patients eventually show some diurnal variation in their responsiveness to levodopa. Often, the patient reports that she or he does best after the first morning dose, and the response is less as the day wears on. An occasional patient will report the opposite – doing better at the end of the day. The mechanism for the poorer response at the end of the day might relate to decreased plasma levels of levodopa with each subsequent dose (Fig. 6.14A). But increasing the dose in the afternoons usually does not help. The patient might not get any improved response, and could develop drowsiness or adverse mental effects instead. Nevertheless, one should try increasing the dosage of afternoon and evening levodopa. If this fails, it is worth adding slow-release levodopa, supplemental dopamine agonist, anticholinergics, or amantadine.

Response varies in relation to meals

Levodopa is absorbed only from the proximal small intestine; absorption is thus dependent on passage of levodopa through the stomach to enter the small intestine. There are at least three variations of levodopa responsiveness in regard to meals. First, a full meal with delayed gastric emptying will result in a delayed and weaker response to levodopa that is ingested after or during the meal compared to taking levodopa about 20 minutes before the meal. Pharmacokinetic studies confirm that levodopa concentrations in plasma are delayed when the medication is taken in the fed state (Contin et al., 1998b). Second, patients who had normally taken levodopa with or after a meal will find that if they now take it before a meal, the response is much greater and they might develop peak-dose dyskinesia. If either of these two variations is present, it can be corrected by accommodating the timing of dosages of levodopa according to the pathophysiology of the particular problem.

A third variation relates to high-protein meals. Competition with other amino acids in the diet can interfere with transport of levodopa across the intestinal mucosa and across the blood–brain barrier (Muenter et al., 1972; Nutt et al., 1984). Only rarely does this competition with other amino acids pose a serious problem for patients. Most accommodate to protein in their diet. In those rare individuals in whom any protein in any meal interferes with their

response to levodopa, it is necessary to plan a meal strategy. Having non-protein meals at breakfast and lunch, and making up for this lack by having higher protein meals at dinner, will usually be effective. If the patient goes "off" at night when he or she can best afford to be "off," the patient can adjust to this situation.

Freezing

The freezing phenomenon (Fahn, 1995) is often listed as a type of fluctuation because the patient transiently has difficulty initiating movement. But this phenomenon probably should be considered distinct from the other types of fluctuations. Freezing takes many forms, and these have different names, such as start hesitation, target hesitation, turning hesitation, startle (fearfulness) hesitation, and sudden transient freezing. However, it is not clear whether any of these types has a different pathophysiologic mechanism. Of major importance is the need to distinguish between "off freezing" and "on freezing." "Off freezing" is best explained as a feature of PD, and its treatment is to keep the patient from going "off." "On freezing" remains an enigma, and this problem tends to be aggravated by increasing the dosage of levodopa. It is not benefited by adding direct-acting dopamine agonists. Rather, it is lessened by reducing the dosage of levodopa. Both the "on" and "off" types of freezing appear to correlate with duration of illness and duration of levodopa therapy (Giladi et al., 1992). Although Narabayashi and colleagues (1986) reported benefit with L-threo-DOPS, supposedly a precursor of brain norepinephrine, Fahn (unpublished data) has not seen any benefit with this drug in the treatment of "on freezing." L-threo-DOPS did not increase norepinephrine in rat brain (Reches et al., 1985) or in human cerebrospinal fluid (Suzuki et al., 1984). Giladi and colleagues (2001a) report some benefit with botulinum toxin injections into the legs of freezers, but we have not been impressed with the results based on personal observations.

Interestingly, in the intravenous infusions of levodopa performed by Shoulson and colleagues (1975), a sudden stimulus, such as tilting the patient upright on a tilt table, resulted in sudden transient worsening of parkinsonism. This can be interpreted to indicate the induction of sudden transient freezing. It might be a useful model for future studies.

Treatment of dyskinesias associated with levodopa therapy

Peak-dose dyskinesias

Choreic movements can occur early in the treatment with levodopa, but the incidence of these involuntary movements increases with continuing treatment (Duvoisin, 1974a). Chorea is more common than dystonia as the type of peak-dose dyskinesia, particularly in the early stages of levodopa therapy, but with continuing treatment individual patients can develop more dystonia and less chorea (Fahn, 2000). Many patients probably end up having a combination of chorea and dystonia. Dystonia is a more serious problem than chorea because dystonia is usually more disabling. In fact, mild chorea is not noticed as much by the patient as by the family.

Overall, except for young-onset Parkinson disease, dyskinesias are troublesome in only about 40% of patients, and only about 10% cannot be managed by medication adjustments (Van Gerpen et al., 2006). Peak-dose dyskinesia is due to too high a dose of levodopa and is representative of an overdosed state. The plasma levels of levodopa are high (Muenter et al., 1977) and there is presumably excess striatal dopamine. Reducing the individual dose can resolve this problem. The patient might need to take more frequent doses at this lower amount because reducing the amount of an individual dose also reduces the duration of benefit (Nutt et al., 1985). It was once believed that chorea appears only in the presence of supersensitive dopamine receptors, but if the dosage of levodopa were high enough, chorea could occur in normal individuals, as has been demonstrated in normal monkeys (Sassin et al., 1972).

Another method to reduce peak-dose dyskinesia is to substitute higher doses of a dopamine agonist while lowering the dose of Sinemet. Dopamine agonists are less likely to cause dyskinesias, and therefore can usually be used in this situation quite safely. If lowering the dose of Sinemet results in more severe "off" states, then the agonists become more important and need to be increased. Sinemet CR can help some patients by keeping the peak plasma levels of levodopa at a lower level. However, there is also the danger of increased dyskinesias at the end of the day as the blood levels become sustained from frequent dosing. Once dyskinesias appear with Sinemet CR, they last for a considerable time because of the slow decay in the plasma.

In some patients peak-dose chorea and dystonia occur at subtherapeutic doses of Sinemet, and lowering the dosage will render a patient even more parkinsonian. Use smaller and more frequent doses, coupled with dopamine agonists or other antiparkinsonian drugs, such as amantadine. Possibly through an antiglutamatergic action, amantadine can be a useful antidyskinetic agent (Rajput et al., 1997; Metman et al., 1998a, 1999; Snow et al., 2000, Luginger et al., 2000), aside from its dopaminergic effect. Its antidyskinetic effect is dose dependent and patients often require at least 400 mg/day. Start with 100 mg twice daily and increase stepwise to 200 mg twice daily as needed. Unfortunately, the antidyskinetic benefit from amantadine is only a few months (Thomas et al., 2004). Other antiglutamatergic agents reported to reduce levodopa-induced dyskinesias are dextromethorphan (Metman et al., 1998b), dextrorphan (Metman et al., 1998c), and riluzole (Merims et al., 1999).

A possible approach is to use clozapine, the atypical neuroleptic that does not aggravate parkinsonism. It is increasingly being utilized as an antipsychotic in patients with dopa-induced psychosis. Clozapine can suppress dopa-induced dyskinesias, while simultaneously increasing "on" time without dyskinesias (Bennett et al. 1993,1994; Durif et al., 1997; Pierelli et al., 1998; Durif et al., 2004). Adverse effects consist of sedation, sialorrhea, and orthostatic hypotension. Clozapine also can reduce dyskinesias from apomorphine (Durif et al., 1997). Olanzapine has greater dopamine D2 receptor antagonism and usually worsens parkinsonism.

Increasing serotonin activity in the substantia nigra could induce or worsen parkinsonism, as is sometimes seen with fluoxetine treatment. A trial of fluoxetine, a selective serotonin uptake inhibitor, was shown to reduce dyskinesias

induced by apomorphine treatment (Durif et al., 1995), suggesting that it be considered for levodopa-induced dyskinesias. The serotonin agonist sarizotan was developed for its possible use (Bara-Jimenez et al., 2005) as an antidyskinesia agent; but a phase III trial was unsuccessful (Goetz et al., 2007). Propranolol is another drug that has been reported to reduced dyskinesias (Carpentier et al., 1996). Buspirone appears to be somewhat effective in reducing the severity of dyskinesias (Bonifati et al., 1994), but because buspirone has resulted in aggravating tardive dyskinesia (LeWitt et al., 1993), it might have some dopamine receptor blocking activity. Mirtazapine is an antidepressant with a novel pharmacologic profile (alpha-2 antagonist, 5-HT$_{1A}$ agonist, and 5-HT$_2$, antagonist). It was tested in a small open-label trial and found to have a modest effect in reducing dopa-induced dyskinesias (Meco et al., 2003). Although opioid antagonists have been found to reduce dopa-induced dyskinesias in parkinsonian monkeys (Henry et al., 2001), high-dose naltrexone was not effective in humans (Manson et al., 2001). Other medications such as cannabis (Carroll et al., 2004), low-dose quetiapine (Katzenschlager et al., 2004), and gabapentin (Van Blercom et al., 2004) were not found to be effective.

Diphasic dyskinesias

Diphasic dyskinesias were first described by Muenter and his colleagues (1977), who labeled them the "D-I-D" phenomenon, for dystonia–improvement–dystonia. Although most of the affected individuals have dystonia as their pattern of dyskinesia, some have choreic movements, and others have a mixture of the two types. Diphasic dyskinesia is a situation in which the dyskinesia develops as the plasma levels of levodopa are rising or falling, but not during the peak plasma level (Muenter et al., 1977; Lhermitte et al., 1978; Agid et al., 1979). Clinically, the involuntary movements predominantly involve the legs (Marsden et al., 1982; Luquin et al., 1992).

This phenomenon is difficult to explain. It is possible that there is a differential sensitivity of at least two dopamine receptors. The more sensitive one would respond to lower levels of levodopa to induce the dyskinetic state. The other receptor would be activated at higher levels and inhibit the dyskinesia. Treatment of the problem is difficult. Although Lhermitte and colleagues (1978) proposed treating this condition with higher doses of levodopa, Fahn's experience (unpublished data) is that higher dosages merely induce peak-dose dyskinesia and possibly other forms of central adverse effects. On the other hand, lowering the dosage is equally unsatisfactory because increasing parkinsonism ensues. The most effective approach is to utilize a dopamine agonist, with its longer duration of action, as the major therapeutic agent, and levodopa as the supplementary drug. The end-of-dose dyskinesia, when it appears at the end of the day at a time when no further levodopa is to be taken, is particularly troublesome for the patients who have diphasic dyskinesias.

"Off" dystonia and "off" painful cramps

Dystonic spasms are not always a sign of levodopa overdosage. This is particularly true in many instances of painful sustained contractions. Painful dystonic cramps most often occur when the plasma level of levodopa is low, particularly in the early morning (Melamed, 1979). A survey of 383 patients with PD revealed that 16% had experienced early morning dystonia (Currie et al., 1998). But this type of dystonia can occur at any time the patient goes "off" (Ilson et al., 1984), and early morning dystonia is a form of "off" dystonia, albeit the most common form. In this sense, "off" dystonia is a pharmacokinetic problem, and it has been correlated with low plasma levels of levodopa after an intravenous infusion was discontinued (Bravi et al., 1993). But why painful dystonic spasms should occur in addition to or instead of classic parkinsonian signs during low plasma levels of levodopa is not clear. This phenomenon may relate to some peculiarity of the dopamine receptors as well as the low plasma levels of levodopa in these patients. de Yebenes et al. (1988) have proposed that dystonia may occur when the ratio of norepinephrine/dopamine is high. However, there are only speculations about the pathophysiology of dystonia in general, and it is difficult to be certain of the explanation of either peak-dose dystonia or of "off" dystonia such as early-morning dystonia. Preventing "offs" is the best way to control "off" dystonia. The use of pergolide is often effective when it is the major dopaminergic agent. Sinemet CR appears to be helpful for a number of patients with early-morning dystonia (Pahwa et al., 1993).

One should not forget that dystonia can also occur as a feature of PD. However, "off" dystonia does not appear to be merely a reflection of the dystonia of parkinsonism. If patients with "off" dystonia are given a drug holiday from levodopa, the painful dystonia will disappear after a few days, and the patient will be left with a baseline parkinsonian state and without painful dystonia (unpublished observations).

Combination of fluctuations and dyskinesias; yo-yo-ing

Many patients with advanced PD have both clinical fluctuations ("wearing-off" or "on–off") and dyskinesias (usually peak-dose and sometimes end-of-dose). Most patients are more troubled by the "off" states in which they are fully or partially immobile than they are by dyskinesias. In other words they prefer having the dyskinesias rather than being unable to move freely. As a result of their discomfort with the "off" states, patients tend to overdose themselves, resulting in the alternating "offs" and dyskinesias. An extreme form of this combination is "yo-yo-ing." The term comes from the repetitive ups and downs of a yo-yo and refers to a condition in which there is little time during the day of an optimally good "on" in which the patient has neither dyskinesia nor "offs." Moreover, in yo-yo-ing the patient usually responds to a dose of levodopa almost immediately with a peak-dose dyskinesia, followed by a predictable wearing-off, with little optimum time in between these two states (Fahn, 1982).

Sudden "offs" and dose failures can further complicate the clinical situation of patients with advanced PD who have combinations of "offs" and dyskinesias (whether with good periods in between or as a yo-yo). Overcoming these highly variable clinical periods is challenging. It is a matter of attempting to smoothly activate the striatal dopamine receptors throughout the entire day. The dopamine receptors are obviously intact, but they are supersensitive to allow the dyskinesias. Hence, there appears to be a pharmacodynamic factor to account for the dyskinesias. At the same time the short plasma half-life and the need for constant bioavailability of levodopa in the plasma accounts for the "off" states. Hence the "offs" are the result of a pharmacokinetic factor. Thus, this condition should be considered as a combined pharmacokinetic and pharmacodynamic problem. Treatment is virtually impossible with tablets of standard Sinemet and is even worse with Sinemet CR. The CR form has an unreliable pharmacokinetic profile. For patients who have both "offs" and dyskinesias, Sinemet CR tends to increase and prolong the dyskinesias; in some patients the dyskinesias may be so severe that the patients have to be put to sleep to "ride them out."

Using medications with a longer biological half-life than levodopa is a preferred method to smooth out the clinical fluctuating state. There has been partial success using direct-acting dopamine agonists as the sole or dominant form of pharmacotherapy, with carbidopa/levodopa used sparingly. In some patients, particularly those with yo-yo-ing, plain levodopa (without carbidopa) may be the preferred supplement instead of carbidopa/levodopa. The presence of carbidopa augments the potency of levodopa, so it is difficult to titrate patients for smaller-dose responses in the presence of carbidopa.

Another, though more cumbersome, approach to smoothly activate the dopamine receptors without severe extremes of peaks and valleys is to place the patient on sips of small doses of liquefied Sinemet throughout the day (Metman et al., 1994). Liquefied Sinemet is not stable at room temperature unless in an acidified solution. In the absence of ascorbic acid, the concentration of levodopa in water declines significantly by 48 hours (Pappert et al., 1996a). Ascorbate prolongs stability to 72 hours. Refrigeration and freezing prevents a significant decline in concentration for a full 7 days. In place of ascorbic acid, carbonated water can be used, which is easier for many patients.

To prepare liquefied Sinemet, a simple method is to dissolve 4 tablets of 25/250 mg strength tablets in a liter of acidified solution (dietetic soda, seltzer or other carbonated water, or ascorbic acid solution), providing a concentration of 1 mg levodopa per milliliter. Prepare it fresh daily and store the liquid in a dark environment to prevent oxidation of levodopa. It can be placed in the refrigerator. Then measure out the number of milliliters needed for a dose, which is equivalent to the milligrams of the dose. Liquefied Sinemet has been found to improve the amount of "on" time (Kurth et al., 1993a; Pappert et al., 1996b). In one double-blind trial comparing the liquid formulation versus standard tablets, no significant advantage of the liquid formulation over tablet therapy was found (Metman et al., 1994), but in another double-blind trial there was an advantage of the liquid preparation and without increasing dyskinesias (Pappert et al., 1996b). The liquid formulation can more quickly resolve "off" states and also facilitate small dose adjustments that are not possible with tablets. It seems particularly valuable for patients who have both fluctuations and dyskinesias.

A more heroic approach is to utilize the infusion of levodopa via an intraduodenal pump (Sage et al., 1989a, 1989b;

Bredberg et al., 1993; Kurth et al., 1993b; Nilsson et al., 1998). Such an approach, utilizing a levodopa gel and a battery-driven pump with insertion of the delivery tube percutaneously through the stomach and inserted in the jejunum, has been developed commercially (Nyholm et al., 2005). This "DuoDopa" treatment has been approved in some European countries, and the results have been positive in reducing fluctuations and in improving quality of live (Antonini et al., 2007, 2008). Subcutaneous infusions of apomorphine (Colzi et al., 1998) and other dopamine agonists, such as lisuride, are also being used in Europe.

The Europeans are reporting long-term experiences with DuoDopa infusion. In France, 102 patients treated with duodenal levodopa infusion since 2003 were analyzed (Devos and French DUODOPA Study Group, 2009). Patients were at advanced stage: mean age was 72.7 years, average disease duration of 17 years, 91% had gait disorders, 65% had visual hallucinations, and 50% had dementia. More than 90% reported an improvement in motor fluctuations, quality of life, and autonomy. There were few severe adverse events. Technical problems were commonplace. In Sweden, 65 cases were analyzed for safety (Nyholm et al., 2008). The mean daily dose of levodopa was reduced by 5%; technical problems with the tube were common. In Italy, six patients were analyzed (Raudino et al., 2009); fluctuations were improved, but two patients had more dyskinesias.

Myoclonus

The lightning-like jerks of myoclonus can occur in untreated PD, but these are rarely disabling and are hardly commented on by patients. Klawans and colleagues (1975) described myoclonus as occurring as a complication of long-term levodopa therapy. They reported the movements as occurring as single unilateral or bilateral jerks in the extremities, most frequently during sleep. They found the serotonin antagonist methysergide helpful in controlling these. Such nocturnal myoclonus is infrequently encountered in our experience, and is rarely disabling. Myoclonus occurs during the day as well. Its presence is usually ominous, indicating the presence of cognitive complications from levodopa, and often representing either toxicity to levodopa in PD or some other form of parkinsonism, such as diffuse Lewy body disease (Crystal et al., 1990).

Other motor complications

Simultaneous somatotopically-specific dyskinesias and parkinsonism

Many patients have different responses to levodopa therapy in different parts of the body. For example, head and neck regions might be more sensitive to levodopa than the legs. When the upper part of the body responds in this situation, the legs might remain parkinsonian and the patient may not be able to walk well. In this example, on higher dosages of levodopa, the legs improve, but the head and neck regions are dyskinetic. This problem might be due to different sensitivities of the striatal dopamine receptors on a somatotopic basis. That is, in the case described, the head and neck areas of the striatum would have more sensitive receptors than the leg area. This problem is difficult to treat, and one can only

titrate the dosage to the optimum response between the two extremes for each individual patient.

Loss of efficacy over time

A debated point in the treatment of parkinsonism is the cause of declining efficacy from continuing treatment with levodopa in many patients (Yahr, 1976). If the postsynaptic dopamine receptors in the striatum are not lost in this disease, why should a patient get less response from medication over time? Progression of the illness with further loss of dopamine storage sites in the presynaptic terminals is the most invoked explanation. However, loss of these structures does not automatically produce a loss of response to levodopa. For example, postencephalitic parkinsonism, with its much greater loss of dopamine in the striatum (Ehringer and Hornykiewicz, 1960; Bernheimer et al., 1973), has more, not less, sensitivity to levodopa (Calne et al., 1969; Duvoisin et al., 1972). This observation is sufficient to argue against the concept that reduction in storage sites for dopamine is responsible for the declining efficacy of levodopa. Perhaps increasing PD is associated with loss of striatal dopamine receptors as well as the presynaptic dopaminergic neuron.

Even so, there may be additional factors contributing in part to the loss of efficacy that is seen with continuous treatment with levodopa. Some decline may arise in part from gradual downregulation of striatal dopamine receptors (Rinne et al., 1980). Not all patients develop this problem, but it appears to be due to the receptors being constantly exposed to high levels of dopamine. Evidence to support this concept comes from the studies of drug holidays from levodopa. After levodopa is eliminated for a short period, restoration of levodopa therapy usually provides enhanced temporary benefit (Direnfeld et al., 1980; Weiner et al., 1980). Unfortunately this enhanced sensitivity is short-lived, and the potential risks of aspiration during the drug holiday render this approach undesirable for the short-term benefit that can be obtained.

It is important to differentiate between loss of response despite a seemingly adequate dosage of medications and insufficient response due to too low a dose because of inability to tolerate adequate dosages. Secondary loss of response implies (1) a parkinsonism-plus syndrome instead of PD, (2) the development of nondopaminergic motor symptoms (flexed posture, freezing, loss of postural reflexes), (3) development of intractable bradykinesia with disease progression that had previously responded to treatment, or (4) end-stage PD. Treatment of end-stage PD requires adjusting the dosages of all medications both up and down to find the optimum level for each.

Increased parkinsonism

A few patients on high-dosage levodopa may become more parkinsonian. This was initially reported unaccompanied by any other features of levodopa toxicity (Fahn and Barrett, 1979). This phenomenon has also been seen accompanied by confusion (Sage and Duvoisin, 1986). In both situations, improvement occurs when the dosage of levodopa is reduced. In fact, the phenomenon of increased parkinsonism without other signs of toxicity probably occurs more often than is recognized. Many physicians, unaware of this complication, are inclined to increase the dosage of antiparkinsonian medication, which does not help. Rather, a reduction of dosage should be tried first to see whether symptoms improve. This problem would appear to be related to reduced receptor sensitivity by high dosages of dopamine present in the striatum.

Increased tachyphemia and increased running gait

A number of patients who are overdosed with levodopa will speak faster, running syllables together, so that it is difficult for the listener to understand what the patient is saying. At the same time as the speech is rapid (tachyphemia), the amplitude is lower so the voice is softer, aggravating the situation. If the patient purposely tries to enunciate each syllable distinctly, he or she is able to do so for a few words, but then the tachyphemia takes over again. With speech therapy, sometimes using a metronome for pacing, a patient can improve the pattern of speaking, but only during the treatment session. There seems to be little carry-over. Associated with tachyphemia are rapid voluntary movements in other parts of the body, displayed as such when the patient is asked to perform rapid successive movements. These are usually very fast and of small amplitude, i.e., tachykinetic and hypokinetic.

This type of tachykinetic problem can also involve walking. Usually the patient moves more rapidly but with smaller steps. Gait in this instance can be mistaken for festination, which it resembles. If postural instability is impaired, such a running gait can lead to falling. Often, lowering the dosage of levodopa will allow the patient to slow down, with a resulting clarity of speech and gait. However, parkinsonian bradykinesia can become more of a problem.

Falling due to loss of postural reflexes

Falling is a common feature of PD as the illness progresses and there is increasing loss of postural reflexes. Since this particular cardinal sign of PD is little benefited by levodopa therapy (Klawans, 1986), this problem persists and worsens despite pharmacotherapy (Agid et al., 1990). Because levodopa may allow the patient to be more mobile, such as allowing the patient to arise more easily from a chair and walk independently, the persistence of postural instability becomes a particular problem because it raises the hazard of increased likelihood of falling. Thus, this complication of levodopa therapy in this particular subpopulation of patients with PD is technically not a true adverse effect of the medication, but a complication of the improvement in mobility in a patient who is at risk for falling, thereby increasing that risk. In this situation, the patient should use physical assistance, such as a walker. An alternative approach is to keep the patient sufficiently parkinsonian that he or she cannot arise without assistance.

Intractable tremor

Persistent tremor, i.e., rest tremor that has been resistant to antiparkinsonian medication, sometimes responds to clozapine (Friedman and Lannon, 1990; Jansen, 1994). If it is unresponsive to any medications, deep brain stimulation of the subthalamic nucleus could still be effective.

Treatment of PD during surgery or prolonged conditions of oral unavailability

Levodopa is absorbed via the small intestine. During periods when the patient is unable to swallow or be allowed oral intake, such as during surgery, a method is needed to keep the patient's parkinsonism from being too severe. Most surgical procedures require only a short period of time for the patient to be without oral liquids or foods, and most patients can suspend taking their medications when liquids are not allowed for these periods without major difficulty. During anesthesia, parkinsonism is not a problem, so even a prolonged operation will not present a problem. It is postoperatively, if the patient is not allowed oral liquids, such as from gastric surgery, that a problem could arise. The resulting rigidity, akinesia, decreased gastrointestinal motility, and respiratory function are dangerous and could complicate the recovery process. In this situation, the four approaches are providing Parcopa to dissolve in the mouth, subcutaneous infusions of apomorphine with rectal domperidone (Galvez-Jimenez and Lang, 1996), enteral administration of levodopa (Furuya et al., 1998) and utilizing rotigotine dermal patch.

Nonmotor features of PD

A discussion of nonmotor features of PD, including the development of nonmotor side effects from treatment of PD, is provided in Chapter 8.

References available on Expert Consult: www.expertconsult.com

CHAPTER **7**

Surgical treatment of Parkinson disease and other movement disorders

Chapter contents

Introduction	157	Deep brain stimulation	164
Functional anatomy of the basal ganglia	157	Deep brain stimulation for hyperkinetic and other disorders	177
Techniques of stereotactic surgery	159	Vagus nerve and other stimulation procedures	179
Thalamotomy	160	Brain grafting	179
Ablative lesions of the pallidum and subthalamic nucleus	160		

Introduction

A variety of surgical treatments for Parkinson disease (PD), including ablation or deafferentation of motor and premotor cortex, cervical cordotomy, and mesencephalic pedunculotomy, were performed in the first five decades of the twentieth century (Meyers, 1968). These procedures generally yielded relief of the movement disorder at the expense of concomitant weakness and other complications. Surgery at the level of the basal ganglia for PD was pioneered by Meyers in 1939 (Meyers, 1968). These open procedures included removal of the head of the caudate and section of the anterior limb of the internal capsule and pallidofugal pathways. After Spiegel and Wycis introduced the principles of stereotactic surgery in clinical practice in 1947, this method was applied for lesioning the pallidum and ansa lenticularis in an attempt to treat the symptoms of PD and other movement disorders (Mundinger and Reichert, 1963; Hassler et al., 1979; Grossman and Hamilton, 1991). Stereotactic thalamotomy for parkinsonian symptoms was introduced by Hassler and Riechert in 1951 (Hassler et al., 1979). Thalamotomies gradually replaced pallidotomies in the late 1950s and early 1960s (Table 7.1) because thalamotomies were thought to produce more sustained control of tremor. The introduction of levodopa in the late 1960s resulted in a marked reduction in the number of functional stereotactic procedures, and only a few specialized centers continued to perform such operations.

The renewed interest in surgical treatment of movement disorders has been stimulated in part by improved understanding of the functional anatomy underlying motor control, as well as refinement of methods and techniques in neurosurgery, neurophysiology, and neuroimaging (Krauss et al., 1998; Gross et al., 1999a; Lang, 2000b; Mazziotta, 2000; Jankovic, 2001; Krauss, et al., 2001a; Walter and Vitek, 2004). Furthermore, important strides have been made in assessments of the outcomes of surgery and in providing useful guidelines for inclusion–exclusion criteria (Defer et al., 1999; Tan and Jankovic, 2000, 2009). As a result of increased awareness about surgical options for patients with PD, the attitudes of clinicians toward referring patients for surgery have been changing, and in one survey, 99.4% of neurologists were aware of surgery for PD (Mathew et al., 1999). Furthermore, there is growing appreciation of the importance of holding surgical trials to as stringent evidentiary standards as other clinical studies, and the notion of double-blind design including "sham" operations is increasingly accepted (Prehn et al., 2006). Although this review focuses primarily on surgical treatment of PD, there is growing interest in the application of surgical intervention in the treatment of a variety of movement disorders (Pollak, 1999; Krauss et al., 2001a). While the interest in surgical treatment of movement disorders is growing, there is a remarkable paucity of well-designed, randomized trials (Stowe et al., 2003).

Functional anatomy of the basal ganglia

Before discussing the indications for and the results of surgery for PD, it is helpful to review the current concepts about the functional anatomy of the basal ganglia (Figs 7.1 and 7.2). The basal ganglia (extrapyramidal system) include the striatum, globus pallidus, substantia nigra, subthalamic

DOI: 10.1016/B978-1-4377-2369-4.00007-X

nucleus (STN) (Hameleers et al., 2006; Benarroch, 2008), and thalamus (Parent and Cicchetti, 1998; Hamani et al., 2004). The caudate and putamen are contiguous and comprise the striatum, and the putamen and globus pallidus are referred to as the lenticular nucleus. The cortical input from the prefrontal supplementary motor area, amygdala, and hippocampus is excitatory, mediated by glutamate. Neurons in the substantia nigra pars compacta provide major dopaminergic input to the striatum. The interaction between the afferent and efferent pathways is mediated by striatal

interneurons that utilize acetylcholine as the main neurotransmitter. The substantia nigra is a melanin-containing (pigmented) nucleus in the ventral midbrain, and it consists of dopaminergic neurons. The striatal output system is mediated by the inhibitory neurotransmitter gamma-aminobutyric acid (GABA). However, the basal ganglia appear to be more complex than is indicated by the current models (Parent and Cicchetti, 1998; DeLong and Wichmann, 2007). For example, it is now well recognized that the STN provides powerful excitatory projection not only to the globus pallidus interna (GPi), but also to the striatum and globus pallidus externa (GPe) and, in turn, receives input from the cerebral cortex, substantia nigra pars compacta, and various brainstem and

Table 7.1 Milestones in the surgical treatment of Parkinson disease

	Ablative	Stimulation	Brain grafts
1950s and 1960s	Pallidotomy (ant.) Thalamotomy		
1987		Thalamic	Adrenal autografts
1992	Posteroventral pallidotomy Gamma knife radiosurgery		Human fetal nigral grafts
1995		Pallidal (GPi)	Porcine fetal nigral xenografts
1996		Subthalamic (STN) Later: cZI, PPN	
2001			Spheramine Trophic factors (CERE-120) Gene delivery (GAD) Stem cells?

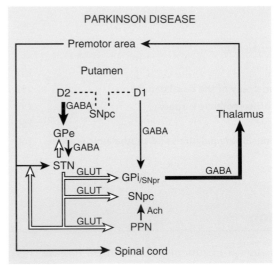

Figure 7.1 Basal ganglia circuitry relevant to PD. Ach, acetyl choline; DA, dopamine; D1, D2, dopamine receptors; GABA, gamma-aminobutyric acid; GLUT, glutamate; GPe, globus pallidus externa; GPi, globus pallidus interna; PPN, pedunculopontine nucleus; STN, subthalamic nucleus; SN, substantia nigra pars compacta (pc) and pars reticularis (pr).

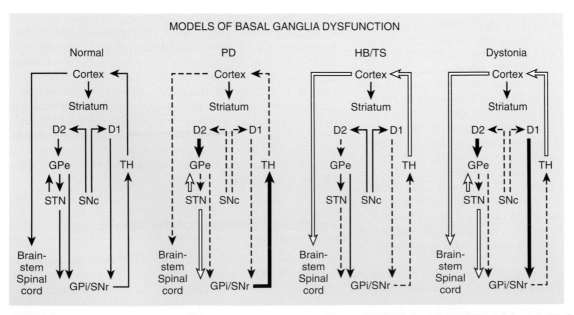

Figure 7.2 Hypothetical models of basal ganglia dysfunction in PD, hemiballism (HB)/Tourette syndrome (TS), and dystonia. TH, thalamus.

thalamic nuclei. Although most reports emphasize the pallidal-thalamic projection, major output from the GPi is to the brainstem nuclei, such as the pedunculopontine nucleus (PPN) (Alam et al., 2011; Jenkinson et al., 2006; Kenney et al., 2007a; Kuo et al., 2008; Zrinzo et al., 2008; Jenkinson et al., 2009; Ferraye et al., 2010; Moro et al., 2010). Some studies have also drawn attention to the role of the PPN in gait and locomotion as PD patients have a markedly reduced number of cholinergic PPN neurons (Rinne et al., 2008).

The reemergence of surgical treatment of PD, particularly pallidotomy and STN/GPi deep brain stimulation (DBS) (see later), has been fueled in part by improved understanding of basal ganglia circuitry, including the recognition that the STN and the GPi are overactive in experimental and human parkinsonism (Bergman et al., 1990; Limousin et al., 1995). Microelectrode guided single-cell recordings in patients with PD showed that the average firing rate in the GPi was 91 ± 52 Hz and that in the GPe it was 60 ± 21 Hz (Magnin et al., 2000). In addition, rhythmic, low-threshold calcium spike bursts are often recorded in the pallidum and medial thalamus; some but not all are synchronous (in phase) with the typical rest tremor. It has been postulated that the low-threshold calcium spike bursts contribute to rigidity and dystonia by activating the supplementary motor area. Apomorphine, a dopamine agonist, has been found to suppress the abnormal hyperactivity of the GPi and STN and to enhance the activity of the GPe on the basis of cellular recordings during surgery (Lozano et al., 2000). However, marked or complete suppression of GPi activity is associated with an emergence of dyskinesias. Indeed, levodopa- or dopamine-induced dyskinesias are associated with decreased firing frequency of the GPi neurons and a modification in the firing pattern (Boraud et al., 2001). This suggests that dopaminergic drugs and pallidotomy improve parkinsonian symptoms through a similar mechanism. Single-cell recording of the STN in patients with PD showed characteristic somatotopic organization, with neurons responding to sensorimotor stimuli localized chiefly in the dorsolateral region, and were of the irregular or tonic type (Rodriguez-Oroz et al., 2001). These two groups of neurons represent 60.5% and 24% of all STN neurons, respectively; only 15.5% of the STN neurons are oscillatory. Oscillatory activity in the basal ganglia is attracting more and more attention on the basis of various surgery-related neurophysiologic studies (Dostrovsky and Bergman, 2004). Microinjection of 10–23 µL of lidocaine into the STN of three patients with PD produced "striking improvements in bradykinesia, limb tremor and rigidity" in all (Levy et al., 2001). Furthermore, microinjections of 5–10 µL of muscimol, a GABA$_A$ receptor agonist, in the region of the STN that showed oscillatory activity resulted in suppression of contralateral tremor in two patients. Simultaneous microelectrode recordings showed suppression of neuronal activity in the near vicinity (up to 1.3 mm) of the injection. In a study designed to explore the effects of GPi on the STN, Sterio and colleagues (2002) showed that GPi stimulation markedly reduced the firing rate of dorsal STN cells in the ventral STN (and substantia nigra pars reticulata). In addition to providing support for STN segregation, this suggests that there is a feedforward GPi–STN interaction that needs to be incorporated in revised models of functional anatomy of the basal

ganglia. The oscillatory nature of human basal ganglia activity in relationship to movement has been recently reviewed (Brown et al., 2004).

The basal ganglia models in dystonia are even less clear; some studies have found that the GPi neuronal activity is increased in dystonia (Sanghera et al., 2003), whereas other studies have failed to find any decrease in basal ganglia output (Hutchison et al., 2003). Neurophysiologic studies performed during STN DBS have found that the STN receives direct input from the supplementary motor area and is thus involved in movement preparation, as demonstrated by recorded activity in the nucleus before voluntary movement (Paradiso et al., 2003).

Posteroventral pallidotomy (PVP) as well as GPi and STN DBS (see later) improve motor performance in patients with PD, presumably by interrupting inhibitory pallidal projections to the ventrolateral thalamus. This is supported by measurements by positron emission tomography (PET) of regional cerebral blood flow showing increased activity of supplementary motor area and premotor cortex (but not in primary motor cortex) after pallidotomy (Grafton et al., 1995; Eidelberg et al., 1996). One possible explanation for the apparent improvement of parkinsonian features after STN or GPi ablation or simulation is that the reduced excitability of the GPe in PD prevents the normal "brake" on STN firing and leads to overactivation of the STN and GPi. Despite lack of clear understanding of the mechanisms, surgical approaches are increasingly used in the treatment of patients with PD who fail to obtain satisfactory relief from pharmacologic therapy (Krauss and Jankovic, 1996; Hallett et al., 1999).

Techniques of stereotactic surgery

Stereotactic surgery is based on a Cartesian coordinate system, which implies that any point in space may be determined by three right-angled planes defined as the x, y, and z axes (Krauss and Jankovic, 1996). Functional stereotactic surgery relies on the acquisition of data from various imaging modalities and its transfer to the Cartesian coordinates referenced to an apparatus, the stereotactic frame, which is rigidly fixed to the patient's head (Hassler et al., 1979; Grossman and Hamilton, 1991). By using computed tomography, magnetic resonance imaging (MRI), or positive-contrast ventriculography, the target coordinates for functional stereotactic surgery are determined by extrapolation referring to the coordinates of the anterior and posterior commissure. The data for the spatial relation of the target to the anterior commissure (AC) and posterior commissure (PC) are derived from stereotactic atlases. For example, the STN target, used chiefly for STN DBS, is 10–12 mm lateral and 2–3 mm posterior to the midcommissural point and 2–4 mm below the AC–PC line. Some surgeons have also advocated the use of the red nucleus as an internal marker for targeting the optimal region of STN stimulation (Andrade-Souza et al., 2005). Various issues related to techniques of stereotactic surgery, particularly related to DBS, have been summarized in several reviews (Gross et al., 2006; Machado et al., 2006; Rezai et al., 2006).

To improve the accuracy despite normal anatomic variability, physiologic verification of the target by microelectrode recordings of spontaneous neuronal activity or by electric stimulation has been considered critical by some (Tasker, 1993; Obeso et al., 1998; Starr et al., 1998; Vitek et al., 2004), but other investigators believe that stereotactic surgery can be performed safely and effectively without microelectrode recording, using MRI-directed targeting (Dewey et al., 2000; Patel et al., 2003b; Hamid et al., 2005).

Different types of stereotactic devices are available. Functional stereotactic operations are generally performed under local anesthesia to allow examination of the patient during the physiologic investigations and during application of the lesions. In some cases, generalized anesthesia may be used safely (Maltete et al., 2004). The choice of the target and the techniques for calculation of the target as well as for physiologic localization differ (Mundinger and Reichert, 1963; Hassler et al., 1979; Grossman and Hamilton, 1991; Tasker, 1993; Tasker and Kiss, 1995). Usually, the target is chosen contralateral to the side that is more severely affected. The stereotactic frame is fixed to the skull with screws. The patient then undergoes stereotactic computed tomography scanning. While the coordinates of the target are calculated, the patient is brought back to the operating room. A small area of the head in the frontal region is shaved. A precoronal parasagittal burrhole is made via a linear incision under local anesthesia. The arch of the stereotactic device is fixed to the frame and the electrode for recording, or stimulation is directed to the precalculated target via a cannula. The tip of the microelectrode that is used for recording has a diameter of 0.01 mm, whereas the tip of the electrode that is used to produce the lesion has a diameter of 1.1 mm. After physiologic localization of the target, one to three lesions are made along the trajectory, heating the tip of the electrode to 75°C for 60 seconds. The symptomatic improvement, particularly the cessation of tremor or levodopa-induced dyskinesia, reduced rigidity, and improved performance of rapid succession movements, is usually noted immediately after placing the lesion. It is advisable to operate when the patient is "off" (before taking his or her morning dose of medication), since the effect of the surgery can be assessed more readily. The duration of the procedure varies between 2–3 hours for a standard thalamotomy and 4–5 hours for a pallidotomy. The hospital stay varies between 2 and 5 days.

Thalamotomy

Prior to the advent of levodopa therapy for PD, thalamotomy offered the most effective means of controlling disabling and embarrassing tremor. Stereotactic thalamotomy has been refined substantially since its introduction in 1947 as a result of improvements in neuroimaging and electrophysiologic and surgical techniques. The application of the procedure has broadened to disorders other than tremor, particularly dystonia, hemiballism, and severe levodopa-induced dyskinesias (Cardoso et al., 1995; Jankovic, 1998; Krauss and Grossman, 1998; Starr et al., 1998; Jankovic et al., 1999c). We analyzed the outcome of 60 patients with medically intractable tremor who underwent a total of 62 stereotactic thalamotomies at Baylor College of Medicine (Jankovic et al., 1995). The ventral intermediate (VIM) nucleus of the thalamus was the target in all patients. The patients were followed for as long as 13 years (mean: 53.4

months) after their surgery. At the most recent follow-up visit, 36 of 42 (86%) patients with PD, 5 of 6 (83%) with essential tremor (ET), 4 of 6 (67%) with cerebellar outflow tremor, and 3 of 6 (50%) with post-traumatic tremor had complete cessation of or moderate to marked improvement in their contralateral tremor. Patients who were taking levodopa ($n = 35$ patients) were able to reduce their daily dose by approximately 156 mg. Immediate postoperative complications, such as contralateral weakness (34%), dysarthria (29%), and confusion (23%), occurred in 58% of the 60 patients; these complications usually resolved rapidly during the postoperative period. These results are consistent with other reports, confirming the beneficial effects of thalamotomy on tremor and rigidity but no effect on bradykinesia in patients with PD (Zirh et al., 1999). Thalamotomy was also considered to be modestly effective in reducing the amplitude of kinetic tremor associated with multiple sclerosis (Alusi et al., 2001; Matsumoto et al., 2001; Thevathasan et al., 2011). In one series, 11 consecutive patients with multiple sclerosis tremor, permanent tremor reduction was observed in 11 of the 18 upper limbs with tremor (Thevathasan et al., 2011). Some authors have suggested that thalamic stimulation in multiple sclerosis promotes local "demyelinative lesioning." Furthermore, thalamotomy may improve levodopa-induced dyskinesia. Improved localization of the cluster of thalamic neurons with the largest amount of tremor discharges, correlated with electromyographic activity, should produce even better results. The likelihood of marked or complete tremor relief is high when the thalamic lesion is made within 2 mm of this site (Lenz et al., 1995). High-frequency stimulation (to be discussed later) rather than lesioning of the thalamic nuclei may be more effective and safer in the treatment of tremor (Schuurman et al., 2000). Since bilateral thalamotomy can cause hypophonia, dysarthria, and dysphagia, DBS is emerging as a useful alternative in those patients who require bilateral procedures. Thalamotomy has the advantage over DBS in that there is no need for hardware; and for patients with disabling bilateral tremor, unilateral thalamotomy in combination with contralateral DBS may offer the optimal tremor control with the fewest adverse side effects. Finally, microinjections of muscimol into the region of VIM thalamus that contains the tremor-synchronous cells consistently reduced tremor, suggesting that GABA agonists might be useful in the treatment of tremor (Pahapill et al., 1999).

Ablative lesions of the pallidum and subthalamic nucleus

Although a common procedure in the 1950s and 1960s, anterior pallidotomy was later abandoned because of inconsistent results, particularly concerning tremor, and because of improved results with posterior pallidotomy and later with DBS (Okun and Vitek, 2004). While some investigators had noted improvement of bradykinesia, this observation was not described by others (Hassler et al., 1979). Most surgeons at that time targeted the anterior dorsal portion of the GPi. More favorable results, with improvement of rigidity, bradykinesia, and tremor, were reported by the group of Leksell, who had chosen a different target, namely, the posterior and ventral aspect of the GPi. After Laitinen had reevaluated Leksell's approach in the early 1990s (Laitinen et al., 1992), pallidotomy was quickly reintroduced in North America and Europe (Sterio et al., 1994; Dogali et al., 1995; Lozano et al., 1995). Lesioning of the most ventral segment of the GPi provides the most antidyskinetic effect (Kishore et al., 2000).

The tentative target in the posteroventral GPi is located most commonly 20–21 mm lateral to the midline, 4–5 mm below the intercommissural line, and 2–3 mm anterior to the midcommissural point. The accurate localization of the target within the pallidum is essential not only for optimal therapeutic results, but also to avoid lesioning of adjacent structures. Single-cell microelectrode recording helps in delineating the borders of the GPi (Alterman et al., 1999). Different neuronal signals are identified along the pathway through the putamen, GPe, and GPi (Grafton et al., 1995). Cells with bursting discharges and low frequency activity interrupted by pauses are characteristic for the GPe, while irregular, high-frequency discharges at a frequency of 60–130 Hz mark the GPi. GPi neurons may change their firing rates on movements of various joints of the limbs. It is particularly important to identify the ventral border of the GPi and the adjacent optic tract, which might be located at a distance of only 2–3 mm from the derived target. Stimulation via the microelectrode, which may elicit visual phenomena, is also helpful in recognizing the optic tract. The mapping might require several trajectories before the final localization for the lesion is determined. Then the radiofrequency lesioning electrode is advanced, and "macrostimulation" is applied to identify whether and at what threshold the electric current spreads to the adjacent internal capsule. If no unwanted responses are encountered, the final lesion is then made.

Because of the importance of proper localization, several reports have raised concerns about the role of gamma knife (GK) in the treatment of various movement disorders (D.P. Friedman et al., 1999; Okun et al., 2001). Okun and colleagues (2001) described eight patients who, over a period of 6 months, were treated with GK surgery for PD and developed serious complications; one died as a result of aspiration pneumonia secondary to dysphagia. Other complications included hemiplegia, hemianopsia, limb weakness, speech and voice impairment, sensory deficit, and uncontrollable laughter. The authors concluded that these complications were related in all cases to missing the intended target and a resultant involvement of adjacent structures. Some problems may also relate to delayed effects of radiation necrosis, which might not have been fully appreciated in earlier reports on GK. Since their report represents only a small subset of patients treated with GK in their institution, the overall frequency of GK-related complications is not known. Nevertheless, this study sounds a loud alarm by drawing attention to the possibility that this procedure, often promoted as safer than the surgical treatment requiring penetration of the skull and brain parenchyma with a lesioning or stimulating electrode, can be associated with serious complications. This study must be interpreted cautiously, however, as this is not a controlled study in which patients are randomized to receive GK, ablative procedure, or DBS. Nevertheless, the report by Okun and colleagues (2001) is important because it highlights two major limitations of GK in the treatment of movement disorders: (1) it does not allow

microelectrode recordings to verify the location of the target, and (2) it is associated with an unacceptably high rate of immediate and delayed complications. Although GK thalamotomy has been reported to improve essential tremor (Niranjan et al., 2000), a study of 18 patients concluded that this procedure provides "only modest antitremor efficacy" (Lim et al., 2010). Nevertheless some reports have suggested that GK thalamotomy is effective in ameliorating action tremor associated with multiple sclerosis (Niranjan et al., 2000) and with other movement disorders (J.H. Friedman et al., 1999).

Lesioning of the posteroventral portion of the GPi (Laitinen et al., 1992; Dogali et al., 1995; Iacono et al., 1995; Lozano et al., 1995; Baron et al., 1996; Lai et al., 1996; Olanow, 1996; Kishore et al., 1997; Lang et al., 1997; Uitti et al., 1997; Kumar et al., 1998b; Masterman et al., 1998; Starr et al., 1998; Bronstein et al., 1999; Dalvi et al., 1999; Gross et al., 1999b; Hallett et al., 1999; Lang et al., 1999; Samii et al., 1999; Schrag et al., 1999; Lai et al., 2000; Counihan et al., 2001) and the STN (Bergman et al., 1990; Guridi et al., 1993; Limousin et al., 1995; Obeso et al., 1998; Barlas et al., 2001; Guridi and Obeso, 2001; Strutt et al., 2009) has an advantage over thalamotomy because this procedure improves not only tremor but also bradykinesia and rigidity. Although some investigators (Subramanian et al., 1995) have suggested that PVP is as effective as thalamotomy in controlling parkinsonian tremor, others (Dogali et al., 1995) feel that pallidotomy provides only partial relief of tremor. The latter authors suggest, however, that thalamotomy has a higher complication rate, particularly with respect to dysarthria and impairment of balance. In our series, only 6 of 60 (10%) patients had persistent dysarthria, and none had persistent loss of balance (Jankovic et al., 1995). However, because the two procedures have never been compared in a controlled fashion, it is difficult to comment on possible differences in efficacy and complication rates.

When a lesion is precisely localized to the GPi by neuroimaging (Krauss et al., 1997; Desaloms et al., 1998; Kondziolka et al., 1999) or by microelectrode recording techniques (Lang et al., 1997), the benefits can be quite dramatic. Subsequent follow-up of 39 patients who were followed for 6 months, 27 who were followed for 1 year, and 11 who were followed for 2 years provided additional evidence of long-term efficacy of this procedure (Lang et al., 1997). There was a 28% reduction in the "off" motor score in 6 months and an 82% improvement in contralateral "on" dyskinesias. The motor improvement was generally sustained during the 2-year follow-up, although the improvement in ipsilateral and axial symptoms gradually waned. In another study of 15 PD patients who were followed postoperatively for 1 year, the total Unified Parkinson's Disease Rating Scale (UPDRS) score improved by 30% at 3 months, and the score remained improved at 1 year ($P < 0.001$) (Baron et al., 1996). In addition, there was a marked improvement in contralateral rigidity, tremor, and bradykinesia as well as improvement in gait, balance, and freezing. Although contralateral dyskinesia and tremor remain improved, all other symptoms of PD usually worsen 3 years after the surgery (Pal et al., 2000).

The most robust beneficial effect of pallidotomy is improvement in levodopa-induced dyskinesia (Jankovic et al., 1999b, 1999c; Fine et al., 2000; Lai et al., 2000; Lang, 2000a; Counihan et al., 2001). At Baylor College of

Medicine, we followed 101 consecutive patients who underwent PVP procedures performed at our center and returned for at least one postoperative evaluation after 3 months (Lai et al., 2000). All had standardized clinical evaluations within 1 week before surgery and every 3–6 months after surgery. Data were collected during "on" and practically defined "off" periods for the UPDRS, Hoehn and Yahr stage, Schwab and England Activities of Daily Living (ADL) scale, and movement and reaction time. In addition, the severity and anatomic distribution of dyskinesia, neuropsychologic status, average percent of "on" time with and without dyskinesia, and clinical global impression were assessed during a longitudinal follow-up. Eighty-nine patients (46 men and 43 women) underwent unilateral PVP, and 12 patients (6 men and 6 women) had staged bilateral PVP. At 3 months after unilateral or staged bilateral PVP, 84 of the 101 patients reported marked or moderate improvement in their parkinsonian symptoms. Postoperative UPDRS mean total motor score improved in the "off" state by 35.5%, and the mean ADL score improved by 33.7% ($P < 0.001$). Rigidity, bradykinesia, and tremor scores also markedly improved after PVP, particularly on the contralateral side. Levodopa-induced dyskinesia was markedly reduced, while daily "on" time increased by 34.5% ($P < 0.001$). Seven patients had transient perioperative complications, including confusion, expressive aphasia, pneumonia, and visual changes. Improvements in parkinsonian symptoms were maintained in both "off" and "on" states in 67 patients at 12 months after PVP and in 46 patients who were followed for a mean period of 26.3 months. Patients who underwent staged bilateral PVP benefited further from the second procedure. Five of 12 patients experienced some adverse event. On the basis of this large series of patients with extended follow-up, we conclude that PVP is an effective and relatively safe treatment for medically resistant PD, especially for dopa-induced dyskinesia, tremor, rigidity, and bradykinesia. Motor fluctuations also improved. Benefits are most noticeable on the side contralateral to the PVP. Sustained (>1 year) improvement in motor function after bilateral pallidotomy has been also demonstrated by others (Counihan et al., 2001). Clinical improvement has been sustained for longer than 2 years. In a "blinded" review of videotapes, Ondo and colleagues (1998b) showed a significant improvement in "off" UPDRS scores in patients undergoing pallidotomy. Unilateral pallidotomy was found to be an effective treatment in a randomized, single-blind, multicenter trial (de Bie et al., 1999). In comparison to a control group that did not receive surgery, the pallidotomy patients improved their UPDRS III "off" motor score from 47 to 32.5, whereas the score in the control group increased from 52.5 to 56.5 ($P < 0.0001$). Furthermore, "on" UPDRS scores improved by 50%, chiefly as a result of marked improvement in dyskinesias. Most important, there was a significant improvement in the quality of life in patients who were treated surgically in comparison to those who were treated medically. In a follow-up study, the investigators showed that the benefits persist for at least 1 year and that patients with 1000 levodopa equivalent units or lower were most likely to improve (de Bie et al., 2001). An improvement in the quality of life, using various measures, has been demonstrated by other pallidotomy series (Martinez-Martin et al., 2000). This improvement may persist for up to 5.5 years (Baron et al., 2000; Fine et al., 2000). Evidence-based analysis of the effects of medical and surgical interventions on health-related quality of life (HRQoL) measures concluded that only unilateral pallidotomy, STN DBS, and rasagiline have been shown to be efficacious in improving HRQoL, but there is "insufficient evidence" that many well-established treatments, including levodopa and dopamine agonists, improve HRQoL (Martinez-Martin and Deuschl, 2007). The longest follow-up, over 10 years, after pallidotomy showed that while the patients clearly benefited from the procedure, the levodopa dosage had to be increased as a result of the disease progression, and most patients gradually became troubled by various mental and medical complications associated with the disease and aging (Hariz and Bergenheim, 2001). In a randomized trial of pallidotomy versus medical therapy, Vitek and colleagues (2003) found pallidotomy more effective as suggested by a 32% reduction in total UPDRS compared to 5% at 6 months.

Pallidotomy improves not only levodopa-induced dyskinesias, but also PD-related bradykinesia. This is best demonstrated by the finding of improved movement time and reaction time during the practically defined "off" state following pallidotomy (Jankovic et al., 1999a). Unilateral pallidotomy was also associated with improved simple and choice reaction times during the optimal "on" period (Hayashi et al., 2003). Kimber and colleagues (1999) suggested that the improvement in bradykinesia after pallidotomy may be explained by "greater efficacy of external cues in facilitating movement after withdrawal of the abnormal pallidal discharge." Pfann and colleagues (1998) also showed that "off" bradykinesia improves after pallidotomy but could not demonstrate any improvement in "on" bradykinesia. We also found a remarkable improvement in freezing contralateral to the lesion in several of our patients as well as objective evidence of benefits in gait and balance (Robert-Warrior et al., 2000; Jankovic et al., 2001). Improvements in gait (Baron et al., 1996; Siegel and Verhagen Metman, 2000) and postural stability (Melnick et al., 1999) were also reported in other pallidotomy series (Bakker et al., 2004).

Pallidotomy requires a multidisciplinary approach involving skilled neurologists, neurosurgeons, neuroradiologists, physiologists, physiatrists, and nurses to obtain optimal results (Bronstein et al., 1999). Even when performed by a team of experienced clinicians, pallidotomy can be associated with potentially serious complications. The reported complications include transient confusion, expressive aphasia, hemiparesis, facial paresis, pneumonia, and visual changes, such as homonymous hemianopia (Laitinen et al., 1992; Shannon et al., 1998).

Cognitive function and various neuropsychologic measures have been studied extensively in patients following surgery for PD, and these domains have been found to be generally preserved, particularly after unilateral pallidotomy (Masterman et al., 1998; Perrine et al., 1998; Rettig et al., 1998; York et al., 1999; Lombardi et al., 2000; Rettig et al., 2000; Saint-Cyr and Trépanier, 2000; Green et al., 2002; Contarino et al., 2007), although subtle changes in verbal fluency and possibly executive functions have been noted after left pallidotomy (Schmand et al., 2000) and after bilateral pallidotomy (Scott et al., 1998). Staged bilateral pallidotomy, although beneficial in most patients, results in increased risk of complications, particularly worsening of speech and other bulbar functions (Intemann et al., 2001).

Bilateral simultaneous pallidotomy may be associated with even more frequent and severe complications, such as depression, obsessive-compulsive disorder, abulia, pseudobulbar palsy, apraxia of eyelid opening, and visual field deficits (Ghika et al., 1999). In a systematic review of morbidity and mortality associated with unilateral pallidotomy, de Bie and colleagues (2002) found that the risk of permanent adverse effects was 13.8%, and symptomatic infarction or hemorrhage occurred in 3.9%; mortality was 1.2%. Several investigators have used implanted DBS electrodes to produce lesions in the thalamus for treating tremor and in the pallidum for treating levodopa-induced dyskinesias (Raoul et al., 2003). Although pallidotomy is used primarily to improve parkinsonian symptoms and levodopa-induced dyskinesias, bilateral pallidal lesions in otherwise normal individuals result in inadequate anticipatory and compensatory postural reflexes, bradykinesia, and other signs of motor impairment (Haaxma et al., 1995). This apparent paradox is difficult to explain with the current models of basal ganglia circuitry, but it suggests that nigrostriatal dopaminergic deficiency causing activation of the GPi is a necessary prerequisite for the beneficial effects of pallidotomy. Pallidotomy has now been essentially abandoned in favor of DBS and prior pallidotomy has been shown to be a poor predictor of outcome from STN DBS (Ondo et al., 2006).

The mechanism by which pallidotomy improves levodopa-induced dyskinesia is not known, but single-cell recordings in the GPi of parkinsonian monkeys show a marked reduction in firing rates only when dyskinesias were present (Papa et al., 1999). The average firing rate decreased from 46 Hz during the "off" state to 26 Hz during the "on" state and to 7.6 Hz during dyskinesia. It has been hypothesized that either overactive GPi (in a parkinsonian state) or low GPi activity (during dyskinesias) results in an abnormal ("noisy") input to the thalamocortical circuit. Pallidotomy tends to eliminate the "noise" and "normalize" the output.

Since pallidotomy has such a robust effect on levodopa-induced dyskinesia, including dystonia, the procedure has been applied in the treatment of primary and secondary dystonia (Jankovic, 1998; Ondo et al., 2001b; Yoshor et al., 2001). In a series of patients with generalized dystonia, about 50% improvement on various dystonia rating scales was observed following pallidotomy (Ondo et al., 1998a). Some patients, particularly those with primary generalized dystonia, however, had a marked improvement, and as a result of the surgery, their dystonia-related disability changed from a dependent state to completely independent functioning.

Since the greatest effect of GPi ablation or DBS is on levodopa-induced dyskinesias, these procedures have been also tried in the treatment of other hyperkinesias, such as generalized dystonia (Jankovic, 1998; Coubes et al., 2000; Ondo et al., 2001b; Albright, 2003; Coubes et al., 2004; Diamond and Jankovic, 2005; Vidailhet et al., 2005; Kupsch et al., 2006; Vidailhet et al., 2007; Tisch et al., 2007; Isaias et al., 2008, 2009; Sensi et al., 2009), cervical dystonia (Krauss et al., 1999; Parkin et al., 2001; Krauss et al., 2002; Hung et al., 2007; Kiss et al., 2007; Moro et al., 2009), cranial-cervical dystonia (Hebb et al., 2007; Ostrem et al., 2007, 2011), chorea and ballism (Thompson et al., 2000; Hashimoro et al., 2001; Krauss and Mundinger, 2001), and tics associated with Tourette syndrome (TS) (Cosgrove

and Rauch, 2001). In a study of 9 patients with primary cervical dystonia, STN DBS resulted in an improvement of the TWSTRS total score from a mean of 53.1 (± 2.57) to 19.6 (± 5.48) (P < 0.001) at 12 months (Ostrem et al., 2011).

High-frequency stimulation of the subthalamic nucleus (STN) has become an accepted treatment option for patients with moderately advanced PD (see later), but subthalamotomy has not been studied extensively (Tarsy, 2009). Because of its key role in the pathogenesis of PD, the STN has become a primary target for surgical treatment of PD. Although hemichorea/hemiballism is a well-recognized complication of a lesion in the STN, such hyperkinesias is very rare when the STN is lesioned (or stimulated) in the setting of PD (Barlas et al., 2001; Guridi and Obeso, 2001). This suggests that as a result of reduced activity of the "direct" GABAergic pathway from the striatum to the GPi, the parkinsonian state increases the threshold for such hyperkinesias. In PD, STN lesion reduces excitation of the GPi and simultaneously further reduces the hypoactivity of the GPe, compensating for the GPi hypoactivity, self-stabilizing the basal ganglia output, and reducing the risk of hemichorea/hemiballism. Alvarez and colleagues (2005) reported their experience in 11 patients after unilateral dorsal subthalamotomy. They found a significant reduction in UPDRS score, which was maintained in four patients for 24 months. Despite the location of the lesion, the procedure was not complicated by hemiballism. They followed up on their initial experience in 89 patients treated with unilateral subthalamotomy, 68 of whom were available for evaluations after up to 36 months (Alvarez et al., 2009). In addition to significant reduction in the UPDRS scores, levodopa daily dose was reduced by 45%, 36%, and 28% at 12, 24, and 36 months after surgery. Postoperative hemichorea-ballism was noted in 14 patients (15%) and it required pallidotomy in eight. Thus subthalamotomy seems to be a useful alternative to STN DBS when the latter is not accessible for economic or other reasons. In another study, unilateral dorsal subthalamotomy, particularly when combined with lesions in the H2 field of Forel and the zona incerta, resulted in a marked improvement in contralateral tremor, rigidity, and bradykinesia (Patel et al., 2003a). In one patient, a lesion confined to the STN produced "dyskinesia" that required H2/zona incerta DBS. In a series of 12 patients who underwent unilateral subthalamotomy, Su and colleagues (2003) showed a 30–38% improvement in UPDRS II and UPDRS III and an 85% improvement in dyskinesia, with 42% reduction in levodopa dosage. The benefits persisted for about 18 months. Complications included three (25%) cases of hemiballism; two of these patients recovered spontaneously, and one died of aspiration pneumonia. In a long-term (>3 years) follow-up of 18 patients with PD, bilateral subthalamotomy was associated with a significant improvement of ADL, reduction of levodopa-related dyskinesia by 50%, and lowering of levodopa dose by 47%, but the response was quite variable (Alvarez et al., 2005). Bilateral subthalamotomy was performed through DBS electrodes in a 60-year-old man with PD as a rescue option for DBS-device-related infection (Deligny et al., 2009). One potential advantage of subthalamotomy compared to pallidotomy is that the latter may adversely affect subsequent response to levodopa, DBS, or other restorative therapies, since these depend on the normal function of the outflow nuclei. Subthalamotomy, however, also seems to reduce the metabolic activity of the ipsilateral GPi, midbrain, pons, and thalamus (Su et al., 2001).

Deep brain stimulation

Ablative procedures have been largely replaced by DBS following the 1987 discovery that high-frequency stimulation of the thalamus mimics the therapeutic effects of lesioning in controlling tremor (Benabid et al., 1987, 1991, 2009). It has long been known that high-frequency (>100 Hz) stimulation employed during thalamotomies at the site of the planned lesion temporarily suppresses tremor (Mundinger and Reichert, 1963; Meyers, 1968; Hassler et al., 1979). Because of the ability to customize the stimulation parameters and the relatively low risk of complications, DBS is now considered the preferred surgical treatment for disabling PD-related tremor, ET, levodopa-related complications, generalized dystonia, and other movement disorders (Tasker, 1998). This application of chronic thalamic stimulation was later adopted for the treatment of chronic pain. Hypothalamic DBS is currently used for the treatment of various pain disorders, including migraines and cluster headaches (Leone et al., 2003). The Food and Drug Administration (FDA) approved DBS for the treatment of ET in 1997, PD in 2002, and granted a special Humanitarian Device Exemption for dystonia in 2003.

Depending on the desired effects, various subcortical nuclei, such as VIM nucleus of the thalamus, GPi, STN, zona incerta, and PPN, and other subcortical nuclei and even cortical areas, have been targeted for stimulation (Benabid et al., 1991; Caparros-Lefebvre et al., 1993; Limousin et al., 1995; Benabid et al., 1996; Koller et al., 1997; Krack et al., 1998a, 1998b; Limousin et al., 1998; Ondo et al., 1998c; Pollak et al., 1998; Starr et al., 1998; Tasker, 1998; Koller et al., 1999; Limousin et al., 1999; Deep-Brain Stimulation for Parkinson's Disease Study Group, 2001; Krause et al., 2001; Lopiano et al., 2001; Volkmann et al., 2001; Kumar, 2002; Okun and Foote, 2005; Perlmutter and Mink, 2006; Halpern et al., 2007; Stefani et al., 2007; Yu and Neimat, 2008; Limousin and Martinez-Torres, 2008) (Tables 7.2 and 7.3; Fig. 7.3).

DBS involves the implantation of the following hardware: (1) a DBS lead with four electrodes that are surgically inserted into the desired target and fixed at the skull with a ring and cap, (2) an extension wire that passes from the scalp area under the skin to the chest, and (3) an implantable pulse generator, a pacemaker-like device (unilateral Soletra or bilateral Kinetra, Medtronic Activa, ITREL model), which can deliver pulses with adjustable parameters (frequency, amplitude, width, modes, and polarities) (Kumar, 2002; Vesper et al., 2002). The implantable pulse generator is placed under the skin in the upper chest area near the collarbone. The patient can activate or deactivate the DBS system by placing a magnet or Access Review Device, a small mouse-like computer, over the chest area overlying the implantable pulse generator. Guidance on how to troubleshoot hardware complications and the utility of measuring impedance need to be better defined (Farris et al., 2008b). In the Medtronic Soletra and Kinetra devices the impedance measurement should be <50 Ω (ohms) and current >250 μA, but for an open circuit the impedance is usually >2000 Ω and current <7 μA for Soletra and >4000 Ω and current <15 μA for Kinetra. In seven patients with poor response to STN DBS, reimplantation of the electrodes presumably corrected misplacement and resulted in improvement in PD symptoms (Anheim et al., 2008).

In addition to appropriate selection of patients, it is critical that the most relevant and sensitive measures are used to assess the response to the therapeutic intervention, especially surgery as this intervention is particularly susceptible to a placebo effect. In this regard, instruments have been developed utilizing questionnaires, such as questions on life satisfaction: "general life satisfaction" (QLSM-A) and "satisfaction with health" (QLSM-G), in which each item is weighted according to its relative importance to the individual. In one study these instruments were validated against the 36-item short form health survey (SF-36) and the EuroQol (EQ-5D) (Kuehler et al., 2003). When the initial

---

Table 7.2 Advantages and disadvantages of deep brain stimulation

Advantages

Immediate symptomatic and functional improvement

Stimulation is adjustable and can be customized

Lower risk of lesion-related complications

Lower risk with bilateral procedure

Disadvantages

Long-term outcome unclear

Replacement of batteries

Implantation of a foreign body (hardware)

Cost to the patient and the neurologist

Limited coverage by Medicare and other insurance carriers

Table 7.3 Targets for deep brain stimulation in the treatment of various movement and other disorders

Thalamus

- Tremor (essential tremor, Parkinson disease, multiple sclerosis, trauma) – VIM
- Dystonia – VIM
- Ballism – VIM
- Myoclonus – VIM
- Tics (Tourette syndrome) – centromedian-parafascicular complex

Globus pallidus interna

- Dyskinesia (levodopa-induced, tardive)
- Dystonia
- Tics (Tourette syndrome)
- Chorea (Huntington disease)

Subthalamic nuclei

- Tremor, rigidity, bradykinesia
- Lower levodopa → ↓dyskinesia

Other targets

- Globus pallidus externa, anterior capsule, caudal zona incerta, pedunculopontine nucleus

VIM, ventral intermediate nucleus of the thalamus.

ZONA INCERTA AND ITS CONNECTIONS

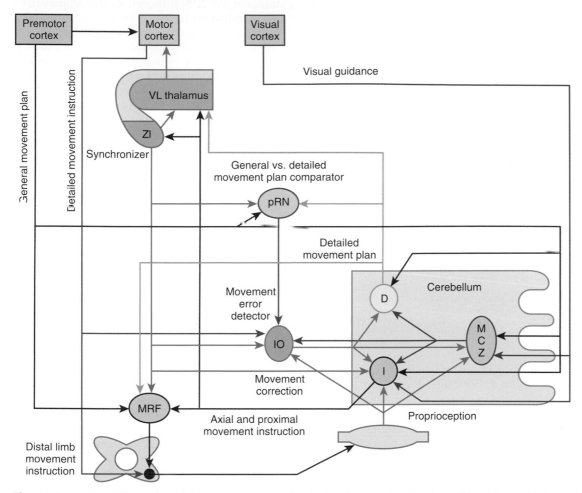

Figure 7.3 Zona incerta (ZI) and its role in various movement disorders. VL, the ventrolateral nucleus of the thalamus; MRF, medial reticular formation; IO, inferior olive; MCZ, microcomplex zone; D, dentate; I, interpositus; pRN, parvocellular red nucleus. *Redrawn from Plaha P, Khan S, Gill SS. Bilateral stimulation of the caudal zona incerta nucleus for tremor control. J Neurol Neurosurg Psychiatry 2008;79:504–513.*

questionnaires were reduced to 12 items for a "movement disorder module" (QLSM-MD), and five items for a "deep brain stimulation module" (QLSM-DBS), psychometric analysis revealed Cronbach's α values of 0.87 and 0.73, and satisfactory correlation coefficients for convergent validity with SF-36 and EQ-5D. Several quality-of-life instruments have been used in assessing the response to DBS (Kuehler et al., 2003; Diamond and Jankovic, 2005; Martinez-Martin and Deuschl, 2007; Diamond and Jankovic, 2008). Using the Sickness Impact Profile (SIP), improvements in various dimensions were maintained at 3–4 years after STN ($n = 45$) or GPi DBS ($n = 20$); 40% of STN DBS and 24% of GPi DBS patients were able to sustain their 6-month improvements at 3–4 years after surgery (Volkmann et al., 2009). In a prospective analysis of 21 patients before and after STN DBS for medically refractory PD, patients experienced an improvement in HRQoL as measured by various items of the movement disorder and health modules of the QLSM; specifically, QLSM items pertaining to energy level/enjoyment of life, independence from help, controllability/fluidity of movement, and steadiness when standing and walking showed significant improvements, although items concerning general

life issues (e.g., occupational function, interpersonal relationships, leisure activities) did not improve (Ferrara et al., 2010). Thus, following STN DBS, symptomatic and functional improvements translate into higher HRQoL, with high satisfaction in domains related to movement disorders and general health. The cost associated with STN DBS has been estimated to be about $60 000 per patient over 5 years (McIntosh et al., 2003).

The mechanism of benefits of DBS produced by the electrical stimulation is not known, but in some cases improvement can be observed even before the stimulator is activated (Table 7.4). This microlesioning effect may last several days or even weeks (Maltete et al., 2009). Besides microlesion effect, the following mechanisms have been suggested to explain the beneficial effects of DBS: (1) disruption of the network ("jamming" of feedback loop from the periphery), (2) depolarization block, (3) functional ablation by desynchronizing a tremorigenic pacemaker, (4) preferential activation of large axons that inhibit GPi neurons, (5) stimulation-evoked release of GABA (Dostrovsky et al., 2002; Garcia et al., 2005), (6) release of adenosine (Bekar et al., 2008), (7) overriding of pathological bursts and

Table 7.4 Possible mechanisms of deep brain stimulation

- Microlesioning
- Disrupts the network ("jamming")
- Depolarization block
- Functional ablation by desynchronizing a tremorigenic pacemaker
- Preferential activation of large axons
- Stimulation-evoked release of GABA, adenosine
- Stimulation-induced (time-locked) modulation of pathological network activity
- Overriding of pathological bursts and oscillations and replacing them with more regular firing
- Activation and excitation of the target nucleus (rather than inhibition as seen with lesioning)
- Marked increase in the release of ATP, resulting in accumulation of its catabolic product, adenosine
    - Adenosine A1 receptor activation depresses excitatory transmission in the thalamus and reduces tremor (and DBS-induced side effects)

Adapted from Hilker R, Voges J, Ghaemi M, et al. Deep brain stimulation of the subthalamic nucleus does not increase the striatal dopamine concentration in parkinsonian humans. Mov Disord 2003;18:41–48 and Bekar L, Libionka W, Tian GF, et al. Adenosine is crucial for deep brain stimulation-mediated attenuation of tremor. Nat Med 2008;14:75–80.

oscillations and replacing them with more regular firing (Birdno and Grill, 2008; Johnson et al., 2008; Hammond et al., 2008), and (8) activation and excitation of the target nucleus (rather than inhibition as seen with lesioning) (Hilker et al., 2008). Studies have shown that electrical stimulation consisting of short (<1 ms) duration pulses preferentially activates axons rather than somas (Nowak and Bullier, 1998). In support of the hypothesis of DBS preferentially activating large axons is the observation in one patient in whom stimulation inhibited GPi firing recorded with another microelectrode 600–1000 μm away (Wu et al., 2001). The effects of stimulation appear to be restricted to an area of 2–3 mm from the macroelectrode (at 2 mA, 2 V and impedance of 1000 Ω). This would be similar to a bipolar stimulation with two adjacent contacts 1.5 mm apart. Unipolar stimulation seems to have a significantly higher efficacy than bipolar stimulation, but this is accompanied by a higher rate of side-effects (19% vs. 0%); approximately 0.4–0.5 V higher amplitude was required for bipolar than unipolar stimulation to achieve the same effect (Deli et al., 2011).

Some studies suggest that the observed 15–30 Hz oscillations of the STN might reflect synchronization with cortical beta oscillation via the corticosubthalamic pathway and might relate to mechanisms of bradykinesia, since stimulation at the 15 Hz rate worsens bradykinesia and dopaminergic drugs promote faster oscillations (about 70 Hz) and improve bradykinesia, similar to the high-frequency stimulation associated with DBS (Levy et al., 2002). Studying the effects of STN DBS in 1-methyl-4-phenyl-1,2,3,6-tetrahydropyridine (MPTP) monkeys, Hashimoto and colleagues (2003) showed that the activation of the STN efferent fibers results in a change in firing pattern of pallidal neurons, and they postulated that this could underlie the beneficial effects of chronic STN DBS. In contrast to the popular notion that DBS inhibits the target nucleus, DBS has

been shown actually to activate the cerebellothalamocortical pathway (Molnar et al., 2004). Indeed, recent studies have suggested that stimulation-induced, time-locked modulation of pathologic network activity represents the most likely mechanism of the effects of DBS (McIntyre et al., 2004). DBS could have a dual effect, switching off a pathologically disrupted activity but also imposing a new discharge (in the upper gamma-band frequency) that results in beneficial effects (Garcia et al., 2005; Hammond et al., 2008). The most suitable target for DBS electrode is probably a region of the brain where DBS can most effectively interfere with spontaneous pathologic patterns by introducing regular rhythmical activity without causing additional adverse effects (Hammond et al., 2008). The frequency of stimulation might markedly influence the effects. For example, low-frequency (0.1–30 Hz) stimulation of STN has been shown to depolarize glutamatergic and GABAergic synaptic terminals, evoking excitatory and inhibitory postsynaptic potentials. Animal studies have shown that STN DBS (130 Hz for 1 hour) increases extracellular dopamine in the ipsilateral denervated striatum (Meissner et al., 2003). Although this has not yet been confirmed in patients, indirect evidence from [^{11}C]raclopride PET studies has not indicated that STN DBS induces dopamine release (Hilker et al., 2003). In untreated parkinsonian animals and patients, the neuronal activity in STN and GPi is dominated by low-frequency (11–30 Hz) oscillation that is increased with levodopa to >70 Hz. The therapeutic effects of high-frequency DBS might be mediated through the same mechanism (Brown et al., 2004). The role of adenosine in the effects of DBS on tremor has been suggested by the observation of a marked increase in the DBS-induced release of ATP from local astrocytes, which metabolizes to adenosine (Bekar et al., 2008). Previous studies have demonstrated that adenosine A1 receptor activation depresses excitatory transmission in the thalamus and reduces tremor, whereas caffeine, a nonselective adenosine receptor antagonist, can trigger or exacerbate tremor. The various mechanisms by which DBS improves neurologic and psychiatric function have been a subject of several reviews (Perlmutter and Mink, 2006; Kringelbach et al., 2007; Tye et al., 2009).

The abnormal motor cortical overactivity associated with PD is reduced with STN DBS (Payoux et al., 2004). Frontal cortex function, as measured by contingent negative variation, has been improved by bilateral STN DBS (Gerschlager et al., 1999). Metabolic changes in ipsilateral premotor cortex and cerebellum bilaterally, measured by [^{18}F]fluorodeoxyglucose and PET, correlated with clinical improvement related to GPi DBS (Fukuda et al., 2001b). Other regional cerebral blood flow studies showed that when the STN DBS is on, the ipsilateral rostral supplementary motor area and premotor cortex are activated during contralateral movement, but there was a reduction in regional cerebral blood flow in primary motor cortex during rest (Ceballos-Baumann et al., 1999). Modulation of cortical activity may be also responsible for improved bladder function with STN DBS (Herzog et al., 2006).

The placement of the electrode can be verified radiographically. Although computed tomography scan, rather than MRI, has been recommended by some, several studies have concluded that standard MRI (Tronnier et al., 1999; Jech et al., 2001) and functional MRI (Arantes et al., 2006) can be safely performed in patients with implanted neuro-stimulation systems, although transient and permanent neurologic deficits have been rarely reported following MRI (Henderson et al., 2005; Rezai et al., 2005; Spiegel et al., 2003).

Using PET, Ceballos-Baumann and colleagues (2001) found that VIM DBS in patients with ET was associated with increased regional cerebral blood flow in the ipsilateral motor cortex and a decrease in regional cerebral blood flow in the retroinsular (parietoinsular vestibular) cortex. They suggested that the latter affects function of the vestibular-thalamic-cortical projections and might therefore explain the frequent occurrence of disequilibrium in patients treated for tremor with VIM DBS, a reversible complication of this therapy. The authors also postulated that the increased synaptic activity in the motor cortex overrides the abnormal tremor-related rhythmic neuronal bursting. In another study (Ceballos-Baumann et al., 2001), the authors suggested that the beneficial effects of VIM DBS are due to nonphysiologic activation of thalamofrontal projections or frequency-dependent neuroinhibition. This has been also confirmed by Perlmutter and colleagues (2002). In another study involving functional MRI during DBS of STN (three patients) and thalamus (one patient), Jech and colleagues (2001) showed an increase in blood oxygenation level-dependent signal in the subcortical regions ipsilateral to the stimulated nucleus. The authors concluded that this effect cannot be simply explained by a mechanism of depolarization blockade; rather, it is caused by "overstimulation" of the target nucleus resulting in the suppression of its spontaneous activity.

DBS in tremor

Thalamic stimulation appears to be particularly effective in the treatment of parkinsonian tremor and ET (Koller et al., 1997; Ondo et al., 1998c; Pollak et al., 1998; Koller et al., 1999; Pahwa et al., 1999; Koller et al., 2001; Krauss et al., 2001b; Rehncrona et al., 2003) (Videos 7.1 and 7.2). In the North American Multi-Center Trial, 25 ET and 24 PD patients were followed for 1 year after implantation (Koller et al., 1997). Combined blinded tremor ratings (0–4) in ET patients randomized to "on" were 0.9 compared to 2.7 for those randomized to "off" stimulation. All subjective functional measures improved, and 9 of 29 patients (31%) had complete tremor cessation. In PD patients, "on" randomized scores were 0.6 compared to 3.2 for those who were randomized to "off." Fifty-eight percent (14 of 24) of patients had complete tremor cessation. Subjective functional measures (UPDRS part II), however, were not significantly improved. Complications were manageable and included paresthesia, headache, disequilibrium, dystonia, and device failure. Results were similar at 1 month and 1 year after implantation. Although some loss of efficacy and device-related complications have been encountered after 2 years of follow-up, the authors concluded that unilateral DBS of the thalamus has long-term efficacy in patients with ET (Koller et al., 2001). In a multicenter European study in which 37 patients with ET were followed for a mean of 6.5 years, unilateral or bilateral VIM DBS offered long-term benefits and safety (Sydow et al., 2003). Our experience at Baylor is similar to that reported in other centers. In a blinded and open-label trial of unilateral thalamic DBS in 33 patients (14

ET and 19 PD) with severe tremor refractory to conventional therapy, ET and PD patients demonstrated an 83% and 82% reduction ($P < 0.0001$), respectively, in observed contralateral arm tremor (Ondo et al., 1998c). All measures of tremor, including writing samples, pouring tests, subjective functional surveys, and disability scores, significantly improved. We found that bilateral thalamic DBS is more effective than unilateral DBS in controlling bilateral appendicular and midline tremors of ET and PD, and thalamic DBS does not seem to improve meaningfully any parkinsonian symptoms other than tremor (Ondo et al., 2001a). Although unilateral VIM DBS can markedly improve midline tremor, this improvement is significantly enhanced by the bilateral procedure (Putzke et al., 2005). Several studies have found that gait and balance may be impaired in some, but not all, patients treated for ET with VIM DBS (Earhart et al., 2009). One long-term study found that bilateral VIM DBS was often associated with dysarthria, loss of balance, and incoordination (Pahwa et al., 2006). Similar findings were reported in a 6-year follow-up of 38 PD patients treated with VIM DBS in a multicenter European study (Hariz et al., 2008b). The authors suggest that unilateral VIM DBS should be reserved for elderly PD patients with predominant unilateral tremor, but STN DBS may be a better choice for other patients with tremor-dominant PD. This recommendation is supported by other studies showing benefit of STN DBS in PD patients with prominent tremor (Fraix et al., 2006; Diamond et al., 2007b). VIM DBS has been found to be associated with modest improvement, rather than tremor augmentation as was previously suggested, in ipsilateral tremor in patients with ET (Ondo et al., 2001c). Other studies have demonstrated bilateral effects of unilateral thalamic DBS (Kovacs et al., 2008). A review of long-term efficacy of VIM DBS in 39 patients (20 PD, 19 ET) showed that the benefits might be maintained for at least 6 months (Rehncrona et al., 2003). In one study, three of eight patients with PD no longer required DBS after 3–5 years because the tremor markedly improved (Kumar et al., 2003). In addition to reducing the amplitude, VIM DBS increased the frequency of ET by 0.5–2 Hz at low inertial loads, made the tremor more irregular, and reduced the tremor-electromyography coherence (Vaillancourt et al., 2003).

To compare thalamic DBS with thalamotomy, Schuurman and colleagues (2000) conducted a prospective, randomized study of 68 patients with PD, 13 with ET, and 10 with multiple sclerosis. They found that the functional status improved more in the DBS group than in the thalamotomy group, and tremor was suppressed completely or almost completely in 30 of 33 (90.9%) in the DBS group and in 27 of 34 (79.4%) in the thalamotomy group. Although one patient in the DBS group died after an intracerebral hemorrhage, DBS was associated with significantly fewer complications than was thalamotomy. Similar results were obtained on this group after a 5-year follow-up, with the outcomes still favoring the DBS group (Schuurman et al., 2008). In one study of VIM DBS, dysarthria worsened when both stimulators were turned on in three of six patients (Pahwa et al., 1999). DBS also has been found to be effective in rare patients with disabling task-specific tremors (Racette et al., 2001). In addition to improving distal tremor associated with PD and ET, VIM DBS can effectively control ET-related head tremor, which usually does not respond to conventional therapy (Koller et al., 1999). Other midline tremors, such as voice, tongue, and face tremor, also may improve with unilateral VIM DBS, although additional benefit can be achieved with contralateral surgery (Obwegeser et al., 2000; Putzke et al., 2005). In addition, VIM DBS appears to improve postural stability (Pinter et al., 1999). Furthermore, unilateral thalamic DBS for ET has been found to be cognitively safe and to improve anxiety and quality of life (QoL) in terms of ADL and psychologic well-being (Tröster et al., 1999). Several studies have demonstrated that VIM DBS improves ADL and QoL, and one study showed that these improvements may be sustained for up to 7 years after implantation (Hariz et al., 2008a).

Several studies have sought to determine the optimal stimulation parameters. Algorithms for programming of the stimulation parameters have been suggested (Volkmann et al., 2006) but programming is generally based on the judgment of the programmer. Charge is the product of pulse width and current (current = voltage/impedance). Charge density is defined as the charge divided by the geometric surface area of the electrode. Short pulse widths require high current but low charge, and are thus more efficient at exciting neural elements and reducing the risk of neural damage. Linear voltage increases above 3 V do not correlate to a linear increase in the volume of neural elements excited, but significantly increase power consumption (Kuncel and Grill, 2002). While the amount of tremor suppression does not substantially increase in frequencies above 100 Hz, power consumption increased markedly at the higher frequencies (Kuncel et al., 2006). Power consumption (and battery drain) is determined by calculating the voltage squared (V^2) times the pulse width (PW) and frequency (F) divided by the impedance (Z).

$$P = \frac{V^2 \times PW \times F}{Z}$$

Bin-Mahfoodh et al. (2003) evaluated 14 implantable pulse generators (IPGs) that needed battery replacement out of 163 single channel batteries implanted over 7 years and found that the higher the total electrical energy delivered as calculated by the power consumption formula, the shorter the battery lifespan. A review of all battery replacements in patients at Baylor College of Medicine found 122 batteries needed replacement in 73 patients. The main predictors of a shorter battery life were greater amplitude, pulse width, and not using exclusive bipolar settings (Ondo et al., 2007). O'Suilleabhain et al. (2003), studied 13 VIM thalamic stimulators (8 for ET and 5 for PD) and measured tremor with an electromagnetic tracker. They randomly programmed 78 combinations of voltages (0, 1, 2, 3, or 4 V), pulse widths (60, 90, or 120 μs), and frequencies (130, 160, or 185 Hz) for both monopolar and bipolar polarity configurations. The voltage response curve for ET was flatter than for PD patients. Monopolar configurations were up to 25% more effective than bipolar but this configuration tended to shorten calculated battery life by 35%. The longest pulse width tested was up to 30% more effective than the shortest, but frequency changes had little effect on tremor amplitude. The authors recommended that there was no need to increase the frequency above 130 Hz and another study concluded that stimulation frequency of 100 Hz is generally the optimal

frequency and that there is little if any additional benefit from a higher frequency (Ushe et al., 2006). Low-frequency (10 Hz) STN DBS has been shown to improve verbal fluency but worsen motor function in a double-blind randomized crossover study of 12 patients with PD (Wojtecki et al., 2006). Moro et al. (2006) studied 44 patients with PD who had a long-term (mean, 3.5 years), stable response to STN DBS. Each underwent reprogramming of their stimulation by a neurologist expert in both PD and DBS, along with medication adjustments. Scores on the UPDRS were compared before reprogramming and up to 14 months thereafter. In half the patients (24, or 54.6%), UPDRS parts II and III scores improved significantly after reprogramming, by 15.0% and 29.5%, respectively. Anti-PD drug use decreased significantly as well, by 29.5%, in these responders. No improvement was seen in 16 patients (36.4%), and the condition of 4 patients (9.1%) worsened. These results suggest that patient outcomes with STN DBS can be improved when a neurologist expert in movement disorders and DBS programming is directly responsible for patient care.

VIM DBS has been found to be useful not only in the treatment of troublesome tremors associated with ET and PD but also in orthostatic tremor (Espay et al., 2008), and cerebellar outflow tremor associated with multiple sclerosis and post-traumatic tremors (Montgomery et al., 1999; Matsumoto et al., 2001; Wishart et al., 2003; Lyons and Pahwa, 2008) (Video 7.3). Thalamic DBS may be also effective in the treatment of levodopa-induced dyskinesia, possibly owing to involvement of the center median and parafascicularis complex (Caparros-Lefebvre et al., 1999). Thalamic DBS, however, does not seem to provide any benefit in PD-related gait difficulty (Defebvre et al., 1996). Bilateral ventralis oralis anterior thalamic DBS has been also reported to be effective in a patient with severe postanoxic generalized dystonia and bilateral necrosis of the basal ganglia (Ghika et al., 2002). Medically intractable myoclonus was reported to improve 80% with VIM DBS in one case of myoclonus–dystonia syndrome (Trottenberg et al., 2001a), and GPi DBS has been found to be effective in relieving myoclonus–dystonia syndrome (Magarinos-Ascone et al., 2005).

In addition to VIM as a target for patients with disabling tremor, STN DBS has been also found to be useful in the treatment of severe proximal tremor (Kitagawa et al., 2000) as well as rest and postural tremor in PD (Sturman et al., 2004).

DBS in Parkinson disease and levodopa-related complications

Several studies have demonstrated that DBS of the GPi and STN improves not only parkinsonian tremor but also other PD-related symptoms and prolongs the "on" time (Pahwa et al., 1997; Limousin et al., 1998; Pollak et al., 1998; Moro et al., 1999; Deep-Brain Stimulation for Parkinson's Disease Study Group, 2001; Lanotte et al., 2002; Alvarez et al., 2005) (Videos 7.4, 7.5). While levodopa improves predominantly finger bradykinesia, STN DBS improves predominantly proximal and axial bradykinesia (Timmermann et al., 2008). Elderly patients (>70 years old) seem to benefit as much as younger patients with respect to a reduction in dyskinesias and motor fluctuations, but during the "off" times, older patients have more difficulties with ADL and axial symptoms, particularly if they had some gait problems before surgery (Russmann et al., 2004b). Depending on the location of the stimulating electrode, pallidal stimulation has a variable effect on parkinsonian features versus levodopa-induced dyskinesias. In one study, stimulation of the dorsal GPi improved parkinsonian features, but stimulation of the posteroventral GPi improved levodopa-induced dyskinesia and worsened gait and akinesia (Bejjani et al., 1997). In another study, stimulation of the most ventral part of the GPi improved rigidity and eliminated levodopa-induced dyskinesia but produced marked bradykinesia, whereas stimulation of the most dorsal contacts improved bradykinesia and induced dyskinesia (Krack et al., 1998a). Best results could be obtained by stimulating the intermediate contacts. Similar results were reported by Durif and colleagues (1999), who found that ventral GPi stimulation was more effective than dorsal stimulation for alleviating rigidity and levodopa-induced dyskinesia. But in contrast to Krack and colleagues (1998a), whose target was posterolateral to the location of the target used by Durif and colleagues (1999), the latter group found that ventral stimulation also improved bradykinesia. They concluded that "chronic stimulation in the anteromedial GPi shows that this is a safe and effective treatment for advanced PD." GPi DBS has been found not only to improve "off" state UPDRS and movement onset time and spatial errors, but also to enhance motor activation responses as measured by concurrent PET recordings of regional cerebral blood flow in the sensorimotor cortex, supplementary motor area, and anterior cingulated gyrus (Fukuda et al., 2001a). Normalization of abnormal pattern of cerebral blood flow and an increase in cerebral blood flow in the supplementary motor area and anterior cingulated cortex has been also found with STN DBS, and this correlated with improvement in bradykinesia (Strafella et al., 2003). This effect was more robust with bilateral than unilateral stimulation. Hershey and colleagues (2003), however, found that STN DBS increased blood flow in the midbrain, globus pallidus, and thalamus but decreased blood flow in cortical areas. They concluded that "STN stimulation appears to drive, rather than inhibit, STN output neurons." This is consistent with the model that increased STN output driven by STN DBS leads to excitation of pallidal neurons, which increases inhibitory output to the thalamus resulting in thalamocortical inhibition. This is supported by the observed decrease in overactivity of SMA and other areas of overactivity presumably recruited to compensate for abnormal motor initiation as measured by resting regional cerebral blood flow (rCBF) (Grafton et al., 2006). In one study, bilateral STN DBS was associated with increased rCBF in both thalami and right midbrain and with decreased rCBF in the right premotor cortex (Karimi et al., 2008). The increased rCBF in the thalami correlated with improved bradykinesia and decreased rCBF in the SMA correlated with improvement in rigidity. It is, however, still not fully understood how rCBF reflects "normalization" of the abnormal pattern of neuronal firing in the target nuclei. 🎥

The localization of STN has been facilitated by the neurophysiologic characterization of the STN (Hutchison et al., 1998). The mean firing rate was found to be 37 Hz. The firing pattern was irregular and movement-sensitive. In addition, tremor cells were identified in the STN and ventral pallidum. Macroelectrode STN stimulation completely suppressed contralateral tremor (Ashby et al., 1999). In a 1-year follow-up of 24 PD patients treated with bilateral STN stimulation, the UPDRS, parts II and III, improved by 60%, and the mean dose of dopaminergic drugs was reduced by half (Limousin et al., 1998). Krack and colleagues (1998b) found a 71% reduction in the UPDRS score in patients treated with STN DBS. Using subjective evaluation of contralateral wrist rigidity, Rizzone and colleagues (2001) studied the effects of various STN stimulation parameters in patients with PD during a drug-free state. They found that stimulus rates higher than 90 Hz and a pulse width larger than 60 μs rarely produce additional benefits and are associated with narrowing of the therapeutic window. On the basis of longitudinal experience in a large number of patients, a monopolar stimulation with 2 V, pulse width 60 μs, and frequency of 100–130 Hz is usually found to provide maximal benefit (Ushe et al., 2004). There is a characteristic pattern of emergence of tremor within minutes of discontinuation of the DBS, followed by slow and steady worsening of axial signs over 3–4 hours, with 90% of the UPDRS score worsening occurring within 2 hours after DBS is turned off (Temperli et al., 2003). When the STN DBS is turned on, a similar but faster rate of improvement is observed. In an analysis of the effects of 25 electrodes used in STN DBS, placement in the dorsolateral STN border was associated with best clinical results and least energy consumption (Herzog et al., 2004) and stimulation of the dorsal border of STN has been associated with the most robust clinical improvement (Maks et al., 2009). Furthermore, ventral stimulation was associated with more adverse cognitive and mood changes (Okun et al., 2009).

Stereotactic surgery is the most effective and predictable treatment for levodopa-induced dyskinesia resistant to pharmacologic therapy (Guridi et al., 2008). In a multicenter, prospective, double-blind, crossover study in 134 patients with advanced PD treated with DBS of STN or GPi, the UPDRS motor scores improved by 49% ($P < 0.001$) and 37% ($P < 0.001$), respectively, in comparison to the nonstimulated state (Deep-Brain Stimulation for Parkinson's Disease Study Group, 2001). Furthermore, 6 months following implantation as compared to baseline, the percent time "on" without dyskinesias increased from 27% to 74% ($P < 0.001$) and from 28% to 64% ($P < 0.001$) with STN and GPi DBS, respectively. While the levodopa dosage remained unchanged in the GPi group, the daily levodopa dose equivalents were reduced by 37% in the STN DBS group ($P < 0.001$). Adverse events included intracranial hemorrhage in seven patients and infection necessitating removal of the leads in two. Although the largest and best-designed study, it was criticized because of methodologic flaws (e.g., absence of true blindness), short follow-up, and underreporting of adverse effects (Obeso et al., 2002). In a blinded assessment at 1 year after implantation of STN DBS in 30 patients, the motor UPDRS decreased by only 30%, but duration of daily wearing-off decreased by 69%, and levodopa requirements decreased by 30% (Ford et al., 2004). In a double-blind study of 7 patients treated with STN DBS, Kumar and colleagues (1998a) found 58% improvement in the UPDRS motor score in a medication-off state when the stimulator was turned on. Furthermore, there was an 83% improvement in levodopa-induced dyskinesias, and the total drug dosage decreased by 40%. In another study involving 23 patients with PD treated with bilateral STN DBS, Houeto and colleagues (2000) showed that the procedure decreased levodopa-induced motor fluctuations, dyskinesias, and daily dose of levodopa by 61–78%. Similarly, Fraix and colleagues (2000) showed in 24 patients with PD treated with bilateral STN DBS that the observed improvement in levodopa-induced dyskinesia was associated with a reduction in levodopa dosage. In another study, the combination of reduced levodopa and STN stimulation reduced the duration of diphasic and peak-dose dyskinesias by 52% and reduced "off" period dystonia by 90% and "off" period pain by 66% (Krack et al., 1999). In another, much smaller study involving only 15 patients with PD treated with bilateral STN DBS, the overall levodopa daily dose was reduced by 80.4%, and levodopa was withdrawn in 8 (53%) patients (Molinuevo et al., 2000). In a long-term follow-up, they showed that 10 of 26 (38%) patients were maintained on STN DBS monotherapy after 1.5 years of treatment (Valldeoriola et al., 2002). Similarly, Vingerhoets and colleagues (2002) found that 21 ± 8 months after implantation of bilateral STN DBS under stereotactic guidance, microelectrode recording, and clinical control in 20 patients, the UPDRS III "off medication" score decreased by 45% and was similar to UPDRS III "on medication" score. Furthermore, medication was reduced by 79%, and 10 (50%) were able to withdraw their medications completely. In a subsequent study of two groups of six STN DBS-treated patients, the investigators showed that patients who were able to discontinue their medication and were subsequently challenged with levodopa had much less severe levodopa-induced dyskinesia than those who had continued on levodopa, thus supporting "dopaminergic stimulation and striatal desensitization as major determinants of levodopa-induced dyskinesia in PD" (Russmann et al., 2004a). In a 2-year follow-up of 20 patients with STN DBS, the 50.9% UPDRS motor score reduction observed at 6 months was maintained during the follow-up period (Herzog et al., 2003). In a 5-year prospective study of the first 49 patients, mean age 55 years, treated with bilateral STN DBS, assessed during "on" and "off" states at 1, 3, and 5 years, the Grenoble group found a 54% improvement in "off" motor function compared to baseline and 49% improvement in ADL (Krack et al., 2003). Speech was apparently the only motor function that did not improve. Except for improved dyskinesia and lower daily levodopa dose, there was no additional improvement in "on" motor function beyond 1 year, and the axial symptoms continued to deteriorate after the first year. Of the initial 49 patients, 7 did not complete the study, 3 died, 4 were lost to follow-up, 3 developed dementia after 3 years, 1 committed suicide, and 1 had a large cerebral hemorrhage. This and other studies provide evidence for the conclusion that STN DBS is no better than levodopa, but it ameliorates levodopa-related motor complications and dyskinesias and "off" period dystonia. In a double-blind, crossover evaluation of STN DBS in 10 patients during practically defined "off" (medications stopped overnight), the mean motor UPDRS score improved from 43 to 26 ($P < 0.04$), and various timed tests (walking and tapping) also improved significantly ($P < 0.04$) (Rodriguez-Oroz et al., 2004). Open-label, 4-year follow-up also showed significant improvement in dyskinesia and levodopa reduction by half. In a 5-year follow-up of 11 patients

treated with bilateral pallidal DBS, dyskinesias remained well controlled, but the initial benefit in "off" motor symptoms and fluctuations as well as ADL gradually declined, and the benefits were restored in 4 patients after replacement of the pallidal electrodes into STN (Volkmann et al., 2004). These results are consistent with many other studies showing long-term benefits of STN DBS in PD (Wider et al., 2008). In a study of 30 patients undergoing STN DBS, levodopa-induced complications based on UPDRS IV and during an acute levodopa challenge improved markedly after 1 year (both on and off stimulation) and still further at 5 years (Simonin et al., 2009). Furthermore, the peak-dose dyskinesia decreased significantly between 1 and 5 years, possibly related to a reduction in levodopa-equivalent dose from 1323 ± 501 mg at baseline to 753 ± 451 mg at year 1, and 850 ± 555 mg at year 5. The DBS parameters at 5-year follow-up were as follows: voltage 2.92 ± 0.73 V, frequency 127 ± 28 Hz and pulse 76 ± 14 μs. Reduction of dopaminergic drugs as a result of STN DBS may unmask restless legs syndrome (Kedia et al., 2004). STN DBS, however, has been reported to improve restless legs syndrome in 6 patients in whom the syndrome accompanied PD (Driver-Dunckley et al., 2006). Bilateral STN DBS has been reported to produce about 78% improvement in the thoracolumbar angle of patients with PD-associated camptocormia (Sako et al., 2009).

Besides reducing the need for levodopa, bilateral STN DBS also reduces the need for other medications, including apomorphine (Varma et al., 2003). Moro and colleagues (2002) showed that while the duration and latency of levodopa response are well maintained in patients with chronic STN DBS, the magnitude of the short-duration response tends to decrease with time. Since improvements in dyskinesia usually require a reduction in levodopa dosage, unilateral STN DBS is impractical because the side of the body contralateral to the unstimulated side would clearly worsen. Many investigators recommend bilateral STN DBS even in markedly asymmetric PD (Kim et al., 2009). Furthermore, bilateral implantation during a single procedure is less inconvenient to the patient than a staged procedure, the neurophysiologic mapping may be facilitated by anatomic symmetry, and implantation of both stimulators can be performed under a single general anesthetic.

Bilateral STN DBS appears to be more effective than unilateral STN DBS in improving parkinsonism, but unilateral STN DBS may be appropriate for patients with asymmetric parkinsonian symptoms, including a high-amplitude tremor (Kumar et al., 1999b; Linazasoro et al., 2003; Sturman et al., 2004; Stover et al., 2005; Diamond et al., 2007b; Fishman, 2008). STN DBS has been shown to have a robust effect not only on levodopa-related motor complications but also on the treatment of PD-related tremor (Diamond et al., 2007b). This marked benefit on tremor is also supported by marked improvement of postural and kinetic tremor with stimulation of the subthalamic area (Hamel et al., 2007; Herzog et al., 2007). Since bilateral STN DBS appears to be associated with less ataxia and dysarthria than VIM DBS (Pahwa et al., 2006), it may be considered as the target of choice in patients with ET requiring bilateral stimulation (Diamond et al., 2007b).

Bilateral STN DBS greatly improves functioning and reduces levodopa-induced dyskinesias, probably by allowing a reduction in total levodopa dosage. STN DBS, however, may also somehow reverse the levodopa sensitization, since levodopa-induced dyskinesias seem to be markedly reduced after continuous bilateral STN stimulation even when the DBS is turned off (Bejjani et al., 2000b). This may be due to the marked reduction in daily levodopa dose permitted by chronic STN DBS. Nutt and colleagues (2001b) suggested that the improvement in motor fluctuations produced by STN and GPi DBS is due to improvement in "off" disability rather than any effects on pharmacodynamics or pharmacokinetics of levodopa. Younger patients with levodopa-responsive PD are considered the best candidates for bilateral STN DBS (Charles et al., 2002; Welter et al., 2002). In a 2-year follow-up of patients with bilateral STN DBS, preoperative response to levodopa was found as the only predictor of a favorable outcome (Kleiner-Fisman et al., 2003). In patients with prior pallidotomy, bilateral (not unilateral) STN DBS may be beneficial (Su and Tseng, 2001; Kleiner-Fisman et al., 2004). The mean firing frequency of STN on the side ipsilateral to the pallidotomy is lower than on the contralateral, intact side (Mogilner et al., 2002). In a randomized trial involving 34 patients with advanced PD the "off" UPDRS score improved significantly more following bilateral STN DBS as compared to unilateral pallidotomy; "on" UPDRS motor and dyskinesia scores also improved more in the DBS group than in the pallidotomy group (Esselink et al., 2004).

Although bilateral STN DBS is clearly effective in improving the cardinal as well as other parkinsonian symptoms, the procedure does not necessarily improve all the symptoms, and as a result of progression of cognitive, speech, and other deficits frequently associated with PD, the QoL might not substantially improve in patients who exhibit these additional features (Hariz et al., 2000; Diamond and Jankovic, 2005), only about half of patients regain their employment, and many experience new marital and socio-professional problems (Schupbach et al., 2006). In one study, only young PD patients were found to have a significant improvement in their quality of life with STN DBS (Derost et al., 2007). Furthermore, preexisting personality disorders and psychiatric disorders might not necessarily improve with STN DBS and might actually worsen and further compromise the patient's quality of life (Houeto et al., 2002), but in carefully selected patients, mood, anxiety, apathy, and quality of life may improve with the procedure (Czernecki et al., 2005; Houeto et al., 2006). Normalization of bladder symptoms associated with PD-related detrusor hyperreflexia was demonstrated in a study of 16 patients with bilateral STN DBS (Seif et al., 2004).

Using the PD Quality of Life Questionnaire in 60 patients, Lagrange and colleagues (2002) showed improvements 1 year after bilateral STN DBS in all dimensions, including motor (+48%), systemic (+34%), emotional (+29%), and social (+63%). Other studies have demonstrated significant improvements in health-related quality of life in patients with advanced PD treated with bilateral STN DBS (Just and Ostergaard, 2002; Lagrange et al., 2002; Martinez-Martin et al., 2002). In another study, Lezcano and colleagues (2004a) applied the UPDRS, PDQ-39, and the scale of quality of life for caregivers (SQLC) in 11 PD patients 2 years after they had undergone bilateral STN DBS and found 62% improvement in PDQ-39 ($P < 0.001$) and 68% in SQLC

($P = 0.002$). In an 18-month follow-up of patients after bilateral implantation of STN DBS, sustained improvements were demonstrated in a variety of measures of health-related quality of life (Siderowf et al., 2006). A cost-effectiveness analysis suggests that DBS could be cost-effective in treating PD quality of life, which improved 18% or more compared with best medical treatment (Tomaszewski and Holloway, 2001). In a European, SPARK, study, the 6-month cost of PD decreased from about $10 000 to $1600 after bilateral STN DBS, largely due to marked reduction in medications (Fraix et al., 2006). In a 6-month study of 156 patients with advanced PD randomized to STN DBS or medical management, the German Parkinson Study Group (Deuschl et al., 2006b) concluded that STN DBS was more effective than medical management. The baseline characteristics, including the mean age of the patients in each group (60.5 vs. 60.8 years, respectively) was similar, but the mean PDQ-39 score, the primary endpoint, decreased from 41.8 to 31.8 in the DBS group (25% improvement) and increased from 39.6 to 40.2 in the medication group (no improvement). The PDQ-39 improvement in the DBS group was significant in the subscales for mobility, ADL, emotional well-being, stigma, and bodily discomfort. The mean UPDRS-III score during "off" time improved from 48.0 to 28.3 (41% improvement) with DBS, but remained unchanged in the medication group (46.8 vs. 46.0) and improved during "on" time from 18.9 to 14.6 (23% improvement) in the DBS group, but remained unchanged in the medication group (17.3 vs. 17.5). Although a total of 39 (50%) adverse events were reported in the DBS group as compared to 50 (64%) in the medication group, there were significantly more serious adverse events reported in the DBS group ($n = 10$, 12.8%), including 3 deaths, as compared to the medication group ($n = 3$, 3.8%) ($P = 0.04$). In another prospective study of 20 patients with early PD, randomized to either STN DBS or medical therapy, the authors found that the quality of life measures improved 24% in the surgical group but not at all in the medical group and after 18 months the severity of parkinsonian motor signs "off" medication, levodopa-induced motor complications, and daily levodopa dose were reduced by 69%, 83%, and 57% in operated patients and increased by 29%, 15%, and 12% in the group with medical treatment only ($P < 0.001$) (Schupbach et al., 2006). The authors concluded that DBS "should be considered a therapeutic option early in the course of PD." A total of 255 patients were enrolled in a randomized, controlled trial, designed to compare the effects of DBS (STN, $n = 60$ or GPi, $n = 61$) and "best medical therapy" ($n = 134$) after 6 months, at seven Veterans Affairs (The Parkinson's Disease Research, Education, and Clinic Center, PADRECC) and six university hospitals (Weaver et al., 2009). Patients treated with DBS gained a mean of 4.6 hours/day of "on" time without troubling dyskinesia compared with 0 hours/day for patients who received best medical therapy ($P < 0.001$). Furthermore, motor function improved by ≥5 points on the motor UPDRS in 71% of DBS and 32% of medical therapy patients. This was accompanied by improvements in the majority of PD-related HRQoL measures and only minimal decrement in neurocognitive testing. The overall risk of experiencing a serious adverse effect, however, was 3.8 times higher in the DBS than in the medical therapy group (40% vs. 11%). While benefits associated with DBS extend beyond what can

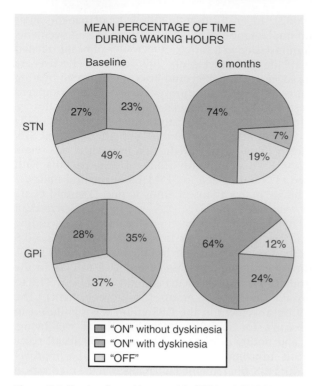

MEAN PERCENTAGE OF TIME DURING WAKING HOURS

Figure 7.4 Results of a multicenter trial of STN and GPi DBS. *Redrawn from Deep-Brain Stimulation for Parkinson's Disease Study Group. N Engl J Med 2001;345:956–963.*

be achieved with medical therapy alone, selection of the appropriate patients and target as well as skills and experience of the DBS team must be considered before referring patients for this surgical treatment (Okun and Foote, 2009). It is also important when selecting candidates for surgery to carefully evaluate all the ethical aspects of DBS, the net benefit, and the long-term burden it may place on the patient and his or her caregiver, especially given the impaired cognition that can follow the implantation of the DBS (Farris et al., 2008a). Although there are many reports concluding that GPi DBS is less effective than STN stimulation, there are only few studies that have objectively compared these two approaches (Okun and Foote, 2005; Okun et al., 2009) (Fig. 7.4). Before addressing this controversy, it is important to point out that GPi is a much larger target than STN (500 mm³ versus 200 mm³) and therefore requires larger density of stimulation. On the other hand, stimulation of the STN, because it is a smaller target, may lead to spreading of current from the intended sensorimotor area to potentially unwanted areas of the nucleus, such as the associative and limbic regions. This might account for a slightly higher frequency of cognitive and behavioral adverse effects with STN DBS (Anderson et al., 2005). Several studies have demonstrated greater antidyskinetic effects of GPi versus STN stimulation, and some studies have suggested that GPi DBS might be especially indicated in patients with a low threshold for dyskinesia (Minguez-Castellanos et al., 2005), and GPi is considered the desirable target for treatment of dystonia and other hyperkinetic movement disorders. The relative safety and efficacy of STN versus GPi DBS have been compared in a few studies (Burchiel et al., 1999; Anderson et al., 2005;

Okun et al., 2009). Although Burchiel and colleagues (1999) found no difference between the two targets, their initial study had insufficient power to detect a difference between the two groups. In their subsequent study involving 23 patients with PD complicated by marked levodopa-related motor fluctuations and dyskinesias, the investigators concluded that there were no significant differences in the overall benefits, although levodopa was decreased more in the STN group and dyskinesia improved more in the GPi group (Anderson et al., 2005). Krause and colleagues (2001) reported results in 6 patients with PD treated with GPi DBS and 12 patients with STN DBS. They found that while GPi DBS was associated with a lower frequency of levodopa-related complications, there was no improvement in bradykinesia or tremor. STN DBS, on the other hand, improved all parkinsonian symptoms and was associated with a reduced daily dose of levodopa. The authors concluded that STN was "the target of choice" for patients with severe PD who have side effects from levodopa. In a retrospective analysis of 16 patients undergoing STN DBS versus 11 treated with GPi DBS, Volkmann and colleagues (2001) showed that STN stimulation was associated with a 65% reduction in medication and required less electric power but required more intensive postoperative monitoring and was associated with a higher frequency of adverse effects related to levodopa withdrawal as compared to GPi DBS. When STN and GPi DBS were compared, no difference between stimulation of the two targets on improvement of rigidity, strength, speed of movement execution, or movement initiation was found (Brown et al., 1999). For most effective results, the upper STN (sensorimotor part) and the subthalamic area containing the zona incerta, fields of Forel, and STN projections should be stimulated (Hamel et al., 2003). However, further controlled, randomized studies are needed to answer the question of which of the two methods is more effective and which patients should be considered the best candidates for either of the two procedures. In the COMPARE trial 52 patients were randomized to unilateral STN or GPi DBS without any significant difference in outcomes except more worsening in letter verbal fluency in patients with STN DBS (Okun et al., 2009). In the a follow-up analysis of the Veterans Affairs Cooperative Studies Program (Weaver et al., 2009) outcomes, STN and GPi DBS were analyzed after 24 months in 299 patients; there were no differences in mean changes in the motor (Part III) UPDRS between the two targets (Follett et al., 2010). Patients undergoing STN required a lower dose of dopaminergic agents than those undergoing pallidal stimulation ($P = 0.02$) and visuomotor processing speed declined more after STN than after GPi stimulation ($P = 0.03$). On the other hand, there was worsening of depression after STN DBS but mood improved after GPi DBS ($P = 0.02$). Slightly more than half of the patients experienced serious adverse events but there was no difference in the frequency of these events between the two groups. As the results of comparative trials become available there is emerging evidence that GPi DBS may be particularly suitable for patients who may have some cognitive or behavioral issues whereas bilateral STN DBS may be the surgical choice for patients in whom reduction in levodopa dosage is the primary goal.

DBS of the STN has been found to be effective in controlling not only parkinsonian tremor (Sturman et al., 2004), but also bradykinesia, gait difficulty, and freezing (Limousin et al., 1995; Allert et al., 2001; Faist et al., 2001; Stolze et al., 2001; Bakker et al., 2004; Ferraye et al., 2010; Moro et al., 2010) and handwriting (Siebner et al., 1999). In addition to improving limb signs and the cardinal signs of PD, bilateral STN DBS has been found to also improve axial parkinsonian symptoms, particularly rising from chair and gait (Bastian et al., 2003; Bakker et al., 2004), as well as speech, neck rigidity, abnormal posture, "off" dystonia, balance and postural instability (Maurer et al., 2003; Colnat-Coulbois et al., 2005; Nilsson et al., 2005; Shivitz et al., 2006), and sensory symptoms (Bejjani et al., 1999; Loher et al., 2002; Rocchi et al., 2002; Krystkowiak et al., 2003). Even sexual functioning has been shown to improve after STN DBS (Castelli et al., 2004). Using static posturography, Rocchi and colleagues (2002) found an improvement in postural sway with bilateral STN DBS but worsening with levodopa. Bilateral STN DBS has been reported to improve PD-related dysarthria in some studies (Gentil et al., 1999; Pollak, 1999). Other studies, however, have found that dysarthria, cognitive impairment, and postural instability fail to improve with STN DBS even in the same PD patient in whom the procedure improved the usual levodopa-responsive symptoms (Jarraya et al., 2003). STN or GPi DBS has been shown to improve gait velocity by increasing stride length with normalization of the gait pattern (Pahwa et al., 1997; Damier et al., 2001; Allert et al., 2001; Faist et al., 2001; Bastian et al., 2003). In one study, the "off" period cadence increased from 117 ± 18.9 steps per minute to 126 ± 9.4 steps per minute (P < 0.05) after GPi DBS (Volkmann et al., 1998). In contrast, bilateral STN DBS increased stride length but not cadence (Allert et al., 2001; Faist et al., 2001). Other studies reported significant improvements in essentially all components of gait (Krystkowiak et al., 2003; Bakker et al., 2004).

The possibility that chronic DBS interferes with STN's excitatory output suggests a potential role of this treatment as a neuroprotective strategy (Piallat et al., 1996; Henderson and Dunnett, 1998; Krack et al., 1998b). This notion is supported by the observation that ablation of STN attenuates the loss of DA neurons in rats exposed to the mitochondrial toxin 3-nitroproprionic acid (3-NP) or the catecholamine toxin 6-hydroxydopamine (6-OHDA) (Nakao et al., 1999). A 20–40% preservation of SN neurons was observed with STN lesion of DBS using MPTP monkeys as a model for PD (Wallace et al., 2007). The animal studies have led some investigators to argue that STN DBS may offer neuroprotection by reducing glutamate excitotoxicity and that performing the procedure early in the course of the disease might prevent motor disability and adverse reactions to levodopa (Mesnage et al., 2002; Schupbach et al., 2007; Wallace et al., 2007).

Effects of ablative surgery versus DBS on various parkinsonian features have not been adequately compared. In one prospective study, 13 patients with PD were randomized to pallidal stimulation versus pallidal ablation (Merello et al., 1999). Although the primary endpoint effects at 3 months on UPDRS and ADL were "comparable," pallidal DBS had more beneficial effects on hand-tapping speed, whereas pallidotomy had more robust effect on levodopa-induced dyskinesias. However, additional blinded comparison studies of STN versus GPi DBS are needed before any definite conclusions about the relative effects of the two targets can be

Table 7.5 Selection of patients for deep brain stimulation surgery

Parkinson disease >5 years (to allow for atypical features to emerge and assess response to dopaminergic therapy)
Dopaminergic responsiveness (>30% reduction in motor UPDRS)
Troublesome dyskinesias despite optimal medical therapy
Disabling medication resistant tremor
Normal MRI
Exclude atypical and secondary parkinsonism
Exclude dementia and depression
Good medical health
Realistic expectations

made. DBS electrodes are increasingly being used to make ablative lesions in the target areas (Raoul et al., 2003). GPe DBS might also provide benefits to patients with PD and with less delay than GPi DBS, although in one study, it was associated with slightly higher frequency of dyskinesia (20% versus 9%) (Vitek et al., 2004).

As with any procedure, appropriate selection of patients as candidates for DBS surgery is critical to ensure optimal outcome (Table 7.5). Screening tools for surgical candidates have been developed and validated (Okun et al., 2004a; Tan and Jankovic, 2009). Many studies have demonstrated that patients with atypical parkinsonism, such as progressive supranuclear palsy, multiple system atrophy, or dementia with Lewy bodies, do not respond well to surgery and their symptoms may substantially worsen after surgery. Patients with atypical parkinsonism, such as multiple system atrophy, are poor candidates for surgery, and STN DBS may aggravate speech, swallowing, and gait (Tarsy et al., 2003; Lezcano et al., 2004b; Shih and Tarsy, 2007).

Since the diagnostic inaccuracy improves with follow-up, it is advisable to consider patients for surgery only when there is a considerable duration of symptoms (at least 5 years). This is reasonable considering the fact that most patients develop complications of fluctuations and dyskinesias, the chief indications for surgery, only after 5–6 years of levodopa therapy.

Besides GPi, GPe, and STN, other targets that are being explored for DBS treatment of PD include the caudal part of the zona incerta (cZI) (Plaha et al., 2006, 2008a, 2008b) and the PPN (Hamani et al., 2007; Stefani et al., 2007). Several groups have reported that the most effective target for treatment of PD lies dorsal/dorsomedial to the STN (region of the pallidofugal fibers and the rostral zona incerta) or at the junction between the dorsal border of the STN and the latter. In a study of 35 patients with PD who underwent MRI-directed implantation of 64 DBS leads into the STN (17), dorsomedial/medial to STN (20), and cZI (27), the mean adjusted contralateral UPDRS III score with cZI stimulation was 3.1 (76% reduction) compared to 4.9 (61% reduction) in the group with target dorsomedial/medial to STN, and 5.7 (55% reduction) in the STN (P value for trend <0.001) (Plaha et al., 2008a). There was a 93% improvement in tremor with cZI stimulation, but no improvement in dyskinesia scores and there was no change in levodopa dosage. The authors concluded that "High frequency stimulation of the cZI results in greater improvement in contralateral motor scores in PD patients than stimulation of the STN." The authors also showed that rest tremor of PD can be induced by 5–40 Hz stimulation of cZI (Plaha et al., 2008a) and that PD tremor, essential tremor, and other tremors may be markedly improved with low-voltage, high-frequency DBS of cZI (Plaha et al., 2008b). A pathologically proven case of cZI DBS provided evidence for effective treatment of PD symptoms with stimulation of this target (Guehl et al., 2008).

Although low-frequency (60 Hz) as compared to the standard high-frequency (130 Hz) STN stimulation has been reported to benefit freezing (Moreau et al., 2008), this PD symptom is usually refractory to both medical and surgical therapy. High-frequency STN DBS does not appear to provide additional benefit on freezing beyond levodopa (Ferraye et al., 2010).

Although PPN DBS has been reported to provide improvement in gait in monkeys, targeting this brainstem nucleus for therapeutic purposes in patients with PD or other movement disorders associated with gait difficulty will be technically challenging (Jenkinson et al., 2006). PPN has been proposed as a potential therapeutic target in patients with gait and balance difficulties, including freezing (Nashatiazadeh and Jankovic, 2008; Strafella et al., 2008; Ferraye et al., 2010; Moro et al., 2010). Six patients with unsatisfactory pharmacologic control of axial signs such as gait and postural stability underwent bilateral implantation of DBS electrodes in the STN and PPN (Stefani et al., 2007). Clinical effects were evaluated 2–6 months after surgery in the off- and on-medication state, with both STN and PPN stimulation on or off, or with only one target being stimulated. Bilateral PPN DBS at 25 Hz in off-medication produced an immediate 45% amelioration of the motor UPDRS subscale score, followed by a decline to give a final improvement of 32% in the score after 3–6 months. In contrast, bilateral STN DBS at 130–185 Hz led to about 54% improvement. PPN DBS was most effective on gait and postural items. In on-medication state, the association of STN and PPN DBS provided a significant further improvement when compared to the specific benefit mediated by the activation of either single target. Moreover, the combined DBS of both targets promoted a substantial amelioration in the performance of daily living activities. The authors felt these findings indicate that in patients with advanced PD, PPN DBS associated with standard STN DBS may be useful in improving gait and in optimizing the dopamine-mediated on-state, particularly in those whose response to STN-only DBS has deteriorated over time and may also prove useful in disorders, such as progressive supranuclear palsy. In another study, involving 6 patients with PD, unilateral PPN DBS was reported to reduce frequency of falls (Moro et al., 2010), but further studies are needed to confirm this initial finding. Patients with significant freezing of gait were not evaluated in this study, but were the subjects of other reports. In one patient, a 63-year-old man with PD-related freezing of gait, postural instability, and marked bradykinesia, PPN DBS resulted in 20% improvement in motor function, associated with increased regional cerebral blood flow in both thalami (Strafella et al., 2008). At Baylor College of Medicine, we assessed the effects of PPN DBS in three patients. Patient 1, a 59-year-old man, underwent bilateral PPN DBS with noticeable improvement in his freezing of gait 2 and 6 weeks postoperatively, but the improvement was not subsequently sustained despite adjustments of stimulating parameters (Nashatiazadeh and Jankovic, 2008). Patient 2, a 76-year-old man, previously received unsuccessful bilateral GPi DBS, but had transient improvement in freezing after DBS of the right PPN. Patient 3, a 66-year-old man, underwent isolated right PPN but developed an increase in his Gait and Balance Scale score without noticeable improvement in freezing. In all three patients DBS setting adjustments were limited by blurry vision and balance problems. Further studies are needed before PPN DBS can be routinely recommended for the treatment of gait and balance problems and freezing of gait. In a study of 6 patients with PD-related freezing of gait PPN DBS resulted in modest improvements with overall results described as "disappointing" (Ferraye et al., 2010).

DBS safety and complications

STN stimulation, while usually well tolerated, may produce ballistic and choreic dyskinesia when the voltage is increased above a given threshold, which is probably different from that produced by levodopa (Moro et al., 1999) (Video 7.6). Except for mild deficit in verbal memory and fluency, STN or GPi DBS does not appear to adversely affect cognitive performance (Pillon et al., 2000; Heo et al., 2008). In a study at Baylor College of Medicine, when 23 patients undergoing bilateral STN DBS were compared with 28 treated medically at 6 months after surgery, the DBS patients were found to have mild but significant declines in verbal recall and fluency and mild decline in frontostriatal cognitive measures, even when good motor outcome was achieved (York et al., 2008). When followed for 2 years, the STN DBS patients demonstrated significant impairments in verbal memory, oral information processing speed, and language (Williams et al., 2010). Additionally, one-third of the STN DBS patients declined on confrontational naming compared to none of the PD patients, and one-third of the STN DBS patients progressed to PD dementia 2 years following STN DBS compared to none in the PD group. These results are consistent with the more recent reports on STN DBS that have found long-term deficits in multiple cognitive domains, including memory, attention, and frontostriatal functioning following STN DBS when more comprehensive neuropsychologic measures were administered (Contarino et al., 2007). In one controlled study 60 patients were randomly assigned to receive STN DBS and 63 to have best medical treatment. After 6 months, DBS-treated patients showed mild but significantly more evidence of impairments in executive function and verbal fluency, irrespective of the improvement in quality of life (Witt et al., 2008). In contrast, anxiety was reduced in the DBS group compared with the medication group. Based on data collected from eight advanced PD patients, mean age 56.5 years, during off-medication periods, significant declines in cognitive and motor function were found under modest dual-task conditions with bilateral but not with unilateral STN DBS (Alberts et al., 2008). Impaired performance in verbal fluency associated with STN DBS has been correlated with decreased regional cerebral blood flow in the left frontotemporal areas as measured by PET (Schroeder et al., 2003). While many studies have concluded that cognitive function is unchanged with STN DBS (Tröster et al., 1997; Ardouin et al., 1999;

Gerschlager et al., 1999; Vingerhoets et al., 1999; Pillon et al., 2000; Daniele et al., 2003), even after 3 years (Funkiewiez et al., 2004), or only slightly declines even after 5 years (Contarino et al., 2007), other studies have found declines in working memory and response inhibition performance (Hershey et al., 2004), impaired frontal executive function, particularly in older patients, reduced verbal fluency, impaired naming speed, reduced selective attention, and delayed verbal recall (Saint-Cyr et al., 2000; Woods et al., 2006). Although the presence of dementia is considered a contraindication to DBS, cognitive function apparently improved in a patient with PD dementia with bilateral stimulation of the nucleus basalis of Meynert and STN (Freund et al., 2009). Further studies, however, are necessary before this approach can be recommended for patients with PD and cognitive deficit.

Several studies have reported changes in mood and behavior after DBS. Emotional lability and psychiatric complications, found in about 9% of patients after STN DBS, have been found in one prospective study with a control group consisting of PD patients without DBS (Smeding et al., 2006). In another study, bilateral STN DBS was associated with moderate improvement in tasks of prefrontal function and obsessive-compulsive behavior (Mallet et al., 2002, 2008) but moderate deterioration in verbal memory and prefrontal and visuospatial function (Alegret et al., 2001). While some patients have experienced euphoria, mania, infectious laughter, and hilarity with STN DBS (Krack et al., 2001; Kulisevsky et al., 2002), others have experienced depression and other mood changes, aggressive behavior (posteromedial hypothalamus), pseudobulbar crying (Okun et al., 2004b), and other psychiatric problems (Bejjani et al., 2002; Berney et al., 2002; Mayberg and Lozano, 2002), and some have noted improvement in psychiatric symptoms, particularly obsessive-compulsive disorder (Mallet et al., 2002, 2008; Tye et al., 2009). STN DBS may occasionally lead to increased impulsivity, similar to pathological gambling seen in patients treated with dopamine agonists, which may possibly be due to impaired ability to self-modulate decision processes and cognitive control (Frank et al., 2007; Stamey and Jankovic, 2008; Hälbig et al., 2009). The neuropsychologic and neuropsychiatric issues of DBS have been of increasing interest and concern and have been the topic of several reviews (Parsons et al., 2006; Saint-Cyr and Albanese, 2006; Voon et al., 2006; Appleby et al., 2007; Heo et al., 2008; Witt et al., 2008; Le Jeune et al., 2009). A meta-analysis of 10-year experience with DBS has concluded that the prevalence of depression was 2–4%, mania 0.9–1.7%, emotional changes 0.1–0.2%, and suicidal ideation/suicide attempt 0.3–0.7% (completed suicide rate was 0.16–0.32% over 2.4 years, compared to 0.02% annual suicide rate in the United States) (Appleby et al., 2007). Other studies have drawn attention to apathy (Le Jeune et al., 2009) and suicidal behavior as a potential hazard of STN DBS (Soulas et al., 2008; Voon et al., 2008). A survey of 75 DBS surgical centers representing four continents, 55 of which responded, indicated that out of a total of 5311 patients, 24 (0.45%) completed and 48 (0.90%) attempted suicide (Voon et al., 2008). The mean interval after surgery for all events was 17.8 months (range 1–48 months for completed suicides, 0.25–100 months for attempts), and 75% of all events occurred within this interval. The suicide rate in the first postoperative year was approximately 10 times the expected rate, adjusted for age, gender, and country, and remained elevated at 4 years. The risk of suicide correlated with postoperative depression, single marital status, and impulse control disorder. Although the rate of suicide following epilepsy surgery is even higher (1%), according to the authors "the baseline suicide rate [among patients with epilepsy] is eight times higher than the general population, [while] baseline Parkinson's disease suicide rates range from the same to as much as ten times lower than the general population." Transient mania also has been reported as an adverse effect of DBS, particularly involving the medial portion of the STN (Raucher-Chéné et al., 2008). STN DBS has been found to also improve autonomic dysfunction, including orthostatic hypotension, associated with PD (Stemper et al., 2006). Psychogenic tremor following DBS surgery for ET has been reported in one case (McKeon et al., 2008).

Hypophonia and dysarthria were reported to be the most frequent long term effects of STN DBS (Romito et al., 2002). Dysarthria, observed as a side effect more with left than right STN DBS (Santens et al., 2003), may develop despite improved oral control of jaw, lips, and tongue movements (Pinto et al., 2003). While some individual components of speech may improve with STN DBS, most studies have shown that speech either fails to improve or deteriorates with STN DBS (Klostermann et al., 2008).

Several studies have now demonstrated a significant weight gain in patients with STN DBS (Montaurier et al., 2007). In one study, there was a 3.4 ± 0.6 kg body weight increase, associated with a significant decrease in energy expenditures, $-7.3 \pm 2.2\%$ in men and $-13.1 \pm 1.7\%$ in women ($P < 0.01$), associated with a gain primarily in fat-free mass in men and fat in women. In another study 32.1% of patients showed about 15% increase in body weight and a mean body mass index increase of 24.7 kg/m^2 in 1 year (Barichella et al., 2003).

While over half of patients initially considered to be DBS failures eventually had good results, 34% had persistently poor outcomes despite optimal management (Okun et al., 2005). In one study of 100 patients who were implanted with a total of 191 STN DBS devices, there were 7 (3.7%) device infections, 1 cerebral infarct, 1 intracerebral hematoma, 1 subdural hematoma, 2 (1%) skin erosions, 3 (1.6%) periprocedural seizures, and 6 (3.1%) brain electrode revisions (Goodman et al., 2006). There were 13 (6.8%) patients with postoperative confusion and 16 (8.4%) had battery failures, but there were no surgical deaths or permanent new neurologic deficits. The frequency of intraoperative complications associated with implantation of DBS was found to be 4.2% (11/262) and during a 3-year follow-up the frequency of hardware-related complications was 13.9% (25/180) (Voges et al., 2006). A total of 319 patients underwent DBS implantation at Baylor College of Medicine, Houston, Texas over a 10-year period, 182 of whom suffered from medically refractory PD; the other patients had essential tremor (113), dystonia (18), and other hyperkinetic movement disorders (6) (Kenney et al., 2007b) (Table 7.6). Intraoperative adverse effects were rare: vasovagal response in 8 patients (2.5%), syncope in 4 (1.3%), severe cough in 3 (0.9%), transient ischemic attack in 1 (0.3%), arrhythmia in 1 (0.3%), and confusion in 1 (0.3%). Perioperative adverse effects included headache in 48

Table 7.6 Safety data related to deep brain stimulation at Baylor College of Medicine and The Methodist Hospital

- Of the 319 patients treated with DBS (Baylor/Methodist) between 1995 and 2005, 182 had PD; the other patients had ET (112), dystonia (19), and other hyperkinetic movement disorders (6)
- Intraoperative adverse events (AEs) included vasovagal response in 8 patients (2.5%), syncope in 4 (1.2%), severe cough in 3 (0.9%), transient ischemic attack in 1 (0.3%), arrhythmia in 1 (0.3%), and confusion in 1 (0.3%)
- Perioperative AEs included headache in 48 patients (15%), confusion in 16 (5%), and hallucinations in 9 (2.8%)
- Intraoperative/perioperative AEs included isolated seizure in 4 patients (1.2%), intracerebral hemorrhage in 2 (0.6%), intraventricular hemorrhage in 2 (0.6%), and a large subdural hematoma in 1 (0.3%)
- Persistent long-term complications of DBS surgery included dysarthria (4%), worsening gait (3.8%), cognitive dysfunction (4%), and infection (4.4%)
- Revisions were required in 25 patients (7.8%) for the following reasons: loss of effect, lack of efficacy, infection, lead fracture, and lead migration
- Hardware-related complications included 12 lead fractures and 10 lead migrations
- Conclusions: based on the 10-year experience, DBS has proven to be safe for the treatment of medically refractory movement disorders

From Kenney C, Simpson R, Hunter C, et al. Short-term and long-term safety of deep brain stimulation in the treatment of movement disorders. J Neurosurg 2007;106:621–625.

patients (15.0%), confusion in 16 (5.0%), and hallucinations in 9 (2.8%). The most serious intraoperative/ perioperative adverse effects occurred in 4 (1.3%) patients with an isolated seizure, 2 (0.6%) patients with intracerebral hemorrhage, 2 (0.6%) patients with intraventricular hemorrhage, and 1 (0.3%) patient with a large subdural hematoma (Kenney et al., 2007b). Long-term complications of DBS surgery included dysarthria (4.0%), worsening gait (3.7%), cognitive decline (4.0%), and infection (4.4%). Hyperhidrosis has been reported in a single case as a complication of thalamic stimulation for essential tremor (Diamond et al., 2007a). Revisions were completed in 25 (7.8%) patients for several reasons: loss of effect, lack of efficacy, infection, lead fracture, and lead migration. In another study of 60 patients who underwent 96 DBS-related procedures, followed over a period of 43.7 months (range 6–78 months), 18 (30%) developed 28 adverse events, requiring 28 electrodes to be replaced (Paluzzi et al., 2006b). The rate of adverse events per electrode-year was 8%. Hardware-related complications included 12 lead fractures and 10 lead migrations. In one study 25.6% of all 215 patients with DBS presented to the emergency department (ED) at least once for various reasons including neurologic (54.6%) such as headache (22.1%), change in mental status (15.1%), and syncope (9.3%), followed by infections/hardware issues (27.9%), orthopedic/focal problems (10.5%), and medical issues (7%) (Resnick et al., 2010). Several other studies have addressed DBS-related complications (Morishita et al., 2010).

Knowledge and skills needed to prevent and troubleshoot problems, such as a non-ideal initial DBS candidate, inadequate multidisciplinary team care, failure of perceived expectations, DBS procedural complication, hardware complication, suboptimal lead placement, programming, access to care, disease progression, and tolerance/habituation, are critical to the optimal response to DBS and to prevent potential "DBS failures" (Okun et al., 2008). Postoperative issues including outcomes and complications have been summarized in recent reviews (Deuschl et al., 2006a; Kleiner-Fisman et al., 2006; Voges et al., 2007; Hariz et al., 2008b; Videnovic and Metman, 2008).

Chronic stimulation appears to be well tolerated, and the risk of local gliosis is minimal (Caparros-Lefebvre et al., 1994; Haberler et al., 2000; Henderson et al., 2002), although more extensive damage has been rarely reported (Henderson et al., 2001). Electron microscopy examination of tissue adherent to the explanted electrode revealed foreign body multinucleate giant cell-type (some larger than 100 μm) reaction, possibly representing a response to the polyurethane component of the DBS electrode (Moss et al., 2004). Very few studies have addressed the rate and type of complications associated with DBS. During a mean follow-up period of 33 months and the cumulative follow-up of 217 patient-years of 84 consecutive cases, Oh and colleagues (2002) found that 20 patients (25.3%) had 26 hardware-related complications involving 23 (18.5%) of the electrodes. These comprised 4 lead fractures, 4 lead migrations, 3 short or open circuits, 12 erosions and/or infections, 2 foreign body reactions, and 1 cerebrospinal fluid leak. In addition, the hardware-related complication rate per electrode-year was 8.4%.

Several studies have addressed the safety concerns related to performance of MRI scans in patients with implanted DBS devices. Standard and functional MRI scans have been performed in many patients with implanted DBS without significant complications (Jech et al., 2001; Tagliati et al., 2009) (Table 7.7). In a survey of medical directors of National Parkinson Foundation Centers of Excellence, data on MRI safety was available on 3304 PD patients with one or more DBS leads; DBS patients had MRI of other body regions. No complications were reported except in one case in which MRI of the brain was associated with an IPG failure with no neurologic sequelae (Tagliati et al., 2009). Diathermy treatment, which involved pulse-modulated radiofrequency to the maxilla, in a 70-year-old patient with PD implanted with ITREL model 7424 in the STN, resulted in permanent diencephalic and brainstem lesions and a vegetative state (Nutt et al., 2001a). This tragic complication probably resulted from induction of radiofrequency current and heating of the electrodes, leading to the edema surrounding the DBS electrode. Although no serious complications have been reported in women with implanted DBS during pregnancy or delivery (Paluzzi et al., 2006a), the use of electrocautery during delivery by cesarean section should be used cautiously.

To improve the safety and efficacy of DBS, it is important to continue advancing our understanding of the mechanisms underlying DBS and to build on and improve DBS technology (e.g., develop directional electrodes, prolonging battery life, allow remote and "smart" programming).

Table 7.7 Results of a safety survey on MRI in patients with DBS devices

- Investigators from 40 of 42 (95%) National Parkinson Foundation Centers of Excellence (COEs) completed the survey
- 23 (58%) reported that they were currently performing brain MRI in DBS patients; 3 (7.5%) had done it in the past
- The 17 COEs currently not performing postoperative MRI for DBS listed the following reasons:
  - Industry guidelines and/or warning (53%)
  - Defer clinical decision to outside department (29%)
  - Liability/risk/safety (18%)
  - No active DBS program (18%)
  - No available MRI (12%)
  - Insurance and reimbursement concerns (6%)
- A total of 3304 PD patients with one or more DBS leads had a brain MRI scan, and 177 DBS patients had MRI of other body regions
- In one case MRI was associated with an IPG failure without neurological sequelae after IPG replacement. No other complications were reported.
- Conclusions: These data provide evidence for a favorable risk/benefit ratio for brain MRI in patients with DBS implants. We suggest that the current safety guidelines be re-examined given this large and positive experience.

From Tagliati M, Jankovic J, Pagan F, et al.; National Parkinson Foundation DBS Working Group. Safety of MRI in patients with implanted deep brain stimulation devices. Neuroimage 2009;47(Suppl 2):T53–T57.

Deep brain stimulation for hyperkinetic and other disorders

Dystonia

GPi DBS also has been reported to be effective in patients with primary generalized dystonia (Krauss et al., 1999; Kumar et al., 1999a; Coubes et al., 2000; Tronnier et al., 2000; Brin et al., 2001; Krack and Vercueil, 2001; Muta et al., 2001; Vercueil et al., 2001; Albright, 2003; Coubes et al., 2004; Diamond et al., 2006; Vidailhet et al., 2005; Jankovic, 2006; Kupsch et al., 2006; Jankovic, 2007; Vidailhet et al., 2007; Kenney and Jankovic, 2008; Isaias et al., 2008, 2009), segmental dystonia (Wohrle et al., 2003), cervical dystonia (Bereznai et al., 2002; Krauss et al., 2002), blepharospasm-oromandibular (cranial) dystonia (Capelle et al., 2003; Foote et al., 2005; Vagefi et al., 2008), tardive dyskinesia (Eltahawy et al., 2004a; Lenders et al., 2005), and tardive dystonia (Trottenberg et al., 2001b, 2005; Cohen et al., 2007; Sako et al., 2008; Gruber et al., 2009). Vercueil and colleagues (2001) described ten patients with bilateral GPi DBS; five had a major improvement, two had a moderated improvement and one had a minor improvement after 14 months. They concluded that GPi DBS is much more effective than thalamic DBS for the treatment of dystonia. In a 2-year follow-up of 31 patients with primary generalized dystonia, Coubes and colleagues (2004) noted a mean improvement in the clinical and functional Burke–Fahn–Marsden Dystonia Rating Scale (BFMDRS) of 79% and 65%, respectively. There was no difference in response between DYT1-positive and DYT1-negative patients, but the magnitude of improvement was greater in children than in adults.

In a presentation during the seventh International Congress of Parkinson's Disease and Movement Disorders in Miami in November 2002, Coubes provided data on 68 patients with generalized dystonia, 78% with primary dystonia, 19 of whom were DYT1-positive, and 29% with secondary dystonia, treated with GPi DBS. The MRI-guided, single-tract, bilateral implantation showed an overall 80% improvement, and this was most robust in primary, DYT1 dystonias and in the pantothenate kinase-associated neurodegeneration cases. Primary dystonia clearly responds better than secondary dystonia to either pallidotomy or GPi DBS, although patients with pantothenate kinase-associated neurodegeneration also experience marked improvement in their dystonia (Coubes et al., 2000; Eltahawy et al., 2004b; Castelnau et al., 2005). Essentially all patients achieved steady state in 6 weeks. The improvement was particularly noticeable in the rapid ("ballistic") dystonic movements, pain, and bradykinesia, but there was no effect on the slow dystonia or associated bradykinesia. Except for implantable pulse generator infection in three patients and lead fracture and other lead problems in two patients, there were no other complications. The stimulating parameters were as follows: pulse rate was 450 µs, frequency was 130 Hz, and amplitude was 0.8–1.6 V. In a prospective, multicenter study of 22 patients with generalized dystonia, 7 of whom had DYT1 mutation, the BFMDRS score improved after bilateral GPi DBS from a mean of 46.3 ± 21.3 to 21.0 ± 14.1 at 12 months ($P < 0.001$) (Vidailhet et al., 2005). A "blinded" review of the videos at 3 months showed improvement with stimulation from a mean of 34.63 ± 12.3 to 24.6 ± 17.7. The improvement in mean dystonia motor scores was 51%, and one-third of the patients improved more than 75% compared to preoperative scores. In addition, there was a significant improvement in health-related quality of life as measured by the SF-36, but there was no change in cognition or mood. Although the sample was rather small, the authors were not able to find any predictors of response such as DYT1 gene status, anatomic distribution of the dystonia, or location of the electrodes. Patients with a phasic form of dystonia improved more than those with tonic contractions and posturing. The maximum benefit was not achieved in some patients until 3–6 months after surgery. In a 3-year follow-up, motor improvement observed at 1 year (51%) was maintained at 3 years (58%) and the authors concluded that "bilateral pallidal stimulation provides sustained motor benefit after 3 years" (Vidailhet et al., 2007). In a study involving French centers, bilateral DBS of ventral GPi was associated with a 42% reduction in the BFMDRS score; whereas DBS of dorsal GPi resulted in less predictable effects (Houeto et al., 2007). In a retrospective review of 40 patients with primary generalized dystonia who had been treated by bilateral GPi DBS followed for up to 8 years, the most important predictors of poor response were high preoperative BFMDRS score, older age at surgery, and small GPi volume, but no significant correlation was found between the electrical parameters used and the mean motor scores (Vasques et al., 2009).

Neurophysiologic studies at the time of the implantation of stimulating electrodes or during chronic stimulation have provided insights into the pathophysiology of dystonia and how DBS alleviates the involuntary muscle contractions. Based on a study of 15 patients with primary dystonia treated with bilateral pallidal stimulation, modulation of oscillatory local field potentials (LFPs) were recorded from pallidal electrodes and were correlated with surface electromyography of the affected muscles (Liu et al., 2008). Dystonic movements were associated with increased theta, alpha and low beta activity and the strength of the contraction correlated with an increase in frequency range of 3–20 Hz; the increase preceded the spasms by about 320 ms. There was a significant decrease in LFP synchronization at 8–20 Hz during sensory modulation, but voluntary movement increased gamma band activity (30–90 Hz). It has been suggested that DBS alleviates the hypertonic activity by desynchronizing these excessive synchronized discharges. In six patients treated for their dystonia with bilateral GPi DBS, the contralateral prefrontal overactivity was reduced (Detante et al., 2004). Kupsch et al. (2006) compared GPi DBS with sham stimulation in a randomized, controlled clinical trial of 40 patients with primary segmental or generalized dystonia. The primary endpoint was the change from baseline to 3 months in the severity of symptoms, according to the movement subscore on the BFMDRS. Two investigators who were unaware of treatment status assessed the severity of dystonia by reviewing videotaped sessions. Three months after randomization, the change from baseline in the mean (±SD) movement score was significantly greater in the neurostimulation group (−15.8 ± 14.1 points) than in the sham-stimulation group (−1.4 ± 3.8 points, $P < 0.001$). Similar results were obtained in other centers (Krause et al., 2004).

Targeting the posteroventral GPi seems to provide the most robust benefits in patients with dystonia (Tisch et al., 2007). It is of interest that an ablative lesion or high-frequency stimulation of the GPi can both produce and improve dystonia, suggesting that it is the pattern of discharge in the basal ganglia rather than the actual location or frequency of discharge that is pathophysiologically relevant to dystonia (Münchau et al., 2000). In one patient, a 49-year-old woman with severe generalized dystonia, bilateral GPi DBS produced an immediate improvement in dystonia, which was associated with a reduction in PET activation in certain cortical motor areas that are usually overactive in dystonia (Kumar et al., 1999a). Bilateral GPi DBS has been found effective not only in distal or generalized dystonia, but also in patients with cervical dystonia (Krauss et al., 1999; Kulisevsky et al., 2000; Parkin et al., 2001). In a report of two patients with cervical dystonia, bilateral GPi DBS produced more improvement in pain than in motor symptoms (Kulisevsky et al., 2000). Parkin and colleagues (2001) reported progressive improvement in pain and posture in three patients with cervical dystonia. A prospective, single-blind, multicenter study assessing the efficacy and safety of bilateral GPi DBS in 10 patients with severe, chronic, medication-resistant cervical dystonia found that the Toronto Western Spasmodic Torticollis Rating Scale (TWSTRS) severity score improved from a mean (SD) of 14.7 (4.2) before surgery to 8.4 (4.4) at 12 months postoperatively ($P = 0.003$) (Kiss et al., 2007). The disability and pain scores also improved, as did general health and physical functioning and depression scores.

GPi DBS has been also reported to improve cranial-cervical dystonia in selected cases (Ostrem et al., 2007; Blomstedt et al., 2008; Pretto et al., 2008; Markaki et al., 2010). While bilateral GPi DBS may improve symptoms of dystonia, motor function in non-dystonic body parts may worsen (Ostrem et al., 2007). Muta and colleagues (2001) described a 61-year-old woman with cranial dystonia manifested chiefly as blepharospasm, facial grimacing, cervical dystonia, and spasmodic dysphonia who had previously failed to improve with bilateral thalamotomy but who had marked improvement in all aspects of her dystonia with bilateral GPi DBS, including complete resolution of blepharospasm and oromandibular dystonia. In a blinded review of videos of 13 patients with segmental dystonia caused by various etiologies and different distributions (4 with cranial dystonia), GPi DBS was associated with global subjective gains and notable objective improvement in 11 of 13, but the response was quite variable and unpredictable (Pretto et al., 2008). The pattern of recurrence of segmental dystonia after discontinuation of GPi DBS was studied in 8 patients (Grips et al., 2007). Phasic dystonia appeared within a few minutes but the tonic form of dystonia recurred with a more variable delay. Some patients obtain optimal improvement with lower-than-usual stimulation frequency (80–100 Hz) (Alterman et al., 2007). GPi DBS is gaining acceptance as the surgical treatment of choice not only in adult patients with dystonia but also in children (Alterman et al., 2007).

Tourette syndrome

There has been increasing interest in DBS as a treatment of medically intractable or malignant Tourette syndrome (TS) (Cheung et al., 2007). Because of prior success with thalamic ablation in the treatment of severe TS reported in 1970 by Hassler and Dieckman, recently translated from French (Rickards et al., 2008), most investigators use the original report as a rationale for selecting the thalamus as the target in ablative and DBS treatment of TS. In 1999, thalamic DBS was introduced for intractable TS, but since then, multiple targets have been used with relatively comparable results (Ackermans et al., 2008). Globus pallidus has been increasingly used as the target in patients with disabling tics because of the long-term experience with this target in the treatment of other hyperkinetic movement disorders, such as dystonia and levodopa-induced dyskinesia (Diederich et al., 2005). In a 16-year-old boy with disabling, medically intractable TS, bilateral GPi DBS resulted in 63% improvement in Yale Global Tic Severity Scale, 85% improvement in Tic Symptom Self Report, and 51% improvement in SF-36, a quality of life measure (Shahed et al., 2007). Furthermore, the patient was able to return to school. Several other reports confirmed that GPi is an effective target for the treatment of TS (Dehning et al., 2008). Although these observations must be confirmed by a controlled trial before DBS can be recommended even to severely affected patients, it suggests that stimulation of certain targets involved in the limbic striato-pallidal-thalamo-cortical system may be beneficial in the treatment of various aspects of TS. In TS, perhaps even more importantly than in other movement disorders, appropriate screening, and accurate and comprehensive assessment of not only tics but also behavioral comorbidities is absolutely critical in patient selection for DBS (Mink et al., 2006). Surgery for treatment of TS is discussed in more detail in Chapter 16 (Porta et al., 2009; Ackermans et al., 2011).

Other Indications for DBS

The expanding use of DBS in the treatment of various disorders could provide insights into the pathophysiology of other disorders (Benabid et al., 2000). In addition to the hyperkinetic movement disorders already discussed, DBS may be useful in patients with severe chorea associated with Huntington disease. Bilateral GPi was found to control chorea and markedly improved the quality of life in a 60-year-old man with a 10-year history of Huntington disease (Biolsi et al., 2008). Bilteral GPi DBS has been also reported to produce about 24.4% improvement in the Burke–Fahn–Marsden scale in adult patients with dystonia–choreoathetosis associated with cerebral palsy (Vidailhet et al., 2009). It has been also found to be helpful in patients with neurodegeneration with brain iron accumulation (NBIA), although not as much as in patients with primary dystonia (Timmermann et al., 2010).

In addition to VIM as a target for patients with disabling tremor, STN DBS has been also found to be useful in the treatment of severe proximal tremor (Kitagawa et al., 2000) as well as rest and postural tremor in PD (Sturman et al., 2004).

The observation that stimulation of the substantia nigra precipitates acute depression (Bejjani et al., 1999) or mania (Ulla et al., 2006) that resolves immediately when the DBS is turned off suggests that the nigrothalamic pathway may play an important role in bipolar disorder. Besides left substantia nigra stimulation (Bejjani et al., 1999), stimulation superior and lateral to the right STN also produced mood changes (dysphoria) (Stefurak et al., 2003). Stimulation of white matter adjacent to the subgenual cingulated region (Brodmann area 25), which is metabolically overactive in treatment-resistant depression, has been found to be effective in treating depression in four of six patients (Mayberg et al., 2005).

Other emerging applications of DBS include treatment of obsessive-compulsive disorder targeting chiefly the ventral anterior limb of the internal capsule and adjacent ventral striatum or STN (Gabriels et al., 2003; Nuttin et al., 2003; Mallet et al., 2008; Greenberg et al., 2010), as well as various pain disorders, including migraines and cluster headaches (Leone et al., 2003) (Table 7.8).

Table 7.8 Current and potential indications for deep brain stimulation

- Suppression of tremor: essential tremor, Parkinson disease, multiple sclerosis, Wilson disease, cerebellar outflow, post-traumatic
- Parkinson disease (bilateral STN, GPi, GPe, cZI, PPN)
  - ↑ "On time" (without dyskinesias)
  - Improves cardinal signs and dyskinesia
  - Improves quality of "off"
  - Improves QoL; ↓levodopa dosage
  - Neuroprotective?
- Dystonia
- Tourette syndrome
- Spasticity
- Epilepsy
- Pain, cluster headaches
- Depression
- Obesity
- Addiction
- Obsessive-compulsive disorder

Vagus nerve and other stimulation procedures

On the basis of the observation that vagus nerve stimulation has a nonspecific "calming" effect in treated epileptic patients and that it suppresses harmaline-induced tremor in rats (Handforth and Krahl, 2001), a multicenter trial was conducted to study the effects of vagus nerve stimulation in patients with essential and parkinsonian tremor, but no meaningful benefit was demonstrated (Handforth et al., 2003). Encouraged by the initial reports of prefrontal rapid-rate, repetitive transcranial magnetic stimulation in PD and despite lack of effect in more recent studies (Ghabra et al., 1999), some investigators have tried extradural motor cortex simulation using a quadripolar electrostimulator and reported bilateral benefits in PD motor signs and in dyskinesias (Canavero and Paolotti, 2000; Arle and Shils, 2008). The results of these preliminary studies, however, must be confirmed by a larger study before this procedure can be considered as a potential treatment in PD.

Brain grafting

Neurotransplantation using fetal nigral tissue as a treatment for PD was introduced after laboratory studies demonstrated that grafts of fetal dopaminergic neurons can survive for long periods in the host striatum, that they are capable of forming synapses with striatal neurons, and that they actually produce dopamine (Freed et al., 1992; Freeman et al., 1995; Collier and Kordower, 1998; Hauser et al., 1999; Lindvall, 1999). Ventral mesencephalic grafts into parkinsonian animal models have been found to improve not only parkinsonian features but also levodopa-induced dyskinesias (Lee et al., 2000). Initial results of clinical trials have been inconsistent, and only moderate improvement has been observed. The variable results have been thought to be due to differences in surgical methods, the age and the amount of donor tissue, methods of storage, the site of implantation, and the distribution of the tissue within the target region (Hauser et al., 1999). Controlled trials designed to determine the efficacy of fetal nigral transplantation are currently underway, but ethical concerns about the justification of sham operations, employed in these trials, have generated a lively controversy. Inclusion of sham surgery in design of clinical trials is, however, gaining more and more acceptance not only among investigators, but also among patients, particularly those who are more educated (Frank et al., 2008). Fetal tissue is generally obtained from elective abortions at postgestational ages ranging between 6 and 9 weeks. The tissue must be screened for infections and is implanted stereotactically in the striatum. Commonly, the putamen is chosen as the target site, sometimes in combination with the caudate. The donor tissue may be delivered via several needle tracts, either unilaterally or bilaterally. Tissue of up to eight fetal donors is grafted per patient. Whether cyclosporine or other immunosuppressants are needed has not yet been determined.

Although the initial results were encouraging, subsequent controlled studies have failed to show any meaningful benefit from neuronal grafting, and in one study, more than half of the implanted patients experienced "off" dyskinesias (Freed et al., 1992; Sawle et al., 1992; Spencer et al., 1992;

Peschanski et al., 1994; Freeman et al., 1995; Wenning et al., 1997; Lindvall, 1998; Hauser et al., 1999; Lindvall, 1999; Freed et al., 2001b; Olanow, 2002; Mendez et al., 2005). Improvement is commonly noted between 1 and 3 months postoperatively. In single patients, functional improvement has been demonstrated up to 46 months postoperatively (Freed et al., 1992). Several patients were able to markedly reduce or even discontinue their dopaminergic drugs. Additional improvements have been noted after sequential bilateral transplantation (Hagell et al., 1999). [^{18}F]fluorodopa PET scans have demonstrated increased uptake following fetal transplants (Sawle et al., 1992; Freeman et al., 1995; Hauser et al., 1999), but this method has been challenged (Martin and Perlmutter, 1994). In one report, a patient received a unilateral fetal implant in 1989, with "gradual, major clinical improvement" over 3 years. Levodopa was withdrawn at 32 months, and immunosuppression was stopped at 64 months (Piccini et al., 1999). In the grafted putamen, the [^{11}C]-raclopride PET had normalized by 3 years with minor increases thereafter, while the untreated side showed gradual decline. While the untreated side showed increased raclopride (D2) binding (indicative of upregulation of receptors), the grafted side showed normal levels of binding. Following administration of amphetamine, which promotes dopamine release, the untreated side showed no decrease in raclopride binding, while the grafted side had a decrease in binding (due to competition from dopamine) equivalent to nondiseased controls.

Freed and colleagues (2001b) reported the results of the first double-blind placebo-controlled trial of fetal graft transplantation for advanced PD. Forty patients, stratified by age into younger than 60 years and older than 60 years, with about a 7-year history of PD symptoms, were randomized to receive either four embryonic mesencephalons delivered via four needle passes to the left and right putamen or a sham operation (four drill holes to the forehead without dural penetration). After 1 year, the "sham" patients were given the option to be implanted and were then followed in an open-label manner; a total of 33 patients received an implant. Overall, there was no difference between the implanted and sham patients with respect to the primary outcome variable, a global rating by the patients (from −3, PD markedly worse, to +3, PD markedly improved). There was, however, a significant improvement in bradykinesia and rigidity, but only in the younger (<60 years old) patients. There was no improvement in freezing or motor fluctuations, and gait actually deteriorated. Although there were more adverse events in the implanted group, these were not considered directly related to the surgery. There was a marked placebo effect, sometimes lasting the whole year. Of the 20 implanted patients, 17 had evidence of fiber outgrowth from the transplanted tissue, as indicated by ^{18}F-fluorodopa PET scans, but there was no correlation between the PET results and the UPDRS, except in the younger patient group. In a 1-year follow-up, a blinded PET study showed that patient age did not affect viability of the implant, but only in the younger group was there significant correlation between ^{18}F-fluorodopa putaminal uptake and an improved UPDRS score for bradykinesia, though not tremor or rigidity (Nakamura et al., 2001). Most important, 5 of 33 patients who eventually received the implant experienced dyskinesias even during "off" periods, which correlates with increased F-dopa uptake

on PET scans (Ma et al., 2002). GPi DBS improved these "runaway dyskinesias" in three of the five patients (Freed et al., 2001a) and in other patients (Graff-Radford et al., 2006). In the second, National Institutes of Health funded, controlled trial of fetal transplants, 34 patients were randomized to receive bilateral grafting into the posterior putamen of four or one fetal tissue per side or sham surgery (partial burr hole without penetration of the dura) (Olanow et al., 2003). All patients received immunosuppression for 6 months after surgery and were followed for 24 months. Thirty-one patients completed the trial; two died during the trial, and three died afterward, from causes unrelated to the procedure. There was no significant overall treatment effect, but the patients with milder PD did show significant improvement ($P = 0.006$). PET results indicated a significant dose-dependent increase versus baseline in fluorodopa uptake, with no change in placebo patients and an approximate one-third increase in patients receiving four tissues. Despite these histochemical and imaging improvements, no significant differences were seen in clinical measures. Increase (worsening) from baseline in the UPDRS motor score while off medication was 9.4 for placebo, 3.5 for one tissue, and −0.72 for four tissues ($P = 0.096$ for four versus placebo). Although treated patients improved for approximately 9 months, they then worsened. There was no difference between implanted and sham patients in "on" time without dyskinesias, total "off" time, ADL scores, or levodopa dose required. No placebo patients, but 13 of 23 (56%) treated patients, developed off-medication dyskinesias. The authors concluded that "Fetal nigral transplantation currently cannot be recommended as a therapy for PD based on these results." The off-medication dyskinesias emerged about 5 months after transplant, with legs being more frequently affected in a stereotypic, repetitive manner, similar to the pattern observed in diphasic dyskinesias (Olanow et al., 2009a). "Off" period dyskinesias were also reported in all 14 PD patients at a mean of 40 months following fetal transplants performed in Europe (Hagell et al., 1999). Many of these patients required GPi DBS, which markedly improved the "off" dyskinesias as well as levodopa dyskinesias (Herzog et al., 2008).

Limitations of both of the National Institutes of Health sponsored studies have been reviewed (Winkler et al., 2005). Subsequent analysis suggested that younger patients and those with milder disease, particularly if immunosuppressed for more than 6 months, had more robust benefit. Both studies demonstrated a marked placebo effect and highlighted the need for controlled trials in assessing surgical interventions (McRae et al., 2004). Survival of the human grafts can be prolonged by administering the lazaroid tirilazad mesylate, a lipid peroxidation inhibitor, into the graft tissue (Brundin et al., 2000) or possibly by immunosuppression, although postmortem studies performed 3–4 years after implants found that the grafts are only mildly immunogenic to the host brain (Mendez et al., 2005). Serious neurologic complications of neurotransplantation have occurred in 1–2% of cases and may include intracerebral hemorrhage (Hauser et al., 1999). There is also a potential risk of transmission of infectious vectors.

Besides the in-vivo evidence of graft survival, neuropathologic studies also provide evidence of graft survival and striatal reinnervation up to 16 years after transplantation of fetal mesencephalic tissue (Kordower et al., 1995; Collier and Kordower, 1998; Kordower et al., 2008a, 2008b; Morley and Duda, 2009). In one case, Lewy-body-like inclusions that stained positively for α-synuclein and ubiquitin were found in nigral neurons grafted into the striatum 14 and 16 years earlier (Kordower et al., 2008a, 2008b; Brundin et al., 2008; Li et al., 2010). These findings suggest that the disease can propagate from host to graft cells and have implications for future cell-based therapies (Braak and Del Tredici, 2008). Furthermore, there is no evidence that the grafted cells will innervate nondopaminergic regions that are known to be damaged in PD (Olanow et al., 2009b). However, no microglial infiltration or any other pathologic changes were noted in five other patients who underwent fetal midbrain suspension grafts (Mendez et al., 2008). Later studies showed that α-synuclein may be transported via endocytosis to neighboring neurons and forms Lewy-like inclusions (Desplats et al., 2009). Furthermore, there is some evidence that α-synuclein acts like a prion (Olanow and Prusiner, 2009). Indeed, the propagation of synuclein pathology from caudal brainstem (Braak and Del Tredici, 2008) has been linked to oligomerization and propagation of beta-sheet, similar to prion, although it is not clear how the spread would skip important brainstem structures such as the oculomotor nuclei, spared in PD.

Observations that cell division can occur in an adult brain have led to speculations that stem cell technology could be applied to neurodegenerative diseases, including PD (Barker, 2002; Bjorklund et al., 2002). One of the most exciting areas of current research is the potential use of cultured, well-characterized stem cells or adult bone marrow cells, with the ability to generate neurons and glia, for therapeutic applications in PD. This interest has been fueled by the encouraging findings from clinical trials utilizing fetal grafts into brains of PD patients (see later). It has become possible to generate central nervous system cells that express neuronal and glial properties by manipulating the tissue cultures with various cytokines and growth factors. When these progenitor cells are injected into an intact striatum, they acquire the characteristics of striatal cells (but when injected into a lesioned brain, they differentiate into glia). In one experiment, neuronal progenitor cells from a neonatal anterior subventricular zone were implanted in an adult rat with unilateral nigrostriatal denervation by 6-OHDA and were found to differentiate into neuronal phenotype as long as 5 months postimplantation (Zigova et al., 1998). Transplanting low-dose undifferentiated mouse embryonic stem cells into the rat striatum results in a proliferation and full differentiation into dopaminergic neurons (Bjorklund et al., 2002; Winkler et al., 2005). These studies suggest the possibility that in PD, the progenitor or stem cells could be eventually used to replace lost or degenerated cells. However, this enthusiasm must be tempered by the two negative studies of fetal transplants (see later) and the findings from animal studies that show that fetal transplants produce more robust motor and behavioral effects than transplanted embryonic stem cells. Other major limitations of stem cells are the lack of effect on nondopaminergic symptoms of PD and the potential for unregulated release of dopamine and cellular growth.

Many questions regarding fetal tissue grafting remain open, and the procedure should be viewed as experimental (Winkler et al., 2005). Ethical concerns on the use of fetal tissue have been raised. Selection criteria for neurotransplantation differ among investigators. It has not yet been determined which patients are the ideal candidates for these procedures. Because of logistic and ethical problems associated with harvesting human fetal mesencephalon, the use of other donor tissues has been explored. The implantation of autologous adrenal medulla into a patient's striatum has been found to be helpful in about one-third of patients, but the limited benefits and the potential risks of complications have resulted in the cessation of these procedures (Jankovic et al., 1989). Porcine (pig) fetal mesencephalic transplants, however, are currently being investigated as a potential therapeutic intervention (Galpern et al., 1996; Deacon et al., 1997). In 12 patients with advanced PD who received embryonic porcine ventral mesencephalic tissue, Schumacher and colleagues (2000) found 19% improvement in total UPDRS 12 months after the surgery. There were no changes in the ^{18}F-dopa PET scans. Preliminary results from a double-blind, randomized, controlled, multicenter trial of fetal porcine implants in 10 patients with PD have not produced encouraging results (Hauser et al., 2001). In addition to human embryonic tissue, other donor sources are currently being investigated, including retinal pigment epithelial cells (Spheramine) (Watts et al., 2003; Bakay et al., 2004). These cells, located in the inner layer of neural retina, produce dopamine. When attached to crosslinked gelatin microcarriers (Spheramine) and implanted stereotactically into the striatum, the cells have improved parkinsonian symptoms in rodents, nonhuman primates, and parkinsonian patients. A pilot open-label study of six patients showed 48% improvement in the UPDRS motor score 12 months after implantation (Bakay et al., 2004). A randomized, controlled trial conducted in selected centers in North America and Europe did not show any benefit, but the full report has not yet been published. In one patient, a 68-year-old man who underwent bilateral surgical implantation of 325 000 retinal pigment epithelium cells in gelatin microcarriers (Spheramine) but died 6 months after surgery, a total of 118 cells (estimated 0.036% survival) were found associated with marked inflammation (Farag et al., 2009).

The use of immortalized neural progenitor cells in repair and as a source of trophic factors is also being investigated in many centers (Martinez-Serrano and Björklund, 1997). Other approaches include transplantation of polymer-coated xenografts, transfected mesencephalic neural cell lines, genetically engineered dopamine-producing fibroblasts, viral vectors modifying host cells by intrusion of the tyrosine hydroxylase gene, and carotid body glomus cells which also express the glial cell line derived neurotrophic factor (GDNF) (Minguez-Castellanos et al., 2007). Alternative approaches also include the intraventricular or intraparenchymal infusion of neurotrophic factors such as GDNF (Gash et al., 1996). A multicenter study of this approach, however, was discontinued because of lack of efficacy. Another approach, involving surgical gene delivery of adeno-associated virus-based vector encoding human neurturin (AAV2-NTN; also called CERE-120), has been tested in parkinsonian animals and is currently undergoing clinical trials. In the phase I study involving 12 patients with Hoehn and Yahr Stage 3–4 PD, neurturin (CERE-120) was infused into their putamina at doses of 1.3×10^{11} and 5.4×10^{11}, respectively (Marks et al., 2008). No adverse effects were observed and there was 29%

improvement in "off" total UPDRS, 36% reduction in the motor UPDRS, and a mean increase of 2.3 hours in "on" time without troublesome dyskinesia. There was no change in other secondary measures or the ^{18}F-L-DOPA PET, and there were no "off" dyskinesias. In a phase 2 multicenter, double-blind, sham-surgery controlled trial, 58 patients with advanced PD were randomly assigned (2 : 1) to receive either AAV2-neurturin (5.4×10^{11} vector genomes) (CERE-120) injected bilaterally into the putamen or sham surgery (Marks et al., 2011). There was no significant difference in the primary endpoint (a change in motor UPDRS after 12 months) in patients treated with AAV2-neurturin compared with control individuals. Serious adverse events occurred in 13 of 38 patients treated with AAV2-neurturin and 4 of 20 control individuals. Three patients in the AAV2-neurturin group and two in the sham surgery group developed tumors. Another trial, currently in progress, is targeting not only the putamen but also the SN (Lewis and Standaert, 2011). The latter strategy is based on the hypothesis that neurturin will be transported from degenerating terminals to their cell bodies in the SN to the striatum, which was observed in MPTP primates. This hypothesis is supported by the post-mortem findings in 2 brains of patients who participated in the above-described phase 2 trial with neurturin-immuno-staining in the targeted striatum (15% of the putamen), but there was no evidence of expression in the SN (Bartus et al., 2011). Unilateral injection of the gene for the enzyme glutamic acid decarboxylase (GAD), which converts gluta-mate to GABA, with adeno-associated virus (AAV) into the subthalamic nucleus (STN) of 12 patients with PD was reported to result in significant improvements in motor UPDRS scores ($P = 0.0015$), predominantly on the side of the body that was contralateral to surgery, noted at 3 months after the gene therapy, and the effects persisted up to 12 months (Kaplitt et al., 2007). This was associated with a substantial reduction in thalamic metabolism measured by ^{18}F-fluorodeoxyglucose PET in the treated hemisphere. The authors concluded that "AAV-GAD gene therapy of the sub-thalamic nucleus is safe and well tolerated by patients with advanced PD," suggesting that in-vivo gene therapy in the adult brain might be safe for various neurodegenerative dis-eases. While this pilot, phase I, study provides evidence for proof-of-principle, it is not clear how this strategy differs from STN stimulation or lesioning, also designed to inhibit impulses from hyperactive STN (Stoessl, 2007). In a double-blind, phase 2, randomized controlled trial, of 66 patients assessed for eligibility, 21 randomly assigned to sham surgery and 16 to AAV2-GAD infusions were analyzed at the 6-month endpoint (LeWitt et al., 2011). The UPDRS score for the AAV2-GAD group decreased by 8.1 points (SD 1.7, 23.1%; $P < 0.0001$) and by 4.7 points in the sham group (1.5, 12.7%; $P = 0.003$); the AAV2-GAD group showed a signifi-cantly greater improvement from baseline in UPDRS scores compared with the sham group ($P = 0.04$). In addition to the relatively small magnitudes of improvement, the study raises some questions about methodology and conduct of the study, such as whether blinding is possible in patients who are awake during the procedure. Furthermore, of the 45 randomized subjects only 37 were analyzed; 6 from the active treatment arm and 2 from the sham group were excluded from the analyses because of missed surgical target or catheter/pump malfunction.

Other genes delivered surgically or via a vector, including genes for vesicular monoamine transporter-2 (VMAT-2) and aromatic L-amino acid decarboxylase (AADC) genes, are cur-rently being investigated in preclinical and early clinical trials (Lee et al., 2006). There are other gene-based therapies that are being pursued in laboratories all over the world such as ProSavin (Oxford Biomedica). Some have started in France, with experts confident of success, such as a lentivec-tor system carrying amino acid decarboxylase (AADC), tyro-sine hydroxylase (TH), and CH1 (GTP-cyclohydrolase) (www.biomedica-usa.com).

References available on Expert Consult: www.expertconsult.com

CHAPTER **8**

Nonmotor problems in Parkinson disease

Chapter contents

Introduction	183	Depression, anxiety, and change in personality	189
Sensory symptoms	184	Cognitive problems	191
Autonomic dysfunctions: bladder and sexual problems	185	Dementia and confusion	192
Other autonomic symptoms	186	Compulsive behaviors	193
Respiratory distress	187	Psychosis: hallucinations and paranoia	194
Difficulties at night and daytime sleepiness	187	Quality of life	196
Fatigue	189		

Introduction

While the motor symptoms of Parkinson disease (PD) dominate the clinical picture – and even define the parkinsonian syndrome – many patients with PD have other complaints that have been classified as *nonmotor* (Chaudhuri et al., 2006a), and a scale has been developed to quantify them (Chaudhuri et al., 2006b). Also, there is an ongoing modification process to update the Unified Parkinson's Disease Rating Scale (UPDRS) to include more nonmotor features of PD (Goetz et al., 2007). These include fatigue, depression, anxiety, sleep disturbances, constipation, bladder and other autonomic disturbances (sexual, gastrointestinal), and sensory complaints. Sensory symptoms, including pain, may occur. Orthostatic hypotension can lead to syncope. Behavioral and mental alterations include changes in mood, lack of motivation or apathy, slowness in thinking (bradyphrenia), and a declining cognitive capacity; and these are frequent causes for concern. In one survey of nondemented PD patients, nonmotor symptoms (NMS) were found to occur in the majority of patients (Table 8.1). Genetic as well as sporadic forms of PD have NMS (Kasten et al., 2010).There is even the suggestion that presentation of nonmotor symptoms that commonly occur in PD patients but without any of the cardinal signs of PD may be considered part of the same disease spectrum (Langston, 2006). Lang (2011) uses the term premotor for nonmotor symptoms that are part of PD and precede the motor symptoms. This is based on the Braak hypothesis discussed in Chapter 5. Braak and his colleagues are now estimating that the disease (pathology of Lewy neurites) begins in the olfactory and autonomic system by approximately 20 years before the onset of the motor

symptoms of PD, and that many nonmotor symptoms appear (Hawkes et al., 2010).

A large collaborative Italian study of more 1072 patients with PD found that 98.6% of patients with PD reported the presence of NMS (Barone et al., 2009). The most common were: fatigue (58%), anxiety (56%), leg pain (38%), insomnia (37%), urinary urgency and nocturia (35%), drooling of saliva (31%), and difficulties in maintaining concentration (31%). The mean number of NMS per patient was 7.8 (range, 0–32). NMS in the psychiatric domain were the most frequent (67%). Frequency of NMS increased along with the disease duration and severity.

Always ask the patient what problems bother him/her; many times a nonmotor symptom is the most troublesome. Helping patients with PD to cope with these difficulties is just as important as manipulating therapy to provide control of their motor symptoms. In addition, antiparkinsonian drugs commonly induce unwanted nonmotor effects and aggravate such complaints. And so-called sensory "offs" are often underappreciated but are usually a greater source of discomfort than are motor "offs." In this chapter, we cover nonmotor problems inherent to the disease and also those induced by medications to treat the disease. Nonmotor symptoms can become disabling with the increasing duration of the disease (see Tables 6.7 and 6.8).

Nonmotor symptoms not uncommonly can be the presenting complaint in PD. In pathologically proven PD 91/433 (21%) of patients presented with nonmotor symptoms, of which the most frequent were pain (53%), urinary dysfunction (16.5%), and anxiety, or depression (12%) (O'Sullivan et al., 2008). Presenting with nonmotor symptoms was associated with a delayed diagnosis of PD. These

DOI: 10.1016/B978-1-4377-2369-4.00008-1

Table 8.1 Frequency of nonmotor symptoms in Parkinson disease

Symptom	Frequency
Depression	36%
Anxiety	33%
Fatigue	40%
Sleep disturbances	47%
Sensory symptoms	63%
No nonmotor symptoms	12%

Data from Shulman LM, Taback RL, Bean J, Weiner WJ. Comorbidity of the nonmotor symptoms of Parkinson's disease. Mov Disord 2001;16:507–510.

Table 8.2 Sensory symptoms in Parkinson disease

Pain
Paresthesias
Numbness
Burning
Akathisia
Restless legs syndrome
Hyposmia
Urgency to urinate

patients were more likely to be misdiagnosed initially and were more likely to have been referred to orthopedic surgeons or rheumatologists than neurologists. Comparing newly diagnosed patients with a control population, Miller and colleagues (2011) found a statistically significant higher number of autonomic and sensory symptoms in the PD group, especially olfaction, urinary, drooling, constipation, and sensory complaints.

With continuing PD, nonmotor symptoms become more common and can become the major troublesome symptom (Hely et al., 2005, 2008). Also medications to treat the motor symptoms of PD can cause nonmotor symptoms, including impulse control problems, confusion, hallucinations, and paranoid psychosis. Behavioral, mood, and cognitive problems can develop as complications of surgery for PD, such as deep brain stimulation (Voon et al., 2006c), and these are covered in Chapter 7.

Nonmotor symptoms as part of PD fit the pattern of the location of Lewy neurites described by Braak and his colleagues (see review by Braak et al., 2006), and presented in detail in Chapter 6. The Braak hypothesis as an early feature of PD is not uniformly accepted (Burke et al., 2008). As more parkinsonologists are focusing on nonmotor symptoms, there are more publications. Three recent reviews on this topic are recommended: Simuni and Sethi (2008), Lim et al. (2009), Chaudhuri and Schapira (2009), Lang (2011).

Two prominent risk factors for mortality in PD are the nonmotor symptoms of psychosis and dementia (Forsaa et al., 2010).

Sensory symptoms

Pain

Many textbooks do not list pain and the other sensory complaints in Table 8.2 as a part of PD, and they are often not considered symptoms of the disease, but they can be (Snider et al., 1976; Koller, 1984; Goetz et al., 1986; Quinn et al., 1986; Ford et al., 1996; Ford, 2010). A constant, boring pain in the initially affected limb may be the first complaint. Aching in the shoulder and arm is a common earlier symptom in PD and is often incorrectly attributed to bursitis or a frozen shoulder. When pain occurs in the hip or leg, it is often attributed to arthritis, whereas this could be a symptom of PD. That such pain is due to the PD is indicated by its relief with antiparkinsonian medication. Once adequate dosing is achieved, whether or not mobility is restored, such pain commonly abates. Of course, patients with PD may also have coincidental joint disease, so if the pain persists, patients require appropriate investigation.

Another initial complaint, particularly in younger patients, may be painful dystonic foot cramps, especially on walking. Rarely, similar painful cramp may occur in the hands. An extended big toe or curling of small toes may be seen with the cramping. In recent surveys, about two-thirds of patients experience chronic pain (Defazio et al., 2008; Nègre-Pagès et al., 2008).

When patients with PD develop fluctuations and dyskinesias, pain may become a major feature. "Off-period" dystonia often is painful. This may manifest as early morning painful cramps, particularly affecting the feet (Melamed, 1979). Similar painful dystonic cramps may emerge during "off" periods during the day, and can be very distressing (Ilson et al., 1984). Some patients may experience more generalized excruciating pain during "off" periods, often a deep-seated aching, but sometimes with a more superficial burning quality. Again, such pains disappear when the patient is switched "on" by appropriate medication to regain mobility. "Off-period" pain may be an indication for the use of rapidly-acting water-soluble preparations of levodopa or apomorphine rescue injections.

Burning, numbness, and paresthesia

Other specific sensory symptoms, such as burning, numbness, and paresthesia, are less common in PD. However, some patients may describe rather nonspecific paresthesia in the affected limbs, but objective sensory signs are not evident (Snider et al., 1976; Koller, 1984). A rare patient may have sensory complaints from levodopa therapy, unaccompanied by dystonia. Electroconvulsive therapy (ECT) can be effective in alleviating the problem. If parkinsonian pain occurs during an "off" or due to parkinsonism, one should increase medications to avoid "offs." (Sensory "offs" are considered later in this chapter.) If pain occurs during peak-dose dystonia, one needs to lower the dose. If pain is secondary to levodopa or dopamine agonists, one needs to reduce or eliminate the causal agent. Occasionally, the ergot dopamine agonists, bromocriptine and pergolide, cause a burning pain with inflammatory skin on parts of the body, known as St Anthony's fire. If this occurs, the agonist needs to be discontinued.

Akathisia

A more common sensory symptom is akathisia or a sense of inner restlessness. This sometimes is focused on the legs with uncomfortable paresthesias and the need to move them to gain relief, in which case it may be termed a true restless legs syndrome (Lang, 1987). More often, there is a sense of generalized inner restless discomfort, demanding walking for relief, when akathisia is the more appropriate description (Lang and Johnson, 1987). Akathisia may be a presenting feature of PD. The symptoms of both restless legs and akathisia may respond to dopamine replacement therapy. Akathisia may also occur during the "off" period (Lang, 1994). It may be difficult for the patient and the clinician to distinguish between akathisia and restless legs syndrome in some patients.

Akathisia probably occurs more often in PD than is commonly recognized. It can be a sensory complaint of the disease itself and also an adverse effect from levodopa. Lang and Johnson (1987) asked patients with PD specifically for complaints of restlessness and found that 86% did have this subjective complaint. Most patients with PD who complained of an inner feeling of restlessness did not overtly manifest any signs such as moving about. From Lang and Johnson's study it was not clear whether akathisia represented an adverse effect from levodopa or was a feature of the disease. In most of their patients it appeared only after the introduction of antiparkinsonian drugs, but a small number had this symptom early in the course of PD, prior to receiving any medication. It is likely that levodopa and other antiparkinsonian agents may also contribute to this complaint, for it has occurred in patients with primary torsion dystonia after starting these drugs.

Restless legs syndrome

Restless legs syndrome (RLS) is encountered fairly often in patients with PD. In one study, 24% of patients with PD had RLS (Peralta et al., 2009). The symptoms are described in Chapter 23. Briefly, it consists of unpleasant crawling sensations in the legs, particularly when sitting and relaxing in the evening, and disappears on walking. Whether RLS is an epiphenomenon of PD, because both respond to dopaminergics, is not clear. Like PD, dopamine transporter binding is reduced in the striatum in sporadic RLS (Early et al., 2011). Sporadic and familial RLS respond to dopamine agonists and levodopa, but these drugs can cause augmentation, a worsening of the restless legs symptoms – more severe unpleasant sensations, occurring earlier in the day, and spread to involve other body parts. This raises the possibility that some cases of RLS in patients with PD may be the result of dopaminergic medications used to treat PD. Fortunately, opioids are effective in treating RLS and periodic movements in sleep, whether in patients with PD or in sporadic and familial RLS (Hening et al., 1986; Kavey et al., 1988), and these can be used safely in PD. Propoxyphene 65 mg late in the day before the onset of symptoms is usually effective. Start with a half-tablet, and titrate up to two tablets if necessary. Other opioids like oxycodone (Walters et al., 1993), tramadol (Lauerma and Markkula, 1999) and methadone (Silver et al., 2011) are effective without the augmentation problem.

Hyposmia

Decreased sense of smell is not a complaint that patients usually make, but if olfaction is tested, decreased olfaction is detected in most patients with PD. In one study, 45% of patients were functionally anosmic, 51.7% were hyposmic, and only 3.3% were normosmic (Haehner et al., 2009). This indicates that 96.7% of PD patients present with significant olfactory loss when compared to young normosmic subjects. This figure falls to 74.5%, however, when adjusted to age-related norms.

Hyposmsia often precedes the onset of motor symptoms (Ponsen et al., 2004; Haehner et al., 2007), and is now being studied to determine if it can predict future PD. Hyposmia is more predictive than is executive dysfunction (Ponsen et al., 2009). One study indicates that it can predict PD in men up to 4 years before onset of motor features (Ross et al., 2008), and an autopsy study showed that those with the greatest reduction of smell were more likely to have incidental Lewy bodies at autopsy (Ross et al., 2006). One problem as a predictive test is that hyposmia is not selective; it is decreased in other neurodegenerative disorders, including corticobasal degeneration (Pardini et al., 2009). Hyposmia has been associated with striatal dopamine deficiency (Wong et al., 2010), but showed a better correlation with decreased cholinergic activity in the cortical and limbic areas (Bohnen et al., 2010).

Autonomic dysfunctions: bladder and sexual problems

The listing in Table 8.1 does not include autonomic symptoms, but PD patients also complain more about these, such as gastrointestinal, urinary, cardiovascular, thermoregulatory, and sexual dysfunction, than a control population, with the greatest differences in the gastrointestinal and urinary domain (Verbaan et al., 2008). These symptoms were found to increase with age, disease severity, and medication use.

The autonomic dysfunctions in patients with PD can be segregated into urogenital problems and those that affect other functions, such as blood pressure, the gastrointestinal tract, and skin (Table 8.3). In this section, we discuss bladder problems in patients with PD.

The prevalence of bladder symptoms in PD is high; the most common complaint is nocturia followed by frequency and urgency (Fitzmaurice et al., 1985; Winge and Fowler, 2006). Of course PD patients are usually of an age at which prostatic problems in the male and stress incontinence in the female can occur anyway. But PD itself affects bladder

Table 8.3 Autonomic dysfunction in Parkinson disease

Bladder problems
Sexual dysfunction
Hypotension
Gastrointestinal
Seborrhea
Sweating
Rhinorrhea
Abdominal bloating

control, owing to detrusor hyperreflexia. As a result, premature uninhibited bladder contractions cause frequency and urgency, which can be particularly troublesome at night and during "off" periods. Araki and Kuno (2000) assessed voiding dysfunction in 203 consecutive PD patients and found that 27% had symptomatic voiding dysfunction. Its severity correlated with the severity of PD and not with disease duration, age, or gender.

Prostatic outflow obstruction can add to the problem in the male. Incontinence not explained by immobility when taken by the urge to micturate or by retention with overflow is not, however, a part of PD. True neurogenic incontinence in someone with parkinsonism suggests a diagnosis of multiple system atrophy (MSA) (Stocchi et al., 1997). In this case, sphincter electromyographic studies usually reveal signs of denervation due to involvement of Onuf's nucleus in the sacral spinal cord, which does not occur in PD.

The diagnosis of significant prostate enlargement in PD is difficult, and prostatectomy by the unwary often leads to disaster. Prostatectomy should be considered only in those with proven outflow obstruction. A simple screening test in patients with PD is noninvasive ultrasonic estimation of post-micturition residual volume, and simple mechanical measurement of urinary flow rate. If there is significant residual volume after urination (>100 mL) or if flow rate is reduced, there may be bladder outlet obstruction and further investigation by more extensive urodynamic studies, and other urologic testing is required. If there is no significant residual volume or reduction of flow rate, urinary frequency and urgency may be helped by a peripheral antimuscarinic drug such as oxybutynin (Ditropan), 5–10 mg at night or 5 mg three times a day. Fluid intake should be reduced at night. A tricyclic antidepressant with anticholinergic properties, such as amitriptyline, may help sleep not only through its sedative actions but also by reducing bladder irritability. Intranasal DDAVP (desmopressin) at night also may reduce nocturia.

Impotence in the male patient with PD causes distress to both partners (as do immobility and other problems in the female). PD itself does not normally cause impotence, although this is a common early complaint in MSA. Loss of libido and failure to gain or sustain erections may have some other cause in this age group, be it psychological, vascular, hormonal or neurogenic, and appropriate investigation is warranted. Some antidepressant drugs, monoamine oxidase inhibitors, and antihypertensive medications can impair sexual performance. Failure of erection can be overcome by a variety of intrapenile or oral medications such as sildenafil (Viagra) (Zesiewicz et al., 2000). Sildenafil can be efficacious in the treatment of erectile dysfunction in both PD and MSA; however, it can unmask or exacerbate hypotension in MSA (Hussain et al., 2001). Parkinsonian symptoms are not affected, but a side benefit of reduced dyskinesias has been reported (Swope, 2000). Hypersexuality, particularly in the male, is a rare and unacceptable side effect of dopamine replacement therapy in PD, both levodopa and dopamine agonists, and usually requires reduction of antiparkinsonian medication.

Levodopa itself can affect the bladder (Brusa et al., 2007). In dopa-naive PD patients challenged with carbidopa/levodopa 50/200 mg, bladder overactivity (neurogenic overactive detrusor contractions) threshold and bladder capacity significantly worsened (32% and 22% of worsening, respectively). But when the same patients were rechallenged after being on levodopa therapy for 2 months, there was improvement of bladder function. Compared to the values obtained earlier, bladder activity and capacity improved 93% and 33%, respectively. Furthermore the sensation of bladder filling had a 120% improvement.

Other autonomic symptoms

Lewy body degeneration affects the autonomic nervous system in PD. Both sympathetic ganglion neurons and para-sympathetic myenteric and cardiac plexi can be involved (Qualman et al., 1984; Kupsky et al., 1987; Wakabayashi et al., 1988). The postganglionic sympathetic nerves to the heart degenerate early and in a centripetal manner, with synuclein accumulation, not only in PD but also in persons with incidental Lewy bodies (Orimo et al., 2008). The loss of these sympathetic neurons is reflected in the reduced cardiac uptake of ^{123}I-meta-iodobenzylguanidine (MIBG), a physiologic analog of norepinephrine, in patients with PD and dementia with Lewy bodies (Oka et al., 2007a). In contrast, postganglionic sympathetic fibers remain intact in MSA, and so MIBG uptake is normal in MSA. Central autonomic nuclei, such as those of the hypothalamus and dorsal motor nucleus of the vagus, can also be affected in Lewy body degeneration (Eadie, 1963).

Orthostasis: Control of blood pressure may be compromised by sympathetic failure with impaired vasoconstriction and inadequate intravascular volume. Faintness on standing (pre-syncope) and frank loss of consciousness on standing (postural syncope) can occur owing to orthostatic hypotension (OH). OH can also cause posturally induced fatigue and weakness, blurring of vision, and "coat-hanger" neck and shoulder aching. Hypotension also may occur postprandially due to gastrointestinal vasodilatation. Levodopa, dopamine agonists, and selegiline (Churchyard et al., 1999) may aggravate postural hypotension. Oka and colleagues (2007b) compared PD patients with and without OH and found a greater association with male gender, older age, longer disease duration, posture and gait instability phenotype, low Mini-Mental State Examination (MMSE) scores, and visual hallucinations. Cardiac ^{123}I-MIBG uptakes were lower in patients with OH.

Prominent early symptoms of postural hypotension are, of course, one of the hallmarks of MSA, so such complaints may raise concern over the diagnosis of PD. The severity of postural hypotension in PD rarely is as severe as that seen in MSA. Nevertheless, treatment might be required. A selective peripheral dopamine antagonist such as domperidone sometimes helps, as does increasing fluid and salt intake, with head-up tilt at night which reduces nocturnal polyuria. Intranasal DDAVP (desmopressin) (5–40 µg) at night also reduces nocturnal polyuria, but can cause hyponatremia. However, a small dose of fludrocortisone (0.1–0.5 mg) (to promote salt retention), or midodrine (ProAmatine) (a selective α-agonist) (2.5–5 mg three times a day), might be required to maintain adequate blood pressure. Pyridostigmine was found to improve orthostatic hypotension, probably due to enhanced sympathetic ganglionic neurotransmission and a vagal shift in cardiac sympathovagal balance (Singer et al., 2006).

Gastrointestinal problems cause significant disability in PD (Edwards et al., 1991, 1992). Dysphagia is due mainly to poor masticatory and oropharyngeal muscular control making it difficult to chew and propel the bolus of food into the pharynx and esophagus (Bushman et al., 1989; Edwards et al., 1994). Soft food is easier to eat, and antiparkinsonian medication improves swallowing.

Parasympathetic failure may contribute to gastrointestinal problems in PD, causing delay in esophageal and gastric motility. A sense of bloating, indigestion, and gastric reflux are common in PD (Edwards et al., 1992). Many factors contribute to delayed gastric emptying, including immobility, parasympathetic failure, constipation, and antiparkinsonian drugs (both anticholinergic and dopamine agonists). Levodopa is absorbed in the upper small bowel, so gastric stasis may slow or prevent levodopa assimilation, leading to "delayed-ons" and "no-ons" (dose failures) after single oral doses (either there is an excessive interval before the drug works, or it does not work at all).

Constipation is another frequent complaint in PD (Edwards et al., 1992, 1994; Kaye et al., 2006), and is multifactorial. Again, immobility, drugs, reduced fluid and food intake, and parasympathetic involvement prolonging colonic transit time may all contribute. In addition, malfunction of the striated muscles of the pelvic floor due to the PD itself can make evacuation of the bowels difficult (Mathers et al., 1988, 1989). Constipation may exacerbate gastric stasis. Anticholinergic drugs should be stopped and physical exercise should be increased. The role of levodopa in causing or treating constipation is uncertain. This drug usually does not relieve the problem, and some patients believe that it worsens the problem. Constipation is ameliorated by adequate fluid intake, fruit, vegetables, fiber, and lactulose (10–20 g/day) or other mild laxatives. The following "rancho recipe" provided by Dr Cheryl Waters has been found useful for many patients: Mix together one cup each of bran, applesauce, and prune juice; take two tablespoons every morning; the mixture can be refrigerated for one week, then should be discarded. Polyethylene glycol powder (marketed as MiraLax) can be effective to overcome constipation; the usual dose is 17 g/day dissolved in a glass of water at bedtime. Refractory constipation may be helped by apomorphine injections to assist defecation (Edwards et al., 1993; Merello and Leiguarda, 1994).

Pyridostigmine by enhancing parasympathetic tone can also aid peristalsis and help in the treatment of constipation. For patients who have *abdominal bloating* due to suppression of peristalsis when they are "off", keeping them "on" with levodopa or other dopaminergics is beneficial.

Excessive sebum (*seborrhea*) probably is due more to facial immobility that to overproduction. The greasy skin contributes to seborrheic dermatitis and dandruff. Medicated soaps and shampoos help. Blepharitis also is common, due in part to reduced blinking. Artificial teardrops can help.

Excessive sweating can be a problem, particularly in the form of sudden drenching sweats (sweating crises). These seem to occur as part of an "off" phenomenon (Sage and Mark, 1995; Swinn et al., 2003; Pursiainen et al., 2007). Sweating can cause physical, social, and emotional impairment.

Excessive salivation (sialorrhea) is due more to failure to swallow saliva frequently than to overproduction (Bateson et al., 1973). Drooling of saliva can be helped by chewing gum (which also helps those with dry mouth) or by using peripherally-acting anticholinergic drugs, which are quaternary ammonium compounds that do not cross the blood–brain barrier. Two such compounds are glycopyrrolate and propantheline. The former was tested in a controlled clinical trial and found to be effective and safe therapy for sialorrhea in PD (Arbouw et al., 2010). If these are unsuccessful, intraparotid injections of botulinum toxin B can sometimes be effective in reducing salivary secretions and drooling (Lipp et al., 2003; Racette et al., 2003; Ondo et al., 2004). Chewing gum has also been found useful to increase swallow frequency, and it decreases latency of swallowing in PD (South et al., 2010), which are common problems in advanced PD and contribute to weight loss in PD.

Rhinorrhea is not infrequent in patients with PD and has been reported to occur in almost 50% (Friedman et al., 2008). Patients with PD with rhinorrhea were older and had a higher Hoehn and Yahr stage. Duration of disease was not different between those with and without rhinorrhea. Most patients with rhinorrhea reported that it worsened with eating.

Respiratory distress

Respiratory distress such as dyspnea can occur as a symptom of PD in some patients, including during the "off" period in some (Ilson et al., 1983). It can also occur as a complication of dystonia, usually peak-dose dystonia (Braun et al., 1983), and with some dopamine agonists, particularly pergolide. Removing the offending drug is required. "Off" period dyspnea is difficult to treat, other than attempting to keep the patient "on." Despite the sensation of dyspnea, oxygen saturation is not affected because the patient will have a voluntary sigh or transient deep breathing when feeling short of breath. Some forms of parkinsonism-plus syndromes may have an accompanying apnea that is life-threatening, such as postencephalitic parkinsonism (Strieder et al., 1967; Efthimiou et al., 1987), frontotemporal dementia (Lynch et al., 1994), MSA (Chester et al., 1988; Salazar-Grueso et al., 1988), Joseph disease (SCA3) (Kitamura et al., 1989), and other familial parkinsonian syndromes (Perry et al., 1990).

Difficulties at night and daytime sleepiness

Table 8.4 lists some of the sleep problems seen in PD. Patients often have troubled nights for many reasons (Factor et al., 1990; Askenasy, 1993; Van Hilten et al., 1994; Bliwise et al., 1995). The most common problem is difficulty with

Table 8.4 Sleep problems in Parkinson disease

Sleep fragmentation
REM sleep behavior disorder
Excessive daytime sleepiness
Altered sleep–wake cycle
Drug-induced sleep attacks

sleep maintenance (so-called sleep fragmentation). Frequent awakenings may be caused by tremor reappearing in the lighter stages of sleep, difficulty in turning in bed due to nocturnal akinesia as the effects of daytime administration of dopaminergic drugs wear off at night, and nocturia. In addition, periodic leg movements in sleep (sometimes associated with restless legs), fragmentary nocturnal myoclonus, sleep apnea, REM sleep behavioral disorders (intense dream-like motor and behavioral problems), and parasomnias (nocturnal hallucinations and nocturnal wandering with disruptive behavior) may all disrupt sleep in PD. Reversal of sleep rhythm with sundowning also is common in PD (Bliwise et al., 1995). Many of these conditions probably occur more frequently in PD than in other aged populations. As a result, PD patients and their caregivers face disrupted nights, which lead to poor quality of life and worse parkinsonism the next day. In fact, along with depression, poor sleep is a major factor in a PD patient's assessment of having a poor quality of life (QoL) (Karlsen et al., 1999b). Rating scales to assess severity of sleep disturbances have been developed (Trenkwalder et al., 2011). A good night's sleep reduces the severity of daytime parkinsonism, and many patients comment on sleep benefit, describing better mobility the morning after a restful night. Indeed, patients with marked sleep benefit might not require antiparkinsonian medication for some hours after they awaken, and some PD patients find that a daytime nap "charges the batteries." These may be the young-onset PD patients with mutations in the *parkin* gene for they typically show sleep benefit (Elibol et al., 2000).

Another cause of disturbed sleep is the return of parkinsonian symptoms during the night after the last dose of medication has worn off. Nocturnal tremor and akinesia due to the PD and nocturia in the elderly can cause arousals. Depression, which is common in PD, can cause insomnia and is a major factor associated with nighttime sleep problems (Verbaan et al., 2008). Drugs given to treat PD symptoms can interfere with sleep.

PD pathology can also be associated with REM sleep behavior disorder (RBD) and parasomnias, especially in patients with incipient or frank dementia. RBD, described initially by Schenck and colleagues (1986), is a condition in which there is lack of somatic muscle atonia, thus enabling such individuals to move while they dream (acting out their dreams). The animal model of REM sleep without atonia indicates that lesions to the perilocus coeruleus disrupt the excitatory connection to the nucleus reticularis magnocellularis in the descending medullary reticular formation and disable the hyperpolarization of the alpha spinal motoneurons (Ferini-Strambi and Zucconi, 2000). The development of RBD may be an early marker for the later onset of PD (Schenck et al., 1996; Tan et al., 1996; Postuma et al., 2006).

RBD may precede or develop after PD. RBD is suspected of arising in the pons–medulla area, and therefore the Braak scheme would have RBD occurring before PD, if RBD is a component of PD. In the survey of their PD patients, Scaglione and colleagues (2005) found that only 33% had RBD. Of these, PD preceded RBD in 73%, an average of 8 years before onset of RBD. In another study, RBD preceded PD in only 22% (De Cock et al., 2007). Postuma and colleagues (2009) followed patients with idiopathic RBD and found that the risk for developing any neurodegenerative disease

(PD, dementia with Lewy bodies, MSA, or Alzheimer disease) is 17.7% by 5 years, 40.6% by 10 years, and 52.4% by 12 years. Only 14 out of 93 developed PD. With longer follow-up, approximately 50% of idiopathic RBD cases will develop PD and the more severe the loss of atonia on baseline polysomnograms, the better the prediction of the development of PD (Postuma et al., 2010).

RBD is usually successfully treated with a bedtime dose of clonazepam (Schenck et al., 1987); 0.5 mg is often sufficient, but sometimes a higher dosage is required to obtain complete relief.

The treatment of sleep disorders in PD is important. Attention to sleep hygiene by avoiding alcohol, caffeine, and nicotine, and excessive fluid intake at night is helpful. Deprenyl (selegiline), which is metabolized to methamphetamine and amphetamine, should not be given at night. Treatment of depression might be required. A sedative antidepressant, such as amitriptyline (10–25 mg at night), mirtazapine, or trazodone, can be very useful, not only to induce and maintain sleep, but also to reduce urinary frequency. A dose of a long-acting levodopa preparation last thing at night may improve nocturnal akinesia (Laihnen et al., 1987; Lees, 1987). However, levodopa given at night may provoke excessive dreaming and disrupted sleep in some patients (Nausieda et al., 1982). A benzodiazepine, especially clonazepam, may lessen REM sleep behavior disorders. A low dose of 0.5 mg at bedtime is usually effective. Propoxyphene is useful for periodic leg movements of sleep and restless legs (Hening et al., 1986). A small bedtime dose of clozapine (Rabey et al., 1995) or quetiapine may be very effective in improving sleep. For patients who have no problem falling asleep, but awaken in 2–3 hours, the short-acting hypnotic zolpidem is useful when taken after the awakening. It helps the patient get back to sleep quickly and still be refreshed in the morning.

Excessive daytime sleepiness (EDS) occurs in about 15% of patients with PD, and is associated with more severe PD and patients with cognitive decline (Tandberg et al., 1999). In one study, EDS was found in 50% of patients (Shpirer et al., 2006). EDS is determined by short sleep latency and sleep-onset REM periods. When studied with tests determining these two criteria, PD patients with EDS were found to correlate not with variables related to disease severity or to total sleep time or sleep stage percentages, but rather those related to primary impairments of waking arousal and REM-sleep expression (Rye et al., 2000). Dopamine agonists are more likely than levodopa to be associated with EDS (Ondo et al., 2001; Gjerstad et al., 2006). The antisoporific agent modafinil can sometimes be beneficial in overcoming EDS in patients with PD (Happe et al., 2001). Oxybate has been reported to reduce EDS (Ondo et al., 2008).

Some patients who sleep a lot during the day may have their problem related to drowsiness following a dosage of levodopa. This phenomenon is usually seen in patients with developing or more pronounced dementia. With post-levodopa drowsiness, patients can sleep during much of the day and are then awake at night. This altered sleep–wake cycle can make life unbearable for the caregiver, who requires adequate sleep at night. If a patient becomes drowsy after each dose of medication, this is a sign of overdosage. Reducing the dosage can correct this problem. Sometimes, substituting Sinemet CR for standard Sinemet will help because this provides for a slower rise in plasma and brain levels of levodopa.

If the patient's sleep problem has advanced to that of an altered sleep–wake cycle, it is important to get the patient onto a sleep–wake schedule that fits with that of the rest of the household. To correct the problem, it might be necessary to use a combination of approaches. Efforts must be made to stimulate the patient physically and mentally during the day and force the patient to remain awake, otherwise he or she will not be able to sleep at night. At night, the patient should then be drowsy enough so that he or she will be able to sleep. If this fails, it might be necessary to use stimulants in the morning and sedatives at night to reverse the altered state. This should be done in addition to prodding the patient to remain awake during the day. Drugs such as methylphenidate and amphetamine are usually well tolerated by patients with PD. A 10 mg dose of either of these two drugs, repeated once if necessary, may be helpful. To encourage sleep at night, a hypnotic might be necessary in addition to using daytime stimulants. It should be noted that strong sedatives, such as barbiturates, are poorly tolerated by patients with PD. Milder hypnotics, such as benzodiazepines, are usually taken without difficulty. Short-acting benzodiazepines would be preferable, but if the patient awakens too early, a longer-acting one might need to be used.

Sleep attacks

Falling asleep while driving and without warning is a serious problem that has been encountered with dopaminergic agents; it seems more likely to occur with pramipexole and ropinirole, but is not limited to just these drugs (Frucht et al., 1999; Ferreira et al., 2000; Hoehn, 2000; Schapira, 2000). The decision about which dopamine agonist to place a patient on was discussed in Chapter 6. Once sleep attacks have occurred, the patient should not drive, except on short trips, or the medication should be changed. Fortunately, modafinil has been reported to be helpful in preventing sleep attacks (Hauser et al., 2000). A review of the literature (Homann et al., 2002) showed that sleep attacks have been reported with all dopaminergic medications, including levodopa, the greatest number being associated with pramipexole and ropinirole. Unfortunately, not all reports refer strictly to sudden attacks without warning; some reports refer to falling asleep from drowsiness, so the interpretation is open to uncertainty.

Sleep and deep brain stimulation of the pedunculopontine (PPN) area

One consequence of the experimental deep brain stimulation in the PPN in an attempt to treat parkinsonian gait disorders has been the effect this procedure has had on sleep. It was found that low-frequency stimulation of the PPN area increased alertness, whereas high-frequency stimulation induced non-rapid eye movement sleep (Arnulf et al., 2010).

Fatigue

Although fatigue can be a symptom of sleepiness or depression, it is also a symptom that may be unassociated with these states. The clinician should probe the patient to distinguish between fatigue and sleepiness. In patients with PD, fatigue is often a complaint during the earliest phase of the disease, before motor symptoms, such as stiffness and slowness, become prominent. As these other features of PD develop, with their important contribution to disability, these become more of a complaint than does fatigue. But when patients are specifically asked, fatigue remains a common feature in PD. In a community study of elderly people in Norway, 44% of PD patients and 18% of healthy controls reported fatigue (Karlsen et al., 1999a). In a Japanese study involving 361 PD patients, fatigue was present in 41.8% and depression was not a contributing factor (Okuma et al., 2009). In newly diagnosed patients with PD, fatigue was discerned in 36% and was less likely to worsen if the patient received levodopa compared to a placebo (Schifitto et al., 2008). Treating depression and daytime sleepiness would be helpful, but when fatigue is an independent symptom, no treatment has been found to be satisfactory. Despite the claimed benefit of amantadine in treating fatigue in multiple sclerosis, neither this drug nor the monoamine oxidase inhibitor selegiline has been found particularly beneficial in treating fatigue in PD. Neither has modafinil in a small controlled trial (Lou et al., 2009). Methylphenidate 30 mg/day has been reported to reduce fatigue in a controlled clinical trial (Mendonça et al., 2007) and in fatigue in patients with prostate cancer (Roth et al., 2010). Oxybate at bedtime has also been reported to help (Ondo et al., 2008). Friedman and colleagues have published a thorough review of fatigue in PD (Friedman et al., 2007).

Depression, anxiety, and change in personality

Loss of motivation

It is common in patients with PD to have a change in personality (Table 8.5), and such change may precede motor symptoms, but usually develops and worsens over the course of PD. Executives with decision-making tasks might find such duties so difficult that they might not be able to continue in their work. Passivity, dependency, and lack of motivation are often more troublesome for the spouse than for the patient. Lack of motivation, as it becomes more severe, becomes apathy; and when apathy becomes more severe, it is abulia. Abulia is a severe form of both mental and motor apathy, with not only a loss of initiative and drive but also a general restriction of activities, including the reticence to speak. Abulia is a recognized clinical syndrome due to

Table 8.5 Personality and behavior in Parkinson disease

Depression
Fearfulness
Anxiety
Loss of assertive drive
Passivity
Dependency
Inability to make decisions
Loss of motivation, apathy
Abulia

caudate and prefrontal dysfunction, so it might well feature in the overall symptomatology of PD. In its milder form (i.e., apathy), the loss of initiative, both mental and motor, is often commented on by the spouse or close relatives, who perceive a change in personality. Spouses particularly complain about the patient's lack of desire to socialize with friends and communicate freely. When the spouse wants to go out, dine, or meet with friends, the apathetic patient just wants to sit at home and not participate in these activities. Such alterations in activity may be due to depression, but not infrequently, there is no change in mood. A direct test for apathy and depression in patients with PD and dystonia (control group) found no apathy in the absence of depression in the dystonic population, whereas apathy in the absence of depression was frequent in PD (29%) (Kirsch-Darrow et al., 2006). Evaluation in 175 untreated PD patients found 37% with depression, 27% with apathy, 18% with sleep disturbance, and 17% with anxiety (Aarsland et al., 2009b). Apathy does not respond to dopamine replacement therapy in the way the motor problems of PD do, nor to antidepressants, unless depression is present and is itself the cause of the apathy.

In one survey of 164 patients with PD, 52 (32%) met diagnostic criteria for apathy (Starkstein et al., 2009). Of these, 83% had comorbid depression and 56% had dementia. Forty of the 164 PD patients had neither depression nor dementia; only 5 (13%) of the 40 had apathy. One study found that apathy appears to be a predictive factor for dementia and cognitive decline over time (Dujardin et al., 2009).

Depression

Depression is common in PD, with at least one-third of patients exhibiting significant depressive symptoms in cross-sectional surveys (Brown et al., 1988; Dooneief et al., 1992). Anguenot and colleagues (2002) reported a higher number of one-half of PD patients having depression. The Geriatric Depression Scale was administered to subjects enrolled in clinical trials for early PD, and 28% were found to have some depression (Ravina et al., 2007). Forty percent did not require treatment. However, depression was a predictor of more impairment in activities of daily living and increased need for symptomatic therapy of PD. In another study, all patients with early PD were found to have executive dysfunction, and those with major depression also had episodic/working memory and language deficits (Stefanova et al., 2006).

However, it is often difficult to distinguish true depression from the apathy (abulia) associated with PD, especially in the presence of the characteristic expressionless face, bowed posture, and slowed movement, which resemble the psychomotor retardation of a primary depressive illness. The critical factor is whether the patient has a true disturbance of mood (dysphoria), with low spirits, loss of interest, bleak outlook, typical depressive sleep disturbance, paranoid ruminations, and sometimes suicidal thoughts. Schrag and colleagues (2007) evaluated a variety of depression rating scales and found many of them satisfactory for use and conclude that it is not necessary to develop new ones.

The reasons for depression in PD are debated. On the one hand, depressive symptoms are not surprising in vulnerable individuals who are faced with the disabilities and handicaps imposed by PD, with reduced activities and independence, and the prospects of a chronic incurable condition. Such reactive depression certainly contributes to the problem. But one study suggests that depression in PD is more strongly influenced by the patients' perceptions of handicap than by actual disability (Schrag et al., 2001). However, there is also the probability that the pathology of PD in itself might predispose to depression, especially that involving serotonergic and noradrenergic systems, which have been implicated in the neurochemical basis of primary depressive illnesses. The substantia nigra, itself, is implicated by the report that deep brain stimulation of this structure in a patient with PD induced acute severe depression (Bejjani et al., 1999).

The recognition and treatment of depression in PD is important because depression has a major impact on the overall disability imposed by the illness. In fact, depression carries a hazard ratio of 2.66 for increased mortality in PD (Hughes et al., 2004). Most antidepressant drugs can be used safely in PD. However, nonselective monoamine oxidase inhibitors are contraindicated in patients who are taking levodopa because of potential pressor reactions. There also have been concerns over the use of selective serotonin reuptake inhibitors (SSRIs), which in a few cases have been reported to interact with levodopa to induce the "serotonin" syndrome (confusion, myoclonus, rigidity, and restlessness) and to worsen PD symptoms. Despite these worries, many depressed patients with PD have been treated safely and successfully with SSRIs, for example fluoxetine or paroxetine (20–40 mg daily). By enhancing serotonergic "tone" and thereby potentially inhibiting dopaminergic neurons in the substantia nigra, there is the potential, especially in the absence of dopaminergic drug treatment, that SSRIs may increase parkinsonian symptoms, but such events are rare (Jansen Steur, 1993; Jimenez-Jimenez et al., 1994; Richard et al., 1999; Ceravolo et al., 2000; Tesei et al., 2000). The traditional tricyclic antidepressants can also be employed, although their sedative and anticholinergic properties may be detrimental in elderly patients. A small double-blind trial comparing paroxetine, nortriptyline, and placebo in 52 patients with PD and depression was carried out over 8 weeks and showed that nortriptyline was superior to placebo but paroxetine was not (Menza et al., 2009). A clinical trial testing the efficacy of pramipexole found the drug to be superior to placebo in treating the depression of PD patients (Barone et al., 2010). A trial of the norepinephrine uptake inhibitor, atomoxetine, found it to be ineffective in treating depression in PD (Weintraub et al., 2010b).

If a severely depressed patient with PD fails to respond to antidepressant drug treatment, electroconvulsive therapy (ECT) can be used (Douyon et al., 1989). Indeed, ECT in itself can temporarily improve mobility in PD. Tranylcypromine, a noncompetitive inhibitor of types A and B monoamine oxidase, is an effective antidepressant (Fahn and Chouinard, 1998), but cannot be give in the presence of levodopa because of the likelihood of hypertension.

Anxiety

Anxiety and panic can be major difficulties in PD (Stein et al., 1990). Many patients, even early in the illness, complain of loss of confidence. In particular, they fear social occasions and public display at work, and they tend to withdraw from outside life. In part, this is due to anxiety over their friends and acquaintances perceiving that they have PD, and to their loss of mobility and their nonverbal emotional responses to social interactions. However, some also develop a generalized and disturbing anxiety state, which might require psychotherapy and anxiolytic drug treatment. Those in the more advanced stages of the illness may experience profound anxiety and even terror during "off" periods (Nissenbaum et al., 1987).

Often, anxiety can be relieved by effective antiparkinsonian drug therapy, but if uncontrolled and pervasive, it might require an antidepressant, and if dysphoria is present, a benzodiazepine (e.g., lorazepam 0.52 mg three times a day) or buspirone. Anxiety and stress worsen tremor, and alprazolam 0.25 mg during those periods can provide relief. However, all these drugs can increase confusion in those who are cognitively impaired.

Many patients have sensory or behavioral "off" periods, either accompanying or instead of a motor "off." The behavioral symptoms can consist of depression, anxiety, dysphoria, and panic; the sensory symptoms consist of pain or akathisia mainly. These sensory or behavioral "offs" are most distressing to the patient. Whereas motoric "offs" represent insufficient dopaminergic "tone" in the neostriatum, the behavioral and sensory "offs" probably represent an insufficient dopaminergic "tone" in the limbic dopaminergic areas of the brain, such as the nucleus accumbens, amygdala, and cingulate cortex. Like motor "offs," these sensory "offs" respond to dopaminergic medication. Keeping the patient "on" all the time would prevent these sensory "offs," but this is a difficult task. It is not clear that deep brain stimulation can overcome sensory "offs." Often patients with sensory "offs" will take more and more levodopa in order to stay "on." This can lead to dopamine dysregulation syndrome, and these patients can be considered as "levodopa addicts."

Cognitive problems

As listed in Table 8.6, slowness of thinking (bradyphrenia) and trouble finding words ("tip of the tongue phenomenon") are common in patients with PD. (Dementia is discussed in the next section.) If these defects are specifically looked for, about two-thirds of patients with early PD will show abnormalities of cognitive function on formal neuropsychological testing (Lees and Smith, 1983; Brown and Marsden, 1990; Levin et al., 1989; Cooper et al., 1991). In particular, such patients are weak in performance of tests that are sensitive to frontal lobe dysfunction (executive function), such as verbal fluency, the Wisconsin card sorting test, the

Tower of London test and its variants, and tests of working memory. Poor performance on tests such as these suggests abnormalities of frontal lobe executive functions, which may be due to defective input from nonmotor basal ganglia regions (via thalamus) into prefrontal cerebral cortical areas. Thus, some patients with early PD may exhibit a frontostriatal cognitive syndrome, which is sometimes rather inaccurately described as a subcortical dementia, in the absence of any major defects in language, episodic memory, or visuospatial functions. The pathologic substrate of such a frontostriatal cognitive syndrome in PD is debatable. Dopamine deficiency in the nonmotor regions of the striatum, especially the caudate nucleus which receives from and projects to prefrontal cerebral cortex, loss of dopamine projections from the midbrain ventral tegmental area to the frontal lobes, loss of cortical cholinergic projections from the substantia innominata, loss of cortical noradrenergic projections from the locus coeruleus, and cortical Lewy body degeneration may all contribute.

The Montreal Cognitive Assessment (MoCA) was found to be a useful screening tool for cognitive dysfunction in PD and more sensitive than the MMSE (Gill et al., 2008; Hoops et al., 2009). Using more formal neuropsychological testing in newly diagnosed PD patients and controls, Aarsland and colleagues (2009) found that 18.9% of patients had mild cognitive impairment, with a relative risk of 2.1. Ultimately most patients with PD have cognition problems and eventually dementia. In one study, 13 out of 126 (10%) newly diagnosed cases of PD had developed dementia at a mean of 3.5 years from diagnosis, corresponding to an annual dementia incidence of 30.0 per 1000 person-years; rapid development of dementia was associated with the postural instability and gait disorder (PIGD) form of PD (Williams-Gray et al., 2007). Hely and colleagues (2005) reported cognitive decline in 84% and dementia in 48% of patients with PD for 15 years. By 20 years, 83% had dementia (Hely et al., 2008). The Hely results are presented in Tables 6.7 and 6.8. Aarsland and colleagues (2003), following patients for 8 years, found that by that time span, 78% had cognitive decline. In another Norwegian study, in which PD patients were followed for 12 years, 60% had developed dementia, with dementia steadily increasing with age, reaching to 80–90% by age 90 years (Buter et al., 2008).

One approach to determine the pathoanatomic correlates with cognitive decline is to measure the functional networks detected by fluorodeoxyglucose positron emission tomography (FDG PET) scanning. Whereas the motor manifestations of PD have been linked to an abnormal covariance pattern involving basal ganglia thalamocortical pathways, a covariance pattern that correlated with impaired memory and executive functioning was found to be metabolic reductions in frontal and parietal association areas and relative increases in the cerebellar vermis and dentate nuclei (Huang et al., 2007). This network of PD cognitive pattern (PDCP) increased stepwise with worsening cognitive impairment (Huang et al., 2008).

The clinical question is to what extent such neuropsychological defects intrude into everyday life in patients with PD. In this context two clinical features of PD deserve further comment, namely bradyphrenia and abulia.

Bradyphrenia or slowness of thought probably is a real component of PD in many patients. For example, patients

Table 8.6 Cognition and dementia in Parkinson disease

Bradyphrenia
"Tip of the tongue" phenomenon
Confusion
Dementia

might comment on a slowing of mental processing and memory retrieval, and examination of neuropsychological test performance might show delay in deciding on choices, although the final decisions are correct. Finding the right word, or the answer to a question may be slow. The "tip of the tongue" phenomenon refers to the patient's knowing the word he or she wants, but not being able to come up with it and say it at that moment, a problem that is often encountered in PD (Matison et al., 1982). Some patients with PD spontaneously volunteer the observation that they have less ability to deal with mental problems, particularly multiple tasks at the same time. However, the extent to which depression might contribute to such problems is controversial. The general concept of bradyphrenia could be considered in the wider issue of abulia.

The overall impression of cognitive dysfunction in nondemented patients with PD may be summarized as follows: (1) Many, but not all, patients with early PD exhibit subtle frontostriatal cognitive impairments, but to begin with, these do not necessarily intrude into everyday life. (2) However, a substantial number of patients with early PD do complain of some cognitive change, in particular a slowing of thought, a difficulty or delay in memory retrieval, and problems in handling multiple tasks. (3) Such cognitive impairments may be due to depression, when there is a change in mood, but often there is no dysphoria. One multicenter survey of nondemented PD patients revealed that 26% had mild cognitive impairment (Aarsland et al., 2010).

Unfortunately, these selective cognitive impairments do not seem to respond to dopamine replacement therapy in the way the motor problems of PD do. Nor do they respond to antidepressants, unless depression is present and is itself the cause of the slowness of thinking. It is important to assess and treat any concurrent depression. It also is important to review current drug therapy. Anticholinergics, amantadine, dopamine agonists, and even levodopa in excess might well impair cognitive function, especially in the elderly PD patient.

Whether these cognitive difficulties are the precursor to frank dementia is uncertain, but obviously, they raise concern. In practice, it is likely that a minority of patients with such complaints in the early stages of PD will progress to frank dementia. Risk factors for developing dementia are low serum epidermal growth factor (Chen-Plotkin et al., 2011), low CSF amyloid-beta (Siderowf et al., 2010), and severity of olfactory impairment (Stephenson et al., 2010).

Dementia and confusion

Unfortunately, a sizable proportion of patients with PD eventually develop a multifocal, pervasive dementia. This typically occurs in elderly patients. Cross-sectional studies suggested that in those with PD aged over 65 years some 20% will be demented, compared to some 10% of non-PD individuals in this age group (Brown and Marsden, 1984). Initial prospective longitudinal studies raised that up to 40% becoming demented as they age (Biggins et al., 1992; Mayeux et al., 1990; Hughes et al., 2000). Aarsland and colleagues (2001) found the incidence rate for dementia to be 95.3 per 1000 person-years, which is a six-fold greater risk than that in non-PD individuals. Following PD patients over an 8-year

period, Aarsland and colleagues (2003) found that 78.2% developed dementia, and that hallucinations and akinetic-dominant or mixed tremor/akinetic PD were high risk factors for dementia. Another study also found that dementia was more likely to occur in the PIGD (postural instability gait disorder) category of patient than in the type presenting with tremor (Burn et al., 2006a). In fact, in studying the incidence of dementia, Alves and colleagues (2006) found that the tremor-dominant subtype did not develop dementia until those patients converted to the PIGD subtype. Other correlations for developing dementia are older age, greater severity and longer duration of PD, and male gender. However, looked at from the opposite perspective, most patients with PD, particularly the young, do not have dementia. Aarsland and colleagues (2004) followed the MMSE and found that the mean annual decline for PD patients was 1 point. However, a marked variation was found. In patients with PD and dementia, the mean annual decline was 2.3, which was similar to the decline observed in patients with Alzheimer disease. The Montreal Cognitive Assessment was found to be more sensitive as a screening tool than the MMSE, but a positive screen using either instrument requires additional assessment due to suboptimal specificity at the recommended screening cutoff point (Hoops et al., 2009).

It is bad enough to develop the debilitating and disabling problem of dementia, but what compounds this development is a lesser response to levodopa therapy in controlling motor symptoms (Alty et al., 2009). In patients without dementia the "off" phase motor function worsened at a yearly rate of 2.2% of the maximum disability score, and the magnitude of the levodopa response was well preserved as the disease progressed. Typically, patients who developed motor fluctuations maintained better "on" phase motor function than non-fluctuators ($P = 0.01$). However, dementia was associated with worse "on" and "off" motor disability scores ($P < 0.001$), and a smaller levodopa response magnitude after 14 years ($P = 0.008$).

The Movement Disorder Society's Task Force on Dementia developed a set of criteria for diagnosing dementia in patients with PD (Emre et al., 2007). PD dementia (PDD) is characterized by impairment in attention, memory, executive and visuospatial functions, and behavioral symptoms such as affective changes, hallucinations, and apathy are frequent. The Task Force proposed clinical diagnostic criteria for "probable" and "possible" PDD (Emre et al., 2007). It also proposed guidelines for assessing such patients (Dubois et al., 2007). Level 1 is for general clinicians; and Level 2 tests are for more sophisticated evaluations and even for clinical trials.

Concurrent Alzheimer disease, probably coincidental, obviously accounts for some of the dementia in PD (Boller et al., 1980). However, in recent years with the use of antisynuclein antibody stains to detect Lewy bodies, it has become apparent that widespread Lewy body degeneration is another common cause of dementia (Byrne et al., 1989), some say second in frequency to Alzheimer disease. In those with prior PD, this may follow the progression and spread of Lewy neurite distribution observed by Braak and colleagues (2003). *PD dementia* (PDD) is now the term applied to those whose PD symptoms began at least one year prior to the onset of dementia. It is called dementia with Lewy bodies (DLB) (McKeith et al., 1996) when the dementia precedes or occurs within 1 year after onset of parkinsonian motor features (Lippa et al., 2007). While there is a clear relationship between the duration of PD prior to the onset of dementia and key neuropathologic and neurochemical characteristics, there is a gradation of these differences across the dementia with Lewy bodies/Parkinson disease dementia spectrum and the findings do not support an arbitrary cutoff between the two disorders (Ballard et al., 2006).

DLB may coexist with the pathologic changes of Alzheimer disease, particularly with amyloid plaques rather than neurofibrillary tangles. One hypothesis is that the two pathologies, Lewy body degeneration in cerebral cortex and the cholinergic substantia innominata, and Alzheimer disease change, coexist by chance but summate to cause dementia. Another hypothesis is that the one predisposes to the other, and it is intriguing that α-synuclein is a component of both plaques (the non-amyloid component) and Lewy bodies. Whatever the pathogenic mechanism, this combination (which some have called the Lewy body variant of Alzheimer disease) is a common cause of dementia in PD. Pure dementia with Lewy bodies probably is less common. But it has been shown pathologically that cortical Lewy bodies can be associated with cognitive impairment independent of Alzheimer disease type pathology (Mattila et al., 2000).

Thus, there are at least three common substrates for dementia in PD: Alzheimer disease, Alzheimer disease with Lewy bodies, and diffuse Lewy body disease (also called dementia with Lewy bodies) (DLB). A fourth possibility is dementia with just the standard pathology of PD (PDD), typically with Lewy bodies in the cerebral cortex. Whether such dementia in patients with PD occurs without the spread of Lewy bodies into the cortex is uncertain. In addition, all the other causes of dementia may occur in patients with PD, including cerebrovascular disease, rarer degenerations such as frontotemporal dementia and Pick disease, cerebral tumors and other intracranial mass lesions, hydrocephalus, and metabolic, endocrine, and vitamin abnormalities. In one pathologic study, the Lewy body score was significantly associated with the rate of cognitive decline (Aarsland et al., 2005).

Parkinson disease dementia (PDD) shares identical clinical features with dementia with Lewy bodies (DLB); both entities can be distinguished from Alzheimer disease (Galvin et al., 2006). A personality trait that distinguishes DLB/PDD from Alzheimer disease is passivity (diminished emotional responsiveness, relinquished hobbies, growing apathy, and purposeless hyperactivity) (Galvin et al., 2007). Neuroimaging with Pittsburgh Compound B (PIB) ligand with PET can reveal the presence of fibrillar Abeta amyloid, which is present in patients with PDD (Brooks, 2009; Burack et al., 2010). This is present in the absence of Alzheimer disease at autopsy.

Accordingly, the first step in assessment of a patient with PD who has dementia is to undertake the usual investigations for known causes, especially those that are treatable. Depression causing a pseudo-dementia also must be carefully assessed. Anticholinergic drugs in PD appear to hasten cognitive decline (Ehrt et al., 2010), and withdrawal of such agents could improve cognitive function.

Having excluded such symptomatic causes of dementia, the clinical picture may give important clues as to the underlying degenerative condition causing the dementia.

Prominent early memory difficulties with language, praxis, and visuospatial problems pointing to temporo-parietal problems suggest Alzheimer disease. A variable, fluctuating course with prominent hallucinations (especially visual), confusion, and an unusual susceptibility to neuroleptics could indicate dementia with Lewy bodies (McKeith et al., 1996, 1999), i.e., diffuse Lewy body disease. Prominent behavioral, speech and memory difficulties could point to frontotemporal dementia or Pick disease.

FDG PET scans were correlated with the dementia score on the UPDRS. A correlation was found with left limbic structures such as the cingulate gyrus, parahippocampal gyrus, and medial frontal gyrus (Wu et al., 2000).

Whatever the pathologic substrate of dementia in PD, the combination poses formidable management problems. These are similar to those discussed in the section entitled "Psychosis; hallucinations, and paranoia." The difficulty is to maintain mobility with adequate doses of antiparkinsonian medication without exacerbating the mental and behavioral problems. Behavioral disturbances, including verbal and physical aggression, wandering, agitation, inappropriate sexual behavior, uncooperativeness, and urinary incontinence, cause major difficulties. General structured care in a familiar environment is essential. Judicious use of daycare facilities and home assistants may be necessary. Drug therapy should be simplified, removing selegiline, anticholinergic agents, amantadine, and dopamine agonists. Depression might require specific treatment, preferably avoiding antidepressants with marked anticholinergic properties. Nocturnal sedation might require quetiapine, which provides both sedation and antihallucinatory effects. Clozapine does the same but requires weekly ascertainment for neutropenia. Other bedtime hypnotics, such as benzodiazepines and zolpidem, can be effective. Donepezil (Aricept), which provides modest benefit in Alzheimer disease, has been found also to provide modest benefit in cognition in those with PD who are demented without aggravating the motoric symptoms of PD (Aarsland et al., 2002; Ravina et al., 2005). Rivastigmine and other centrally active cholinesterase inhibitors were found to provide some improvement in apathy, anxiety, delusions, and hallucinations in patients with DLB (McKeith et al., 2000) and can improve dementia (Giladi et al., 2003). In a large multicenter, controlled clinical trial, rivastigmine was found to provide moderate improvement in dementia associated with PD (Emre et al., 2004). Memantine was found to be superior to a placebo in a couple of small studies (Aarsland et al., 2009a; Leroi et al., 2009). An evidence-based review of treatment of PD dementia and psychosis was conducted by the American Academy of Neurology (Miyasaki et al., 2006).

Dementia, with or without a frank confusional state, is the commonest cause of final nursing home placement in those with PD, and shortens life expectancy (Goetz and Stebbins, 1993).

Compulsive behaviors

A large multicenter, cross-sectional evaluation of impulse control disorders (ICDs) assessed 3090 patients with PD (Weintraub et al., 2010a). The point prevalence estimates of four ICDs were 5.0% with pathological gambling, 3.5% with hypersexuality, 5.7% with compulsive buying, and 4.3% with binge-eating. ICDs were more common in patients treated with a dopamine agonist than in patients not taking a dopamine agonist (17.1% vs. 6.9%; odds ratio, 2.72; $P < 0.001$). ICD frequency was similar for pramipexole and ropinirole (17.7% vs. 15.5%). ICDs have become a problem, particularly for young individuals on a dopamine agonist. A screening questionnaire for ICDs has been validated (Weintraub et al., 2009).

In the category of compulsive behaviors, the most newsworthy has been *pathologic gambling* (Driver-Dunckley et al., 2003), which is now being more widely recognized. It is possibly related to dopaminergic stimulation in the mesolimbic system (Gschwandtner et al., 2001). Treatment of PD with a dopamine agonist increases the lifetime risk of a PD patient to have pathologic gambling from 3.4% to 7.2% (Voon et al., 2006a). In a PD clinic in Scotland, pathologic gambling occurred in 8% of patients on dopamine agonists (Grosset et al., 2006b). Patients with a younger age at PD onset, higher novelty seeking traits, and a personal or family history of alcohol use disorders were found to have a greater risk for pathologic gambling with dopamine agonists (Voon et al., 2007). Pathologic gambling is not limited to patients with PD on dopamine agonists. It has also been seen in patients with restless legs syndrome treated with these drugs (Tippmann-Peikert et al., 2007). In a PET study of PD patients during gambling, those with pathologic gambling had greater decreases in raclopride binding in the ventral striatum during gambling (13.9%) than control patients (8.1%), likely reflecting greater dopaminergic release (Steeves et al., 2009).

In a survey of other reward-seeking behaviors in 297 patients with PD, pathologic *hypersexuality* lifetime prevalence was 2.4%, and *compulsive shopping* was 0.7% (Voon et al., 2006b); combined with pathologic gambling data, the lifetime prevalence of these behaviors was found to be 6.1% and increased to 13.7% in patients on dopamine agonists. In another survey of 272 patients with PD, these compulsive behaviors were found to have occurred in 6.6% (Weintraub et al., 2006). Dopamine agonists and a history of ICD symptoms prior to PD onset were found to be risk factors.

Compulsive eating with weight gain has also been reported with dopamine agonist therapy, especially pramipexole (Kumru et al., 2006; Nirenberg and Waters, 2006). This is in contrast to the typical weight loss often seen in patients with PD. In one analysis, patients with PD were found to have lost a mean of 7.7% of body weight over a mean of 13.1 years with PD (Uc et al., 2006).

The term *punding* has been used to describe an abnormal motor behavior in which there is an intense fascination with repetitive handling and examining of mechanical objects, such as picking at oneself, taking apart watches and radios, or sorting and arranging of common objects, such as lining up pebbles, rocks, or other small objects. Punding has been reported with levodopa (Fernandez and Friedman, 1999) and dopamine agonists (McKeon et al., 2007), including for the treatment of restless legs syndrome (Evans and Stegeman, 2009).

A common form is repetitive cleaning/rearranging/ordering behaviors, which can be disabling. These have associated features of hypomania, occur during motor "on" periods, and often occur nocturnally (Kurlan, 2004). The repetitive

behavior responds poorly to serotonin reuptake inhibitors, but may benefit from atypical antipsychotics (Kurlan, 2004). Punding, a term that was first used in amphetamine abusers, is considered a dopamine dysregulation disorder (Evans et al., 2004). This behavior would appear to be a form of compulsive disorder. In this age of technology, excessive use of the computer is a particular form of repetitive behavior reported to be caused by levodopa therapy (Fasano et al., 2006). Punding incidence is lower than other compulsive behaviors (Miyasaki et al., 2007).

In a small cross-over study, amantadine was found to reduce pathologic gambling (Thomas et al., 2010), however two reviews of databases showed that pathologic gambling and other ICDs are more often associated with patients on amantadine (Weintraub et al., 2010c; Lee et al., 2011).

Psychosis: hallucinations and paranoia

Criteria for diagnosing psychosis in PD and differentiating it from other causes of psychosis were established by an NIH working group (Ravina et al., 2007). These criteria were in the style of the Diagnostic and Statistical Manual of Mental Disorders IV-TR (Table 8.7).

Hallucinations occur in a significant proportion of those with PD, especially in elderly patients. In a community study

---

Table 8.7 Proposed diagnostic criteria for PD-associated psychosis

Characteristic symptoms

Presence of at least one of the following symptoms (Criterion A) (specify which of the symptoms fulfill the criteria):
Illusions
False sense of presence
Hallucinations
Delusions

Primary diagnosis

UK brain bank criteria for PD

Chronology of the onset of symptoms of psychosis

The symptoms in Criterion A occur after the onset of PD

Duration

The symptom(s) in Criterion A are recurrent or continuous for 1 month

Exclusion of other causes

The symptoms in Criterion A are not better accounted for by another cause of parkinsonism such as dementia with Lewy bodies, psychiatric disorders such as schizophrenia, schizoaffective disorder, delusional disorder, or mood disorder with psychotic features, or a general medical condition including delirium

Associated features (specify if associated):

With/without insight
With/without dementia
With/without treatment for PD (specify drug, surgical, other)

From Ravina B, Marder K, Fernandez HH, et al. Diagnostic criteria for psychosis in Parkinson's disease: report of an NINDS, NIMH work group. Mov Disord 2007;22(8):1061–1068.

in Norway, 10% of PD patients had hallucinations with insight retained, and another 6% had more severe hallucinations or delusions (Aarsland et al., 1999). Forsaa and colleagues (2010b) followed Norwegian PD patients over 12 years, and found that 60% developed hallucinations or delusions, with an incidence rate of 79.7 per 1000 person-years. Risk factors were higher age at onset, dopaminergic dose, and RBD at baseline.

Psychotic features appear to be due to a complex interaction between the progressive and widespread pathology of the illness (diffuse cortical Lewy body degeneration, concurrent Alzheimer plaques and tangles, and cortical cholinergic, noradrenergic, and serotonergic denervation), the unwanted effects of drugs (anticholinergics, levodopa, and dopamine agonists), and intercurrent illness (such as infections or metabolic disturbances)

Isolated visual hallucinations are fairly common (Naimark et al., 1996; Sanchez-Ramos et al., 1996). Auditory hallucinations are very uncommon (Inzelberg et al., 1998). Visual hallucinations often take the form of familiar humans or animals, which the patients know are false (pseudo-hallucinations). Even when the hallucinations do not disturb the patient because the visual images are friendly and not frightening (benign hallucinations), these milder forms can worsen to a more malignant type of hallucination (Goetz et al., 2006). Such hallucinations may progress to a delusional paranoid state (often concerning infidelity) or a frank confusional state with impairment of attentiveness and disorientation. FDG PET reveals that PD patients with visual hallucinations have a reduced metabolic rate in the occipitotemporoparietal regions, sparing the occipital pole (Boecker et al., 2007).

When such symptoms occur, although antiparkinsonian drug therapy is the most likely cause, it is wise first to search for some intercurrent illness, such as a stroke or intracranial mass lesion, a chest or urinary infection, disturbance of electrolytes, renal or hepatic dysfunction, anemia, or endocrine dysfunction. Psychosis due to antiparkinsonian medications can usually be counteracted by atypical antipsychotics, drugs that usually do not aggravate parkinsonism at a dosage that has a therapeutic benefit in treating the psychosis, namely quetiapine (Seroquel) and clozapine (Clozaril). Quetiapine appears to be effective only for milder psychosis, such as hallucinations, but not in more severe forms of psychosis, as demonstrated by its failure in controlled trials (Ondo et al., 2005; Kurlan et al., 2007; Rabey et al., 2007). Quetiapine had a similar clinical benefit to clozapine in one study (Merims et al., 2006). Because quetiapine does not cause agranulocytosis and does not require blood count monitoring (Fernandez et al., 1999; Juncos et al., 2004) as does clozapine, it is practical to start therapy with quetiapine if the hallucinations are mild. A dose of 25–50 mg at night can often control confusion and psychosis without worsening the parkinsonism. Because of the potential for drowsiness, it is best initially to use a small dose of such drugs at night, thereafter gradually increasing the dose to that required to control the confusion without worsening the parkinsonism. The benefit of aiding sleep at night is an advantage, but try to avoid a dose that might extend the drowsiness to daytime. Quetiapine can be utilized as a hypnotic in older patients with PD to take advantage of suppressing the development of hallucinations in this susceptible population.

If quetiapine is ineffective or produces too much daytime drowsiness or other adverse effects, including worsening of parkinsonism, clozapine (Clozaril) should be tried next, starting with 12.5 mg at night to avoid daytime drowsiness and increasing the dose until benefit or adverse effects are encountered. It is more effective than quetiapine, but its use requires regular monitoring of blood counts to prevent the 1–2% risk of agranulocytosis (Scholz and Dichgans, 1985; Friedman and Lannon, 1990; Pfeiffer et al., 1990; Wolters et al., 1990; Kahn et al., 1991; Factor and Brown, 1992; Greene et al., 1993; Pinter and Helscher, 1993; Factor et al., 1994; Diederich et al., 1995; Rabey et al., 1995; Factor and Friedman, 1997; Ruggieri et al., 1997; Friedman et al., 1999; Pollak et al., 2004). In one open-label comparative trial, quetiapine and clozapine appeared equally effective; interestingly both also reduced the severity of dyskinesias as well as controlling psychosis (Morgante et al., 2004).

Other so called atypical antipsychotics appear to be so designated for marketing purposes. Olanzapine can be effective, but easily increases parkinsonism and so needs to be used in small doses to avoid a worsening of parkinsonism (Wolters et al., 1996; Friedman, 1998; Jimenez-Jimenez et al., 1998; Goetz et al., 2000); therefore, it is relegated to third choice. Risperidone more closely resembles a typical, rather than an atypical antipsychotic, and worsens PD. Aripiprazole has also worsened parkinsonism (Fernandez et al., 2004). A more thorough discussion of atypical antipsychotics is found in Chapter 19. Molindone, pimozide, or other relatively weak antipsychotics might also be considered.

An alternative to atypical antipsychotics are the centrally active anticholinesterase drugs that are used in the treatment of dementia. They have been reported to have similar efficacy on psychosis as quetiapine (Van Laar et al., 2001; Bergman and Lerner 2002; Reading et al., 2002; Burn et al., 2006b).

If psychosis continues without adequate benefit from the antipsychotics, selegiline, anticholinergics, and amantadine should be withdrawn. The need for anxiolytics and antidepressants should be reconsidered. If the symptoms persist, dopamine agonists should be reduced or stopped. If necessary, the dose of levodopa should be tapered. However, more often than not, as drugs are reduced to improve the mental state, mobility deteriorates. A brittle balance is reached at which the patient either is mobile but confused, paranoid or hallucinating, or is mentally clear but immobile. More dopamine replacement therapy is required to maintain mobility, but this causes a recurrence of the confusion, and it is very difficult to achieve a compromise. In this situation, a limited drug holiday, withdrawing dopaminergic drugs for 1–2 days each week, might help to dispel psychotoxicity, allowing a reasonable dose of medication to maintain mobility on other days. Sustained withdrawal of levodopa provokes unacceptable parkinsonism and, sometimes, particularly if the levodopa is withdrawn suddenly, a "neuroleptic" malignant syndrome (Friedman et al., 1985; Hirschorn and Greenberg, 1988). When it comes to balancing drug-induced psychosis and parkinsonism, keep in mind that an intact mental function is more important than an intact motor function.

The serotonin 5HT$_3$-receptor antagonist ondansetron blocks nausea and vomiting due to anticancer drugs. It has been reported to reduce hallucinations, paranoia, and confusion in PD (Zoldan et al., 1995). Fifteen out of the 16 patients treated with 12–25 mg/day for up to 8 weeks showed moderate to marked improvement of visual hallucinations and paranoid delusions. There was no worsening of the parkinsonism. However, this was not replicated by Eichhorn and colleagues (1996), who failed to find benefit in most patients, and found waning of benefit in the few for whom the drug was initially beneficial.

Quality of life

Measuring quality of life (QoL) in 124 patients with PD, Schrag and colleagues (2000) showed that it significantly deteriorated with increasing disease severity, as measured by the PDQ-39, the EQ-5D, and the physical summary of the SF 36. The greatest impairment was seen in the areas related to physical and social functioning, whereas reports of pain and poor emotional adjustment had similar prevalence in patients with PD and the general population. The impairment of QoL was seen in all age groups and was similar for men and women, but the differences between patients with PD and the general population were most marked in the younger patient groups.

From the QoL survey of patients with PD conducted in Norway by Karlsen and her colleagues (1999b), the three most important factors impacting QoL were depression, sleep disorders, and a sense of low degree of independence. The first two were addressed in this chapter, and their prominence in QoL indicates the importance of the nonmotor symptoms of PD. Independence would be affected by gait and balance disorders predominantly. Sexuality is part of quality of life, and patients with PD are more dissatisfied with their sexual functioning and relationship than controls (Jacobs et al., 2000).

Falls and fractures also impact QoL. Compared to an equal number of age- and sex-matched non-PD subjects, PD patients were found to be at a 2.2-fold increased risk of fractures generally and a 3.2-fold greater risk of hip fractures specifically (Melton et al., 2006). Adjusting for age, the independent predictors of overall fracture risk in the PD subjects were female gender and dementia, both with hazard ratios of 1.6. Interestingly, chronic depression was associated with a reduced risk (hazard ratio 0.4). Perhaps depressed patients are more cautions in walking. Hip fractures were predicted by dementia (hazard ratio 2.2). Sato and colleagues (2006, 2007) showed that the incidence of fractures could be reduced by treating with risedronate, ergocalciferol (Sato et al., 2007), and lendronate and vitamin D2 (Sato et al., 2006).

Patients with PD tend to forget to take their medication or are late in the timing of a dose, which usually affects the patients with wearing-off. Erratic intake was shown to be an emerging and more common problem, which is likely to affect motor control and QoL adversely (Grosset et al., 2005). Electronic monitoring of tablet administration provides the most accurate methodology for determining accurate compliance (Grosset et al., 2006a). Improved QoL might be better achieved with better compliance of timing of medication in those who are fluctuators.

References available on Expert Consult:
www.expertconsult.com

Atypical parkinsonism, parkinsonism-plus syndromes, and secondary parkinsonian disorders

Chapter contents

Introduction	197
Progressive supranuclear palsy	197
Multiple system atrophy	208
Corticobasal degeneration	218
Parkinsonism–dementia syndromes	222
Frontotemporal dementias and other tauopathies	225
Parkinsonism–dementia–amyotrophic lateral sclerosis complex of Guam	232
Heredodegenerative parkinsonism	233
Secondary parkinsonism	233
Appendix	240

Introduction

Most patients who are referred to specialized movement disorder clinics with hypokinetic disorders are diagnosed clinically as having Parkinson disease (PD) (Table 9.1) (Jankovic et al., 2000). The second most common group of parkinsonian patients is categorized clinically as having parkinsonism-plus disorders and pathologically as having multiple system degenerations (Fahn, 1977; Jankovic, 1989; Stacy and Jankovic, 1992; Jankovic, 1995b; Jankovic et al., 2000; Litvan et al., 2003; Abdo et al., 2006) (Fig. 9.1). There is, however, a growing body of evidence to support the emerging classification of neurodegenerative disorders according to pathogenetic mechanisms into (1) amyloidoses (e.g., Alzheimer disease, or AD), (2) ubiquitin-proteasome disorders (e.g., PD, parkin PD), (3) synucleinopathies (e.g., PD, multiple system atrophy, or MSA), (4) tauopathies (e.g., frontotemporal dementia (FTD) with parkinsonism, or FTDP; progressive supranuclear palsy, or PSP; corticobasal degeneration, or CBD), (5) polyglutamine expansion diseases (e.g., Huntington disease, spinocerebellar atrophies (SCAs)), and (6) prion diseases (e.g., Creutzfeldt–Jakob disease) (Jankovic, 2008). As our understanding of the mechanisms of these diseases advances, refinements in this classification and new categories of disease will undoubtedly emerge. Besides parkinsonian findings, patients with these disorders exhibit additional ("plus") features. For example, supranuclear ophthalmoparesis typifies patients with PSP; dysautonomia and ataxia are typically present in MSA; laryngeal stridor occurs in striatonigral degeneration (SND); a combination of apraxia, cortical myoclonus, and "alien hand" occurs in CBD; dementia-parkinsonism occurs not only in PD dementia (PDD), but also in dementia with Lewy bodies (DLB) and AD; and dementia coupled with motor neuron disease occurs in parkinsonism–dementia–amyotrophic lateral sclerosis complex of Guam (Table 9.1). As there are no biologic markers for any of these disorders, the diagnostic criteria are based on the presence of certain clinical features and neuropathologic confirmation (Cummings, 2003; Litvan et al., 2003). While levodopa continues to be the most effective drug for the treatment of motor symptoms associated with PD, a minority (about a third) of patients with atypical parkinsonism also respond to levodopa, although "responsiveness" has not been well defined in the literature (Constantinescu et al., 2007).

Rarely, psychogenic causes have been implicated in the pathogenesis of parkinsonism (Lang et al., 1995). This chapter focuses only on the sporadic (nongenetic) forms of multisystem degenerations. The secondary and heredodegenerative causes of parkinsonism are covered elsewhere in this book and in other reviews.

Progressive supranuclear palsy

Clinical features and natural history

First described by Steele, Richardson, and Olszewski (Steele et al., 1964; Steele, 1972; Williams et al., 2008) in 1964, progressive supranuclear palsy (PSP) has become a well-characterized, distinct clinical-pathologic entity (Jankovic et al., 1990a; Golbe, 1993; Collins et al., 1995; Litvan, 1998b; Golbe et al., 2007; Golbe and Ohman-Strickland, 2007; Houghton and Litvan, 2007; Azher and Jankovic, 2008). The first volume solely devoted to PSP was published

© 2011 Elsevier Ltd, Inc, BV
DOI: 10.1016/B978-1-4377-2369-4.00009-3

Table 9.1 Classification of parkinsonism

I. Primary (Idiopathic) parkinsonism

Parkinson disease

Juvenile parkinsonism (Ishikawa and Miyatake, 1995)

II. Multiple system degenerations (parkinsonism-plus)

Progressive supranuclear palsy

Multiple system atrophy

Lytico–bodig or parkinsonism–dementia–ALS complex of Guam

Corticobasal degeneration

Progressive pallidal atrophy (primary pallidal degeneration)

Parkinsonism–dementia complex

Pallidopyramidal disease (PARK15) (Remy et al., 1995; Horstink et al., 2010)

III. Heredodegenerative parkinsonism

Hereditary juvenile dystonia–parkinsonism (Ishikawa and Miyatake, 1995)

Autosomal dominant Lewy body disease (Wszolek et al., 1995)

Huntington disease

Wilson disease

Hereditary ceruloplasmin deficiency

Neurodegeneration with brain iron accumulation

- Aceruloplasminemia
- Neuroferritinopathy
- Pantothenate kinase associated neurodegeneration (PKAN)
- PLA2G6 associated neurodegeneration (PLAN)
- Fatty acid hydroxylase associated neurodegeneration (FAHN)
- ATP13A2 mutation (Kufor–Rakeb disease) and lysosomal disorders
- Woodhouse–Sakati syndrome (WSS)

Spinocerebellar ataxia (SCA) type 2, 3, 6, 12, 21

Frontotemporal dementia

Progressive autosomal dominant parkinsonism with central hypoventilation, depression, apathy, and weight loss (Perry syndrome) (Tsuboi et al., 2002)

Gerstmann–Strausler–Scheinker disease

Familial progressive subcortical gliosis (FPSG) (Lanska et al., 1994)

Lubag (X-linked dystonia–parkinsonism) (Wilhelmsen et al., 1991)

Familial basal ganglia calcification (bilateral striopallidodentate calcinosis; Fahr's disease) (Manyam et al., 2001; Brodaty et al., 2002; Oliveira et al., 2004)

Mitochondrial cytopathies with striatal necrosis

Juvenile neuronal ceroid lipofuscinosis (Åberg et al., 2000)

Juvenile parkinsonism with neuronal intranuclear inclusions (O'Sullivan et al., 2000)

Familial parkinsonism with peripheral neuropathy

Parkinsonian–pyramidal syndrome (Nisipeanu et al., 1994)

Neuroacanthocytosis (Rinne et al., 1994)

Hereditary hemochromatosis (Nielsen et al., 1995; Costello et al., 2004)

Fragile X-associated tremor/ataxia syndrome (FXTAS) (Hagerman et al., 2008)

Autosomal dominant striatal degeneration with dysarthria and gait disorder (5q13–5q14) (Kuhlenbaummer et al., 2004)

Progressive external ophthalmoplegia and parkinsonism associated with *POLG1* mutation (Hudson et al., 2007; Milone and Massie, 2010)

Sensory ataxic neuropathy dysarthria and ophthalmoparesis (SANDO) with parkinsonism and dystonia with *POLG1* mutation (McHugh et al., 2010)

Progressive encephalopathy with rigidity (with glycine receptor antibodies)

IV. Secondary (acquired, symptomatic) parkinsonism

Infectious: postencephalitic, AIDS, subacute sclerosing panencephalitis, CJD, prion diseases

Immunologic and paraneoplastic: voltage-gated potassium channel autoimmunity

Drugs: dopamine receptor-blocking drugs (antipsychotic, antiemetic drugs), reserpine, tetrabenazine, α-methyl-dopa, lithium, flunarizine, cinnarizine, ecstasy (MDMA), cyclosporine, (Mintzer et al., 1999)

Toxins: 1-methyl-4-phenyl-1,2,3,6-tetrahydropyridine, CO, Mn, Hg, CS2, cyanide (Rosenow et al., 1995), methanol, ethanol, organophosphates (Bhatt et al., 1999)

Vascular: multi-infarct, Binswanger disease, Sjögren syndrome

Trauma: pugilistic encephalopathy

Other: parathyroid abnormalities, hypothyroidism, hepatocerebral degeneration (Burkhard et al., 2003), alcohol-induced coma and respiratory acidosis with bilateral pallidal lesions (Kuoppamaki et al., 2005), brain tumor, brain stem astrocytoma (Cicarelli et al., 1999), normal pressure hydrocephalus (NPH), noncommunicating hydrocephalus, syringomesencephalia, hemiatrophy-hemiparkinsonism, wasp sting, peripherally induced tremor and parkinsonism, and psychogenic

in 1993 (Litvan and Agid, 1993), and a summary of the 1999 "First Brainstorming Conference on PSP" was published (Litvan et al., 2000). The diagnosis of PSP should be considered in any patient with progressive parkinsonism and disturbance of ocular motility (Jankovic, 1984a; Maher and Lees, 1986; Jankovic et al., 1990a; Friedman et al., 1992; Cardoso and Jankovic, 1994).

PSP is considered to be a sporadic disorder, but familial PSP has been reported (Brown et al., 1993; de Yebenes et al., 1995; Tetrud et al., 1996; Rojo et al., 1999; Kaat et al., 2009). The supranuclear ophthalmoparesis was not well documented in the familial cases, and the presence of atypical features, such as early cognitive decline in the family reported by Brown and colleagues (1993) and the relatively early age at onset (53 years) in the de Yebenes and colleagues (1995) kindred, suggested that these families had a neurodegenerative disorder

that was distinct from idiopathic PSP. Furthermore, no linkage to the *tau* gene has been identified in any of these families, although linkage to 1q31.1 has been demonstrated in one large Spanish family (Ros et al., 2005). In a comprehensive epidemiologic-genetic study, 33% of individuals with PSP were found to have at least one first-degree relative with dementia or parkinsonism and 12 families with PSP were identified (5 cases were pathologically confirmed), but the intrafamily phenotype was very variable, the P301L *MAPT* mutation was identified in only one patient, and there were other limitations in obtaining the family and medical information (Kaat et al., 2009). While it is possible that homozygous mutations occur, such as deletion at codon 296 in *MAPT* gene identified in one atypical case of PSP (Ferrer et al., 2003), the presence of subhaplotypes overrepresented in individuals with PSP increases the risk of the disease.

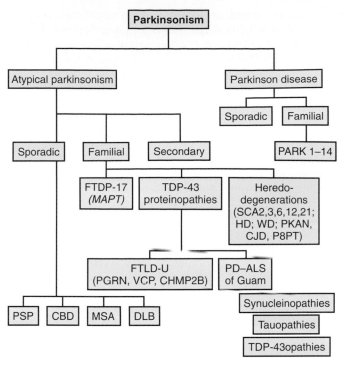

Figure 9.1 Classification of parkinsonism. SCA, spinocerebellar degeneration; WD, Wilson disease; PKAN, pantothenate kinase associated neurodegeneration; CJD, Creutzfeldt–Jakob disease. *Redrawn from Jankovic J. Parkinson's disease and movement disorders: moving forward. Lancet Neurol 2008;7:9–11.*

In a review of 126 PSP patients, unsteadiness of gait, frequent falling, monotonous speech, loss of eye contact, slowness of movement and of mentation, sloppy eating habits, and nonspecific visual difficulty were the most typical presenting features (Jankovic et al., 1990a). The earliest and most disabling symptom of PSP usually relates to gait and balance impairment, as a result of which patients frequently fall and sustain injuries. The average period from onset of symptoms to the first fall in PSP is 16.8 months, as compared to 108 months in PD, 42 months in MSA, 54 months in dementia with Lewy bodies, and 40.8 months in vascular parkinsonism (Williams et al., 2006). The marked instability is presumably a result of visual-vestibular impairment, axial rigidity, and bradykinesia (Jankovic et al., 1990a). Using computerized posturography, we demonstrated that measures of balance impairment can reliably differentiate between PSP and PD even in early stages of the disease (Ondo et al., 2000). In contrast to the short and shuffling steps, stooped posture, narrow base, and flexed knees that are typically seen in PD, PSP patients have a stiff and broad-based gait, with a tendency to have their knees (and trunk) extended and arms slightly abducted. Instead of turning en bloc, they tend to pivot, which further compromises their balance (Video 9.1). Some PSP patients may present with the syndrome of pure akinesia, also referred to by some as *motor blocks* (Matsuo et al., 1991; Giladi et al., 1992; Riley et al., 1994) and *gait ignition failure* (Atchison et al., 1993; Nutt et al., 1993), which is manifested chiefly by akinesia of gait (start hesitation, freezing, motor blocks, festination, disequilibrium with frequent falling), marked impairment of speech (stuttering, stammering, hypophonia), handwriting difficulty

(micrographia), and eyelid motor disturbance (blepharospasm, eyelid freezing) without rigidity, tremor, or dementia and without response to levodopa. Primary progressive freezing of gait or pure akinesia with gait freezing may be the initial, main, or the only presentation of PSP (Compta et al., 2007; Williams et al., 2007b; Facheris et al., 2008; Williams and Lees, 2009). Some of the patients with pure freezing may also have PD, pallidonigroluysian degeneration (Ahmed et al., 2008), CBD, and diffuse Lewy body disease (DLBD) (Factor et al., 2006; Williams et al., 2007b). In addition to PSP, frontal gait disorder may be the initial manifestation of AD and CBD (Rossor et al., 1999). Although the PSP may be associated with ataxia and the gait may appear ataxic, the patients usually do not exhibit prominent cerebellar findings. The uncompensated loss of postural reflexes and motor blocks (freezing) especially on turning, coupled with a peculiar lack of insight into the difficulties with equilibrium (possibly secondary to frontal lobe dysfunction), leads to frequent falling. There is, however, also emerging evidence of cerebellar abnormalities, both clinically and pathologically, in PSP (Kanazawa et al., 2009). Abnormal otolith-mediated reflexes may also contribute to the falls of PSP (Liao et al., 2008). Loss of insight, particularly inability to accurately predict performance on future tasks (anticipatory awareness), is a common feature not only in PSP but also in patients with FTD and CBD (O'Keeffe et al., 2007). This is often present even in the early stages of the disease and helps to differentiate PSP from PD (Litvan et al., 1996c). Although the motor subscale of the Unified Parkinson's Disease Rating Scale (UPDRS) has been found to reliably assess most aspects of PSP (Cubo et al., 2000), the PSP Rating Scale (PSPRS) has been found to be sensitive to disease progression, increasing at a mean rate of about 1 point per month (Golbe and Ohman-Strickland, 2007). PSPRS, along with the Quality of Life Scale (Schrag et al., 2006b), should be used in future clinical trials investigating novel therapeutic interventions. 🎥

Along with postural instability, supranuclear ophthalmoparesis typically manifested by paralysis of downgaze is the most important distinguishing sign of PSP (Litvan et al., 1997c) (Video 9.2). The predictability of these two features with regard to the final pathologic diagnosis was confirmed by a clinical-pathologic study of 24 autopsy-proven cases of PSP (Litvan et al., 1996b). About one-third of PSP patients complain of blurred vision, diplopia, and eye discomfort, but most eventually lose their ability to read or maintain eye contact (Friedman et al., 1992). Involuntary persistence of ocular fixation is a typical, though rarely mentioned, feature of PSP. Other oculomotor abnormalities that are seen in patients with PSP include impairment of saccades, optokinetic nystagmus, and the presence of square wave jerks (Rascol et al., 1991). In early stages of PSP, patients might have only mild limitation of voluntary downgaze and inability to converge, but slowing of horizontal and vertical saccades (also demonstrated by optokinetic nystagmus) appears to be the earliest oculomotor sign of PSP (Video 9.3). Indeed, slowing of vertical saccades, even in the presence of normal vertical saccade amplitude, was found to be an early sign of an autopsy-proven PSP (Hardwick et al., 2009). One study compared saccades, optokinetic nystagmus, and other ophthalmologic signs in six patients with PSP compared to PD and normal control (Garbutt et al., 2004). All PSP patients showed slowing of vertical saccade and quick phase of nystagmus; square wave jerks were more frequent and larger during fixation; vertical optokinetic nystagmus showed impaired slow wave response, and quick phases were slowed and combined with square wave jerks. Deficient generation of the motor command by midbrain burst neurons has been suggested as the primary mechanism for the slow vertical saccades (Bhidayasiri et al., 2001). Slowing of vertical saccades might help to differentiate PSP from other parkinsonian disorders, including PD, MSA, and CBD, although some slowing of vertical saccades can be seen occasionally also in these parkinsonian disorders (Vidailhet et al., 1994; Rivaud-Péchoux et al., 2000; Bhidayasiri et al., 2001). In addition to slow vertical saccades, bilateral impairment of the antisaccade task (the patient is instructed to look in the direction opposite to the visual stimulus) correlates well with frontal lobe dysfunction in PSP (Vidailhet et al., 1994) and other neurodegenerative and frontal lobe disorders (Condy et al., 2004; Munoz and Everling, 2004; Zee and Lasker, 2004). Abnormalities in antisaccades imply a dysfunction of the dorsolateral prefrontal cortex and the superior colliculus (Condy et al., 2004). Later, limitation of vertical and then lateral eye movements follows. The ophthalmoparesis can be overcome by the oculocephalic (doll's eye) maneuver (Videos 9.1, 9.2, and 9.4), but with disease progression and brainstem involvement, vestibulo-ocular reflexes can be lost, suggesting additional nuclear involvement (Ishino et al., 1974).

Several clinical-pathologic studies have attempted to establish criteria that separate PSP from other, related disorders. In 60 cases of patients clinically diagnosed with PSP, 47 (78%) of which were pathologically proven, false-positive diagnoses included PD combined with cortical Lewy body pathology or AD, MSA, CBD, Pick disease, motor neuron disease, cerebrovascular disease, and FTD (Osaki et al., 2004). The application of NINDS-SPSP diagnostic criteria (Litvan et al., 1996a) and other criteria improved the accuracy of initial clinical diagnosis only marginally. On the basis of an analysis of 103 pathologically confirmed consecutive cases of PSP, Williams and colleagues (2005) divided PSP into two categories: Richardson syndrome, characterized by the typical features described in the original report, and PSP-P, in which the clinical features overlap with PD and the course is more benign. The latter group, representing about a quarter of all patients with PSP (Williams et al., 2005), has less tau pathology than the classic Richardson syndrome (Williams et al., 2007a, 2008; Williams and Lees, 2009). The mean 4R-tau/3R-tau ratio of the isoform composition of insoluble tangle-tau isolated from the pons was significantly higher in Richardson's syndrome (2.84) than in PSP-P syndrome (1.63). Further studies are needed to confirm or refute this classification. Another subgroup of PSP that has been identified is the so-called "frontal" PSP, representing about 20% of all PSP patients (Kaat et al., 2007). These patients initially present with behavioral and cognitive symptoms, with or without ophthalmoparesis, and then they evolve into typical PSP.

Pathologically documented cases of PSP without ophthalmoparesis have been reported (Davis et al., 1985; Collins et al., 1995; Daniel et al., 1995). When PSP patients with ophthalmoparesis were compared with those without ophthalmoparesis, no differences in the pathology of the two groups were noted, and there was no correlation between the severity of clinical symptoms and degenerative changes (Daniel et al., 1995). In another pathologic study, brains of patients with PSP who had gaze palsy had two-fold greater loss of neurons in the substantia nigra pars reticulata (SNr) (Halliday et al., 2000). Since SNr projects to the superior colliculi, degeneration of SNr might contribute to the limitation of eye movements. Supranuclear ophthalmoparesis may occur also in DLB (Lewis and Gawel, 1990; Fearnley et al., 1991; De Bruin et al., 1992; Daniel et al., 1995; Brett et al., 2002), CBD (Gibb et al., 1990), postencephalitic parkinsonism, prion disease, Wernicke encephalopathy, dorsal midbrain syndrome, paraneoplastic syndrome, progressive subcortical gliosis, Whipple disease (Jankovic, 1986; Simpson et al., 1995; Averbuch-Heller et al., 1999), Niemann–Pick and Gaucher disease (Shulman et al., 1995; Uc et al., 2000), Kufor-Rakeb syndrome (PARK9; secondary to mutation in *ATP13A2* gene on chromosome 1p36) (Hampshire et al., 2001; Schneider et al., 2010), stiff-person syndrome (Oskarsson et al., 2008), primary pallidal degeneration, and other disorders (Calabrese and Hadfield, 1991).

Pseudobulbar symptoms in PSP patients are characterized chiefly by dysarthria, dysphagia, and "emotional incontinence" (Video 9.5). Rigidity, bradykinesia, and hypertonicity of the facial muscles produce deep facial folds and a typical worried or astonished facial expression (Jankovic, 1984b) (Fig. 9.2). The worried appearance is partly due to contraction of the procerus (and possibly corrugator) muscle, the so-called "procerus signs" (Romano and Colosimo, 2001) (Videos 9.1 and 9.2). Speech in PSP is characterized by a spastic, hypernasal, hypokinetic, ataxic, monotonous, low-pitched dysarthria (Kluin et al., 1993) (Videos 9.1, 9.4, and 9.5). The speech rate may be slow or fast, and some patients have severe palilalia and stuttering. An "apraxia of phonation" has been reported in one patient who was aphonic except during periods of excitement or during sleep (Jankovic, 1984b). In contrast, some patients have almost continuous involuntary vocalizations, including loud groaning, moaning, humming, and grunting sounds (Jankovic et al., 1990a). Progressive dysphagia causes most patients to modify their diet, and some eventually need a feeding gastrostomy to maintain adequate nutrition. As a result of chewing difficulties, inability to look down, and poor hand coordination, PSP patients are often described as "sloppy eaters."

In a review of dystonia in pathologically proven cases of PD, MSA, and PSP, Rivest and colleagues (1990) found dystonia to be an uncommon feature, noted in only 15 of 118 (13%) cases. They regarded the frequently reported neck extension as a form of axial rigidity rather than dystonia. In another study, the increased neck muscle tone was thought to have features of both dystonia (tonic shortening reaction) and rigidity (antagonist muscle contraction indicative of increased tonic stretch reflex) (Tanigawa et al., 1998). Neck extension, although often noted in published reports, is actually an uncommon sign in PSP. Indeed, neck flexion, usually associated with MSA (Quinn, 1994), can occasionally be seen in PSP (Daniel et al., 1995). In contrast to the typical presence of neck rigidity, truncal muscle tone is only slightly increased, and distal limbs may actually seem hypotonic (Tanigawa et al., 1998). In some patients, however, distal dystonia can be seen (Barclay and Lang, 1997).

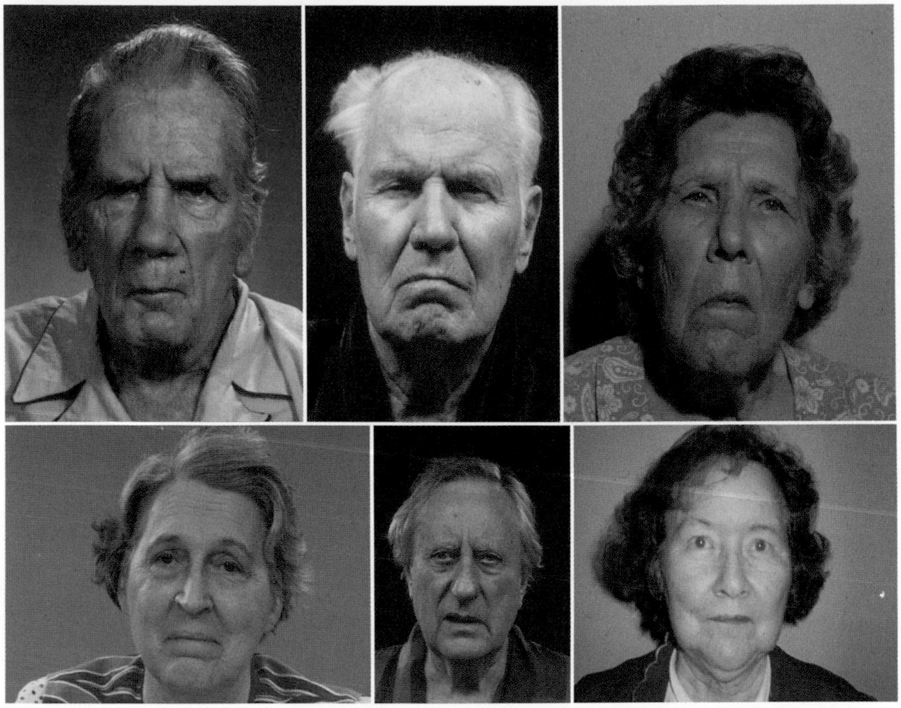

Figure 9.2 Faces of PSP.

Although PSP is usually a symmetrical disorder, dystonia represents an occasional exception in that unilateral dystonia may be present, particularly in the more advanced stages of the disease. The most common form of dystonia in PSP is blepharospasm. In one study, 29% of patients had involuntary orbicularis oculi contractions producing blepharospasm, and over one-third had "apraxia" of eyelid opening, eyelid closure, or both (Friedman et al., 1992). Although some (Lepore and Duvoisin, 1985) have hypothesized that these lid abnormalities are due to involuntary supranuclear inhibition of levator palpebrae, others have drawn attention to the similarity of this disorder of eyelid motor control to the parkinsonian phenomenon of sudden transient freezing, hence suggesting the term *lid freezing* (Jankovic, 1995a). Other terms that are used to describe this condition include *pretarsal blepharospasm* (Elston, 1992) and *focal eyelid dystonia* (Krack and Marion, 1994). In one study of 83 patients with PSP, 38 (46%) had some form of dystonia, 22 (24%) had blepharospasm, 22 (27%) had limb dystonia, and 14 (17%) had axial dystonia (Barclay and Lang, 1997). Sometimes, spontaneous arm levitation, a well-recognized sign in CBD, is also seen in patients with PSP and may be wrongly attributed to dystonia (Barclay et al., 1999).

In their original monograph, Steele, Richardson, and Olszewski (1964) indicated that mild dementia was present during early stages of the disease. Though some investigators have reported severe cognitive impairment in this population (Pillon and Dubois, 1993), others have attributed these deficits, at least in part, to poor visual processing (Fisk et al., 1982; Rafal et al., 1988; Jankovic et al., 1990a; Daniel et al., 1995). Despite a relative preservation of short-term memory, cognitive slowing, impairment of executive (goal-directed) functions, and subcortical dementia with deficits in tasks requiring sequential movements, conceptual shifts, and rapid retrieval of verbal knowledge are typically present in patients with PSP (Johnson et al., 1991; Pillon and Dubois, 1993; Litvan et al., 1998e). The memory disturbance that is found in patients with PSP is similar to that of patients with PD and Huntington disease, but it is markedly different from that of patients with AD (Pillon et al., 1994). The apathy, with or without depression, and other hypoactive behaviors that are typically seen in PSP have been attributed to a dysfunction in the frontal cortex and associated circuitry (Litvan et al., 1998e). This is in contrast to Huntington disease, in which behaviors such as agitation, anxiety, and irritability have been related to hyperactivity of the medial and orbitofrontal cortical circuitry. Sparing of olfactory function in PSP, in contrast to that in PD, is another clinical difference between the two neurodegenerative disorders (Doty et al., 1993). Litvan and colleagues (1996d) studied the neuropsychiatric aspects of PSP in 22 patients and found that apathy occurred in 91%, disinhibition in 36%, dysphoria in 18%, anxiety in 18%, and irritability in fewer than 9%. Another sign of frontal lobe dysfunction in PSP is the "applause sign" (*signe de l'applaudissement*), which probably represents a perseveration of automatic behavior (Dubois et al., 1995, 2005) (Video 9.6). This sign, characteristically present in patients with PSP (but also present in some patients with FTD with parkinsonism and CBD), is manifested by persistence (perseveration) of clapping after the patient is instructed to clap consecutively three times as quickly as possible. In a study of patients with various neurologic disorders evaluated at Baylor College of Medicine, the applause sign was present in 77.8% of 9 patients with CBD, 53.9% of 13 patients with MSA, 52.6% of 19 patients with PSP, 20% of 10 patients with Huntington disease, and 12.5% of 24 patients with PD (Wu et al., 2008). Although the test differentiated patients with CBD from those with PD ($P < 0.005$) and HD ($P < 0.005$), it failed to discriminate patients with PSP from other parkinsonian groups, but had a 100% specificity in distinguishing parkinsonian patients from normal subjects. 🎥

After idiopathic PSP, the most common cause of PSP is a multi-infarct state. Multi-infarct or vascular PSP can be difficult to differentiate clinically from the more common idiopathic variety (Dubinsky and Jankovic, 1987; Stern et al., 1989; Winikates and Jankovic, 1994; Rektor et al., 2006). In addition to a much higher frequency of stroke risk factors and abnormal imaging studies, the vascular PSP patients are more likely to have asymmetric and predominantly lower-body involvement, cortical and pseudobulbar signs, dementia, and bowel and bladder incontinence (Winikates and Jankovic, 1994). The concept of vascular PSP is supported by the observation by Ghika and Bogousslavsky (1997), who found that 81% of patients with clinically diagnosed PSP had hypertension. A clinical-pathologic study of four patients who were clinically diagnosed with PSP but found to have vascular PSP at autopsy showed that vascular PSP is characterized by asymmetric signs, falls within 1 year of onset, and vascular lesions on magnetic resonance imaging (MRI) (Josephs et al., 2002). In addition, three of the four patients carried the H2 tau haplotype, whereas 93.7% of patients with idiopathic PSP carry the H1 tau haplotype (78.4% of controls carry this haplotype) (see later). Reported causes of secondary PSP include exposure to organic solvents (McCrank et al., 1989), paraneoplastic syndrome (Jankovic, 1985), mesencephalic tumor (Siderowf et al., 1998), surgery on aorta (Mokri et al., 2004), and other rare and often unsubstantiated causes.

The relentlessly progressive course leads to death, usually from aspiration, within 10 years of onset in the majority of cases. In one clinical-pathologic study of 24 patients with PSP, the median survival from onset was 5.6 years, and this was shorter in men and in patients who experienced falls during the first year of symptoms and with early dysphagia or supranuclear palsy (Litvan et al., 1996c; Litvan, 2003). Overall, the median latency from onset to chairbound state is 5 years and to death is 7 years (Golbe and Ohman-Strickland, 2007).

In another clinical-pathologic study involving 16 cases of PSP, Birdi and colleagues (2002) found the mean survival to be 8.6 years (range: 3–24) years, and the mean age at death was 72.3 years (range: 60–89). The early onset, presence of falls, slowness, and early downward gaze palsy correlated with a rapid progression (Santacruz et al., 1998). In a review of 187 cases, those with early bulbar features had around 5 years less life expectancy than those who had no or late bulbar features (Nath et al., 2003). Similar to other series, the median survival in this study was 5.7 years. Since this figure is based on deceased cases, it might be too pessimistic because slowly progressive cases are still being followed. In another study of 50 PSP patients, Goetz and colleagues (2003) found the median survival from the onset of first symptom to be 7.9 years (6.5 years in the 21 patients who were followed to death). In addition to the short survival, PSP is associated with many symptoms that have a serious impact on the quality of life (Schrag et al., 2006b).

Epidemiology

About 6% of all parkinsonian patients who are evaluated in a specialized clinic fulfill the clinical criteria for PSP. On the basis of a medical record review of the Rochester Epidemiology Project, the average annual incidence rate has been estimated to be 5.3 new cases per 100 000 person-years (Bower et al., 1997). The prevalence, after age adjustment to the US population, has been estimated to be 1.39 per 100 000 (Golbe et al., 1988). In a review of computerized records of 15 general practices in and around London, Schrag and colleagues (1999) found an age-adjusted prevalence for PSP of 6.4 per 100 000. In other studies carried out in the United Kingdom, the prevalence of PSP ranged from 1 to 6.5 per 100 000 (Nath et al., 2001). Similar to the European studies, a prevalence of 5.82 per 100 000 has been reported in Yonago, Japan (Kawashima et al., 2004).

Like PD, PSP occurs more often in men, but its onset at a mean age of 63 years is about 10 years later than the typical onset of PD. Although no well-designed epidemiologic studies have been performed in PSP, one case-control study found that PSP patients were more likely to live in areas of relatively sparse population (Davis et al., 1988). Another study by the same investigators failed to identify any risk factor, except for low likelihood of completing at least 12 years of education, that would differentiate patients with PSP from a matched control population (Golbe et al., 1996).

Neurodiagnostic studies

Electrophysiologic studies have been helpful in documenting other abnormalities, such as sleep difficulties and seizures. Polysomnographic evaluation of 10 patients with moderate to severe PSP revealed marked sleep abnormalities; all had significant periods (2–6 hours) of insomnia (Aldrich et al., 1989). Sleep problems were correlated with worsening dementia. Another study showed marked reduction in percentage of REM sleep (Montplaisir et al., 1997). The same study also showed frontal electroencephalogram (EEG) slowing in patients with PSP. In a review of 62 patients seen over a 9-year period, Nygaard and colleagues (1989) noted seizures in 7 patients and suggested a higher-than-expected frequency of seizures in this population. This has not been our observation, but the relatively high frequency of seizures reported by Nygaard and colleagues (1989) might have been secondary to cortical infarcts. Abnormalities in motor and frontal sensory evoked potentials have been found in 8 of 13 patients with the clinical diagnosis of PSP (Abbruzzese et al., 1991).

The typical findings on computed tomography or MRI scans of patients with PSP include generalized and brainstem, particularly midbrain, atrophy (Stern et al., 1989; Soliveri et al., 1999). Measuring the anteroposterior diameter of the suprapontine midbrain, Warmuth-Metz and colleagues (2001) found that in contrast to PD patients (mean 18.5 mm), PSP patients had a significantly lower diameter (13.4 mm) on axial T2-weighted MRI, and as a result, the authors concluded that this finding reliably differentiates between PD and PSP and recommended that this evaluation "should be incorporated into the diagnostic criteria for PSP." In another study, utilizing midsagittal MRI, the average midbrain area of patients with PSP was 56 mm^2, which was significantly smaller than that of patients with PD (103 mm^2) or MSA-P (97.2 mm^2), and this parameter, particularly the ratio of the area of the midbrain to the area of the pons, was found to reliably differentiate among the three disorders

THE BIRDS OF PSP

Hummingbird   Penguin

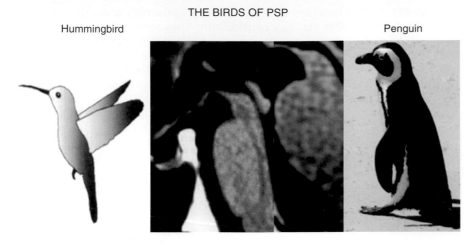

Figure 9.3 MRI characteristics of PD: the birds of PSP. Center image shows sagittal MRI of a brainstem of a PSP patient with characteristic atrophy of the midbrain with preservation of the pons giving the appearance of a hummingbird or penguin. *From Kato N, Arai K, Hattori T: Study of the rostral midbrain atrophy in progressive supranuclear palsy. J Neurol Sci 2003;210:57–60; from Oba H, Yagishita A, Terada H, et al. New and reliable MRI diagnosis for progressive supranuclear palsy. Neurology 2005;64:2050–2055, with permission.*

(Oba et al., 2005). On the midsagittal view of the MRI, as a result of atrophy of the rostral midbrain tegmentum, the most rostral midbrain, the midbrain tegmentum, the pontine base, and the cerebellum appear to correspond to the bill, head, body, and wing, respectively, of a hummingbird (Kato et al., 2003) or penguin (Oba et al., 2005; Sitburana and Ondo, 2009) (Fig. 9.3). The "hummingbird sign" was demonstrated in all 8 MRI scans of PSP patients but not in any of the 12 scans of PD patients or 10 scans of normal controls (Kato et al., 2003). The "morning glory sign," a peculiar MRI finding of midbrain atrophy with concavity of the lateral margin of the midbrain tegmentum, resembling the lateral margin of the morning glory flower, is observed in PSP patients with supranuclear gaze palsy (Adachi et al., 2004). Using diffusion-weighted MRI (DWI-MRI), Seppi and colleagues (2003) were able to differentiate between PSP and PD with 90% sensitivity and 100% specificity, but this technique could not differentiate between PSP and MSA. Using diffusion tensor imaging and voxel-based morphometry in PSP, Padovani et al. (2006) provided evidence of both gray and white matter degeneration even in early stages of PSP. Using voxel-based morphometry in 15 patients with clinically proven PSP and 14 with CBD, distinct patterns of atrophy were observed that differentiated between the two disorders with 93% accuracy (Boxer et al., 2006). CBD patients had marked asymmetric (L > R) pattern of atrophy involving premotor cortex, superior parietal lobules, and striatum, whereas PSP was characterized by atrophy of the midbrain, pons, thalamus, and striatum.

Stroke risk factors and a multi-infarct state on computed tomography or MRI have been noted in patients with PSP with a higher frequency than in those with PD (Dubinsky and Jankovic, 1987). One etiology for a subgroup of PSP might be small vessel disease producing subcortical ischemia with reduction of regional cerebral blood flow, cerebral hypometabolism, and a multi-infarct state. MRIs in patients with PSP, MSA, and other parkinsonian syndromes have been associated with putaminal hypointensity on T2-weighted MRI, but this finding is less consistently noted in PSP than in the other parkinsonism-plus syndromes (Drayer et al., 1989; Stern et al., 1989). In one study, PSP could be differentiated from MSA by the presence of marked atrophy and hyperintensity of the midbrain as well as atrophy of the frontal and temporal lobes (Schrag et al., 2000).The "eye

of the tiger" sign on brain MRI, typically associated with neurodegeneration with brain iron accumulation type 1 (NBIA1), formerly Hallervorden–Spatz disease (see later), has been also reported in PSP (Davie et al., 1997). PSP is associated with dorsal midbrain atrophy, and as a result of degeneration of superior colliculi, the floor of the third ventricle is flattened on sagittal MRI images (Savoiardo et al., 1994).

Positron emission tomography (PET) scanning has revealed decreased metabolic activity in the caudate, putamen, and prefrontal cortex (Foster et al., 1988; Goffinet et al., 1989; Blin et al., 1990), but the earliest sign of PSP appears to be decreased glucose metabolism in the midbrain (Mishina et al., 2004). Uptake of ^{18}F-dopa is usually reduced in PSP but may be normal in early stages (Bhatt et al., 1991). This suggests that the parkinsonian findings in early PSP are related more to postsynaptic receptor changes than to a loss of presynaptic dopamine terminals. In another study, ^{18}F-dopa uptake was markedly reduced in the caudate as well as in the anterior and posterior putamen of PSP patients (Brooks et al., 1990a). In contrast, the uptake was reduced only in the posterior putamen in PD patients. Similarly, dopamine transporter, imaged by [^{11}C]-WIN PET, showed a relatively uniform reduction involving the entire striatum, whereas patients with PD had involvement chiefly of the posterior putamen (Ilgin et al., 1999). F-dopa and F-deoxyglucose PET were abnormal in 5 (33%) individuals among 15 subjects at risk of familial PSP even though they did not (yet) exhibit any symptoms (Piccini et al., 2001). Using ^{11}C-raclopride as a D2 ligand, Brooks and colleagues (1992) showed a 24% reduction in D2 density in the caudate and a 9% reduction in the putamen of patients with PSP. A discriminant analysis of striatal ^{18}F-dopa PET studies indicates that this technique can reliably differentiate between PD and PSP, but it is less accurate in differentiating between PD and MSA (Burn et al., 1994). By using [^{11}C]diprenorphine, significantly reduced opioidergic binding has been demonstrated in both caudate and putamen, whereas the binding is essentially normal in PD and reduced in the putamen but not the caudate in SND (Burn et al., 1995). The cortical muscarinic acetylcholine receptors, as measured by PET and [^{11}C]N-methyl-4-piperidyl benzilate, were found to be normal in a series of patients with PSP (Asahina et al., 1998). Using [^{123}I]β-CIT SPECT, Pirker and colleagues (2000) showed marked reduction of striatal binding in PD, PSP, MSA, and CBD, but the pattern of abnormality (reduction in overall binding and asymmetry) did not allow a differentiation between the various disorders. Using the receptor ligand $[^{18}F]$altanserin, PET scans in 8 patients with PSP showed upregulation of 5-HT$_{2A}$ receptors in the substantia nigra and to a lesser degree in the striatum, as compared to 13 controls, and these changes significantly correlated with the UPDRS-III and PSP-Rating Scale (Stamelou et al., 2009).

In addition to imaging studies, analysis of the CSF may also be helpful in evaluation of patients with PSP. One study, for example, found a low ratio of light (33 kDa) to heavy (55 kDa) tau protein in the CSF of patients with PSP, which differentiated (without any overlap) this group from other tauopathies such as AD, CBD, and FTD and from synucleinopathies such as PD and DLB (Borroni et al., 2008). This finding had an 87% sensitivity and 86% specificity and was validated against MRI voxel-based morphometry of brainstem gray matter.

Neuropathology, neurochemistry, and pathogenesis

The motor, neurobehavioral, and neuro-ophthalmic findings seen in patients with PSP reflect marked neuronal degeneration in the basal nucleus of Meynert, pallidum, subthalamic nucleus, superior colliculi, mesencephalic tegmentum, substantia nigra pars compacta (SNc) and SNr, locus coeruleus, red nucleus, reticular formation, vestibular nuclei, cerebellum, and spinal cord (Steele et al., 1964; Steele, 1972; Zweig et al., 1987; Juncos et al., 1991; Jellinger and Bancher, 1993; Hardman et al., 1997a, 1997b; Kanazawa et al., 2009). In addition, in contrast to PD, both the globus pallidus interna (GPi) and externa (GPe) are markedly affected in PSP, and this may contribute to thalamic inhibition and some of the parkinsonian features (Hardman and Halliday, 1999a, 1999b). Along with the degeneration of the SNc and the pedunculopontine tegmental nucleus, the glutamatergic caudal intralaminar thalamic nuclei are involved in both PSP and PD (Henderson et al., 2000). In addition there is a widespread loss of A10 dopamine neurons, clearly more severe than in PD (Murphy et al., 2008). Atrophy of the superior cerebellar peduncle has been found to be a frequent finding in the brains of patients with PSP, and this correlates with the duration of the disease (Tsuboi et al., 2003b). In one pathologic study, marked atrophy of the GPi differentiated PSP from PD and DLB (Cordato et al., 2000). Cerebellar degeneration and tau-positive inclusion bodies have been demonstrated in the Purkinje cells of patients with PSP, particularly when associated clinically with ataxia (Kanazawa et al., 2009). Although bladder dysfunction has not been considered a prominent feature in patients with PSP, the finding of neuronal loss in Onuf's nucleus in patients with PSP suggests that bladder function should be carefully evaluated in patients with PSP (Scaravilli et al., 2000).

On the basis of a workshop sponsored by the National Institutes of Health, the following neuropathologic criteria were proposed: (1) high-density neurofibrillary tangles (NFTs) and neuropil threads in the basal ganglia and brainstem and (2) tau-positive astrocytes or their processes in areas of involvement (Hauw et al., 1994; Litvan et al., 1996a). Using rather crude pathologic criteria, De Bruin and

Lees (1994) demonstrated that the clinical manifestations of PSP can vary considerably. They reviewed 90 cases reported in the literature between 1951 and 1992 that met the following two criteria: subcortical neurofibrillary degeneration and exclusion of other recognized nosologic entities. There were 51 men and 34 women (in 5 cases, the gender was not specified), with an average age at onset of 62 years and mean age at death of 67 years. The most common symptoms were unsteady gait (70.7%), stiffness (67.4%), slurred speech (67.4%), falls (60.6%), dysphagia (57.3%), and blurring of vision (21%). Vertical gaze palsy was the most common sign but was noted in only 68.5% of all cases, followed by bradykinesia in 67.4%, dysarthria in 67.4%, rigidity in 58.4%, axial dystonia in 48.3%, segmental dystonia in 20.2%, and tremor in 16.8%.

Microscopic examination reveals NFTs, granulovacuolar degeneration, gliosis, and rare Lewy bodies (Steele et al., 1964; Steele, 1972; De Bruin and Lees, 1994). One pathologic study showed no evidence of increased Lewy bodies in PSP (Tsuboi et al., 2001). The NFTs in PSP differ from those seen in AD and other neurodegenerative disorders in that PSP tangles consist of 15 nm straight tubules rather than 20–24 nm wide paired helical filaments (PHF) (Joachim et al., 1987; Jellinger and Bancher, 1993; Dickson, 1997). PHFs are composed of the microtubule-associated protein tau (MAPT) in a hyperphosphorylated state (Goedert et al., 1996). In contrast to the other neurodegenerative diseases with tau pathology, such as AD, Pick disease, CBD, and the parkinsonism–dementia complex of Guam, which are characterized by flame-shaped NFTs, the NFTs in PSP are predominantly of the globose type. The tau-containing astrocytic inclusions ("tufted astrocytes") are more common in the basal ganglia and the brainstem of PSP, whereas they are more common in the cortex of brains of CBD. Tau inclusions in PSP oligodendrocytes are described as "coiled bodies." Tsuboi and colleagues (2003a) showed that APOE ε4 is a risk factor for Alzheimer-type pathology in PSP. Some brains of patients with Guam parkinsonism–dementia complex also contain deposits of the TDP-43 protein (TAR-DNA binding protein 43), which binds ubiquitin, suggesting that a common pathogenic mechanism through conformational changes in this protein links this disease with FTDP, ALS, and related neurodegenerative diseases (Hasegawa et al., 2007).

The clinical and pathologic overlap between PSP, CBD, and AD provides evidence that these disorders are closely related, although the absence of amyloid deposits in PSP and CBD suggests a clear difference between the two disorders and AD (Feany and Dickson, 1996; Litvan et al., 1999; Rossor et al., 1999; Boeve et al., 2003a; Wakabayashi and Takahashi, 2004; Galpern and Lang, 2006). Among 180 cases of clinically diagnosed PSP that came to autopsy, only 137 (36%) met the pathologic criteria for PSP (Josephs and Dickson, 2003). The other diagnoses included CBD, MSA, DLBD, and Creutzfeldt–Jakob disease (CJD). The following features were seen more frequently in non-PSP cases than in PSP cases: tremor, psychosis, early dementia, asymmetric findings, absence of H1 haplotype, and presence APOE ε4. The various disorders can be differentiated by a careful histologic examination. For example, the tau in NFTs of AD shows marked ubiquitin immunoreactivity, whereas the NFT-tau from PSP does not (Flament et al., 1991; Shin et al.,

MICROTUBULE ASSOCIATED PROTEIN TAU (MAPT)

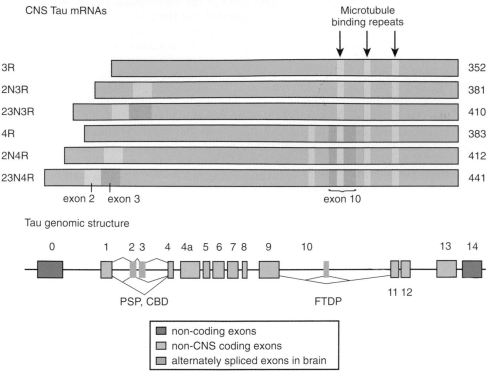

Figure 9.4 Tau gene and protein. The top of panel shows that the microtubule associated protein tau (MAPT) can contain three or four microtubule binding repeat domains depending on whether exon 10 is spliced in (4 repeats) or out (3 repeats). The tau genomic structure (bottom) shows alternative splicing of exon 10 (as well as exons 2 and 3). *Redrawn from Bird and Tapscott, in: Bradley WG, Daroff RB, Fenichel GM, Jankovic J, eds. Neurology in Clinical Practice, 5th edition. Elsevier, Philadelphia PA, 2007.*

1991). While the abnormal tau in AD consists chiefly of 55, 64, and 68 kDa forms, the PSP tau consists only of 64 and 68 kDa forms (Conrad et al., 1997) (Fig. 9.4). Cdk5, a kinase that is physiologically involved in the phosphorylation of tau protein, is overexpressed in PSP brains (Borghi et al., 2002). PSP and CBD also overlap with FTD in clinical, pathologic, biochemical, and genetic aspects (Boeve et al., 2003a). Tuft-shaped astrocytes seem to be more indicative of PSP than CBD, with prominent tuft-shaped astrocytes in the precentral gyrus and premotor cortex, caudate, putamen and globus pallidus, red nucleus, and superior colliculus in PSP brains (Hattori et al., 2003). Another pathologic evidence of overlap between PSP and CBD is the abundance of pathologic tau in the white matter in both disorders (Zhukareva et al., 2006). The histopathologic features of PSP also overlap closely with those of postencephalitic parkinsonism (Litvan et al., 1998c) and the parkinsonism–dementia complex of Guam, but the pallidum and the subthalamic nucleus are usually spared in the former, and the cortex seems to be more involved in the latter. Rarely, cases with clinical presentation nearly identical to that of PSP have been reported to have the pathologic picture of pallidonigroluysial atrophy (PNLA) (Kosaka et al., 1981; Ahmed et al., 2008). Of 400 cases of PSP, 8 (2%) were found to have pathologic features of PSP and PNLA is now considered a rare variant of PSP, with the latter usually presenting at a younger age, with gait and handwriting abnormalities in early stages, and having slower progression (Ahmed et al., 2008). In one study, 54% of pathologically proven cases of PSP had coexistent AD and PD, providing evidence for

overlap between these neurodegenerative disorders (Gearing et al., 1994). Calbindin-D_{28k} immunoreactivity, normally found in the medium-sized neurons and neuropil of the striatal matrix, GP, and SNr, is reduced in the GP of patients with PSP (and in striatum and SNr of patients with SND) (Ito et al., 1992). This finding suggests that calcium cytotoxicity might play a role in the marked neuronal degeneration that is found in these structures.

PSP and CBD also share pathologic tau doublet (64 and 69 kDa) as well as the predominance of 4R tau isoforms with argyrophilic grain disease (AGD). This sporadic neurodegenerative disease, which accounts for about 5% of all cases of dementia, is manifested by late-onset episodic memory loss and progressive dementia along with personality changes, irritability, agitation, delusions, and apathy. Neither clinical nor neuroimaging features can reliably differentiate between AGD and AD, and the diagnosis of AGD is based on autopsy findings. Pathologically, aggregated tau proteins are found in limbic structures in the shape of distinct argyrophilic grains and coiled bodies (Tolnay et al., 2002; Liang et al., 2005; Ferrer et al., 2008). Because of overlap in pathologic features with not only PSP and CBD, but also AD and other neurodegenerative diseases, questions have been raised whether AGD represents a distinct entity. Argyrophilic grains are present in 4–9% of adult brains and the incidence increases with age. Besides aging, oxidative stress appears to play a critical role in the development of the pathologic changes, including activation of tau kinases, which facilitate tau hyperphosphorylation in some neurons. The abnormal tau apparently binds to p62 and, after ubiquitation, aggregates, forming grains and tangles. Thrombin, which accumulates in the grains, has been thought to facilitate tau truncation, which further increases oxidative stress and contributes to the toxicity.

Molecular misreading of the ubiquitin-B (*UBB*) gene results in a dinucleotide deletion in ubiquitin-B mRNA, which in turn leads to accumulation of the mutant protein ubiquitin-B+1 in AD, Pick disease, FTD, PSP, and AGD, but not in synucleinopathies (PD or MSA) (Fischer et al., 2003) (Fig. 9.1). This finding provides evidence that the ubiquitin-proteasome system is impaired in these tauopathies and that ubiquitin-B+1 protein serves as a marker for these diseases. Unique haplotype in 17q21, found in 16% of Spanish as well as American PSP patients but not in any of the controls, provides further evidence that PSP is a form of a tauopathy (Pastor et al., 2004). Better understanding of the molecular pathways that are altered in various neurodegenerative disorders could be helpful in differential diagnosis based on postmortem examination of brain tissue. Using microarray technology in substantia nigra (SN) samples from six patients with PD, two patients with PSP, one patient with FTDP, and five controls, Hauser and colleagues (2005) found 142 genes that were differentially expressed in PD cases and controls, 96 in the combination of PSP-FTDP, and 12 genes that were common to all three disorders.

The marked reduction in striatal D2 receptors in PSP, demonstrated by PET studies, has also been documented in postmortem studies (Ruberg et al., 1993). In contrast to the D2 receptors, the striatal D1 receptors are spared (Pierot et al., 1988; Pascual et al., 1992). Biochemical studies show that in addition to degeneration of the nigrostriatal dopaminergic system, the cholinergic and GABAergic systems seem to be particularly affected. Cholinergic neurons have been found to degenerate in the Edinger–Westphal nucleus, the rostral interstitial nucleus of Cajal (possibly contributing to the extensor nuchal rigidity), the medial longitudinal fasciculus (contributing to vertical gaze palsy), the superior colliculus, and the pedunculopontine nucleus (Zweig et al., 1987; Juncos et al., 1991). Autoradiographic study of 18 brains of patients with pathologically confirmed PSP showed marked reduction in M2 and M4 receptors in the posterior striatal cholinergic interneurons and a reduction of M4 receptors on medium spiny projection neurons, confirming marked cholinergic dysfunction in PSP compared to Lewy body dementia ($n = 45$), Alzheimer disease ($n = 39$), and normal controls ($n = 50$) (Warren et al., 2007). Using the technique of an in-situ hybridization of GAD_{67} messenger RNA, Levy and colleagues (1995) demonstrated 50–60% reduction in the number of neurons expressing GAD_{67} messenger RNA in the caudate nucleus, ventral striatum, and both segments of the GP in three brains of patients with PSP. They suggest that the marked destruction of the basal ganglia output nuclei might explain the poor response to dopaminergic therapy in this disorder.

The most striking neurochemical abnormality found in PSP brains is a marked reduction in striatal dopamine, dopamine receptor density, choline acetyltransferase activity, and loss of nicotinic, rather than muscarinic, cholinergic receptors in the basal forebrain (Young, 1985; Pierot et al., 1988; Ruberg et al., 1993). Normal dopamine levels in the nucleus accumbens suggest that the mesolimbic system is relatively spared. Because of the relative sparing of the mesocorticolimbic dopaminergic system in contrast to the severe degeneration of the mesostriatal system, some investigators have suggested that the primary site of pathology in PSP is the striatum and that the changes observed in the SN are simply a result of a retrograde degeneration (Ruberg et al., 1993). The cholinergic neurons are, however, also markedly affected and may be primarily involved in PSP. The cholinergic innervation of the thalamus is particularly affected in PSP, and this finding helps to differentiate PSP from PD (Shinotoh et al., 1999). Also, reduction in acetylcholine vesicular transporter has been found to differentiate PSP from other types of neurodegenerative disorders (Suzuki et al., 2002). Suzuki and colleagues (2002) were able to correlate reductions in acetylcholine vesicular transporter and choline acetyltransferase activity in the striatum of postmortem brains of patients with PSP, but choline acetyltransferase was also significantly reduced in the inferior frontal cortex. Glutamate has been found to be increased in the striatum, pallidum, nucleus accumbens, and occipital and temporal cortex. In contrast to PD, glutathione was found to be increased in the SN of PSP patients (Perry et al., 1988). The observation that multiple neurotransmitters, particularly dopamine and acetylcholine, are affected in PSP suggests that PSP is not a primary neurotransmitter disease but a disorder in which multiple subpopulations of neurons degenerate for yet unknown reasons.

The cause of PSP is unknown, but oxidative damage, mitochondrial dysfunction, and abnormal protein (e.g., tau) processing have received the most attention (Albers and Augood, 2001). Decreased rates of adenosine triphosphate production were found in a preliminary study of muscle mitochondria function in patients with PSP, suggesting impaired mitochondrial respiratory chain activity in PSP (Di Monte et al., 1994). Further support for mitochondrial defect in PSP was later provided by additional studies. Using cybrid lines expressing mitochondrial genes, Swerdlow and colleagues (2000) found a 12.4% decrease in complex I activity ($P < 0.005$) in cybrid (cytoplasmic hybrid) cells but no change in complex IV activity. Cybrid cells also had significantly increased levels of several antioxidant enzymes. This study suggests a mtDNA-encoded electron transport chain enzyme defect in PSP. Further evidence for a defect in mitochondrial oxidative metabolism is the finding of significantly reduced levels of phosphocreatine and Mg^{2+} and increased levels of adenosine diphosphate and inorganic phosphate using phosphorus magnetic resonance spectroscopy of the brain and calf muscle in five PSP patients (Martinelli et al., 2000). Using proton magnetic resonance spectroscopic imaging, Tedeschi and colleagues (1997) found a reduced N-acetylaspartate/creatine-phosphocreatine ratio in the brainstem, centrum semiovale, and frontal and precentral cortex and N-acetylaspartate/choline in the lentiform nucleus in patients with PSP.

Research into mechanisms and treatment of PSP has been hampered by paucity of suitable animal models. Rats that are exposed systemically and chronically to annonacin, a lipophilic mitochondrial complex I inhibitor extracted from tropical fruit plants, have been shown to produce neurodegeneration resembling PSP, providing further evidence of mitochondrial dysfunction in PSP (Champy et al., 2004). Another potential animal model of PSP is a transgenic mouse (TgT34) which overexpresses wild-type human tau

(T34 *tau* isoform) driven by the astrocyte-specific glial fibrillary acidic protein promoter (Forman et al., 2005). These transgenic mice accumulate tau in astrocytes, similar to what occurs in PSP, leading to focal neuronal degeneration. Another potential animal model of PSP is the JNPL3 mouse in which the human four repeat *tau* with the P301L mutation is expressed resulting in a severe phenotype within 5–6 months but without motor defects (Lewis et al., 2000).

Recent studies have drawn attention to abnormal phosphorylation of tau proteins as an important mechanism of neurodegeneration in PSP. Tau exon 10 + 16 mutation in the *tau* gene (MAPT, IVS10, C-U, +16) was found in a case of young-onset (age 40 years) of PSP phenotype with neuropathologic features of FTD (Morris et al., 2003). Tau is phosphorylated by serine, threonine, and tyrosine kinases, and this phosphorylation might lead to abnormal aggregation. There is growing support for the notion of altered regulation of *tau* gene expression in PSP (Rademakers et al., 2005). The relationship between abnormalities in tau and PSP is described in detail in the section on tauopathies.

Treatment

Although in the early stages, mild improvement in parkinsonian symptoms may be noted with levodopa or dopamine agonists (e.g., pergolide, pramipexole), most PSP patients fail to reach and maintain any meaningful improvement with these drugs (Jankovic, 1983; Litvan and Chase, 1993; Nieforth and Golbe, 1993; Jankovic, 1994; Weiner et al., 1999). The most likely reason is that in PSP, there is a marked loss of the postsynaptic receptors, particularly the D2 receptors, secondary to the loss of the postsynaptic striatal neurons (Pierot et al., 1988). Idazoxan, an experimental, potent and selective α-2 presynaptic inhibitor that increases norepinephrine (NE) transmission, was shown in a double-blind crossover study to improve motor function in nine PSP patients (Ghika et al., 1991). Physostigmine has been shown to have variable clinical effects on cognitive deficits (Blin et al., 1995). Furthermore, PSP patients have been found to be unusually sensitive to cholinergic blockade with anticholinergic drugs (Litvan et al., 1994); therefore, these drugs should be avoided in patients with PSP. On the other hand, the cholinergic drug donepezil has not been found to be beneficial in a placebo-controlled trial of 21 patients with PSP, and it might actually worsen motor function (Litvan et al., 2001b). Other drugs, including methysergide and amitriptyline, although anecdotally reported to be beneficial, have been generally disappointing (Newman, 1985). Besides amitriptyline and serotonin uptake inhibitors, AVP-923 (Zenvia), a combination of dextromethorphan and quinidine developed by Avanir, has been used to treat involuntary emotional expression disorder (IEED), or pseudobulbar affect, also known as emotional lability or incontinence (Panitch et al., 2006; Rosen and Cummings, 2007). Zolpidem, a GABA agonist and a short-acting hypnotic drug, was found to improve moderately voluntary saccadic eye movements and motor function in a small (*n* = 10) group of patients with PSP as compared to placebo (Daniele et al., 1999). Blepharospasm, with or without eyelid freezing, and other forms of focal dystonias, can be effectively treated with botulinum toxin injections (Jankovic and Brin, 1991; Jankovic, 2004) (Video 9.7). Electroconvulsive therapy, while helpful in some patients with PD, markedly exacerbated motor and mental symptoms in one patient with PSP (Hauser and Trehan, 1994). Cricopharyngeal myotomy is almost never performed, but severe dysphagia in advanced stages of the disease often necessitates the placement a feeding gastrostomy. There is no evidence, however, that tube feeding prevents aspiration (Finucane et al., 1999).

Only symptomatic therapy has been used thus far, albeit with disappointing results, but it is hoped that better understanding of the pathogenesis of neuronal degeneration in PSP will lead to more effective, hypothesis-driven therapeutic interventions. It is possible, for example, that since cross-linking of tau protein by transglutaminase stabilized tau filaments into NFTs, inhibitors of transglutaminase may prevent the formation of NFTs and may have a neuroprotective effect on the disease (Zemaitaitis et al., 2000). For example, drugs such as lithium and valproic acid that inhibit abnormal phosphorylation of the tau protein by blocking the enzyme GSK-3β (also known as tau protein kinase I) might possibly exert neuroprotective effects (Chen et al., 1999). Lithium has been found to induce phosphorylation of the serine 9 residue of the glycogen synthase kinase (GSK-3β), inhibiting tau phosphorylation on the PHF-1 epitope and, therefore, this GSK-3β inhibitor may have neuroprotective properties in various tauopathies including PSP. Besides GSK-3β, lithium also inhibits inositol monophosphatase and the proteasome, protects cultured neurons against amyloid beta toxicity, prevents NFT accumulation, and causes downregulation of tau proteins by reducing tau mRNA (Rametti et al., 2008). By limiting tau phosphorylation, valproate would be expected to prevent the disturbed microtubule function, disrupted intracellular protein trafficking, formation of NFTs, and neuronal death. Valproate might also prevent elevations of intracellular calcium, increase levels of the antiapoptotic protein Bcl-2, act as a histone deacetylase inhibitor (which might interfere with apoptosis), and inhibit GSK-3β (Phiel et al., 2001; Qing et al., 2008). Other kinase inhibitors, such as noscovitine and olomoucine, might also play a role as potential therapeutic strategies in PSP.

Because of some evidence of mitochondrial complex I dysfunction in PSP (Di Monte et al., 1994), mitochondrial enhancers, such as coenzyme Q10 (CoQ10), have been studied in PSP. One randomized, placebo-controlled, phase II trial involving 21 patients with PSP showed slight but significant improvements in the scores of the total PSP Rating Scale and Frontal Assessment Battery in the group treated with a nanoparticular emulsion of CoQ10 (lipophilic emulsion, nanoQuinon, 5 mg/kg) compared to placebo (Stamelou et al., 2008). This was accompanied by a significant reduction in adenosine diphosphate (ADP) on magnetic resonance spectroscopy (MRS) in the occipital lobe and right basal ganglia. These encouraging findings from the initial study must be confirmed by a larger, phase III, clinical trial. Another drug, methylene blue (Urolene Blue), an old drug used for the treatment of urinary tract infections, thought to prevent formation of tangles in Alzheimer disease at doses of 60 mg three times a day of methylthioninium chloride (Rember, made by TauRx Therapeutics), may be potentially helpful in PSP. It is not clear whether the drug acts as a kinase inhibitor, but it has been shown to increase mitochondrial complex IV and to have a variety of antioxidant properties (Atamna et al., 2008). Another drug that is currently investigated in PSP is davunetide, an analog of vasoactive intestinal peptide which enhances the synthesis of the activity-dependent neuroprotective protein, of which Davunetide is a fragment (also known as NAP), administered as a nasal spray. This neurotrophic factor has been shown to stimulate neurite elongation and synapse formation, prevent toxicity from amyloid beta peptides, and limit tau hyperphosphorylation (Shiryaev et al., 2009).

Multiple system atrophy

Clinical features and natural history

Historically, the first case that James Parkinson described in his 1817 "Essay on the Shaking Palsy" had associated autonomic features and might have been the first case of MSA. First coined by Graham and Oppenheimer in 1969 (Graham and Oppenheimer, 1969), the term *multiple system atrophy* describes a syndrome characterized clinically by parkinsonism, dysautonomia, and other features previously reported as Shy–Drager syndrome (SDS), SND, and sporadic olivopontocerebellar atrophy (OPCA). The term *Shy–Drager syndrome* is still occasionally used in the literature, particularly by some American clinicians, as a tribute to Dr Shy, a neurologist from University of Pennsylvania and Columbia University, and Dr Drager, a urologist at Baylor College of Medicine, who first drew attention to this disorder in 1960 (Shy and Drager, 1960). In their initial report, Shy and Drager described two men who presented with symptoms of orthostatic syncope, impotence, and bladder dysfunction. They later developed parkinsonian features, including gait disturbance, mild tremor, dysarthria, constipation, and bowel and bladder incontinence. In addition to the combination of parkinsonism and autonomic failure, patients with SDS also frequently manifest cerebellar (60%) and pyramidal signs (50%). Other features described by Shy and Drager as part of the "full syndrome," such as rectal incontinence, fasciculations, and iris atrophy, are seen rarely. The term *striatonigral degeneration* was introduced in the 1960s by Adams, Van Bogaert, and Van de Eecken (Aotsuka and Paulson, 1993). In an attempt to characterize SND, Gouider-Khouja and colleagues (1995) used the following clinical criteria: (1) onset after 40 years; (2) disease duration less than 10 years; (3) parkinsonian syndrome poorly responsive or unresponsive to levodopa; (4) autonomic failure; and (5) absence of family history, dementia, apraxia, supranuclear ophthalmoplegia, and "detectable focal lesions on neuroimaging study." Dejerine and Thomas (1900) introduced the term *olivopontocerebellar atrophy* to describe a group of heterogeneous disorders characterized clinically by the combination of progressive parkinsonism and cerebellar ataxia and pathologically by neuronal loss in the ventral pons, inferior olives, and cerebellar cortex (Berciano, 1992). OPCA may be inherited, usually in an autosomal dominant pattern (Currier and Subramony, 1993; Rosenberg, 1995; Berciano et al., 2006), but only the sporadic OPCAs are included in the classification of MSA (Berciano, 1992; Gilman and Quinn, 1996; Wenning et al., 2004a). Although considered a sporadic disease, families with a phenotype suggestive of autosomal recessive MSA have been described (Hara et al., 2007).

It is possible, however, that these familial cases represent either some forms, yet to be identified, of spinocerellar ataxia (SCA) or familial OPCA. A rating scale, the Unified Multiple System Atrophy Rating Scale (UMSARS), that assesses all important symptoms and signs of MSA has been developed and validated against related rating scales, such as the UPDRS and the International Cooperative Ataxia Rating Scale (Wenning et al., 2004b). The UMSRARS Motor Examination score seems to be the best outcome measure for future therapeutic trials (May et al., 2007).

The discovery by Papp and colleagues (1989) that the pathologic hallmark shared by all three disorders is the presence of filamentous α-synuclein-containing glial cytoplasmic inclusions (GCI) led to the recognition that these disorders are manifestations of the same pathologic process. MSA has therefore been redefined as a sporadic, progressive, adult-onset disorder characterized clinically by autonomic dysfunction (MSA-A), parkinsonism (MSA-P), and cerebellar ataxia (MSA-C) in any combination (American Academy of Neurology, 1996; Consensus Committee of the AAS and AAN, 1996; Gilman et al., 1998; Gilman, 2002; Osaki et al., 2002; Watanabe et al., 2002; Gilman et al., 2008). A second consensus statement in the diagnosis of MSA simplified the prior criteria (Consensus Committee of the AAS and AAN, 1996) and proposed the following diagnostic criteria (Gilman et al., 2008): "Definite MSA requires neuropathologic demonstration of CNS α-synuclein-positive glial cytoplasmic inclusions with neurodegenerative changes in striatonigral or olivopontocerebellar structures. Probable MSA requires a sporadic, progressive adult-onset disorder including rigorously defined autonomic failure and poorly levodopa-responsive parkinsonism or cerebellar ataxia. Possible MSA requires a sporadic, progressive adult-onset disease including parkinsonism or cerebellar ataxia and at least one feature suggesting autonomic dysfunction plus one other feature that may be a clinical or a neuroimaging abnormality." Features that would argue against the diagnosis of MSA include: age at onset >75 years, the presence of typical PD rest tremor, neuropathy, sporadic hallucinations, dementia, white matter lesions in MRI suggestive of multiple sclerosis, and a family history of ataxia or parkinsonism.

Until the mid-1990s, the literature still used the terms SND and OPCA, and we continue to use the term OPCA for disorders that do not fit the nosology of MSA-C, such as some sporadic or autosomal dominant ataxias and other disorders such as certain hereditary, metabolic, or degenerative disorders with pathologic features of OPCA (Berciano et al., 2006).

Fearnley and Lees (1990) reviewed 10 patients, ranging in age from 47 to 50 years, with autopsy-proven SND (MSA-P). Five of these patients were misdiagnosed as having PD, largely because of good response to levodopa. Features that were helpful in differentiating SND from other parkinsonian disorders included early-onset falling, severe dysarthria and dysphonia, excessive snoring and sleep apnea, respiratory stridor, hyperreflexia, and extensor plantar responses. Cerebellar or pyramidal tract signs were present in two patients each, while autonomic symptoms were present in seven. Duration of illness ranged from 3 to 8 years, and no difference in survival was seen in levodopa responders compared to non-levodopa responders. In another series, tremor was found in only 6% of SND patients and in 71% of PD patients;

the predominant features were rigidity and hypokinesia, present at onset in 84% of all SND (MSA-P) patients (Van Leeuwen and Perquin, 1988). Besides lack of tremor, the symmetrical onset of SND (MSA-P) is sometimes helpful in differentiating SND from PD, although 6 of 10 patients described by Fearnley and Lees (1990) had asymmetrical onset. In a study comparing 16 patients with pathologically proven MSA of the SND (MSA-P) variety with PD and PSP, a set of clinical criteria reliably differentiated MSA from PD but not from PSP (Colosimo et al., 1995). In addition to cerebellar and pyramidal signs, early instability with falls, and relative preservation of cognition, the following features were more typically present in MSA than in PD: autonomic dysfunction (69% versus 5%), absence of rest tremor (87% versus 40%), rapid progression (mean disease duration 7.1 years versus 13.6 years), and poor or unsustained response to levodopa (31% versus 0%). In contrast to other reports, only 43.7% of the MSA patients in this series had a symmetric onset. As in PD, PSP, and other subcortical neurodegenerative disorders, the cognitive deficit in SND consists chiefly of mild impairment of memory and executive functions, which has been attributed to "inefficient planning of memory processes" and "frontal lobe-like syndrome related to a dysfunction of the supervisory attentional system" (Pillon et al., 1995b). While pseudobulbar affect associated with emotional incontinence is typically seen in patients with PSP, pathologic laughter and crying has been also described in autopsy-proven cases of MSA, particularly the MSA-C type (Parvizi et al., 2007). Cognitive impairment, particularly associated with prefrontal dysfunction, is more severe in patients with MSA-P than those with MSA-C (Kawai et al., 2008).

MSA appears to be more common in men than in women, with symptoms first beginning in the sixth decade; death usually occurs 7–8 years after the initial symptoms and approximately 4 years after the onset of neurologic impairment (McLeod and Tuck, 1987a, 1987b). In a review of 188 pathologically proven cases of MSA, 28% patients had involvement of all four systems (parkinsonism, cerebellar dysfunction, corticospinal signs, and dysautonomia); 18% had the combination of parkinsonism, pyramidal, and autonomic findings; 11% had parkinsonian, cerebellar, and autonomic findings; another 11% had parkinsonism and dysautonomia; 10% had only parkinsonism; and parkinsonism was absent in 11% of all cases (Quinn, 1994). The clinical features and natural history of MSA were analyzed in 100 cases with probable MSA, of which 14 were confirmed at autopsy (Wenning et al., 1994b). The population consisted of 67 men and 33 women, with a median age at onset of 53 years (range: 33–76). Autonomic symptoms were present at onset in only 41% of the patients, but 97% developed autonomic dysfunction during the course of the disease. Whereas impotence was the most frequent autonomic symptom in males, urinary incontinence predominated in women. Some evidence of orthostatic hypotension was present in 68% of patients, but severe orthostatic hypotension was noted in only 15%. In contrast to PD and other parkinsonian disorders in which the latency to onset of orthostatic hypotension is usually several years, patients with MSA usually develop symptomatic orthostatic hypotension within the first year after onset of symptoms (Wenning et al., 1999), and urinary dysfunction may occur even earlier (Sakakibara et al., 2000a,

2000b). Parkinsonism was the predominant motor disorder in SND, while gait ataxia was the usual presentation of the OPCA type of MSA. Tremor was present in only 29% and was typical "pill-rolling" in only 9%. Although 29% of all patients had initial good or excellent response to levodopa, this benefit was usually short-lived; only 13% maintained a good response to levodopa. Facial dystonia (often asymmetrical) was a typical levodopa-induced complication in patients with MSA. In another study of 16 autopsy-proven cases of MSA, Litvan and colleagues (1997d) identified early severe autonomic failure, absence of cognitive impairment, early cerebellar symptoms, and early gait problems as the best predictors of the diagnosis of MSA. In a study designed to validate the clinical criteria for MSA, Litvan and colleagues (1998a) found that the accuracy was best when at least six of the following eight features were present: sporadic adult onset, dysautonomia, parkinsonism, pyramidal signs, cerebellar signs, no levodopa response, no cognitive dysfunction, and no downward gaze palsy. Wenning and colleagues (1997) examined the clinical features of 203 pathologically proven cases of MSA reported in 108 publications. The male:female ratio was 1.3:1, dysautonomia was present in 74%, parkinsonism in 87%, cerebellar ataxia in 54%, and pyramidal signs in 49%. The progression and prognosis were analyzed in 230 Japanese patients with MSA; the median time from onset to aid-requiring walking, confinement to wheelchair, bedridden state, and death were 3, 5, 8, and 9 years, respectively (Watanabe et al., 2002). MSA-P patients had more rapid deterioration than MSA-C patients. When patients present with parkinsonism alone, without other evidence of MSA, their MSA might be difficult to differentiate from PD during the first 6 years (Albanese et al., 1995). In one study, the following features were found to be the best predictors of MSA: dysautonomia, poor response to levodopa, speech or bulbar dysfunction, falls, and absence of dementia and of levodopa-induced confusion (Wenning et al., 2000). Early development of autonomic dysfunction has been found to be an independent predictor of poor prognosis (Tada et al., 2007). It should be noted, however, that pure autonomic failure (PAF) might herald the onset not only of MSA, but also of PD and DLB (Kaufmann et al., 2004; Mabuchi et al., 2005). In PAF, orthostatic hypotension and sudomotor dysfunction followed by constipation are the typical initial symptoms, whereas in MSA, the initial presentation usually consists of urinary problems, followed by sudomotor dysfunction or orthostatic hypotension, with subsequent progression to respiratory dysfunction (Mabuchi et al., 2005; Benarroch, 2007)). A study of 115 patients with MSA showed that autonomic dysfunction, motor impairment, and depression were most closely related to poor outcome in measures of health-related quality of life (Schrag et al., 2006a).

Prior to reclassification of sporadic OPCA as MSA-C, there were many attempts to characterize the different forms of OPCA. Approximately one-quarter of patients with sporadic OPCA, particularly those with older-onset ataxia, develop parkinsonian features and evolve into MSA-C (Gilman et al., 2000). Berciano (1992) reviewed 133 (68 familial and 65 sporadic) pathologically proven cases of OPCA. While there was a nearly 2:1 male preponderance in familial OPCA, no gender difference was found in the sporadic form. Age at onset was more variable in this disorder than in the other parkinsonism-plus syndromes, ranging from infancy to 66 years. Cerebellar ataxia was the presenting symptom in 73% of all patients; 8.2% began with parkinsonian symptoms, and the remainder presented with nonspecific symptoms. Dementia, gaze impairment, dysarthria, dysphagia, incontinence, and upper and lower motor neuron signs usually become apparent within a few years after onset. In one large Japanese family with OPCA, the oculomotor abnormalities consisted of limitation of upgaze and convergence, horizontal gaze nystagmus, relative sparing of pupil reactivity, and loss of vestibulo-ocular responses (Shimizu et al., 1990). Autopsy of one patient in this series revealed degeneration of the oculomotor nucleus with sparing of the Edinger–Westphal nucleus. Neuropsychological evaluation in patients with clinically diagnosed OPCA revealed emotionality, anxiety, and a tendency toward depression without cognitive decline (Brent et al., 1990). Other studies, however, noted some degree of dementia in up to 80% of patients (Berciano, 1992).

While this review focuses on the sporadic forms of OPCA, it is worth pointing out that the classification of familial cerebellar ataxias has been markedly facilitated by the discoveries of specific mutations associated with the different phenotypes. Of the autosomal dominant cerebellar ataxias with known genetic defects, SCA1, SCA2, SCA3 (Machado–Joseph disease) (Kawaguchi et al., 1994; Lu et al., 2004), SCA6, SCA12, and SCA21, and dentatorubral-pallidoluysian atrophy (DRPLA) (Komure et al., 1995; Warner et al., 1995) are associated with extrapyramidal features, including parkinsonism (Rosenberg, 1995). Young-onset, levodopa-responsive parkinsonism may be the presentation of SCA2 and may precede the onset of ataxia by 25 years (Furtado et al., 2002; Lu et al., 2002; Payami et al., 2003; Furtado et al., 2004; Lu et al., 2004). Interruption of the SCA2 CAG/CAA repeat expansion has been found to be associated with autosomal dominant parkinsonism (Charles et al., 2007).

Although rarely pathologic features of sporadic MSA are found in the autosomal dominant form of SCA (Gilman et al., 1996b), the typical sporadic MSA is genetically distinct from the inherited forms of SCA and OPCA (Bandmann et al., 1997). These disorders should be differentiated from cortical cerebellar atrophy and SCA, in which cerebellar signs are unaccompanied by autonomic features (Bürk et al., 1996; Dürr et al., 1996; Gilman and Quinn, 1996; Hammans, 1996; Osaki et al., 2002). Pathologically, there might be some similarities between the central disorders, including the presence of GCIs in rare cases of SCA, but the spinal cord is usually more atrophied in SCA than in MSA. Some features of MSA overlap with the syndrome of fragile X-associated tremor/ataxia syndrome caused by permutations of the fragile X mental retardation 1 gene (*FMR1*), and fragile X-associated tremor/ataxia syndrome may be a rare cause of MSA (Biancalana et al., 2005).

Several clinical studies have addressed the differentiation between MSA-P and parkinsonism and a collection of "red flags" has been generated and recently validated as having high diagnostic specificity (Kollensperger et al., 2008; Stefanova et al., 2009) (Table 9.2). The red flags were grouped into the following six categories: (1) early instability, (2) rapid progression, (3) abnormal postures (includes Pisa syndrome, disproportionate anterocollis, and/or contractures of hands or feet), (4) bulbar dysfunction (includes severe

---

Table 9.2 "Red-flag" features suggestive of MSA

2 out of the following 6 needed for diagnosis of probable MSA-P:

1. Early instability (wheelchair within 5 years)
2. Rapid progression
3. Abnormal postures: Pisa syndrome, anterocollis and/or contractures
4. Bulbar dysfunction: severe dysphonia, dysarthria, and/or dysphagia
5. Respiratory dysfunction: diurnal or nocturnal inspiratory stridor and/or inspiratory sighs
6. Emotional incontinence: inappropriate crying and/or laughing

and

- Early autonomic dysfunction
- Myoclonus, jerky tremor
- "Cold hands/feet" (Raynaud phenomenon)
- REM sleep behavior disorder, sleep apnea
- Poor response to levodopa, orofacial dystonia

From Kollensperger M, et al. (European MSA Study Group). Red flags for multiple system atrophy. Mov Disord 2008;23:1093–9.

---

dysphonia, dysarthria, and/or dysphagia), (5) respiratory dysfunction (includes diurnal or nocturnal inspiratory stridor and/or inspiratory sighs), and (6) emotional incontinence (includes inappropriate crying and/or laughing). They proposed that a combination of two out of these six red flag categories were used as additional criteria for the diagnosis of probable MSA-P. Movement disorders other than parkinsonism that are seen in patients with MSA include dystonia, stimulus-sensitive cortical myoclonus, hemiballism, and chorea, unrelated to dopaminergic therapy (Chen et al., 1992; Steiger et al., 1992; Salazar et al., 2000). Dystonia is relatively rare in MSA patients (Rivest et al., 1990), but in one study, 46% of patients with MSA were found to have dystonia, particularly if anterocollis is considered a form of cervical dystonia (Boesch et al., 2002). Some investigators, however, believe that the neck flexion, often associated with anterior sagittal shift, is due to disproportionally increased tone in the anterior neck muscles leading to secondary fibrotic and myopathic changes (van de Warrenburg et al., 2007). Although dystonia is frequently considered to be a cause of the MSA-associated anterocollis, the mechanism of progressive neck flexion, so characteristic of MSA, particularly MSA-P, may be multifactorial. In some cases, the neck flexion has been attributed to neck extensor weakness as part of "dropped head" syndrome associated with axial myopathy (Suarez and Kelly, 1992; Oerlemans and de Visser, 1998; Askmark et al., 2001), motor neuron disease (Gourie-Devi et al., 2003), or other causes. Neck flexion, however, is not unique to MSA and can be also seen in patients with otherwise typical PD (Djaldetti et al., 1999). In some cases of PD, more frequently than in MSA, the axial postural abnormality may lead to severe flexion of the trunk, the so-called bent spine syndrome, or camptocormia (Umapathi et al., 2002; Azher et al., 2005). Another abnormal posture frequently encountered in MSA is the "Pisa syndrome" manifested by leaning of the body to one side reminiscent of the leaning tower of Pisa (Ashour et al.,

2006) (Video 9.8). Besides anterocollis, another form of dystonia that is relatively frequently encountered in patients with MSA is facial and oromandibular dystonia associated with levodopa therapy. As was noted earlier in the chapter, inspiratory stridor may be a variant of laryngeal dystonia (Merlo et al., 2002). In addition to action myoclonus (Video 9.8), focal reflex myoclonus, induced by pinprick, may be seen in MSA patients (Clouston et al., 1996; Salazar et al., 2000). This form of myoclonus has a longer latency than that seen in patients with CBD (see later). In 9 of 11 patients with MSA and myoclonic tremulous movements, jerk-locked averaging technique showed premyoclonic potential, suggesting that the jerk-like movements represent a form of cortical myoclonus (Okuma et al., 2005).

Although dysautonomia is a cardinal feature of MSA, this neurodegenerative disorder should be differentiated from PAF, which has no central component (Mathias, 1997). Autonomic dysfunction is essential for the diagnosis of MSA, and in many cases of MSA, autonomic failure, particularly impotence, precedes other neurologic symptoms or signs by several years. In contrast to PD associated with dysautonomia, in which there is predominantly peripheral (ganglionic and postganglionic) involvement, including myocardial (Goldstein et al., 2002), sympathetic denervation, the peripheral autonomic system appears to be spared in MSA and the primary lesion is preganglionic (Lipp et al., 2009). In fact, some persistence of central autonomic tone might be responsible for the frequently observed supine hypertension in MSA (Parikh et al., 2002). MSA patients also have more autonomic symptoms at baseline and more progression to global anhidrosis than patients with PD (Lipp et al., 2009). The "cold hands" sign, manifested by cold, dusky, violaceous appearance of the hands, is another characteristic feature of MSA (Klein et al., 1997). Some patients have the "cold feet" sign (Video 9.9). Liquid meal, consisting chiefly of glucose and milk, markedly reduces blood pressure in patients with MSA but not in those with PD (Thomaides et al., 1993) (Video 9.9). Respiratory disturbance, including severe obstructive sleep apnea, and vocal cord paralysis with stridor may be found in more advanced stages of the disease (Munschauer et al., 1990), but respiratory insufficiency may be the presenting symptom of MSA (Glass et al., 2006). Inspiratory stridor due to the paradoxical movement of the vocal cords (also known as Gerhardt syndrome) has been described in MSA (Eissler et al., 2001). The observation that stridor improves with botulinum toxin injections into the adductor laryngeal muscles suggests that this symptom of MSA could be due to focal laryngeal dystonia (Merlo et al., 2002). The occurrence of nocturnal or daytime stridor carries a poor prognosis, particularly when it is associated with central hypoventilation (Silber and Levine, 2000). Occasionally, however, vocal cord abductor paralysis can be seen even in the initial stages of the disease, and it has been associated with nocturnal sudden death (Isozaki et al., 1996). Early diagnosis can be made by laryngoscopy during sleep. Hypoxemia with increased alveolar-arterial oxygen gradient, associated with laryngopharyngeal movements, however, has been demonstrated in MSA patients even during wakefulness (Shimohata et al., 2007). The presence of impaired hypoxic ventilatory response has helped to differentiate MSA-C from idiopathic late-onset cerebellar ataxia (Tsuda et al., 2002).

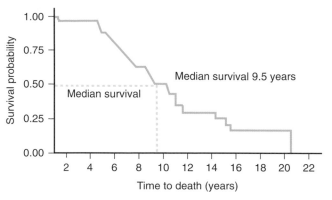

Figure 9.5 Natural history of MSA. *Redrawn from Wenning GK, Shlomo YB, Magalhaes M, et al. Clinical features and natural history of multiple system atrophy: An analysis of 100 cases. Brain 1994;117:835–845.*

The natural history of MSA has been the subject of several recent studies. In contrast to the approximately 1.5% annual decline in UPDRS-III noted in patients with PD (Jankovic and Kapadia, 2001), the average annual decline in MSA-P is 28.3% (Seppi et al., 2005). Since most of the studies were based on pathologically proven cases, the prognosis in these series has been worse than otherwise predicted. In one study of 59 patients with MSA that included 25 with SDS, 24 with OPCA, and 10 with SND, the survival was poorest in SDS, followed by SND and OPCA (Saito et al., 1994). On the basis of a meta-analysis of 433 reported cases of MSA, Ben-Shlomo and colleagues (1997) found survival to range from 0.5 to 24 years (mean: 6.2 years), and cerebellar features were associated with marginally better survival. In one study of 100 patients clinically diagnosed with probable MSA (14 of whom were pathologically confirmed), nearly half of all the patients were markedly disabled or wheelchair bound within 5 years after onset, and the median survival was 9.5 years (Wenning, et al., 1994b) (Fig. 9.5). This is similar to the median survival of 8.6 years for men and 7.3 years for women in a group of 22 patients with pathologically proven MSA followed prospectively (Schrag et al., 2008). In another study, the investigators analyzed 35 pathologically confirmed cases of MSA and confirmed a direct correlation between severity of disease and nigrostriatal cell loss (Wenning et al., 1995). Although marked degeneration in the olivopontocerebellar system, particularly the cerebellar vermis, was noted in 88% of the brains, the cerebellar pathology did not correlate with the presence of cerebellar signs. Although some authors have suggested that the earlier and the more severe the involvement of the autonomic nervous system, the poorer the prognosis (Saito et al., 1994), this has not been confirmed by other studies (Ben-Shlomo et al., 1997). MSA patients usually die from aspiration, sleep apnea, or cardiac arrhythmia. Survival data and clinically relevant milestones – namely: frequent falling, cognitive disability, unintelligible speech, severe dysphagia, dependence on wheelchair for mobility, the use of urinary catheters, and placement in residential care – were determined based on a retrospective chart review of pathologically confirmed cases of PSP ($n = 110$) and MSA ($n = 42$) (O'Sullivan et al., 2008). Patients with PSP had an older age of onset ($P < 0.001$) and reached their first clinical milestone earlier than patients with MSA ($P < 0.001$). Patients with PSP generally had a less favorable prognosis than those with MSA, and rarely autonomic failure in MSA was associated with shorter survival.

Epidemiology

The average annual incidence rate for MSA has been estimated to be 3 new cases per 100 000 person-years. (Bower et al., 1997), and the age-adjusted prevalence has been estimated at 4.4 per 100 000 (Schrag et al., 1999). Some studies have shown that, similar to PD, smoking is significantly less frequent in patients with MSA, and farming is an independent risk factor for MSA (Vanacore et al., 2005).

Neurodiagnostic studies

In addition to tests of autonomic function, patterns of plasma levels of catecholamines and their metabolites may be helpful in differentiating the various forms of autonomic failures (Cohen et al., 1987; Goldstein et al., 1989; Polinsky, 1993; Mathias, 1995; American Academy of Neurology, 1996; Parikh et al., 2002). These studies are designed primarily to localize the site of autonomic impairment and include investigation of neurogenic bladder (Fowler, 1996), sphincter electromyography (EMG) (Stocchi et al., 1997), and other investigations designed to test the integrity of the autonomic nervous system. Neurogenic sphincter electromyography, however, can be also seen in other disorders, including PD, PSP, Huntington disease, and a variety of common urologic problems (Colosimo et al., 1999; Giladi et al., 2000; Vodusek, 2001). Although anorectal dysfunction does not differentiate MSA from PD, external anal sphincter electromyography denervation is a very sensitive measure of anorectal dysfunction (Tison et al., 2000), and this abnormality occurs much earlier in MSA than in PD (Stocchi et al., 2000). Patients with SDS show a deficit in the central component of the baroreflex, whereas peripheral sympathetic pathways are affected primarily in the syndrome of PAF. While the peripheral sympathetic neurons are spared in MSA, there is some evidence that they lack the normal preganglionic activation (Parikh et al., 2002). Furthermore, the relatively well-preserved sympathetic tone is probably responsible for the supine hypertension that is seen in most patients with MSA. In neurogenic orthostatic hypotension, the rise in NE levels is minimal or absent despite a marked drop in blood pressure after either head-up tilt or an upright position. Clonidine has been found to increase growth hormone (GH) in normal controls, patients with PAF, and patients with PD but not patients with MSA (Thomaides et al., 1992; Kimber et al., 1997). Whether this clonidine-GH test can reliably differentiate between MSA and PD, as Kimber and colleagues (1997) suggested, awaits further clinical-pathologic studies. In a study of 69 MSA patients, 35 PD patients, and 90 healthy controls, the GH response to arginine was found to be significantly lower in MSA patients as compared to PD or healthy controls, a finding with over 90% sensitivity and specificity (Pellecchia et al., 2006).

While somatosensory, visual, and auditory evoked responses are often abnormal, motor evoked potentials are usually normal (Abele et al., 2000). In one study, 73% of patients with SDS had abnormal brainstem auditory evoked responses (Sinatra et al., 1988). In a study comparing polysomnograms of seven patients with SDS with those of seven control patients, significant obstructive sleep apnea without oxygen desaturation was seen in four of the five nontracheotomized SDS patients; three of these patients later died suddenly during sleep (Munschauer et al., 1990). In a more recent study, Plazzi and colleagues (1997) demonstrated that 90% of MSA patients experience some form of REM sleep behavioral disorder (RBD). A strong relationship between RBD and subsequent MSA has been demonstrated by a number of other studies.

Using PET scan technology to measure 6-[^{18}F]fluoro-dopamine-derived radioactivity in myocardium, Goldstein and colleagues found normal rates of cardiac spillover of NE and normal production of levodopa, dihydroxyphenyl-glycol, and dihydroxyphenylacetic acid suggestive of intact cardiac sympathetic terminals in patients with SDS (Goldstein et al., 1997). This is in contrast to absent radio-activity in patients with PAF, indicating loss of postganglionic sympathetic terminals in this peripheral autonomic disorder. The value of this test in diagnosing MSA has been questioned (Mathias, 1997), however, since both sympathetic and parasympathetic failure have been associated with MSA. Neurochemical changes seen in MSA are similar to those present in PAF, and some suggest that MSA represents a central progression from PAF (McLeod and Tuck, 1987a, 1987b). Pharmacologically, these two conditions may be distinguished by supine and standing plasma NE levels. In PAF, both standing and supine NE levels are low, while in MSA, only the standing value is diminished. Besides decreased NE, acetylcholine and cerebrospinal fluid (CSF) acetylcholinesterase (AChE) levels are also reduced (Polinsky et al., 1989). This is consistent with the notion that postganglionic sympathetic neurons are intact in MSA but their function is markedly impaired in PAF.

Another imaging study used [^{11}C]DTBZ PET and [^{123}I]iodo-benzovesamicol single-photon emission computed tomography (SPECT), and showed that RBD in patients with MSA correlates with nigrostriatal dopaminergic deficit. Furthermore, obstructive sleep apnea in MSA is related to a thalamic cholinergic deficit, possibly owing to decreased pontine cholinergic projections (Gilman et al., 2003a). The same group used PET with [^{11}C]PMP and that subcortical AChE activity was significantly more decreased in MSA-P and PSP than in PD. The authors suggested that this reflects greater impairment in the pontine cholinergic group (PPN) and may account for the greater gait disturbances in the early stages of these two disorders compared to PD (Gilman et al., 2010). Carbon-11-labelled 2-[2-(2-dimethylaminothiazol-5-yl)ethenyl]-6-[2-(fluoro)ethoxy]benzoxazole PET, believed to image α-synuclein, in 8 patients with MSA showed high distribution volumes in the subcortical white matter, putamen and posterior cingulate cortex, globus pallidus, primary motor and anterior cingulate cortex, and substantia nigra compared to the normal controls (Kikuchi et al., 2010). Since these areas are also rich in glial cytoplasmic inclusions, the carbon-11-labelled 2-[2-(2-dimethylaminothiazol-5-yl)ethenyl]-6-[2-(fluoro) ethoxy] benzoxazole PET may be a potential surrogate marker for progression of synucleinopathies.

Neuroimaging techniques, including MRI, transcranial sonography, functional imaging (PET and SPECT), and imaging cardiac sympathetic innervation, can be very helpful in differentiating MSA from other parkinsonian disorders and neuroimaging criteria have been proposed (Brooks et al., 2009). Neuroimaging specifically designed to assess putaminal integrity may prove helpful in differentiating MSA from PD and in predicting levodopa response (Drayer et al., 1989; Stern et al., 1989). MRI in patients with SDS sometimes reveals areas of decreased signal bilaterally in the posterolateral putamen on T2-weighted images (Pastakia et al., 1986). Although increased levels of iron may contribute to this hypointensity, reactive microgliosis and astrogliosis may also play an important role. In addition to striatal (putaminal) hypointensity on T2-weighted MRI scans, a characteristic finding in patients with MSA, particularly MSA-P, is the slit-hyperintensity in the lateral margin of the putamen (Savoiardo et al., 1994; Sitburana and Ondo, 2009). This abnormality was found in 17 of 28 (61%) of patients with clinically diagnosed MSA (Konagaya et al., 1994). Although not all MSA patients with this slit-hyperintensity had parkinsonism, none of the 25 patients with clinically diagnosed PD demonstrated this finding on MRI. Linearization of putaminal margin was found in 88.8% of patients with MSA-P, but only in 8.3% of patients with MSA-C, 7.9% of patients with PD, and 7.4% of healthy subjects (Ito et al., 2007). Although hyperintense putaminal rim is quite specific for MSA, putaminal hypointensity was not found to be a useful discriminator in one study (Schrag et al., 1998). The combination of increased signal on T2 or FLAIR in the lateral putamen (indicating iron deposition) and the slit-hyperintensity at the posterolateral border of the putamen on T2-weighted images provides a sensitivity for MSA of 97% (von Lewinski et al., 2007). Using DWI-MRI, Schocke and colleagues (2002) found that regional apparent diffusion coefficients values are increased in the putamen of patients with MSA, and this evidence of striatal degeneration apparently reliably differentiates MSA from PD. DWI imaging showing abnormal signal in the middle cerebellar peduncle is apparently relatively specific for MSA-C and is not seen in PSP or PD (Nicoletti et al., 2006; Paviour et al., 2007). Ghaemi and colleagues (2002) found that both multitracer PET and three-dimensional MRI-based volumetry are very sensitive measures and that they reliably differentiate MSA from PD by demonstrating decreased putaminal volume, glucose metabolism, and postsynaptic D2 receptor density in patients with MSA. These techniques, when applied to the imaging of the midbrain, did contribute additional gain in diagnostic accuracy. In one study, however, the typical "hot cross bun" sign in the pons was present on MRI in 63% of patients (Watanabe et al., 2002). Other studies have highlighted the "hot cross bun" sign as a characteristic feature of MSA (Sitburana and Ondo, 2009). This study also drew attention to the involvement of the cortex in MSA. T2*-weighted gradient echo was more sensitive in demonstrating hypointense putaminal changes than T2-weighted fast spin echo MRI (Kraft et al., 2002) (Fig. 9.6). A diagnostic algorithm based on brain MRI has been proposed (Bhattacharya et al., 2002).

Using proton magnetic resonance spectroscopy, Davie and colleagues (1995) showed a significant reduction in the N-acetylaspartate (NAA)/creatine ratio from the lentiform nucleus in six of seven patients with MSA and in only one of nine patients with PD. Similar abnormalities were found in some patients with OPCA and most likely reflect regional neuronal loss. Further studies are needed to determine whether this technique can reliably differentiate between MSA and PD. Brain parenchyma sonography has been used in one study to differentiate PD from atypical parkinsonism, mostly MSA (Walter et al., 2003). The investigators found that 24 of 25 (96%) patients with PD exhibited hyperechogenicity, whereas only 2 of 23 (9%) patients with atypical parkinsonism showed a similar pattern. They concluded that brain parenchyma sonography might be highly specific in differentiating between PD and atypical parkinsonism. Computed tomography and MRI scans in patients with OPCA (MSA-C) typically show pancerebellar and brainstem atrophy, enlarged fourth ventricle and cerebellopontine angle cisterns, and demyelination of transverse pontine fibers on T2-weighted MRI images (Berciano, 1992). Although the MRI findings in MSA are highly specific, they have low sensitivity (Schrag et al., 2000). In a cross-sectional study of 15 MSA-P patients and 17 PD patients matched for age and disease duration, there were lower activity ratios of striatal to frontal uptake on iodobenzamide (IBZM)-SPECT; and on DWI, there were similar differences in the regional apparent diffusion coefficients (rADC). The findings from DWI were more accurate when compared to IBZM-SPECT based on the higher specificity, predictive accuracy, and positive predictive values of both the methods. Further studies using DWI validating these changes with disease progression are needed (Seppi et al., 2004).

PET scanning has revealed decreased striatal and frontal lobe metabolism (De Volder et al., 1989; Brooks et al., 1990b; Eidelberg et al., 1993) and a reduction in D2 receptor density in the striatum (Brooks et al., 1992; Antonini et al., 1997). Using [18F]fluorodeoxyglucose, [18F]fluorodopa, and [11C]raclopride (RACLO) PET scans, Antonini and colleagues (1997) showed that the combination of [18F] fluorodeoxyglucose and [11C]raclopride scans reliably differentiated between MSA and PD, but [18F]fluorodopa PET scans could not distinguish between the different forms of parkinsonism. In a study of 167 patients [18F]fluorodeoxyglucose PET was found to have high specificity and sensitivity in distinguishing between parkinsonian disorders (Tang et al., 2010). In a study of three patients with SDS, the two with more advanced stages of the disease showed reduced 18F-6-fluorodopa uptake, indicating nigrostriatal dysfunction (Bhatt et al., 1990). Gilman and colleagues (1999) found significantly reduced specific binding to the type 2 vesicular monoamine transporter using PET and [11C]dihydrotetrabenazine as a type 2 vesicular monoamine transporter ligand in striatal monoaminergic presynaptic terminal of patients with MSA. PET scans in patients with MSA-C show a reduced metabolic rate in the brainstem and cerebellum (Gilman, 2002), and these changes can be detected even before the onset of extrapyramidal features (Gilman et al., 1996a). A study of 10 patients with the sporadic OPCA form of MSA showed that the 18F-fluorodopa uptake was reduced by a mean of 21% in the putamen, and 11C-diprenorphine uptake was reduced by a mean of 22% (Rinne et al., 1995). Although the authors suggest that these findings support "subclinical" nigrostriatal dysfunction, all of the patients were clinically impaired, and some were disabled by severe ataxia and autonomic dysfunction. The reduced 11C-diprenorphine uptake suggests that in addition to involvement of the nigrostriatal projection, some MSA patients have a loss of intrinsic striatal

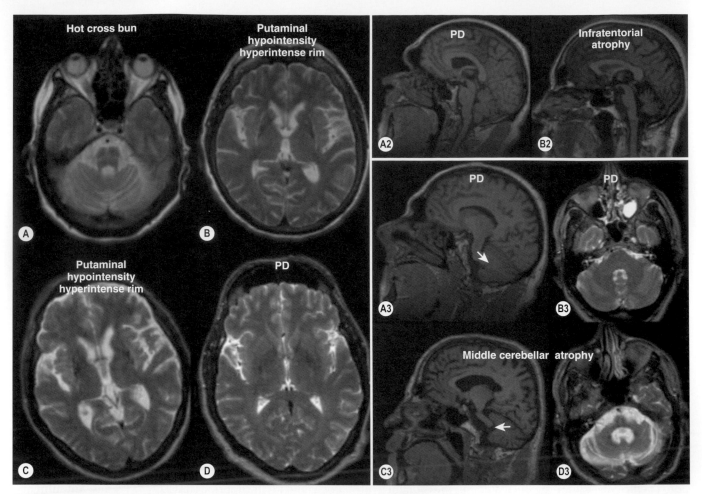

Figure 9.6 Radiologic features of MSA versus PD. **A** Hot cross bun sign in a patient with MSA-C on T2-weighted images. **B** Hyperintense rim, putaminal hypointensity in comparison with the globus pallidus, and putaminal atrophy in a patient with MSA-P on T2-weighted images. **C** Hyperintense putaminal rim, putaminal hypointensity in comparison with the globus pallidus, and putaminal atrophy at both sides in a patient with MSA-C on T2-weighted images. **D** No relevant abnormalities in the basal ganglia in a patient with PD on T2-weighted images. **A2** No relevant brainstem atrophy in a patient with PD on midsagittal T1-weighted image. **B2** Infratentorial atrophy in a patient with MSA-P on midsagittal T1-weighted image. **A3, B3** No relevant atrophy of the middle cerebellar peduncle (arrow) in a patient with PD on sagittal T1-weighted images and on axial T2-weighted images. **C3, D3** Atrophy of the middle cerebellar peduncle (arrow) in a patient with MSA-P on sagittal T1-weighted images and on axial T2-weighted images. *From Brooks DJ, Seppi K; for the Neuroimaging Working Group on MSA. Proposed neuroimaging criteria for the diagnosis of multiple system atrophy. Mov Disord 2009;24:949–964, with permission.*

neurons that contain presynaptic and postsynaptic mu, kappa, and delta opioid receptors.

Besides neuroimaging, transcranial ultrasonography has been reported to provide high diagnostic yield in differentiating PD from atypical parkinsonian disorders. Sonographic studies in 102 patients with PD, 34 with MSA, and 21 with PSP found marked unilateral or bilateral hyperechogenicity in 89% of 88 patients with PD, 25% of 32 patients with MSA-P, and 39% of 18 patients with PSP (Behnke et al., 2005).

Neuropathology, neurochemistry, and pathogenesis

The spectrum of pathologic changes in MSA includes cell loss, gliosis, and demyelination in the striatum (caudate and putamen), SN, locus coeruleus, inferior olives, pontine nuclei, dorsal vagal nuclei, Purkinje cells of the cerebellum,

intermediolateral cell columns, and Onuf's nucleus of the caudal spinal cord. Involvement of at least three of these areas, including the putamen and SN, is required for the pathologic diagnosis of MSA (Quinn, 1994; Ito et al., 1996). In one pathologic study of 100 MSA cases (46 men and 54 women), 34% were categorized as SND, 17% were categorized as OPCA (MSA-C), and the remainder (49%) had a mixed pathology (Ozawa et al., 2004). On the basis of the distribution of GCIs and correlation of the clinicopathologic changes, the study showed that GCIs might be contributing to neuronal damage in the MSA-C type more than the in MSA-P type, suggesting the possibility of different mechanisms of cell death in the subtypes of MSA. The brunt of the pathology in MSA brains is in the dorsolateral portion of the striatum and ventrolateral portion of the globus pallidus and SN, and the degree of response to levodopa seems to correlate inversely with the severity of the striatal efferent involvement (Ito et al., 1996). The putamen is the most prominently affected, with neuronal cell loss and deposition of iron, producing brownish pigmentation (O'Brien et al., 1990). Cholinergic neurons in the pedunculopontine nucleus and laterodorsal tegmentum and noradrenergic neurons in locus coeruleus were found to be markedly depleted in the brains of patients with MSA, whereas the serotonergic rostral raphe neurons are well preserved (Benarroch et al., 2002). Lewy bodies or NFTs are not common. Using calcineurin immunostaining, Goto and colleagues (1996) found marked neuronal loss particularly in the caudal and lateral portion of the putamen, with corresponding degeneration of GPi, GPe, and ventrolateral portion of the SNr. The same group (Goto et al., 1990b) noted selective degeneration of the met-enkephalin-containing neurons in the putamen and GPe, with relative preservation of the caudate nucleus. Previous studies have noted low levels of dopamine and increased activity of dopamine β-hydroxylase, the NE-synthesizing enzyme, in the midbrain. Vasomotor impairment in SND has been attributed to selective loss of tyrosine hydroxylase-immunoreactive neurons in the A1 and A2 regions of the medulla oblongata (Malessa et al., 1990). Loss of arginine-vasopressin synthesizing neurons in the hypothalamic suprachiasmatic nucleus has been demonstrated in the brains of patients with MSA (Benarroch et al., 2006). Calbindin-D_{28k} immunoreactivity in the striatal projection system is markedly decreased in the brains of patients with SND (Ito et al., 1992) and in Purkinje cells of the cerebellum in patients with MSA (Wüllner et al., 2000). In the early stages of MSA-P, the medium spiny neurons staining for calbindin (localized to the matrix), but not those staining for calcineurin (localized striasomes), appear to be depleted first (Sato et al., 2007). Reduced calcium-binding capacity in these neurons might affect the bcl-2 family of proteins and lead to apoptosis of selected neuronal regions not only in PD, but also in other neurodegenerative diseases, such as MSA. The small myelinated fibers innervating the vocal cord are lost in nearly all patients with MSA, but when the large myelinated fibers of the recurrent laryngeal nerve become affected, as is seen in some patients with SND, vocal cord paralysis becomes evident and may be life-threatening (Hayashi et al., 1997).

The fundamental pathologic changes in OPCA (MSA-C), whether familial or sporadic, are a loss of Purkinje cells in the cerebellar cortex, particularly in the vermis, and degeneration of the olivopontine nuclei (Wenning et al., 1996). In addition to cerebellar atrophy, SN degeneration and depigmentation, neuronal loss in other brainstem nuclei, and demyelination of corticospinal tracts and posterior columns are seen (Koeppen et al., 1986; Matsuo et al., 1998). One clinical-pathologic study found a strong correlation between the frequency of neuronal cytoplasmic inclusions exclusively found in the pontine nucleus and the severity of olivopontocerebellar degeneration. The immunohistochemical and ultrastructural features of the neuronal inclusions were identical to those of the glial inclusions (Yokoyama et al., 2001). Detailed morphometric and biochemical studies of OPCA brains correlated reductions in aspartic and glutamic acid with Purkinje cell loss in the cerebellar cortex and with neuronal cell loss in the inferior olives (aspartic acid) (Bebin et al., 1990). In addition, quisqualate receptors appear to be decreased, while quinolinic acid metabolism is increased (Makoweic et al., 1990; Kish et al., 1991). The increased

quinolinic acid phosphoribosyl-transferase activity in OPCA has been interpreted as a compensatory mechanism designed to protect quinolinic acid-sensitive granule cells (Kish et al., 1991). In addition, low glutamate dehydrogenase activity has been found in most, but not all, studies; however, this defect probably is not disease-specific (Berciano, 1992; Kostic et al., 1989). In a study of 14 brains of patients with OPCA, Kish and colleagues (1992) found a 53% reduction in dopamine in the putamen, 35% in the caudate, and 31% in the nucleus accumbens. Only two patients had severe neuronal loss in the SN and a corresponding dopamine depletion in the striatum. Mitochondrial deoxyribonucleic acid abnormalities have been postulated to be important in the pathogenesis of OPCA in some patients (Truong et al., 1990). A mitochondrial DNA G11778 mutation has been identified in a family with levodopa-responsive parkinsonism and multisystem degeneration (Simon et al., 1999).

Degeneration of the catecholaminergic neurons in the intermediate reticular formation of the rostral ventrolateral medulla seems to correlate well with autonomic failure in patients with MSA (Benarroch et al., 1998, 2000). The medial spiny neurons that give rise to both the direct pathway from the striatum to the GPi and the indirect pathway from the striatum to the GPe are affected. Gliosis, however, seems to be much more prevalent in GPe than in GPi. Upregulation of D1 receptors, determined by dopamine-stimulated adenylyl cyclase, has been demonstrated in brains of patients with PD as compared to PSP and MSA ($n = 10$ each); it is actually reduced in MSA (Tong et al., 2004). While the median CSF concentration of the neurotransmitter metabolites 5-hydroxyindolacetic acid and 3-methoxy-4-hydroxyphenylethyleneglycol was reduced significantly (49–70%) in MSA compared to PD, several brain-specific proteins (tau, neuron-specific enolase, myelin basic protein) were elevated (130–230%) in MSA compared with those in PD (Abdo et al., 2004). Although a combination of CSF tau and 3-methoxy-4-hydroxyphenylethyleneglycol significantly discriminated PD from MSA, it is too early to recommend routine use of CSF in differentiating these two disorders.

The discovery in 1989 by Papp and Lantos (Papp et al., 1989) of the characteristic histologic marker, the GCIs, led to improved characterization of MSA as a clinical-pathologic entity. These inclusions are particularly concentrated in the oligodendrogliocytes and have been found in all autopsied brains of patients with SDS, SND, and sporadic OPCA. This shared pathologic feature strongly argues in support of the notion that these three disorders should be regarded as variants of the same disease entity, namely, MSA (Kato and Nakamura, 1990; Arima et al., 1992; Murayama et al., 1992; Papp and Lantos, 1992; Lantos and Papp, 1994; Quinn, 1994; Wenning et al., 1994a). GCIs, argyrophilic, perinuclear inclusions with a diameter varying from 4 μm to 20 μm, are found particularly in the oligodendrogliocytes in the supplementary motor cortex, anterior central gyrus, putamen, pallidum, basal pons, and medullary reticular formation. They are composed of 20–30 nm straight tubules, and they contain ubiquitin, tau protein, α- and β-tubulin, MAP-5, αB-crystallin, and α-synuclein. Several studies have documented the presence of α-synuclein in the GCI (Spillantini et al., 1998; Tu et al., 1998; Wakabayashi et al., 1998), but the significance of this finding is uncertain (Mezey et al., 1998). Although very characteristic of MSA, GCIs have been rarely found in other disorders, such as CBD, PSP, and autosomal dominant spinocerebellar ataxia (Gilman et al., 1996b). The characteristics and distribution of the inclusions, however, may be slightly different from the typical GCIs that are seen in MSA. Originally, α-synuclein was identified as the precursor protein for the non-Aβ component (NAC) of Alzheimer disease of amyloid plaques and these plaques have been found to contain fragments of the α-synuclein protein (NAC precursor protein, or NACP). NACP/α-synuclein accumulates not only in Lewy bodies, but also as small granules in neurons and as diffuse deposits in neuronal process in PD brains (Shoji et al., 2000). In addition, NACP accumulates in cortical astrocytes. The distribution and cell type of NACP accumulation are similar in DLB, but in MSA, NACP accumulates chiefly in the oligodendroglia and olivary neurons. α-Synuclein is selectively and extensively phosphorylated at serine 129, especially by casein kinase 1 and 2, in various synucleinopathies, including MSA (Fujiwara et al., 2002). Recently, p39 immunoreactive GCIs have been reported as the hallmark of GCI in MSA (Honjyo et al., 2001). A cdk5 (cyclin-dependent kinase) activator in oligodendrocytes, p39 induces formation of GCIs in the oligodendrocytes. Midkine, a neurotrophic factor, has also been identified in the GCI, indicating a rescue of neurons via oligode (Burn and Jaros, 2001). Because of increasing evidence of dysregulation of myelin basic protein and p25α, also called tubulin polymerization promoting protein, in MSA, there is an emerging notion that MSA represents an oligodendrogliopathy (Wenning et al., 2008). Only 10% of the MSA cases are found to have Lewy bodies (Ozawa et al., 2004). A significant correlation has been found between the frequency of GCIs, severity of neuronal cell loss, and disease duration (Ozawa et al., 2004).

The autonomic failure in MSA has been largely attributed to the depletion of sympathetic preganglionic neurons in the spinal intermediolateral cell column (IML) and its afferent medullary catecholaminergic and serotonergic neurons. In 12 MSA patients who had died within 3.5 years after disease onset, 4 died suddenly and 8 died as a result of established causes (Tada et al., 2009). The investigators found that the spinal IML and medullary catecholaminergic and serotonergic systems were involved even in the early stages of MSA, and their degeneration may be responsible for sudden death in patients with MSA.

Using antibodies against certain components of myelin basic protein, several investigators found evidence of extensive myelin degeneration in MSA, thus supporting the notion of widespread oligodendroglial dysfunction in MSA (Castellani, 1998; Matsuo et al., 1998). Diffuse degeneration of the white matter, particularly involving the central tegmental tract associated with vacuolation, has been an increasingly recognized pathologic feature of MSA (Armstrong et al., 2007). Other studies found evidence of apoptosis in the glia, but not neurons, of MSA brains (Probst-Cousin et al., 1998). Furthermore, microglial activation involving translocation of NF-kappaB/Rel A to the nucleus was found to be particularly prominent in affected brain regions (Schwarz et al., 1998).

In addition to the typical findings in the brain, there is a marked loss of neurons in the lateral horns of the spinal cord, but these pathologic changes correlate poorly with dysautonomia (Gray et al., 1988). Substance P-like immunoreactivity was markedly decreased in laminae I + II of fourth thoracic and third lumbar spinal cord segments in 10 of 11 SDS patients, and all had a decrease in small and large myelinated fibers in the fourth thoracic ventral roots (Tomokane et al., 1991).

The cause of MSA is unknown, and genetic factors probably do not play an important role. Recent findings link MSA to PD and related neurodegenerative disorders as "α-synucleinopathies" (Jaros and Burn, 2000; Galvin et al., 2001). To test whether variations in the gene coding for α-synuclein (SNCA) are associated with increased risk in MSA, a candidate single nucleotide polymorphism (SNP) association study was performed on 384 most-associated SNPs in a genome-wide association study of PD in 413 MSA cases and 3974 control subjects. The 10 most significant SNPs were then replicated in an additional 108 MSA cases and 537 controls (Scholz et al., 2009). The study found that SNPs at SNCA were associated with increased risk for the development of MSA at an odds ratio of 6.2 ($P = 5.5 \times 10^{-12}$).

While many studies have investigated the putative role of environmental toxins in the pathogenesis of idiopathic PD, the possible role of such toxins in MSA has received little attention. We reported on 10 patients whose clinical features were consistent with MSA and in whom toxins were suspected to play an etiologic role (Hanna et al., 1999). One patient with pathologically confirmed MSA was exposed to high concentrations of various toxins, including formaldehyde, malathion, and diazinon. The other MSA patients had a history of heavy exposure to various agents, such as n-hexane, benzene, methyl-isobutyl-ketone, and pesticides. The pathologic case revealed extensive advanced glial changes, including GCIs, which were seen particularly in the deep cerebellar white matter, brainstem, cortex (superior frontal, insula, and hippocampus), and putamen. Additionally, there was notable neuronal cell loss with depigmentation of the SN and locus coeruleus. Although a cause-and-effect relationship cannot be proven, these cases suggest that environmental toxins could play a role in the pathogenesis of some cases of MSA. The inverse relationship between PD and smoking has been also found with MSA but not with PSP (Vanacore et al., 2000).

Although there is no experimental model of MSA, intraperitoneal injection of 3-acetylpyridine in rats produces neurochemical and histologic changes that are consistent with OPCA (Deutch et al., 1989). In addition to causing degeneration of the nigrostriatal dopaminergic pathway, this neurotoxin causes degeneration of the climbing fibers, which normally originate in the inferior olive and terminate in the cerebellum. Another possible animal model of MSA is the "double lesion" rat model in which an initial 6-OHDA substantia nigra lesion is followed by a quinolinic acid induced lesion in the striatum (Kollensperger et al., 2007). Transgenic mice overexpressing human wild-type α-synuclein in oligodendrocytes exhibit many of the features of MSA (Yazawa et al., 2005).

Treatment

About two-thirds of patients with MSA respond to levodopa. Parkinsonian symptoms accompanying SDS are difficult to treat, because dopaminergic drugs frequently exacerbate the already prominent symptoms of orthostatic hypotension.

The addition of liberal salt, fludrocortisone, and elastic stockings can improve standing blood pressures (Mathias and Kimber, 1998). However, parkinsonian patients have difficulty putting on elastic stockings, such as the Jobst stockings. In addition, physical maneuvers such as leg-crossing and squatting can alleviate orthostatic lightheadedness (Van Lieshout et al., 1992). In a double-blind, placebo-controlled study of 97 patients with various causes of autonomic failure, including 18 patients with SDS and 22 patients with PD, midodrine, a peripheral α-adrenergic agonist, has been found to be effective in the treatment of orthostatic hypotension (Jankovic et al., 1993a, 1993b). The safety and efficacy of midodrine were later confirmed by a larger controlled study involving a total of 171 patients with orthostatic hypotension (Low et al., 1997). Wright and colleagues (1998) showed dose-dependent increases in standing systolic blood pressure with midodrine in patients with MSA. In patients with neurally mediated recurrent syncope, midodrine reduced frequency of syncope from 67% (8 of 12) to 17% (2 of 12) when compared to placebo (Kaufmann et al., 2002). The most frequent side effects associated with the drug included piloerection, scalp pruritus, urinary retention, and supine hypertension. The effects of subcutaneous injections of octreotide, a somatostatin analog, were tested in a group of nine patients with MSA (Bordet et al., 1995). The drug improved orthostatic hypotension, and it allowed patients to maintain an upright posture for a longer period of time as compared to placebo. Because fludrocortisone and midodrine, particularly when combined with liberal salt intake, increase the risk of supine hypertension, patients should be instructed to place their beds in the reverse Trendelenburg position. The use of nighttime nitroglyceride or clonidine patches has been suggested for the treatment of supine hypertension, but these measures are not always successful. Although this modest improvement was attributed to a release of NE by octreotide during maintenance of erect posture, no increase in plasma NE levels could be demonstrated.

Other agents that are used to increase standing blood pressure include indomethacin, ibuprofen, pseudoephedrine and other sympathomimetics, caffeine and dihydroergotamine, yohimbine, and NE precursors, such as 3,4-dihydroxyphenyl serine, also known as L-threo DOPS or droxidopa (McLeod and Tuck, 1987a, 1987b; Polinsky, 1993; Senard et al., 1993; Freeman et al., 1999). Droxidopa appears to increase NE in the brains of normal and NE-depleted animals, suggesting that droxidopa acts as an NE precursor. The drug may also act in the peripheral nervous system as evidenced by increased heart rate and elevated blood pressure. In 32 patients (26 MSA, 6 PAF) with symptomatic orthostatic hypotension, droxidopa (up to 300 mg twice daily) reduced the fall in systolic blood pressure during orthostatic challenge (by a mean of 22 ± 28 mmHg) and 78% of the patients were considered clinically improved. There were no reports of supine hypertension (Mathias et al., 2001). However, carbidopa blunted the effects of droxidopa and thus the drug may have limited value in patients with PD or MSA who also take carbidopa/levodopa (Kaufmann et al., 2003). Phase III studies are currently under way to determine the safety and efficacy profile of droxidopa.

Bladder problems, particularly urinary retention and incontinence, are relatively common and often troublesome manifestations of MSA (Scientific Committee of the First International Consultation on Incontinence, 2000). Increased urinary frequency due to overactive bladder is less common and often improves with 5 mg of antimuscarinic oxybutynin (Ditropan) three to four times per day and 2 mg of tolterodine (Detrol) three times per day. The latter drug may be better tolerated because it has eight times less affinity for the salivary gland, thus causing much lower frequency of dry mouth. Use of 0.4 mg of the α-blocker tamsulosin (Flomax) twice a day may be effective if the urinary frequency is associated with benign prostatic hypertrophy; this condition must be excluded prior to the use of antimuscarinic agents. Prazosin and moxisylate are specific antagonists of bladder α-adrenergic receptors. In a controlled study in 49 patients, there was improvement of symptoms in 47.6% in the prazosin group and 53.6% in the moxisylate group. Orthostatic hypotension was seen in about 23% in the prazosin group and 11% in moxisylate group. More than 35% of patients had reduction in residual volume, and there was improvement in urinary urgency, frequency, and incontinence. The dosage used was 1 mg of prazosin and 10 mg of moxisylate three times a day in an oral form (Sakakibara et al., 2000a, 2000b). The combination of intravesical prostaglandin E2 and oral bethanechol chloride has been found to be of limited usefulness in treating urinary retention (Hindley et al., 2004). Sildenafil citrate (Viagra) has been found to be safe and effective in the treatment of erectile dysfunction associated with PD, but it may unmask orthostatic hypotension in patients with MSA (Zesiewicz et al., 2000; Hussain et al., 2001; Farooq et al., 2008). Constipation represents the most frequent gastrointestinal manifestations of MSA. Psyllium (Metamucil) was found to increase stool frequency and weight but did not alter colonic transit or anorectal function. Other effective treatments for constipation include polyethylene glycol (Miralax), bisacodyl (Dulcolax), magnesium sulfate, and macrogol 3350 (Movicol). Mosapride citrate, a novel 5-HT$_4$ agonist and partial 5-HT$_3$ antagonist, has been found to ameliorate constipation in parkinsonian patients (Liu et al., 2005). Other recently introduced drugs for constipation include lubiprostone (Amitiza), which locally activates intestinal ClC-2 chloride channels and increases intestinal fluid secretion without altering serum electrolyte levels, and tegaserod maleate (Zelnorm), a novel selective serotonin receptor type-4 (5-HT$_4$) partial agonist that stimulates upper gastrointestinal motility (Sullivan et al., 2006).

Despite the marked involvement of the striatum, many patients with MSA do improve with levodopa, at least initially (Fearnley and Lees, 1990). Although patients with MSA often respond to dopaminergic therapy (levodopa or apomorphine), in contrast to PD, the MSA patients may experience dyskinesias without concomitant improvement in motor functioning (Hughes et al., 1992b). The levodopa-induced dyskinesias that are seen in MSA patients seem to be more dystonic, often involving the face, rather than the choreic or stereotypic movements that are characteristically seen in patients with PD. Furthermore, MSA patients do not seem to notice a recurrence of parkinsonian symptoms until several days after levodopa withdrawal. In one study, only four of eight patients with MSA had a moderate response to levodopa; in contrast, all eight control patients with PD had a consistently good response to levodopa (Parati et al., 1993). Ataxia, present in patients with the OPCA type of

MSA, does not respond to pharmacologic therapy and has to be treated by physical means, such as a cane or a walker. In a study of 20 patients with MSA, Iranzo and colleagues (2000) found vocal cord abduction dysfunction in 14 (70%); and in 3 of 3 patients, continuous positive airway pressure completely eliminated laryngeal stridor, obstructive apnea, and hemoglobin desaturation. In another study, continuous positive airway pressure effectively ameliorated nocturnal stridor in 13 patients with MSA (Iranzo et al., 2004). Tracheostomy or other airway restoration techniques must be sometimes performed in patients who have vocal cord abductor paralysis (Isozaki et al., 1996). Stridor has been reported to improve with botulinum toxin injections into the adductor laryngeal muscles (Merlo et al., 2002).

Corticobasal degeneration

Clinical features and natural history

In 1968, Rebeiz and colleagues (1968) reported three patients of Irish descent with parkinsonism, myoclonus, supranuclear palsy, and apraxia who were found at autopsy to have "corticodentatonigral degeneration with neuronal achromasia." The full spectrum of clinical manifestations of this complex neurodegenerative disorder was not fully recognized until quite recently. Since cerebellar deficit is not a feature of the disorder, the term *corticobasal ganglionic degeneration* has been used to describe the predominant involvement of the cortex and the basal ganglia; the term *corticobasal degeneration* is also used, particularly in the European literature (Mahapatra et al., 2004). Since the initial description of CBD was based on clinical-pathologic characteristics, some have suggested the term corticobasal syndrome to draw attention to the marked clinical heterogeneity and to emphasize that CBD pathology may be encountered in PSP, FTD, speech apraxia, primary progressive aphasia, and the posterior cortical atrophy syndrome (Wadia and Lang, 2007). The most striking features of CBD include marked asymmetry of involvement; focal rigidity and dystonia with or without contractures, and hand, limb, gait, and speech apraxia (Video 9.10), although a symmetric form of CBD has been described (Hassan et al., 2010). This series of five pathologically proven patients, however, had many atypical features such as absence of limb dystonia, myoclonus, apraxia, or alien hand and 40% had positive family history, suggesting the possibility of a disorder other than CBD, despite its pathologic overlap, or the concept of CBD as a distinct clinical-pathologic entity needs to be revisited. In addition, some patients manifest coarse rest and action tremor, and cortical-type focal myoclonus (Video 9.8); and parkinsonism, and in some cases cognitive decline may precede these classic features (Bergeron et al., 1998). Other features include cortical sensory deficit, language and speech alterations (Özsancak et al., 2000), frontal lobe symptomatology, depression, apathy, irritability, and agitation (Litvan, et al., 1998b). 🎥

The asymmetric onset differentiates CBD from most other neurodegenerative disorders, and some patients who have been categorized as having "asymmetric cortical degenerative syndrome" (Caselli, 2000) might have CBD. In a study of 14 patients with pathologically confirmed CBD, Wenning and colleagues (1998) found that asymmetric hand clumsiness was the most common presenting symptom, noted at onset in 50% of the patients. At the time of the first neurologic visit, about 3 years after onset, the following signs were present: unilateral limb rigidity (79%), bradykinesia (71%), ideomotor apraxia (64%), postural imbalance (45%), unilateral limb dystonia (43%), and cortical dementia (36%). The mean age at onset was 63 ± 7.7 years; the mean duration of symptoms from onset to death was 7.9 ± 0.7 years (range: 2.5–12.5). Patients with early bradykinesia, frontal syndrome, and two of the following three – tremor, rigidity, and bradykinesia – had a poor prognosis. These clinical features are similar to those described earlier by Rinne and colleagues (1994b), who reviewed 36 patients (20 females and 16 males), with a mean age at onset of 60.9 ± 9.7 years (range: 40–76). In the patients reported by Riley and colleagues (1990), the mean age at onset was 60 years (range: 51–71), and men were more commonly affected than women (3:2). Two patients died 7 and 10 years after disease onset. In a series of 147 cases collected from eight centers, the following features were most common: parkinsonism (100%), higher cortical dysfunction (93%), dyspraxia (82%), gait disorder (80%), dystonia (71%), tremor (55%), myoclonus (55%), alien limb (42%), cortical sensory loss (33%), and dementia (25%) (Kompoliti et al., 1998). In one clinical-pathologic study, the presence of varying combinations of early frontal-lobe type behavioral symptoms, nonfluent language disturbance, orobuccal apraxia, and utilization behavior were predictive of CBD rather than Alzheimer pathology (Shelley et al., 2009).

The typical features of CBD can be categorized into movement disorders (akinesia, rigidity, postural instability, limb dystonia, cortical myoclonus, and postural/intention tremor) and cortical signs, such as cortical sensory loss, apraxias (ideational and ideomotor) (Video 9.10), and the alien limb phenomenon (Video 9.11) (Riley et al., 1990; Rinne et al., 1994b; Fitzgerald et al., 2007; Brainin et al., 2008). The alien hand syndrome occurs not only in CBD but also in other disorders including strokes involving the genu or anterior rostrum of the corpus callosum and the contralateral frontomedial cortical and subcortical region (Brainin et al., 2008). Ideomotor apraxia, possibly secondary to involvement of the supplementary motor area and characterized by not knowing "how to do it" (as opposed to not knowing "what to do" in ideational apraxia), is the most typical form of apraxia (Leiguarda et al., 1994; Leiguarda and Marsden, 2000; Zadikoff and Lang, 2005; Wheaton and Hallett, 2007). This apraxia may improve with tactile stimulation, such as the use of the appropriate tool (Graham et al., 1999). Using the De Renzi ideomotor apraxia test, Soliveri and colleagues (2005) compared limb apraxia in patients with CBD ($n = 24$) and PSP ($n = 25$). They found that "awkwardness errors," conceptually appropriate but clumsily executed actions because of fine finger motility, were the most common apraxic errors in patients with CBD, followed by spatial errors, characterized by incorrect orientation or trajectory of the arm, hand, or digits in space or in relation to the body. Sequence errors, incorrect sequences of actions or inappropriate repetition of movements, were least impaired in CBD. The order of impairment was reversed in patients with PSP. Overall, apraxia, particularly ideational or limb-kinetic apraxia, was more frequent and more severe in patients with CBD than in those with PSP, in whom ideomotor apraxia appears more common. Limb contractures, often preceded by the alien hand phenomenon, are more common in this condition than in the other parkinsonism-plus syndromes (Doody and Jankovic, 1992; Leiguarda et al., 1994; Leiguarda and Marsden, 2000). This anterior or motor alien hand syndrome must be differentiated from sensory or posterior syndrome associated with a lesion in the thalamus, splenium of corpus callosum, and temporal-occipital lobe (Hakan et al., 1998). In autopsy-proven cases of CBD, the following were found to be the best predictors of the diagnosis of CBD: limb dystonia, ideomotor apraxia, myoclonus, and asymmetric akinetic-rigid syndrome with late onset of gait or balance disturbance (Litvan et al., 1997a; Wenning et al., 1998). In some cases of CBD, the alien hand phenomenon is associated with spontaneous arm levitation and either tactile avoidance or tactile pursuit or both, each in the opposite limb (Fitzgerald et al., 2007). Arm levitation has been also described in PSP, another feature overlapping these two disorders (Barclay et al., 1999). In our study of 66 patients diagnosed clinically with CBD, 39 (59%) had dystonia (Vanek and Jankovic, 2001). 🎥

Neurologic examination often reveals asymmetrical apraxia, oculomotility disturbance particularly manifested by impaired convergence and vertical and horizontal gaze palsy, bulbar impairment, focal myoclonus, mirror movements, hyperreflexia, Babinski sign, but no ataxia. In contrast to PSP, the vertical saccades are only slightly impaired in CBD and usually involve only upward gaze; furthermore, there is a marked increase in horizontal saccade latency in CBD, which correlates well with an "apraxia score" (Vidailhet et al., 1994). Focal myoclonus, usually involving one arm, present at rest and exacerbated by voluntary movement or in response to sensory stimulation, resembles typical cortical myoclonus but differs in several features. In contrast to the typical reflex cortical myoclonus, which is characterized by long latency (50 ms in the hand), enlarged somatosensory evoked responses (SEP), and cortical discharge preceding the movement, the reflex myoclonus associated with CBD is usually not associated with enlarged SEP and has a shorter latency from stimulus to jerk (40 ms) (Thompson et al., 1994). This suggests that the characteristic short-latency reflex myoclonus in CBD represents enhancement of a direct sensory-cortical pathway, whereas the more typical reflex cortical myoclonus involves abnormal sensorimotor cortical relays (Strafella et al., 1997). Using transcranial magnetic stimulation, Valls-Solé and colleagues (2001) found evidence of enhanced excitability, or reduced inhibition, in the motor area of the hemisphere contralateral to the alien hand sign in patients with CBD. [^{18}F]fluorodeoxyglucose PET scanning in patients with CBD and upper limb apraxia showed marked hypometabolism in the superior parietal lobule and supplementary motor area (Peigneux et al., 2001). In another study of a 70-year-old right-handed man who had alien hand syndrome-related right parietal infarction, functional MRI identified selective activation of contralateral primary motor cortex (M1), presumably released from conscious control by intentional planning systems (Assal et al., 2007).

Although considered by some as "the most common presentation" of CBD (Grimes et al., 1999), in our experience, dementia is a late feature of CBD, and semantic memory is usually well preserved (Graham et al., 2003a, 2003b; Murray

et al., 2007). This has been also suggested by a clinical-pathologic study of 15 patients with CBD followed longitudinally. Despite the persistence of apraxia, impaired executive functioning, and worsening language performance, memory remained relatively preserved (Murray et al., 2007). CBD-type syndrome, however, may be the main clinical manifestation of AD (Chand et al., 2006) and some patients with clinical presentation consistent with FTD have been found to have CBD at autopsy (Mathuranath et al., 2000b). The full spectrum of clinical features typically seen in CBD can be also present in patients with documented Pick disease, but the latter disorder is usually dominated by cognitive, behavioral, and language disturbances, such as progressive nonfluent aphasia or primary progressive aphasia (PPA) and semantic dementia (Kertesz et al., 1994; Bond et al., 1997; Litvan et al., 1997b; Hodges, 2001; Rossor, 2001; Graham et al., 2003b; Kertesz and Munoz, 2003; McMonagle et al., 2006; Rohrer et al., 2008). There are three PPA syndromes: (1) progressive nonfluent aphasia (PNFA), characterized by effortful speech with agrammatism and speech apraxia; (2) semantic PPA or semantic dementia (SemD), which involves fluent speech with loss of word and object meaning; and (3) logopenic progressive aphasia (LPA), characterized by word-finding pauses, moderate anomia, and impaired repetition of sentences (Mendez, 2010). In a clinicopathologic study of 18 patients followed in the Lille Memory Clinic over a 15-year period, patients with anarthria had a tauopathy, the agrammatics had a ubiquitin-positive, TDP-43 proteinopathy, the jargon and LPA patients had Alzheimer disease, those with typical SemD had a ubiquitin-positive TDP proteinopathy, and those with atypical SemD had either corticobasal degeneration or argyrophilic grain disease (Deramecourt et al., 2010).

Maurice Ravel, the well-known French composer, was thought to have PPA, which later evolved to right hand apraxia and other features of CBD (Amaducci et al., 2002). Another patient with PPA, a scientist with an interest in visual arts, became fascinated with Ravel's Bolero and during the evolution of her own PPA, transformed the musical elements of the piece into visual form ('transmodal art") (Seeley et al., 2008). Despite severe degeneration in the left inferior frontal-insular, temporal and striatal regions, this new creativity was associated with increased gray matter volume and hyperperfusion in her right posterior neocortex on various neuroimaging studies. This form of synesthesia has been described in a variety of disorders, present to a variable degree in up to 4% of normal individuals (Simner, 2007), but also has been found in patients with thalamic lesions (Ro et al., 2007) and new or increased creativity has been reported in patients with temporal lobe lesion, PD, FTD, and other neurodegenerative disorders (Pollak et al., 2007; Griffiths, 2008; Mesulam et al., 2008).

Neuropsychological testing in patients with CBD typically shows deficits in frontal-striatal-parietal cognitive domains, including attention/concentration, executive functions, verbal fluency, praxis, language, and visuospatial functioning (Pillon et al., 1995a). Patients also typically exhibit impaired graphesthesia and may present with visuospatial dysfunction (Tang-Wai et al., 2003). This profile depends on which hemisphere is primarily affected. Usually presenting as word-finding disturbances (anomia), this language disorder then evolves into impairment of the grammatical structure (syntax) and comprehension (semantics) (Mesulam, 2003). Some patients with PPA present as the "foreign accent syndrome" (Luzzi et al., 2008). In one study of 10 patients with PPA who were followed prospectively until they became nonfluent or mute, Kertesz and Munoz (2003) found that at autopsy, all had evidence of FTD: CBD in 4, Pick body dementia in 3, and tau and synuclein negative ubiquinated inclusions of the motor neuron disease in 3. Although no mutations were found in the *tau* gene in 25 patients with PPA, there was a significant overrepresentation of the tau H1/H1 genotype, also found in PSP and CBD (Mesulam, 2003; Sobrido et al., 2003). Imaging studies have shown that PPA is often associated with atrophy in the left frontotemporal region, and other areas such as the fusiform and precentral gyri and intraparietal sulcus are activated, possibly as a compensatory neuronal strategy (Sonty et al., 2003). These and other studies provide evidence that PPA is related to dissociation for grammatical and working memory aspects of sentence processing within the left frontal cortex (Grossman, 2002). In one study of 55 patients, CBD was divided into "motor onset" (*n* = 19) and "cognitive onset" (*n* = 36) and it was found that language was more impaired in the latter, but there was no correlation between side of atrophy or motor impairment and the severity of language dysfunction (McMonagle et al., 2006). Tau-positive pathology was present in 85% of the 19 brains and the pathologic diagnosis of CBD was confirmed in 58%.

PPA is sometimes confused with the syndrome of slowly progressive anarthria that is seen in the late anterior opercular syndrome (see later), but in the latter syndrome, there is no associated language or cognitive deficit. The majority of patients with CBD have been found to have aphasia (e.g., anomic, Broca's, and transcortical motor aphasia) (Frattali et al., 2000) with phonologic (e.g., spelling) impairment even without clinically observable aphasia (Graham et al., 2003b). Another disorder that progresses rapidly to a nonambulatory state and muteness is motor neuron disease-inclusion body dementia (MND-ID) (Josephs et al., 2003; Kleiner-Fisman et al., 2004). This entity, a subtype of FTD, which is confirmed only pathologically, usually begins in the patient's mid-forties and shares some features of CBD. Typically, the patients have early dysphagia suggestive of bulbar palsy but without fasciculations. Pathologically, the brains show severe caudate atrophy, with intracytoplasmic inclusions that stain with antibodies against heavy and light subunits of neurofilaments and against ubiquitin. Families with clinical features of Pick disease and the pathologic picture of CBD have been described (Brown et al., 1996). In contrast, apraxia and parkinsonism, if present, are usually late findings in Pick disease, whereas personality changes, aggressive behavior, disinhibition, cognitive deficits, elements of Klüver–Bucy syndrome, and other features of FTD are common (Cherrier and Mendez, 1999; Nasreddine et al., 1999). CBD is probably most frequently confused with PSP, chiefly because of the overlapping oculomotor findings. The CBD patients, however, have much more marked asymmetry in their motor deficits, less severe ophthalmoparesis, and more prominent apraxia and myoclonus (see Table 9.1). The neuropsychological studies show a pattern of deficits that is different from that seen in PSP or AD. When 21 patients with CBD were compared with a group of patients with AD, the CBD patients performed significantly better than the AD

patients on tests of immediate and delayed recall of verbal material, whereas the AD patients (with or without extrapyramidal symptoms) performed better on tests of praxis, finger-tapping speed, and motor programming (Massman et al., 1996). The CBD and AD groups all displayed prominent deficits on tests of sustained attention/mental control and verbal fluency and exhibited mild deficits on confrontation naming. The CBD patients endorsed significantly more depressive symptoms on the Geriatric Depression Scale. A similar neuropsychological pattern was demonstrated in another study of 15 patients with CBD (Pillon et al., 1995a). The spectrum of neuropsychological deficits in CBD is broadening (Bergeron et al., 1997).

In addition to parkinsonian, aphasia, neuropsychological, and oculomotor deficits, patients with CBD may also present with progressive spasticity (Hasselblatt et al., 2007).

Neurodiagnostic studies

Computed tomography scans were abnormal in 14 of the 15 patients in one series; 8 had asymmetrical parietal lobe atrophy corresponding to the most affected side, and 6 had bilateral parietal atrophy (Riley et al., 1990). Asymmetric frontoparietal atrophy helps to differentiate CBD from PSP (Soliveri et al., 1999; Sitburana and Ondo, 2009). Another radiographic abnormality that is occasionally encountered in CBD is the "eye of the tiger" sign on brain MRI, characteristically seen in NBIA1 (formerly Hallervorden–Spatz disease) (Molinuevo et al., 1999). One patient with typical CBD clinically was found to have basal ganglia calcification, similar to Fahr disease, on MRI (Manyam et al., 2001; Brodaty et al., 2002; Warren et al., 2002; Oliveira et al., 2004). In a clinical-radiologic study of 8 patients with CBD compared to 36 controls, Yamauchi and colleagues (1998) found atrophy of the corpus callosum, especially the middle portion, which correlated with cognitive impairment and cerebral cortical metabolism measured by ^{18}F-fludeoxyglucose PET. Hyperintensity in the subcortical white matter in the rolandic region on FLAIR images with asymmetric atrophy in the cerebral peduncle, and atrophy in the midbrain tegmentum also have been described as typical MRI findings in patients with CBD (Koyama et al., 2007). Marked asymmetry of the motor pathways (corticospinal and transcallosal fibers) in CBD can be also demonstrated by diffusion tensor tractography using MR diffusion tensor imaging (DTI) (Boelmans et al., 2009). Despite these reported abnormalities, no specific neuroimaging picture of CBD has emerged, and there is no correlation between antemortem MRI and pathologically confirmed CBD (Josephs et al., 2004). PET scans show reduced [^{18}F]fluorodopa uptake in the caudate and putamen and markedly asymmetrical cortical hypometabolism, especially in the superior temporal and inferior parietal lobe (Eidelberg et al., 1991; Sawle et al., 1991; Blin et al., 1992). In one study, [^{123}I]β-CIT SPECT showed marked asymmetry in reduced striatal binding in patients with CBD, similar to PD, but this did not allow reliable differentiation between PD, PSP, MSA, and CBD (Pirker et al., 2000). In two CBD patients with myoclonus, SEP showed a reduced N20 amplitude but without giant SEP (Brunt et al., 1995). Although the other neurophysiologic studies were consistent with cortical reflex myoclonus, the unusual absence of SEP may be explained either by cortical parietal atrophy or by pathologic hyperexcitability of the motor cortex due to a loss of inhibitory input from the sensory cortex (Lu et al., 1998).

Neuropathology, neurochemistry, and pathogenesis

Despite marked asymmetry in clinical findings, autopsy studies of CBD brains show predominantly bilateral atrophy of the precentral gyrus without significant asymmetry of neuropathologic changes (Cordato et al., 2001). Pathologic features in this disease include neuronal degeneration in the precentral and postcentral cortical areas, degeneration of the basal ganglia, including the SN, and the presence of achromatic neural inclusions seen not only in the cortex, but also in the thalamus, subthalamic nucleus, red nucleus, and SN (Gibb et al., 1990; Lippa et al., 1991; Lowe et al., 1992; Kumar et al., 2002). These ballooned neurons, characterized by perikaryal swelling, dispersion of Nissl substance, eccentrically located nucleus, cytoplasm vacuolation, and achromasia, show strong diffuse cytoplasmic immunoreactivity with anti-αB crystallin, a protein that is homologous with the small cell stress proteins. They also show weak, diffuse immunoreactivity with anti-ubiquitin (not present in swollen neurons in infarcted brain). While ballooned neurons are not specific for CBD and have been found in Pick disease, PSP, AD, FTD, and argyrophilic grain disease, as well as Creutzfeldt–Jakob disease, tau-containing distal astrocytic processes producing "astrocytic plaques" have been suggested by Feany and Dickson (1996) to be a distinctive pathologic feature of CBD. These cortical plaques, which are amyloid- and microglia-negative, represent clusters of miliary-like tau-positive structures within the distal processes of the astrocytes. In one review of clinical-pathologic studies, 83% of the patients with the clinical syndrome of CBD (CBS) had evidence of tauopathy in autopsied brains (Wadia and Lang, 2007). Abnormal phosphorylation of tau is not specific for CBD; it can be seen in a variety of neurodegenerative disorders. In the CBD brain, however, tau accumulates as two 64 and 68 kDa polypeptides that are not recognized by antibodies specific to the adult tau sequences encoded by exons 3 and 10 of the *tau* gene (Bergeron et al., 1998; Kumar et al., 2002). In contrast to the 80 nm periodicity of twisted filaments in AD, the periodicity is about 290 nm in CBD. Tau immunostains usually show granular neuronal deposits, neuropil threads, and glial inclusions. In addition, NFTs and Pick bodies, spherical cortical intraneuronal inclusions, are usually present in the cortical areas but, in contrast to Pick disease, not in the hippocampus. Another characteristic finding of CBD is the presence of corticobasal inclusions, which consist of round, fibrillary or homogeneous basophilic tau-positive inclusions that displace cellular pigment into the periphery, similar to globose neurofibrillary tangles seen in PSP (Kertesz et al., 2009). Neuronal inclusions in CBD are found predominantly in cortical pyramidal and nonpyramidal neurons and may have a distinctive perinuclear, coiled filamentous appearance. In addition to the different distribution, the Pick bodies of Pick disease and the Pick-like bodies of CBD have distinct staining characteristics. While Pick bodies are strongly argentophilic with Bodian and Bielschowsky stains but negative with the Gallyas stain, the Pick-like bodies of CBD stain

with Gallyas stain but are not strongly argentophilic. Furthermore, typical Pick bodies usually do not stain with the anti-tau antibody 12E8, which detects phosphorylation at SER 262/356, while the CBD inclusions are recognized by the 12E8 antibody. Astrocytic plaques, different from thorn-shaped astrocytes that are typically seen in PSP, are also typically present in the brains of patients with CBD. In addition, coiled bodies, ubiquitin-negative, tau-immunoreactive inclusions and oligodendroglial inclusions that consist of filaments coiled around a nucleus and extend into the proximal part of the cell process are also typically present in CBD. These inclusions are found not only in CBD but also in PSP and Pick disease; they are particularly numerous in CBD and PSP.

The apparent overlap in clinical and pathologic features between CBD, PSP, and Pick disease needs clarification from further pathologic studies (Kosaka et al., 1991; Woods and McKee, 1992; Lang et al., 1994; Mori et al., 1994; Jendroska et al., 1995; Schneider et al., 1997; Boeve et al., 1999; Cordato et al., 2001; Boeve et al., 2003a; Wadia and Lang, 2007). In one study of 13 patients with clinically diagnosed CBD, pathologic examination found evidence of CBD in 7 patients; AD in 2 patients; and PSP, Pick disease, CJD, and nonspecific neurodegenerative disorder in 1 patient each (Boeve et al., 1999). This indicates marked pathologic heterogeneity and argues for a need to examine the brain before the diagnosis of CBD can be confirmed. Asymmetric parietofrontal cortical degeneration was the most consistent pathologic abnormality in this autopsy series. One of the most important studies addressing the clinical and pathologic overlap between CBD and PSP was based on 35 cases from the Queen Square Brain Bank in which there were 21 clinically and 19 pathologically diagnosed cases of corticobasal syndrome (CBS) or degeneration (CBD) (Ling et al., 2010). Of 19 pathologically confirmed CBD cases, only 5 had been diagnosed correctly in life (sensitivity = 26.3%). All had a unilateral presentation, clumsy useless limb, limb apraxia, and myoclonus, 4 had cortical sensory impairment and focal limb dystonia, and 3 had an alien limb. Eight cases of CBD had been clinically diagnosed as PSP, all of whom had vertical supranuclear palsy, and 7 had falls within the first 2 years. Of 21 cases with CBS, only 5 had CBD (positive predictive value of 23.8%); 6 others had PSP pathology, 5 had AD, and the remaining five had other non-tau pathologies. Forty-two percent of CBD cases presented clinically with a PSP phenotype and 29% of CBS cases had underlying PSP pathology. The authors suggested the CBD–Richardson syndrome for the overlap cases and concluded that CBD "is a discrete clinico-pathological entity but with a broader clinical spectrum than was originally proposed."

Pathologic features of CBD have been reported in one family with tauopathy in which all three siblings and their grandmother exhibited parkinsonism with levodopa response in one member of the family (Uchihara and Nakayama, 2006). Since frontal lobe dysfunction was also present this family may have had FTDP rather than CBD. The clinical features of CBD, including PPA, have been described in two cases with *LRRK2* G2019S mutation (Chen-Plotkin et al., 2008).

A relationship between CBD, Pick disease, and PSP is suggested by the presence of ballooned neurons and nigral

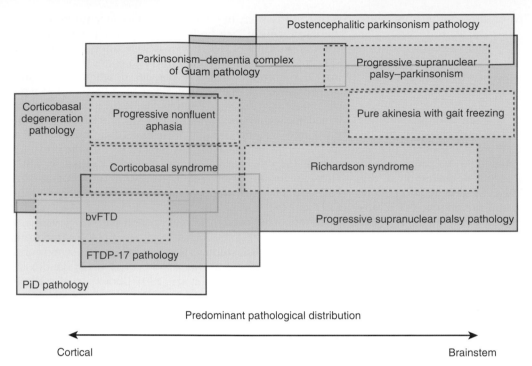

Figure 9.7 Overlap between PSP, CBD, FTDP, and Parkinsonism–dementia complex of Guam (PDCG). bvFTD, behavioral variant of frontotemporal dementia. *Redrawn from Williams DR, Lees AJ. Progressive supranuclear palsy: clinicopathological concepts and diagnostic challenges. Lancet Neurol 2009;8:270–9.*

basophilic inclusions, which are usually present in all three disorders. Although these disorders are clinically and pathologically similar, there are some distinguishing pathologic features. While "parietal Pick disease" has been reported, the vast majority of pathologically documented Pick cases exhibit degenerative changes predominantly in the frontotemporal distribution with "knife-edge" atrophy of the gyri. In addition, ballooned neurons and Pick bodies, strongly argentophilic and homogeneously ubiquitinated intraneuronal inclusions, are typically present in Pick disease. However, neither of the two histologic hallmarks is absolutely required for the neuropathologic diagnosis of Pick disease (Growdon and Primavera, 2000). Kertesz and colleagues (1994) proposed the concept of "Pick complex" for certain focal cortical degenerations such as PPA (with or without amyotrophic lateral sclerosis, or ALS), frontal lobe dementia, and CBD. He and his colleagues (Kertesz et al., 2000b) later suggested that there is a clinical and pathologic overlap between CBD, FTD, and PPA (Williams and Lees, 2009) (Fig. 9.7).

Dopamine concentration was reduced in the CBD brains throughout the striatum and SN when compared with age-matched controls (Riley et al., 1990).

Treatment

To date, no effective treatment has been found, although myoclonus may improve with clonazepam, and painful rigidity and dystonia may improve with botulinum toxin injections (Jankovic and Brin, 1991). Dopaminergic drugs are rarely, if ever, effective. Although levodopa rarely provides any improvement in patients with CBD (Kompoliti et al., 1998), levodopa-induced dyskinesia has been reported

in rare autopsy-proven cases (Frucht et al., 2000). Rehabilitation has been reported to improve ideomotor apraxia following stroke, but it is not known whether similar strategies improve apraxia associated with CBD (Hanna-Pladdy et al., 2003).

Parkinsonism–dementia syndromes

Clinical features and natural history

Cognitive impairment is common in parkinsonian disorders, and characteristic psychological profiles can differentiate PD from atypical parkinsonian syndromes (Pillon et al., 1996; Litvan, 1998a; Emre, 2003; Galvin et al., 2006; Lippa et al., 2007; Aarsland et al., 2008). Significant dementia occurs in 30% of patients with PD, a six-fold increase over the risk of dementia in non-PD controls ((Emre et al., 2007; Aarsland et al., 2008). This risk of dementia increases during the course of the illness, reaching 80%, and with estimated incidence ranging from 2.7%/year at ages 55–64 to 13.7%/ year at ages 70–79 (Braak et al., 2005; Galvin et al., 2006; Aarsland et al., 2008). Clinical diagnostic criteria for possible and probable dementia associated with PD (PDD) have been formulated but it is not clear how sensitive and specific these criteria are in differentiating PDD from DLB (Emre et al., 2007). In one prospective study, the incidence of dementia was 19% over 54 months of observation (Biggins et al., 1992). Patients with PD have nearly twice the risk for developing dementia as controls (Marder et al., 1995), and siblings of demented PD patients have an increased risk for AD (Marder et al., 1999). Poor performance on tests of verbal fluency appears to be predictive of incipient dementia in patients who are in early phases of PD (Jacobs et al., 1995). Cognitive decline seems to be more prominent in patients with older onset and the postural instability with dysfunctional gait form of PD (Jankovic et al., 1990b; Biggins et al., 1992; Galasko et al., 1994a). In addition to the Mini-Mental State Examination (Dufouil et al., 2000), other tests have been developed and validated to assess the cognitive (e.g., the Addenbrooke's Cognitive Examination) (Mathuranath et al., 2000a) and frontal lobe function (e.g., the Frontal Assessment Battery) (Dubois et al., 2000) in patients with dementia with or without parkinsonism. About 15–45% of patients with AD develop parkinsonism, and the presence of such motor impairment markedly increases the burden on the patient and increases the cost of patient care (Murman et al., 2003). Except for tremor, parkinsonian and other motor signs increase during the course of the disease (Scarmeas et al., 2004).

PD dementia (PDD) is defined as cognitive impairments that include cognitive and motor slowing, executive dysfunction, and impaired memory retrieval. The relationship of PDD to AD and other dementing disorders such as DLB has not yet been well defined. While some investigators suggest that clear clinical-pathologic separation is possible between the three disorders, the differences in neuropathologic and neurochemical characteristics suggest that there is a continuum and that the disorders are difficult to differentiate clinically and pathologically (Ballard et al., 2006; Lippa et al., 2007). While longer duration of PD symptoms appears to be associated with less Alzheimer pathology and less cortical α-synuclein, the cholinergic deficit is more severe, probably due to LB pathology in the nucleus basalis of Meynert present in both PDD and DLB (Ballard et al., 2006; Lippa and Emre, 2006; Lippa et al., 2007). Extrapyramidal signs have been reported in about one-third of patients with AD (Chen et al., 1991), and their presence correlates with greater cognitive impairment and worse prognosis as compared to AD patients without extrapyramidal signs (Funkenstein et al., 1993; Merello et al., 1994; Stern et al., 1994; Clark et al., 1997; Kurlan et al., 2000; Wilson et al., 2003). Using [^{11}C]β-CFT PET scans to image striatal dopamine reuptake sites, Rinne and colleagues (1998) showed a significant reduction in the dopamine transporter in patients with AD, and the reduction correlated with the severity of the extrapyramidal symptoms. Pathologically, the parkinsonian signs in AD correlate best with the presence of NFTs rather than Lewy bodies in the SN (Liu et al., 1997) and with the presence of iron in the SN (Brar et al., 2009). Other studies have shown that AD patients with parkinsonism have PD-like pathology in their SN (Burns et al., 2005). In a prospective clinicopathologic study by the Consortium to Establish a Registry for Alzheimer's Disease (CERAD), 16 (20.5%) of the 78 cases of AD had coexistent PD pathology (Hulette et al., 1995). Research into molecular, cellular, and genetic mechanisms of AD will undoubtedly provide insight not only into AD but also into other neurodegenerative disorders.

Current research has been focusing on the role of the amyloid-β (Aβ) amyloid precursor protein (APP) in the pathogenesis of AD. Elevated levels of APP have been found to correlate with cognitive decline (Näslund et al., 2000). For example, mice expressing mutations in the APP gene develop Aβ deposits, and this process is accelerated by coexpression of mutant senilin genes and by apolipoprotein E (Emilien et al., 2000). In addition to the gene mutation in 21q21.2 that produces mutant APP and is responsible for early-onset AD, mutations in other genes (e.g., 1q41,12p, 14q24.3, and 19q13.2) affect the formation of Aβ. Currently, the most sensitive and specific biologic markers for AD are reduced levels of Aβ42 amyloid protein and sulfatide and increased levels of tau and phosphorylated tau in the CSF. Using PET with radiolabeled Pittsburgh Compound-B (14C-PIB) in 10 patients with PD, 12 with PDD, 13 with LBD, and 41 age-matched controls, amyloid load was significantly increased in over 80% of DLB subjects, but amyloid pathology was infrequent in PDD (Edison et al., 2008a, 2008b). These findings were confirmed by other (Gomperts et al., 2008) but not all studies (Rowe et al., 2007). This noninvasive technique has been validated by postmortem as well as biopsy findings as an indicator of amyloid deposits (Leinonen et al., 2008).

Several genetic markers have been identified in patients with the combination of parkinsonism and dementia, including overexpression of α-synclein due to mutplication of SNCA (Ross et al., 2008) and high beta-amyloid load associated with APOE genotype (Lashley et al., 2008). Similar to PSP, H1/H1 is also associated with PDD (Goris et al., 2007).

Consensus guidelines for the clinical and pathologic diagnosis of DLB have been proposed (McKeith et al., 1996; Hohl et al., 2000; Lopez et al., 2002; McKeith et al., 2005). These criteria have been reformulated by the Consortium on DLB by adding the presence of extrapyramidal signs (McKeith et al., 1996; Mega et al., 1996). In addition to progressive cognitive decline, two of the following criteria are required for the diagnosis of probable DLB (one for a "possible" diagnosis): (1) fluctuating cognition with pronounced variations in attention and alertness; (2) recurrent, typically well-formed, visual hallucinations; and (3) motor features of parkinsonism. Supportive features, not required for the diagnosis, include repeated falls, syncope, transient loss of consciousness, neuroleptic sensitivity, systematized delusions, and hallucinations in other modalities. Using these clinical criteria in 18 cases of pathologically diagnosed AD, the authors found 100% specificity with high interrater reliability (Mega et al., 1996). In a review of 31 pathologically proven cases of DLB, Louis and colleagues (1997) found that the presence of myoclonus, absence of rest tremor, no response to levodopa, or no perceived need to treat with levodopa was highly predictive of the diagnosis of DLB. REM sleep behavior disorder has been described at onset in a group of patients with DLB (Boeve et al., 1998), and REM sleep behavior disorder and depression were added as additional features that are supportive of the diagnosis of DLB during the second DLB workshop (McKeith et al., 1999).

Dementia with Lewy bodies (DLB), considered by some as a variant of AD or an overlap between AD and PD, is now well recognized, but its clinical and pathologic criteria have not yet been fully defined (Burkhardt et al., 1988; Crystal et al., 1990; Sage and Mark, 1993; McKeith et al., 1994, 1996; Mega et al., 1996; Litvan et al., 1998d; Gomez-Isla et al., 1999; Verghese et al., 1999; Lopez et al., 2002; Pompeu and Growdon, 2002; McKeith et al., 2005; Galvin et al., 2006). Also referred to variably as diffuse Lewy body disease, senile dementia of Lewy body type, and Lewy body variant of AD, DLB has emerged as the second most common cause of degenerative dementia in the elderly. Although it is usually a sporadic disorder, a few families with DLB have been described (Tsuang et al., 2002). Differentiation of AD and DLB on clinical findings alone can be difficult, but the following features are significantly more frequent in DLB than in AD and serve to differentiate the two disorders: cognitive fluctuations, visual and auditory hallucinations, depression, and sleep disturbance (Galvin et al., 2006). DLB and Parkinson disease dementia (PDD), however, share identical clinical features and DLB is believed to represent the most common form of PDD, accounting for 38% of pathologic cases of PDD; PD-AD was seen in 32% (Galvin et al., 2006). Crystal and colleagues (1990) reviewed the course of six patients with DLB, three with AD, and one with PD with autopsy-confirmed diagnosis, and found that DLB patients were more likely to have gait impairment, rigidity, and resting tremor early in the course of the illness. In another study of 30 patients with DLB, psychosis and dementia were often found to precede parkinsonism (Burkhardt et al., 1988). Agitation, hallucinations, delusions, and abnormal EEGs were more common in the DLB than in the AD patients (Burkhardt et al., 1988). Complex visual hallucinations, even in the early stages of the disease, are particularly characteristic of DLB (Manford and Andermann, 1998) and the presence of visual hallucinations is the strongest positive predictor of the diagnosis of DLB (Tiraboschi et al., 2006). Visual hallucinations in DLB seem to correlate with the presence of Lewy bodies in the temporal lobe (Harding et al., 2002). Indeed, the presence of hallucinations should suggest Lewy body pathology as non-Lewy body parkinsonism is only infrequently associated with hallucinations. In a study of 15 patients (14 men) diagnosed at Mayo Clinic with RBD, all had clear histories of dream enactment behavior, and 10 had RBD confirmed by polysomnography; the neuropathologic diagnoses were LBD in 12 patients (neocortical in 11 and limbic in 1) and MSA in 3 patients (Boeve et al., 2003a). The clinical and pathologic literature therefore suggests that when associated with a neurodegenerative disorder, RBD tends to occur in certain disorders (e.g., DLB, PD, and MSA) and rarely if ever occurs in others (e.g., PSP, CBD, AD, FTD). The RBD Screening Questionnaire (RBDSQ) seems to be a sensitive instrument that captures most of the characteristics of RBD (Stiasny-Kolster et al., 2007). In another study, the authors showed that in the setting of dementia or parkinsonism, the presence of RBD often reflects synucleinopathy (Boeve et al., 2003b). No differences were found with respect to age, gender, or disease progression between autopsy-proven cases of AD and DLB (Gibb et al., 1989). On neurologic examination, rigidity, bradykinesia, and action tremor were more frequent in the DLB patients, while impairment of upgaze was surprisingly more common in the AD group. Fluctuations, particularly when associated with disturbed arousal and disorganized speech, are very characteristic of DLB and serve to differentiate it from AD (Ferman et al., 2004). Although DLB patients might not respond as well to levodopa as do those with typical PD, many do obtain satisfactory improvement with levodopa and benefit from chronic treatment (Bonelli et al., 2004). Using voxel-based morphometry, patients with DLB were found to have more cortical atrophy on MRI than patients with PDD, thus arguing that the two disorders are two separate subtypes of Lewy body disease (Beyer et al., 2007). There are, however, many limitations to this study, including small sample size, lack of more sophisticated MRI, such as diffusion tensor MRI, lack of pathologic confirmation of the cortical gray matter atrophy or pathologic diagnosis (Seppi and Rascol, 2007).

In addition to the expected Lewy bodies in the SN, patients with parkinsonism and dementia have cortical pathology, including Lewy bodies in neocortex, the density correlating with the severity of dementia (Hurtig et al., 2000). Diffuse Lewy body disease is the most common pathologic finding in patients with PD who later developed dementia (Apaydin et al., 2002). But Braak and colleagues (2005), in their detailed clinical-pathologic studies, attribute cognitive decline in PD to "the cumulative effects of the progressive PD pathology," although cognitively impaired PD patients also had a greater degree of AD pathology than those who were cognitively unimpaired.

Differentiation between DLB and the other parkinsonism-plus syndromes, particularly PSP, can be particularly difficult when a patient with parkinsonism and dementia is also found to have oculomotor disturbance, as has been noted in some patients with DLB (Lewis and Gawel, 1990). Since orthostatic hypotension and other autonomic symptoms can be seen in DLB, this disorder may at times be difficult to differentiate from MSA (Thaisetthawatkul et al., 2004). In contrast to AD, in which urinary incontinence usually occurs late in the course of the dementia, urinary incontinence may precede severe cognitive decline in DLB (Del-Ser et al., 1996). The relationship between AD and other dementing disorders such as DLB, CBD, and Pick disease is illustrated by the observation of rapidly progressive aphasia, apraxia, dementia, myoclonus, and parkinsonism in an autopsy-proven case of AD (Wojcieszek et al., 1994). Medial temporal lobe atrophy (MTA) on MRI failed to differentiate between DLB and AD, although the latter had more severe MTA (Barber et al., 1999).

Until a disease-specific biologic marker that differentiates the various neurodegenerative disorders is identified, the clinical categorization of the various dementing diseases will continue to present a diagnostic challenge. In this regard, the study of various risk markers might provide clues to the pathogenesis of the various disorders. The frequency of the ApoE ε4 allele, a major risk factor for AD, in nondemented controls is 10–15% (Roses, 1995). The finding that the frequency of ApoE ε4 allele was increased to a similar extent in autopsy-proven cases of AD and the Lewy body variant of AD (40% and 29%, respectively) (Galasko et al., 1994b) and that ApoE ε4 allele is strongly associated with increased neuritic plaques in both disorders (Olichney et al., 1996) suggests that the two disorders are related and that they are different from DLB, in which the frequency of the ApoE ε4 allele was significantly lower (6.2%). The frequency of ApoE ε4 genotype did not differ between demented and nondemented patients with clinically diagnosed PD and was similar to that in controls, thus suggesting that the PD-related dementia is pathogenetically different from AD (Koller et al., 1995). Mutations in the β-synuclein gene have recently been linked to cases of DLB (Ohtake et al., 2004).

Frontotemporal dementias and other tauopathies

Clinical features and natural history

The FTDs, along with PSP, CBD, PPA, Pick disease, and other neurodegenerative disorders, are examples of a group of neurologic disorders that are referred to as tauopathies (Sha et al., 2006; Snowden et al., 2007). The prototype tauopathy is an inherited parkinsonism–dementia disorder, initially described as the Wilhelmsen–Lynch disease (disinhibition–dementia–parkinsonism–amyotrophy complex), linked initially by Lynch and colleagues (1994) to a locus on 17q21–q22. Another family with autosomal dominant parkinsonism–dementia was later described by Muenter and colleagues (1998). Clinically, the affected individuals had young-onset, rapidly progressive, levodopa-responsive parkinsonism and mild dysautonomia, later associated with dementia. Some members of the family had isolated postural tremor, phenomenologically identical to essential tremor. Pathologically, the brains showed features similar to those of primary PD. Subsequently other families with the hereditary parkinsonism–dementia have been described, and the disorder is now referred to as *frontotemporal dementia and parkinsonism linked to chromosome 17* (FTDP-17) (Lendon et al., 1998; Poorkaj et al., 1998; Stevens et al., 1998; Cherrier and Mendez, 1999; Foster, 1995; Nasreddine et al., 1999; van Swieten et al., 1999; Spillantini and Goedert, 2000; Yasuda et al., 2000; Kertesz et al., 2000a; Lee et al., 2001; McKhann et al., 2001; Morris et al., 2001). In a study of nine British families with pathologically and genetically proven FTD, disinhibition was the most common presenting symptom, followed by frontal dysexecutive symptoms, apathy, impairment of episodic memory, and depression (Janssen et al., 2002). Subsequently, essentially all patients develop personality and behavioral changes, memory impairment, language deficits, ritualistic behavior, hyperphagia, hyperorality, parkinsonism, and neuroleptic sensitivity. Semantic dementia, a term coined by Snowden and associates in their description of patients with fluent PPA and impaired word comprehension, is one of the main features of FTD (Hodges and Patterson, 2007). Stereotypies, such as rubbing and self-injurious behavior, similar to those seen in patients with autism and intellectual disability, are also characteristically seen in patients with FTD (Mendez et al., 2005).

The overall prevalence of FTD has been estimated to be 16%, but it is the most common cause of presenile dementia, equal in prevalence to AD in patients younger than 65 years old; it accounts for >3% of those with dementia onset after 70 years. About 40% of FTD cases are of genetic origin and 60% are sporadic. Several studies have demonstrated that 11–50% of all patients with familial FTD have mutations in the *tau* gene (Morris et al., 2001). The majority of testing for the various mutations in the *MAPT* gene is done on a research basis, but information about commercially available testing can be found at http://www.genetests.org. Furthermore, *MAPT* gene sequence analysis screening mutations in seven exons (1, 7, 9, 10, 11, 12, and 13) is available through Mayo Foundation (the panel list price = $900) (http://cancercenter.mayo.edu/mayo/research/hutton_lab/

Table 9.3 Classification of tauopathies

3R tauopathies
Pick disease

4R tauopathies
Progressive supranuclear palsy
Corticobasal degeneration
Argyrophilic grain disease

3R and 4R tauopathies
Tangle-predominant dementia

Dementia lacking distinctive histopathology (no inclusions)

Dementia with motor neuron disease-type inclusions (FTD-MND)

tau.cfm). While mutations in the *tau* gene on chromosome 17q21 account for many of these diseases, similar phenotypes have been attributed to mutations in other genes such as *p97* (also known as valosin-containing protein) on chromosome 9p21–p12 and *CHMP2B* (charged multivesicular body protein 2B) on the pericentromeric region of chromosome 3 (Skibinski et al., 2005; Parkinson et al., 2006), and *progranulin* (*PRGN*) on chromosome 17q21 (1.5 Mb centromeric of *tau*) (Goedert and Spillantini, 2006; Baker et al., 2006; Cruts et al., 2006; Boeve, 2010). The number of different types of frontotemporal lobar degenerations, classified according to genetic mutations or tau pathology, is growing (Josephs, 2008) (Table 9.3).

The following diagnostic criteria for FTD were formulated by an international group of clinical and basic scientists (McKhann et al., 2001):

1. The development of behavioral or cognitive deficits manifested by either:
   a. early and progressive change in personality, characterized by difficulty in modulating behavior, often resulting in inappropriate responses or activities, or
   b. early and progressive changes in language, characterized by problems with expression or severe naming difficulty and problems with word meaning.
2. The deficits in 1a and 1b cause significant impairment in social or occupational functioning and represent a significant decline from previous level of functioning.
3. The course is characterized by gradual onset and continuing decline in function.
4. Other causes are excluded.

Pathologically defined frontotemporal lobar degeneration (FTLD) includes a heterogeneous group of clinical syndromes such as FTD, PPA, progressive apraxia (PAX), semantic dementia (SD), and frontotemporal dementia with motor neuron disease (FTD/MND). Based on examination of pathologic material from 79 FTLD brains, blind to clinical diagnosis, tau pathology was found in half of FTD and all PAX cases, but in no FTD/MND or SD cases. FTD/MND, SD, and PPA cases were ubiquitin and TDP-43 positive. SD cases were associated with dystrophic neurites without neuronal cytoplasmic or intranuclear inclusions (FTLD-U, type 1), FTD/MND with numerous neuronal cytoplasmic inclusions (FTLD-U, type 2) and PPA with neuronal cytoplasmic inclusions, dystrophic neurites, and neuronal intranuclear inclusions (FTLD-U, type 3). *MAPT* mutations were linked to FTD and *PGRN* mutations to FTD and PPA.

The presence of tau pathologic findings (neuronal loss and glial tau deposition) strongly predicts the presence of *tau* mutation, whereas FTD with ubiquitin inclusions or with neuronal loss and spongiosis essentially excludes mutation in *tau*. The neuropathologic examination shows tau-positive neuronal and glial inclusions (Lantos et al., 2002).

FTDP-17 joins a growing list of tauopathies such as AD, Pick disease, PSP, CBD, ALS–dementia complex (lytico-bodig disease of Guam), pallidopontonigral degeneration, Niemann–Pick disease type C, Gerstmann–Sträussler–Scheinker disease with tangles, prion protein amyloid angiopathy, familial multiple system tauopathy, hereditary dysphasic disinhibition–dementia, and familial progressive subcortical gliosis (Lee and Trojanowski, 1999; Morris et al., 1999b; Hutton, 2001; Kuzuhara et al., 2001). Although FTDP-17 is heterogeneous in its presentation, typical clinical features include personality changes (withdrawal, apathy, depression, aggressive and addictive behavior, alcoholism, excessive craving of sweets, childishness, apathy, loss of empathy, abulia, Klüver–Bucy syndrome, hypersexuality, and other evidence of disinhibition), defective executive functions (e.g., drawing to command), language deficits eventually leading to muteness, seizures (Sperfeld et al., 1999), pyramidal signs, and amyotrophy. Some have suggested that "FTD patients do not do things they should do, but do many things they shouldn't do." Parkinsonian features include bradykinesia, rigidity, and gait difficulty, but there is usually no tremor and no response to levodopa. The age at onset is usually in the sixth and seventh decade, but the symptoms can begin as early as age 27 and as late as age 75. The family history suggests autosomal dominant inheritance. There are two major phenotypes of FTDP-17: type 1 (late age at onset, dementia, cortical pathology, missense mutations) and type 2 (earlier onset, parkinsonism, basal ganglia pathology). Besides the tau locus, there are probably other genetic loci in which mutations can produce a clinical-pathologic phenotype that is similar to that of FTD-17 (Kertesz et al., 2000b). Reduction in striatal dopamine transporter correlates with the severity of parkinsonian symptoms in patients with FTDP-17 (Rinne et al., 2002).

Genetics

Although FTD is relatively common, only a small percentage of these patients have an autosomal dominant FTDP-17, caused by a coding or intronic mutation in the *tau* gene. After sequencing the tau gene, located in the 17q21.11 locus, Hutton (1999) and colleagues (1998) found three missense mutations and three mutations in the 5′ splice site of exon 10. This results in increased usage of the 5′ splice, causing an increase in exon 10 messenger RNA, consequently increasing the portion of tau containing four microtubule-binding repeats. Three types of mutations in the *tau* gene have been subsequently identified: intronic mutations in a presumed stem-loop splice site that alters expression of tau isoforms,

missense mutations in sites that bind microtubules, and missense mutations in or near phosphorylation sites. The numerous mutations that have been identified in the microtubule-binding domain of the *tau* gene are localized to the following areas: exon 9 (Gly272Val), exon 10 (Pro-301Leu), exon 12 (Val337Met) or in the splice region immediately following exon 10. Mutations outside of exon 10 and its flanking region tend to result in AD-like pathology (NFTs consisting of PHFs made up of all six isoforms of tau). Exon 10 mutations result in a four-repeat tau pattern, typically seen in PSP and FTDP-17, in which the ratio is at least 3 : 1 in favor of the four-repeat tau. About 30 different mutations have been identified in more than 60 separately ascertained families. One of the earliest families identified, a large American family with pallidopontonigral degeneration (Wszolek et al., 1995), has been found to have N279K mutation in exon 10 (Clark et al., 1998). This, the third most common mutation, is characterized by rapidly progressive, levodopa-nonresponsive, parkinsonism-predominant phenotype with supranuclear palsy (Tsuboi et al., 2002a). A novel mutation, consisting of a C-to-T transition at position +12 of the intron following exon 10, has been also described (Yasuda et al., 2000). This resulted clinically in FTD; pathologically, the brains of patients with this disorder had tau aggregates in degenerating neurons and glia with overproduction of tau isoforms with four microtubule-binding repeats. Thus, instead of the normal 1 : 1 ratio of the three-repeat and four-repeat isoforms, the brains of patients with FTDP-17 have an increased proportion of exon 10+ mRNA and a corresponding increase in the proportion of four-repeat tau. Intronic mutations, however, also destabilize a stem-loop structure that sequesters the 5′ splice downstream of exon 10 in tau pre-mRNA, leading to increases in U1 small nuclear ribonucleoprotein (snRNP) binding and in splicing between exons 10 and 11. As a result of the altered structure, the 5′ splice site mutations increase recognition of exon 10 by the U1 snRNP splicing factor, increasing the proportion of exon 10+ mRNA and four-repeat tau (Hutton, 2000). Thus, mutations close to the 5′ splice site appear to disrupt a stem-loop-type secondary structure in the tau pre-mRNA around the exon–intron junction and eventually lead to abnormal aggregation of the tau protein. An extended tau haplotype (H1), known to be associated with PSP, has been found to interact with the ε2 allele of APOE to increase the risk of FTD (Verpillat et al., 2002).

Mutations in exons 9, 10, 12, and 13 of *MAPT* are associated with prominent dementia, whereas intronic and exonic mutations are associated with overproduction of four-repeat tau and predominant parkinsonism-plus phenotype. The phenotypic variation related to the type of mutation is illustrated by one study, which found that the average age at onset of symptoms was greatest in patients with the R406W mutation (59.2 years) as compared with the other mutations P301L (51.4 years), G272B (47.6 years), and delta-K280 (53 years) (van Swieten et al., 1999). The R406W mutation was also associated with a longer duration of illness and later development of mutism. The presenting symptoms, such as disinhibition, loss of initiative, and obsessive-compulsive behavior, did not seem to differ between the four tau mutations. Additional studies are needed to explain the intrafamilial variation or differences in genotype. Expression of human tau containing the most common FTDP-17 mutation

(P301L) in transgenic mice results in motor and behavioral deficits similar to those in human tauopathies, along with formation of NFTs and Pick body-like neuronal inclusions in the amygdala, hippocampus, brainstem, cerebellum, and basal ganglia (Lewis et al., 2000). Further studies in humans as well as in mouse and *Drosophila* models of tauopathies will undoubtedly provide greater insight into the phenotypic variability of tauopathies and clarify the question of whether the observed tau aggregates are the cause or the result of neurodegeneration (de Silva and Farrer, 2002). Clinico-pathologic studies have shown that FTDs that are manifested chiefly by behavioral symptoms and semantic dementia have a broad specific range of pathologic changes, whereas those associated with motor neuron disease have predominantly ubiquitinated inclusions; parkinsonism and apraxia are associated with corticobasal pathology, and nonfluent aphasia predicted Pick bodies (Hodges et al., 2004). Although 18F-dopa PET is usually normal in patients with motor neuron disease (ALS), SPECT studies have shown that parkinsonism in these patients correlates with decreased blood flow in the frontotemporal areas, suggesting that the parkinsonism in these patients is due to cortical lesions rather than nigrostriatal damage (Hideyama et al., 2006).

These disorders not only have in common genetic abnormalities in the *tau* gene, but also overlap in neuropathologic abnormalities (Munoz et al., 2003; Goldman et al., 2004). The human gene that encodes MAPT occupies over 100 kb on chromosome 17q21 and contains 16 exons (Lee et al., 2001). Tau is a low-molecular-weight protein that has a number of functions, including stabilization of polymerization of microtubules in the brain, facilitating axonal transport, and contributing to cytoskeletal stability (Buee et al., 2000). In certain disorders, such as PSP, AD, CBD, and Pick disease (tauopathies), the normally soluble tau protein becomes hyperphosphorylated and forms ordered filamentous assemblies; these deposits of filamentous tau are the characteristic pathologic features of tauopathies. Alternative splicing of tau mRNA from 11 of the 16 exons produces six tau isoforms ranging in size from 352 to 441 amino acids. These three- and four-carboxy-terminal tandem repeat forms are further differentiated by tau isoforms without (0N) or with either 29 (1N) or 58 (2N) amino acid inserts located on the N-terminal half; an additional 31 amino acid insert is located on the C-terminal half. Inclusion of the latter, which is encoded by exon 10 of the *tau* gene, gives rise to the three isoforms with four microtubule-binding repeats each; the other three isoforms have three repeats each. While all six tau isoforms are found in the abnormal filaments in AD, only four-repeat tau isoforms are found in PSP and CBD, and there is a preponderance of three-repeat isoforms in Pick disease. Splicing, a process in which introns are excised and the remaining exons are joined together to generate mRNA, is regulated in part by unique proteins, such as the neuro-oncologic ventral antigen 1 (NOVA-1) (Dredge et al., 2001). The six major tau protein isoforms that are found in the normal adult brain are generated by alternative splicing of exons 2, 3, and 10; exons 9–12 encode four microtubule-binding domains that are imperfect repeats of 31 or 32 amino acid residues. Exon 10 encodes the second of four microtubule-bindings domains in the C-terminal half of the protein. Alternative splicing of exon 10 generates isoforms with either four or three microtubule-binding domains; the inclusion of exon 10 results in isoforms with four repeats, and the exclusion of exon 10 results in three repeats. Mutations in the splice-donor site of exon 10 lead to increased incorporation of exon 10 and therefore an increase in levels of four-repeat tau. The presence of three or four microtubule-binding repeats in the C-terminal region depends on whether E10 is spliced out or in (Goedert et al., 1998). The tau protein occurs in equal proportions of two isoforms, one with three repeats and the other with four repeats of microtubule-binding peptide domain, but the 1N-insert tau isoform is more abundant than the 0N isoform.

There are four tau microtubule-binding domains localized to the C-terminus of the protein. In the longest isoform, there are 79 serine and threonine sites to accept phosphorylation, about 30 of these sites being phosphorylated under normal circumstances (Buee et al., 2000). Overall tau phosphorylation is high during brain development but declines after birth. Abnormally high levels of tau phosphorylation in adult brains are associated with a variety of neurodegenerative disorders (Brich et al., 2003). A new proteinopathy, termed *neuronal intermediate filaments inclusion disease*, has been described with the identification of the novel intermediate filament protein α-internexin (DeKosky and Ikonomovic, 2004). This is the fourth of the phosphorylated neurofilament proteins that have been found to accumulate in various degenerative disorders; the others include light, medium, and heavy neurofilament triplet proteins (Cairns et al., 2004). The clinical phenotype is very similar to that of other FTDs. Different N-terminally cleaved tau fragments have been found in brains of patients with PSP and CBD; a 33 kDa band predominated in the low-molecular-weight tau fragments in PSP, whereas two closely related bands of approximately 37 kDa predominated in CBD (Arai et al., 2004). This suggests that the two disorders have different proteolytic processing of abnormal tau. Some, but not all (e.g., AD), diseases characterized by tau phosphorylation are associated with mutations in the *tau* gene. These sites flank the microtubule-binding domains. Since phosphorylation decreases microtubule binding, regulating tau phosphorylation might be of therapeutic value in neurodegenerative disorders associated with an abnormality of tau, including PSP. A number of serine- and threonine-protein kinases, including glycogen synthase kinase 3β (GSK-3β) and cyclin-dependent kinases 2 (cdk2) and 5 (cdk5), have been identified as possible regulators of tau phosphorylation (Buee et al., 2000). Valproate has been found to inhibit these protein kinases regulating phosphorylation of tau, including GSK-3β (Mora et al., 1998), suggesting that it might have a modifying effect on the course of PSP.

The role of tau in neurodegeneration is unknown, but one hypothesis suggests that the hyperphosphorylated tau loses its affinity for microtubules and becomes resistant to proteases, thus leading to aggregation. Tau is also the main component of NFTs, and tau pathology is observed in neurons, C4d-positive oligodendrocytes, and glial fibrillary acidic protein-positive and CD44-positive astrocytes (Ikeda et al., 1998). Another hypothesis suggests that under oxidative conditions, the cysteine 322 residue on tau forms intermolecular bridges between tau proteins (Schweers et al., 1995). Tau immunoblotting has shown that four-repeat tau predominates in insoluble fractions of NFTs from PSP brains, particularly the basal ganglia (Sergeant et al., 1999).

Although case-control studies have failed to show that family history is a significant risk factor, research involving the *tau* gene suggests that certain polymorphisms or mutations in this gene increase an individual's susceptibility to PSP, but the penetrance of this "risk allele" is low. The genetic association between PSP and an intronic short tandem repeat polymorphism within the *tau* gene indicates that *tau* is a candidate gene for PSP. In a family with phenotypically heterogeneous PSP, Stanford and colleagues (2000) found a novel mutation in the *tau* gene that does not change the amino acid sequence in the tau protein, but it causes a 4.8-fold increase in the splicing of exon 10, disrupting the RNA stem loop and resulting in a tau that contains four microtubule-binding repeats (Stanford et al., 2000). In another report, after screening 96 PSP patients for MAPT for mutations, Poorkaj and colleagues (2002) found a single point mutation, which they concluded caused PSP by a gain-of-function mechanism.

There is growing evidence that mRNA for a tau protein isoform that contributes to NFTs is overexpressed in the brainstem of patients with PSP but not patients with AD. Chambers and colleagues (1999) showed that, compared to control brains, PSP brains had elevated levels of four microtubule-binding domains (4R) mRNA in the brainstem but not in frontal or cerebellar cortex. They found that the regional distribution of the increases in 4R tau mRNA expression in PSP correlated with the selective vulnerability for NFT in the disease and they concluded that: "The genetic as well as pathologic studies have provided powerful evidence that overexpression of 4R tau isoforms plays an important role in the formation of NFTs and in the pathogenesis of PSP and that PSP is a repeat tauopathy." The *tau* genetic markers associated with PSP are therefore probably related to a defect within an intron yet to be sequenced. Zemaitaitis and colleagues (2000) have hypothesized that "transglutaminase-induced cross-linking may be a factor contributing to the abnormal polymerization and stabilization of tau in straight and PHFs leading to NFT formation in neurodegenerative diseases, including PSP and AD." Atypical PSP was found to be due to homozygosity for the delN296 mutation in the *tau* gene (Pastor et al., 2001).

An association of a particular *tau* genetic marker with PSP was initially reported by Conrad and colleagues (1997). In their study, they found that 95% of 22 PSP patients were homozygous for the A0 tau allele, whereas only half of controls and AD patients were homozygous for this particular allele. In another study, Morris and colleagues (1999a) found the A0 allele in 91% and the A0/A0 genotype in 84% of patients with PSP and in 73% (allele) and 53% (genotype) of controls ($P < 0.001$ and $P < 0.01$, respectively). The A0 allele and A0/A0 genotype was more frequent in patients with PSP than in controls, but this is also true for asymptomatic relatives of patients with PSP (Hoenicka et al., 1999). This finding, suggesting that PSP is associated with a genetic alteration in tau, is further supported by the demonstration that the tau a1 allele and the tau a1a1 genotype are overrepresented in patients with PSP and that the tau polymorphism is in linkage disequilibrium with the PSP disease locus using a disease model of recessive inheritance (Higgins et al., 1998). Although some studies have demonstrated an increased frequency of the A0 allele and the A0/A0 genotype in PSP versus controls (Bennett et al., 1998; Oliva et al., 1998), this finding could not be confirmed in

Japanese patients (Conrad et al., 1998). Furthermore, this finding does not seem to be specific for PSP, and a higher frequency of the A0/A0 genotype has been also demonstrated in PD (Pastor et al., 2000). Other studies showed that the H1 haplotype (93.7% vs. 78.4%) and the H1/H1 genotype (87.5% vs. 62.8%) are significantly overrepresented in patients with PSP compared to controls (Baker et al., 1999). In addition to the overrepresentation of the H1 haplotype, other genotypes have been found (e.g., extended, 670 kb, haplotype H1E) to be overrepresented, thus suggesting that changes in the *tau* gene could increase the genetic susceptibility to PSP (Pastor et al., 2002). Patients with PSP who are H1/H2 heterozygotes may display a lesser tau burden at autopsy than H1/H1 homozygotes, but the Richardson disease and PSP-parkinsonism phenotypes do not differ with regard to H1 haplotype frequency (Williams et al., 2007b). The H1c haplotype, which is more specifically associated with PSP than other H1 subhaplotypes, increases expression of tau, especially of the four-repeat variant, which includes the product of exon 10, the location of one of the microtubule-binding repeat domains (Myers et al 2007). The H1 haplotype extends beyond the outer edges of *MAPT* and displays considerable variability, whereas the H2 haplotype is relatively conserved and seems to play a protective role in both PSP and CBD (Kalinderi et al., 2009).

Both H1 and H1/H1 are also overrepresented in CBD compared to controls, strongly supporting the conclusion that PSP and CBD are genetically and pathologically related, suggesting a common pathogenic mechanism involving tau dysfunction, although other risk factors must be present to explain the divergent clinical and pathologic presentation (Houlden et al., 2001). The observation that the haplotype that is overrepresented in PSP is the common tau haplotype present in a homozygous form in about 55% of normal white individuals suggests that the *tau* gene is a susceptibility gene for PSP but that other genetic and environmental factors must play an important role in the pathogenesis of this neurodegenerative disorder. Some studies, however, failed to demonstrate that the H1 haplotype has a major influence on the biochemical or pathologic phenotype of PSP (Liu et al., 2001), and neither H1/H1 nor A0/A0 genotype predicts the prognosis of PSP (Litvan et al., 2001a).

Subsequently, other "susceptibility" haplotypes have been identified in PSP patients (Higgins, 1999; Pastor and Tolosa, 2002). In a follow-up study of 52 patients with PSP and 54 age-matched controls, Higgins and colleagues (2000), found that an extended 5'-tau haplotype consisting of four single nucleotide polymorphisms (SNPs) in tau exons 1, 4A, and 8 has a 98% sensitivity and a 67% specificity, suggesting that this susceptibility haplotype is a sensitive marker for sporadic PSP. The four SNPs formed two homozygous 5'-tau haplotypes (HapA and HapC) or a heterozygous genotype. Fifty-one (98%) patients with PSP had HapA haplotype, same as the H1 haplotype found originally by Hutton's group (Baker et al., 1999), whereas only 33% of controls had the same haplotype. While the *tau* mutations in FTD and parkinsonism linked to chromosome 17 (FTDP-17) (see later) affect microtubule-binding domains of the C-terminus of the tau protein, the PSP variants affect domains that interact with the neural plasma membrane. The clinically typical PSP is most likely associated with the tau PSP susceptibility genotype (H1/H1) and doublet tau protein pattern (64 and 69 kDa) (Morris et al., 2002).

There are only two common extended haplotypes, H1 and H2, that cover the entire *tau* gene. In certain neurodegenerative disorders, termed *tauopathies*, this normal ratio is altered: NFTs found in PSP, CBD, and FTDP-17 (see later) contain only four-repeat tau isoforms, whereas NFTs in AD contain all six, and those in Pick disease contain only three isoforms. Other tauopathies include postencephalitic parkinsonism and ALS-dementia-parkinsonism syndrome. It has been proposed that an increase in the available pool of free tau, not bound to microtubules, leads to NFT formation. An increase in the 4R tau isoform mRNA has been demonstrated in PSP. Furthermore, phosphorylated tau protein is unable to interact with the microtubules. Free unbound tau protein can form tau polymers via crosslinking by transglutaminase. These insoluble complexes become resistant to proteolysis and can eventually accumulate and lead to neurodegeneration. If this hypothesis is correct, transglutaminase inhibitors, such as cystamine and monodansyl cadaverine, could potentially have a neuroprotective effect in these neurodegenerative disorders.

It is possible that the four-repeat tau leads to pathologic increase in tau aggregation as has been noted not only in FTDP-17, but also in other neurodegenerative diseases such as PSP (Chambers et al., 1999; Stanford et al., 2000). Tau *gene* mutation has been associated with early dementia and PSP-like syndrome (Soliveri et al., 2003). Despite identical missense mutations in the tau gene involving exon 10, various family members exhibit marked clinical and genetic heterogeneity, suggesting the influence of additional environmental and/or genetic factors (Bird et al., 1999). Biochemically and pathologically confirmed Pick disease also has been associated with mutations in the *tau* gene (Neumann et al., 2001). The unifying theme of all these tauopathies is that the mutated *tau* cannot interact with microtubules, thus inappropriately freeing the mutant *tau*, resulting in an accumulation of the aberrant tau.

Even though genetically engineered mice that make no tau seem healthy, an animal model that reproduces neuronal tau pathology is now available. These transgenic mice of human tau with four tubulin-binding repeats (4R) containing three missense mutations associated with FTD-17, G272V, P301L, and R406W develop intracellular filaments composed of hyperphosphorylated 4R tau mainly concentrated in the apical dendrites and distributed in the cortex, hippocampus, and basal forebrain (Lim et al., 2001). This and other models (Lewis et al., 2000) can be used to study the effects of oxidative stress or toxins to clarify the role of tau pathology in neurodegeneration.

Besides tauopathies (PSP, CBD, Pick disease, dementia pugilistica, FTDP-17, postencephalitic parkinsonism, and ALS-dementia-parkinsonism syndrome), there are synucleinopathies (PD, MSA, DLB, and neurodegeneration with brain iron accumulation type 1, NBIA). There is growing evidence, however, that tau and α-synuclein affect each other, which might explain the overlap in clinical and pathologic features of the two types of neurodegenerative disease (Lee et al., 2004). Some patients with ALS-dementia-parkinsonism of Guam (ADPG) have been found to have both tau and synuclein inclusions. Genome-wide analysis, however, has not identified any mutations in patients with

ADPG (Morris et al., 2004). One form of FTD, associated with ALS, has been linked to chromosome 9q21–q22 (Hosler et al., 2000).

In addition to abnormalities in the *tau* gene, FTD has been associated with mutations in the gene for progranulin (*PGRN*), which is located 1.7 Mb centromeric to the *tau* gene at 17q21.31. The function of the gene product is not fully understood, but it appears to act as a growth factor involved in cell proliferation and repair (Rowland, 2006; Mukherjee et al., 2006; Cruts et al., 2006; Baker et al., 2006; Goedert and Spillantini, 2006; Snowden et al., 2006; Boeve et al., 2006; Masellis et al., 2006; Davion et al., 2007). *PGRN* also mediates proteolytic cleavage of TDP-43, a ubiquitin-binding protein, and mutations (or siRNA suppression) of *PGRN* result in caspase-dependent accumulation of TDP-43 fragments that can be inhibited with caspase inhibitor treatment (Zhang et al., 2007). Plasma and CSF levels of progranulin have been found to be nearly four-fold reduced in affected and unaffected subjects with *PGRN* mutations and low (75% reduction) plasma progranulin levels may be used as a screening tool for *PGRN* mutations (Ghidoni et al., 2008; Sleegers et al., 2009; Finch et al., 2009).

Families with *PGRN* mutations have clinical features indistinguishable from other cases of FTD, including "hereditary dysphasic disinhibition dementia (HDDD)" (Mukherjee et al., 2006), PPA which may evolve into CBD (Mesulam et al., 2008), and other abnormalities such as parkinsonism, stuttering dysarthria, oculomotor abnormalities and orolingual dyskinesia (Wider et al., 2008). Pathologically they are similar to Pick disease, but differentiated by the presence of cytoplasmic and intranuclear ubiquitin inclusions and AD pathology in areas other than the frontal lobes without tau pathology (FTLD-U). In addition to ubiquitin, tau, and synclein pathology, some brains of patients with *PGRN* mutations also stain with antibodies to the TDP-43 protein (TAR-DNA binding protein 43) (Leverenz et al., 2007). The TDP-43 proteinopathies are now recognized to represent a continuum of clinical and pathologic syndromes with various phenotypes ranging from FTLD-U to motor neuron disease (Geser et al., 2009). Other genes in which mutations have been associated with FTD include those coding for "charged multivesicular body protein 2B" (CHMP2B), DJ-1, and other proteins, such as valosin, synuclein, TDP-43, and prion protein (Rowland, 2006). The nuclear protein TDP-43 has been found to be present in both FTD and ALS inclusions, providing a biochemical link between the two neurodegenerative disorders (Neumann et al., 2006). In addition to *MAPT*, *PGRN*, *CHMP2B*, the other gene associated with FTD is valosin-containing protein gene *VCP* (Tolnay and Frank, 2007). The identification of TDP-43 as the major disease protein in the pathology of both FTLD with ubiquitin inclusions and ALS provides the first molecular link for these diseases. TDP-43 is the pathologic substrate of neuronal and glial inclusions in frontotemporal lobar degeneration with ubiquitin-positive inclusions (FTLD-U) and in amyotrophic lateral sclerosis (ALS) (Neumann et al., 2007). Mutations in the progranulin gene (*PGRN*) have been shown to cause familial FTLD-U, but there is no evidence that it plays a genetic role in PD (Nuytemans et al., 2008). The relationship between progranulin and TDP-43 and their respective roles in neurodegeneration is unknown. Suppression of *PGRN* expression with small interfering RNA leads to caspase-dependent accumulation of TDP-43 fragments that can be inhibited with caspase inhibitor treatment. The results suggest that abnormal metabolism of TDP-43 mediated by progranulin may play a pivotal role in neurodegeneration. Brains of patients with CBD apparently show TDP-43 inclusions, but these are not seen in brains of patients with clinically diagnosed PSP (Trojanowski, personal communication).

Neurodiagnostic studies

There are no diagnostic studies, including PET scans, that can reliably differentiate between PD, AD, and DLB (Tyrell et al., 1990). PET metabolic studies in patients with FTDP-17 show marked frontal hypoactivity. Using SPECT to image [^{123}I] iodobenzovesamicol, Kuhl and colleagues (1996) have found that, in contrast to nondemented PD patients, those who have coexistent dementia have extensive cortical reduction in the binding of this cholinergic marker, suggesting that the integrity of the cholinergic neurons is impaired in PD patients with dementia in a pattern similar to that of early AD.

In one series of 37 AD patients, concentrations of CSF homovanillic acid and biopterin were noted to be significantly lower in the AD patients with extrapyramidal signs than in the group without extrapyramidal signs matched for age and dementia severity (Kaye et al., 1988). It is not yet clear whether apolipoprotein E genotyping will be useful in the differential diagnosis of the parkinsonism–dementia syndrome (Roses, 1995). Plasma TDP-43 and PGRN determined by ELISA are being developed as diagnostic tools (Rademakers, personal communication).

Neuropathology, neurochemistry, and pathogenesis

The development of new immunocytochemical staining techniques using antibodies directed against ubiquitin, a highly conserved protein that is produced by cells in response to stress, has dramatically improved the identification of Lewy bodies. A ubiquitin-like epitope of PHFs is also present in Lewy bodies and may represent a common link between Lewy bodies and NFTs (Dickson et al., 1989). About one-third of patients with AD have both cortical and SN Lewy bodies at autopsy (Forstl et al., 1992; Galasko et al., 1994a), and essentially all patients with PD have Lewy bodies in the cortex (Hughes et al., 1992a). Patients with DLB, however, seem to have a greater neuronal loss in the SN, substantia innominata, and locus coeruleus and have lower cortical choline acetyltransferase levels than the AD patients (Gibb et al., 1989). In addition to the diffuse distribution of Lewy bodies throughout the basal forebrain, brainstem, and hypothalamus, the lack of NFTs in DLB helps to differentiate it from AD (Burkhardt et al., 1988; Gibb et al., 1989). Though Gibb and colleagues (1989) found no Lewy bodies in the hippocampus or cortex in AD, Burkhardt and colleagues (1988) reported "Lewy-like" bodies in the limbic system and neocortex. Others report different antigenic components of the Lewy body in DLB and PD, tau protein being present only in the dementing disorder (Galloway et al., 1989). Pathologic changes in AD

have been well characterized: neuritic plaques containing β-amyloid protein have been demonstrated in both sporadic and familial AD; and NFTs consist of the PHF tau. The abnormal phosphate substitution is thought to interfere with normal neurotubule formation (Kosic, 1991). The NFTs in AD are found predominantly in the hippocampus, but extrapyramidal signs are more likely associated with the presence of NFTs in SN (Gibb et al., 1989). Tabaton and colleagues (1988) noted antigenic similarities between the tangles of PSP and AD when they were derived from neurons of similar populations and postulated that anatomic location, rather than disease specificity, was the determining factor for antigenicity. In a study contrasting PD dementia and AD, de la Monte and colleagues (1989) found similar reductions in the cross-sectional areas of the globus pallidus–putamen; but greater cell loss was noted in the amygdala of PD dementia brains, while AD was associated with prominent cortical atrophy. However, the relative frequencies of Lewy bodies, neuritic plaques, and NFTs were not discussed.

In contrast to PD, no reductions in dopamine transporter sites, tyrosine hydroxylase, and D2 autoreceptors were found in the SN of patients with AD or AD–parkinsonism (Murray et al., 1995). The brains of patients with pure AD, however, had loss of dopamine transporter sites in the nucleus accumbens, and those with AD–parkinsonism had additional loss, particularly in the rostral caudate and putamen. Since bradykinesia and rigidity, but not tremor, are usually the chief parkinsonian features of AD–parkinsonism, the observed biochemical alterations are consistent with the hypothesis that the presence of tremor correlates with dopamine depletion in the caudal, rather than rostral, caudate nucleus. The pathologic findings suggest that in AD–parkinsonism, the loss of dopaminergic striatal terminals is not simply a reflection of nigral dopaminergic neuronal loss.

The tauopathies are neurodegenerative disorders that are manifested pathologically by neuronal and glial inclusions consisting of hyperphosphorylated, insoluble tau. The mutated tau presumably prevents proper binding to the microtubules, which could either destabilize the microtubules, interfering with axoplasmic transport, or lead to an excess of free-floating, toxic tau. In-vitro experiments have shown that four repeats preferentially form into straight-filament NFTs. All the identified mutations appear to destabilize the self-aggregating stem loop structure at the exon 10 splice site, leading to overproduction of four (rather than three) repeat isoforms of tau (Morris et al., 1999b). The four-repeat tau is insoluble, and it aggregates to form neuronal and glial inclusions. These inclusions contain "twisted ribbon" filaments rather than the PHFs and straight filaments that are typically observed in AD (Poorkaj et al., 1998; Hutton, 1999, 2000). In contrast, missense mutations outside exon 10, which affect all tau isoforms, result in neuronal inclusions that consist of both three- and four-repeat tau, with morphology similar to that of AD. In addition to the abnormal tau, brains of patients with FTDP-17 have pronounced frontotemporal atrophy, neuronal loss, gliosis, granulovacuolar degeneration, and cortical spongiform changes. Silver-positive, spheroidal enlargements of the presynaptic terminals have been found within the neuropil of the vulnerable regions (Zhou et al., 1998).

These neuropil spheroids are immunopositive cytoskeletal proteins, including tau, and probably represent dystrophic changes associated with retrograde degeneration. In a study of 90 brains with clinically diagnosed FTD, tauopathies were found in 46%, frontotemporal lobar degeneration with ubiquitin-positive inclusions in 29% (often associated with motor neuron disease), and AD in 17% (Forman et al., 2006).

There are many disorders that resemble AD–parkinsonism clinically but that can be differentiated from pure AD only at autopsy. These include not only DLB, as discussed previously, but also Pick disease, CJD, and sporadic or familial progressive subcortical gliosis (Lanska et al., 1994). Autosomal dominant subcortical gliosis, with prominent white matter changes on MRI and at autopsy, may present as frontotemporal dementia (Swerdlow et al., 2009).

NBIA1, formerly known as Hallervorden–Spatz disease, is an autosomal recessive disorder characterized by dystonia, parkinsonism, dementia, and brain iron accumulation (Thomas and Jankovic, 2003). Because of Julius Hallervorden's terrible past and his shameless involvement in active euthanasia during World War II (Shevell, 2003), the eponym carrying his name has been replaced by the new term NBIA1. Characterized by childhood-onset progressive rigidity, dystonia, choreoathetosis, spasticity, optic nerve atrophy, and dementia, NBIA1 has been also associated in some cases with acanthocytosis (Racette et al., 2001; Thomas and Jankovic, 2003). NBIA1 can present as an adult-onset parkinsonism–dystonia–dementia syndrome (Jankovic et al., 1985). Linkage analyses initially localized the *NBIA1* gene on 20p12.3–p13; subsequently, 7 bp deletion and various missense mutations were identified in the coding sequence of gene *PANK2*, which codes for pantothenate kinase (Taylor et al., 1996; Zhou et al., 2001; Hayflick et al., 2003), hence the term pantothenate kinase-associated neurodegeneration. Pantothenate kinase is an essential regulatory enzyme in coenzyme A biosynthesis. It has been postulated that as a result of phosphopantothenate deficiency, cysteine accumulates in the globus pallidus of brains of patients with NBIA1. It undergoes rapid auto-oxidation in the presence of nonheme iron, which normally accumulates in the GPi and SN, generating free radicals that are locally neurotoxic. Interestingly, atypical subjects were found to be compound heterozygotes for certain mutations for which classic subjects were homozygous. Most, but not all, patients with NBIA1 phenotype have mutations in the *PANK2* gene (Thomas and Jankovic, 2003). On the basis of an analysis of 123 patients from 98 families with NBIA1, Hayflick and colleagues (2003) found that "classic Hallervorden–Spatz syndrome" was associated with *PANK2* mutation in all cases and one-third of "atypical" cases (late onset, slowly progressive disorder characterized by palilalia, dysarthria, dystonia, perseverative behavior and movements, freezing, and dementia) had the mutations within the *PANK2* gene. Those who had the *PANK2* mutation were more likely to have dysarthria and psychiatric symptoms, and all had the typical "eye of the tiger" abnormality on MRI with a specific pattern of hyperintensity within the hypointense GPi.

Another disorder that can cause NBIA1 is the Kufor-Rakeb syndrome (PARK9), caused by mutations in the *ATP13A2* gene on chromosome 1p36 (Hampshire et al., 2001; Schneider et al., 2010). These rare cases usually present with early-onset behavioral disturbances and levodopa-responsive, asymmetric dystonia, akinetic-rigid parkinsonism with pyramidal signs and eye movement abnormalities. Although they usually do not have typical tremor at rest they may exhibit a "jerky," myoclonic tremor, particularly involving the face and fingers. Brain MRI revealed generalized atrophy and putaminal and caudate iron accumulation bilaterally.

Adult-onset, levodopa-responsive dystonia–parkinsonism, a variant of NBIA1, has been described and categorized as PARK14 (Paisan-Ruiz et al., 2008). Inherited in an autosomal recessive fashion, this subtype of NBIA1 is due to mutations in the *PLA2G6* gene, located on chromosome 22q13.1, which encodes a calcium-independent phospholipase A2 enzyme that catalyzes the hydrolysis of glycerophospholipids. *PLA2G6*-associated neurodegeneration (PLAN) is an early-childhood-onset syndrome with axial hypotonia, spasticity, bulbar dysfunction, ataxia, and dystonia, associated with MRI changes indicative of iron deposition in GP and SN (Kurian et al., 2008). Previously diagnosed as infantile neuroaxonal dystrophy, a form of NBIA1 (NBIA2) and in the past referred to as Karak syndrome, PLAN may also present as adult-onset, levodopa-responsive dystonia–parkinsonism without iron on brain imaging (Paisan-Ruiz et al., 2008). The dystonia–parkinsonism syndrome occurs when arginine is replaced by glutamine in both copies of the gene, but when it is replaced by tryptophan either the classic infantile neuroaxonal dystrophy or more insidious NBIA1 will develop, but there is marked phenotypic variability even within the same family. One mechanism that both PANK2 and PLAN share may be an abnormality in the deactylation–reacetylation cycle of repair to polyunsaturated fatty acids damaged by reactive oxidative species resulting in secondary damage to the inner mitochondrial membrane, rich in these fatty acids. Regression of symptoms after 6 months of iron chelation with deferiprone has been reported in some patients with NBIA1 (Forni et al., 2008).

The syndrome of early-onset, progressive parkinsonism, variably responsive to levodopa, with pyramidal tract signs previously referred to as pallido-pyramidal or parkinsonian-pyramidal syndrome, has been found to be due to mutation in the *FBXO7* gene on chromosome 22q12–q13 and nominated as PARK15 (Di Fonzo et al., 2009). The gene codes for F-box only protein 7 with unknown function. Both homozygous and compound heterozygous mutations have been identified, suggestive of autosomal recessive inheritance.

Other disorders that are associated with abnormal brain iron accumulation include PD, MSA, AD, Huntington disease, human immunodeficiency encephalopathy, neuroferritinopathy (caused by a mutation in the gene coding for ferritin light polypeptide on chromosome 19q13.3) (Curtis et al., 2001), aceruloplasminemia (caused by mutations in the gene coding ceruloplasmin) (Miyajima, 2002; Nittis and Gitlin, 2002), and other inborn errors of metabolism (Sedel et al., 2008). A novel mutation in the ferritin light chain gene was reported in a French Canadian family with Dutch ancestry manifested chiefly by atypical postural instability with dysfunctional gait, parkinsonism with blepharospasm and oromandibular dystonia, and putaminal hyperintensity on T2-weighted MRI (Mancuso et al., 2005).

Treatment

While the parkinsonian features might improve with dopaminergic therapy, there is little that one can do to improve the cognitive deficit. With the introduction of cholinesterase inhibitors such as donepezil (Aricept) and rivastigmine (Exelon), it is possible that cognition, orientation, and language function will improve and that such improvement will lead to a meaningful improvement in function. Rivastigmine inhibits not only acetylcholinesterase but also butyrylcholinesterase, which, in contrast to its relative absence in normal brain, accounts for 40% of cholinergic activity in the cortex and 60% in the hippocampus in AD brains. In a randomized, double-blind, placebo-controlled, multicenter study of 120 patients with probable DLB, McKeith and colleagues (2000) found the drug to be safe and to effectively ameliorate apathy, anxiety, delusions, and hallucinations. The efficacy of cholinesterase inhibitors in DLB has been attributed to relative preservation of cortical muscarinic M1 receptors. In addition to the usual side effects of cholinesterase inhibitors, such as nausea, vomiting, anorexia, and weight loss, four patients noted emergent tremor without a significant worsening of the UPDRS. Hallucinations, a frequent complication of dopaminergic drug therapy, may be controlled with clozapine, but potentially serious side effects, including agranulocytosis, require weekly monitoring of the white blood cells (Kahn et al., 1991; Chacko et al., 1993). Olanzapine (Zyprexa), another atypical neuroleptic, has been reported to exert an antipsychotic effect similar to that of clozapine but without the risk of agranulocytosis (Wolters et al., 1996). In several studies, however, olanzapine was associated with exacerbation of parkinsonian motor disability (Ondo et al., 2002b). Quetiapine fumarate (Seroquel), a dibenzothiazepine that blocks not only D1 and D2 receptors but also 5-HT_{1A} and 5-HT_2 receptors, has also been found to have a beneficial effect in PD patients with hallucinations described previously with the other atypical neuroleptics (Fernandez et al., 1999). Indeed, quetiapine is our drug of choice for psychosis in patients with PD, followed by clozapine and olanzapine.

Parkinsonism–dementia–amyotrophic lateral sclerosis complex of Guam

Clinical features and natural history

The combination of parkinsonism, dementia, and motor neuron disease was first noted in a population of Guam, where it is known as *lytico-bodig* (Hirano et al., 1961), and the associated dementia is known among the Chamorros, the native inhabitants of Guam, as *Mariana dementia* (Galasko et al., 2002). Guam dementia is more common than the parkinsonism–dementia complex and is strongly associated with age and low education (Galasko et al., 2007). In a review of 363 Chamorro and 3 Filipino immigrants with this disease, men were affected twice as frequently as women, but no differences in age of onset (57 years) or death (62 years) were seen between the genders (Zhang et al., 1990). Besides parkinsonism, supranuclear ocular motility disorder has been reported in all 37 patients in one series (Lepore et al., 1988) (Video 9.12). Patients with parkinsonism usually present later than those with ALS, possibly because patients presenting with motor neuron disease do not survive long enough to develop extrapyramidal symptoms (Zhang et al., 1990; Rowland and Shneider, 2001). Furthermore, basal ganglia signs might be masked by the motor neuron disease. Environmental etiology of the parkinsonism–dementia–ALS complex of Guam (PDACG) is suggested not only by its restricted geographic distribution but also by its declining incidence (Galasko et al., 2002). Among 194 Chamorros evaluated between 1997 and 2000, Galasko and colleagues (2002) found 10 with ALS, 11 with PD, 90 with parkinsonism–dementia complex, and 83 with late-life dementia. They suggest that the rapid decline in incidence of these disorders in Guam strongly supports the role of environmental factors in their pathogenesis. In a report of 13 patients diagnosed with motor neuron disease who exhibited some clinical features of coexistent parkinsonism, Qureshi and colleagues (1996) suggested that motor neuron disease and parkinsonism have common pathogenetic mechanisms because the onset of the two disorders was closely temporally related.

Another geographically determined PSP-like disorder was described in 1999 by Caparros-Lefebvre and colleagues (1999) on the Caribbean island of Guadeloupe. The case-control survey found that the disease is associated with the use of an indigenous plant (*Annona muricata*; synonyms: soursop, corossol, guanbana, graviola, and sweetsop) that contains the mitochondrial complex I and dopaminergic neuronal toxins reticuline, corexime, and annonacin (Hoglinger et al., 2003; Lannuzel et al., 2007; Lannuzel et al., 2008). Custard apple is also considered to be one of the foods containing annonaceous benzyltetrahydroisoquinoline alkaloids that might be responsible for the neurotoxicity leading to these geographically specific tauopathies (Steele et al., 2002), associated in some cases with unusual asymptomatic retinopathy (Campbell et al., 1993; Jano-Edward et al., 2002). Patients with the Guadeloupean tauopathy have usually levodopa-resistant parkinsonism, tremor, rest and action myoclonus, subcortical dementia, and ophthalmoparesis with predominant cortical dysfunction demonstrated by various neurophysiologic studies (Apartis et al., 2008). About a third of parkinsonian patients in Guadeloupe had typical PD, one-third had a PSP-like syndrome, and one-third had parkinsonism–dementia complex. The PSP-like syndrome differs from the typical PSP in that the majority have tremor and hallucinations and half have dysautonomia (Lannuzel et al., 2007). A similar clinical syndrome has been reported in Afro-Caribbean and Indian immigrants in England who regularly consumed imported Annonaceae products (Chaudhuri et al., 2000). The Guadeloupean parkinsonism was later characterized as a PSP-like tauopathy, although no mutation of the *tau* gene was found (Caparros-Lefebvre et al., 2002; Steele et al., 2002). It has been postulated that the high prevalence of atypical parkinsonism resembling PSP on the island of Guadeloupe is related to consumption of Annonaceae fruit and teas that contain high levels of mitochondrial complex I inhibitors such as benzyl-tetrahydroisoquinolines (TIQs, reticuline) and tetrahydroprotoberberine (coreximine). In addition to Guam and Guadeloupe, another geographic area where ALD–dementia–parkinsonism complex has been identified is the Kii peninsula of Japan (Kuzuhara et al.,

2001). Although the *tau* gene failed to show any mutations, an analysis of insoluble protein extracted from the brain of one of the affected family members showed a 60, 64, 68 kDa triple, suggesting that this disorder might be a variant of a tauopathy. While no mutations in the *tau* gene have been identified, Poorkaj and colleagues (2001) suggested that the *tau* gene might be a modifying gene because of linkage disequilibrium between PDACG and certain tau polymorphisms.

Neurodiagnostic studies

PET scanning in patients with the parkinsonian form of this disease reveals decreased presynaptic [^{18}F]fluorodopa uptake similar to that in patients with PD, while those with ALS have a picture intermediate between that of PD and that of control populations, suggesting a preclinical lesion (Snow et al., 1990). Reduced [^{18}F]fluorodopa uptake on PET scans of patients with advanced ALS has provided evidence in support of basal ganglia involvement in ALS.

Neuropathology, neurochemistry, and pathogenesis

The increased prevalence of this neurodegenerative disorder on the island of Guam suggests a possible environmental etiology (Hirano et al., 1961). The neurotoxins methyl-azoxymethanol β-D-glucoside (cycasin) and β-N-methylamino-L-alanine (BMAA), compounds that are found in the cycad plant and are believed to be in high concentrations in flour made from this plant, produce a similar spectrum of neurologic decline in rats (Shen et al., 2010) and monkeys (Spencer et al., 1987; Kisby et al., 1992). However, an analysis of the β-N-methylamino-L-alanine content of cycad flour suggests that the quantities of β-N-methylamino-L-alanine that are normally consumed by the inhabitants of the endemic areas were not sufficient to produce neurologic toxicity (Duncan et al., 1990). Cox and Sacks (2002) have hypothesized that the consumption of flying foxes by the Chamorro people might have generated sufficiently high cumulative doses of plant neurotoxins (Banack and Cox, 2003; Cox et al., 2003). The Chamorro eat flying foxes (*Pteropus mariannus*) boiled in coconut cream in ceremonial feasts. The bats eat the seeds of cycad trees (*Cycas micronesia*), which contain neurotoxin β-N-methylamino-L-alanine. Flying foxes, like the disease, are now rare. Other hypotheses concerning abnormalities in mineral metabolism and hypomagnesemia or hypocalcemia have also been suggested, but supporting evidence is lacking (Garruto and Yase, 1986; Ahlskog et al., 1995). The most recent epidemiologic evidence supports the association between the Guamanian syndrome and the picking, processing, and eating of foods by young adults containing flour called "fadang," made from the seeds of a plant, *Cycas cicinalis*, which contains cycasin and BMAA (Borenstein et al., 2007).

Pathologically, this condition resembles AD more than PD. Tau-containing NFTs are present, particularly in the hippocampus (Gilbert et al., 1988; Shankar et al., 1989), and other brain and spinal cord areas (Matsumoto et al., 1990). Beta-amyloid protein-containing NFTs have been identified in the brains of patients with PDACG (Ito et al., 1991). Immunohistochemical studies of autopsied brains of patients with PDACG showed marked reduction in the number of dopaminergic neurons in both the lateral and medial SN (Goto et al., 1990a). Despite marked reduction of nigrostriatal dopamine concentration, the striatal output system was well preserved, and glutamate, GABA, choline acetyltransferase, and serotonin were spared. One study provided evidence for nigrostriatal dopaminergic dysfunction in patients with familial ALS, but patients without the copper/zinc superoxide dismutase mutations were more likely to have the abnormality than those with the mutation (Przedborski et al., 1996). This suggests that the mutation is more cytotoxic to motor neurons than to the dopaminergic neurons.

Heredodegenerative parkinsonism

Parkinsonism may be an associated feature or the dominant clinical feature in some heredodegenerative disorders, as listed in Table 9.1. Most of these disorders are discussed elsewhere. There are currently 15 types of genetic parkinsonism, categorized as PARK1–PARK15, many of which are associated with atypical features. An X-linked dystonia–parkinsonism (XDP, DYT3 (MIM 314250)) that is seen almost exclusively in male adults with maternal roots from the Philippine island of Panay may, in addition to dystonia (intermittent twisting referred to as Lubag, sustained posturing referred to as Wa-eg) and parkinsonism with bradykinesia and shuffling gait (referred to as Sud-sud), manifest a wide spectrum of movement disorders. These include tremor, myoclonus, chorea, and myorhythmia. Linkage analyses and linkage disequilibrium studies have assigned the disease locus to a 260 kb interval on Xq13.1, and five disease-specific sequence changes (DSCs) were described in the "multiple transcript system" (MTS) in the DYT3 critical region. Recently, a disease-specific SVA (short interspersed nuclear element, variable number of tandem repeats, and Alu composite) retrotransposon insertion related to reduced neuron-specific expression of the TATA-binding protein-associated factor 1 gene (*TAF1*) was reported in some DYT3 patients (Deng et al., 2008).

Secondary parkinsonism

Parkinsonism, the clinical syndrome that is manifested chiefly by tremor, bradykinesia, rigidity, and postural instability, may be the sole manifestation of a disorder, such as PD, it may be a component of a more complex disorder such as one of the multiple system degenerations or heredodegenerations, or it may result from pharmacologic, physiologic, or pathologic abnormalities with different etiologies (see Table 9.1). Although the "secondary" parkinsonian disorders are produced by different mechanisms, they all seem to produce parkinsonian symptoms by interfering with normal dopaminergic production or transmission. Only the most important secondary types of parkinsonism are reviewed here.

Infections

An exposure to an infectious agent, such as the one (or more) responsible for the 1917–1928 pandemic of encephalitis lethargica (von Economo's encephalitis), has long been recognized as a cause of parkinsonism (Krusz et al., 1987, Calne and Lees, 1988; Takahashi and Yamada, 1999; Dale et al., 2004). Indeed, postencephalitic parkinsonism was once thought to be the primary cause of PD (Litvan et al., 1998c). The clinical presentation often involved fever, somnolence, ophthalmoplegia, and CSF lymphocytic pleocytosis (50–100 lymphocytes). About 40% of the affected individuals died during the acute illness. Parkinsonism occurred in 50% of the survivors within 5 years and 80% within 10 years. In addition to the typical parkinsonian features, which were usually levodopa responsive, there were many other neurologic and movement disorders that helped to differentiate this postencephalitic syndrome from idiopathic PD. The accompanying features included oculogyric crises, blepharospasm, palilalia, and various hyperkinesias such as dystonia, chorea, tics, and hiccups.

The pathologic finding of the acute disorder consisted chiefly of midbrain and periventricular inflammation. The delayed-onset movement disorder was characterized by marked depletion of neurons in the SN and NFTs in the residual neurons (Litvan et al., 1998c). No virus was ever documented as the cause of postencephalitic parkinsonism, but there has been a recent reemergence of interest in the influenza A virus as a possible etiologic agent. This virus displays preferential tropism to the brainstem (especially the nigral neurons), cerebellum, and limbic system, and it produces changes (e.g., phosphorylation of cytoskeletal proteins and alterations in intermediate filaments) that could lead to the formation of Lewy bodies (Takahashi and Yamada, 1999). The mechanism of the latency between the acute illness and the subsequent development of parkinsonism has never been elucidated. The syndrome of postencephalitic parkinsonism, however, serves as a model for other delayed-onset movement disorders (Saint Hilaire et al., 1991; Scott and Jankovic, 1996).

Sporadic cases of postencephalitic parkinsonism have been reported since the 1917–1928 pandemic (Howard and Lees, 1987). Japanese encephalitis not only may involve the cortex, thalamus, brainstem, and spinal cord, but in some cases may be associated pathologically with predominant involvement of the SN and clinically with otherwise typical parkinsonism (Pradham et al., 1999). West Nile encephalitis has been associated with tremor, myoclonus, and parkinsonism during the acute illness with complete recovery in some patients (Sejvar et al., 2003). We reported on a 21-year-old man with viral encephalitis of the SN and reviewed the world literature of similar cases (Savant et al., 2003). More recently, West Nile encephalitis involving the SN has been increasingly recognized as a cause of acute parkinsonism (Bosanko et al., 2003). When it affects other brainstem areas and spinal cord, West Nile infection can present as acute poliomyelitis (Agamanolis et al., 2003). Poststreptococcal acute disseminated encephalomyelitis (PSADEM), a poststreptococcal disorder that may include parkinsonism and dystonia, has been described in association with the anti-basal ganglia antibodies (Dale et al., 2001). Dale and colleagues (2004) also described 20 patients with the clinical picture of encephalitis lethargica; in 55%, the onset was preceded by pharyngitis. MRI showed inflammatory changes in the deep gray matter in 40% of patients. Laboratory investigation suggested poststreptococcal etiology in that the

anti-streptolysin O titer was elevated in 65% of patients and Western immunoblotting showed that 95% of the patients had autoantibodies reactive against human basal ganglia antigens, compared to 2–4% of these antibodies in controls ($n = 173$, $P < 0.0001$). One case that was examined at autopsy showed striatal encephalitis with perivenous B- and T-lymphocytic infiltration. The methodology of the study and the specificity of the antibodies, however, have been questioned (Vincent, 2004). Other infectious causes of parkinsonism include human immunodeficiency virus and associated infections (Nath et al., 1987).

Prion diseases

The elegant studies of Prusiner and his collaborators have drawn attention to a group of disorders known as *prion diseases*, and because of their growing scientific importance as well as their potential impact on public health, Prusiner was awarded the 1997 Nobel Prize for Medicine (Prusiner, 1997, 2001; Glatzel et al., 2005). These transmissible spongiform encephalopathies, some of which are associated with parkinsonian features, consist of five conditions: (1) CJD and its variant (see later), (2) kuru (Kompoliti et al., 1999), (3) Gerstmann–Sträussler–Scheinker (GSS) disease, protease-sensitive prionopathy (PSPr) (Gambetti et al., 2008), and (5) familial or sporadic fatal insomnia (Haywood, 1997; Gambetti and Parchi, 1999; Mastrianni et al., 1999; Collins et al., 2004). CJD can present with rapidly progressive parkinsonism, often accompanied by dementia, myoclonus, and gait disorder (Shinobu et al., 1999). In a series of 232 cases of sporadic CJD that was shown to be experimentally transmitted, cognitive decline was present in 100%, myoclonus in 78%, cerebellar signs in 71%, pyramidal signs in 62%, and extrapyramidal signs, including parkinsonism, in 56% (Brown et al., 1994). Prominent amyotrophy is also occasionally present in patients with CJD (Worrall et al., 2000). Periodic EEG was recorded in only 60% of the cases, and this pattern was rarely present in the familial cases. Periodic complexes are relatively specific for CJD, with only a 9% false positive rate (Steinhoff et al., 2004). On the basis of a study involving 300 cases of sporadic CJD, the authors proposed a classification of six phenotypic variants with a variable degree of rapidly progressive dementia, myoclonus, ataxia, insomnia, and typical EEG (Parchi et al., 1999). The "new-variant" CJD, caused by bovine spongiform encephalopathy prions, differs dramatically from the more common sporadic form in that the patients' age is usually in the twenties, about three or four decades earlier than that in the sporadic disease, and many patients present with prominent affective symptoms, including dysphoria, irritability, anxiety, apathy, loss of energy, insomnia, and social withdrawal. Evidence of focal cortical syndrome, such as alexia without agraphia, may be the presenting feature of CJD (Adair et al., 2007). Symptoms that are typically seen in the sporadic disease, such as cognitive impairment, dysarthria, gait abnormalities, and myoclonus, are late features.

A definite diagnosis of these disorders can be made only by examination of the brain tissue, but one study showed that neuron-specific enolase can be a potentially useful biochemical marker for CJD (Zerr et al., 1995). Diagnostic criteria for sporadic CJD include immunohistochemistry with antibodies against the prion protein (Kretzschmar et al.,

1996). When the CSF of 58 patients with definite or probable CJD was examined and compared with that of 29 control subjects, the level was significantly higher in the former group ($P < 0.001$), and when a cutoff of 35 ng/mL was used, the optimum sensitivity was 80%, and specificity was 92%. More recently, two studies have detected two disease-specific proteins, p130/131, in the CSF of patients with CJD (Hsich et al., 1996; Zerr et al., 1996). Several studies showed that the presence of 14-3-3 protein in the CSF improved the diagnosis of CJD (Poser et al., 1999; Aksamit, 2003). Although the sensitivity of this test may be as high as 97% and its specificity may be as high as 87% (Lemstra et al., 2000; Castellani et al., 2004), particularly in the classic variety of sporadic CJD, some studies have found the sensitivity to be as low as 53% (Geschwind et al., 2003). False positives include stroke, meningoencephalitis, vasculitis, paraneoplastic disorders, FTD, and AD (Chapman et al., 2000). When added to the diagnostic criteria, the presence of 14-3-3 protein in the CSF markedly increased the sensitivity of diagnostic criteria and increased the estimated incidence of CJD (Brandel et al., 2000; Zerr et al., 2000). Subsequent studies, however, showed that the 14-3-3 test does not differentiate between CJD and other neurodegenerative disorders associated with dementia (Burkhard et al., 2001). In addition to the positive 14-3-3 immunoassay, over 70% of patients with the new variant of CJD who were homozygous for methionine at codon 129 of the prion protein gene had bilateral pulvinar high signal on MRI (Will et al., 2000). More recently, CSF tau-protein assay by enzyme-linked immunosorbent assay, already readily available in routine laboratories, has been found to have a 92% positive predictive value in diagnosing CJD; 74 of 77 patients with probable CJD had tau protein greater than 1300 pg/mL, whereas only 2 of 28 patients with AD had such high levels, and the percentage was even lower in other dementias (Otto et al., 2002). The National Prion Disease Pathology Surveillance Center at Case Western Reserve University offers, free of charge, a variety of diagnostic tests, including Western blots on frozen brain tissue to detect protease-resistant prion protein (PrP), immunohistochemical tests for PrP on fixed tissue, analysis of DNA extracted from blood or brain tissue for *PRNP*, and analysis of CSF for 14-3-3 protein. Parchi and colleagues (1999) classified the six types of CJD according to homozygosity or heterozygosity of methionine (M) and valine (V) at codon 129 of the prion protein gene: the MM1 and MV1 correlate with the phenotype of classical sporadic CJD (rapidly progressive dementia with periodic EEG), whereas others are more atypical, with slower progression and young age at onset (VV1) or ataxia (MV2 and VV2).

Imaging can also be very helpful in the diagnosis of CJD. DWI-MRI has the highest sensitivity for the detection of signal intensity abnormalities in CJD. Increased signal intensity is typically seen bilaterally in the striatum, thalamus, and cortex ("cortical ribbon") (Murata et al., 2002; Mendez et al., 2003; Tschampa et al., 2003; Shiga et al., 2004; Geschwind et al., 2007). In an analysis of 19 reported cases of CJD with DWI-MRI lesions, CSF protein 14-3-3 was negative in 6 cases and positive in 2 others (Mendez et al., 2003). The authors concluded that "multifocal cortical and subcortical hyperintensities confined to gray matter regions in DWI-MRI may be a more useful noninvasive diagnostic marker for CJD than CSF protein 14-3-3." Furthermore, high

T2-weighted signal in the basal ganglia correlated with VV or MV codon 129 genotypes (Meissner et al., 2004).

The prion diseases appear to be related to an abnormal metabolism of a normal cellular constituent, the prion protein (PrP), which is normally encoded by a gene on the short arm of chromosome 20 (Haywood, 1997; Prusiner, 1997). When the normal PrP^c protein, which has an α-helical structure, undergoes a conformational change to a β-pleated structure, the resulting abnormal PrP^{Sc} (Sc = scrapie) isoform leads to development of the disease. There is growing evidence that the fundamental process in prion propagation involves seeded aggregation of misfolded host proteins (Collinge, 2005). A substantial percentage of patients with sporadic or iatrogenic CJD share methionine or valine homozygosity in codon 129, indicating increased susceptibility of this population. In sporadic CJD, an increase of relative risk for CJD with codon 129 genotypes (Met/Met:Val/Val:Met/Val) was assessed at 11:4:1. The molecular strain characteristics of nvCJD are clearly different from those of previously recognized human prion strains, but it closely resembled those seen in bovine spongiform encephalopathy. None of the patients with nvCJD had mutations in the *PRNP* gene, but all so far reported have been methionine homozygotes at codon 129.

Point missense mutations and insertional mutations have also been instructive in classifying familial CJD. In other human prion diseases, mutations causing familial forms of disease have been identified. In Gerstmann–Sträussler–Scheinker disease, *PRNP* mutations were found in codons 102, 117, 198, and 217. In fatal familial insomnia (FFI), a *PRNP* mutation is present in codon 178. Clinicopathologic diversity of FFI overlaps widely with CJD, and it has been proposed that molecular diagnostics (*PRNP* mutation at codon 178, polymorphism at codon 129) might separate those two entities. Point mutations in the prion protein gene segregate with the familial prion diseases. For example, a mutation at codon 210, coupled with some genetic and environmental factors, is associated with CJD (Pocchiari et al., 1993). The risk of developing CJD in Libyan Jews with the *PRNP* gene codon 200 point mutation is virtually 100% by age 80 years (Chapman et al., 1994; Goldfarb and Brown, 1995). A mutation in codon 200 accounts for three geographic clusters that have been described in Slovakia and in Chile. Insertional mutations of additional copies of an octapeptide (24–216 base pairs) in the *PRNP* gene have been described in CJD patients worldwide.

Mutations in the prion protein gene (*PRNP*) have been found not only in patients with CJD, but also in fatal familial insomnia and Gerstmann–Sträussler–Scheinker disease, manifested by autosomal dominantly inherited progressive ataxia and dementia (Panegyres et al., 2001). Prion protein abnormalities, however, do not seem to be associated with either idiopathic parkinsonism or with MSA (Jendroska et al., 1994). Experimental therapeutics of CJD and other transmissible spongiform encephalopathies is an emerging area of basic science research that is soon to be translated into clinical trials. Some novel therapies that are currently being tested in experimental animals include a variety of anti-infectious agents, immunomodulating drugs, compounds designed to eliminate misfolded membrane-bound prion proteins, and neutralizing antibodies (Brown, 2002). Detection of pathologic PrP^{Sc} in the olfactory epithelium in nine patients with sporadic CJD but not in any controls suggests that the olfactory pathway might be the route of infection by the prions; this finding suggests that olfactory biopsy might be of diagnostic importance (Zanusso et al., 2003).

There is no treatment for CJD, but there might be some rationale for using the antimalarial drug quinacrine because of its protease resistance of PrP peptide aggregates, although there is little hope that this drug will significantly alter the natural course of the fatal disease (Barret et al., 2003). Flupirtine, a centrally acting nonopioid analgesic antiapoptotic drug, was found to have beneficial effects on cognitive functioning of patients with CJD (Otto et al., 2002). Improved understanding of the molecular mechanisms of prion diseases may eventually lead to effective therapies, but current therapeutic strategies do not seem to offer meaningful improvements in the symptoms or progression of the disease (Stewart et al., 2008).

Drugs

Although drug-induced parkinsonism might be the most common form of parkinsonism, it is not commonly encountered in movement disorder clinics (see Table 9.1). Parkinsonian symptoms and findings, often indistinguishable from those seen in patients with PD, may be evident within the first few days of neuroleptic therapy; nearly all cases become evident within 3 months after initiation of treatment (Hardie and Lees, 1988; Jankovic, 1995c). In addition, chronically treated patients may develop parkinsonian findings when the dose of a neuroleptic is increased. The prevalence of neuroleptic-induced parkinsonism has been reported to range from 10% to 60% of patients treated with antipsychotics. Advanced age, female gender, and possibly genetic predisposition, such as the presence of essential tremor, have been identified as potential risk factors. About one-third of all patients referred to our movement disorder clinics with drug-induced movement disorders, such as tardive dyskinesia, have parkinsonian findings (Jankovic, 1995c). While two-thirds of all patients recover within 7 weeks after stopping the offending drug, the symptoms may persist for more than 18 months. In one study, 11% of patients who recovered from neuroleptic-induced parkinsonism were later found to have the characteristic pathologic findings of PD at autopsy (Rajput et al., 1982). This suggests that parkinsonism that persists even after the offending drug is withdrawn may represent subclinical, latent PD. Evidence for persistent dysfunction in patients with drug-induced parkinsonism has been provided by the demonstration of reduced [^{18}F]fluorodopa uptake in some patients and by depression of platelet mitochondrial complex I activity (Burkhardt et al., 1993; Burn and Brooks, 1993). In a study of 20 patients with drug-induced parkinsonism, 11 had abnormal β-CIT SPECT scans indicating underlying nigrostriatal deficiency, suggesting that even though the patients were taking neuroleptics, their parkinsonism may have been due to exacerbation of underlying PD (Lorberboym et al., 2006). There were no differences in clinical features between the 11 patients who had abnormal SPECT scans and 9 patients with normal scans.

Besides the neuroleptics there are many other drugs that may cause parkinsonism, including valproate, lamotrigine, zonisamide, vigabatrin and other anticonvulsants (Zadikoff et al., 2007; Jamora et al., 2007). Also certain cardiac drugs, such as amiodarone (Werner and Olanow, 1989), may cause parkinsonism.

Toxins

Our knowledge of the mechanisms and treatment of parkinsonism has expanded dramatically as a result of the discovery that the neurotoxin 1-methyl-4-phenyl-1,2,3,6-tetrahydropyridine (MPTP) can induce parkinsonism (Langston et al., 1983; Bloem et al., 1990). MPTP can produce parkinsonism in animals (particularly primates) and humans that can be clinically indistinguishable from idiopathic PD. However, in contrast to PD, which affects chiefly the putamen, MPTP impairs dopaminergic function in both the caudate and putamen (Snow et al., 2000).

There are several other toxins that can cause parkinsonism, but only carbon monoxide and manganese are reviewed here. Carbon monoxide exposure can result in acute intoxication, which is associated with about 35% mortality rate, progressive akinetic-mute state, or delayed-relapsing encephalopathy (Sohn et al., 2000). The latter syndrome usually develops after a 3-week recovery period. The delayed relapsing type of carbon monoxide sequelae is characterized by slow, short-stepped gait; start hesitation; freezing; body bradykinesia; and rigidity but little or no tremor. In addition, these patients often develop akinetic mutism and other peculiar behaviors. They usually do not improve with levodopa. In a review of 8 patients with progressive sequelae and 23 patients with the delayed relapsing sequelae, Lee and Marsden (1994) could not identify any reliable predictors of eventual outcome following acute intoxication. During a 1-year follow-up, 50% of the patients with the progressive type of carbon monoxide encephalopathy died, and another 50% remained severely disabled; some developed contractures in the advanced stages (Lee and Marsden, 1994). Of the patients with the delayed relapsing type of carbon monoxide sequelae, 61% subsequently improved, and 13% died. Delayed-onset parkinsonism has been documented not only after carbon monoxide poisoning, but also after anoxia, trauma, and other brain injuries (Bhatt et al., 1993; Scott and Jankovic, 1996; Li et al., 2000).

Because certain metals, such as iron, copper, and manganese, can facilitate oxidative reactions, there is growing interest in these transitional metals in the pathogenesis of neurodegenerative disorders. Manganese was first reported to cause a parkinsonian syndrome in 1837, only 20 years after James Parkinson described the disease that now bears his name (Calne et al., 1994). Since that time, there have been many reports of manganese intoxication causing psychiatric problems ("manganese madness"), usually followed in a few months by motor symptoms. These consist of dystonia, parkinsonism, retropulsion, and a characteristic gait called cock-walk, which is manifested by walking on the toes with elbows flexed and the spine erect. There is usually no tremor, and the motor deficits rarely improve with levodopa therapy. Manganese intoxication has been reported in miners, smelters, welders, workers involved in the manufacture of dry batteries, chronic accidental ingestion of potassium permanganate, and incorrect concentration of manganese in parenteral nutrition. Welders with PD were found to have their onset of PD on the average 17 years earlier than a control population of PD patients, suggesting

MANGANESE-INDUCED PARKINSONISM

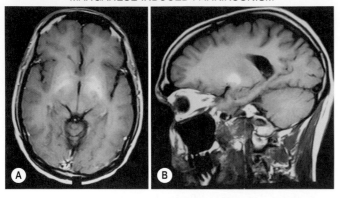

Figure 9.8 Manganese parkinsonism showing typical increased signal intensity in the globus pallidus on T1-weighted images.

that welding, possibly by causing manganese toxicity, is a risk factor for PD (Racette et al., 2001). Besides welding and manganese mining, manganese toxicity may occur with long-term parenteral nutrition. Although it has been postulated that manganese causes parkinsonism because of pallidal damage, some studies, including β-CIT SPECT scans, indicate a presynaptic form of parkinsonism associated with a reduction in striatal dopamine transporter (Kim et al., 2002). Manganese intoxication has been suggested as a possible cause of some of the neurologic abnormalities and abnormal MRI imaging (abnormal signal hyperintensity in the globus pallidus and SN on T1-weighted images) associated with chronic liver failure (Hauser et al., 1994; Racette et al., 2005; Sitburana and Ondo, 2009) (Fig. 9.8). The abnormal imaging studies and the lack of response to levodopa are consistent with the pathologic findings in humans and experimental primates of marked neuronal loss and gliosis in the globus pallidus and SNr (Olanow et al., 1996). Despite a growing number of publications, there is little evidence that welding causes manganese-induced parkinsonism or PD (Jankovic, 2005; Kieburtz and Kurlan, 2005). The associated marked accumulation of iron and aluminum suggests that oxidant stress plays an important role in manganese neurotoxicity. One piece of evidence that has been used to link welding with manganese-induced parkinsonism are the occasional reports of increased T1 basal ganglia signal on MRI of the brain (Sadek et al., 2003; Josephs et al., 2005). In one report from the Mayo Clinic, eight male career welders with such MRI findings exhibited parkinsonism (three patients), myoclonus and limited cognitive impairment (two patients), vestibular-auditory dysfunction (two patients), and minor subjective cognitive impairment, anxiety, and sleep apnea (one patient) (Josephs et al., 2005). The broad spectrum of clinical manifestations, however, argues against a direct cause-and-effect relationship. In contrast to PD, fluorodopa PET scans are normal in patients with manganese parkinsonism (Lu et al., 1994), and raclopride (D2 receptor) binding is only slightly reduced in the caudate but is normal in the putamen (Shinotoh et al., 1997). β-CIT SPECT scans, however, may be abnormal, indicating degeneration of presynaptic dopaminergic terminals in some patients with manganese parkinsonism (Kim et al., 2002).

There are other toxins, such as certain hydrocarbons (Pezzoli et al., 2000) and organophosphates (Bhatt et al., 1999), that have been implicated in the pathogenesis of parkinsonian syndromes. Many of the cases are complicated by legal issues; therefore, it is not always easy to prove a cause-and-effect relationship. If the parkinsonian syndrome occurs in a cluster, then it is more likely that the putative toxin is responsible.

Vascular

Parkinsonism due to strokes or other vascular causes can mimic idiopathic neurodegenerative disorders, such as PD or PSP. In a systematic review of 25 articles, patients with vascular parkinsonism were older, with a shorter duration of illness, presented with symmetrical gait difficulties, were less responsive to levodopa, and were more prone to postural instability, falls, and dementia (Kalra et al., 2010). Pyramidal signs, pseudobulbar palsy, and incontinence were more common in vascular parkinsonism while tremor was not a main feature. Structural neuroimaging was abnormal in 90–100% of vascular cases, compared to 12–43% of PD cases. In contrast to PD, there is usually no abnormality in presynaptic striatal dopamine transporters as measured by SPECT in vascular parkinsonism. Winikates and Jankovic (1999) compared a group of patients who satisfied the clinical, radiographic, or pathologic criteria for vascular parkinsonism with a group of patients with PD to determine which clinical variables differentiate these two forms of parkinsonism. Patients with vascular parkinsonism were older, were more likely to present with gait difficulty than with tremor, and were less likely to respond to levodopa than patients with PD. Vascular patients were also significantly more likely to have predominant lower-body involvement, postural instability, a history of falling, dementia, corticospinal findings, incontinence, and pseudobulbar effect. "Lower-body" parkinsonism, a condition in which upper-body motor function is relatively preserved while gait is markedly impaired, has previously been linked to multiple lacunar infarctions (Fitzgerald and Jankovic, 1989). Only about one-third of patients with vascular parkinsonism respond to levodopa (Demirkiran et al., 2001). A clinical-pathologic study of 17 patients concluded that vascular disease per se can cause parkinsonism without invoking coexistent neurodegenerative disease (Zijlmans et al., 2004a). Binswanger disease, a form of leukoencephalopathy caused by hypoxia-ischemia of distal watershed periventricular territories associated with aging, hyperviscosity, and increased fibrinogen levels (Roman, 1999), can rarely present as levodopa-responsive parkinsonism (Mark et al., 1995). Alternatively, about 10% of patients with small deep infarcts and white matter lesions have been found to have a parkinsonian syndrome (van Zagten et al., 1998). It is possible that some of the familial forms of vascular parkinsonism represent the entity CADASIL, an autosomal dominant arteriopathy associated with stroke and dementia, caused by mutations in the *Notch3* gene on chromosome 19p13.2 (Joutel et al., 2000; Wang et al., 2000). Because of multiple mutations, patients who are suspected to have this syndrome should first be screened for mutations in exons 4, 5, and 6, and if the tests are negative, a skin biopsy should be carried out searching for thickened basal lamina distorted by irregular deposits of granular osmophilic material, coupled with MRI T2 scanning (Markus et al., 2002). Vascular parkinsonism has been also described in moyamoya (Tan et al., 2003). A substantial number of patients with vascular parkinsonism improve with levodopa, particularly those with vascular lesions in or close to the nigrostriatal pathway (Zijlmans et al., 2004b). About one-third of patients with vascular parkinsonism, particularly those who respond to levodopa and do not have vertical gaze palsy or freezing, have a transient improvement in their gait after removal of 35–40 mL of CSF (Ondo et al., 2002a). CADASIL, the most common heritable cause of stroke and vascular dementia in adults, may also cause vascular parkinsonism (Chabriat et al., 2009).

Trauma

Although no definite link between trauma and PD can be established, there is convincing evidence for the concept of posttraumatic parkinsonism (Factor and Weiner, 1991; Goetz and Stebbins, 1991; Stern, 1991; Jankovic, 1994). Parkinsonism is a rare complication of a single trauma to the head unless the injury is severe enough to result in a comatose or vegetative state or causes a penetrating injury to the brainstem or a subdural hematoma with compression of the brainstem. However, parkinsonism is a well-recognized sequela of repeated head trauma, such as is seen in the "punch-drunk" syndrome or pugilistic dementia in boxers. In addition to typical parkinsonian symptoms, other neurologic consequences of boxing include dementia, paranoia, loss of inhibitions, and bradyphrenia. One of the reasons for the initial underrecognition of boxer's parkinsonism and other progressive neurologic problems has been the long latency, lasting several years or even decades, between cessation of competitive boxing and the development of neurologic symptoms and signs. The evidence indicates that it is the number of bouts (and presumably repetitive subconcussive blows) rather than the number of knockouts that correlates best with the development of chronic brain damage (Lampert and Hardman, 1984). A study of 86 amateur boxers found no evidence of cognitive impairment, suggesting that only a small minority of boxers have brain damage (Butler et al., 1993).

Most of the blows to the head that boxers sustain result in rotational (angular) acceleration, which can cause not only subdural hematoma, petechial hemorrhages, and diffuse axonal injury to the long fiber tracts, but also injury to the medial temporal cortex and rostral brainstem, particularly the SN. Marked neuronal degeneration, especially in the lateral and intermediate cell groups, depigmentation, gliosis, and NFTs have been well documented in the SN of boxers' brains (Lampert and Hardman, 1984). Although initial pathologic studies of brains of boxers with dementia pugilistica emphasized the presence of numerous NFTs without plaques, subsequent reexamination of the brains with immunocytochemical methods has provided evidence that the β-amyloid protein present in brains of patients with AD is also present in the boxers' brains and that dementia pugilistica and AD share common pathogenic mechanisms (Roberts et al., 1990). One study showed increased severity of neurologic deficits in boxers with the APOE ε4 allele, suggesting that genetic predisposition may play a role in the

neurologic impairments associated with chronic traumatic brain injury (Jordan et al., 1997).

Parkinsonism can result not only from injury to the central nervous system, but also from peripheral trauma (Cardoso and Jankovic, 1995). In 21 patients, the onset of movement disorder began within 2 months after injury; in 6 patients, the tremor started 3–5 months after the trauma; and the onset was delayed by 1 year in 1 patient. The mean age at onset of the movement disorder was 46.5 ± 14.1 years. Among the parkinsonian patients, high-dose levodopa failed to ameliorate the symptoms in 4 of the 10 patients, and the others had only modest improvement. None of the patients achieved spontaneous remission; in 19 patients, the movement disorder worsened or remained unchanged. The PET scans showed decreased fluorodopa uptake in the striatum of three patients who were tested, and the raclopride binding in the striatum was symmetrical and slightly increased in two of the three patients. While it is possible that the parkinsonism in these patients occurred by chance alone, the young age at onset, the anatomic and temporal relationship to severe local injury, and the atypical clinical and pharmacologic features suggest that peripherally induced parkinsonism should be added to the growing list of peripherally induced movement disorders.

Hemiparkinsonism–hemiatrophy

Hemiparkinsonism–hemiatrophy syndrome is a rare form of secondary parkinsonism that begins usually in the third or fourth decade; it is characterized by unilateral body atrophy and ipsilateral parkinsonian findings, dystonia, slow progression, and poor response to levodopa (Jankovic, 1988; Giladi et al., 1990; Wijemanne and Jankovic, 2007). Contralateral cortical hemiatrophy is usually present, and there is often a history of perinatal asphyxia or other perinatal injury (Scott and Jankovic, 1996; Wijemanne and Jankovic, 2007). In contrast to a presynaptic involvement in PD, PET studies have provided evidence of presynaptic and postsynaptic nigrostriatal dopaminergic dysfunction in patients with hemiparkinsonism–hemiatrophy syndrome (Przedborski et al., 1994). One patient with hemiparkinsonism–hemiatrophy was found to have a mutation in the *parkin* gene on chromosome 6 (Pramstaller et al., 2002).

Normal pressure hydrocephalus

Normal pressure hydrocephalus (NPH) should be considered in the differential diagnosis of all patients with progressive gait disturbance and other parkinsonian features (Curran and Lang, 1994; Vanneste, 2000; Palm et al., 2009). Since the CSF pressure is not always normal and the disorder seems to be quite heterogeneous in terms of age at onset and clinical presentation, the term chronic hydrocephalus has been proposed (Bret et al., 2002). The gait and parkinsonian features associated with NPH include short steps, wide base, stiff legs, start hesitation, and freezing ("magnetic gait"). In contrast to other parkinsonian disorders associated with freezing, the gait of patients with NPH usually does not improve with visual clues (Lai and Jankovic, 1995). In addition to the characteristic gait disturbance, the NPH patients frequently exhibit bradykinesia, flexed posture, and loss of postural reflexes as well as cognitive decline and urinary incontinence. In contrast to PD, patients with NPH have near normal leg function in supine and sitting positions, and they tend to have less tremor. Some patients with NPH may later develop PD (Curran and Lang, 1994). Shunting may be considered for patients with NPH in whom gait disturbance precedes mental impairment and the mental impairment is of recent origin and mild. Other predictors of favorable outcome after shunting include a known cause of NPH, absence of white matter lesions on MRI, a substantial clinical improvement after CSF tap, 50% occurrence of B-wave on intracranial pressure recording, and resistance to CSF outflow of at least 18 mmHg per minute during CSF infusion test.

Patients with short history, a known cause of hydrocephalus, predominant gait disorder, and imaging studies suggestive of hydrodynamic hydrocephalus without cortical atrophy and without white matter involvement, are considered the best candidates for shunting, and 50–70% experience substantial improvement after surgery (Vanneste, 2000). In one study of 55 patients treated with shunting for NPH, the improvement was sustained during the mean follow-up of 5.9 ± 2.5 years, with gait and cognitive function improving the most (Pujari et al., 2008). NPH is sometimes difficult to differentiate from vascular parkinsonism or subcortical arteriosclerotic encephalopathy (SAE). The CSF sulfatide concentration was markedly increased in patients with arteriosclerotic encephalopathy (mean: 766 nmol/L, range: 300–3800 nmol/L) and this test distinguished between patients with arteriosclerotic encephalopathy and those with NPH with a sensitivity of 74% and a specificity of 94%, making it an important diagnostic marker (Tullberg et al., 2000). Obstructive hydrocephalus, with or without aqueductal stenosis, can also result in parkinsonism that may respond to levodopa (Jankovic et al., 1986; Zeidler et al., 1998; Racette et al., 2004). Most patients with disabling symptoms of hydrocephalus-associated parkinsonism require ventriculoperitoneal shunting. Despite aggressive marketing directly to patients by various companies promoting their shunting devices (e.g., Codman), NPH is actually quite uncommon and even well-selected patients do not always obtain satisfactory results from shunting (http://www.ninds. nih.gov/disorders/normal_pressure_hydrocephalus/normal_pressure_hydrocephalus.htm).

Other secondary parkinsonian disorders

It is beyond the scope of this review to discuss all other causes of parkinsonism. Brain tumors and gliomatosis cerebri, even when they spare basal ganglia, may cause parkinsonism (Krauss et al., 1995; Cicarelli et al., 1999; Pohle and Krauss, 1999; Tagliati et al., 2000). Familial basal ganglia calcification (bilateral striopallidodentate calcinosis or Fahr disease) is another diagnosis that should be considered in any patient with parkinsonism unresponsive to levodopa, ataxia, and personality changes (Manyam et al., 2001; Brodaty et al., 2002; Warren et al., 2002; Oliveira et al., 2004). The basal ganglia, cerebellar, paraventricular, and cortical calcification may be missed on MRI and may not become apparent until a CT scan of the head is obtained.

Other causes of parkinsonism include paraneoplastic degeneration of the SN manifested by parkinsonism and dystonia (Golbe et al., 1989), central pontine and extrapontine myelinolysis (Seiser et al., 1998), wasp sting (Leopold et al., 1999), Sjögren syndrome (Walker et al., 1999), and others. There is growing interest in autoimmunity as a mechanism of some atypical forms of parkinsonism and other movement disorders. For example, the clinical spectrum of voltage-gated potassium channelopathies (VGKC), with autoantibodies detected in the blood, neurons, glia, and muscle, includes parkinsonism, tremor, myoclonus, and chorea (Tan et al., 2008). Other features of this paraneoplastic syndrome include cognitive impairment, seizures, dysautonomia, peripheral neuropathy and the presence of certain cancers.

Parkinsonism and pyramidal signs associated with speech and orofacial apraxia slowly progressing to anarthria and muteness without other language or cognitive deficits should suggest the possibility of late anterior opercular syndrome (Broussolle et al., 1996; Bakar et al., 1998). This syndrome resembles Foix–Chavany–Marie syndrome, also known as Worster–Drought syndrome (Christen et al., 2000), which is characterized by bilateral facioglossopharyngomasticatory paresis (pseudobulbar palsy) associated with bilateral lesions in the frontal and parietal opercula. The anterior opercular syndrome is a severe form of pseudobulbar palsy in which patients with bilateral lesions of the perisylvian cortex or subcortical connections become completely mute. These patients can follow commands involving the extremities but not of the cranial nerves; for example, they might be unable to open or close their eyes or mouth or smile voluntarily, yet they smile when amused, yawn spontaneously, and even utter cries in response to emotional stimuli. The syndrome is usually seen in patients who have had multiple strokes, but rare cases of progressive disease, as in the syndrome of primary progressive anarthria, may occur. A related cheiro-oral syndrome (sensory disturbance in one hand and the ipsilateral oral corner) has been associated with rostral brainstem lesions. Similar to CBD, imaging studies usually show markedly asymmetrical (L > R) cortical atrophy and reduced metabolism, especially involving the posterior inferior frontal lobe, particularly the operculum (the cerebral cortex and subcortical white matter covering the insula). One of our patients with this syndrome also exhibited pseudobulbar palsy, vertical ophthalmoparesis, and postural instability similar to that of PSP. Supranuclear ophthalmoparesis has been described in some previously reported cases of the anterior opercular syndrome. Some of the cases that came to autopsy showed focal frontal (particularly left opercular) cortical atrophy with spongiform changes in layers II and III and SN degeneration without Lewy bodies. Although this syndrome is considered to be due to some yet-unknown neurodegeneration, phenotypically similar cases have been documented to be due to herpes simplex encephalitis (McGrath et al., 1997), cortical infarcts, trauma, meningitis, benign epilepsy of childhood with rolandic spikes, and developmental dysplasia (Weller, 1993). Antiphospholipid syndrome has been associated with chorea and other movement and neurologic disorders, including parkinsonism (Huang et al., 2008).

Rapidly progressive autosomal dominant parkinsonism with central hypoventilation, depression, apathy, weight loss, and poor response to levodopa, referred to as Perry syndrome, has neuropathology similar to PD, but without Lewy bodies (Wider and Wszolek, 2008). TDP-43-positive neuronal inclusions, dystrophic neurites, and axonal spheroids in a predominantly pallidonigral distribution, sparing the neocortex and motor neurons, were demonstrated in autopsied brains of patients with this autosomal dominant neurodegenerative disorder (Wider et al., 2008). This genetic disorder has been found to be caused by mutations in the CAP-Gly domain of dynactin (encoded by the *DCTN1* gene) resulting in impaired microtubule binding and formation of intracytoplasmic inclusions (Farrer et al., 2009). Parkinsonism, frontal dementia, peripheral neuropathy, neurogenic bladder, and upper motor neuron signs have been described in adult polyglucosan body disease (Robertson et al., 1998). There is a growing number of mitochondrial disorders described with a broad phenotype, including parkinsonism. These include the *POLG1* mutation syndromes that may also include intellectual disability, epilepsy, migraines, ataxia, neuropathy, myopathy, ophthalmoparesis, dementia, dystonia, focal myoclonus, and liver disease (Hudson et al., 2007; McHugh et al., 2010). The symptoms and liver failure may be markedly exacerbated by valproate. Inherited in an autosomal recessive or dominant mitochondrial pattern, the disease, referred to also as Alper syndrome, is due to mutations in *POLG1*, a nuclear gene which encodes for the catalytic subunit of the mtDNA polymerase gamma, essential for mtDNA replication (Milone and Massie, 2010). A single point mutation in mitochondrial 12SrRNA has recently been reported to be associated with parkinsonism, deafness, and neuropathy (Thyagarajan et al., 2000). Encephalopathy and parkinsonism have been reported in children with leukemia who have been treated with bone marrow transplantation, amphotericin, immunosuppressants, and total body irradiation (Mott et al., 1995).

Juvenile parkinsonism (onset before age 20 years), often characterized by prominent gait and balance difficulties, dystonia, and improvement after sleep, may occur sporadically or as an autosomal recessive disorder (Ishikawa and Miyatake, 1995; Ishikawa and Tsuji, 1996; Shimoda-Matsubayashi et al., 1997). One form of juvenile parkinsonism (onset age <20 years) is neuronal intranuclear inclusion disease, a rare disorder characterized by asymmetric-onset, levodopa-responsive parkinsonism, associated with gaze-evoked nystagmus, early-onset dysarthria and dysphagia, and oculogyric crises. At autopsy, there were widespread neuronal hyaline intranuclear inclusions, immunoreactive for ubiquitin, which can be also found on rectal biopsy, as well as neuronal depletion in the substantia nigra, locus coeruleus, and, to a lesser extent, in the frontal cortex, and inclusions were particularly prominent in these areas (O'Sullivan et al., 2000; Lai et al., 2010).

Some causes of secondary parkinsonism in childhood were reviewed by Pranzatelli and colleagues (1994). Although the heredogenerations are reviewed elsewhere, some of the genetic forms of parkinsonism with known genetic defects are listed in Table 9.1.

Appendix

CurePSP
Foundation for PSP, CBD and Related Brain Diseases
30 E. Padonia Road, Suite 201
Timonium, Maryland 20193
Website: http://www.psp.org

SDS/MSA support group websites
http://www.shy-drager.org
http://www.msatrust.org.uk
http://groups.yahoo.com/group/shydrager
http://www.emedicine.com/neuro/topic671.htm

References available on Expert Consult: www.expertconsult.com

CHAPTER 10

Gait disorders
Pathophysiology and clinical syndromes

Chapter contents

Balance	241	Gait disorders	244
Gait	242	Therapeutic considerations	249

Gait is a fundamental skill. It permits movement from place to place, and, as anthropologists are fond of pointing out, that humans do it on two legs frees up the arms for other skilled tasks. The ability to walk is basic to quality of life. However, walking on two legs is a difficult motor task involving the ability to balance and execute a complex motor program at the same time. Many movement disorders affect gait and this becomes an important aspect of the disorder. The nature of the gait disorder, conversely, of course, can be a clue to the diagnosis of the movement disorder. This chapter will first briefly review the physiology of balance and gait, and then consider the different gait disorders.

Balance

It is important to distinguish between balance and stance. Stance is the posture of standing. It is normally upright on two legs with a distance between the feet approximately equal to pelvic width. An example of abnormal stance would be the stooped posture seen in Parkinson disease. Balance is the ability to maintain stance without falling or excessive lurching (Benvenuti, 2001). If balance is poor, sometimes persons modify their stance; the most common manifestation is increasing the distance between the feet to widen the base of support (BOS).

From standard Newtonian physics, for an object to maintain its position, its center of mass (COM) must be over its BOS. In the case of a human standing, the COM is generally somewhere in the abdomen and the BOS is the area between and including the feet. Since the BOS is relatively small and the COM relatively high above the BOS, it takes considerable skill to maintain the BOS above the COM. Recently, it was recognized that the ability to remain upright cannot be explained best by just the simple need to maintain the BOS above the COM. This is a static requirement, and the body or body parts are constantly moving. This movement must be taken into account. A "dynamic model" of balance

includes consideration of the velocity of COM (Pai et al., 1998). The general principle is that the balance mechanisms of the body (such as the postural muscles) must be able to counteract any large velocities of the COM, even if the COM is currently over the BOS, since if they cannot, the COM will soon be beyond the BOS.

The body is constantly moving and this movement is called sway. Each body part can have its own movement, but the important "summary" of these movements would be movement of the COM for the reasons already described. Neurologists are used to doing a visual analysis of sway, but this is not very exact, of course. Instrumental methods have been developed. The position of the COM can be estimated although it is generally somewhat difficult. The position of the different body parts can be determined with video methods, and if their individual masses are estimated, then the COM can be calculated. This is generally done only in research laboratories. An alternative method, generally called posturography, comes from the ability to record forces that the body exerts on the floor with devices called force plates (Kaufman et al., 2001). The devices measure force in three directions, vertical, forward/backward, and side-to-side, and the two-dimensional center of action of the forward/backward and side-to-side force is called the center of pressure (COP). In the static situation, the COM is directly over the COP. Movements of the COM cause deviance of the matching of the COM and COP, but if the movements are small and slow, the deviance is not much. For this reason, sway is often measured with movements of the COP.

Generally it is thought that more sway means less good balance. This is often but not always true. In some circumstances, because the balance is bad, patients stiffen up, voluntarily or involuntarily, and the sway might decrease. This might be true in Parkinson disease, for example (Panzer et al., 1990). When a patient is "off," balance is poor and patients are very stiff, often swaying little. When the patient is "on," balance is better, the patient is more relaxed and sway might increase. Sway markedly increases with

DOI: 10.1016/B978-1-4377-2369-4.00010-X

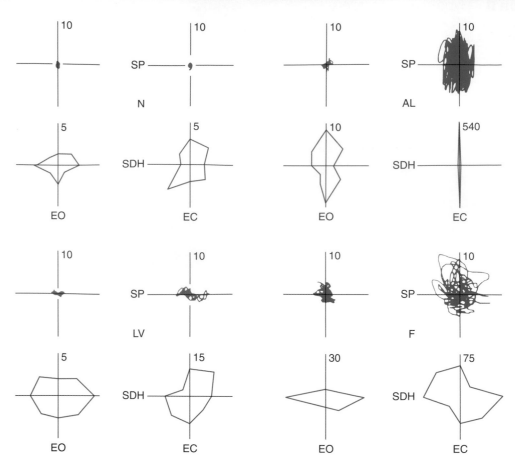

Figure 10.1 Examples of posturography, the path of the COP while standing. In each part of the figure, SP is the sway path and SDH is the sway direction histogram. The upper left, N, is the normal pattern; the upper right, AL, is from a cerebellar patient with anterior lobe dysfunction; the lower left, LV, is from a cerebellar patient with lower vermis dysfunction; the lower right, F, is from a patient with Friedreich ataxia. EO, eyes open; EC, eyes closed. *From Diener HC, Dichgans J, Bacher M, Gompf B. Quantification of postural sway in normals and patients with cerebellar diseases. Electroencephalog Clin Neurophysiol 1984;57:134–142, with permission.*

dyskinesias (characteristic of the "on" state and good balance). In most circumstances, however, increased sway does indeed indicate poor balance and posturography can be employed to make this assessment quantitatively. A surer way to assess balance is to see what happens with a perturbation to stance. If patients can remain upright, then balance is good; if they fall, balance is defective. This is the logic of the pull test.

The pull test is done by having the patient stand and having the investigator stand behind the patient and give a sudden pull backward. The patient is told to maintain balance. The best ability is to deal with the perturbation by body movements without moving the feet. A second-level ability is to maintain balance by taking a timely step backward. Failure, of course, is a fall, and that is the reason that the test is a pull rather than a push; the patient can fall into the examiner. Balance is virtually always better in the forward direction than the backward direction. With poor balance, patients tend to fall backward. All the reasons for this are not clear, but one is likely that when standing, the COM is closer to the back of the foot than the front. In any event, because of this, the pull test is often only done in the backward direction. A related test called the push and release test has been suggested, and it might be more sensitive and consistent than the pull test, but it has not been much utilized (Jacobs et al., 2006).

Good balance depends on good motor control abilities, but also good sensory feedback about what the exact body position and velocity are at any time. Feedback comes from vision, proprioception, and vestibular sensation. When one sensory modality is impaired, generally the others can compensate. When two modalities are impaired, there is more of a problem. This is the source for the popular Romberg test. Sway is assessed when the eyes are closed. If there is a problem with proprioception, in the absence of vision, sway will be increased.

Abnormalities in posturography have been reported in many disorders. The best studied has been cerebellar disturbances (Diener et al., 1984; Gatev et al., 1996); the findings are reviewed in detail in Chapter 2 and illustrated as an example here (Fig. 10.1).

Gait

Human gait is a complex, rhythmic, cyclic movement (Winter, 1991). The movements are generated to some extent by a locomotor generator in the spinal cord, but they are under control by supraspinal mechanisms. The spinal cord generator can produce only simple, primitive stepping and react to perturbations in stereotypic fashion (Burke, 2001). Supraspinal mechanisms are required for a person to go in desired directions, with desired velocities and to deal well with perturbations. An important supraspinal control center is the mesencephalic locomotor region, which includes the pedunculopontine nucleus (PPN). The PPN is an important integrator of activity from basal ganglia, cerebellum, and motor cortex and projects to reticular nuclei in the brainstem. The fastigial nucleus of the cerebellum seems also important (Mori et al., 2001). Supraspinal control signals are conveyed to the spinal cord by reticulospinal and vesti-bulospinal tracts.

There are a number of terms that are useful in describing gait, and many of them are defined below.

Stance phase: When the foot is on the floor.
Swing phase: When the foot is in the air.
Stance time: The time that the foot is on the floor, measured as the time between heel strike and toe or heel off, whichever is last.
Swing time: The time that the foot is in the air, measured as the time between toe off and heel strike.
Cadence: The number of steps per minute.
Step length: The distance advanced by one foot compared to the position of the other.
Stride length: The sum of two consecutive step lengths or the distance advanced by one foot compared to its prior position.
Step time: The time from heel strike of one foot to the subsequent heel strike of the contralateral foot.
Gait cycle: One complete cycle of events, often looked at as the time between two consecutive heel strikes of the same foot. Hence, a gait cycle would begin at the beginning of stance phase of one foot, go through stance and swing, and end at the end of swing (which is the beginning of the next stance phase).
Stride time: The time for a full gait cycle.
Average gait velocity: The stride length divided by the stride time.

A gait cycle for the right leg is illustrated in Figure 10.2. Note that the gait cycle for the left leg is not exactly 180° out of phase. For this reason, and because stance phase is longer than swing phase, there are several periods where both feet are on the ground, and these are called double support. (In normal walking, there are no periods of simultaneous swing; that is, no "flying," but this may occur with running.) With normal gait, when the foot contacts the ground, the heel contacts first and then the foot rotates to flat with the heel as the point of rotation. When the foot leaves the floor for swing, the foot rotates over the toe and the heel leaves the ground first.

The joint angles of a normal gait cycle are illustrated in Figure 10.3. The ankle shows a brief plantar flexion at heel strike, followed by a gentle dorsiflexion in stance as the body moves over the foot. The ankle then shows a brisk plantar flexion producing push-off lasting from heel off to toe off. During swing there is a dorsiflexion of the ankle to avoid hitting the toe on the ground and to prepare for heel strike. The knee shows a slight flexion during stance and a more pronounced flexion during swing. The hip extends in stance and flexes during swing.

Muscle activities during gait are illustrated in Figure 10.4. During the gait cycle, the triceps surae (gastrocnemius-soleus) is active primarily at the end of stance to push off for the swing phase. The tibialis anterior muscle is active in the beginning of stance to slow the plantarflexion of the foot so that it does not slap onto the floor. Then it is active again during swing to produce the dorsiflexion of the ankle mentioned above.

Gait initiation

The initiation of gait is a special problem (Elble et al., 1994). Not only does it pose a unique biomechanical problem, it also causes some patients particular difficulty (Mancini et al., 2009). The task is to get the body moving forward and to get the first foot off the ground into a "swing phase." In quiet standing, there is a very slight tonic activation of the

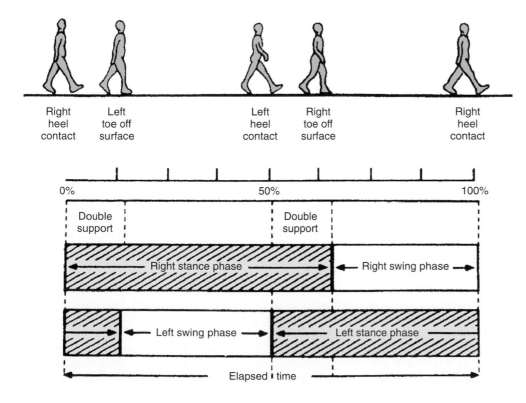

Figure 10.2 Diagram of the gait cycle; see text for detailed description. *From Sudarsky L. Geriatrics: gait disorders in the elderly. N Engl J Med 1990,322(20):1441–1446, with permission.*

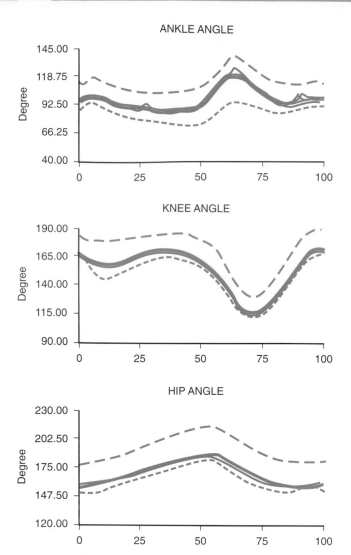

Figure 10.3 Changes of the ankle, hip, and knee angles during a full gait cycle beginning with the start of stance phase. The solid lines are multiple trials from a single, healthy subject showing the excellent reproducibility from cycle to cycle. The dashed lines are the normal limits from a group of 10 healthy subjects. *Modified from Palliyath S, Hallett M, Thomas SL, Lebiedowska MK. Gait in patients with cerebellar ataxia. Mov Disord 1998;13(6):958–964, with permission.*

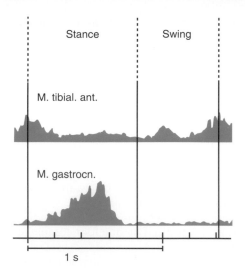

Figure 10.4 EMG activity in the tibialis and gastrocnemius muscles during a full gait cycle. The figure shows rectified activity in a healthy subject. *Modified from Conrad B, Meinck HM, Benecke R. Motor patterns in human gait: adaptation to different modes of progression. In: Bles W, Brandt T, eds. Disorders of Posture and Gait. Amsterdam: Elsevier Science Publishers BV; 1986: pp. 53–67, with permission.*

Table 10.1 **Frequency of etiologies of neurologically referred undiagnosed gait disorders**

Sensory deficits	18.3%
Myelopathy	16.7%
Multiple infarcts	15.0%
Unknown	14.2%
Parkinsonism	11.7%
Cerebellar degeneration	6.7%
Hydrocephalus	6.7%
Psychogenic	3.3%
Other	7.5%

"Other" etiologies include metabolic encephalopathy, antidepressant and sedative drugs, toxic disorders, brain tumor, and subdural hematoma.
From Sudarsky L. Clinical approaches to gait disorders of aging. In: Masdeu J, Sudarsky L, Wolfson L, eds. Gait Disorders of Aging: Falls and Therapeutic Strategies. Philadelphia: Lippincott-Raven; 1997, pp. 147–158, with permission.

triceps surae. This prevents the body from falling forward since the COM is anterior to the ankle joints. The first event is a diminution of activity in the triceps surae muscles, more prominent on the side of the leg that will become the stance leg for the first step. This by itself would cause the body to start moving forward, rotating around the ankle. Then, the tibialis anterior muscles contract, which actively rotates the body forward around the ankle. These events get the body moving.

The next set of events is like a mini-step. The leg that will become the stance leg briefly flexes slightly at the knee and hip, just like in a swing phase. This helps drive the COP toward the swing leg. Then, the swing leg makes a large burst of electromyographic (EMG) activity in the triceps surae producing the push-off force for the swing phase. This force, coupled with a slight abduction of the hip, drives the COP toward the stance leg, which it accepts as it serves a full stance function during the swing of the other leg.

Gait disorders

Epidemiology

Gait problems are a major neurologic problem, particularly in elderly people (Sudarsky, 2001). In this population, common causes for problems are stroke, peripheral neuropathy, brain or spinal cord trauma, and Parkinson disease. The term "senile gait" is sometimes used, but it likely does not exist as a distinct entity. Multiple medical problems accumulate with age, including visual difficulties and arthritis, that become additive.

Sudarsky (1997) evaluated a series of patients referred for an unknown gait disorder. After careful neurologic evaluation, he was able to make a diagnosis in most (Table 10.1).

The most frequent entities were sensory deficits, myelopathy, multiple infarcts, parkinsonism, and unknown.

Evaluation of gait

Of course, the gait itself should be observed, but special attention should be paid to different aspects including: nature of the steps including stride length and cadence, deviations from the direction of progression, width of the feet from each other during periods of double support, variability of the stepping, and angular movements at the joints. Any stiffness of motion should be indicated. Additionally, the ability to initiate stepping and the ability to turn should be noted. Looking for more subtle abnormalities, individuals can be asked to walk a straight line, heel to toe. In the case of dystonia, the patients might be asked to walk backward to see if this improves performance. Balance should be assessed as well, observing quiet standing with eyes open and eyes closed, and performing the pull test. Of course, it is critical to evaluate patients for non-neurologic features such as arthritis, limitation of motion, pain (antalgic gait), and asymmetries of leg length.

There are a number of important observations that have implications for the differential diagnosis (Nutt et al., 1993):

Weakness. Weakness should ordinarily be noted on general neurologic examination. Depending on the muscles affected there will be certain patterns identified such as steppage and waddling, which will be described further below. Weakness is commonly due to neuropathy or myopathy.

Dysmetria of stepping. Steps that are abnormal by virtue of being the wrong length or direction and are also highly variable. This is characteristic of ataxia and chorea. Ataxia looks mostly clumsy, while chorea often has a dancing quality.

Stiffness or rigidity. This is characterized by reduction of joint movement. It is seen with spasticity, parkinsonism, and dystonia.

Veering. Deviations from a direct line of progression are due to either vestibular or cerebellar disorders.

Freezing. Freezing is also known as motor blocks and is characterized by lack of movement with the feet looking like they are glued to the floor (Snijders et al., 2008; Browner and Giladi, 2010). Patients often look like they are trying to move, but they cannot. This may be due to inability to generate sufficient postural shifting to initiate forward movement (Elble et al., 1996; Mancini et al., 2009). Freezing can occur when trying to initiate gait, in which circumstance it has also been called "start hesitation." Freezing can also interrupt walking, and in this circumstance is sometimes precipitated by a sensory stimulus such as a doorway, the ring of a doorbell, or a street light changing color. Curiously, sensory stimuli can also be used to improve freezing. They appear to act in this regard by providing external triggers for movement.

The pathophysiology of freezing is not clear, but there are a number of associated abnormalities. Patients show defective bilateral coordination of stepping (Plotnik et al., 2008). There is an association of freezing with loss of frontal lobe executive function (Amboni et al., 2008). Another possible factor is the sequence effect where sequential movements become progressively smaller (Iansek et al., 2006; Chee et al., 2009). One study showed that freezing would occur when the demands for rapid stepping were high (Moreau et al., 2008a). Yet another factor contributing to freezing is the excessive dependence on external stimuli in patients with PD (Hallett, 2008). Imaging studies suggest that freezing is associated with abnormalities of the mesencephalic locomotor region (Snijders et al., 2011).

In addition to the absence of movement, another form of freezing is characterized by rapid, side-to-side shifting of weight, but no lifting of the feet and no forward progression. This has been called the "slipping clutch syndrome." In this situation, physiologic studies show co-contraction activity in antagonist muscles, apparently not permitting effective forward movement (Yanagisawa et al., 2001).

Freezing is very common in idiopathic PD, but is also seen in other parkinsonian states such as progressive supranuclear palsy, vascular parkinsonism, and normal pressure hydrocephalus. It seems less common in multiple system atrophy and drug-induced parkinsonism (Giladi, 2001).

Marché à petit pas. Walking with very short, often shuffling, steps. This is most typical of a multi-infarct state, but can be seen with parkinsonism.

Festination. This is where short steps become progressively more rapid. This extension of marché à petit pas is also characteristic of parkinsonism. The stepping may even become much more rapid than normal. This can also be called a propulsive gait.

Anatomic/physiologic classification

Gait disorders, like gait itself, are very complex. This chapter will follow the classification of Nutt, Marsden, and Thompson, proposed in 1993, since that has been the most commonly used (Nutt et al., 1993). There have been some more recent refinements suggested (Jankovic et al., 2001; Nutt, 2001).

Lowest level

This refers to elemental disorders such as those resulting from muscle, nerve, or root disorders. This would also include the consequences of sensory deficits such as peripheral neuropathy, vestibular or visual disorder. Severe sensory loss can produce a gait similar to that of cerebellar ataxia; these patients have particular difficulty walking in the dark. An example is the GALOP syndrome, characterized by gait "ataxia" and peripheral neuropathy associated with a monoclonal IgM specific for galopin, a central nervous system white matter antigen (Alpert, 2004).

One set of examples relates to disturbances generated by particular patterns of weakness. For example, the steppage gait is the result of a foot drop. The hip and knee have to be excessively flexed to bring the leg up high enough so the toes do not scrape the floor. Another example is the waddling gait, where weakness of the hip abductors leads to dropping of the pelvis toward the swing leg and compensatory lean toward the stance leg.

Middle level

The level refers to central nervous system disorders arising from standard parts of the motor system.

Hemiparetic gait

Because of a unilateral lesion of the corticospinal tract, most commonly seen with stroke, there is a stiff extended leg that circumducts during swing with scraping of the toe (Video 10.1). Typically, of course, there should be some weakness in a "pyramidal" distribution and increased reflexes. The earliest sign might be reduced knee flexion during swing (Kerrigan et al., 2001).

Treatment of the spasticity might be useful, but this must be done carefully since without spasticity, the leg might collapse and not provide support. Oral agents or intrathecal baclofen can be used. Botulinum toxin directed to the triceps surae has been used very successfully, particularly in the setting of cerebral palsy (Simpson, 1997; Flett et al., 1999).

Paraparetic gait

The gait is a bilateral hemiparetic gait and shows stiffness of both legs with scissoring (excessive hip adduction) (Video 10.2). Conditions where this is prominent include spinal cord injury, hereditary spastic paraparesis, and primary lateral sclerosis.

Stiff-legged gait

This term includes the spastic syndromes of hemiparetic and paraparetic and also the disorder seen with the stiffperson syndrome (Video 10.3). There is particular stiffness of the spine with hyperlordosis, but all joints of the lower extremity will have reduced range of motion as well.

Ataxic gait

Patients with cerebellar ataxia have difficulty with motor control by virtue of dysmetria, dyssynergia, variability of performance, and poor balance. All these features contribute to their disorder of gait (Ilg et al., 2008). Clinically, the gait is characterized by irregularity of stepping, in direction, distance, and timing. Patients may lurch in different directions. Stability of upright stance is poor and patients may fall. Just as with standing balance, the base, or distance between the feet, is said to be broad (Video 10.4).

Palliyath et al. (1998) studied the gait pattern in 10 patients with cerebellar degenerations. Gait at natural speed was studied using a video-based kinematic data acquisition system for measuring body movements. Patients showed a reduced step and stride length with a trend to reduced cadence. Heel off time, toe off time, and time of peak flexion of the knee in swing were all delayed. Range of rotation of ankle, knee, and hip were all reduced, but only ankle range of rotation reached significance. Multijoint coordination was impaired as indicated by a relatively greater delay of plantar flexion of the ankle compared with flexion of the knee and a relatively late knee flexion compared with hip flexion at the onset of swing. The patients also showed increased variability of almost all measures. While some of the deviations from normal were due simply to the slowness of walking, the gait pattern of patients with cerebellar degeneration showed incoordination similar to that previously described for their multijoint limb motion. A wide base was not seen in this study, but it was seen in another one (Hudson and Krebs, 2000).

Patients with essential tremor have a mild gait abnormality that is ataxic in type (Stolze et al., 2001b). This forms part of the evidence that essential tremor results from cerebellar dysfunction.

Parkinsonian gait

Parkinson patients often have a stooped posture and stand and walk on a narrow base (Morris et al., 2001a, 2001b). Sometimes there is marked flexion of the trunk, called camptocormia, a condition also seen in dystonia and in psychogenic conditions (Azher and Jankovic, 2005). Balance is poor and patients often fall (Kerr et al., 2010). They have short, shuffling steps, the marché à petit pas, and this can be associated with festination. They turn en bloc, and important associated signs are lack of arm swing and tremor of the hands. Freezing is common and can occur in both the "off" and "on" states. Freezing is seen in about one-quarter of patients by 4 years (Rascol et al., 2000). Abnormalities of EMG pattern have been described (Nieuwboer et al., 2004).

Gait speed in Parkinson disease is slow. If trying to walk faster, patients increase step rate proportionally more than stride length (compared with normal subjects) (Morris et al., 1994, 1998). EMG and kinematic studies have illuminated the pathophysiology (Albani et al., 2003; Svehlik et al., 2009; Nanhoe-Mahabier et al., 2011).

Variability of stride length is a gait feature that has been associated with falls. Stride time and variability were studied in patients with Parkinson disease and compared with other clinical measures (Schaafsma et al., 2003). Variability was independent of tremor, rigidity, and bradykinesia, but somewhat responsive to levodopa. Gait variability markedly increases with a simultaneous cognitive task, and this certainly would make patients more prone to falls (Hausdorff et al., 2003a). Those patients with more freezing also have more variability, suggesting that this might be a factor in the etiology of freezing (Hausdorff et al., 2003b).

Since gait does require some attention, if patients are asked to do a second task while walking, the gait performance can deteriorate (Plotnik et al., 2009). Patients can even fall. Patients realize this, at least subconsciously, and may well stop walking to answer a question. This is the basis of the "stops walking when talking" test (Lundin-Olsson et al., 1997).

Treatment of the parkinsonism with dopaminergic therapy or deep brain stimulation (DBS) improves gait, but often not as much as other motor symptoms (Lubik et al., 2006; Ferraye et al., 2008). Freezing particularly is generally difficult to treat, but off-freezing may well improve with dopaminergic medication. Another approach is the use of methylphenidate (Auriel et al., 2006; Devos et al., 2007; Pollak et al., 2007) although there is some negative evidence (Espay et al., 2011). On-freezing is a particularly difficult problem, and may even respond to lowering the dopaminergic medication. It was suggested that botulinum toxin might improve gait freezing (Giladi et al., 2001), but this was not confirmed in a double-blind trial (Wieler et al., 2005). Parkinsonian gait can also be improved by rhythmic visual or auditory clues (Suteerawattananon et al., 2004; Ledger et al., 2008; Arias and Cudeiro, 2010). Mental singing while walking may also improve gait performance (Satoh and Kuzuhara, 2008). Physical therapy can help, but may have only a short-term benefit (Ellis et al., 2005; Kwakkel et al., 2007; Frazzitta et al., 2009; Morris et al., 2010). One component of therapy should have the patients concentrate on making "big" steps (Werner and Gentile, 2010). Action observation may improve freezing of gait in Parkinson patients (Pelosin et al., 2010). Treadmill training can be helpful as well (Bello et al., 2010; Mehrholz et al., 2010). Dance therapy may have some longer lasting effects (Hackney et al., 2007; Hackney and Earhart, 2009). Transcranial magnetic stimulation may have benefit (Lomarev et al., 2006).

Indeed, it is now often the case that problems with balance and gait are continuing despite improvements in bradykinesia after DBS. This has led to attempts to improve DBS. One approach is to change the stimulation parameters (Moreau et al., 2008b). There has also been considerable interest in the pedunculopontine nucleus (PPN) as a DBS target (Stefani et al., 2007; Pereira et al., 2008).

Dystonic gait

An early common manifestation of dystonic gait is the inversion of the foot with walking. The great toe can be flexed or extended. It is an action dystonia and would not be present at rest. As the dystonia worsens, there can be more abnormal posturing of the legs, trunk, and arms. Sometimes there is so much abnormal movement that the gait looks like the dancing gait of chorea. The disorder is task-specific so that walking backward may be much better than walking forward, and running can be spared (Video 10.5). Dystonic gaits can look very unusual and care is needed to distinguish them from psychogenic. Camptocormia, flexion of the spine, is one such abnormal posture where a principal differential diagnosis is psychogenic. 🎥

Choreic gait

This gait is often called dancing gait and represents the superimposition of chorea on the locomotor movements. Stepping is also uncoordinated and appears dysmetric like an ataxic gait (Video 10.6). 🎥

Bouncing gait (myoclonus)

When myoclonus affects stance and gait, it gives rise to a characteristic bouncing (Video 10.7). The appearance is due more to frequent negative myoclonus than to positive myoclonus. 🎥

Highest level

The highest-level disorders come from malfunction of the cerebral hemispheres, and include disorders arising from psychiatric origin, including cautious gait and psychogenic gait. These disorders are not completely distinct from each other; patients may have characteristics of more than one or may progress from one to another (Jankovic et al., 2001; Nutt, 2001; Thompson, 2001).

Subcortical disequilibrium

This is a severe impairment of balance (Masdeu, 2001). The disorder arises from dysfunction at midbrain, basal ganglia, or thalamic levels, and is often a feature of parkinsonism-plus disorders. It has been called thalamic astasia. This entity, by its etiology, is really misplaced and belongs in the middle-level category. Perhaps it really represents a combined basal ganglionic and cerebellar balance disorder.

The next three conditions, frontal disequilibrium, isolated gait ignition failure, and frontal gait disorder, are frequently

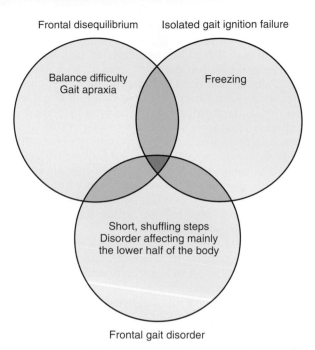

Figure 10.5 Relationship of the three different types of higher-level gait disorders arising from frontal lobe dysfunction. See text for more detail.

difficult to separate from each other and might be considered varied presentations of a frontal lobe dysfunction of gait (Figure 10.5).

Frontal disequilibrium

This is also characterized by a loss of balance, but is accompanied by disordered stepping that is difficult to describe. Some have called the stepping disorder "apraxia" (Gerstmann and Schilder, 1926) and others have called it "ataxia" (Bruns, 1892). The concept of apraxia comes from the observation that leg movements unrelated to walking seem reasonably good. It is also associated with frontal lobe signs, and it is this feature that suggests the frontal origin.

Isolated gait ignition failure

This is the particular difficulty in initiating and sustaining locomotion. The patient has freezing, particularly of the type getting started. The term primary progressive freezing gait has also been used (Factor et al., 2002). Balance can be good, and while steps begin short, they gradually increase in amplitude. Hence, the patient may say that they walk normally once they get started. This gradual increase differs from festination in that with festination, the stepping is never really normal looking.

Frontal gait disorder

These patients at first look like they have a parkinsonian gait, with short, shuffling steps, poor balance, initiation failure, and hesitations on turns (Video 10.8). Differentiating features are a more upright stance, lack of tremor, frontal lobe signs, and apparent involvement of only the lower part of the body (Thompson, 2001). This last feature gives rise to the term "lower half parkinsonism" or "lower body parkinsonism." The disorder can evolve to a frontal disequilibrium with the difficult-to-describe stepping disorder. The disorder does not respond to levodopa. 🎥

As noted, frontal disequilibrium, isolated gait ignition failure, and frontal gait disorder often overlap. Their etiologies are also similar and include subcortical arteriosclerotic encephalopathy (Binswanger disease), multi-infarct state, anterior cerebral artery stroke, normal pressure hydrocephalus, Pick disease, Alzheimer disease, frontotemporal dementia, subdural hematoma, brain tumor, multiple sclerosis, progressive supranuclear palsy (PSP), and corticobasal degeneration (Thompson, 2001). Older patients are more likely to have gait dysfunction if they have more white matter lesions on MRI (Franch et al., 2009). Two patients have been described with lesions predominant in the supplementary motor area (SMA) (Nadeau, 2007).

The gait in normal pressure hydrocephalus has been the most studied. These patients have freezing and gait apraxia. Quantitative gait studies show decreased stride length and reduced foot floor clearance (Stolze et al., 2000, 2001a). It is, of course, critical to make this diagnosis since it is a treatable disorder (McGirt et al., 2008). The diagnosis can be tricky at times and laboratory data must be used thoughtfully (Relkin et al., 2005). An evidence-based review suggested that the best test is prolonged external lumbar drainage in excess of 300 mL, which is associated with high sensitivity (50–100%) and high positive predictive value (80–100%) (Marmarou et al., 2005). The features of gait most responsive to lumbar drainage are walking speed, number of steps for turning, and tendency for falls (Ravdin et al., 2008). MRI features can be helpful, but are not as good as lumbar drainage (Lee et al., 2010). Identification of increased pulsatility of intracranial pressure might well also be of value (Eide and Sorteberg, 2010). One study has shown that the white matter lesions in patients will improve with shunting, suggesting that this aspect may play a role in the pathophysiology of the disorder (Akiguchi et al., 2008).

Increased ventricular dilation, even independent of a formal diagnosis of normal pressure hydrocephalus, is associated with gait impairment (Palm et al., 2009). An increased ratio of ventricular volume compared with sulcal cerebrospinal fluid volume predicted gait speed; this was independent of white matter hyperintensity volume.

In the series of 30 patients reported by Factor et al. (2002) under the name of primary progressive freezing gait, they found a clinically distinct, progressive neurologic disorder that primarily affected gait, initially resulting in freezing and later in postural instability. A wheelchair-bound state often developed within 5 years. It was accompanied by other parkinsonian features, particularly bradykinesia, but was unresponsive to dopaminergic medications. Because of its stereotyped manner, they suggested that it be considered a specific entity within the parkinsonism-plus disorders. Such patients may well have progressive supranuclear palsy (Williams et al., 2007).

Another classification of frontal gait disorders has been proposed: three main types based on presumptive sites of anatomical damage: (a) ignition apraxia, where damage is predominantly in the supplementary motor area and its connections, with good responses to external clues; (b) equilibrium apraxia, where damage is predominantly in the premotor area in its connections, with poor responses to external cues; and (c) mixed gait apraxia (Liston et al., 2003).

The authors of this proposal studied 13 patients with cerebral multi-infarct states and higher-level gait disorder and diagnosed 7 with ignition apraxia and 6 with equilibrium apraxia.

In some patients with frontal gait disorder at least one component of the difficulty may be due to orthostatic myoclonus–jerking of the legs only when standing (Glass et al., 2007). In 13 of 15 patients with postural unsteadiness due to this type of myoclonus, there was also a frontal gait disorder. Some of these patients improved with clonazepam.

While the term frontal gait disorder is used, it is not completely clear where the relevant pathology is. There is, in fact, some evidence for frontal dysfunction. For example, relevant white matter lesions leading to poor gait were largely in the frontal lobe (Srikanth et al., 2010). One study looked at SPECT scanning in patients with subcortical chronic vascular encephalopathy with and without walking. In those patients with gait dysfunction, there was less activation of the medial frontal gyrus bilaterally (as well as the anterior lobes of the cerebellum) (Carboncini et al., 2009). Dysfunction of the basal ganglio-thalamo-cortical loop may also play a role (Iseki et al., 2010).

Cautious gait

This is a common disorder, particularly in the elderly or with patients who have already experienced a fall for some reason (Kurlan, 2005; Sudarsky, 2006). The term "space phobia" has been used. Patients become cautious because of anxiety that they will fall. The gait is like what it would be for normal persons who are walking on ice. There is a wide base with slow, short steps; turns are en bloc. Arms are tense. Patients try to find support and when they have it, there is marked improvement. These individuals do not have overt freezing or shuffling.

Psychogenic gait

A gait disorder is a common way for psychogenic movement disorders to present (Lempert et al., 1991; Hayes et al., 1999; Bhatia, 2001; Morris et al., 2006; Sudarsky, 2006; Baik and Lang, 2007) (Video 10.9) This is also called astasia–abasia or acrobatic gait. There are unusual patterns of stance and gait, often inconsistent, often dramatic, with lurching, but only rarely falls (and then without hurting themselves). Sudden knee buckling without falling is a common pattern (Lempert et al., 1991). Extreme slow motion can be seen, and there is a sense that energy is being wasted. Camptocormia is one of the patterns that is commonly psychogenic (Skidmore et al., 2007). Careful observation will show that the person typically demonstrates excellent balance. There may well be wide fluctuations over short periods of time. As with other psychogenic movement disorders, positive psychiatric features are frequent and can be important in making a clear diagnosis. A possible clue to this is a suffering or strained facial expression, with moaning and hyperventilation (Lempert et al., 1991). 🎥

It was mentioned earlier, but worth noting again at this point, that disorders of gait are often multifactorial, particularly in elderly patients. It is useful to continue searching for etiologies even after one has been identified. This is certainly true of psychogenic gait as well since many of these patients have an organic neurologic disturbance.

Therapeutic considerations

As with other aspects of movement disorders, etiologic considerations come first. Is there a treatable neuropathy? Can vision be improved? Parkinson disease can be treated, as can normal pressure hydrocephalus. The second consideration would be symptomatic treatments. Physical therapy can help with strengthening exercises or practice with elemental coordination. There are a variety of walking aids from canes to walkers. There are weighted walkers and rolling walkers that help in special circumstances. It is also critical to know when to suggest that the patient no longer should be trying to walk without assistance. Falls are potentially disastrous, with broken hips and subdural hematomas as possible consequences.

References available on Expert Consult: www.expertconsult.com

CHAPTER 11

Stiffness syndromes

Chapter contents

Spasticity	250	Syndromes of continuous muscle activity	255
Stiff-person (stiff-man) syndrome	252		

Muscle stiffness may be the presenting symptom in many disorders of the motor nervous system and muscles (Table 11.1) (Rowland, 1985; Thompson, 1993, 1994; Brown and Marsden, 1999). Spasticity is the most classic, and the others must be distinguished from it. In this chapter, therefore, spasticity will be considered first. The stiff-person syndrome and its variants is perhaps the major entity confronting the movement disorder specialist, and it will be considered next. Stiffness can arise not only from dysfunction of the central nervous system but also from disorders where there is continuous muscle activity where the pathology lies in the muscle, nerve, or anterior horn cell. These conditions will be considered last.

Stiffness is assessed by the amount of force needed to get a movement. Tone, the more general clinical term, can be defined as the resistance to passive stretch of a joint. Normal tone is very low, and it is difficult to appreciate a decrease in tone, but some authorities say that they can detect a hypotonia in cerebellar dysfunction. Increased tone, hypertonia, is characteristic of several different states and can come from three theoretical mechanisms: (1) altered mechanical properties of the muscle or joint; (2) background co-contraction of muscles acting on the joint; and (3) increase in reflex response to the stretch opposing the movement (Hallett, 1999, 2000). A clear example of altered mechanical properties is contracture. Increased background contraction is often seen with difficulty in relaxation, such as commonly characterizes Parkinson's disease. There are many different reflexes that can occur in response to stretch and these can help differentiate different states of hypertonia. In differentiating spasticity and rigidity, in simple terms, spasticity shows exaggerated short latency reflexes and rigidity shows exaggerated long latency reflexes.

Spasticity

Spasticity is a form of hypertonia with a number of characteristic features (Benecke et al., 2002; Sheean, 2002; Sanger et al., 2003). The increased resistance to stretch is velocity sensitive; there is more resistance the faster the joint is moved. There may be a clasped-knife phenomenon where the resistance increases and then suddenly gives way. There are also several other "positive" features such as increased tendon jerks, clonus, increased flexor reflexes, spontaneous flexor spasms, and abnormal postures (spastic dystonia). Importantly, there are also "negative" features including weakness (in a "pyramidal distribution"), fatigue, loss of coordination, and a decrease of some cutaneous reflexes. It can be noted that the increased stiffness can be valuable to a patient with significant weakness, as it might, for example, allow the patient to stand.

Loosely, neurologists usually say that spasticity arises from a lesion in the pyramidal tract or that it is from damage to the "upper motor neuron." The first seems false and the second is vague. Supraspinal control of movement is complicated and consists of many tracts. Briefly, those fibers that go through the pyramid arise from the cortex and go to the spinal cord and can be called also the corticospinal tract (Wiesendanger, 1984; Davidoff, 1990). Approximately 30% of those fibers arise from the primary motor cortex; there are also significant contributions from premotor cortex and sensory cortex. The fibers largely cross in the pyramid, but some remain uncrossed. Some terminate as monosynaptic projections onto alpha-motoneurons, and others terminate on interneurons including those in the dorsal horn. Other cortical neurons project to basal ganglia, cerebellum, and brainstem; these structures can also originate spinal projections. Particularly important is the reticular formation that originates several tracts with different functions (Nathan et al., 1996). The dorsal reticulospinal tract may have particular relevance for spasticity and is normally inhibitory onto the spinal cord (Habaguchi et al., 2002; Takakusaki et al., 2001, 2003). Thinking about the cortical innervation of the reticular formation, it is possible to speak of a cortico-reticulo-spinal tract. Lesions of the primary motor area alone and lesions of the pyramid alone do not cause spasticity (Sherman et al., 2000). It appears that premotor damage is

DOI: 10.1016/B978-1-4377-2369-4.00011-1

Table 11.1 Causes of muscle stiffness, cramps, spasms, rigidity, or contracture

Cerebral – brainstem

Encephalitis lethargica

Torsion dystonia

Akinetic–rigid syndromes

Spinal cord

Stiff-person syndrome (also supraspinal abnormalities)

Toxins

    Tetanus

    Strychnine poisoning

    Black widow spider bite

Inflammatory myelitis

    Progressive encephalomyelitis with rigidity

    Subacute myoclonic spinal neuronitis

    Borrelia burgdorferi infection

Traumatic myelopathy

Spinal cord neoplasm (intrinsic)

Ischemic myelopathy

Spinal arteriovenous malformation

Cervical spondylotic myelopathy

Peripheral nerve

Neuromyotonia (myokymia with impaired muscle relaxation)

    Idiopathic

    Isaacs syndrome

    Paraneoplastic syndrome

    Hereditary motor and sensory neuropathies

    Inflammatory neuropathies

    Toxic neuropathies

    Radiation plexopathies

    Paroxysmal ataxia and myokymia

Morvan syndrome (Morvan's fibrillary chorea)

Episodic ataxia type 1

Hereditary distal muscle cramps without neuropathy

Tetany (hypocalcemia, hypomagnesemia)

Cramps

    Post-exertion

    Dehydration/Salt depletion

Pregnancy

Denervation (motor neuron disease, motor neuropathies)

Cause unknown

Muscle

Myotonic syndromes

    Myotonic dystrophy

    Myotonia congenita

    Paramyotonia congenita

Metabolic myopathies

    Myophosphorylase deficiency (McArdle disease)

    Phosphofructokinase deficiency

    Ca^{2+} ATPase deficiency (Brody disease)

Inflammatory myopathies

    Polymyositis

Endocrine myopathies

    Hypothyroidism

    Addison disease

Congenital myopathies

    Stiff-spine syndrome

    Emery–Dreifuss muscular dystrophy

    Bethlem muscular dystrophy

Schwartz–Jampel syndrome

Other conditions presumed to be muscular in origin

    Rippling muscle disease

    Rolling muscle disease

Unknown origin

Satoyoshi syndrome

Contracture

Bone (ankylosis)

    Arthritis

    Ankylosing spondylitis

Soft tissue

    Volkmann ischemic contracture

---

necessary and likely involvement of cortico-reticulo-spinal pathways. Dysfunction of the dorsal reticulospinal tract will disinhibit the spinal cord and may give rise to the hyperexcitability characteristic of spasticity. The term "corticofugal syndrome" has been suggested to indicate that "spasticity" has important negative as well as positive features and that the lesions involve descending tracts other than the corticospinal tracts, but it is not commonly accepted (Thilmann, 1993).

The clinical and physiologic features of spasticity differ to some degree depending on whether the lesion is cortical or spinal. Spasticity seen in hemiparesis differs from that seen with spinal cord lesions. For example, exaggeration of flexor reflexes is much more likely with spinal lesions. This certainly must come from the difference in the exact pattern of damage to the descending tracts.

The neurologic syndromes where spasticity can be seen are numerous. These include stroke, spinal cord injury, brain trauma, cerebral palsy, and demyelinating illnesses such as multiple sclerosis. Spasticity can also be a part of degenerative disorders such as amyotrophic lateral sclerosis. In primary lateral sclerosis or hereditary spastic paraplegia, spasticity is the primary feature. A variety of degenerative movement disorders such as the ataxias often include some spasticity.

Clinical features of spasticity that help with the diagnosis, in addition to the velocity-dependent increased tone, include brisk tendon reflexes, the Babinski sign, Hoffman reflex (indicating brisk finger flexor reflexes), and loss of cutaneous abdominal reflexes. The negative features will often be seen as well, with weakness in the lower extremities of flexors more than extensors and in the upper extremities of extensors more than flexors. In the clinical neurophysiology laboratory, there will be increased H reflexes, identified with an increase of the maximum amplitude H reflex compared to the M wave (muscle response to direct supramaximal stimulation of the nerve), called the H/M ratio (Hallett, 1999, 2000; Benecke et al., 2002). There is also a diminished decrease of the H reflex with vibration of the body part. Characteristics of the tonic stretch reflex can also be assessed for threshold and gain to stretches of varying velocity. In spasticity, there is some controversy, but both lowered velocity threshold and an increased gain have been found (Powers et al., 1988; Katz and Rymer, 1989; Thilmann et al., 1991; Ibrahim et al., 1993; Musampa et al., 2007). It is important to recognize that there are both reflex and nonreflex contributions to spastic hypertonia (Chung et al., 2008).

There are many methods to treat spasticity, but this must be done carefully as correction of the positive features may not be all that helpful, and, as noted before, may even be detrimental. For many patients, the much more important aspects of their corticofugal syndrome are the negative features such as the weakness and these cannot be dealt with easily. Increased tone can be improved with a variety of oral agents including benzodiazepines, baclofen, and tizanidine (Krach, 2001; Abbruzzese, 2002; Ronan and Gold, 2007; Kamen et al., 2008). Baclofen can be given intrathecally by pump, and this can be much more efficacious, likely because of the ability to increase the dose at the target tissue without side effects (Ivanhoe et al., 2001; Albright et al., 2003; Dykstra et al., 2007; Rietman and Geertzen, 2007; Saval and Chiodo, 2010). Tolperisone has been evaluated in patients after stroke (Stamenova et al., 2005) and might be another consideration (Quasthoff et al., 2008).

Direct blockade of muscle contraction with agents such as phenol has been used for some time and the introduction of botulinum toxin for this purpose has been welcomed with enthusiasm (Boyd and Hays, 2001; Moore, 2002; Barnes, 2003; Mancini et al., 2005; Mohammadi et al., 2009). An evidence-based review gave botulinum toxin its highest recommendation for treatment in both adults and children (Simpson et al., 2008). For post-stroke spasticity, there is very good evidence for reduction of spasticity. Evidence is developing for an increase in functional ability (Elia et al., 2009; McCrory et al., 2009; Foley et al., 2010; Fridman et al., 2010; Sun et al., 2010), but often this is rather limited (Kaji et al., 2010). Children with cerebral palsy can be much improved (Baird and Vargus-Adams, 2009; Kanellopoulos et al., 2009; Lukban et al., 2009; Coutinho Dos Santos et al., 2011), but are a vulnerable population and need to be treated with care (Albavera-Hernandez et al., 2009). Several evidence-based reviews document the utility of botulinum toxin for this indication (Delgado et al., 2010; Hoare et al., 2010). It is interesting to note that the effect of botulinum toxin is mediated not only on the alpha motoneuron neuromuscular junction but also via the gamma motoneuron effect on the muscle spindle (Trompetto et al., 2008). Surgical methods such as rhizotomy can also be used in some cases for symptomatic relief of severe spasticity (Lazorthes et al., 2002).

Stiff-person (stiff-man) syndrome

The stiff-person syndrome (originally called the stiff-man syndrome) (Table 11.2) consists of progressive fluctuating muscular rigidity (Moersch and Woltman, 1956; Blum and Jankovic, 1991; Thompson, 1993, 1994; Stayer and

Table 11.2 Criteria for the diagnosis of the stiff-person syndrome

Clinical

Gradual onset of aching and tightness of axial muscles

Slow progression; stiffness spreads from axial muscles to limbs (legs > arms)

Persistent contraction of thoracolumbar paraspinal and abdominal muscles

Abnormal hyperlordotic posture of lumbar spine

Board-like rigidity of abdominal muscles

Rigidity abolished by sleep

Stimulus-sensitive painful muscle spasms

No other abnormal neurologic signs

Intellect normal

Cranial muscles rarely (if ever) involved

Neurophysiologic

Continuous motor unit activity at rest

EMG activity abolished by sleep, peripheral nerve block, spinal or general anesthesia

Normal peripheral nerve conduction

Normal motor unit morphology

Disturbed exteroceptive reflexes and reciprocal inhibition

Exaggerated startle reflex

Other observations that may be helpful but are of uncertain diagnostic specificity

Autoantibodies directed against GABAergic neurons, in particular to GAD

Increased CSF IgG and oligoclonal bands in some

Association with autoimmune endocrine disease (e.g., diabetes, pernicious anemia, vitiligo, hypothyroidism)

Epilepsy in 10%

Meinck, 1998; Brown and Marsden, 1999; Levy et al., 1999; Thompson, 2001; Meinck and Thompson, 2002). Typically, the rigidity affects axial muscles of the back, abdomen, hips, and shoulders, causing excessive lordosis with prominent contraction of paraspinal muscles, a "board-like" abdomen, and stiffness of the legs on walking (Fig. 11.1) (Video 11.1). Superimposed upon this continuous stiffness are spasms provoked by excitement, anxiety, voluntary movement, sudden noise, or peripheral stimuli. These spasms can be intensely painful and forceful such as to fracture bones or dislocate joints. Voluntary movement can provoke similar spasms that sometimes may cause falls "like a wooden man."

The syndrome usually begins in the fourth and fifth decades and affects men and women equally. The onset of the illness usually is gradual with increasing painful tightness, stiffness, clumsiness of the trunk and legs, and limitation of range of motion (Fig. 11.2). On examination there is continuous muscular contraction of the paraspinal and abdominal muscles, but there are no other neurologic signs, other than brisk reflexes. The illness is slowly progressive with stiffness spreading from the trunk to hip and then shoulder muscles, but the face and distal limbs usually are spared. Sphincter function is normal. While the onset of the disorder seems typically spontaneous, one case has been

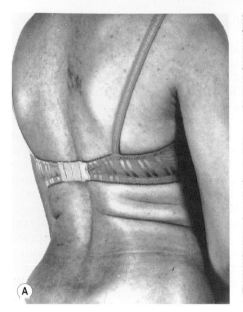 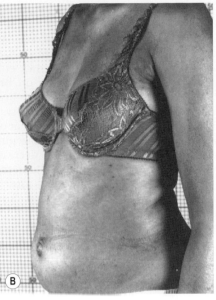

Figure 11.1 Patient with stiff-person syndrome. Note the marked lumbar lordosis (**A**) and the prominent abdomen (**B**). *Photos courtesy of Dr M. Dalakas.*

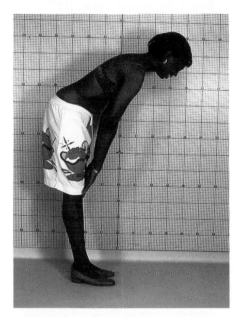

Figure 11.2 Patient with stiff-person syndrome. Note the limitation in bending forward. *Photo courtesy of Dr M. Dalakas.*

reported where the onset appears to have been triggered by West Nile fever (Hassin-Baer et al., 2004). There has also been a report of a father and daughter, each with anti-GAD-positive stiff-person syndrome (Burns et al., 2003).

Electromyography shows continuous normal motor unit activity, despite attempted relaxation, with no signs of denervation and normal peripheral motor and sensory nerve conduction velocity. Other physiologic abnormalities include exaggerated, non-habituating exteroceptive or cutaneomuscular reflexes, brainstem myoclonus, and an exaggerated startle reflex ("jerking stiff-man") (Leigh et al., 1980; Meinck et al., 1983; Matsumoto et al., 1994; Meinck et al., 1995; Stayer and Meinck, 1998; Brown and Marsden, 1999).

Insulin-dependent diabetes mellitus occurs in up to two-thirds of patients. Diabetic ketoacidosis is the commonest

cause of death in such patients. Other autoimmune endocrine diseases include thyroid disease, pernicious anemia, and vitiligo (Solimena et al., 1990). Epilepsy occurs in 10% of cases, although this is debatable.

A central, perhaps spinal cord origin for the spasms, rigidity, and continuous motor unit activity is suggested by their disappearance after peripheral nerve block, sleep, and general anesthesia. Other neurophysiologic tests suggest that spinal motoneuron excitability is normal and that the condition is due to defective input of inhibitory pathways onto motoneurons. To test inhibitory spinal circuits in patients, Floeter et al. (1998) used H-reflexes to test reciprocal inhibition in the forearm and thigh, vibration-induced inhibition of flexor carpi radialis and soleus H-reflexes, recurrent inhibition, and nonreciprocal (1b) inhibition of soleus H-reflexes. Vibration-induced inhibition of H-reflexes was diminished in eight of nine patients tested, but the presynaptic period of reciprocal inhibition was normal in most patients. Both circuits are presumed to involve presynaptic inhibition and GABAergic interneurons. Presumed glycinergic circuits, including the first period of reciprocal inhibition and nonreciprocal (1b) inhibition, showed occasional abnormalities. Recurrent inhibition was normal in all five patients tested. It appears that some, but not all, populations of GABAergic neurons are affected. The involvement of presumptive glycinergic circuits in some patients could point to impairment of non-GABAergic neurons, unrecognized involvement of GABAergic neurons in these inhibitory circuits, or, more likely, alterations of supraspinal systems that exert descending control over spinal circuits. Studies of cortical excitability with transcranial magnetic stimulation show decreased intracortical inhibition likely due to loss of GABA function at this level (Sandbrink et al., 2000). Hyperexcitability of the brainstem has been demonstrated by increased R2 recovery in the blink reflex recovery curve (Molloy et al., 2002). Direct measurement of GABA with magnetic resonance spectroscopy shows a deficiency in the sensorimotor cortex (Levy et al., 2005). There is also a cortical loss of flumazenil binding, a measure of postsynaptic benzodiazepine receptors associated with GABA receptors (Perani et al., 2007; Galldiks et al., 2008).

The significance of the association of insulin-dependent diabetes mellitus with the stiff-person syndrome has been emphasized by the discovery of antibodies directed against glutamic acid decarboxylase (GAD), the enzyme responsible for the synthesis of GABA, in both blood and cerebrospinal fluid in 60% or more of patients (Solimena et al., 1990; Walikonis and Lennon, 1998). The great majority of these patients also have antibodies directed against pancreatic islet cells, as well as gastric parietal cells and the thyroid. The anti-GAD antibodies are the same as those found in insulin-dependent diabetes mellitus, but it appears that the antibodies do have subtle differences (Lohmann et al., 2000). Currently the best test is the radioimmunoassay for GAD65 (Walikonis and Lennon, 1998). The luciferase immunoprecipitation technology (LIPS) seems also to be very good for this purpose (Burbelo et al., 2008). Present evidence raises the possibility that the anti-GAD antibodies may destroy GABAergic inhibitory mechanisms in the spinal cord, but, alternatively, they may be secondary to some other process leading to an appropriate immunologic response (Raju et al., 2005; Raju and Hampe, 2008). Anti-GAD antibodies have been demonstrated to block GABAergic neurotransmission in rat cerebellar slices (Ishida et al., 1999; Mitoma et al., 2000). One study reported that motor cortex excitability correlated with antibody levels suggesting an etiologic role (Koerner et al., 2004). In a study of 18 patients with stiff-person syndrome and serum antibodies, all had high titers as well in the cerebrospinal fluid (CSF) and 11 of 13 patients had an increased anti-GAD(65)-specific IgG index (Dalakas et al., 2001b). In the same study, the mean level of GABA in the CSF was found to be lower in patients than in controls. On the other hand, the levels of antibodies do not correlate with the severity of the disorder (Rakocevic et al., 2004).

The role of anti-GAD antibodies continues to be somewhat confusing, in part because they are not specific to stiff-person syndrome. In one study of 61 neurologic patients with high antibody titers, 22 (36%) had stiff-person syndrome and 17 (28%) had cerebellar ataxia (Saiz et al., 2008). Intrathecal synthesis of antibody gives more assurance that the antibody might be relevant (Jarius et al., 2010).

Another antibody found in a large number of patients is that directed against GABA(A) receptor-associated protein (GABARAP) (Raju et al., 2006; Dalakas, 2008, 2009). This has been identified in up to 65% of patients. Such antibodies would inhibit GABA(A) receptor expression on GABAergic neurons and certainly would be pathophysiologically relevant.

Stiff-person syndrome can also be seen in association with anti-amphiphysin I antibodies in patients with breast cancer (Saiz et al., 1999; Wessig et al., 2003). Anti-amphiphysin antibodies can block GABAergic neurotransmission (Geis et al., 2010). A report of 11 patients with anti-amphiphysin antibodies found that all were women, and 10 had breast cancer (Murinson and Guarnaccia, 2008). Average age was 60, and cervical involvement was particularly prominent. Marked improvement was seen in three of five patients with tumor excision and chemotherapy. Other neurologic disorders such as sensory neuropathy, cerebellar ataxia, and opsoclonus may be present as well, and the syndrome can occur with other tumor types (Antoine et al., 1999). Another antibody in some cases is directed against 17-beta-hydroxysteroid dehydrogenase type 4 (Dinkel et al., 2002).

Oligoclonal bands have been reported in the CSF in a number of cases (Meinck and Ricker, 1987; Williams et al., 1988; Meinck et al., 1994), and white matter lesions have been seen on brain MRI. However, so far no consistent pathology has been demonstrated in the few cases that have come to autopsy.

The treatment of this condition relies upon a combination of benzodiazepines and baclofen in high dosage. These drugs may decrease the superimposed severe spasms, but are not entirely effective in controlling the background sustained continuous muscle hyperactivity. Sodium valproate and tizanidine have also been reported to be beneficial (Meinck and Conrad, 1986; Stayer and Meinck, 1998). Intrathecal baclofen has been used (Silbert et al., 1995; Stayer et al., 1997; Stayer and Meinck, 1998). Patients have been reported to respond to steroid therapy (Blum and Jankovic, 1991), intravenous human immunoglobulin (IVIg) infusions (Khanlou and Eiger, 1999; Souza-Lima et al., 2000), and plasmapheresis (Vicari et al., 1989; Blum and Jankovic, 1991; Brashear and Phillips, 1991; Hayashi et al., 1999), but others have gained no benefit from plasmapheresis (Harding et al., 1989). A double-blind, placebo-controlled study documented the value of IVIg (Dalakas et al., 2001a). Another study has shown improvement in quality of life with IVIg (Gerschlager and Brown, 2002). Rituximab has been reported to be useful in a few patients (Bacorro and Tehrani, 2010; Dupond et al., 2010; Katoh et al., 2010).

Progressive encephalomyelitis with rigidity, sometimes known as spinal interneuronitis, may present with similar clinical features to the stiff-person syndrome. However, such patients go on to develop a relentless and progressive course, with the emergence of cranial nerve dysfunction producing bulbar symptoms and disorders of eye movement, along with cognitive impairment and long tract signs (Whiteley et al., 1976; Howell et al., 1979; Brown and Marsden, 1999; Gouider-Khouja et al., 2002). The condition may be isolated, or may occur in the setting of neoplasia associated with the pathologic changes of paraneoplastic encephalomyelitis (Roobol et al., 1987; Bateman et al., 1990).

The condition may start at any age in adults (Kraemer and Berlit, 2008). Initial symptoms may be those of pain, dysesthesia or sensory loss in the limbs, or weakness, stiffness, clumsiness, and rigidity. Extensor trunk spasm and/or brainstem myoclonus may be striking (Video 11.2). The tendon reflexes often are absent and the plantar responses are extensor. Nystagmus, opsoclonus, ophthalmoplegia, deafness, dysarthria, and dysphagia can occur. The illness usually leads to death within about 3 years. As in the stiff-person syndrome, there is continuous motor unit activity with particular involvement of trunk muscles, which disappears after a peripheral nerve or spinal nerve root block, or general anesthesia. EMG exploration may reveal evidence of denervation of muscles. A few have reticular reflex myoclonus. Progressive myoclonus with rigidity and myoclonus has been called PERM. Some of these patients may also exhibit anti-GAD (Burn et al., 1991), or antineuronal (anti-Ri) antibodies (Casado et al., 1994). The CSF may contain a lymphocytic pleocytosis, elevated protein and immunoglobulin levels, and oligoclonal IgG bands. MRI may show brainstem atrophy and altered signal in the brainstem and spinal cord.

Pathologic examination has shown widespread encephalomyelitis with perivascular lymphocytic cuffing and infiltration, associated with neuronal loss throughout the brainstem and spinal cord, mainly involving interneurons. The relation of progressive encephalomyelitis with rigidity to the classic stiff-person syndrome, particularly in those with anti-GAD antibodies, remains to be established (Brown and Marsden, 1999). Antibodies to the glycine receptor have also been described (Hutchinson et al., 2008; Mas et al., 2010). A model of the disease in mice can be produced by glutamic acid decarboxylase-specific CD4(+) T cells, and this suggests that cellular immunity may play an important role (Burton et al., 2010).

As with the stiff-person syndrome, treatment is with high doses of diazepam and baclofen. One case, with evidence of myelitis on spinal cord biopsy, improved on steroids (McCombe et al., 1989). Rituximab has also been used (Saidha et al., 2008).

Spinal alpha rigidity is a related condition resulting from isolation of spinal motor neurons from inhibitory interneuronal control (Gelfan and Tarlov, 1959). Examples have been described with trauma, cord vascular disease, cord tumors, and syringomyelia, as well as with myelitis. Most of these lesions have involved the cervical cord. Characteristically, there are stimulus-induced spasms, rigidity and abnormal limb postures involving rigid adduction, extension, and internal rotation of the affected body parts. These postures are produced by continuous motor activity which is not influenced by voluntary effort. In addition, there is wasting, weakness and loss of tendon reflexes in the arms, with long tract signs in their legs.

A variant of the stiff-person syndrome has been recognized, namely the *"stiff leg" syndrome* (Brown et al., 1997; Barker et al., 1998; Brown and Marsden, 1999; Fiol et al., 2001; Gurol et al., 2001; Bartsch et al., 2003). In contrast to the classic stiff-person, where continuous motor unit activity affects the back and thighs, those with the stiff-leg syndrome present with stiffness and painful spasms of one or both legs, which are rigid and dystonic. EMG findings are characteristic with continuous motor unit activity at rest, spasms of repetitive grouped discharges, and abnormal cutaneomuscular reflexes. Anti-GAD antibodies are present in about 15% of cases. Whether this is a partial syndrome or a separate disorder is debated. The prognosis is generally relatively benign with absence of other neurologic symptoms and signs for up to 16 years, but other cases can progress to the syndrome of progressive encephalomyelitis with rigidity (Gouider-Khouja et al., 2002).

Syndromes of continuous muscle activity

Continuous muscle fiber activity or neuromyotonia

A variety of disorders of peripheral nerve origin may produce continuous muscle activity causing stiffness and cramps (Table 11.3). This condition has been described as "continuous muscle fiber activity or Isaacs syndrome" (Isaacs, 1961), "neuromyotonia" (Mertens and Zschocke, 1965), "myokymia with impaired muscle relaxation" (Gardner-Medwin and Walton, 1969), or "pseudomyotonia and myokymia"

Table 11.3 Neuromyotonia

Clinical
Gradual onset of muscle stiffness at rest
Continuous twitching (fasciculation) or rippling (myokymia)
Cramps and delayed relaxation (pseudomyotonia)
Mainly distal (carpopedal)
Sweating
Possible peripheral neuropathy
Treatment: carbamazepine, phenytoin, procainamide, plasmapheresis

EMG
Continuous motor unit activity
Persists in sleep and after nerve block
Fasciculations
Grouped high-frequency discharges
After discharges
Denervation changes
Nerve conduction studies abnormal

Causes
Idiopathic (autoimmune, K^+ channels of nerve membrane)
Paraneoplastic
Peripheral neuropathies
Hereditary motor and sensory neuropathy, types I and II
Inflammatory
Toxic
Radiation plexopathies

(Hughes and Matthews, 1969). This variable terminology reflects the overlap between the clinical and electromyographic use of terms such as myokymia (a wave-like rippling of muscle or motor unit discharges in doublets or triplets) and neuromyotonia (delayed muscle relaxation or high-frequency EMG discharges).

The characteristic and fairly stereotyped clinical picture of this condition is the gradual onset of muscle stiffness at rest, with continuous twitching (fasciculation) or rippling (myokymia) of muscles, with cramps following voluntary contractions due to delay in muscle relaxation (pseudomyotonia). Pain is rare, but muscle aching is common. The distribution of muscle contraction often is predominantly distal (in contrast to the axial involvement in stiff-person syndrome), producing a pseudo-tetany picture. However, proximal and cranial muscles can be affected. Involvement can be focal, as exemplified by one patient who presented with finger flexion that resembled focal hand dystonia (Jamora et al., 2006). The symptoms of muscle contraction, often accompanied by profuse sweating, persist during sleep, and following peripheral nerve or spinal nerve root block, or general anesthesia. The continuous muscle fiber activity is abolished by peripheral neuromuscular blockade with curare, indicating its origin at the neuromuscular junction.

In many cases there are clinical signs and electrophysiologic findings of a peripheral neuropathy. Muscles may be wasted and weak as well as exhibiting rippling myokymia and fasciculations. Sometimes there is muscular hypertrophy. Despite the pseudomyotonia, there is no percussion myotonia. The tendon reflexes are absent and there may be appropriate sensory loss. The serum creatine phosphokinase is raised.

The condition can be inherited (Ashizawa et al., 1983; Auger et al., 1984), or sporadic (Isaacs, 1961; Gardner-Medwin and Walton, 1969), may occur as a result of a paraneoplastic process (Walsh, 1976; Lahrmann et al., 2001), or thymoma with acetylcholine receptor antibodies with or without myasthenia gravis (Halbach et al., 1987; Garcia-Merino et al., 1991), or be associated with many types of inherited (Vasilescu et al., 1984b; Hahn et al., 1991), inflammatory (Valenstein et al., 1978; Vasilescu et al., 1984a), or metabolic (Wallis et al., 1970; Vasilescu and Florescu, 1982) peripheral neuropathies. A case has been described in the setting of lupus (Taylor, 2005). A search for a remote neoplasm is required.

An autoimmune basis for neuromyotonia has been demonstrated in those with no obvious precipitating cause, on the basis of antibodies to specific nerve membrane voltage-gated potassium ion channels (VGKC) (Sinha et al., 1991; Shillito et al., 1995; Nagado et al., 1999; Hart, 2000; Hayat et al., 2000; Arimura et al., 2002; Vernino and Lennon, 2002; Lang and Vincent, 2003; Newsom-Davis et al., 2003). Indeed, it seems that the autoimmune production of antibodies to voltage-gated potassium channels is the common thread for all the etiologies (Rueff et al., 2008).

Electrophysiologically, the hallmark of the syndrome is the presence of continuous motor unit activity that persists during sleep and usually following peripheral nerve block. This continuous muscle activity may originate in proximal nerve segments (when distal nerve block suppresses activity) or distal segments (when nerve block has no effect). The motor unit activity often is increased by hyperventilation or ischemia. Fasciculations and grouped high-frequency discharges are evident on electromyography, with repetitive bursts of motor units of normal appearance (myokymia) (Fig. 11.3) and also bizarre high-frequency (150–300 Hz) discharges (neuromyotonia) (Fig. 11.4). Prolonged high frequency after discharges following nerve stimulation, voluntary contraction, or muscle percussion are characteristic. Evidence of muscle denervation and reinnervation may be found, and measurement of peripheral nerve motor and sensory conduction may confirm the presence of peripheral neuropathy.

Carbamazepine and phenytoin may be successful in abolishing most of the symptoms of neuromyotonia and continuous muscle fiber activity. When the disorder is autoimmune, plasmapheresis may be effective (Hayat et al., 2000; Nakatsuji et al., 2000) as may IVIg (Alessi et al., 2000).

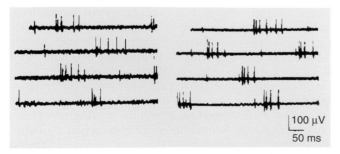

Figure 11.3 Two examples of myokymic discharges as might be seen in patients with neuromyotonia. *From Kimura J. Electrodiagnosis in Diseases of Nerve and Muscle: Principles and Practice. Philadelphia: F.A. Davis; 1984, with permission.*

Neuromyotonia without malignancy or peripheral neuropathy may prove to be relatively benign (Isaacs and Heffron, 1974; Wilton and Gardner-Medwin, 1990). Focal neuromyotonia can be treated with injection of botulinum toxin (Hobson et al., 2009).

Myokymia is also a feature of episodic ataxia type 1 (EA-1). In this disorder, the myokymia is prominent around the eyes or lips or in the fingers. See Chapters 21 and 22 for more details.

Morvan syndrome (Morvan's fibrillary chorea) is a disorder related to neuromyotonia (Kleopa et al., 2006). It is characterized by generalized myokymia, burning pain, cramping, weakness, pruritus, hyperhidrosis, weight loss, sleeplessness, and hallucinations (Madrid et al., 1996; Bajaj and Shrestha, 2007). Some cases are of unknown cause, but others are associated with mercury intoxication, chrysotherapy, thymoma, and other remote neoplasms. In one case with thymoma, muscle histopathology disclosed chronic denervation and myopathic changes and in-vitro electrophysiology demonstrated both presynaptic and postsynaptic defects in neuromuscular transmission (Lee et al., 1998). Probably most cases are associated with increased antibodies to voltage-gated potassium channels (Liguori et al., 2001; Kleopa et al., 2006). Other serum antibodies, such as those to acetylcholine receptors, titin, and N-type calcium channels, can also be detected. Plasmapheresis (Liguori et al., 2001), thymectomy, and long-term immunosuppression may induce a dramatic resolution of symptoms.

Rippling muscle disease is an autosomal dominant inherited disorder of skeletal muscle in which patients present with muscle cramps, pain, stiffness especially on exercise, and exhibit a characteristic lateral rolling movement of muscle after contraction and balling of muscle on percussion (Stephan et al., 1994; Vorgerd et al., 1999; Torbergsen, 2002). In one family with 11 affected members, muscle stiffness and myalgia were the most prominent symptoms (So et al., 2001). Muscle rippling was present in only 6 of affected family members, whereas persistent muscle contraction to muscle percussion was present in all affected adults. Phenotypes clearly vary in the same family (Jacobi et al., 2010). Curiously, EMG shows normal recruitment and motor unit potentials. One hypothesis is that the abnormal muscle contractions are evoked by "silent" action potentials traveling in the muscle's tubular system (Lamb, 2005). In a genetic study of five families, a genome-wide linkage analysis identified a locus on chromosome 3p25 with missense mutations in *CAV3* (encoding caveolin 3) (Betz et al., 2001). Other cases with mutations in the same gene have been found (Vorgerd et al., 2001; Lorenzoni et al., 2007; Traverso et al., 2008). Mutations in *CAV3* have also been described in limb-girdle muscular dystrophy type 1C (LGMD1C) and other neuromuscular syndromes, again demonstrating that different phenotypes can come from mutations in the same gene (Sotgia et al., 2003; Woodman et al., 2004; Aboumousa et al., 2008; Gazzerro et al., 2010). This disorder can be associated with myasthenia gravis and might be improved with immunosuppression (Muller-Felber et al., 1999; Schoser et al., 2009). Indeed, it appears that rippling muscle disease can be immune-mediated without a mutation in the *CAV3* gene (Schulte-Mattler et al., 2005).

Schwartz–Jampel syndrome (chondrodystrophic myotonia) is a rare familial condition, usually occurring with an

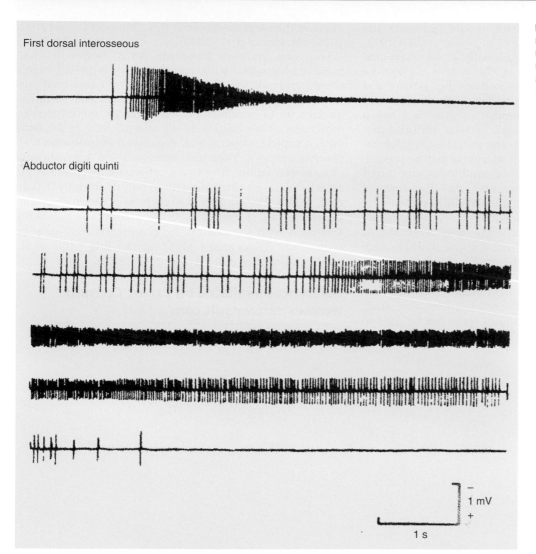

First dorsal interosseous

Abductor digiti quinti

1 mV

1 s

Figure 11.4 Two examples of neuromyotonic discharges as might be seen in patients with neuromyotonia. *From AAEM. Glossary of terms in electromyography. Muscle Nerve 1987;10(8S):G1–G60, with permission.*

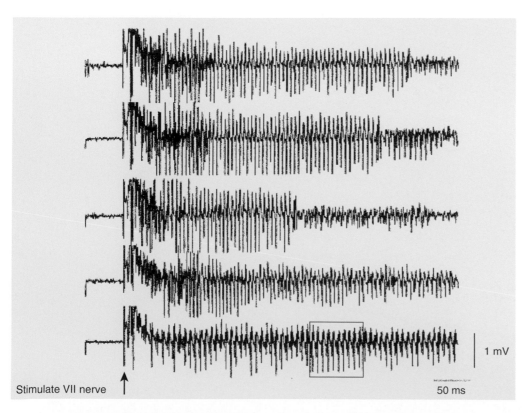

Stimulate VII nerve

50 ms

1 mV

Figure 11.5 Example of EMG discharge from a patient with Schwartz–Jampel syndrome. The discharge is triggered by stimulation of the seventh nerve. *From Thompson PD. Stiff people. In: Marsden CD, Fahn S, eds. Movement Disorders 3. Oxford: Butterworth-Heinemann; 1994, pp. 373–405, with permission.*

autosomal recessive pattern of inheritance (Schwartz and Jampel, 1962; Taylor et al., 1972; Fowler et al., 1974; Fontaine et al., 1996), but occasionally as an autosomal dominant trait (Pascuzzi et al., 1990; Spaans, 1991). The typical picture is of continuous muscle fiber activity and muscle stiffness, especially of the face, with an abnormal facial appearance (blepharophimosis, a small jaw and a puckered chin, and low-set ears), skeletal abnormalities (spondylo-epiphyseal dysplasia), and short stature (Nahara-jakumar et al., 2006). Percussion myotonia may be present. The muscle stiffness is due to semi-continuous motor unit discharges, with high frequency and after-discharges of muscle fibers (Fig. 11.5). These abnormalities persist after ischemia and curare (Spaans et al., 1990). An abnormality of muscle fiber sodium channels has been demonstrated (Lehmann-Horn et al., 1990). Procainamide abolishes such abnormal muscle activity (Lehmann-Horn et al., 1990). In a number of patients, a mutation in the gene for perlecan, the major proteoglycan of basement membranes, has been identified (Nicole et al., 2000; Arikawa-Hirasawa et al., 2002; Stum et al., 2006). Botulinum toxin can be used to improve the blepharospasm in this condition (Vargel et al., 2006; Aburahma et al., 2009).

Satoyoshi syndrome (Satoyoshi, 1978) begins in childhood or adolescence with severe intermittent painful muscle spasms and twitches, twisting the body into abnormal postures. The spasms last up to a few minutes and occur frequently, up to hundreds per day. They are precipitated by movement or stimulation of the affected area. At the same time, complete alopecia and intestinal malabsorption with diarrhea develops. There also is metaphyseal dysplasia with growth retardation. It may also affect adults (Ikeda et al., 1998). One case had manifestations only unilaterally (Uddin et al., 2002). The etiology is likely to be a systemic autoimmune disorder (Heger et al., 2006; Matsuura et al., 2007). Treatment with steroids can be effective (Wisuthsarewong et al., 2001; Endo et al., 2003), as can IVIg (Arita et al., 1996) and methotrexate (Heger et al., 2006).

References available on Expert Consult: www.expertconsult.com

CHAPTER **12**

Dystonia
Phenomenology, classification, etiology, pathology, biochemistry, and genetics

Chapter contents

Historical highlights	259	Dopa-responsive dystonia (DRD)	280
Impact and overview of genetic discoveries	261	Rapid-onset dystonia–parkinsonism (RDP)	283
Phenomenology of dystonic movements	262	Myoclonus–dystonia	284
Epidemiology	265	Secondary dystonias	285
Classification of torsion dystonia	266	Lubag (X-linked dystonia–parkinsonism, XDP)	286
Pseudodystonia	277	Pathophysiology and pathoanatomy of primary dystonia	287
Oppenheim dystonia (DYT1)	277	Biochemistry and neuroimaging	291

In the course of the last five years I have repeatedly observed an affliction, whose meaning and classification caused great difficulties. When examining the first cases I was trying to decide between a diagnosis of hysteria, and idiopathic bilateral athetosis; but then I soon realized that neither of these diagnoses was appropriate, and that this was a new condition, or at least a new type of condition.

… the disease has something quite unique; namely the severe tonic cramps, particularly in the neck, head and the proximal sections of the extremities. The unique "torqued" gait is practically pathological. The prognosis is bad. All therapeutic attempts are as of yet unsuccessful. …

During my efforts to delineate the methodology of the disease through an incisive name, I have selected the titles dysbasia lordotica progressiva and dystonia musculorum deformans and would prefer the latter.

Hermann Oppenheim, 1911
From his description of generalized dystonia

Historical highlights

In 1908, Schwalbe published his dissertation on a family with three affected children who are now recognized to have had primary generalized dystonia. An English translation of Schwalbe's paper is available (Truong and Fahn, 1988). Three years later Oppenheim (1911) described the same disorder in four patients and coined the word "dystonia" to

indicate that in this disorder, there would be hypotonia on one occasion and tonic muscle spasms on another, usually but not exclusively elicited on volitional movements. Oppenheim called this syndrome by two different names: "dystonia musculorum deformans" and "dysbasia lordotica progressiva." The first name relates to the spasms and to the postural deformities that develop in these children; the second name emphasizes the dromedary gait and the progressive nature of the illness. Oppenheim described muscle spasms; bizarre walking with bending and twisting of the torso; rapid, sometimes rhythmic jerking movements; and progression of symptoms leading eventually to sustained fixed postural deformities.

Oppenheim, however, failed to recognize the inherited nature of the disorder, which was emphasized by Flatau and Sterling (1911) later that year; they suggested the name "progressive torsion spasm," which perhaps would have been the preferred one, according to the full syndrome recognized today. The word "dystonia," however, was immediately adopted by neurologists and has been used to describe both a distinctive motor phenomenology and a clinical syndrome in which these motoric features are present. Over time, different meanings were used for "dystonia" (for historical details, see Fahn et al., 1987). To clarify the definition, an ad hoc committee of the Dystonia Medical Research Foundation considered the clinical features described by Oppenheim (1911), Flatau and Sterling (1911) and other early observers, and developed the following definition: *Dystonia is a syndrome of sustained muscle contractions, frequently causing twisting and repetitive movements, or abnormal postures* (Fahn et al., 1987; Fahn, 1988). To emphasize the twisting quality of the abnormal movements and postures, the term "torsion" is often placed in front of the word "dystonia."

DOI: 10.1016/B978-1-4377-2369-4.00012-3

Such twisting is one feature that distinguishes dystonic movements from those of other dyskinesias, such as chorea, and distinguishes dystonic postures from other syndromes of increased muscle tone, such as rigidity, stiff-person syndrome, and neuromyotonia (Fahn, 1999). Exceptions to twisting are around joints that do not allow such torsion. Thus, dystonia involving the jaw, focusing on the temporomandibular joint, are jaw-opening and jaw-closing dystonias, rarely lateral jaw dystonia, but not twisting of the jaw.

The early observers described dystonia as a specific disease entity, but by the next decade, dystonia was recognized to be a feature in other neurologic disorders, such as Wilson disease and cerebral palsy, and following encephalitis. Soon, dystonia as a specific entity (today known as primary dystonia) was lost. It was Herz (1944a, 1944b, 1944c) who, in a masterful series of three papers, resurrected torsion dystonia as a specific neurologic entity as well as its presence within other neurologic diseases, who described the motor phenomenology and compared the duration of its contractions with those of chorea and athetosis, who utilized the analysis of cinematography to distinguish these differences in various movement disorders, and who showed the characteristic simultaneous contractions of agonist and antagonist muscles in dystonia. Another major pioneer in dystonia was Zeman (1970), who, along with his colleagues (Zeman et al., 1959, 1960; Zeman and Dyken, 1967), carried out the first epidemiologic study, emphasized the autosomal dominant pattern of inheritance, described the focal dystonias as formes frustes of generalized dystonia, and found the pathologic anatomy to be normal in primary torsion dystonia (PTD). The disparate varieties of focal dystonias were not linked as focal dystonias until Marsden placed them together (1976). Still, patients with dystonia, both generalized and focal, were often considered to be hysterical, i.e., to have a psychogenic disorder and not an organic one, as Lesser and Fahn (1978) pointed out, often with tragic consequences, as described in Cooper's book (1976). Better awareness of the organic nature of dystonia, both generalized and focal (for torticollis and writer's cramp were often considered hysterical), began to come about with the holding and publication of the first international symposium on dystonia (Eldridge and Fahn, 1976). The final proof came with the discovery of the gene locus for Oppenheim dystonia (Ozelius et al., 1989) and the discovery that dystonia in the Ashkenazi Jewish population was inherited in an autosomal dominant pattern (Bressman et al., 1989).

Other important events in the development of our understanding of dystonia are the formation of the Dystonia Medical Research Foundation in 1976, the creation of four international symposia on dystonia with their subsequent publications (Eldridge and Fahn, 1976; Fahn et al., 1988, 1998b, 2004), and the investigations of clinical and molecular genetics that are leading to the discovery of the mutated genes and clarifying the classification and clinical features of the dystonias (Bressman et al., 1989, 1994a; Ozelius et al., 1989, 1997; Nygaard et al., 1993; Ichinose et al., 1994). The advances in genetics have led to a better etiologic classification of the dystonias (Fahn et al., 1998a) and to the labeling of many of the dystonias using a "DYT" classification, as displayed in Table 12.1.

A number of reviews covering the historical aspects are available to which the reader is referred for more details than are provided in this chapter (Fahn, 1984a; Fahn et al., 1987; Fahn and Marsden, 1987; Rothwell and Obeso, 1987; Fahn et al., 1988; Fahn, 1989a, 1990; Tsui and Calne, 1995; Jankovic and Fahn, 1998; Nemeth, 2002; Stacy, 2007; Breakefield et al., 2008). A collection of historical photographs about dystonia is available for perusal (Goetz et al., 2001).

Table 12.1 Genetic classification of the dystonias

DYT1 = 9q34, *TOR1A*, torsinA, AD, young-onset, limb-onset (Oppenheim dystonia) (Ozelius et al., 1997)

DYT2 = AR, unconfirmed (Gimenez-Roldan et al., 1988; Khan et al., 2003, Moretti et al., 2005)

DYT3 = Xq13.1, lubag in Filipino males (X-linked dystonia-parkinsonism), a multiple transcript system (Müller et al., 1994; Nolte et al., 2003), now believed to be due to a *TAF1* mutation (Makino et al., 2007)

DYT4 = a whispering dysphonia family (Parker, 1985; Elwes and Saunders, 1986)

DYT5 = 14q22.1, GTP cyclohydrolase 1 (*GCH1*), AD (known as dopa-responsive dystonia) (Ichinose et al., 1994); also tyrosine hydroxylase deficiency = 11p11.5, AR, can respond to levodopa (Knappskog et al., 1995)

DYT6 = 8q21–q22, *THAP1*, AD, mixed type, first recognized in the Mennonite/Amish population, now universal (Bressman et al., 2009; Djarmati et al., 2009; Fuchs et al., 2009)

DYT7 = 18p, AD, familial torticollis, but localization is now in doubt (Leube et al., 1996)

DYT8 = 2q34, AD, paroxysmal nonkinesigenic dyskinesia (PNKD1) (FDP1) (Mount–Rebak syndrome) (Fink et al., 1996; Fouad et al., 1996), *MR1* gene, myofibrillogenesis regulator 1

DYT9 = 1p21, AD, paroxysmal dyskinesia with spasticity (CSE) (Auburger et al., 1996) (possibly the gene for GLUT1; see DYT18)

DYT10 = 16p11.2–q12.1, AD, paroxysmal kinesigenic dyskinesia (PKD) (EKD1) (Tomita et al., 1999) (another PKD on this chromosome is at 16q13–q22.1) (Valente et al., 2000) (also PED with infantile convulsions on 16p12–q11.2 (Szepetowski et al., 1997)

DYT11 = 7q21–q23, *SGCE* gene, epsilon-sarcoglycan, AD, myoclonus-dystonia (Zimprich et al., 2001)

DYT12 = 19q12–q13.2, *ATP1A3* gene, Na-K-ATPase α3 subunit, AD, rapid-onset dystonia–parkinsonism (Kramer et al., 1999; de Carvalho Aguiar et al., 2004)

DYT13 = 1p36.13–p36.32, AD, cranial-cervical-brachial (Valente et al., 2001; Bentivoglio et al., 2004)

DYT15 = 18p11, AD, myoclonus–dystonia (Grimes et al., 2002)

DYT16 = 2q31.2, *PRKRA* gene, protein activator of interferon-induced protein kinase, AR, dystonia-parkinsonism (Camargos et al., 2008)

DYT17 = 20p11.2–q13.12, AR, juvenile onset with torticollis, spreading to segmental and generalized (Chouery et al., 2008)

DYT18 = 1p35–p31.3, AD, paroxysmal exertional dyskinesia (PED) associated with hemolytic anemia, *SLC2A1* gene affecting the glucose transporter 1 (GLUT1) (Weber et al., 2008)

DYT19 = 16q13–q22.1, AD, paroxysmal kinesigenic dyskinesia without epilepsy (EKD2) (Valente et al., 2000)

DYT20 = 2q31, AD, paroxysmal nonkinesigenic dyskinesia (PNKD2) (Spacey et al., 2006)

DYT21 = 2q14.3-q21.3, AD, adult onset mixed dystonia (Holmgren et al., 1995; Norgren et al., 2011)

AD, autosomal dominant; AR, autosomal recessive.

Impact and overview of genetic discoveries

Perhaps the greatest advance in dystonia in the past 10 years has been the continual unraveling of an increasing number of distinct genetic forms of dystonia based on gene mapping and cloning. In turn, this has led to the beginning of molecular biology research in the dystonias and a more comprehensive classification of the dystonias based on etiology. The first genetic form of dystonia whose gene was mapped was the form described by Oppenheim (1911), which he called dystonia musculorum deformans and which is now called Oppenheim dystonia (Fahn et al., 1998a) and also DYT1 dystonia (because the mapped gene was given that designation). The gene for Oppenheim dystonia has been identified and cloned, but not before the gene responsible for another genetic form of dystonia was identified, namely, dopa-responsive dystonia (DYT5), or DRD, caused by a mutation in the gene for the enzyme guanosine triphosphate (GTP) cyclohydrolase I (GCH1). As genes are being mapped, the clinicians are able to use this information to better define the clinical features of each genetic type. Table 12.1 lists the currently known genetic designations for the dystonias. The last two genes identified in this nomenclature are those of NA-K-ATPase responsible for rapid-onset dystonia-parkinsonism (RDP) (DYT12) (de Carvalho Aguiar et al., 2004) and TAF1 (TATA box-binding protein-associated factor 1) for lubag (DYT3) (Makino et al. 2007). The official nomenclature committee has labeled 20 DYTs, but omitted other genetic forms of dystonia, which are listed in this section after the first 20. Moreover, clinical neurologists usually consider DYT8, DYT9, and DYT10 to be part of the category of movement disorders known as paroxysmal dyskinesias, and not the dystonia category. These are covered in Chapter 22. Also, the designation of DYT14 for a new form of DRD was incorrect. The family with "DYT14" was thought not to have the DYT5 gene deletion in GCH1 (Grotzsch et al., 2002), but subsequently a mutation in GCH1 was found (Wider et al., 2008). DYT14 has been eliminated in Table 12.1.

A number of other dystonias are known to be genetic, but have not received a "DYT" classification. Two new families with suspected DYT2 dystonia were reported (Khan et al., 2003; Moretti et al., 2005). Siblings from two families with consanguinity developed autosomal recessive childhood-onset generalized dystonia. Gene studies for other known genetic forms of dystonia were negative.

The gene causing lubag (DYT3) was reported to involve a multiple transcript system (Nolte et al., 2003). It was not initially possible to say which mutant protein (and there may be up to six from this mutation) is actually responsible for the disease. However, Makino and colleagues (2007) have subsequently found the mutation for lubag to be in the TAF1 gene.

The gene causing DYT6 was reported in 2009 as the THAP1 gene (Fuchs et al., 2009). Its function is unknown. Subsequently a search was made for familial dystonia with young onset and many more mutations were discovered in this gene, and the age at onset expanded to 49 years, with the majority still being young onset (Bressman et al., 2009). Screening for focal dystonia, singleton cases revealed far fewer cases, with a phenotype of young-onset spasmodic

dysphonia that later spread to become generalized dystonia (Djarmati et al., 2009). The THAP1 gene was analyzed in a series of 362 British, genetically undetermined, primary dystonia patients, and nine mutations were found (Houlden et al., 2010). The main clinical presentation was early-onset (<30 years) dystonia in the craniocervical region or the limbs (8 of 9 patients); laryngeal or oromandibular dystonia was present in 3 cases. Thus, early-onset dystonia that includes involvement of the larynx or face should arouse suspicion of a THAP1 mutation. A search for THAP1 mutations in 1114 patients with adult-onset primary dystonia revealed different THAP1 sequence variants to be associated with varied anatomical distributions and onset ages of both familial and sporadic primary dystonia (Xiao et al., 2010).

de Carvalho Aguiar and colleagues (2004) reported the identification of missense mutations in the gene for the Na+/K+-ATPase $\alpha 3$ subunit (ATP1A3) as a cause of RDP (DYT12).

A fuller description of the phenotype of DYT13 (craniocervical-brachial dystonia) has been reported in the only known family with this disorder (Bentivoglio et al., 2004). Age at onset ranged from 5 to 43 years. Onset occurred either in the craniocervical region or in the upper limbs. Progression was mild, and the disease course was benign in most affected individuals; generalization occurred in only two cases. There was no anticipation of age at onset or of disease severity through generations. Most subjects presented with jerky, myoclonic-like dystonic movements of the neck or shoulders. DYT13 is an autosomal dominant disease, with incomplete penetrance (58%).

Two independent studies searched for mutations in the ϵ-sarcoglycan gene in patients with familial and sporadic myoclonus–dystonia and did not find any (Han et al., 2003; Valente et al., 2003). This finding, plus the report of one family having a mutation on a different chromosome, 18p11 (DYT15), provides additional evidence for genetic heterogeneity in myoclonus–dystonia.

Two unrelated consanguineous Brazilian families with early-onset dystonia–parkinsonism were found to have a mutation in the PRKRA gene for protein kinase, interferon-inducible double-stranded RNA-dependent activator and it has been labeled as DYT16 (Camargos et al., 2008).

DYT17 is the designation given to a large consanguineous Lebanese family in which three sisters had primary torsion dystonia beginning with torticollis at ages 14, 17, and 19 years, spreading to segmental and generalized in one of the sisters (Chouery et al., 2008).

DYT18, DYT19, and DYT20 are paroxysmal dyskinesias and are covered in Chapter 22. DYT21 is an autosomal dominant family from northern Sweden of adult onset manifesting combinations of focal, segmental and generalized dystonia (Holmgren et al., 1995; Norgren et al., 2011).

A number of dystonic conditions are not labeled as "DYT," but dystonia is part of their features (Table 12.2).

The association with a polymorphism in the D5 receptor gene (DRD5) for primary focal dystonias could not be confirmed in German and French patients (Sibbing et al., 2003), but was seen in Italian patients (Brancati et al., 2003).

The autosomal recessive disorder of early-onset cerebellar ataxia with oculomotor apraxia associated with a mutation of the aprataxin gene on chromosome 9p13 can also cause generalized dystonia (Sekijima et al., 2003). Adult-onset craniocervical dystonia preceded ataxia in a case with

Table 12.2 Unlabeled as "DYT" but dystonia is present as well as other neurologic features in some of these disorders

Deafness–dystonia (Mohr–Tranebjaerg syndrome), X-linked recessive (Hayes et al., 1998; Jin et al., 1996; 1999; Koehler et al., 1999; Tranebjaerg et al., 2000). Torticollis and writer's cramp also seen in female carriers (Swerdlow and Wooten, 2001); faulty assembly of the DDP1/TIMM8a–TIMM13 complex (Roesch et al., 2002)

Intellectual disability, seizures, and infantile spasms, X-linked recessive (Stromme et al. 2002). Some also with dystonia

Adult-onset bilateral striopallidodentate calcinosis, also known as idiopathic basal ganglia calcification (IBGC) and improperly called Fahr disease, AD, 14q (Geschwind et al., 1999; Wszolek et al., 2006)

Aromatic amino acid decarboxylase (AADC) deficiency; AR (Swoboda et al., 2003; Brun et al., 2010)

6-Pyruvoyltetrahydropterin synthase deficiency, AR (Hyland et al., 1998; Porta et al., 2009)

Pterin-4a-carbinolamine dehydratase deficiency, AR (Hyland et al., 1998)

Dihydropteridine reductase deficiency; AR (Hyland et al., 1998)

Sepiapterin reductase deficiency; AR (Blau et al., 2001, Neville et al., 2005)

Neurodegeneration with brain iron accumulation type 1 (NBIA1) (formerly called Hallervorden–Spatz syndrome), *PANK2*, pantothenate kinase 2, AR, 20p12.3–p13 (Taylor et al., 1996; Zhou et al., 2001); recently renamed as pantothenate kinase-associated neurodegeneration (PKAN) (Hayflick et al., 2003)

Neurodegeneration with brain iron accumulation type 3 (NBIA2) (neuroferritinopathy), 19q13.3, ferritin light polypeptide (*FTLI*), AD (Curtis et al., 2001; Mir et al., 2005)

Neurodegeneration with brain iron accumulation type 2 due to infantile neuroaxonal dystrophy (INAD) with dystonia, parkinsonism and ataxia, AR, *(PLA2G6)* phospholipase A2, designated as PARK14, 22q12.3–q13.2 (Kurian et al., 2008)

Neurodegeneration with brain iron accumulation due to aceruloplasminemia with dystonia, bradykinesia, tremor, cognitive change, anemia and diabetes, AR, ceruloplasmin gene (Fasano et al., 2008)

Familial torticollis, dopamine D5 receptor gene as a susceptibility factor (Placzek et al., 2001)

Familial blepharospasm, dopamine D5 receptor gene as a susceptibility factor (Misbahuddin et al., 2002)

Familial mild focal and segmental cranio-cervical-brachial dystonia on a Dutch island, no linkage yet (Contarino et al., 2008).

Hereditary spastic paraplegia with dystonia mapped to chromosome 2q24–q31 (Gilbert et al., 2009)

AD, autosomal dominant; AR, autosomal recessive.

spinocerebellar ataxia type 1 (SCA1) (Wu et al., 2004). Cervical dystonia was also seen in SCA10 (Gatto et al., 2007), and spasmodic dysphonia has been reported in SCA17 (Hagenah et al., 2004, 2007).

Some patients with adult-onset dystonia have been found to have a missense mutation in the mitochondrial complex I gene (Simon et al., 2003). In addition to dystonia, spasticity and core-type myopathy are present.

A screen for a combination of dystonia with cerebellar atrophy identified eight such families (Le Ber et al. 2006), which raises the possibility that the cerebellum could be involved in dystonia (Jinnah and Hess, 2006), but more likely these families suggest a phenotype of a newly recognized neurodegenerative disease.

Although the GAG mutation in torsinA (TOR1A) is rare and causes young-onset limb-onset dystonia, two polymorphisms in or near the *TOR1A* gene have been discovered to be common in idiopathic focal dystonia, raising the possible association of a risk factor for this gene and the common adult-onset focal dystonias (Kamm et al., 2006).

Phenomenology of dystonic movements

With few exceptions, the four clinically unifying, consistent, and predominant features of dystonic contractions are (1) their relatively long duration (compared to myoclonus and chorea), although short-duration contractions can occur in dystonia; (2) their simultaneous contractions of agonists and antagonists; (3) their resulting in a twisting of the affected body part; and (4) their continual contractions of the same muscle groups (called patterned movements, see Chapter 1). One exception to the twisting nature of dystonia is that dystonias in facial muscles are rarely twisting; they are patterned and involve sustained contractions of forehead, eyelids, and lower face. As it turns out, twisting facial muscles that move the mouth to one side or the other or back and forth to each side are usually psychogenic (see Chapter 25).

Although the durations of the patterned contractions are usually more sustained than those of chorea, sometimes they can be very short. The range from very short to very prolonged contractions results in the appearance of a wide range in the speed of the patterned dystonic movements from rapid to slow. The movements can be so fast that they have the appearance of repetitive myoclonic jerking. The term "myoclonic-dystonia" has been applied to such dystonia (Davidenkow, 1926; Obeso et al., 1983; Kurlan et al., 1988; Quinn et al., 1988), and the rapid jerks may respond to alcohol (Quinn et al., 1988). In some families, the phenomenology of the combination of myoclonus and dystonia is a major feature, and these families are genetically distinct from those of the originally described PTD (i.e., Oppenheim dystonia) (Wahlström et al., 1994) and have been called by different names, initially dystonia–myoclonus (Fahn et al., 1998a), but now *myoclonus–dystonia* (Klein et al., 1999; Nygaard et al., 1999). The relationship of familial myoclonus–dystonia and hereditary essential myoclonus, which can also include patients with some dystonic features, is not clear (Fahn and Sjaastad, 1991; Quinn, 1996), but will soon be settled, as the identification of a gene (ε-sarcoglycan) for myoclonus–dystonia has been discovered (Zimprich et al., 2001).

Primary dystonia almost always begins by affecting a single part of the body; this is *focal dystonia* (Video 12.1). Most patients' dystonia remains as a focal dystonia without spreading to other parts of the body. However, even within that single body part, multiple muscles can be affected. Thus, in patients with dystonia of the neck (cervical dystonia, or torticollis) a combination of muscles are involved (Video 12.2). Moreover, even if the neck is postured to a stable position, there can be changes in muscle contraction patterns that can be detected with EMG recordings (Munchau et al., 2001a). In a sizeable minority of patients, dystonia that starts in one body part can spread to involve other parts of the body. Most often, the spread is to contiguous body parts; hence, the spread is from focal dystonia to *segmental dystonia*.

Table 12.3 Usual progression of the primary dystonias

Steps of progression	Sites affected	With action or rest	Sensory tricks
Earliest phase	One site of body affected (focal dystonia); most adult-onset dystonias plateau at this level	Usually during a specific task (task-specific dystonia; action dystonia) and not present at rest or when a particular placement in space of the body part (position-specific dystonia). (Note: paradoxical dystonia = present at rest and disappears with action; often seen in focal cranial dystonias, such as blepharospasm, which can present initially either with action or at rest)	Usually effective
Next phase	Contiguous site(s) become involved (segmental dystonia). Many adult- and juvenile-onset dystonias plateau at this level.	Other (non-specific, multiple) actions of the involved body part activate the dystonia	Usually effective
Next phase	Other body sites become involved (multifocal or generalized dystonia). Many childhood-onset dystonias go to this level	Voluntary motor actions at other parts of the body, including talking, bring out dystonia in the originally involved site ("overflow" dystonia).	Partially effective
Next phase	Dystonic movements or postures are more severe and interfere with function	Dystonia is present when the involved body part is at rest – can be either clonic or tonic dystonia	Usually ineffective
Next phase		Dystonia is present when the involved body part is at rest and during light sleep	Ineffective
Most advanced		Dystonia manifests as a fixed posture; i.e., difficult for the examiner to move the limb or other involved body parts	Ineffective

The pattern of spread of adult-onset focal dystonias has been analyzed, especially blepharospasm (Fahn, 1985; Weiss et al., 2006), as has the spread of childhood-onset dystonia (Greene et al., 1995). In blepharospasm, spread to other body parts is faster in patients who carry at least one T allele in a polymorphism site on the *TOR1A* gene (Defazio et al. 2009). As a general rule, the younger the age at onset, the more likely it is that the dystonia will spread; for example, childhood onset with leg involvement usually leads to eventual *generalized dystonia* (Marsden et al., 1976; Fahn, 1986; Greene et al., 1995). Regardless of genetic etiology, the phenotypes of primary dystonias are affected by age at onset, with a caudal-to-rostral change in the site of onset as a function of age (O'Riordan et al., 2004). The severity of dystonia can be quantified by using clinical rating scales for generalized dystonia and the various focal dystonias (Burke et al., 1985; Fahn, 1989b; Comella et al., 1997, 2003).

Dystonic movements are almost always aggravated during voluntary movement. The appearance of dystonic movements with voluntary movement is referred to as "action dystonia." Primary dystonia commonly begins with a specific action dystonia, that is, the abnormal movements appear with a special action (i.e., *task-specific* action) and are not present at rest, in contrast to secondary dystonias which are more likely to begin with dystonia at rest (Svetel et al., 2004). For example, a child who develops primary dystonia might have the initial symptom in one leg, but only when walking forward. It could be absent when the child runs or walks backward (Video 12.3). Other common examples are the task-specific dystonias that are seen with writing (writer's cramp) (Video 12.4), playing a musical instrument (musician's cramp) (Video 12.5), chewing (Video 12.6), and speaking, including auctioneering (Scolding et al., 1995).

Often, these task-specific dystonias produce occupational disability; e.g., musicians usually no longer can play their instrument professionally. Robert Schumann's career as a pianist was impaired, probably because of musician's cramp (de Yebenes, 1995). Musician's cramp and other occupational cramps can occur in any part of body that is engaged in repetitive, highly skilled tasks (Altenmüller and Jabusch, 2010). Embouchure (the pattern of lip, jaw, and tongue muscles used to control the flow of air into a mouthpiece) dystonia has been seen in horn and woodwind players (Frucht and Estrin, 2010). Patients with embouchure dystonia can be separated into several groups, including embouchure tremor, involuntary lip movements, and jaw closure (Frucht et al., 2001). The dystonia can spread to other oral tasks, often producing significant disability. Musician's dystonia, like other focal dystonias (discussed below in pathophysiology of primary dystonia), is associated with increased sensorimotor activation (Haslinger et al., 2010). Focal *task-specific tremors* might be a form of focal dystonia rather than a manifestation of essential tremor (Soland et al., 1996b). Several reviews of musician's cramps were presented at an international symposium on dystonia (Brandfonbrener and Robson, 2004; Charness and Schlaug, 2004; Frucht, 2004; Jabusch and Altenmuller, 2004; Pesenti et al., 2004).

As the dystonic condition progresses, less specific voluntary motor actions of the involved limb can bring out the dystonic movements (see Table 12.3). In the above example, the affected leg might also activate the dystonia when it is tapping the floor. With further evolution, actions in other parts of the body can induce dystonic movements of the involved leg, so-called "overflow." Talking is the most common mechanism for causing overflow dystonia in other body parts. Such activation of involuntary movements by talking is also particularly common with levodopa-induced dyskinesias and in cerebral palsy. With still further worsening, the affected limb can develop dystonic movements while it is at rest. Eventually, the leg can have sustained posturing. Thus, dystonia at rest is usually a more severe form than pure action dystonia. Whereas primary dystonia often begins as action dystonia and may persist as the kinetic (clonic) form, symptomatic dystonia often begins as sustained postures (tonic form). Sustained postures may appear in specific placements of the body. For example, the trunk may be in normal posture when the patient is lying supine or prone, but develop into kyphosis, scoliosis, or lordosis when sitting or standing. Thus, this dystonia is not a fixed dystonia (non-changing with a change in body posture and unable to be altered by the examiner applying normal strength to move the affected body part). Fixed postures, with or without pain, are often psychogenic in origin (Fahn and Williams, 1988; Lang, 1995; Sa et al., 2003; Schrag et al., 2004), although there may be organic cases. Transcranial magnetic stimulation studies revealed similar physiologic alterations in the cerebral cortex as seen in patients with mobile dystonia (Avanzino et al., 2008), but as Espay and colleagues (2006) have shown, and as discussed in Chapter 25, the changes in the brain can be secondary to the abnormal psychogenic postures or sensory abnormalities.

Much less common than action dystonia or overflow dystonia is the reverse phenomenon, i.e., for dystonia at rest to be improved by talking or by other voluntary active movements, so-called *paradoxical dystonia* (Fahn, 1989c). With paradoxical dystonia the patient is usually observed moving the affected or non-affected body part. The patient does this to obtain relief of the dystonia. When the paradoxical dystonia involves the trunk, the observer can easily mistake the patient's moving about as being due to restlessness or akathisia, which is the most common differential diagnosis (Video 12.7). The focal dystonia that is most commonly decreased by voluntary motor activity is blepharospasm (Fahn et al., 1985). About 60% of patients with blepharospasm obtain relief when talking; about 40% worsen with talking. 🎥

Dystonia usually is present continually throughout the day whenever the affected body part is in use; and as a sign of more severity, also when the body part is at rest. A notable phenomenologic feature of DRD is that of diurnal variation in many of the patients, with the dystonia being worse at the end of the day, and minimal in the morning hours (Segawa et al., 1976). Dystonic movements tend to increase with fatigue, stress, and emotional states; they tend to be suppressed with relaxation, hypnosis, and sleep (Fish et al., 1991). Dystonia may be precipitated or exacerbated by pregnancy (dystonia gravidarum) (Lim et al., 2006). Unless it is extremely severe, dystonia often disappears with deep sleep. For patients who appear to have persistent postural abnormalities that cannot be overcome by manual manipulation, it might be necessary to put them to sleep with anesthesia to determine whether a contracture is already present (Fahn, 2006). Propofol anesthesia, however, does not entirely suppress dystonia because recurrences occur even under deep propofol anesthesia (Zabani and Vaghadia, 1996).

One of the characteristic and almost unique features of dystonic movements is that they can often be diminished by tactile or proprioceptive "sensory tricks" (*geste antagoniste*).

Thus, touching the involved body part or an adjacent body part can often reduce the muscle contractions (Video 12.8). For example, patients with torticollis will often place a hand on the chin or side of the face to reduce nuchal contractions, and orolingual dystonia is often helped by touching the lips or placing an object in the mouth (Blunt et al., 1994; Lo et al., 2007). In a study of 50 patients with cervical dystonia who were known to have at least one sensory trick, 54% of them had two to five different tricks and 82% had a reduction of head deviation by at least 30%, with a mean of 60% (Muller et al., 2001). In cervical dystonia, applying the trick when the head is in a neutral or even contralateral position was most effective, while no reduction of muscle activity occurs during trick application at the maximum dystonic head position (Schramm et al., 2004). Sometimes a mechanical device can be utilized therapeutically, especially for cervical dystonia (Krack et al., 1998) (Video 12.9). Greene and Bressman (1998) found that in some patients with torsion dystonia, simply thinking about a sensory trick or task affects the dystonia in the same way as actually performing the activity. A positron emission tomography (PET) study has shown that the sensory trick brings about a normalization of the abnormal cortical physiology that is seen in dystonia, and results in increasing activation of the ipsilateral superior and inferior parietal lobule and decreasing activity of the contralateral supplementary motor area and the primary sensorimotor cortex (Naumann et al., 2000). The presence of a sensory trick is not specific for primary dystonias; it can sometimes occur in secondary dystonias, including psychogenic dystonia (Munhoz and Lang, 2004). 🎥

Pain is uncommon in dystonia except in cervical dystonia; 75% of patients with cervical dystonia (spasmodic torticollis) have pain (Chan et al., 1991). The pain perception threshold appears to be lower in patients with primary cervical dystonia (Lobbezoo et al., 1996). Dystonia in most parts of the body rarely is accompanied by pain; when it is, it is not clear whether the pain is due to painful contractions of muscles or some other factor. The high incidence of pain in cervical dystonia appears to be due to muscle contractions because this pain is usually relieved by injections of botulinum toxin (Greene et al., 1990). It is believed that the posterior cervical muscles are rich in pain fibers, and that continual contractions of these muscles results in pain. On the other hand, because no correlation was found between the severity of motor signs and pain, some investigators hypothesize that central mechanisms are also involved (Kutvonen et al., 1997). Quality of life is negatively affected with cervical dystonia (Camfield et al., 2002). It has been difficult to explain fixed painful postural torticollis following trauma, but recent analysis indicates that many of these cases appear to be psychogenic (Sa et al., 2003). Fixed dystonia in other parts of the body is also usually associated with a peripheral injury and overlaps with chronic regional pain syndrome (reflex sympathetic dystrophy); many of these individuals fulfill strict criteria for a somatoform disorder or psychogenic dystonia (Schrag et al., 2004).

Patients with PTD sometimes have rhythmical movements, particularly in the arms (Video 12.10) and neck, manifested as a tremor (Yanagisawa et al., 1972; Jankovic and Fahn, 1980). In one survey, 68% of patients with cervical dystonia had head tremor (Pal et al., 2000). Two basic types of tremors are seen in dystonic patients: (1) an accompanying postural/action tremor of the upper limbs that resembles essential tremor or enhanced physiologic tremor and (2) a tremor that is a rhythmic expression of rapid dystonic movements (Yanagisawa and Goto, 1971); these occur at the site of the tremor, such as arms, neck, or jaw (Schneider and Bhatia, 2007). The latter can usually be distinguished from the former by showing that the tremor appears only when the affected body part is placed in a position of opposition to the major direction of pulling by the abnormal dystonic contractions and disappears when the body part is positioned where the dystonia wants to place it. Dystonic tremor appears to be less regular than essential tremor (Jedynak et al., 1991). Tremor of the hands in patients with cervical dystonia tends to be irregular and therefore dystonic, rather than an accompanying essential tremor (Shaikh et al., 2008). Sometimes, it is very difficult to distinguish between the two types, particularly with writing tremor and cervical tremor. Primary writing tremor can sometimes represent task-specific dystonia or task-specific essential tremor (Cohen et al., 1987; Rosenbaum and Jankovic, 1988; Elble et al., 1990). A family history of tremor (and stuttering) is increased in PTD (Fletcher et al., 1991a).

Although accompanying essential tremor is recognized in patients with dystonia (Lou and Jankovic, 1991), there is uncertainty as to how common this occurrence is. Tremor of the hands can be seen fairly often in patients with cervical dystonia (spasmodic torticollis) (Couch, 1976). Deuschl and colleagues (1997) analyzed this tremor in 55 patients with cervical dystonia. The mean amplitudes of postural tremor were only slightly higher than those of the controls and much smaller than those found in classic essential tremor; analytic measurements showed evidence of physiologic tremor mechanisms only. In another study, arm tremor in patients with cervical dystonia was found to develop either before or simultaneously with onset of the torticollis; such temporal relationships do not correspond to either dystonic tremor or tremor in the presence of dystonia (Munchau et al., 2001c).

What can be mistaken for tremor or rhythmic jerky movements is the tendency for patients with dystonia to fight the abnormal pulling of dystonic muscles into a sustained posture. Asking the patient not to resist the pulling of the muscles and just relax and let the muscles go where they seek to go will usually enlighten the examiner that those jerky movements are actually a directional pulling with the patient trying to overcome the pull. One can position the affected body part into different postures to determine if there is a "null point" where the jerky movements or tremor ceases, indicating the position the involved muscles are seeking.

Tics are another type of involuntary movement that appears to occur more commonly in patients with dystonia than in the general population (Shale et al., 1986; Stone and Jankovic, 1991; Damasio et al., 2011).

Although this is rare, some children and adolescents with primary and secondary dystonia can develop a crisis of sudden marked increase in the severity of dystonia, which has been called *dystonic storm* (Dalvi et al., 1998) and *status dystonicus* (Manji et al., 1998). It can cause rhabdomyolysis and myoglobinuria, with a threat of death by renal failure (Jankovic and Penn, 1982; Paret et al., 1995). Placing the patient in an intensive care unit and narcotizing him or her with barbiturates is usually necessary to treat this crisis.

Intrathecal baclofen might be necessary if the dystonic storm persists and continues to be present when the patient is allowed to awaken (Jankovic and Penn, 1982; Dalvi et al., 1998). More recently, pallidotomy or pallidal stimulation has been utilized in place of intrathecal baclofen.

A case of orthostatic hemidystonia has been reported (Sethi et al., 2002). The patient developed hemidystonia on rising from the sitting position. It was due to poor vascular perfusion in the contralateral frontoparietal cortex and was the result of occlusion of the contralateral internal carotid artery and near-total occlusion of the ipsilateral internal carotid artery.

Dystonia patients are relatively free of psychopathology, as measured in patients with writer's cramp (Sheehy and Marsden, 1982) and blepharospasm (Scheidt et al., 1996). However, a recent study reports a prevalence of obsessive-compulsive disorder in 20% of patients with primary focal dystonias (Cavallaro et al., 2002). Attentional-executive cognitive deficits have been found in patients with primary dystonia by using the Cambridge Neuropsychological Test Automated Battery (Scott et al., 2003), but not by using a host of other tests (Jahanshahi et al., 2003). Obsessive-compulsive disorder and alcohol dependence are not uncommon in individuals who carry the DYT11 gene for myoclonus–dystonia (Saunders-Pullman et al., 2002), and the DYT1 gene has been associated with an increase in depression, whether the person is a manifesting or nonmanifesting carrier (Heiman et al., 2004).

Site of body involvement is characteristic for many types of dystonia. Children usually have onset equally in a leg or an arm, at least for Oppenheim dystonia. Adult-onset dystonia is typically in the upper body, cranial, cervical, or brachial. A few adult patients may have focal truncal dystonia. Foot onset in adults is uncommon, but does occur (Schneider et al., 2006b). Isolated foot dystonia following exercise in adults is sometimes seen as the first symptom of Parkinson disease. This has now been verified in a patient with neuroimaging by using dopamine transporter single photon emission computed tomography (SPECT). Childhood-onset dystonia that begins in the cranial region is usually non-DYT1 dystonia (Bressman et al., 2000; Fasano et al., 2006). Dystonia may be the presenting or dominant feature of many parkinsonian disorders besides Parkinson disease (Jankovic, 2005; Ashour and Jankovic, 2006). Sometimes dystonia involving the foot can resemble a Babinski sign. This pseudo-Babinski (striatal toe) can be a dystonic phenomenon and should be differentiated from a true Babinski sign seen with pyramidal tract lesions (Horstink et al., 2007).

Epidemiology

Zeman and his colleagues (Zeman and Dyken, 1967; Zeman et al., 1959, 1960) carried out the first epidemiologic study in dystonia in the population of the state of Indiana and emphasized the autosomal dominant pattern of inheritance in PTD. They considered only generalized dystonia to be PTD, and viewed other types as formes frustes. Today, those other forms are viewed as focal and segmental dystonia, and part of the spectrum of PTD. An epidemiologic study of PTD in the population living in Rochester, Minnesota, found the prevalence of generalized PTD to be 3.4 per 100 000 population, and the prevalence of focal dystonia to be 30 per 100 000 (Nutt et al., 1988). In a study of dystonia in Israel, Zilber and colleagues (1984) estimated the prevalence of generalized dystonia among Jews of Eastern European ancestry to be 1/15 000 or 6.8/100 000, which is double the prevalence in the general population of Rochester. However, the analysis by Risch and colleagues (1995) indicates that the frequency in the Ashkenazim is much higher (between 1/6000 and 1/2000), and they suggest that the Ashkenazi population with PTD descends from a limited group of founders of the DYT1 mutation. These investigators also have traced the origin of the mutation to the northern part of the historic Jewish Pale of settlement (Lithuania and Byelorussia), approximately 350 years ago. In Japan, the DYT1 mutation was looked for in 178 patients with various forms of dystonia and was found in 6 (3.4%) (Matsumoto et al., 2001) and phenotypically resembled Oppenheim dystonia seen in other populations.

In Japan the prevalence rate of focal dystonias was found to be 6.12 (Nakashima et al., 1995), 10.1 (Matsumoto et al., 2003), 13.7 (Fukuda et al., 2006), and 14.4 (Sugawara et al., 2006) per 100 000 population, all of which is considerably lower than the 30/100 000 found by Nutt et al. (1988) in Rochester, Minnesota. The prevalence of focal limb dystonia in India was higher, 49.06/100 000 (Das et al., 2007). In the north of England, the prevalence of focal dystonias was found to be 12 per 100 000, and the prevalence of generalized dystonia was found to be 1.6 per 100 000 (Duffey et al., 1998). A European consortium of investigators published their findings of 11.7 per 100 000 for focal dystonia and 3.5 per 100 000 for segmental and generalized primary dystonias (Warner et al., 2000). A survey of primary blepharospasm in the Puglia region of southern Italy found a prevalence of only 13.3 per 100 000 (Defazio et al., 2001). The incidence rate of primary blepharospasm was found to be 1.2 per 100 000 population per year in Olmsted County, Minnesota (Bradley et al., 2003). Incidence for cervical dystonia was higher in white individuals (1.23/100 000/year) than in persons of other ethnicities (0.15/100 000/year) (Marras et al., 2007).

In Belgrade, the prevalence rate for focal, segmental, and multifocal dystonia was 13.6 per 100 000 population (Pekmezovic et al., 2003). It was almost twice as common (25.4 per 100 000 population) in Oslo (Le et al., 2003). Gender appears to play a role in both the prevalence and the age at onset of focal dystonia, women being more at risk and having an earlier age at onset for writer's cramp, but men having an earlier age at onset for cervical dystonia, blepharospasm, and laryngeal dystonia (Epidemiologic Study of Dystonia in Europe (ESDE) Collaborative Group, 1999; Marras et al., 2007).

Table 12.4 lists epidemiologic studies of PTD.

Classification of torsion dystonia

Table 12.5 presents the three ways to classify patients with torsion dystonia: by age at onset, by body distribution of abnormal movements, and by etiology. This method allows physicians and health-care providers some understanding of the nature of the dystonia, including prognosis.

Classification by age at onset

Classification by age at onset is useful because this is the most important single factor related to prognosis of primary dystonia (Marsden et al., 1976; Fahn, 1986; Greene et al., 1995). Even for secondary dystonias, such as tardive dystonia, age is commonly a factor in the location of the dystonia. As a general rule, the younger the age at onset, the more likely it is that the dystonia will become severe and will spread to involve multiple parts of the body. In contrast, the older the age at onset, the more likely it is that the dystonia will remain focal. Onset of dystonia in a leg is the second most important predictive factor (Greene et al., 1995) (Video 12.11). Because a bimodal age distribution is seen with primary dystonia, the age classification consists of two categories: (1) age 26 years or below and (2) above age 26 (Bressman, 2004).

Classification by distribution

Since dystonia usually begins by affecting a single part of the body (focal dystonia) and since dystonia can either remain focal or spread to involve other body parts, it is useful to classify dystonia according to its distribution of involvement of the body. Body distribution is one method of defining the severity of dystonia, and knowing the body distribution of dystonia is very important in planning a therapeutic strategy (Fahn, 1995).

Focal dystonia indicates that only a single area of the body is affected. Frequently seen types of focal dystonia tend to have specific labels, such as blepharospasm, torticollis, oromandibular dystonia, spastic dysphonia, writer's cramp, and occupational cramp. Adult-onset focal dystonias are much more common than generalized dystonias (Fahn, 1986; Marsden, 1986) (Table 12.6). If dystonia spreads, it most commonly does so by next affecting a contiguous body part. When dystonia affects two or more contiguous parts of the body, it is referred to as *segmental dystonia*. Some of the primary focal dystonias, such as blepharospasm and cervical dystonia, affect females more than males, while the reverse is seen for writer's cramp (Soland et al., 1996a).

Generalized dystonia is defined as representing a combination of segmental crural dystonia (i.e., both legs or legs plus trunk) plus involvement of any other area of the body (Videos 12.12, 12.13, 12.14, and 12.15). The term *multifocal dystonia* fills a gap in the above designations. It applies to the involvement of two or more non-contiguous parts of the body. Dystonia affecting one-half of the body is called *hemidystonia*. Almost always, hemidystonia indicates that the dystonia is symptomatic rather than primary (Narbona et al., 1984; Marsden et al., 1985; Pettigrew and Jankovic, 1985). A review of hemidystonia (Chuang et al., 2002) found that the most common etiologies were stroke, trauma, and perinatal injury; the mean age of onset was between 20 and 26 years; the mean latency from insult to dystonia was between 2.8 and 4.1 years, the longest latencies occurring after perinatal injury; and basal ganglia lesions were identified in 48–60% of the cases, most commonly involving the putamen. When there is a delay by a few years between time of insult and time of onset of dystonia, the condition is named delayed-onset dystonia (Burke et al., 1980).

Table 12.4 Prevalence of primary torsion dystonia

Authors	Population	Prevalence	Remarks
Zeman and Dyken (1967)	Indiana	1/200 000	Essentially a white, non-Jewish population Generalized dystonia only
Zilber et al. (1984)	Israel: Jews of Eastern Europe Afro-Asian Jews	1/15 000 1/117 000	Generalized dystonia only Generalized dystonia only
Nutt et al. (1988)	Generalized dystonia Focal dystonia	1/29 400 1/3400	Olmsted County, Minnesota From Mayo Clinic records
Risch et al. (1995)	New York area, Ashkenazi Jewish	Disease 1/6000; gene 1/2000	Based on cases seen at Columbia University Medical Center
Nakashima et al. (1995)	Focal dystonia	1/16 129	Japan
Duffey et al. (1998)	General dystonia Focal dystonia	1/62 000 1/8000	North of England survey
Warner et al. (2000)	Generalized and segmental dystonia Focal dystonia	1/28 500 1/8500	European consortium survey
Defazio et al. (2001)	Blepharospasm	1/7519	Puglia region, southern Italy
Pekmezovic et al. (2003)	Focal dystonia, cervical dystonia	1/8929	Belgrade, Serbia
Le et al. (2003)	Focal and segmental dystonia	1/3534	Europeans in Oslo, Norway
Matsumoto et al. (2003)	Focal dystonia	1/9900	Kyoto, Japan
Bradley et al. (2003)	Blepharospasm	Incidence: 1.2/100 000/year	Olmsted County, Minnesota
Sugawara et al. (2006)	Generalized dystonia Focal dystonia	1/147 000 1/6900	Akita Prefecture, Japan
Fukuda et al. (2006)	Focal dystonia	1/7300	Tottori Prefecture, Japan
Asgeirsson et al. (2006)	Focal dystonia Segmental dystonia Multifocal dystonia Generalized dystonia	1/3077 1/32 258 1/44 667 1/333 333	Iceland
Das et al. (2007)	Focal dystonia (mostly limb)	1/2038	Kolkata, India
Frédéric et al. (2007)	DYT1 (*TOR1A*) mutations in newborns	Incidence: 1/12 000/year	Hérault, France
Marras et al. (2007)	Cervical dystonia, multiethnic population	Incidence: 1.07/100 000/year	Northern California

Table 12.5 Three ways to classify torsion dystonia

1. By age at onset

A. Early-onset: ≤26 years
B. Late-onset: >26 years

2. By distribution

A. Focal
B. Segmental
C. Multifocal
D. Generalized
E. Hemidystonia

3. By etiology

A. Primary (also known as idiopathic) dystonia
B. Dystonia-plus
C. Secondary dystonia (environmental insult)
D. Heredodegenerative dystonia (usually presents as dystonia-plus)
E. A feature of another neurologic disease (e.g., dystonic tics, paroxysmal dyskinesias, PD, progressive supranuclear palsy)

Table 12.6 Distribution of dystonia by body parts

	No.	Percentage
Focal	1230	50
Segmental	837	34
Generalized	383	16
	2450	100

Data from the Center for Parkinson Disease and Other Movement Disorders, Columbia University Medical Center, New York City.

Detailed clinical descriptions as to how dystonia manifests itself in the different regions of the body have been summarized by Fahn (1984a). The most common primary focal dystonia seen in a movement disorder clinic is cervical dystonia (torticollis), followed by dystonias affecting cranial musculature, such as blepharospasm and spasmodic

Table 12.7 Distribution of focal dystonias

Type of dystonia	No.	Percentage
Torticollis	447	44.4
Spasmodic dysphonia	257	25.5
Blepharospasm	140	13.9
Right arm	96	9.5
Oromandibular	31	3.1
Left arm	20	2.0
Left leg	6	0.6
Trunk	5	0.5
Right leg	4	0.4
	1006	100

Data from the Center for Parkinson Disease and Other Movement Disorders, Columbia University Medical Center, New York City.

Table 12.8 Distribution of segmental dystonias

Type of dystonia	No.	Percentage
Segmental cranial	167	42.8
Cranial + brachial	56	14.4
Cranial + axial	14	3.6
Segmental brachial	83	21.3
Segmental axial	31	7.9
Segmental crural	13	3.3
Multifocal	26	6.7
	390	100

Data from the Center for Parkinson Disease and Other Movement Disorders, Columbia University Medical Center, New York City.

Table 12.9 Five categories of the etiologic classification of dystonia

A. Primary (also known as idiopathic) dystonia
B. Dystonia-plus
C. Secondary dystonia
D. Heredodegenerative diseases (usually present as dystonia-plus)
E. A feature of another neurologic disease (e.g., dystonic tics, paroxysmal dyskinesias, Parkinson disease, progressive supranuclear palsy)

seling, but also because it should lead to understanding the pathophysiology of the illness and how to prevent dystonia. The etiologic classification (Fahn et al., 1998a) divides the causes of dystonia into five major categories: primary (or idiopathic), secondary (environmental causes) (or symptomatic), dystonia-plus syndromes, heredodegenerative diseases in which dystonia is a prominent feature, and the presence of dystonia as a feature of another neurologic disease (Table 12.9).

Primary dystonia is characterized as a pure dystonia (with the exception that tremor can be present) and excludes a symptomatic cause. Dystonia-plus syndromes, such as DRD and myoclonus–dystonia, were previously considered to be variants of primary dystonia (Fahn, 1989c). But because symptoms and signs other than dystonia, namely, parkinsonism and myoclonus, respectively, are present, these entities are placed in the dystonia-plus category. Another concept is that dystonia-plus syndromes, like the primary dystonias, are not neurodegenerative disorders, but neurochemical ones (Fahn et al., 1998a). Secondary dystonias are those due to environmental insult, while heredodegenerative dystonias are due to neurodegenerative diseases that are usually inherited.

Primary dystonia

Primary dystonia consists of familial and nonfamilial (sporadic) types. Although most patients with torsion dystonia have a negative family history for this disorder, the presence of other affected family members allows the family to be investigated in terms of localizing the abnormal gene(s) for dystonia. In primary dystonia, the only neurologic abnormality is the presence of dystonic postures and movements, with the exception of tremor that can resemble essential tremor and can even be essential tremor in some individuals. There is no associated loss of postural reflexes, amyotrophy, weakness, spasticity, ataxia, reflex change, abnormality of eye movements, disorder of retina, dementia, or seizures except where they may be the result of a concomitant problem such as a complication from a neurosurgical procedure undertaken to correct the dystonia, or the presence of some other incidental neurologic disease. Since many of the secondary dystonias have these neurologic findings, the presence of any of these findings in a patient with dystonia immediately suggests that one is dealing with a secondary dystonia, a dystonia-plus syndrome, or a heredodegenerative disorder (Table 12.9). However, the absence of such neurologic findings does not necessarily exclude the possibility of a secondary dystonia, which may rarely present as a pure dystonia.

As discussed above in the phenomenology section, tremor in the primary dystonias may be due to a dystonic tremor

dysphonia (Table 12.7). The most common primary segmental dystonia involves the cranial structures, and these are commonly referred to as cranial-cervical dystonia and sometimes as Meige syndrome (Tolosa and Klawans, 1979; Tolosa et al., 1988a) (Table 12.8). Details of cervical dystonia have been reviewed (Dauer et al., 1998). Primary axial dystonia that presents in adulthood is much less common than the cranial-cervical dystonias. In 9 of the 18 patients collected by Bhatia and colleagues (1997), onset was in the back, with the other half spreading to the back from the cranial-cervical region. Probably because of the age at onset, it does not spread to the legs. About one-third of their patients improved with high-dose anticholinergics with or without antidopaminergics.

Classification by etiology

Awareness of etiology is an ultimate aim in the clinical evaluation of dystonia, not only for treatment and genetic coun-

(Fahn, 1984b) that results from rhythmic group action potentials that occur in dystonia (Yanagisawa and Goto, 1971). It remains to be elucidated whether tremor that mimics essential tremor and enhanced physiologic tremor that is seen in many patients with dystonia as well as in members of their families (Zeman et al., 1960; Yanagisawa et al., 1972; Couch, 1976; Deuschl et al., 1997) is actually a component of idiopathic dystonia (i.e., dystonic tremor). Hand tremor in patients with cervical dystonia more closely resembles enhanced physiologic tremor than dystonic tremor or essential tremor (Deuschl et al., 1997).

Within the primary dystonias are a variety of genetic disorders, some of which have had their genes already mapped to DYT1, DYT2, DYT4, DYT6, DYT7, and DYT13. Other familial primary dystonias have not yet been mapped. But most primary dystonias are sporadic and with an onset during adulthood, usually presenting as one of a variety of focal and segmental dystonias (Tables 12.7 and 12.8); these are discussed below. DYT1 (Oppenheim dystonia) is discussed in more detail later in the chapter. Here we comment on some of the other primary familial dystonias listed in Table 12.10.

In the Mennonite and Amish populations, a mixed type of autosomal dominant dystonia has been seen in which onset can be either in childhood or adulthood, with involvement of limbs and the cervical and cranial regions and designated DYT6. Dysphonia and dysarthria are often the most

---

Table 12.10 Detailed etiologic classification of the dystonias

A. Primary (also known as idiopathic) dystonia

1. Oppenheim dystonia (originally called dystonia musculorum deformans)

   Genetics

   a. Autosomal dominant
   b. Penetrance rate between 30% and 40%
   c. Deletion of one of a pair of GAG triplets (codes for glutamic acid) in the DYT1 gene (also called *TOR1A*) located on chromosome 9q34.1
   d. DYT1 codes for the heat-shock, ATP-binding protein, torsinA, an AAA+ protein
   e. In the Ashkenazi Jewish population, there is a characteristic extended haplotype due to a founder's effect in which the mutation entered this population approximately 350 years ago
   f. Gene prevalence is 1/2000 in the Ashkenazi Jewish population
   g. Commercial gene testing is available

   Clinical phenotype

   a. Early onset (age <40)
   b. Limbs usually affected first
   c. Spread to other sites is related to age at onset and site of onset
   d. Pure dystonia (no other neurologic feature except action tremor may be present)
   e. No known consistent pathology
   f. MRI normal
   g. FDG PET: increased lenticular and decreased thalamic metabolic activity consistent with increased direct striatopallidal activity

2. Childhood and adult onset, familial cranial and limb (DYT6)

   Genetics

   a. Autosomal dominant
   b. Mutation in the *THAP1* gene on 8p11.21

   Clinical phenotype

   a. Childhood and adult onset
   b. Site of onset in arm or cranial (including laryngeal), occasionally leg or neck
   c. Usually remains as upper body involvement
   d. Large pedigree in the Mennonite and Amish populations, but is more widespread

3. Adult-onset familial torticollis

   Genetics

   a. Autosomal dominant
      (1) DYT7 = a north German family: 18p (Leube et al., 1996). Platelet complex 1 activity may be decreased
      (2) Gene specificity is uncertain in other torticollis patients in northern Germany (Leube and Auburger, 1998; Klein et al., 1998b), and findings appear to be limited to one family
      (3) Other families with autosomal dominant torticollis that are not DYT1, DYT7, or DYT13, and their gene mappings have not yet been published

   Clinical phenotype

   a. Mostly adult onset, occasionally in adolescence
   b. Limited to neck in 85%
   c. Occasional involvement of arm

4. Adult-onset familial cervical-cranial predominant (DYT13)

   Genetics

   a. Autosomal dominant
   b. Not DYT1
   c. One family has been mapped to chromosome1 p36.13–p36.32

   Clinical phenotype

   a. Mostly adult onset, occasionally in childhood
   b. Site of onset usually in neck, which predominates
   c. Usually remains segmental as cranial-cervical
   d. Occasional involvement of arm

5. Other familial types to be identified as distinct entities

6. Sporadic, usually adult onset
   a. Could be genetic, but uncertain
      (1) In patients with cervical dystonia, a search of polymorphisms in the dopamine receptor (D1 to D5) and dopamine transporter genes found an increased number of polymorphisms in allele 2 of the D5 receptor gene, and a decrease in allele 6 of this gene compared to controls (Placzek et al., 2001). Adult-onset dystonia typically is not associated with the DYT1 gene, whereas almost all young-onset, limb-onset individuals have the DYT1 mutation
   b. Classify by age at onset:

      childhood onset (<13)

      adolescent onset (13–20)

      adult onset (>20)
   c. No known pathology

Continued

Table 12.10 Continued

B. Dystonia-plus syndromes

1. Dystonia with parkinsonism
   a. Dopa-responsive dystonia (DRD)
   (1) GTP cyclohydrolase I deficiency (DYT5). First step in tetrahydrobiopterin (BH4) synthesis

   Genetics

   (a) Autosomal dominant with different mutations of the gene for GTP cyclohydrolase I (GCH) located at 14q22.1

   Clinical phenotype

   (b) Childhood onset (<16) with leg and gait disorder
   (c) Girls > boys
   (d) May be diurnal (no symptoms in morning, worse at night)
   (e) Parkinsonian signs present (bradykinesia, loss of postural reflexes, rigidity)
   (f) Markedly improves with low dose levodopa
   (g) Must differentiate from juvenile Parkinson disease
   (h) Adult onset with parkinsonism or a focal dystonia of neck, cranial, or arm involvement
   (i) No pathological neurodegeneration
   (j) Normal FDOPA PET and β-CIT SPECT
   (k) Abnormal phenylalanine loading test in GCH defect

   (2) Autosomal recessive with mutation of tyrosine hydroxylase gene on chromosome 21; infantile onset
   (3) Other biopterin deficient diseases; infantile or adult onset
       (a) 6-Pyruvoyltetrahydropterin synthase deficiency (second step in BH4 synthesis); autosomal recessive
       (b) Pterin-4a-carbinolamine dehydratase deficiency (required for BH4 regeneration after oxidation); autosomal recessive
       (c) Dihydropteridine reductase deficiency (required for BH4 regeneration after oxidation); autosomal recessive
       (d) Sepiapterin reductase deficiency; autosomal recessive

   b. Dopamine agonist-responsive dystonia
   (1) Aromatic amino acid decarboxylase (AADC) deficiency
   (2) Autosomal recessive

   c. Rapid-onset dystonia–parkinsonism (RDP)
   Genetics

   (1) Autosomal dominant
   (2) Mutation found in the α3 subunit of the gene for the Na$^+$/K$^+$-ATPase (ATP1A3)

   Clinical phenotype

   (1) Adolescent and adult onset
   (2) Progresses to generalized over hours to a few weeks
   (3) Parkinsonian signs present
   (4) Tends to plateau
   (5) Speech involvement
   (6) No known pathology
   (7) Normal dopamine nerve terminal imaging (Zanotti-Fregonara et al., 2008)

   d. Early-onset dystonia with parkinsonism (DYT16)
   Genetics

   (1) Autosomal recessive
   (2) Mutation and a deletion in the *PRKRA* gene for protein kinase, interferon-inducible double-stranded RNA-dependent activator

Clinical phenotype

(1) Childhood-onset
(2) Begins in the legs and spreads to become generalized dystonia
(3) Orofacial dystonia and facial grimacing are prominent
(4) Some patients also had bradykinesia, one with tremor

2. Dystonia with myoclonic jerks that respond to alcohol
   a. Myoclonus–dystonia
   Genetics

   (1) Autosomal dominant
   (2) Gene mapped to chromosome 7q21
   (3) Mutations in the epsilon-sarcoglycan gene
   (4) Another locus on 18p11, gene not identified
   (5) SCA14 can present with a similar phenotype (Foncke et al., 2010)

   Clinical phenotype

   (1) Alcohol-responsive, lightning-like jerks present
   (2) Upper part of body affected, legs usually spared
   (3) Childhood, adolescent and adult onset
   (4) Slowly progressive
   (5) Tends to plateau
   (6) Pathology unknown
   (7) May be same disorder as hereditary essential myoclonus

C. Secondary dystonia

1. Perinatal cerebral injury
   a. Athetoid cerebral palsy
   b. Delayed onset dystonia
   c. Pachygyria
2. Encephalitis, infectious and postinfectious
   a. Reye syndrome
   b. Subacute sclerosing leukoencephalopathy
   c. Creutzfeldt–Jakob disease
   d. HIV infection
3. Head trauma
4. Thalamotomy and thalamic lesions
5. Lenticular nucleus lesions
6. Primary antiphospholipid syndrome
7. Focal cerebral vascular injury
8. Arteriovenous malformation
9. Hypoxia
10. Brain tumor
11. Multiple sclerosis
12. Brainstem lesion, including pontine myelinolysis
13. Posterior fossa tumors
14. Cervical cord injury or lesion, including syringomyelia
15. Lumbar canal stenosis
16. Peripheral injury
17. Electrical injury
18. Drug-induced
    a. Levodopa
    b. Dopamine D2 receptor blocking agents
        (1) Tardive dystonia
        (2) Acute dystonic reaction
    c. Ergotism
    d. Anticonvulsants

Table 12.10 Continued

19. Toxins: Mn, CO, carbon disulfide, cyanide, methanol, disulfiram, 3-nitroproprionic acid, wasp sting (Leopold et al., 1999)
20. Metabolic: hypoparathyroidism
21. Immune encephalopathy: Sjögren syndrome, multiple myeloma, Rasmussen syndrome
22. Psychogenic

D. Heredodegenerative diseases (typically not pure dystonia)

1. X-linked recessive
   a. Lubag (X-linked dystonia-parkinsonism) (DYT3)
   Genetics
   (1) X-linked autosomal recessive
   (2) DYT3 gene mapped to centromere; Xq13, *TAF1* gene

   Clinical phenotype
   (1) Filipino males
   (2) Occasional Filipino female carriers affected; manifesting chorea or dystonia
   (3) Young adult onset
   (4) Cranial (oromandibular and lingual) dystonia or generalized dystonia
   (5) Parkinsonism can appear at onset and be only feature or develop after and replace dystonia
   (6) Steadily progressive → disabling
   (7) Pathology: mosaic gliosis in striatum
   (8) PET: normal FDOPA; hypometabolic in striatum

   Pathology
   Mosaic pattern of gliosis in the striatum

   b. Deafness–dystonia syndrome (Mohr–Tranebjaerg syndrome) (Tranebjaerg et al., 2000; Ujike et al., 2001)
   Genetics
   (1) X-linked recessive
   (2) Mutations in DDP1 (deafness-dystonia peptide 1)
   (3) DDP1 acts with human Tim13 in a complex in the intermembrane space of mitochondria (Rothbauer et al., 2001)

   Clinical phenotype
   (1) Deafness and dystonia in males
   (2) Torticollis and writer's cramp also seen in female carriers (Swerdlow and Wooten, 2001)
   (3) Pelizaeus–Merzbacher disease
   (4) Intellectual disability, seizures and infantile spasms
       Mutations in Aristaless related homeobox gene, *ARX* (Stromme et al., 2002)

2. X-linked dominant
   a. Rett syndrome
3. Autosomal dominant
   a. Juvenile parkinsonism (presenting with dystonia)
   b. Huntington disease (usually presents as chorea)
      Gene: IT15 located at 4p16.3 for protein named huntingtin
   c. Neurodegeneration with brain iron accumulation type 3 (neuroferritinopathy), *FTLI* mutation (Chinnery et al., 2007)
   d. Machado–Joseph disease (SCA3)
   e. Dentatorubro-pallidoluysian atrophy
   f. Other spinocerebellar or cerebellar degenerations (Le Ber et al., 2006)

g. Creutzfeldt–Jakob disease (Hellmann and Melamed, 2002)
h. Familial basal ganglia calcifications, gene on 14q (Geschwind et al., 1999)
i. Familial basal ganglia calcifications, gene not on 14q (Wszolek et al., 2006)

4. Autosomal recessive
   a. Wilson disease (can also present with tremor or parkinsonism)
      Gene: Cu-ATPase located at 13q14.3
   b. Niemann–Pick type C (dystonic lipidosis) (sea-blue histiocytosis) defect in cholesterol esterification; gene mapped to chromosome 18
   c. Juvenile neuronal ceroid-lipofuscinosis (Batten disease)
   d. GM1 gangliosidosis (Kobayashi and Suzuki, 1981; Campdelacreu et al., 2002)
   e. GM2 gangliosidosis
   f. Metachromatic leukodystrophy
   g. Lesch–Nyhan syndrome (Jinnah et al., 2006)
   h. Homocystinuria (Sinclair et al., 2006)
   i. Glutaric acidemia
   j. Triosephosphate isomerase deficiency
   k. Methylmalonic aciduria
   l. Hartnup disease
   m. Ataxia telangiectasia
   n. Friedreich ataxia (Hou and Jankovic, 2003)
   o. Neurodegeneration with brain iron accumulation type 1 (formerly called Hallervorden–Spatz syndrome), recently renamed as pantothenate kinase-associated neurodegeneration (PKAN) (Hayflick et al., 2003)
   p. Neurodegeneration with brain iron accumulation type 2, infantile neuroaxonal dystrophy (*PLA2G6* mutation) (PARK14)
   q. Neurodegeneration with brain iron accumulation type 3, aceruloplasminemia
   r. Neurodegeneration with brain iron accumulation (FAHN) (FA2H mutation)
   s. Neuroacanthocytosis
   t. Neuronal intranuclear hyaline inclusion disease
   u. Hereditary spastic paraplegia with dystonia
   v. Sjögren–Larsson syndrome (ichthyosis, spasticity, intellectual disability) (Cubo and Goetz, 2000).
   w. Ataxia–amyotrophy–intellectual disability–dystonia syndrome (Wilmshurst et al., 2000)
   x. Biotin-responsive basal ganglia disease (SLC19A3 mutation) (Debs et al., 2010)
5. Probable autosomal recessive
   a. Progressive pallidal degeneration
6. Mitochondrial
   a. Leigh disease
      Genes: nuclear and mitochondrial DNA
   b. Leber disease
      Gene: mitochondrial DNA
   c. Other mitochondrial encephalopathies (Sudarsky et al., 1999)
7. Associated with parkinsonian syndromes
   a. Parkinson disease
   b. Progressive supranuclear palsy
   c. Multiple system atrophy
   d. Cortical-basal ganglionic degeneration

Adapted from Fahn S, Bressman SB, Marsden CD. Classification of dystonia. In: Fahn S, Marsden CD, DeLong MR, eds. Dystonia 3. Advances in Neurology vol. 78. Lippincott-Raven, Philadelphia, 1998, pp. 1–10, with more recent additions.

Table 12.11 Comparisons of the focal dystonias

Feature	Blepharospasm	Dysphonia	Cervical dystonia	Hand dystonia
Prevalence per million	17–133	11–59	23–130	3.8–80
Predominant gender	Female	Female	Female	Male
Age at onset, mean	55.7	43	40.7	38
% spread by 5 years	58%	9–19%	12–35%	13%
Sensory trick	Yes	No	Yes	Yes
Task specificity	No	Yes	No	Yes
Possible risk factors	Dry eyes, irritation	Sore throat	Neck-trunk trauma	Repetitive task

Adapted from Defazio G, Berardelli A, Hallett M. Do primary adult-onset focal dystonias share aetiological factors? Brain 2007;130(Pt 5):1183–1193.

disabling features, and when present with segmental or generalized dystonia, one should suspect the possibility that the disorder may be DYT6. The mutation was found on the *THAP1* gene on 8p11.21 (Fuchs et al., 2009). Since this gene discovery, the *THAP1* mutation has been found in populations other than the Mennonite/Amish sect.

Several families with adult-onset familial torticollis have been reported, with one of them (Family K in northwest Germany) mapped to chromosome 18p, this locus being designated DYT7 (Leube et al., 1996). Investigation of more families and of apparently sporadic cases of torticollis from this region showed that most have inherited the same mutation as Family K from a common ancestor and, in fact, owe their disease to autosomal dominant inheritance at low penetrance (Leube et al., 1997a, 1997b). However, subsequent information from these authors now questions whether their findings are incorrect (Leube and Auburger, 1998; Klein et al., 1998b). Other families with torticollis have been excluded from the chromosome 18p region and from DYT1 (Bressman et al., 1996; Cassetta et al., 1999; Jarman et al., 1999).

Cervical-cranial predominant dystonia is another form of autosomal dominant primary dystonia; it has been seen in non-Jewish families that do not link to DYT1 (Bressman et al., 1994b, 1996; Bentivoglio et al., 1997). The site of onset is usually in the neck, which continues to dominate, but dystonia often spreads to involve the cranial structures as well, and occasionally the arm. Onset may be in childhood (Bentivoglio et al., 1997) or adulthood (Bressman et al., 1994b). An autosomal dominant Italian family described by Bentivoglio and colleagues (1997, 2004) with predominantly early onset with cervical-cranial or brachial dystonia has been mapped to chromosome1p36.13–p36.32 and has been categorized as DYT13 (Valente et al., 2001).

Two unrelated consanguineous Brazilian families with early-onset dystonia–parkinsonism were found to have a mutation in the *PRKRA* gene for protein kinase, interferon-inducible double-stranded RNA-dependent activator (Camargos et al., 2008). Onset began with abnormal gait and leg pain around age 12 years. Later the upper body became involved with dysphagia, spasmodic dysphonia, torticollis, upper limb dystonia, and opisthotonus. Orofacial dystonia and facial grimacing were prominent features. Some patients also had bradykinesia, one with tremor.

Subsequently, a deletion in this gene was discovered in a German boy, whose dystonia began in the legs and became generalized (Seibler et al., 2008).

Adult-onset focal dystonias

These are the most common forms of dystonias. Their appearance varies depending on which body part is affected. Although most cases remain focal, there can be contiguous spread to a neighboring segment, thus becoming segmental myoclonus. Seemingly distinct from each other (Table 12.11), the focal dystonias do have some overlap in that when they spread, they affect a contiguous body part and therefore exist in the same patient. This observation and some shared physiological changes have suggested to Defazio and his colleagues (2007) that the different focal dystonias probably share common genetic factors in a multifactorial disease.

The most common focal dystonia involves the neck musculature, known as *spasmodic torticollis* or *cervical dystonia* (Table 12.7). The head can turn (rotational torticollis), tilt, or shift to one side, or bend forward (antecollis) or backwards (retrocollis). Any combination of head positions can be found in individual patients. About 10% have a remission within a year, but relapses usually occur, even many years later (Friedman and Fahn, 1986; Lowenstein and Aminoff, 1988; Jahanshahi et al., 1990; Chan et al., 1991). The average age at onset is between 20 and 50 years. The muscles involved are innervated by cranial nerve (CN) XI and the upper cervical nerve roots. Some cervical dystonias are manifested as a static pulling of the head into one direction, but most have a jerky, irregular rhythmic feature. Some patients try to fight the pulling of the neck muscles and the physician can be misled by seeing or feeling contracted muscles, thinking that these are the dystonic muscles, when in fact they could be the compensatory muscles contracting. To distinguish between involuntary and compensatory/voluntary contractions, the patient should be told to let the movements occur without trying to overcome them. Then the true direction of which muscles are involved by the dystonia is revealed. This is especially important when deciding which muscles to inject with botulinum toxin. Hypermetabolism of dystonic muscles was detected by fluorodeoxyglucose (FDG) PET (Sung et al., 2007), but it is not certain that a compensating muscle would not show the same pattern. Common sensory tricks to reduce dystonia are touching the face or the back of the head. The variety of sensory tricks have been enumerated (Ochudło et al., 2007). Mechanical devices to place cutaneous pressure on the occiput can sometimes be used to advantage. Pain in the neck muscles is common in cervical dystonia (Chan et al., 1991).

Blepharospasm usually occurs in older individuals, women more than men. It begins as excessive blinking, and many patients complain of eye irritation or dryness, although dry eyes from Sjögren disease are usually ruled out. This blinking phase then leads to some longer closing of the eyes, even to very long durations, which has been mistaken for weakness of the levator palpebrae (ptosis) instead of contraction of the orbicularis oculi. Usually there is a combination of eyelid closing and blinking. The muscles involved are the orbicularis oculi innervated by CN VII, and the contractions are symmetrical in the two eyes, quite distinct from hemifacial spasm, which is unilateral. Another interesting difference is that usually in hemifacial spasm the eyebrow may elevate due to simultaneous contraction of the frontalis muscles (known as "the other Babinski sign" – Devoize, 2001; Stamey and Jankovic, 2007), whereas in blepharospasm the eyebrows come down. Dystonia can spread from the upper face causing blepharospasm, to the lower face with movements around the mouth. Common sensory tricks to reduce blepharospasm are touching the corner of the eye, coughing, and talking. Bright light notoriously aggravates blepharospasm and patients have difficulty being in sunlight or bright light and they often wear sunglasses most of the time. Driving at night is very difficult because of oncoming headlights. Blepharospasm tends to spread from upper face to involve lower face, and may spread to involve muscles innervated by CN V, tongue, and neck (Fahn, 1985). Spread of blepharospasm is more common than with other adult-onset dystonias (Svetel et al., 2007; Abbruzzese et al., 2008). Blepharospasm needs to be differentiated from so-called apraxia of eyelid opening in which the lids fail to open due to either "freezing," levator inhibition, or dystonia, and is often seen in atypical parkinsonian disorders, such as progressive supranuclear palsy. Injection of botulinum toxin into the Riolan muscle can be effective in treating lid "apraxia," believed to be analogous to a sensory trick (Inoue and Rogers, 2007). About 4% of patients with blepharospasm also have eyelid-opening apraxia (Peckham et al., 2011).

Ormandibular dystonia (OMD) (jaw muscles innervated by CN V) is often associated with lingual dystonia (tongue muscles by CN XII), and is less frequent than blepharospasm. Jaw-opening dystonia is where the jaw is pulled down by the pterygoids; in jaw-clenching dystonia the masseters and temporalis muscles are the prime movers. The jaw can also be moved laterally. It is important to distinguish the latter from facial muscle pulling the mouth to one side, which is often due to psychogenic etiology. OMD can markedly affect chewing and swallowing. Some OMDs appear only with action and are not present at rest. Such actions can involve talking or chewing. Often a patient attempts to overcome jaw-opening and jaw-closing dystonias by purposefully moving the jaw in the opposite direction. This maneuvering has often led to misdiagnosis of tardive dyskinesia because the movements superficially appear rhythmic. To distinguish between OMD and tardive dyskinesia, the patient should be told to let the movements occur without trying to overcome them. In this manner, the true direction of where the dystonia wants to take the jaw is revealed, and the rhythmic movements stop in OMD. Sensory tricks that have been useful are the placing of objects in the mouth or biting down on an object, such as a tongue blade or pencil. Dental implants have sometimes helped by the physical application of a continual sensory trick. Pure lingual dystonia, with protrusion of the tongue, can affect speech and sometimes swallowing and breathing (Schneider et al., 2006a).

Embouchure dystonia is an action dystonia involving the muscles around the mouth (embouchure) that may develop in professional musicians who play wind instruments. More common are *musician's cramps* involving the fingers in instrumentalists such as pianists, guitarists and violinists. This is a form of occupational cramp, the most common being *writer's cramp*. These are task-specific dystonias. In writer's cramp, only the action of writing brings out the dystonic tightening of the finger, hand, forearm, and arm muscles, such as the triceps. If the dystonia progresses, other actions of the arm, like finger-to-nose maneuver, buttoning or sewing, bring out the dystonia. Ultimately, dystonia at rest can develop, but usually does not. About 15% of patients with writer's cramp have spread to the other arm. Otherwise, the patient can learn to write with the uninvolved arm. Sensory tricks that have been useful are the placing of the pen/pencil in between other fingers, using specially designed larger writing implements, and placing the non-writing hand on top of the writing hand.

Dystonia of the vocal cords come in two varieties: adduction or abduction of the cords with speaking. The former produces a tight, constricted, strangulated type of voice with frequent pauses breaking up the voice, and it takes longer to complete what the patient is trying to say. The latter produces a whispering voice. With dystonic adductor dysphonia, the patient is still able to whisper normally, and may present this way to the physician, who needs to be aware that this is a compensating mechanism. A major differential diagnosis is vocal cord tremor, seen fairly commonly in patients with essential tremor.

Focal trunk dystonia can present in adults, both as primary dystonia and as tardive dystonia. The dystonia is usually absent when the patient is lying or sitting, and appears on standing and walking. This is an uncommon form of adult-onset focal dystonia.

Dystonia-plus syndromes

Dystonia-plus syndromes represent a group of dystonias that are associated with parkinsonism or myoclonus without known degeneration or loss of neurons; these include dopa-responsive dystonia, dopamine agonist-responsive dystonia, and myoclonus–dystonia. These are therefore considered neurochemical disorders instead of neurodegenerative ones. A neurodegenerative disease is a neurologic disorder due to progressive dying and loss of neurons in the central nervous system (CNS), visible by light microscopy, and often accompanied by gliosis and by intracellular inclusions. Many neurodegenerative diseases are inherited, and some are known to have specific metabolic causes; but all produce visible pathologic changes in the brain. A neurochemical disease is a neurologic disorder due to a primary biochemical defect that alters CNS function and is not associated with a loss of neurons.

Details of DRD (including GTP cyclohydrolase 1 deficiency, tyrosine hydroxylase (TH) deficiency, and pterin synthesis deficiencies), rapid-onset dystonia–parkinsonism (RDP), and myoclonus–dystonia are presented in their own sections below.

A disorder that is analogous to DRD is *dopamine agonist-responsive dystonia*, which is considered here briefly. It was first described by Hyland and colleagues (1992) (Video 12.16) and a second family was described by Maller and colleagues (1997). It is due to an autosomal recessive disorder beginning in the first few months of life with hypotonia, hypokinesia, and developmental delay. Eventually, the patient experiences autonomic dysfunction (hyperhidrosis, miosis, and ptosis), dystonia–parkinsonism, episodes of oculogyria, and other paroxysmal movements and bouts of deep sleep (Hyland et al., 1992; Pons et al., 2004). It is the result of reduced activity of aromatic L-amino acid decarboxylase (AADC), so there is reduced metabolism of dopa to dopamine and 5-hydroxytryptophan to serotonin (Hyland et al., 1992). There is reduced concentration of the metabolites of dopamine and serotonin in urine, namely, homovanillic acid and 5-hydroxyindoleacetic acid, respectively. AADC deficiency is one of the pediatric CSF neurotransmitter disorders (Patterson, 2010). The symptoms respond partially to dopamine agonists plus a monoamine oxidase inhibitor. Mild cases do occur. Two siblings presenting with fatigability, hypersomnolence, and dystonia had an excellent response to treatment with dopamine agonist and MAO inhibitor (Tay et al., 2007). The variability of response from excellent to almost none (Pons et al., 2004) is unexplained. The diagnosis depends on reduced CSF biogenic amines, metabolites and plasma AADC levels. CSF 3-O-methyldopa is elevated (Tay et al., 2007). Direct sequencing of the AADC gene should be performed. 🎥

In a series of 78 patients with AADC deficiency (46 reported previously), symptoms (hypotonia 95%, oculogyric crises 86%), and developmental delay (63%) became clinically evident during infancy or childhood (Brun et al., 2010). A total of 24 mutations in the AADC gene were detected in that series. No autopsies have been performed, so there remains uncertainty whether this is a neurochemical rather than a neurodegenerative disease; but without an autopsy to determine this, it is placed now in the dystonia-plus category.

A similar clinical presentation occurs with several pterin disorders (Hyland et al., 1998). The autosomal recessive biopterin deficiency states that are listed with the dopa-responsive dystonias in Table 12.10 should be mentioned here because they also manifest features of decreased norepinephrine and serotonin in addition to dystonia and parkinsonism. In this way they more closely resemble the phenotype of aromatic amino acid decarboxylase deficiency. Their clinical features include miosis, oculogyria, rigidity, hypokinesia, chorea, myoclonus, seizures, temperature disturbance, and hypersalivation. The clinical syndrome can present at any age with generalized dystonia–parkinsonism and with marked diurnal fluctuation (Hanihara et al., 1997). These pterin enzyme deficiencies cause hyperphenylalaninemia, and they may respond partially to levodopa and 5-hydroxytryptophan. There are no neuropathologic

observations, and they have arbitrarily been listed in the dystonia-plus syndrome category rather than as a neurodegeneration. But intellectual disability or delay is common. Dihydropteridine reductase deficiency can respond partially to levodopa without inducing dyskinesias despite long-term therapy (Sedel et al., 2006). Indicating this is a neurochemical disorder rather than a neurodegenerative one is the lack of dopaminergic cell loss as suggested by normal PET imaging of the dopamine transporter (Sedel et al., 2006). Sepiapterin reductase deficiency can be associated with hypersomnolence (Friedman et al., 2006), as seen also in aromatic decarboxylase deficiency syndrome.

In DYT16, onset begins with abnormal gait and leg pain around age 12 years (Camargos et al., 2008). Later the upper body becomes involved with dysphagia, spasmodic dysphonia torticollis, upper limb dystonia, and opisthotonus. Orofacial dystonia and facial grimacing are prominent features. Some patients also had bradykinesia, one with tremor. Subsequently, a deletion in this gene was discovered in a German boy, whose dystonia began in the legs and became generalized (Seibler et al., 2008).

Secondary dystonia and heredodegenerative diseases

Secondary dystonias

The secondary dystonias are subdivided into several categories. Those that are due to environmental causes are mainly due to lesions causing structural brain damage, and many result in hemidystonia. See the discussion of hemidystonia (almost always secondary dystonia) in the section "Classification by distribution." But the secondary dystonias also include psychogenic dystonia (Fahn et al., 1987; Calne and Lang, 1988; Fahn and Williams, 1988; Table 12.10). The heredodegenerative disorders are those conditions associated with various hereditary neurologic disorders, and those in which neuronal degeneration is present. Most secondary dystonias due to structural lesions in the brain are due to insults to the basal ganglia, particularly the putamen, or its afferent and efferent connections, but brainstem lesions can also result in dystonia (Loher and Krauss, 2009).

Clinicians have recognized that dystonia could become worse if an affected limb is casted and immobilized. Okun and colleagues (2002) reported on four patients who developed segmental dystonia following removal of a cast, which the authors attribute to the trauma of prolonged immobilization (Okun et al., 2002).

Dystonia is perhaps the most common movement disorder (often with hypokinesia seen with disorders causing striatal necrosis). Some of these causes are Wilson disease, toxins, metabolic acidosis (such as from 3-oxothiolase deficiency, propionic acidemia, methylmalonic acidemia, isovaleric acidemia, and glutaric adiduria type 1), HIV and other infections, Leigh disease and other mitochondrial encephalopathies, anoxia, wasp sting encephalopathy (Leopold et al., 1999), hemolytic uremia, vascular disease, and head trauma.

A major portion of the clinical investigation of dystonia (Fahn et al., 1987) concerns the tests that are required to uncover the etiology of secondary and heredodegenerative dystonias. Almost yearly, new etiologies of these types of dystonia are reported. These include mildewed sugar cane ingestion containing the mitochondrial toxin 3-nitroproprionic acid (Ludolph et al., 1992), toxoplasmosis (in AIDS) (Tolge and Factor, 1991), disulfiram intoxication (Krauss et al., 1991), Creutzfeldt–Jakob disease (Sethi and Hess, 1991; Hellmann and Melamed, 2002), primary antiphospholipid syndrome (Angelini et al., 1993), spinal cord lesions (Uncini et al., 1994; Madhusudanan et al., 1995), lumbar canal stenosis resulting in foot dystonia on standing or walking (Blunt et al., 1996), ataxia telangiectasia (Koepp et al., 1994), alternating hemiplegia of childhood (Andermann et al., 1994), organophosphorus insecticide poisoning (Senanayake and Sanmuganathan, 1995), pure thalamic degeneration (Yamamoto and Yamashita, 1995), midbrain hemorrhage (Munoz et al., 1996), bilateral lesions of the mesencephalon and vermis (Rousseaux et al., 1996), posterior fossa tumors (Krauss et al., 1997), electrical injury (Adler and Caviness, 1997), intracerebral arteritis from herpes zoster ophthalmicus (Burbaud et al., 1997), childhood-onset (Uc et al., 2000) or adult-onset Niemann–Pick type C disease (Lossos et al., 1997), adult GM1 gangliosidosis (Kobayashi and Suzuki, 1981; Hirayama et al., 1997; Campdelacreu et al., 2002), optic glioma (Vandertop et al., 1997), neuroferritinopathy (Curtis et al., 2001; Mir et al., 2005; Chinnery et al., 2007), dystonia in spinocerebellar ataxia type 1 (Wu et al., 2004) and in type 6 (Sethi and Jankovic, 2002), familial dystonia associated with cerebellar atrophy (Le Ber et al., 2006), hand dystonia due to neurofibromatosis type 1 (Di Capua et al., 2001), striatal necrosis-induced dystonia with acidosis from 3-oxothiolase deficiency (Yalcinkaya et al., 2001), and striatal necrosis-induced dystonia from hereditary biotin deficiency (Debs et al., 2010). From HIV, there can be dystonia from striatal necrosis (Abbruzzese et al., 1990) or from secondary infections, such as toxoplasmosis (Tolge and Factor, 1991). Homocystinuria can result in recurrent dystonia (Sinclair et al., 2006). It is due to cystathionine β-synthase deficiency. Two biochemical markers for homocystinuria, homocystine and methionine, were markedly elevated during periods when dystonia is manifested. In Lesch–Nyhan disease, although originally described as a choreathetotic disorder, when more carefully analyzed, the major movement disorder is dystonia (Jinnah et al., 2006).

Onset of dystonia and chorea of the limbs in adolescence and associated with alopecia, hypogonadism, diabetes mellitus, intellectual disability and sensory neural deafness is known as the Woodhouse–Sakati syndrome (Schneider and Bhatia, 2008). It is an autosomal recessive disorder.

Dystonia can present in patients with pyruvate dehydrogenase deficiency (Head et al., 2004). The main clue to the biochemical diagnosis is a raised concentration of lactate in the cerebrospinal fluid. These patients can respond to levodopa.

If dystonia occurs in the first year of life, the leading cause is cerebral palsy or a metabolic error, such as glutaric aciduria (Kyllerman et al., 1994). A number of cases of symptomatic dystonias, so-called *delayed-onset dystonia*, appear months to years after the cerebral insult (Burke et al., 1980). Often such a delayed onset is seen with perinatal or early childhood asphyxia (Saint-Hilaire et al., 1991). In a series of long-term follow-up of patients with perinatal asphyxia, only about 1% develop delayed-onset dystonia (Cerovac et al., 2007).

Delayed onset of dystonia can be seen also with central pontine myelinolysis (Tison et al., 1991; Maraganore et al., 1992), cyanide intoxication (Valenzuela et al., 1992), head trauma (Lee et al., 1994), and a variety of other static brain lesions (Scott and Jankovic, 1996). Ingestion causes striatal necrosis and coma, and the dystonia evolves as the patient comes out of the coma (He et al., 1995). Dystonia from severe head trauma is usually delayed. Of 221 patients who survived severe head trauma with a Glasgow Coma Score of ≤8, 4% later developed dystonia (Krauss et al., 1996). The dystonia appeared with a latency of 2 months to 2 years. Delayed-onset generalized dystonia due to cerebral anoxia can worsen over time, and show a delay in magnetic resonance imaging (MRI) changes in the globus pallidi (Kuoppamaki et al., 2002). The delayed-onset dystonia from the ingestion of mildewed sugar cane containing the *Arthrinium*-produced mycotoxin 3-nitroproprionic acid (3-NP) is not the same phenomenon. 3-NP is a mitochondrial toxin that irreversibly inhibits complex II (Beal, 1995).

Neurodegenerations with brain iron accumulation (Table 12.12)

The gene for autosomal recessive neurodegeneration with brain iron accumulation type 1 (NBIA) (formerly known as Hallervorden–Spatz syndrome) has been identified as pantothenate kinase (PANK2) (Zhou et al., 2001; Hartig et al., 2006; Valentino et al., 2006). In 49 families with typical phenotype and MRI for NBIA, Hayflick and colleagues (2003) found that all had the PANK2 deficiency; in another 49 families with an atypical phenotype, only 17 had the enzyme deficiency. In another study, looking at 10 families with MRI positive for iron accumulation, only four were found to have a mutation on *PANK2* (Thomas et al., 2004). The presence of a mutation in the *PANK2* gene was associated with younger age at onset and a higher frequency of

Table 12.12 Neurodegenerations with brain iron accumulation (NBIAs)

Condition or acronym	Synonym	Gene	Chromosome
PKAN	NBIA1	*PANK2*	20p13
PLAN	INAD, NBIA2, PARK14	*PLA2G6*	22q12
FAHN	SPG35	*FA2H*	16q23
Aceruloplasminemia		*CP*	3q23
Neuroferittinopathy		*FTL*	19q13
Kufor-Rakeb	PARK9	*ATP13A2*	1p36
SENDA syndrome		?	?

PKAN, pantothenate kinase-associated neurodegeneration; *PANK2*, pantothenate kinase 2; PLAN, PLA2G6-associated neurodegeneration; INAD, infantile neuroaxonal dystrophy; *PLA2G6*, phospholipaseA2; SPG, spastic paraplegia; *FA2H*, fatty acid 2-hydroxylase; *CP*, ceruloplasmin; FAHN, fatty acid hydroxylase neurodegeneration; *FTL*, ferritin light chain; SENDA, static encephalopathy of childhood with neurodegeneration in adulthood.
From Schneider SA, Bhatia KP. Three faces of the same gene: FA2H links neurodegeneration with brain iron accumulation, leukodystrophies, and hereditary spastic paraplegias. Ann Neurol. 2010;68(5):575–577.

Table 12.13 Imaging features of neurodegenerations with iron accumulation

PKAN (*n* = 26)	Neuroferritinopathy (*n* = 21)	INAD (*n* = 4)	Aceruloplasminemia (*n* = 10)
T2*: Eye-of-the-tiger sign in GP in all. Hypointensity of SN (80%); dentate (20%)	T2*: Hypointensity of dentate (95%), SN (81%), cerebral cortex (71%), GP (38%), putamen (28%), thalamus (19%), CN (14%). Hyperintensity as a confluent area between GP and putamen in 52%	T2*: Hypointensity of GP, SN, and dentate in all. No eye-of-the-tiger sign	T2*: Hypointensity of GP, SN, putamen, CN, dentate, thalamus, and cerebral cortex in all. Cerebellar cortex in 50% of cases

CN, cranial nerve; GP globus pallidus; SN, substantia nigra.
Data from McNeill A, Birchall D, Hayflick SJ, et al. T2* and FSE MRI distinguishes four subtypes of neurodegeneration with brain iron accumulation. Neurology 2008;70(18):1614–1619.

dystonia, dysarthria, intellectual impairment, and gait disturbance. Parkinsonism was seen predominantly in adult-onset patients whereas dystonia seemed to be more frequent in the earlier-onset cases. In the most comprehensive study, involving 72 patients with NBIA, 48 (67%) were found to have a *PANK2* mutation (Hartig et al., 2006). No strict correlation between the "eye-of-the-tiger" sign and *PANK2* mutations was found. Not all patients with *PANK2* deficiency have the eye-of-the-tiger sign on MRI; there is a report of one child whose eye-of-the-tiger sign disappeared on the MRI scan over time (Baumeister et al., 2005). Although the "eye-of-the-tiger" sign is very characteristic of *PANK2* mutation, it may also be seen in patients with other NBIA syndromes, such as neuroferritinopathy and aceruloplasminemia, and in corticobasal degeneration and progressive supranuclear palsy (Kumar et al., 2006).

Another iron-accumulating dystonia presenting as infantile neuroaxonal dystrophy (NBIA2) can also present in older individuals, including adult-onset dystonia–parkinsonism with pyramidal tract signs and ataxia. When it presents in adults, it can be without iron accumulation (Kurian et al., 2008; Paisan-Ruiz et al., 2009, 2010). It is due to mutations in a phospholipase gene, *PLA2G6*, and has been labeled PARK14 and as NBIA2, and also called PLAN. Its pathology can show widespread Lewy bodies and hyperphosphorylated tau (Paisan-Ruiz et al., 2010).

Neurodegeneration with brain iron accumulation type 3 is also called neuroferritinopathy. Chinnery and colleagues (2007) studied a large pedigree. Symptoms began in adulthood, and manifested first as chorea in 50%, lower limb dystonia in 42.5%, and parkinsonism in 7.5%. Serum ferritin levels were low in the majority of males and postmenopausal females, but within normal limits for premenopausal females. MR brain imaging was abnormal on all affected individuals and one presymptomatic carrier. A gradient echo brain MRI identified all symptomatic cases.

A fourth neurodegeneration with brain iron accumulation (NBIA4) is aceruloplasminemia, an autosomal recessive disorder affecting the ceruloplasmin gene. NBIA is also seen with a mutation in the fatty acid hydroxylase gene (*FA2H*), manifested with ataxia, spasticity, and dystonia and referred to as FAHN (Kruer et al., 2010). It was originally referred to as a leukodystrophy and as part of the hereditary spastic paraparesis syndromes (Edvardson et al., 2008; Dick et al., 2010). McNeill and colleagues (2008) evaluated gradient

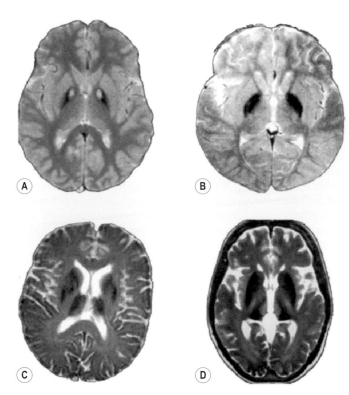

Figure 12.1 Images of four neurodegenerations with iron accumulation. **A** Pantothenate kinase-associated neurodegeneration (PKAN). Note eye-of-the-tiger sign in globus pallidus. **B** Infantile neuroaxonal dystrophy (INAD). **C** Neuroferritinopathy. **D** Aceruloplasminemia.

and fast spin echo MRI scans and showed that the pattern of hypointensities from accumulated iron and hyperintensities differ in the four subtypes of hereditary neurodegenerations with brain iron accumulation, namely pantothenate kinase-associated neurodegeneration (PKAN), neuroferritinopathy, infantile neuroaxonal dystrophy (INAD), and aceruloplasminemia (Table 12.13 and Fig. 12.1).

Other movement disorders in which dystonia can be present

There are some movement disorders, including Parkinson disease and Parkinson-plus syndromes, dystonic tics, and

Table 12.14 Other movement disorders in which dystonia may be present

A. Tic disorders with dystonic tics
B. Paroxysmal dyskinesias with dystonia:
    paroxysmal kinesigenic dyskinesia
    paroxysmal nonkinesigenic dyskinesia
    paroxysmal exertional dyskinesia
    benign infantile paroxysmal dyskinesias
C. Hypnogenic dystonia (sometimes these are seizures)

Table 12.15 Pseudodystonias

(These are not classified as dystonia, but can be mistaken for dystonia because of sustained postures)

1. Sandifer syndrome
2. Stiff-person syndrome
3. Isaacs syndrome
4. Satoyoshi syndrome
5. Rotational atlanto-axial subluxation
6. Soft tissue nuchal mass
7. Bone disease
8. Ligamentous absence, laxity, or damage
9. Congenital muscular torticollis
10. Congenital postural torticollis
11. Juvenile rheumatoid arthritis
12. Ocular postural torticollis
13. Congenital Klippel–Feil syndrome
14. Posterior fossa tumor
15. Syringomyelia
16. Arnold-Chiari malformation
17. Trochlear nerve palsy
18. Vestibular torticollis
19. Seizures manifesting as sustained twisting postures
20. Inflammatory myopathy
21. Torticollis from arteriovenous fistula at craniocervical junction

paroxysmal dyskinesias, in which dystonia is present, but that are not typically classified as dystonia (Table 12.14). Hypnogenic dystonia is commonly a manifestation of frontal lobe epilepsy (Sellal et al., 1991; Meierkord et al., 1992; Montagna, 1992) (see Chapter 22).

Pseudodystonia

There are other neurologic syndromes in which sustained abnormal postures may be present, but that are not considered true dystonias, hence are called pseudodystonia (Table 12.15). These include stiff-person syndrome, Isaacs syndrome, Satoyoshi syndrome (Merello et al., 1994), chronic inflammatory myopathy with involuntary complex repetitive discharges of muscle (Preston et al., 1996), and many others (Table 12.15). It has been found that congenital torticollis not only might be due to thickening and tightness of the sternomastoid muscle (labeled congenital muscular torticollis in Table 12.15), but is even more commonly associated with a palpable sternomastoid tumor (Cheng et al., 2001) and may also be due to other causes, including ocular problems. Most commonly, this is due to weakness of the superior oblique muscle, but it can also be due to paresis of the lateral rectus muscle or nystagmus (Williams et al., 1996). Non-dystonic torticollis may be due to inflammation of joints (Uziel et al., 1998), soft tissue (Shale et al., 1988), and arteriovenous fistula at the craniocervical junction (Bayrakci et al., 1999). Treatment of congenital muscular torticollis by manual stretching is usually safe and effective; surgical treatment is necessary if this noninvasive treatment fails (Cheng et al., 2001).

Following are discussions of a few of the specific entities listed in Table 12.10, in the order presented in the table.

Oppenheim dystonia (DYT1)

Clinical

The phenotypes of Oppenheim dystonia (also known as DYT1 dystonia) was characterized in the Ashkenazi Jewish population when detection of individuals with the DYT1 mutation became possible because of the identification of the special genetic haplotype around the DYT1 gene in this population (Bressman et al., 1994a). The mean ($\pm$ SD) age at onset of symptoms is 12.5 ± 8.2 years. In 94% of patients, symptoms begin in a limb (arm or leg equally) (Videos 12.17 and 12.18); rarely the disorder starts in the neck (3.3%) or larynx (2.2%). Even in the non-Jewish population the same gene is responsible for most cases of early-onset and limb-onset PTD (Kramer et al., 1994). Over time, as diagnostic laboratory examinations for DYT1 have become available, some variations of the phenotype have been observed (Edwards et al., 2003). The phenotype varies from generalized to focal dystonia even in the same family as has been reported in two large families with proven DYT1 gene mutation (Opal et al., 2002; Kostić et al., 2006). The proband of this family died with a dystonic storm, while other family members carrying the same mutation either were asymptomatic or displayed dystonia that was focal, segmental, multifocal, or generalized in distribution. One family member had onset of her dystonia at age 64 years.

The phenotypes in families with non-DYT1 dystonia overlap with each other but differ from those with DYT1 dystonia. In the majority of non-DYT1 families, the dystonia most commonly begins in the cranial-cervical region (Bentivoglio et al., 1997), whereas this site of onset is rare in DYT1 dystonia (Bressman et al., 1994a). Only in DYT6 dystonia in the Mennonite population is there some clinical phenotypic overlap with Oppenheim dystonia (Almasy et al., 1997).

Sequence learning of motor tasks is reduced in manifesting and nonmanifesting gene carriers (Ghilardi et al., 2003). PET imaging obtained during motor task testing showed increased activation in the left premotor cortex and right supplementary motor area, with concomitant reduction in the posterior medial cerebellum. During motor sequence learning, nonmanifesting DYT1 carriers overactivated the lateral cerebellum and the right inferotemporal cortex, and had relative deficits in the dorsolateral prefrontal cortex bilaterally, left anterior cingulate, and the dorsal premotor cortex (Carbon et al., 2008a). These findings suggest that abnormalities in motor behavior and brain function exist in clinically nonmanifesting DYT1 carriers. Similarly, depression has been found in both manifesting and nonmanifesting DYT1 carriers (Heiman et al., 2004). However, evaluation of manifesting and nonmanifesting DYT1 carried out with a comprehensive neuropsychological test battery found no differences from controls on cognitive tests evaluating verbal and nonverbal abstract abilities, attention, information processing speed, and spatial organization (Balas et al., 2006).

Genetics

Previously, Eldridge (1970) proposed that dystonia in the Ashkenazi Jewish population was inherited as an autosomal recessive disorder, while non-Jews inherited dystonia as an autosomal dominant disorder. Reanalysis of Eldridge's data by segregation analysis has shown that dystonia in the Jewish population was also inherited as autosomal dominant (Pauls and Korczyn, 1990). A detailed analysis of the clinical course of dystonia was compared in the Jewish and non-Jewish populations with inherited dystonia, and no major difference was found (Burke et al., 1986). The prevalence of dystonia among Jews of Eastern European ancestry has been estimated to be 1 per 15 000 (Zilber et al., 1984), while for non-Jews the prevalence is 1 per 200 000 (Zeman and Dyken, 1967).

In both Jewish (Bressman et al., 1989) and non-Jewish groups (Zeman and Dyken, 1967), Oppenheim dystonia is inherited as an autosomal dominant disorder, and the gene has been localized to the long arm of chromosome 9 (9q34.1) (Ozelius et al., 1989; Kramer et al., 1990). This abnormal gene has been given the name DYT1, but has been officially renamed *TOR1A*. The mutation that causes the disease has been identified as a deletion of one of a pair of GAG triplets (codes for glutamic acid) in exon 5 near the carboxy terminal in a previously unknown protein, designated torsinA (Ozelius et al., 1997). The GAG deletion is the only sequence change that has been found thus far to be associated uniquely with the disease status, regardless of ethnic origin. Mutations causing this deletion are uncommon, but a few have been encountered (Klein et al., 1998a; Valente et al., 1999), and the unique haplotype found in North American and Russian Ashkenazi Jews with DYT1 has also been seen in Great Britain as well (Valente et al., 1999).

Not every non-Jewish family with dystonia has the DYT1 gene, so dystonia is genetically heterogeneous (Bressman et al., 1994b, 1994c). But all Ashkenazi Jewish families with dystonia with limb onset and onset below the age of 49 in at least one member have so far been found to have the DYT1 gene. Also most cases of non-Jewish individuals with limb-onset and childhood-onset have DYT1 dystonia (Kramer et al., 1994). Intrafamilial correlation for age at onset of dystonia is low (Fletcher et al., 1991b). There is some evidence that dystonia in the Ashkenazi Jewish population tends to begin on the dominant side (Inzelberg et al., 1993). The penetrance rate of gene expression in the Ashkenazi Jewish population is approximately 30% (Bressman et al., 1989; Risch et al., 1990). Variations in the *TOR1A* gene are at least one factor associated with the susceptibility in expressing the disease (Risch et al., 2007). *THAP1* encodes a transcription factor that regulates the expression of *TOR1A*. Wild-type *THAP1* represses the expression of *TOR1A*, whereas DYT6-associated mutant *THAP1* results in decreased repression of *TOR1A* (Gavarini et al., 2010; Kaiser et al., 2010). These observations suggest that transcriptional dysregulation may be a cause of dystonia.

With the availability of direct testing for the DYT1 mutation, Bressman and her colleagues (2000) have developed an algorithm as to which individuals who have the clinical diagnosis of PTD should be tested. They suggest testing in conjunction with genetic counseling for patients with PTD with onset before age 26 years, as this single criterion detected 100% of clinically ascertained carriers, with specificities of 43–63%. Testing patients with onset after age 26 years also may be warranted in those having an affected relative with early onset. The DYT1 gene rarely is found in patients with musician's cramp (Friedman et al., 2000) or in patients with sporadic or familial writer's cramp (Kamm et al., 2000).

The relationship between essential tremor and dystonia has been debated (Lou and Jankovic, 1991; Lang et al., 1992). The finding that families with essential tremor do not have the DYT1 gene by linkage analysis (Conway et al., 1993; Durr et al., 1993) indicates that the two disorders are not genetically identical.

Brain networks and pathways

Neuroimaging studies on Oppenheim dystonia are discussed in the section "Biochemistry and neuroimaging." Based on FDG PET scans and on physiologic monitoring during pallidal surgery in patients with dystonia, there appears to be a disruption of activity within the globus pallidus interna (GPi), suggesting excessive inhibitory input from the striatum. As measured by diffusion tensor imaging, all mutation carriers had reduced connectivity in the cerebellothalamic pathways, with connectivity reduced by approximately 50% compared to normal controls (Argyelan et al., 2009). The reduction was localized to the cerebellar outflow pathway in the white matter of lobule VI, adjacent to the dentate nucleus. Both manifesting and nonmanifesting carriers had reduced connectivity in the proximal segment of the cerebellothalamocortical pathway (i.e., the cerebellothalamic segment), but the nonmanifesting carriers had an additional disruption in the distal, thalamocortical, segment of the pathway. The investigators suggested that perhaps the benefit from pallidal surgery is by affecting the distal connections, bringing the patients to a state resembling nonmanifesting carriers.

Molecular biology

TorsinA is related to homologous proteins throughout the multicellular animal kingdom (Breakefield et al., 2001). It is a 332-amino acid protein and has a molecular weight of 37 813. The torsin family is a member of the AAA+ family of proteins. Their structures indicate that they are heat-shock and ATP-binding proteins. The DYT1 mutation is the first example of a role for any heat-shock protein in a human disease. It suggests a susceptibility to a "second hit." This might explain the low penetrance rate of 30–40% in gene carriers and why many patients with Oppenheim dystonia experience a stress situation prior to the development or exacerbation of the dystonia, e.g., influenza, trauma, surgery, or casting of a body part. Normal torsinA

Table 12.16 Localization of torsinA

Intense expression

Substantia nigra pars compacta dopamine neurons

Locus coeruleus

Cerebellar dentate nucleus

Purkinje cells

Basis pontis

Numerous thalamic nuclei

Pedunculopontine nucleus

Oculomotor nucleus

Hippocampal formation

Frontal cortex.

Moderate expression

Cholinergic neurons in the caudate-putamen

Numerous midbrain and hindbrain nuclei

Weak expression

Noncholinergic striatal neurons

Globus pallidus

Subthalamic nucleus

Data from Augood SJ, Martin DM, Ozelius LJ, et al. Distribution of the mRNAs encoding torsinA and torsinB in the normal adult human brain. Ann Neurol 1999;46(5):761–769.

appears to protect against oxidative stress (Kuner et al., 2003), and torsinA is increased following exposure to the toxin 1-methyl-4-phenyl-1,2,3,6-tetrahydropyridine (MPTP) (Kuner et al., 2004). A malfunctioning torsinA would have difficulty carrying out its chaperoning of damaged proteins that had been altered by a variety of stress factors.

TorsinA mRNA has been mapped in normal human brain and found to be localized in specific regions (Augood et al., 1998, 1999), which are listed in Table 12.16. A similar localization was found by using immunostaining for an antibody raised against torsinA (Augood et al., 2003). Although its location within dopamine neurons, among other types, has suggested to some investigators that dopamine is implicated in Oppenheim dystonia, clinical pharmacology has not yet seen a relationship, and biochemically, dopamine concentration is normal except for a 50% reduction in the rostral portions of the putamen and caudate nucleus in a single case (Furukawa et al., 2000) and a possible increase in striatal dopamine turnover in three cases (Augood et al., 2002). A morphometric analysis of the pigmented substantia nigra pars compacta (SNc) neurons found no difference in neuron number, but the average size of neuronal cell bodies was increased, and dopaminergic SNc neurons were arranged in much closer apposition to each other than was observed in control tissue (Rostasy et al., 2003).

Antibodies to torsinA have been prepared in several laboratories. The normal protein is widely distributed in human, rat, and mouse brain (Shashidharan et al., 2000a; Konakova et al., 2001; Konakova and Pulst, 2001; Walker et al., 2001) and is found in endoplasmic reticulum (ER) (Hewett et al., 2000; Kustedjo et al., 2000). TorsinA immunohistochemistry investigation of a brain from a patient with Oppenheim dystonia failed to show any difference from control brains (Walker et al., 2002; Rostasy et al., 2003). The cholinergic

neurons in rat striatum have a high content of torsinA during development, but then this concentration fades as the animal gets older (Oberlin et al., 2004). This temporal and anatomical pattern could fit with some clinical features of Oppenheim dystonia: young onset with usual sparing after age 28 years, and response to high-dosage antimuscarinic agents.

The AAA+ family of proteins is believed to serve as a chaperone in the processing and repair of damaged proteins. Six torsinA proteins are thought to join together to form a ring, with each of these six proteins bound to its neighbor by ATP. This structure is believed to function to repair other proteins that have been damaged. If the repair is unsuccessful, the damaged proteins can aggregate or die by apoptosis. In neural cultures (Hewett et al., 2000), the normal protein is found throughout the cytoplasm and neurites with a high degree of co-localization with the ER. In contrast, overexpression the mutant protein in transgenic mice showed an accumulation of the protein in multiple, large inclusions in the cytoplasm around the nucleus. These inclusions were composed of membrane whorls, apparently derived from the ER. If disrupted processing of the mutant protein leads to its accumulation in multilayer membranous structures in vivo, these may interfere with membrane trafficking in neurons.

Immunohistochemical studies showed that torsinA is present in Lewy bodies (Shashidharan et al., 2000b; Sharma et al., 2001). A role of torsinA in α-synuclein, a major component of the Lewy body, was subsequently sought. Overexpression of wild-type torsinA dramatically reduced the number of transfected cells containing α-synuclein aggregates, whereas mutant torsinA failed to suppress α-synuclein aggregation (McLean et al., 2002).

TorsinA immunohistochemistry investigation of brains from patients with DYT1 dystonia failed to show any difference from control brains (Walker et al., 2002; Rostasy et al., 2003). A morphometric analysis of the pigmented SNc neurons found no difference in neuron number, but the average size of neuronal cell bodies was increased, and dopaminergic SNc neurons were arranged in much closer apposition to each other than was observed in control tissue (Rostasy et al., 2003). Other evidence for a role in preventing protein aggregation comes from studies of the torsinA homolog in *Caenorhabditis elegans*, TOR-2 (Caldwell et al., 2003). TOR-2 also appears to be an ER protein. Overexpression of either TOR-2 or human wild-type torsinA significantly suppressed the aggregation of a polyglutamine repeat protein, whereas a mutant form of TOR-2 failed to reduce protein aggregation (Caldwell et al., 2003).

Wild-type torsinA is distributed throughout the cell, and is particularly enriched in the lumen of the ER (Hewett et al., 2000; Kustedjo et al., 2000). Mutant torsinA concentrates in large clumps that are largely or completely segregated from the ER. The clumps of mutant torsinA immunostaining are not insoluble aggregates (Kustedjo et al., 2000), and they appear to be composed of whorled double-membrane structures, apparently derived from the ER (Hewett et al., 2000). This DeltaE302/303 mutation appears to be a stable protein, and not toxic. The DeltaE302/3 mutation causes a striking redistribution of torsinA from the ER to the nuclear envelope (Goodchild and Dauer, 2004; Gonzalez-Alegre and Paulson, 2004; Naismith et al., 2004; Hewett et al., 2004). Oppenheim dystonia, therefore, appears to be a previously uncharacterized nuclear envelope disease and the first to selectively affect CNS function. Goodchild and Dauer (2005) found that normal torsinA binds a substrate in the lumen of the nuclear envelope (NE), and the DeltaE mutation enhances this interaction. They identified lamina-associated polypeptide 1 (LAP1) as a torsinA-interacting protein. Goodchild and her colleagues (2005) went on to show that genetic animal models without torsinA or with abnormal torsinA have severely abnormal nuclear membranes in neurons, whereas non-neuronal cell types appear normal. These observations demonstrate that neurons have a unique requirement for nuclear envelope localized torsinA function and suggest that loss of this activity is a key molecular event in the pathogenesis of DYT1 dystonia.

The mutant torsinA has also been shown to have a reduction of its normal ATPase activity (Konakova and Pulst, 2005). Membranous inclusions, which were found to occur in cells transfected with the mutant torsinA (Hewett et al., 2000), have now also been found in patients with Oppenheim dystonia (McNaught et al., 2004). They are present in the perinuclear region within brainstem cholinergic and other neurons in the pedunculopontine nucleus, cuneiform nucleus, and griseum centrale mesencephali. The inclusions stain positively for ubiquitin, torsinA, and the nuclear envelope protein lamin A/C. No inclusions were detected in the SNc, striatum, hippocampus, or selected regions of the cerebral cortex. McNaught and colleagues (2004) also noted tau/ubiquitin-immunoreactive aggregates in pigmented neurons of the SNc and locus coeruleus.

A novel protein, printor, interacts and co-distributes with torsinA in multiple brain regions and co-localizes with torsinA in the endoplasmic reticulum. The interaction of printor with torsinA is abolished by the DYT1 mutant torsinA (Giles et al., 2009).

Genetic models

Homozygous DYT1 knock-in and knock-out mouse models point to a loss-of-function mutation as animals die shortly after birth, suggesting that torsinA is indispensable for specific developmental processes in mammalian brain (Goodchild et al., 2005). Transgenic mice overexpressing either the wild type or the mutant develop neurologic dysfunction (Grundmann et al., 2007). In the former mice, both dopamine and serotonin are reduced in the striatum, whereas the mutant transgenic mice have reduced serotonin in the brainstem. In other transgenic mutant mice studies, most studies on dopamine function in the striatum were normal, including concentration of dopamine and its metabolites, function of the dopamine transporter and the vesicular monoamine transporter, and the D1 and D2 receptors (Balcioglu et al., 2007). However, a reduction of amphetamine-induced release of dopamine was impaired.

Dopa-responsive dystonia (DRD)

It should be mentioned, that in addition to the genetic types described in this section, some patients with focal dystonias, including familial cases, might respond to levodopa therapy. A report of two families with a total of four members with childhood-onset cervical dystonia, all of whom who had an excellent response to levodopa, illustrates this point

(Schneider et al., 2006c). Genetic testing on these patients showed that they did not have any of the genetic types discussed in this section. It is possible that these cases may represent new forms of dopa-responsive dystonia.

Classic dopa-responsive dystonia (DRD)

Segawa and his colleagues (1976) described a syndrome of dystonia in children that has a diurnal pattern. The children may be relatively free of dystonic movements and postures in the morning and be severely afflicted in the late afternoon, evening, and night (Videos 12.19, 12.20, and 12.21). Segawa and colleagues (1976) called this disorder hereditary progressive dystonia with diurnal variation; they also mentioned that it responds to levodopa. Independently, Allen and Knopp (1976) described a form of childhood hereditary dystonia that had features of parkinsonism that showed sustained control by levodopa and anticholinergic medication. This was the same disorder.

Over time, several clinical features have been distinguished as highlighting this disorder: (1) Many patients with onset of dystonia in childhood have features of parkinsonism, including rigidity, bradykinesia, flexed posture, and loss of postural reflexes. (2) The disorder usually, but not exclusively, begins in childhood with a presentation of a peculiar gait, namely a tendency to walk on the toes. (3) The disease can begin in infancy, thereby resembling cerebral palsy (Nygaard et al., 1994) (Videos 12.22 and 12.23), and there has now been a report of a neonatal onset of rigidity, tremor, and dystonia (Nardocci et al., 2003) (Video 12.24). (4) When the disorder begins in adulthood, it can present as a focal dystonia of arm, neck, or cranium, or present as parkinsonism, mimicking Parkinson disease (Nygaard et al., 1992). (5) The patients respond remarkably well to low-dosage levodopa. (6) Not all patients with childhood-onset dystonia have the diurnal fluctuation pattern. (7) Writer's cramp can be brought out with continued writing (Deonna et al., 1997). (8) Cerebellar signs have also been seen, with response to levodopa (Chaila et al., 2006). The term *dopa-responsive dystonia* (DRD) appears to be the preferred label for this disorder (Nygaard, 1989; Nygaard et al., 1990), because response to levodopa is the consistent finding, and the term also highlights the appropriate treatment. Moreover, the term *hereditary progressive dystonia* could apply to many genetic forms of dystonia, and certainly to the more virulent Oppenheim dystonia.

If levodopa therapy is delayed for a great many years, patients still respond to low doses of levodopa (Harwood et al., 1994) (Video 12.25). Even if the onset is in adulthood presenting as parkinsonism, and resembling Parkinson disease, it responds to low doses of levodopa and without adverse effects of response fluctuations (Nygaard et al., 1992; Harwood et al., 1994). Long-term treatment with levodopa does not cause the wearing-off phenomenon. Worsening of dystonia does not occur until 29 hours or more after levodopa withdrawal; the subjective feeling of wearing-off that is experienced by patients with DRD might be from one of the nonmotor effects of levodopa, such as mood elevation (Dewey et al., 1998).

DRD is inherited in an autosomal dominant pattern and needs to be recognized because it is so easily treated. The gene causing DRD has been mapped to chromosome 14q

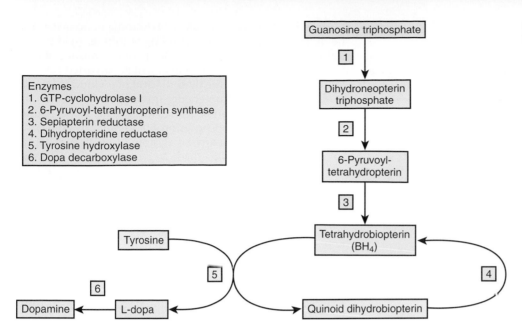

Figure 12.2 Metabolic pathway for the synthesis of tetrahydrobiopterin.

by Nygaard et al. (1993) and identified by Ichinose et al. (1994) as the gene for the enzyme GTP cyclohydrolase I (GCH), the rate-limiting enzyme in the biosynthesis of tetrahydrobiopterin (BH4) (Fig. 12.2), which is the cofactor of monoamine-synthesizing enzymes TH for dopamine and norepinephrine and tryptophan hydroxylase for serotonin (and also phenylalanine hydroxylase). The genetic designation DYT5 has been assigned to this form of dystonia (Table 12.1). Clinically, only dystonia and parkinsonism are manifested. Approximately 40–50% of patients with DRD have no known mutations (Furukawa and Kish, 1999). GCH1 point mutations occur in approximately 54% of DRD patients, and deletions in 8% (Zirn et al., 2008). Different families have different mutations on the same GCH gene (Ichinose et al., 1995; Hirano et al., 1995; Bandmann et al., 1996; Furukawa et al., 1996; Ichinose and Nagatsu, 1997; Jarman et al., 1997; Thony and Blau, 1997; Furukawa et al. 1998b; Steinberger et al., 1998; Tamaru et al., 1998), and spontaneous mutations have been identified. The multiple mutations are scattered over the entire coding region for the six exon-containing GCH gene.

Phenylalanine hydroxylase also requires the cofactor BH4 for its activity, and homozygous mutations and compound heterozygous mutations have been found in the GCH gene to cause the rare autosomal recessively inherited form of hyperphenylalaninemia (Thony and Blau, 1997; Furukawa et al., 1998a). Such mutations are therefore clinically similar to the compound heterozygous or homozygous mutations spread over all six exons encoding 6-pyruvoyl-tetrahydropterin synthase, which manifests as an autosomal recessively inherited variant of hyperphenylalaninemia, along with a deficiency of dopamine and serotonin. Hyperphenylalaninemia may be mild and go undetected neonatally; the child can develop dystonia later in childhood, along with developmental delay and seizures. The condition is treatable with levodopa, 5-hydroxytryptophan, and tetrahydrobiopterin (Demos et al., 2005). The other autosomal recessive pterin deficiency disorders also respond to levodopa, and they often have developmental delay, oculogyria, and dysautonomic features.

Sepiapterin reductase deficiency appears to be fairly common in Malta (Neville et al., 2005). Although dystonia can respond to levodopa, cognitive impairment does not.

In some pedigrees with DRD a mutation in the GCH gene has not been found. This fact, plus the multiple mutations in the GCH gene that have been discovered so far, indicated that genetic testing will not be an easy method to determine the presence of the molecular defect. Ichinose and Nagatsu (1997) found that GCH activity in lymphocytes was decreased to less that 20% of the mean value of healthy controls, and in unaffected carriers was 37%. The enzyme had normal activity in juvenile parkinsonism. These authors suggest that assay of GCH in blood cells might become a useful biochemical marker for the gene defect. A deficiency of neopterin is found in CSF, but this is reduced in juvenile parkinsonism also.

PET scans for FDOPA uptake and dopamine transporter are normal, whereas those for the D2 receptor show increased binding, reflecting supersensitivity (Rinne et al., 2004). Network analysis, using FDG PET, shows that DRD has a unique metabolic architecture that differs from other inherited forms of dystonia (Asanuma et al., 2005a). The characteristic features are increases in metabolism in the dorsal midbrain, cerebellum, and supplementary motor area and reductions in motor and lateral premotor cortex and in the basal ganglia.

There has been a report of a patient with DRD who had a remission (Di Capua and Bertini, 1995), which perhaps should not come as a surprise because not every carrier of the mutation has symptoms. In fact, affected females outnumber affected males by a ratio of approximately 4:1 (Ichinose and Nagatsu, 1997). This ratio has been explained by the observation that males have a higher GCH activity normally, so missing one of the two genes by a mutation may still leave sufficient enzyme intact to avoid symptoms. There is also a report that SSRI antidepressants reversed the benefit from levodopa therapy (Mathen et al., 1999).

The phenotype of DRD is not always easily distinguished from juvenile parkinsonism, but features that help in the

Table 12.17 Differential features between juvenile parkinsonism, dopa-responsive dystonia, and primary torsion dystonia

Clinical feature	Juvenile PD	DRD	Childhood PTD
Age onset	Rare <8 years	Infancy to 12 years	Uncommon <6 years
Gender	Predominantly male	Predominantly female	Equal
Initial sign	Foot dystonia or PD	Foot, leg dystonia, gait disorder	Arm or leg dystonia
Dystonia	At onset	Throughout	Throughout
Diurnal	Perhaps	Sometimes	No
Sleep benefit	Yes	Sometimes	No
Bradykinesia	Present	Present	No
Pull test	Abnormal	Abnormal	Normal
Gait	Abnormal	Abnormal	Abnormal if leg or trunk are affected
Anticholinergic response	Yes	Yes	Yes
Dopa responsive	Yes	Yes	No, or mild
Dopa dosage	Moderate to high	Very low	High
"Off" episodes	Fluctuations	Stable	Unknown
Dyskinesias	Prominent	With high-dose dopa	Unknown
Fluorodopa PET	Decreased	Normal or borderline	Normal
β-CIT SPECT	Decreased	Normal	Normal
CSF HVA	Decreased	Decreased	Normal
CSF neopterin	Moderately decreased	Markedly decreased	Normal
Phenylalanine test	Normal	Abnormal	Normal
Prognosis	Progressive	Plateaus	Usually worsens

differential diagnosis are presented in Table 12.17. Fluorodopa PET scanning reveals a normal or modest reduction of dopa uptake (Sawle et al., 1991; Nygaard et al., 1992; Snow et al., 1993; Turjanski et al., 1993), in contrast to the marked reduction in juvenile parkinsonism. A similar result is seen with β-CIT SPECT (Naumann et al., 1997; Jeon, 1997) or other dopamine transporter ligands (Huang et al., 2002). Another important difference is that long-term treatment with levodopa in DRD is not associated with the motor complications that are seen with levodopa therapy in juvenile (and adult) Parkinson disease (Nygaard et al., 1991, 1992; Harwood et al., 1994).

An early sign of dopa-responsive dystonia in neonates may be difficulty with feeding, including vomiting, rigidity, and opisthotonus (Chieng et al., 2007). One unusual phenotypic expression is myoclonus, which occurred in one kindred and preceded the dystonia and bradykinesia (Leuzzi et al., 2002). Molecular genetics investigation found a missense mutation in exon 6 of the *GCH1* gene. Another phenotype of DRD is adult-onset oromandibular dystonia and no obvious family history of dystonia, which was found in one individual who had a mutation of *GCH* and who responded positively to treatment with levodopa (Steinberger et al., 1999). An adult with exercise-induced limb and trunk dystonia and with diurnal variation was found to respond to levodopa (Regula et al., 2007).

The first report of the pathology of a case of DRD-GCH type revealed decreased neuromelanin in the substantia nigra, but otherwise normal nigral cell counts and morphology (Rajput et al., 1994). Biochemically, this patient had reduced concentrations of dopamine and its metabolite, homovanillic acid, in both the caudate and putamen. Furukawa and his colleagues (1999) carried out more extensive postmortem biochemistry in two patients with typical DRD. One had two GCH mutations, but the other had no mutation in the coding region of this gene. Striatal biopterin and neopterin levels were markedly reduced. Both had severely reduced (<3%) TH protein levels and normal concentrations of dopa decarboxylase protein, dopamine transporter, and vesicular monoamine transporters. The authors suggested that the reduction of TH protein might be explained by reduced enzyme stability/expression consequent to congenital BH4 deficiency.

A second autopsy report of DRD was on a patient with a presumed different genetic locus, chromosome 14q13, and called DYT14 by Grotzsch and colleagues (2002). An autopsy in the elderly proband revealed a normal number of cells in the substantia nigra and locus coeruleus, which is typical of DRD and not Parkinson disease, and there was a decrease in neuromelanin. No Lewy bodies were seen. These pathologic features are typical for DRD. Subsequently more careful and thorough genetic analysis revealed that this family had a deletion in *GCH1*, so was just another pedigree with DYT5 dystonia (Wider et al., 2008). Deletions are harder to detect and care must be made to search for them (Gasser, 2008).

Intracortical inhibition of the primary motor cortex was studied in DRD patients and found to be normal, in contrast to adult-onset focal dystonia (see below in the pathophysiology section) (Hanajima et al., 2007). It is difficult to explain why loss of striatal dopamine in PD produces parkinsonian features while such a loss in DRD produces predominantly dystonic features. Using a transgenic mouse model for DRD, Sato and colleagues (2008) showed that dopamine loss is mainly anteriorly in the putamen affecting the striosomes. They propose that in PD, the major loss of dopamine is in the posterior putamen affecting mainly the matrix, and that this differential loss results in the different phenomenology between the two disorders (Fig. 12.3).

Tyrosine hydroxylase (TH) deficiency

TH deficiency is usually a more serious form of dopa-responsive dystonia, and is transmitted as an autosomal

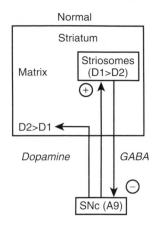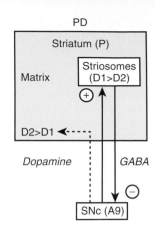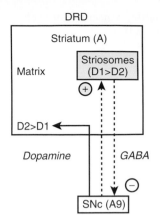

Figure 12.3 Differential loss of putaminal dopamine in DRD and PD. In PD, the loss is primarily in the posterior putamen affecting the matrix. In DRD, the loss is in the anterior putamen affecting the striosomes. *From Sato K, Sumi-Ichinose C, Kaji R, et al. Differential involvement of striosome and matrix dopamine systems in a transgenic model of dopa-responsive dystonia. Proc Natl Acad Sci USA 2008;105(34):12551–12556.*

recessive disorder. The presence of dystonia and parkinsonism in infancy is the clinical clue that this disorder should be suspected. Biochemical analysis of CSF will provide some evidence, but ultimately testing for the gene mutation is required to establish the diagnosis. Decreased CSF concentrations of homovanillic acid and 3-methoxy-4-hydroxyphenylethylene glycol, with normal 5-hydroxyindoleacetic acid CSF concentrations, are the biochemical hallmark of TH deficiency.

At least 10 different point mutations have now been discovered in the human TH gene, and more are reported regularly (Knappskog et al., 1995; Lüdecke et al., 1995, 1996; van den Heuvel et al., 1998; Swaans et al., 2000; de Rijk-van Andel et al., 2000; Janssen et al., 2000; Furukawa et al., 2001; Giovanniello et al., 2007). Many of the reports are in Dutch families. The clinical features range from a mild syndrome of juvenile DRD to a more severe parkinsonism, dystonia, and oculogyric crises (all three representing dopamine deficiency) and also ptosis, miosis, oropharyngeal secretions, and postural hypotension (all representing norepinephrine deficiency). In the most severe form, the infant was virtually immobile, rigid, drooling saliva, with a tremor in tongue and hands. She responded dramatically to levodopa. The severity appears to be associated with the amount of loss of TH activity. Genetically, there can be homozygous mutations to heterozygous mutations. Compound heterozygotes have presented as spastic paraparesis, with a complete or very good response to levodopa (Furukawa et al., 2001; Giovanniello et al., 2007). Some patients with a mild form of the disorder live a normal life with a response to low-dose levodopa, into adulthood. One reported problem is hypersensitivity to levodopa (Grattan-Smith et al., 2002). Hoffmann and colleagues (2003) reported four patients with TH deficiency and emphasized that most patients with this disorder have an encephalopathy that is not predominantly dystonia, but a progressive, often lethal encephalopathic disorder, which can be improved but not cured by levodopa. The DRD of TH deficiency can be as responsive to levodopa as is DYT5 with GCH involvement. Schiller and colleagues (2004) report sustained benefit, and excellent response to levodopa even when treatment was delayed for 20 years. Most patients with tyrosine hydroxylase deficiency can be successfully treated with levodopa.

A review of the literature and a report of 36 cases of TH deficiency divides the disorder into two phenotypes: an infantile-onset, progressive, hypokinetic-rigid syndrome with dystonia (type A), and a complex encephalopathy with neonatal onset (type B) (Willemsen et al., 2010). The homovanillic acid concentrations and homovanillic acid/5-hydroxyindoleacetic acid ratio in cerebrospinal fluid correlate with the severity of the phenotype.

A phenylalanine-loading test has been recommended as a means to distinguish between DRD with GCH deficiency and that with TH deficiency (Hyland et al., 1997). In the former, phenylalanine is not metabolized rapidly and the blood levels remain elevated for a prolonged period. In TH deficiency, this test would be normal. One other potential method of differentiating GCH-deficient DRD from other DRDs or juvenile parkinsonism is the exquisite sensitivity to centrally acting anticholinergics. Some of the trihexyphenidyl responders reported by Fahn (1983) had responded to small doses, such as 6 mg/day. These patients were subsequently determined to have DRD. When trihexyphenidyl was first reported for the treatment of Parkinson disease, some papers pointed out that small doses could have a dramatic benefit in some children with dystonia (Corner, 1952; Burns, 1959). These children had diurnal fluctuations of their dystonia. Jarman and colleagues (1997) screened some of their patients with responsiveness to anticholinergics and found that some had a GCH mutation.

Rapid-onset dystonia–parkinsonism (RDP)

RDP is an autosomal dominant movement disorder characterized by sudden onset of persistent dystonia and parkinsonism, generally during adolescence or early adulthood (Dobyns et al., 1993). Symptoms evolve over hours or days and generally stabilize within a few weeks, with slow or no progression. Members of a family who are wide apart in age may develop symptoms around the same time. Further follow-up of the original family revealed two members to have a more gradual progression of their disorder over 6–18 months. One of them experienced a rapid progression of symptoms 2 years after an initial stabilization of his condition. The phenotype therefore shows considerable variability (Brashear et al., 1996). Two other, seemingly unrelated, kindreds were subsequently reported (Brashear et al., 1997; Pittock et al., 2000). Variability occurs within a kindred, with some members in a kindred becoming stable after their worsening and others having fluctuating worsening or even improving over time (McKeon et al., 2007).

Now that the gene responsible for RDP has been discovered (de Carvalho Aguiar et al., 2004), it is possible to test a wide clinical spectrum of dystonia and determine the expanded phenotype (Brashear et al., 2007). The mutation is in the *ATP1A3* gene responsible for the α3 subunit of Na-K-ATPase. The phenotype of 36 affected individuals from 10 families included abrupt onset of dystonia with features of parkinsonism, a rostrocaudal gradient, and prominent bulbar findings. Other features found in some mutation carriers included common reports of triggers, minimal or no tremor at onset, occasional mild limb dystonia before the primary onset, lack of response to dopaminergic medications, rare abrupt worsening of symptoms later in life, stabilization of symptoms within a month, and minimal improvement overall. Tremor at onset of symptoms, a reversed rostrocaudal gradient, and significant limb pain excluded a diagnosis of RDP. A positive family history is not required.

Although there is little or no response to levodopa or dopamine agonists, a low concentration of homovanillic acid in the CSF in patients has been reported (Brashear et al., 1998). PET studies indicate no loss of dopaminergic nerve terminals in RDP (Brashear et al., 1999), suggesting that this disorder results from a functional deficit rather than being a neurodegenerative disease. An autopsied case revealed no neurodegeneration (Pittock et al., 2000). These findings suggest RDP is a neurochemical rather than a neurodegenerative disorder. Deep brain stimulation has not been helpful (Kamm et al., 2008).

The *ATP1A3* gene for RDP is on chromosome 19q13 (Kramer et al., 1999). Functional studies and structural analysis of the protein suggest that these mutations impair enzyme activity or stability. This finding implicates the Na$^+$/K$^+$ pump, a crucial protein that is responsible for the electrochemical gradient across the cell membrane. The authors suggest that the rapid onset that is seen in the disorder is related to an inability to "keep up with a high demand for ion transport activity" in response to stressful situations. However, there is genetic heterogeneity because one large family with the RDP phenotype was found not to have a mutation in the *ATP1A3* gene (Kabakci et al., 2005). Although most patients have been of European descent, at least one Asian (Korean) has been reported, and with the typical phenotype (Lee et al., 2007).

Now that at least one gene for RDP has been found, genetic analysis can be carried out in dopa-nonresponsive parkinsonism. After being stable for 2.5 years, one patient thought to have Parkinson disease developed overnight oromandibular dystonia and more severe parkinsonian symptoms; he was found to have a missense mutation in the *ATP1A3* gene (Kamphuis et al., 2006).

Myoclonus–dystonia

Myoclonic movements were mentioned early in the description of the phenomenology of dystonia. Although lightning-like movements can occur in Oppenheim dystonia, they can also be seen in a distinct autosomal dominant disorder. Both conditions have unfortunately been called myoclonic dystonia, and in both, the myoclonic jerks can respond to alcohol. It has been recommended that when myoclonic jerks are part of Oppenheim dystonia, it be referred to as dystonia with lightning-like jerks or as myoclonic dystonia (Quinn et al., 1988). The autosomal dominant myoclonus–dystonia that is a distinct entity has been mapped to chromosome 7q21 and the mutated gene has been identified as the gene for ε-sarcoglycan (Zimprich et al., 2001; Asmus et al., 2002). The report of a mutation in the gene for the dopamine D2 receptor in a single family (Klein et al., 1999) has now been recognized to most likely represent a polymorphism (Klein et al., 2000a). This family has since been found to have genetic linkage to 7q21–q31 like the other families (Klein et al., 2000b). Whether myoclonus–dystonia is an entity separate from hereditary essential myoclonus (Fahn and Sjaastad, 1991; Quinn, 1996) remains to be determined through genetic studies. At least one family originally published as familial essential myoclonus has been reported to have a mutation in the ε-sarcoglycan gene and thus has myoclonus–dystonia (Korten et al., 1974; Foncke et al., 2006).

The onset can be in childhood or in adulthood. Age at onset is highly associated with gender; the median age onset for girls is 5 years versus 8 years for boys (Raymond et al., 2008). The myoclonus and dystonia are located predominantly in the arms and neck (Videos 12.26 and 12.27), and the symptoms tend to plateau after a period of progression (Kyllerman et al., 1990). There is clinical heterogeneity, and leg involvement can occur (Nardocci et al., 2008). Obsessive-compulsive disorder (OCD) and alcohol dependence are not uncommon in individuals who carry the gene (Saunders-Pullman et al., 2002; Hess et al., 2007). Psychiatric problems also include substance abuse, anxiety/panic/phobic disorders, and psychosis (Doheny et al., 2002). Cognitive testing showed impaired verbal learning and memory in one family, impaired memory in the second family, and no cognitive deficits in the third family. In a large Dutch family, there was no cognitive deficit, nor OCD, but there was depression and anxiety with panic attacks (Foncke et al., 2009).

In *SGCE* mutation carriers, there is hyperresponsiveness in contralateral inferior parietal cortical areas, ipsilateral premotor and primary somatosensory cortex, and ipsilateral cerebellum during the motor task compared with healthy control subjects (Beukers et al., 2010). This is similar to that in DYT1 and DYT6 dystonia and points to a disorganized sensorimotor integration.

There is markedly reduced penetrance if the parent carrying the mutation is the mother (penetrance about 5–10%), whereas if the father carries the mutation, the penetrance is about 90%. This pattern of phenotypic expression of myoclonus–dystonia is called maternal imprinting. As Asmus and Gasser (2004) explained, if the mutated allele is inherited from the father, inactivation of the maternal allele due to imprinting leads to complete ε-sarcoglycan deficiency, and hence to the development of clinical symptoms. If, on the other hand, the mutated allele is inherited from the mother, the intact paternal allele is sufficient to sustain ε-sarcoglycan function. Making the inheritance pattern more complicated is one report of reduced penetrance in which the mutated gene was inherited from the father (Muller et al., 2002). Deletions in the maternal allele, as well as point mutations, of the *SCGE* gene occur, and these can cause phenotypic variations, depending on the size of the deletion, with the largest deletion causing a split-hand/split-foot malformation and sensorineural hearing loss (Asmus et al., 2007).

Another gene locus has been found for one family with myoclonus–dystonia on chromosome 18p11 (Grimes et al., 2002). In a study of Dutch families with myoclonus–dystonia, only 7 of 31 patients had carried a mutation in the ε-sarcoglycan gene (Gerrits et al., 2006). In one large Dutch family, originally published as essential myoclonus (Korten et al., 1974), the onset of myoclonus can be delayed as late as 75 years (Foncke et al., 2006), and although emphasis was made that the myoclonus was mainly distal in the arms in contrast to an assumption that myoclonus is usually proximal in this disorder, our personal experience is that myoclonus is commonly distal.

A phenotype similar to myoclonus–dystonia has been encountered with the SCA14 mutation (Foncke et al., 2010).

Secondary dystonias

In a movement disorders center, primary dystonias are much more common than secondary dystonias. A screen for the DYT1 gene in Ashkenazi Jewish patients with secondary dystonia failed to find any evidence that the DYT1 mutation contributes to secondary dystonia (Bressman et al., 1997), including tardive dystonia and other environmental insults. The most common secondary dystonias seen at the Dystonia Clinical Research at Columbia University Medical Center are presented in Table 12.18.

Tardive dystonia

Tardive dystonia is the most common form of symptomatic dystonia seen at the Movement Disorders Center at Columbia University Medical Center (Table 12.18). It can manifest exactly like PTD, but there is often accompanying classic tardive dyskinesia or tardive akathisia, which establishes the

Table 12.18 Common causes of torsion dystonia

Cause	No.
Primary	1762
Tardive dystonia	184
Birth injury	83
Psychogenic	64
Peripheral trauma	51
Head injury	39
Stroke	27
Encephalitis	24
Miscellaneous	164
Total	**2398**

Data from the Center for Parkinson Disease and Other Movement Disorders, Columbia University Medical Center, New York City.

diagnosis. One form of clinical presentation seems more common in tardive dystonia. Many patients have retrocollis and extension of the elbows with internal rotation of the shoulders and flexion of the wrists. Tardive dystonia is a persistent dystonia as a result of a complication of drugs that block dopamine receptors. Clinical features of tardive dystonia are discussed in detail in Chapter 19.

Acute dystonic reactions

Acute dystonic reactions can occur from drugs that block dopamine receptors; these reactions are widely recognized and easily treated with antihistaminics and anticholinergics. Acute dystonia has also been reported with exposure to domperidone (Bonuccelli et al., 1991), amitriptyline (Ornadel et al., 1992), fluoxetine (Dave, 1994), clozapine (Kastrup et al., 1994; Thomas et al., 1994), and dextromethorphan (Graudins and Fern, 1996). Since domperidone is a peripherally-acting dopamine receptor blocker, the acute dystonic reaction suggests that some of the drug entered the CNS, at least in the affected patient, who had polycystic ovary syndrome. Amitriptyline would ordinarily not be expected to produce such a reaction; the clinical description is that typical for acute dystonia after a neuroleptic, but no such drug was known to have been taken by the patient.

The so-called atypical antipsychotics drugs have been shown to have less risk for causing acute dystonic reactions. In one study evaluating a population of patients consecutively admitted to a psychiatric intensive care unit, 1337 cases were treated with antipsychotics (Raja and Azzoni, 2001). The authors observed 41 cases (3.1%) of acute dystonic reactions. Four occurred with risperidone monotherapy, one with olanzapine, and one with quetiapine. The remaining cases were with medications labeled as typical antipsychotics.

Serotonergic agents have also been reported to induce acute dystonic reactions (Lopez-Alemany et al., 1997; Madhusoodanan and Brenner, 1997; Olivera, 1997). Serotonergic agents, such as fluoxetine, can inhibit dopaminergic neurons in the substantia nigra, worsening parkinsonism (Baldessarini and Marsh, 1992). This might somehow be related to the development of the dystonic reaction. How clozapine induces an acute dystonic reaction is unknown; it could relate to binding to the D2 receptor, the D4 receptor, or the 5-HT2 receptor.

Other secondary dystonias

A large number of injuries to the nervous system can result in secondary dystonia (Table 12.10). Head trauma and peripheral trauma, including dental procedures (Schrag et al., 1999), can induce generalized and segmental dystonia and focal dystonia, respectively. Neck trauma can result in cervical dystonia, and in one child, also camptocormia (Shuper et al., 2007). Retrocollis is more commonly associated with tardive dystonia, but can also be the result of head or neck trauma (Papapetropoulos et al., 2007a). Delayed-onset focal dystonia can follow electrical injury (Lim and Seet, 2007). Trauma may provoke the onset of PTD in an individual who carries the gene for this disorder (Fletcher et al., 1991c). Segmental axial dystonia was described with a closed head injury with small areas of encephalomalacia, including the caudate nucleus (Jabbari et al., 1992). Cervical dystonia can sometimes be secondary to lesions in the CNS, such as lacunar infarction in the putamen (Molho and Factor, 1993), and to lesions in the upper cervical spinal cord (Klostermann et al., 1993; Cammarota et al., 1995), including syringomyelia (Hill et al., 1999). Torticollis has also been reported to occur after electrocution (Colosimo et al., 1993) and in Moya-Moya disease (Yasutomo et al., 1993). Strokes can occasionally lead to delayed-onset hemidystonia. Perhaps in this category is the primary antiphospholipid syndrome (PAPS), an immune-mediated vascular disorder that has been found to result in hemidystonia in children (Angelini et al., 1993). Sjögren syndrome, also considered an autoimmune disorder, has been associated with dystonia (van den Berg, et al., 1999). X-linked agammaglobulinemia can result in a fatal dementing, dystonia–parkinsonism syndrome (Papapetropoulos et al., 2007b).

Encephalitis, usually from severe equine encephalitis, results in permanent dystonia. The common Asian encephalitis known as Japanese encephalitis can cause severe dystonia (Kalita and Misra, 2000; Murgod et al., 2001). Occasionally, dystonia can be psychogenic in origin (see Chapter 25), and it is reasonable to consider psychogenic dystonia as one of the many etiologies of secondary dystonia. Sometimes psychogenic dystonia occurs following trauma. When associated with pain, it may be diagnosed as reflex sympathetic dystrophy or complex regional pain syndrome, but many of the patients have a psychogenic mechanism (Ochoa, 1999); this syndrome has also been called causalgia–dystonia (Bhatia et al., 1993a).

Clues that dystonia might be secondary

In examining patients with dystonia, there are some clues in the history and neurologic examination that would suggest to the clinician that the patient's dystonia is secondary rather than primary (Table 12.19).

Perhaps the most difficult form of dystonia to diagnose is *psychogenic dystonia*, which can occur in up to 5% of children presenting with what otherwise appears to be primary dystonia. Clues suggesting a psychogenic etiology are false (give-way) weakness, false sensory findings, inconsistent movements with changing patterns of involvement, incongruent movements not fitting with typical organic dystonia, self-inflicted injuries, deliberate slowness of movement, and

multiple types of abnormal dyskinesias that do not fit into a single organic etiology (Fahn and Williams, 1988). Table 12.20 lists the clinical situations that provide clues that the clinician might be encountering a psychogenic movement disorder.

Lubag (X-linked dystonia–parkinsonism, XDP)

While both DRD and classic PTD, as well as focal dystonias (Waddy et al., 1991), are inherited as autosomal dominant disorders, there is a form of dystonia that is inherited as an X-linked recessive trait. This is present in males from the island of Panay in the Philippines (Lee et al., 1976; Fahn and Moskowitz, 1988). The disease can begin with either dystonia or parkinsonism; with progression, parkinsonism develops eventually, even in those who had dystonia earlier (Lee et al., 1991). Pure parkinsonism has been considered a more benign phenotype (Evidente et al., 2002). The symptoms may begin in the big toe with abnormal movements. Dystonia typically spreads from the limbs to axial musculature. Some patients with older onset may have focal dystonia involving the tongue and jaw (Videos 12.28 and 12.29). The

---

Table 12.19 Clues that dystonia is secondary

1. History of possible etiologic factor; e.g., head trauma, peripheral trauma, encephalitis, toxin exposure, drug exposure, perinatal anoxia
2. Presence of neurological abnormality; e.g., dementia, seizures, ocular, ataxia, weakness, spasticity, amyotrophy
3. Presence of false weakness or sensory exam, or other clues of psychogenic etiology (see Table 12.20)
4. Onset of rest instead of action dystonia
5. Early onset of speech involvement
6. Hemidystonia
7. Abnormal brain imaging
8. Abnormal laboratory work-up

Table 12.20 Clues suggesting psychogenic dystonia (see also Chapter 25)

A. Clues relating to the movements

1. Abrupt onset
2. Inconsistent movements (changing characteristics over time)
3. Incongruous movements and postures (movements don't fit with recognized patterns or with normal physiological patterns)
4. Presence of additional types of abnormal movements that are not consistent with the basic abnormal movement pattern or are incongruous with a known movement disorder, particularly:
   rhythmical shaking
   bizarre gait
   deliberate slowness carrying out requested voluntary movement
   bursts of verbal gibberish
   excessive startle (bizarre movements in response to sudden, unexpected noise or threatening movement)
5. Spontaneous remissions
6. Movements decrease or disappear with distraction
7. Response to placebo, suggestion or psychotherapy
8. Presence as a paroxysmal disorder
9. Dystonia beginning as a fixed posture
10. Twisting facial movements which move the mouth to one side or the other (note: organic dystonia of the facial muscles usually do not move the mouth sideways)

B. Clues relating to the other medical observations

1. False weakness
2. False sensory complaints
3. Multiple somatizations or undiagnosed conditions
4. Self-inflicted injuries
5. Obvious psychiatric disturbances
6. Employed in the health profession or in insurance claims
7. Presence of secondary gain, including continuing care by a "devoted" spouse
8. Litigation or compensation pending

families with this disorder refer to the condition as *lubag* (twisting in Filipino). Female heterozygotes have been discovered who manifest mild dystonia or chorea (Waters et al., 1993b). Evidente and colleagues (2004) reported eight more affected women. Six of the eight had parkinsonism, and only one had dystonia. The initial symptom was focal tremor or parkinsonism in four, chorea in three, and focal dystonia (cervical) in one. Seven of eight patients had slow or no progression of their symptoms and required no treatment. The patient with disabling parkinsonism was responsive to carbidopa/levodopa. 🎥

With the aid of molecular genetics for identification, the phenotype has been extended to also include tremor, myoclonus, chorea, and myorhythmia (Evidente et al., 2002). Deoxyglucose and fluorodopa PET scans show decreased metabolism in the striatum and no or little decrease of dopa uptake (Eidelberg et al., 1992). Treatment is not satisfactory, but antimuscarinics and clonazepam appear to be somewhat helpful, as does zolpidem (Evidente, 2002). The abnormal gene that causes lubag has been localized near the centromere of the X chromosome at Xq13.1 (Kupke et al., 1990; Wilhelmsen et al., 1991; Kupke et al., 1992; Graeber et al., 1992; Haberhausen et al., 1995; Makino et al., 2007) and has been given the designation DYT3. The gene involves a multiple transcript system (Nolte et al., 2003). The mutation has been identified in the coding portion of DNA (i.e., an exon). However, this region of DNA is extremely complex, with genes being made from both strands, and multiple different RNAs (each encoding a different protein product) being made from each strand. Thus, while the investigators appear to have identified a specific mutation, they were not able to say which mutant protein (and there may be up to six from this mutation) is actually responsible for the disease. Subsequently, Makino and colleagues (2007) reported that it is the *TAF1* gene in this region that is particularly affected and its decreased function is likely the primary factor resulting in the disease.

The pathology of lubag has been reported (Altrocchi and Forno, 1983; Waters et al., 1993a). The neostriatum shows astrocytosis in a multifocal or mosaic pattern, due to islands of normal striatum sharply demarcated by gliotic tissue. The lateral part of the putamen was most severely gliotic, and the astrocytosis in this region was confluent rather than mosaic-like. The gliotic areas also exhibited neuronal loss involving both large and small populations in the putamen. In the body and head of the caudate nucleus, the gliosis was less extensive and neuronal loss was equivocal. The tail of the caudate was also affected, showing a mild diffuse astrocytosis and loss of nerve cells. No areas of striatum seemed to be spared. The myelinated fiber bundles in caudate and putamen were thinned in affected foci. The brainstem was normal. In particular, there were no Lewy bodies or neurofibrillary tangles. In addition to the pathologic observations in the two Filipino men, a very similar pathologic finding was reported in a non-Filipino youth with progressive generalized dystonia with marked orolingual and pharyngeal involvement (Gibb et al., 1992) and in a non-Filipino man with a combination of psychiatric symptoms, craniocervical dystonia, bulbar dysfunction, and parkinsonism (Factor and Barron, 1997). The similar pathology and clinical features of dystonia suggest that lubag might be present in other populations beside Filipinos. An Italian family with a mutation on the

DYT3 gene could be another case (Fabbrini et al., 2005). Lubag is now a confirmed neurodegenerative disorder and deserves much more intensive study. The mechanism of its pathogenesis might shed light on normal basal ganglia function, as well as leading to a better understanding of the pathophysiologic mechanisms underlying dystonia and parkinsonism.

Toward that end, Goto et al. (2005) found that with the dystonia phenotype, the striosomes in the striatum are severely depleted, while the matrix compartment of the striatum is relatively spared. But as the disease progresses, and the matrix becomes involved, the clinical features become parkinsonian. This suggests that dystonia may result from an imbalance in the activity between the striosomal and matrix-based pathways.

Treatment is difficult, because the response to anticholinergics, baclofen, and benzodiazepines is limited. Levodopa is not effective. Bilateral deep brain stimulation in the GPi has been reported to be of benefit (Evidente et al., 2007).

Pathophysiology and pathoanatomy of primary dystonia

Pathophysiology

A major characteristic of dystonic movements is the presence of sustained simultaneous contractions of agonists and antagonists (Herz, 1944a; Yanagisawa and Goto, 1971; Rothwell et al., 1983; Rothwell and Obeso, 1987). There are also contractions of adjoining and distant muscles, so-called "overflow," particularly during a voluntary movement. Also, rhythmical contractions frequently occur on voluntary movement. None of these physiologic features is specific for dystonia. Increasing muscle spindle activity by the tonic vibration reflex maneuver induced dystonic postures or movements typical of those seen during writing in 11 out of 15 patients with writer's cramp, but not in normal individuals (Kaji et al., 1995). The cutaneous EMG silent period during isometric contraction was studied in primary brachial dystonia. The duration of the silent period was significantly prolonged in dystonia and in Parkinson disease in both affected and unaffected arms compared with controls (Pullman et al., 1996).

Some physiologic reflexes, such as blink reflexes, have been found to be abnormal in primary cranial and cervical dystonias (Berardelli et al., 1985; Tolosa et al., 1988b). The R1 and R2 blink responses have increased amplitude and duration. This finding implies excess physiologic excitatory drive to the midbrain region. In a physiologic study, a sensory trick that reduced blepharospasm was found to decrease the R2 blink response (Gomez-Wong et al., 1998).

In limb dystonia, there is an abnormality of the normal reciprocal inhibition between agonist and antagonist. The second, longer phase of reciprocal inhibition is much reduced or even absent in affected limbs in dystonia (Nakashima et al., 1989). This has been interpreted as evidence for reduced presynaptic inhibition of muscle afferent input to the inhibitory interneurons as a result of defective descending motor control. Reduced reciprocal inhibition is a feature that is seen with other types of dystonia (Valls-Sole and Hallett, 1995). The early and late long-latency reflex responses are often abnormal in primary focal dystonia (Naumann and Reiners, 1997), and this can be influenced by botulinum toxin injections, indicating their influence by peripheral afferents. Cooling the affected limb in writer's cramp has been shown to reduce the dystonia and improve writing performance (Pohl et al., 2002). In addition to adult-onset focal dystonia, abnormal physiologic studies have been found in both DYT1 manifesting and nonmanifesting carriers (Fiorio et al., 2007). The temporal discrimination threshold was increased in the DYT1 carriers, similar to focal dystonias. Whether these physiologic alterations are epiphenomena or part of the underlying pathophysiology is unclear, but Espay and colleagues (2006) found analogous abnormalities in psychogenic dystonia. Cortical abnormalities with transcranial magnetic stimulation in fixed dystonia (Avanzino et al., 2008) could also be secondary to the abnormal postures, rather than primary.

There is a report of decreased N30 amplitude in somatosensory evoked potentials in patients with cervical dystonia (Mazzini et al., 1994). The excitability of the motor cortex was studied in 11 patients with task-specific dystonia and 11 age-matched controls by delivering transcranial magnetic stimuli at different stimulus intensities (Ikoma et al., 1996). With increasing stimulus intensity the increase in the motor evoked potentials in the flexor carpi radialis muscles was greater in patients than in normal subjects, suggesting that cortical motor excitability is increased in dystonia. Transcranial magnetic stimulation has become a popular tool to study cortical excitability and inhibition. The paired-pulse technique has been proposed as a useful technique (Bohlhalter et al., 2007).

Blepharospasm has been studied in some detail, recording EMGs simultaneously from both orbicularis oculi (OO) and levator palpebrae superioris (LPS) (Aramideh et al., 1994). Some patients had contractions only of the OO and simultaneous reciprocal inhibition of LPS; others had combined simultaneous contractions of both OO and LPS; and others had gradual cessation of LPS inhibition along with OO contraction (combination of blepharospasm, LP motor impersistence); a fourth group had a combination of blepharospasm and involuntary LP inhibition; a fifth group had involuntary inhibition of LPS activity, without any dystonic discharges in OO ("apraxia of eyelid opening"). Krack and Marion (1994) suggest that this so-called apraxia of lid opening is actually a dystonic phenomenon.

The cerebral cortex appears to play a physiologic role in dystonia. An animal model of producing focal dystonia by training overusage of a limb resulted in receptive fields in the sensorimotor cortex that were 10–20 times larger than normal (Byl et al. 1996) without local signs of tendon or nerve inflammation (Topp and Byl, 1999). A current concept is that in dystonia there is a loss of surround inhibition in the cerebral cortex (Hallett, 2004; Sohn and Hallett, 2004). Surround inhibition is considered a major function of the basal ganglia to allow accurate voluntary movements (Mink, 1996). In writer's cramp, abnormal sensorimotor integration was found by studying contingent negative variation (Ikeda et al., 1996), and premotor cortex and supplementary motor area (SMA) have increased blood flow as determined with PET blood flow scans (Playford et al., 1998). These results might represent a release of the thalamus from the normal inhibitory influence of the GPi. Both the internal and external segments of the globus pallidus show a reduced neuronal firing pattern in dystonia, including "off" period dystonia in Parkinson disease (Hashimoto, 2000). PET scans that measured sensorimotor activation revealed that DYT1 manifesting, but not nonmanifesting, carriers abnormally increased motor activation responses in the former group (Carbon et al., 2010). The presence of elevated normal motor-related activation pattern expression in the nonmotor condition suggests that abnormal integration of audiovisual input with sensorimotor network activity is an important trait feature of this disorder (Carbon et al., 2010).

The interstitial nucleus of Cajal in the midbrain has been reported to function as a neural integrator for head posture (Klier et al., 2002). A bilateral imbalance in this structure, through either direct damage or inappropriate input, could be one of the mechanisms underlying torticollis.

New insights about occupational cramps, such as musician's cramp, which are associated with repetitive movements, have emerged. Studies in primates support the notion that repetitive motions of the hand can induce plasticity changes in the sensory cortex, leading to degradation of topographic representations of the hand (Chen and Hallett, 1998). Hand dystonia is represented by an abnormality of the normal homuncular organization of the finger representations in the primary somatosensory cortex (Bara-Jimenez et al., 1998). Patients with focal hand dystonia have a decreased performance in sensory detection, suggesting a role for sensory dysfunction in the pathophysiology of dystonia (Bara-Jimenez et al., 2000). Functional magnetic resonance imaging was utilized to study tactile stimulation in patients with focal hand dystonia. These patients, compared to normal controls, have a nonlinear interaction between the sensory cortical response to individual finger stimulation (Sanger et al., 2002). Levy and Hallett (2002) used two-dimensional J-resolved magnetic resonance spectroscopy to reveal GABA levels and found them decreased in sensorimotor cortex and lentiform nuclei contralateral to the affected hand in patients with writer's cramp. This finding correlates with physiologic studies showing reduced intracortical inhibition. Even with hand movement that does not induce dystonic movements, there is reduced cortical sensorimotor integration, suggesting that this abnormal physiology is inherent in dystonia and not secondary to it (Wu et al., 2010).

In addition to focal hand dystonia, focal facial dystonia (blepharospasm) has been studied physiologically. Suprathreshold transcranial magnetic stimuli was applied over the optimal representation of the relaxed abductor digiti minimi muscle of the dominant hand in both groups of subjects following conditioning stimuli (Sommer et al., 2002). Intracortical inhibition was reduced in both patient groups. Physiologic markers of primary dystonia, including cortical inhibition and cutaneous silent period, although abnormal when compared to healthy controls, however, were not different when patients with psychogenic and organic dystonia were compared, suggesting that these abnormal findings represent a consequence, rather than a cause of dystonia, or that they are endophenotypic abnormalities that predispose to both types of dystonia (Espay et al., 2006).

A brief summary of the pathophysiology of dystonia is presented in Table 12.21, in part, taken from Berardelli and colleagues (1998) and Hallett (2009). Briefly, dystonia is

Table 12.21 Highlights of pathophysiology of torsion dystonia

1. Reduced and irregular neuronal firing rate in the internal and external segments of the globus pallidus
2. Reduced pallidal inhibition of the thalamus with consequent overactivity of medial and prefrontal cortical areas and underactivity of the primary motor cortex during movements
3. Cortical abnormalities:
   a. Reduced preparatory activity in the EEG before the onset of voluntary movements
   b. Enhanced premotor and supplementary motor cortical excitability
   c. Reduced primary motor cortex activity
   d. Enlarged, overlapping cortical sensory fields in focal dystonias (Nelson et al., 2009; Hallett, 2009)
   e. Disorganized sensorimotor integration
   f. Increased plasticity (Quartarone et al., 2006, 2009)
4. Loss of surround inhibition
5. Reduced spinal cord and brainstem inhibition is seen in many reflex studies (long-latency reflexes, cranial reflexes, and reciprocal inhibition)
6. Co-contraction and overflow of EMG activity of inappropriate muscles is characteristic
7. Reduced inhibition and increased plasticity are seen in unaffected muscles of patients with focal dystonia. Thus they are thought to be primary abnormalities rather than secondary to dystonic muscle contraction. However, patients with psychogenic dystonia have the same abnormalities of short and long interval intracortical inhibition (SICI and LICI), cortical silent period and spinal reciprocal inhibition as patients with primary dystonia (Espay et al., 2006; Quartarone et al., 2009). Although psychogenic dystonia shows similar cortical inhibition, plasticity (paired associative stimulation) is abnormally high only in the organic group, while there is no difference between the plasticity measured in psychogenic patients and healthy controls (Quartarone et al., 2009). Synaptic plasticity in the motor cortex is induced by repetitive transcranial magnetic stimulation (TMS). Increased plasticity is measured as an increased response to TMS. The finding of reduced cortical inhibition occurs also in psychogenic dystonia and implies that central nervous system inhibition may follow the abnormal usage of a limb or other affected body part, and not necessarily be the cause or the epiphenomenon.

characterized by two main pathophysiological abnormalities: "reduced" excitability of inhibitory systems at many levels of the sensorimotor system, and "increased" plasticity of neural connections in sensorimotor circuits at a brainstem and spinal level (Quartarone et al., 2009).

Pathoanatomy

A number of pathologic studies have been carried out on patients who died with PTD. When these were reviewed by Zeman (1970), who also added his own cases, he concluded that whereas environmental etiologies leave their mark with alterations in the basal ganglia, the hereditary forms are without tangible pathologic abnormalities detectable by light microscopy. He felt that the earlier reports of positive findings could be explained as nonspecific alterations or as artifacts due to the agonal state prior to death. There have been few reports since then. Zweig and colleagues (1988)

described the histology of the brainstem in four patients with PTD (Table 12.22). Two of them started in childhood or adolescence (Cases 1 and 2), Case 1 was Jewish and Case 2 was non-Jewish. Case 1 had numerous neurofibrillary tangles (NFTs) in the locus coeruleus, along with mild neuronal loss and extracellular neuromelanin in this nucleus. There were rare NFTs in the SNc, pedunculopontine nucleus, and dorsal raphe.

The inconsistency of the histology in patients with primary dystonia makes it difficult to interpret the significance of the observations by Zweig and his colleagues (1988). Clearly, there is a large need to have many more cases studied pathologically. Bhatia and colleagues (1993b) found no abnormalities in a patient with orofacial dystonia and rest tremor.

McNaught and colleagues (2004) used special stains for a combination of ubiquitin, torsinA, and lamin in four brains of patients with Oppenheim dystonia. Inclusions were present in the perinuclear region within brainstem cholinergic and other neurons in the pedunculopontine nucleus, cuneiform nucleus, and griseum centrale mesencephali. No inclusions were detected in the substantia nigra pars compacta, striatum, hippocampus, or selected regions of the cerebral cortex. McNaught and colleagues (2004) also noted tau/ubiquitin-immunoreactive aggregates in pigmented neurons of the SNc and locus coeruleus. When this technique was applied to six adult-onset dystonia brains, the results were negative (Holton et al., 2008).

Although primary dystonia is not associated with any known degenerative lesion, the volume of the putamen is increased about 10% (Black et al., 1998). In primary cervical dystonia, an increase in gray matter density bilaterally in the motor cortex and in the cerebellar flocculus and unilaterally in the right GPi was found by using voxel-based morphometry (Draganski et al., 2003). Voxel-based morphometry in patients with blepharospasm showed gray matter increase in the putamina bilaterally and decrease in the left inferior parietal lobule (Etgen et al., 2006). In writer's cramp voxel-based morphometry found decreased gray matter in the hand area of the contralateral primary sensorimotor cortex and bilateral thalamus, and cerebellum (Delmaire et al., 2007). Obermann et al. (2007) evaluated voxel-based morphometry in patients with blepharospasm and cervical dystonia. They found that blepharospasm subjects had increased gray matter in the caudate head and cerebellum bilaterally and a decrease in the putamen and thalamus bilaterally. In cervical dystonia, they found increased gray matter in the thalamus, caudate head bilaterally, superior temporal lobe, and left cerebellum, while gray matter was decreased in the putamen bilaterally. One study assessed patterns of voxel-based morphometry in different types of primary dystonia: generalized dystonia, cervical dystonia, and focal hand dystonia (FHD) as well as in age- and gender-matched controls. There was a common pattern of gray matter changes, namely gray matter volume increase bilaterally in the GPi, nucleus accumbens, and prefrontal cortex, and unilaterally in the left inferior parietal lobe (Egger et al., 2007).

Although no consistent cerebral anatomical abnormality has been reported in primary focal hand dystonia, a voxel-based morphometry study showed a significant bilateral increase in gray matter in the hand representation area of primary somatosensory and, to a lesser extent, primary motor cortices in 36 patients with unilateral FHD compared

Table 12.22 Description of brainstem pathology in four patients with primary torsion dystonia

Case	Ethnicity	Age at onset	Age at death	Site at onset	Final classification	Clinical remarks	Pathology of interest
1	Jewish	14	29	Right foot	Generalized	Bilateral thalamotomies, head injury at age 23, seizures	Numerous NFTs, mild neuronal loss, and extracellular neuromelanin in locus coeruleus. Rare NFT in substantia nigra pars compacta, dorsal raphe and PPN
2	Non-Jewish	4	10	Feet	Segmental crural (trunk and both legs)	Initially improved with anticholinergics	No notable abnormality found
3	Not stated	33	68	Eyelids	Cranial and cervical (face, jaw, tongue, and neck)	Initial diagnosis was postencephalitic, but no history of encephalitis. Marked improvement with baclofen and valproate	Depigmentation of substantia nigra and locus coeruleus. Occasional NFT in nucleus basalis. Moderate to marked neuronal loss in substantia nigra pars compacta, dorsal raphe, PPN, and locus coeruleus. Extracellular pigment in substantia nigra and locus coeruleus
4	Not stated	47	50	Neck	Cervical	Intention tremor developed in right arm. Clonazepam was beneficial. Developed status epilepticus	No notable abnormality found

NFT, neurofibrillary tangles; PPN, pedunculopontine nucleus.
Case 2 had no notable abnormality. Cases 3 and 4 had adult-onset cranial-cervical dystonia and cervical dystonia, respectively. Case 3 had remarkable neuronal loss in the substantia nigra pars compacta, dorsal raphe, PPN, and locus coeruleus. The pigmented nuclei had extracellular pigment. There was occasional NFT in the nucleus basalis and infrequent NFT in the substantia nigra. Case 4, like Case 2, had no notable abnormality.
Data from Zweig RM, Hedreen JC, Jankel WR, et al. Pathology in brainstem regions of individuals with primary dystonia. Neurology 1988;38:702–706.

with 36 controls (Garraux et al., 2004). The presence of anatomical changes in the perirolandic cortex for the unaffected hand as well as that for the affected hand suggested to the investigators that these disturbances might be, at least in part, primary. It has been proposed, based on animal models, that the cerebellum plays a role in dystonia (Neychev et al., 2008), and reduced connectivity in the cerebellothalamic pathway has been found in Oppenheim dystonia (Argyelan et al., 2009). Electrophysiologic studies in patients with cervical dystonia and focal hand dystonia using eyeblink conditioning reflex found differences between the patients and healthy controls (Teo et al., 2009). Since this is mediated via the olivocerebellar pathway, it also suggests that the cerebellum may play a role in dystonia.

In secondary dystonia, however, the basal ganglia, particularly the putamen, is involved (Burton et al., 1984). Lesions in the pallidum also can result in dystonia, often with parkinsonism (Munchau et al., 2000b). Actually, lesions can involve not only the basal ganglia, but also connections to and from these nuclei, such as the thalamus and the cortex (Marsden et al., 1985). A survey of secondary cervical dystonia found that structural lesions were most commonly localized to the brainstem and cerebellum, and fewer cases were in the cervical spinal cord and basal ganglia (LeDoux and Brady, 2003).

In an MRI study of eight patients with secondary unilateral dystonia, lesions associated with dystonic spasms were located in the putamen posterior to the anterior commissure in all patients and extended variably into the dorsolateral part of the caudate nucleus, the posterior limb of the internal capsule, or the lateral segment of the globus pallidus (Lehericy et al., 1996). In imaging studies of dystonia developing after a stroke, focal lesions were seen in the striatopallidum and in different parts of the thalamus (Karsidag et al., 1998; Krystkowiak et al., 1998). A characteristic dystonic tremor following a stroke is commonly localized to the thalamus by imaging studies (Cho and Samkoff, 2000).

However, one should not assume that the basal ganglia are always the site of physiologic pathology in primary dystonia. It has been shown, for example, that the rostral brainstem (Jankovic and Patel, 1983; Kulisevsky et al., 1993), pontine tegmentum (Aramideh et al., 1996), and thalamus (Miranda and Millar, 1998) can be pathologically damaged in some cases of secondary blepharospasm. Lesions from stroke, multiple sclerosis, and encephalitis have all been seen. Moreover, as mentioned in the section on Oppenheim dystonia, there is reduced connectivity in the cerebellothalamic pathway in that disorder.

An abnormality in the striatum in PTD is suggested by finding prolonged MRI T2 times in the lentiform nucleus in patients with primary cervical dystonia (Schneider et al., 1994). Findings on FDG and spiperone PET studies (discussed below) also support this implication. Intraoperative recordings for stereotactic surgery for dystonia show an abnormal firing pattern in the internal segment of the globus pallidus (Lenz et al., 1998).

Biochemistry and neuroimaging

Although no consistent morphologic abnormalities in PTD are seen on brain imaging (Rutledge et al., 1987) or histologic examination (Zeman, 1976; Zweig et al., 1988), some changes have been reported on postmortem biochemical analysis. Hornykiewicz and colleagues (1986) examined the biochemistry of the brain in two patients with childhood-onset generalized primary dystonia, and Jankovic and colleagues (1987) studied a single case of adult-onset primary cranial segmental dystonia. There were changes in norepinephrine, serotonin, and dopamine levels in various regions of brain. It is not clear which, if any, of these alterations, is related to the pathophysiology of dystonia. In a patient with symptomatic dystonia due to neuroacanthocytosis, de Yebenes and colleagues (1988) found large increases in norepinephrine in caudate, putamen, globus pallidus, and dentate nucleus. Again, it is not clear whether norepinephrine is related to dystonia. Many more biochemical studies need to be carried out.

Eidelberg and colleagues (1995) evaluated FDG PET in 11 patients with predominantly right-sided Oppenheim dystonia and 11 age-matched controls. They found that global and regional metabolic rates were normal in PTD. But the Scaled Subprofile Model analysis of the combined groups of PTD patients and controls revealed a significant topographic profile characterized by relative bilateral increases in the metabolic activity of the lateral frontal and paracentral cortices, associated with relative covariate hypermetabolism of the contralateral lentiform nucleus, pons, and midbrain. Subject scores for this profile correlated significantly with Fahn–Marsden disease severity ratings ($r = 0.67$, $P < 0.02$). Thalamic metabolism was decreased. Thus, in contrast to parkinsonism, lentiform and thalamic metabolism were dissociated in dystonia. In Parkinson disease, both regions show increased metabolism; in dystonia the lentiform is increased while the thalamus is decreased. These authors concluded that PTD is characterized by relative metabolic overactivity of the lentiform nucleus and premotor cortices. The presence of lentiform-thalamic metabolic dissociation suggests that in this disorder hyperkinetic movements may arise through excessive activity of the direct putamino-pallidal inhibitory pathway, resulting in inhibition of the GPi. In direct physiologic recordings during surgery, both the internal and external segments of the globus pallidus show a reduced neuronal firing pattern in dystonia, including "off" period dystonia in Parkinson disease (Hashimoto, 2000).

Eidelberg and colleagues utilized FDG PET in nonmanifesting DYT1 carriers using a network analytical approach and identified a pattern of abnormal regional glucose utilization in two independent cohorts (Eidelberg et al., 1998; Trost et al., 2002). They found increased metabolism in the posterior putamen/globus pallidus, cerebellum, and supplementary motor area (SMA). This abnormal torsion dystonia-related pattern (TDRP) was also present in clinically affected patients, persisting even following the suppression of involuntary dystonic movements by sleep induction, and also in non-DYT1 patients who had just essential blepharospasm (Hutchinson et al., 2000). This shows that TDRP expression is not specific for the DYT1 genotype. In fact, these investigators found the same TDRP expression in the primary dystonia (DYT6) that has been reported in the Amish/Mennonite population (Trost et al., 2002). The investigators propose that the TDRP feature in the resting state represents a metabolic trait of primary dystonia.

In other FDG PET studies Galardi and colleagues (1996) found hypermetabolism in the lentiform, thalamus, premotor and motor cortices, and cerebellum in patients with primary cervical dystonia; this did not reveal the lentiform-thalamic metabolic dissociation. Magyar-Lehmann and colleagues (1997) also found lentiform hypermetabolism bilaterally in cervical dystonia.

Carbon and colleagues (2004c) found bilateral hypermetabolism in the presupplementary motor area and parietal association cortices of affected carriers of both DYT1 and DYT6 dystonia, compared with their respective nonmanifesting counterparts. But differences were seen between manifesting DYT1 and DYT6 carriers. Increases in metabolism were found in the putamen, anterior cingulate, and cerebellar hemispheres of DYT1 carriers, while hypometabolism of the putamen and hypermetabolism in the temporal cortex occurred in DYT6-affected patients.

Fluorodopa PET reveals mild reduction of uptake or normal uptake in familial PTD (Playford et al., 1993). PET scans using a ligand to bind to striatal dopamine D2 receptors showed a trend to higher uptake in the contralateral striatum in subjects showing lateralization of clinical signs (Leenders et al., 1993). Spiperone PET scans in primary focal dystonia revealed a 29% decrease in binding in the putamina (Perlmutter et al., 1997a), and suggest an involvement of the D2 receptor. SPECT scans evaluating epidepride binding of the D2 receptors also showed decreased binding in both striata in patients with torticollis (Naumann et al., 1998). Eidelberg and colleagues (Carbon et al., 2004b; Asanuma et al., 2005b) used ^{11}C-raclopride and PET in a cohort of nonmanifesting DYT1 gene carriers, and found significant reductions in binding in both the putamen and caudate (18% and 12% of control values, respectively). In a subsequent study, Carbon and colleagues (2009) found a reduction of D2 receptor binding in both manifesting and nonmanifesting carriers of both DYT1 and DYT6 gene mutations. Todd and Perlmutter (1998) suggest that the pathophysiology of dystonia involves decreased D2 receptor inhibition. In a mouse model of DYT1 dystonia, the effect of decreased D2 function is enhanced GABA transmission from the striatum due to decreased D2 presynaptic function resulting in disinhibition of GABA efferents (Sciamanna et al., 2009). The reductions in D2 receptor sensitivity in the striatum in all these studies suggest that this might be a component in the pathophysiology of primary dystonias. However, spiperone bonds to both D2 and D3 receptors. Perlmutter's lab has now found no decrease in binding when he used a more highly selective D2 receptor binding ligand, and concluded that a defect in D3, rather than D2, receptor expression may be associated with primary focal dystonia (Karimi et al., 2011).

Tempel and Perlmutter (1993) measured blood flow with PET in patients with writer's cramp. Subjects had blood flow scans at rest and during vibration of either the affected or unaffected hand. Vibration produced a consistent peak response in primary sensorimotor area and supplementary motor area, both contralateral to the vibrated hand. Both responses were significantly reduced approximately 25% in patients with writer's cramp whether the affected or unaffected hand was vibrated. This indicates that patients with unilateral writer's cramp have bilateral brain dysfunction. These investigators performed an analogous study in patients with blepharospasm (Feiwell et al., 1999). They found decreased activation of blood flow in the primary sensorimotor cortical area, both ipsilateral and contralateral to the side of facial stimulation.

Following the injection of MPTP into baboons, the animals transiently developed ipsilateral turning and contralateral hemidystonia involving arm and leg. This transient dystonia preceded hemiparkinsonism and corresponded temporally with a decreased striatal dopamine content and a transient decrease in D2-like receptor number (Perlmutter et al., 1997b).

By the use of diffusion tensor MRI, the microstructure of white matter pathways (fractional anisotropy) was assessed in mutation carriers and control subjects. Axonal integrity was found to be reduced in the subgyral white matter of the sensorimotor cortex of DYT1 carriers, and the changes were greater in manifesting than in nonmanifesting carriers (Carbon et al., 2004a). In a subsequent study, both DYT1 and DYT6 dystonic patients and nonmanifesting DYT1 carriers were evaluated. Both groups of dystonic patients had a significant reduction in fractional anisotropy in the pontine brainstem in the vicinity of the left superior cerebellar peduncle and bilaterally in the white matter of the subcortical sensorimotor region (Carbon et al., 2008b). Nonmanifesting DYT1 carriers showed only a slight reduction of fractional anisotropy compared to controls. These data suggest there may be a disturbance in cerebellothalamocortical pathways in these two types of manifesting dystonia.

Diffusion tensor imaging in patients with primary cervical dystonia and in patients with blepharospasm has also been carried out (Fabbrini et al., 2008). There were regional differences in patients with cervical dystonia and healthy controls, but no difference between patients with blepharospasm and controls.

A biochemical study investigating copper proteins in PTD found Wilson protein and ceruloplasmin were increased in the lentiform nuclei in two patients with focal dystonia and reduced in the patient with generalized dystonia, and Menkes protein was reduced in all three patients (Berg et al., 2000). In another biochemical study, plasma concentration of homocysteine was elevated in patients with PTD compared with age- and sex-matched controls (Muller et al., 2000). Naumann and colleagues (1996) studied transcranial sonography (TCS) of the basal ganglia in 86 patients with dystonic disorders, including primary dystonia (generalized and focal). The majority of primary and secondary dystonias had a hyperechogenic lesion of the middle segment of the lenticular nucleus on the side opposite to the clinical dystonic symptoms. Becker and colleagues (1997) found a similar result in patients with idiopathic torticollis. These changes support the proposal of increased copper content in the lentiform nuclei in primary focal dystonia (Becker et al., 2001). Although this increase was suggested to be due to reduced levels of the Menkes protein, a membrane ATPase exporting copper out of the cells, genetic analysis has failed to find an alteration in the genes for this Menkes protein, the Wilson protein (another copper ATPase), or the intracellular copper chaperone, ATOX1, in patients with primary focal dystonia (Bandmann et al., 2002).

In a study of platelet mitochondria, Benecke and colleagues (1992) found a defect in complex I in patients with primary dystonia, most of whom had torticollis (DYT7). However, Reichmann and colleagues (1994) could not replicate this. Schapira and colleagues (1997) found that platelet complex I activity is normal in familial dystonia (including DYT1 dystonia), but is decreased in sporadic torticollis.

References available on Expert Consult: www.expertconsult.com

CHAPTER **13**

Treatment of dystonia

Chapter contents

Physical and supportive therapy	294		Botulinum toxin	298
Dopaminergic therapy	295		Surgical treatment of dystonia	306
Antidopaminergic therapy	295		Other therapies	309
Anticholinergic therapy	296		Therapeutic guidelines	309
Other pharmacologic therapies	296		Appendix	310

Despite the paucity of knowledge about the cause and pathogenesis of dystonic disorders, the symptomatic treatment of dystonia has markedly improved, particularly since the introduction of botulinum toxin. In most cases of dystonia, the treatment is merely symptomatic, designed to improve posture and function and to relieve associated pain. In rare patients, however, dystonia can be so severe that it can produce not only abnormal postures and disabling dystonic movements, sometimes compromising respiration, but also muscle breakdown and life-threatening hyperthermia, rhabdomyolysis, and myoglobinuria. In such cases of dystonic storm or status dystonicus, proper therapeutic intervention can be life-saving (Jankovic and Penn, 1982; Vaamonde et al., 1994; Manji et al., 1998; Dalvi et al., 1998; Jankovic, 2006, 2009a).

The assessment of various therapeutic interventions in dystonia is problematic for the following reasons: (1) Dystonia and its effects on function are difficult to quantitate; therefore, most trials utilize crude clinical rating scales, many of which have not been properly evaluated or validated; (2) dystonia is a syndrome with different etiologies, anatomic distributions, and heterogeneous clinical manifestations producing variable disability; (3) some patients, perhaps up to 15%, may have spontaneous, albeit transient, remissions; (4) many studies have used dosages that may have been insufficient or too short a duration to provide benefit; (5) the vast majority of therapeutic trials in dystonia are not double-blind, placebo-controlled; and (6) most studies, even those that have been otherwise well designed and controlled, have utilized small sample sizes, which makes the results difficult to interpret, particularly in view of a large placebo effect demonstrated in dystonia (Lindeboom et al., 1996). A variety of instruments have been used to assess the response in patients with cervical dystonia; the most frequently used is the Toronto Western Spasmodic Torticollis Rating Scale (TWSTRS) (Consky and Lang, 1994; Comella et al., 1997). TWSTRS (range: 0–87) consists of three subscales: severity (range: 0–35), disability (range: 0–23), and pain (range: 0–20). In addition, visual analog scale, global assessment of change, and pain analog assessments have been used in various clinical trials. Various scales, such as the Fahn–Marsden scale and the Unified Dystonia Rating Scale, have also been used to assess patients with generalized dystonia (Burke et al., 1985a; Ondo et al., 1998; Comella et al., 2003). Another scale designed to capture the burden of dystonia on patients is the Cervical Dystonia Impact Profile scale (Cano et al., 2004). The Jankovic Rating Scale was initially used in the original study of botulinum toxin (BTX) in patients with cranial dystonia which led to the approval of BTX by the Food and Drug Administration (Jankovic and Orman, 1987) and in subsequent studies (Roggenkamper et al., 2006) to assess the severity and frequency of involuntary eyelid contractions in patients with blepharospasm (Jankovic et al., 2009). Subsequent studies have refined the clinical rating scales and included quality-of-life scales (Lindeboom et al., 1996). Health-related quality-of-life instruments, such as the Craniocervical Dystonia Questionnaire (CDQ-24), are increasingly used to assess the function and the impact of treatment in patients with cranial, cervical, and other dystonias on activities of daily living and other measures of quality of life (Muller et al., 2004; Reimer et al., 2005; Hall et al., 2006).

The selection of a particular choice of therapy is guided largely by personal clinical experience and by empirical trials (Greene et al., 1988; Greene, 1995; Jankovic, 1997; Brin, 1998; Jankovic, 2004a, 2006; Albanese et al., 2006; Tinter and Jankovic, 2007) (Table 13.1). An evidence-based review concluded that except for BTX in cervical dystonia and

DOI: 10.1016/B978-1-4377-2369-4.00013-5

Table 13.1 Medical therapy of dystonia

- Levodopa
- Anticholinergics
- Baclofen: oral, intrathecal
- Tetrabenazine
- Anticonvulsants (carbamazepine, pregabalin, levetiracetam)
- Muscle relaxants:
  - Benzodiazepines (clonazepam, lorazepam, diazepam, alprazolam)
  - Other relaxants (tizanidine, cyclobenzaprine, metaxalone, carisoprodol, methocarbamol, orphenadrine)
- Sodium oxybate (salt of gamma-hydroxybutyrate)
- Clozapine
- Botulinum toxin

high-dose trihexyphenidyl in young patients with segmental and generalized dystonia (level A, class I–II), none of the methods of pharmacologic intervention have been confirmed as being effective according to evidence-based criteria (Balash and Giladi, 2004). The patient's age, the anatomic distribution of dystonia, and the potential risk of adverse effects are also important determinants of choice of therapy. The identification of a specific cause of dystonia, such as drug-induced dystonias or Wilson disease (Svetel et al., 2001), may lead to a treatment that is targeted to the particular etiology. It is therefore prudent to search for identifiable causes of dystonia, particularly when some atypical features are present. The diagnostic approach to patients with dystonia is based on being aware of the multiple causes of torsion dystonia, which was covered in Chapter 12 and in other reviews (Jankovic, 2007).

Physical and supportive therapy

Before reviewing pharmacologic and surgical therapy of dystonia, it is important to emphasize the role of patient education and supportive care, which are integral components of a comprehensive approach to patients with dystonia. Various paramedical treatments reported to be useful in patients with primary dystonia have been systematically reviewed (Delnooz et al., 2009). Physical therapy and well-fitted braces are designed primarily to improve posture and to prevent contractures. Although braces are often poorly tolerated, particularly by children, they may be used in some cases as a substitute for a sensory trick. For example, some patients with cervical dystonia are able to construct neck–head braces that seem to provide sensory input by touching certain portions of the neck or head in a fashion similar to the patient's own sensory trick, thus enabling the patient to maintain a desirable head position. Various hand devices have been developed in an attempt to help patients with writer's cramp to use their hands more effectively and comfortably (Ranawaya and Lang, 1991; Tas et al., 2001). In one small study of five professional musicians with focal dystonia, Candia and colleagues (1999) reported success with immobilization by splints of one or more of the digits other than the dystonic finger followed by intensive repetitive

exercises of the dystonic finger. It is not clear, however, whether this therapy provides lasting benefits. In one study of eight patients with idiopathic occupational focal dystonia of the upper limb, immobilization with a splint for 4–5 weeks resulted in a significant improvement at a 24-week follow-up visit, based on the Arm Dystonia Disability Scale (0 = normal; 3 = marked difficulty in playing) and the Tubiana and Champagne Score (0 = unable to play; 5 = returns to concert performances); the improvement was considered marked in four and moderate in three, but the initial improvement disappeared in one (Priori et al., 2001). The splint was applied for 24 hours every day except for 10 minutes once a week when it was removed for brief local hygiene. Immediately on full removal of the splint, all patients reported marked clumsiness and weakness, which resolved in 4 weeks. There was also some local subcutaneous and joint edema and pain in the immobilized joint, and nail growth stopped; none of the patients developed contractures. While the mechanisms of action of immobilization are unknown, the authors have postulated that removing all motor and sensory input to a limb might allow the cortical map to "reset" to the previous normal topography. One major concern about immobilization of a limb, particularly a dystonic limb, is that such immobilization can actually increase the risk of exacerbating or even precipitating dystonia, as has been well demonstrated in dystonia following casting or other peripheral causes of dystonia (Jankovic, 2001a). In one study of 21 patients with writer's cramp, after 4 weeks of immobilization, "retraining" for 8 weeks using drawing and writing exercises was associated with significant improvement relative to baseline as assessed by the Writer's Cramp Rating Scale (Zeuner et al., 2008). A variation of the immobilization therapy, constraint-induced movement therapy, has been used successfully in rehabilitation of patients after stroke and other brain insults, and the observed benefit has been attributed to cortical reorganization (Taub et al., 1999; Levy et al., 2001; Taub and Morris, 2001; Taub et al., 2002; Wolf et al., 2002).

Another technique, using a repetitive task during regional anesthesia of a weak arm in patients following stroke, was also associated with improved hand function (Muellbacher et al., 2002). Some patients find various muscle relaxation techniques and sensory feedback therapy useful adjuncts to medical or surgical treatments. Since some patients with dystonia have impaired sensory perception, it has been postulated that sensory training may relieve dystonia. In a study of 10 patients with focal hand dystonia, Zeuner and colleagues (2002) showed that reading Braille for 30–60 minutes daily for 8 weeks improved spatial acuity and dystonia that was sustained for up to 1 year in some patients (Zeuner and Hallett, 2003). Sensory training to restore sensory representation of the hand along with mirror imagery and mental practice techniques has also been reported to be useful in the treatment of focal hand dystonia (Byl and McKenzie, 2000; Byl et al., 2003).

Siebner and colleagues (1999) showed that using repetitive transcranial magnetic stimulation (rTMS) delivered at low frequencies (≤1 Hz) for 20 minutes can temporarily (8 of 16 patients reported improvement that lasted longer than 3 hours) improve handwriting impaired by dystonic writer's cramp, presumably by increasing inhibition (and thus reducing excitability) of the underlying cortex. Despite some encouraging results from open-label pilot studies it remains to be seen whether rTMS or transcranial direct current stimulation (tDCS) will enter the mainstream of therapeutics of dystonia (Wu et al., 2008).

Other stimulation techniques are also being studied in patients with dystonia. Long-term neck muscle vibration of the contracting muscle might have a therapeutic value in patients with cervical dystonia. This is suggested by transient (minutes) improvement in head position in one patient who was treated for 15 minutes with muscle vibration (Karnath et al., 2000). Transcutaneous electrical stimulation has been found to improve dystonic writer's cramp for at least 3 weeks in a double-blind, placebo-controlled trial (Tinazzi et al., 2005). Also, acoustic and galvanic vestibular stimulation was reported beneficial in one patient with cervical dystonia (Rosengren and Colebatch, 2006). Such observation is consistent with the notion that proprioceptive sensory input affects cervical dystonia.

Dopaminergic therapy

Pharmacologic treatment of dystonia is based largely on an empirical rationale rather than a scientific one. Unlike Parkinson disease, in which therapy with levodopa replacement is based on the finding of depletion of dopamine in the brains of parkinsonian animals and humans, our knowledge of biochemical alterations in idiopathic dystonia is very limited. One exception is dopa-responsive dystonia (DRD), in which the biochemical and genetic mechanisms have been elucidated by molecular DNA and biochemical studies in patients (Ichinose et al., 1994) and by studies of postmortem brains (Furukawa et al., 1999). Decreased neuromelanin in the substantia nigra with otherwise normal nigral cell count and morphology and normal tyrosine hydroxylase immunoreactivity were found in one brain of a patient with classic DRD (Rajput et al., 1994). There was a marked reduction in dopamine in the substantia nigra and the striatum. These findings suggested that in DRD, the primary abnormality was a defect in dopamine synthesis. This proposal is supported by the finding of a mutation in the GTP cyclohydrolase I gene on chromosome 14q that indirectly regulates the production of tetrahydrobiopterin, a cofactor for tyrosine hydroxylase, the rate-limiting enzyme in the synthesis of dopamine (Ichinose et al., 1994; Tanaka et al., 1995; Steinberger et al., 2000). Another form of DRD has been described in four cases belonging to two unrelated families of dopa-responsive cervical dystonia, presenting between 9 and 15 years of age and similar to classic DRD manifesting diurnal variation but no levodopa-induced dyskinesia (Schneider et al., 2006).

DRD usually presents in childhood with dystonia, mild parkinsonian features, and pseudopyramidal signs (hypertonicity and hyperreflexia) predominantly involving the legs. Many patients have a family history of dystonia or Parkinson disease. At least half of the patients have diurnal fluctuations, with marked progression of their symptoms toward the end of the day and a relief after sleep. Many patients with this form of dystonia are initially misdiagnosed as having cerebral palsy. Some patients with DRD are not diagnosed until adulthood, and family members of patients with typical DRD may present with adult-onset levodopa-responsive

parkinsonism (Harwood et al., 1994). The take-home message from these reports is that a therapeutic trial of levodopa should be considered in all patients with childhood-onset dystonia, whether they have classic features of DRD or not.

Most patients with DRD improve dramatically even with small doses of levodopa (100 mg of levodopa with 25 mg of decarboxylase inhibitor), but some might require doses of levodopa as high as 1000 mg per day. In contrast to patients with juvenile Parkinson disease (Ishikawa and Miyatake, 1995), DRD patients usually do not develop levodopa-induced fluctuations or dyskinesias. If no clinically evident improvement is noted after 3 months of therapy, the diagnosis of DRD is probably an error, and levodopa can be discontinued. In addition to levodopa, patients with DRD also improve with dopamine agonists, anticholinergic drugs, and carbamazepine (Nygaard et al., 1991). In contrast to patients with DRD, patients with idiopathic or other types of dystonia rarely improve with dopaminergic therapy (Lang, 1988). While dopaminergic therapy is remarkably effective in treating DRD, this strategy is not useful in the treatment of primary dystonia. Apomorphine, however, may ameliorate dystonia, perhaps by decreasing dopamine as well as serotonin release (Zuddas and Cianchetti, 1996).

Antidopaminergic therapy

Although dopamine receptor-blocking drugs were used extensively in the past, most clinical trials have produced mixed results with these drugs. Because of the poor response and the possibility of undesirable side effects, particularly sedation, parkinsonism, and tardive dyskinesia, the use of these drugs in the treatment of dystonia should be discouraged (Jankovic, 1995b). Clozapine, an atypical neuroleptic, has been reported in a small open trial to be moderately effective in the treatment of segmental and generalized dystonia, but its usefulness was limited by potential side effects (Karp et al., 1999). Although antidopaminergic drugs have been reported to be beneficial in the treatment of dystonia, the potential clinical benefit is usually limited by the development of side effects. Dopamine-depleting drugs, however, such as tetrabenazine, have been found useful in some patients with dystonia, particularly those with tardive dystonia (Jankovic and Orman, 1988; Jankovic and Beach, 1997). Tetrabenazine, a vesicular monoamine transporter 2 (VMAT2) inhibitor, has the advantage over other antidopaminergic drugs in that it does not cause tardive dyskinesia, although it may cause transient acute dystonic reaction (Burke et al., 1985b; Jankovic and Beach, 1997; Kenney and Jankovic, 2006). Tetrabenazine is not readily available in the United States, but it is dispensed by prescription under the trade name Nitoman or Xenazine 25 in other countries, including the United Kingdom. It is possible that some of the new atypical neuroleptic drugs will be useful not only as antipsychotics but also in the treatment of hyperkinetic movement disorders. Risperidone, a D2 dopamine receptor-blocking drug with a high affinity for 5-HT$_2$ receptors, has been reported to be useful in a 4-week trial of five patients with various forms of dystonia (Zuddas and Cianchetti, 1996). Clozapine, a D4 dopamine receptor blocker with relatively low affinity for the D2 receptors and high affinity for the 5-HT$_{2A}$ receptors, has been reported to ameliorate the symptoms of tardive dystonia (Trugman et al., 1994). The treatment of tardive dystonia and other tardive syndromes is discussed in Chapter 19 and in other reviews (Jankovic, 1995b).

Anticholinergic therapy

High-dosage anticholinergic medications, such as trihexyphenidyl, for dystonia were introduced by Fahn (1983) and confirmed by several groups (Marsden et al., 1984; Greene et al., 1988; Jabbari et al., 1989; Hoon et al., 2001), including a double-blind study (Burke et al., 1986). Although helpful in all types of dystonias, the supremacy of botulinum toxin therapy for focal dystonias has relegated anticholinergic therapy to be most useful in the treatment of generalized and segmental dystonia. In the experience of Greene and colleagues (1988), patients with blepharospasm, generalized dystonia, tonic (in contrast to clonic) dystonia, and onset of dystonia at age younger than 19 years seemed to respond better to anticholinergic drugs than other subgroups, but this difference did not reach statistical significance. Except for short duration of symptoms before onset of therapy, there was no other variable, such as gender or severity, that reliably predicted a favorable response. Treating patients within the first 5 years of disease onset was statistically significantly more successful than delaying treatment in both children and adults regardless of severity (Greene et al., 1988). Thus, starting treatment early is important.

This therapy is generally well tolerated when the dose is increased slowly. We recommend starting with a 5 mg preparation, half-tablet at bedtime, and adding a half-tablet a week, advancing up to 10 mg in four divided doses by the end of 4 weeks. Because there is a lag between reaching a dose and seeing a benefit, we hold this dose for a month, and then continue to increase at the same rate over the next 4 weeks until the dose is 20 mg in four divided doses. We continue to increase until there is adequate benefit or adverse effects that limit higher doses. Some patients require up to 60–140 mg/day, but may experience dose-related drowsiness, confusion, or memory difficulty that limit the dose. Children usually tolerate the very high dosages, whereas adults do not. In one study of 20 cognitively intact patients with dystonia, only 12 of whom could tolerate 15–74 mg of daily trihexyphenidyl, drug-induced impairments of recall and slowing of mentation were noted, particularly in the older patients (Taylor et al., 1991). Diphenhydramine, a histamine H$_1$ antagonist with anticholinergic properties, has been reported to have an antidystonic effect in three of five patients (Truong et al., 1995). However, the drug was not effective in 10 other patients with cervical dystonia, and it was associated with sedation and other anticholinergic side effects in most patients. Pyridostigmine, a peripherally acting anticholinesterase, and eye drops of pilocarpine (a muscarinic agonist) often ameliorate many of the peripheral side effects, such as urinary retention and blurred vision. Pilocarpine (Salagen) 5 mg four times per day, Cevimeline (Evoxac) 30 mg three times per day, and synthetic saliva (Glandosane, Salagen, Salivart, Salix) have been found effective in the treatment of dry mouth.

Other pharmacologic therapies

Many patients with dystonia require a combination of several medications and treatments (Jankovic, 2004b, 2006). High-dosage oral baclofen appears to be the next most effective agent for dystonia, particularly in combination with high-dosage anticholinergic treatment. Baclofen is a GABA$_b$ autoreceptor agonist that is used to treat spasticity. It has been found to produce substantial and sustained improvement in 29% of children at a mean dose of 92 mg/day (range: 40–180 mg/day) (Greene, 1992; Greene and Fahn, 1992a). Although baclofen was initially effective in 28 of 60 (47%) of adults with cranial dystonia, only 18% continued baclofen at a mean dose of 105 mg/day after a mean of 30.6 months (Fahn et al., 1985a).

Benzodiazepines (diazepam, lorazepam, or clonazepam) may provide additional benefit for patients whose response to anticholinergic drugs is unsatisfactory. Clonazepam might be particularly useful in patients with myoclonic dystonia. Muscle relaxants that are useful in the treatment of dystonia include cyclobenzaprine (Flexeril, 30–40 mg/day), metaxalone (Skelaxin, 800 mg two to three times per day), carisoprodol (Soma), methocarbamol (Robaxin oral and patch), orphenadrine (Norflex), and chlorzoxazone (Parafonforte). Structurally and pharmacologically similar to amitriptyline, cyclobenzaprine has been found at doses of 30–40 mg/day to be superior to placebo but equal to diazepam. Sodium oxybate, a salt of gamma-hydroxybutyrate, has been also reported to be effective in the myoclonus–dystonia syndrome, similar to alcohol (Frucht et al., 2005).

Narayan and colleagues (1991) first suggested that intrathecal baclofen (ITB) might be effective in the treatment of dystonia in 1991 in a report of an 18-year-old man with severe cervical and truncal dystonic spasms who was refractory to all forms of oral therapy and to large doses of paraspinal BTX injections. Muscle-paralyzing agents were necessary to relieve these spasms, which compromised his respiration. Within a few hours after the institution of ITB infusion, the patient's dystonia markedly improved, and he was able to be discharged from the intensive care unit within 1–2 days. The subsequent experience with intrathecal infusions has been quite encouraging, and studies are currently in progress to further evaluate this form of therapy in patients with dystonia and other motor disorders (Penn et al., 1995; Dressler et al., 1997; van Hilten et al., 1999). In some patients who were treated with intrathecal baclofen for spasticity, the benefits persisted even after the infusion was stopped (Dressnandt and Conrad, 1996). Ford and colleagues (1996) reviewed the experience with ITB in 25 patients and concluded that this form of therapy may be "more effective when dystonia is associated with spasticity or pain." ITB could have a role in selected patients with dystonic storm (Dalvi et al., 1998) and in secondary dystonias associated with pain and spasticity (Ford et al., 1998a). For example, Albright and colleagues (1998) found improvement in dystonia scores in 10 of 12 patients with cerebral palsy using an average daily dose of ITB of 575 µg; the improvement was sustained in 6 patients. In a subsequent study involving 86 patients aged 3–42 years (mean: 13 years) with generalized dystonia (secondary to cerebral palsy in 71% of patients), external infusion or bolus-dose screening was positive in approximately 90% of patients (Albright et al., 2001). Programmable pumps were implanted in 77 patients. Infusion began at 200 μg/day and increased by 10–20% per day until the best dose was achieved. The median duration of ITB therapy was 26 months. The mean dose increased over time, from 395 μg at 3 months to 610 μg at 24 months to 960 μg at 36 months. Patients and care-givers rated quality of life and ease of care as having improved in approximately 85% of patients. Seven patients, including four with cerebral palsy, lost their response to ITB during the study, usually during the first year. The most common side effects were increased constipation (19%), decreased neck and trunk control, and drowsiness. Surgical and device complications occurred in 38% of patients, including infections and catheter breakage and disconnection. Complication rates decreased over time. The authors conclude, "In our opinion, ITB is the treatment of choice for severe, generalized secondary dystonia after oral medications have been shown to be ineffective." One potentially serious complication of ITB is life-threatening intermittent catheter leakage, which might not be detectable by standard noninvasive methods (Bardutzky et al., 2003).

In a long-term (6 years) follow-up of ITB in 14 patients, 5 patients were found to have improvement in their rating scale scores, although only 2 patients had sustained "clear clinical benefit" (Walker et al., 2000). Hou and colleagues (2001) provided a follow-up on long-term effects of ITB in 10 patients (2 males and 8 females; mean age: 43.2 years; range: 21–66 years) with severe segmental or generalized dystonia who responded unsatisfactorily to oral medications and BTX injections. Three patients had peripherally induced dystonia, all with reflex sympathetic dystrophy, two were idiopathic (one with reflex sympathetic dystrophy), two suffered brain injury, two had static encephalopathy, and one had an unknown neurodegenerative disorder. Anatomically, three patients suffered segmental dystonia involving the neck, arms, or abdominal muscles. Seven others had generalized dystonia. The average duration of dystonia prior to implantation was 11 years (range: 1.7–35 years). All patients received test doses of bolus ITB before implantations. Two had relatively poor initial response to the test dose, but still received implantations for continuous infusion. Neurologic assessments were conducted immediately after the implantations, 1 month later, and every 3 months thereafter. The average duration of follow-up was 4.7 years (range: 0.7–11.1 years). Only one patient abandoned the pump after 22 months. Initially, five improved markedly, two improved moderately, two improved mildly, and one had no improvement. Both patients who failed to respond to the initial test of ITB improved on continuous infusion with pump. In four patients, the improvement lessened over time, although the patients were still better than they had been preoperatively. All 10 patients needed to continue oral medications, and 8 continued BTX injections at similar doses. Hou and colleagues (2001) concluded that patients with secondary (spastic) dystonia involving primarily legs and trunk appeared to be the best candidates for continuous ITB infusion. Continuous ITB has been found to be safe and effective in other series of patients with reflex sympathetic dystrophy and dystonia (van Hilten et al., 2000). It is not yet clear whether ITB can induce lasting remissions in patients with dystonia. The American Academy for Cerebral Palsy and Developmental Medicine has published a systematic review of the use of ITB for spastic and dystonic cerebral palsy (Butler et al., 2000). The limited published data show that ITB reduced spasticity and dystonia, particularly in the lower extremities.

There are other medications that are used in the treatment of dystonia. For example, slow-release morphine sulfate has been shown to improve not only pain but also dystonic movement in some patients with primary and tardive dystonia (Berg et al., 2001). Besides clonazepam, gamma-hydroxybutyrate, used in the treatment of alcohol abuse, has been found to be beneficial in the treatment of myoclonus–dystonia syndrome (Priori et al., 2000). It is not known whether acamprosate, another drug that is used in the treatment of alcohol abuse, is useful in the treatment of myoclonus–dystonia. Anticonvulsants, such as levetiracetam (Keppra) and zonisamide (Zonegran), have been reported to be effective in the treatment of cortical myoclonus, but it is not clear whether these drugs play a role in the treatment of dystonia. An open-label trial in 10 patients with segmental and generalized dystonia showed no evidence of efficacy (Hering et al., 2007).

Peripheral deafferentiation with anesthetic was previously reported to improve tremor (Pozos and Iaizo, 1992), but this approach might also be useful in the treatment of focal dystonia, such as writer's cramp (Kaji et al., 1995a) or oromandibular dystonia (Yoshida et al., 1998) that is unresponsive to other pharmacologic therapy. An injection of 5–10 mL of 0.5% lidocaine into the target muscle improved focal dystonia for up to 24 hours. This short effect can be extended for up to several weeks if ethanol is injected simultaneously. The observation that blocking muscle spindle afferents reduces dystonia suggests that somatosensory input is important in the pathogenesis of dystonia (Hallett, 1995; Kaji et al., 1995b). Mexiletine, an oral derivative of lidocaine, has been found to be effective in the treatment of cervical dystonia at doses ranging from 450 to 1200 mg/day (Ohara et al., 1998). Two-thirds of the patients, however, experienced adverse effects, including heartburn, drowsiness, ataxia, and tremor. On the basis of a review and a rating of videotapes by a "blind" rater, Lucetti and colleagues (2000) reported a significant improvement in six patients with cervical dystonia who had been treated with mexiletine.

Local electromyograph (EMG)-guided injection of phenol is currently being investigated as a potential treatment of cervical dystonia, but the results have not been very encouraging because of pain associated with the procedure and unpredictable response (Ruiz and Bernardos, 2000; Massey, 2002). Chemomyectomy with muscle-necrotizing drugs, such as doxorubicin, has been tried in some patients with blepharospasm and hemifacial spasm (Wirtschafter, 1991), but because of severe local irritation, it is doubtful that this approach will be adopted into clinical practice.

Attacks of kinesigenic paroxysmal dystonia may be controlled with anticonvulsants (e.g., carbamazepine, phenytoin) (Table 13.2). The nonkinesigenic forms of paroxysmal dystonia are less responsive to pharmacologic therapy, although clonazepam and acetazolamide may be beneficial. Treatment of paroxysmal dyskinesias is covered in Chapter 22 and in other reviews (Fahn, 1994; Demirkiran and Jankovic, 1995). Table 13.3 lists the common medications and procedures utilized for dystonia.

Table 13.2 Treatment of paroxysmal dyskinesias

PKD	PNKD	PED	PHD	Episodic ataxia
16p11.2–q12.1 (ICCA) X-chromosome (*MCT8*) Anticonvulsants	2q33–q35 (myofibrillio genesis regulator 1, *MR-1*) 10q22 (a-subunit of a Ca-sensitive K channel, *KCNMA1*) Clonazepam	16p12–q12 (ICCA) 1p35–p31 BBB glucose transporter type 1 (*SLC2A1*) Anticonvulsants, levodopa, botulinum toxin	20q13.2–q13.3 (nicotinic receptor alpha 4 subunit, *CHRNA4*) Tetrabenazine	EA-1: 12p13 (K channel *KCNA1*) EA-2: 19p13 (Ca channel *CACNL1A4*)

PKD, Paroxysmal kinesigenic dyskinesia; PNKD, paroxysmal nonkinesigenic dyskinesia; PED, paroxysmal exertional dyskinesia; PHD, paroxysmal hypnogenic dyskinesia; ICCA, infantile convulsions with paroxysmal dyskinesias.
Updated from Demirkiran M, Jankovic J: Paroxysmal dyskinesias: Clinical features and classification. Ann Neurol 1995;38:571–579.

Table 13.3 Treatment of dystonia

Focal dystonias

Blepharospasm

Clonazepam, lorazepam

Botulinum toxin injections

Orbicularis oculi myectomy

Oromandibular dystonia

Baclofen

Trihexyphenidyl

Botulinum toxin injections

Spasmodic dysphonia

Botulinum toxin injections

Voice and supportive therapy

Cervical dystonia

Trihexyphenidyl

Diazepam, lorazepam, clonazepam

Botulinum toxin injections

Tetrabenazine

Cyclobenzaprine

Baclofen (oral)

Peripheral surgical denervation

Task-specific dystonias (e.g., writer's cramp)

Trihexyphenidyl

Botulinum toxin injections

Occupational therapy

Segmental and generalized dystonias

Levodopa (in children to young adults)

Trihexyphenidyl

Diazepam, lorazepam, clonazepam

Baclofen (oral, intrathecal)

Carbamazepine

Tetrabenazine

Intrathecal baclofen (ITB) infusion (axial dystonia)

Deep brain stimulation of GPi (in distal dystonia or hemidystonia)

acupuncture (56%), relaxation techniques (44%), homeopathy (27%), and massages (26%) (Junker et al., 2004).

The involuntary muscle contraction can lead to "status dystonicus" or "dystonic storm" resulting in breakdown of the muscle and a life-threatening myoglobinuria (Opal et al., 2002; Mariotti et al., 2007). In a review of 37 cases of status dystonicus or dystonic storm, the following treatment approach has been used with some success: early admission to the intensive care unit, monitor for evidence of myoglobinuria, avoid respiratory and renal compromise, sedation with intravenous midazolam (initially up to 10 µg/kg/min and subsequently at 30–100 µg/kg/hour), possible barbiturate anesthesia combined with endotracheal intubation and mechanical ventilation, continuous intrathecal baclofen, bilateral pallidotomy, or globus pallidus interna (GPi) deep brain stimulation (DBS) (Mariotti et al., 2007; Jech et al., 2009). Although administration of propofol has been also suggested, we would caution against it as this drug has been demonstrated to cause or exacerbate levodopa-related dyskinesia (Krauss et al., 1996).

Botulinum toxin

The introduction of BTX into clinical practice in the late 1980s revolutionized treatment of dystonia. The most potent biologic toxin, BTX has become a powerful therapeutic tool in the treatment of a variety of neurologic, ophthalmic, and other disorders that are manifested by abnormal, excessive, or inappropriate muscle contractions (Jankovic and Brin, 1991; Jankovic and Hallett, 1994; Brin et al., 2002; Thant and Tan, 2003; Jankovic, 2004a). In December 1989, after extensive laboratory and clinical testing, the Food and Drug Administration approved this biologic (BTX-A or Botox) as a therapeutic agent in patients with strabismus, blepharospasm, and other facial nerve disorders, including hemifacial spasm. In December 2000, the Food and Drug Administration approved Botox and BTX-B (Myobloc) as treatments for cervical dystonia. Although its widest application is still in the treatment of disorders manifested by abnormal, excessive, or inappropriate muscle contractions, the use of BTX is rapidly expanding to include treatment of a variety of ophthalmologic, gastrointestinal, urologic, orthopedic, dermatologic, secretory, painful, and cosmetic disorders (Tintner and Jankovic, 2001b; Jankovic and Brin, 2002; Thant and Tan, 2003; Jankovic, 2004a) (Fig. 13.1; Tables 13.4 and 13.5).

In addition to conventional forms of therapy described previously, many patients with dystonia seek complementary or alternative forms of therapy. In one survey of 180 members of the German Dystonia Group, 131 (73%) patients used some form of alternative treatments, such as

BOTULINUM TOXIN TARGETS AT THE NERVE TERMINAL

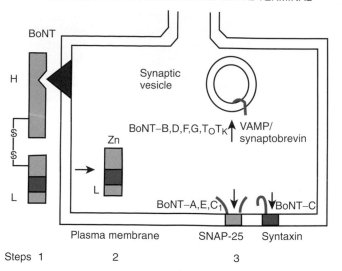

Figure 13.1 Mechanism of action of botulinum toxin. *Redrawn from Jankovic J. Botulinum toxin in clinical practice. J Neurol Neurosurg Psychiatry 2004;75:951–957.*

Few therapeutic agents have been better understood in terms of their mechanism of action before their clinical application or have had greater impact on patients' functioning than BTX. The therapeutic value of BTX is due to its ability to cause chemodenervation and to produce local paralysis when injected into a muscle. There are seven immunologically distinct toxins that share structurally homologous subunits. Synthesized as single-chain polypeptides (molecular weight of 150 kDa), these toxin molecules have relatively little potency until they are cleaved by trypsin or bacterial enzymes into a heavy chain (100 kDa) and a light chain (50 kDa). The 150 kDa protein, the active portion of the molecule, complexes with one or more nontoxin proteins that support its structure and protect it from degradation. Type A is the only serotype that forms the 900 kDa complex. Types A, B, C1, and hemagglutinin-positive D form the 500 kDa complex and 300 kDa complex; types E, F, and hemagglutinin-negative D form only the 300 kDa complex (Melling et al., 1998). The three-dimensional structure of the BTX complex is known (Hanson and Stevens, 2002). When linked by a disulfide bond, these dichains exert their paralytic action by preventing the release of acetylcholine. BTX therefore does not affect the synthesis or storage of acetylcholine, but it interferes with the release of acetylcholine from the presynaptic terminal. This is a three-step process that involves binding to the acceptors on presynaptic membrane (heavy chain), internalization (endocytosis), and an enzymatic action (light chain). BTX serotypes bind to different acceptors, which contain both protein components and gangliosides with more than one neuraminic acid residue. BTX-A has been found to enter neurons by binding to the synaptic vesicle protein SV2 (isoform C) which acts as the BTX-A receptor (Dong et al., 2006; Mahrhold et al., 2006). The neural membrane proteins synaptotagmin I and II act as receptors for BTX-B and for BTX-G (Mahrhold et al., 2006). While the heavy chain of the toxin binds to the presynaptic cholinergic terminal, the light chain acts as a zinc-dependent protease that selectively cleaves proteins that are critical for fusion of the presynaptic vesicle with the

presynaptic membrane. Thus, the light chains of BTX-A and BTX-E cleave SNAP-25 (synaptosome-associated protein), a protein that is needed for synaptic vesicle targeting and fusion with the presynaptic membrane. The light chains of BTX-B, BTX-D, and BTX-F prevent the quantal release of acetylcholine by proteolytically cleaving synaptobrevin-2, also known as VAMP (vesicle-associated membrane protein), an integral protein of the synaptic vesicle membrane. BTX-C cleaves syntaxin, another plasma membrane-associated protein. A three-dimensional study showed that syntaxin 1a forms a complex with neuronal-Sec1, forming a recognition site for the arriving vesicle through a Rab protein, and the subsequent formation of the syntaxin–VAMP–SNAP-25 complex promotes membrane fusion (Misura et al., 2000) (Fig. 13.1).

BTX-A has been studied most intensely and used most widely, but the clinical applications of other types of toxins, including BTX-B and BTX-F, are also expanding (Greene and Fahn, 1992b; Mezaki et al., 1995; Sheean and Lees, 1995; Figgit and Noble, 2002; Jankovic, 2004a). BTX-A is harvested from a culture medium after fermentation of a high-toxin-producing strain of *Clostridium botulinum* that lyses and liberates the toxin into the culture (Schantz and Johnson, 1992). The toxin is then extracted, precipitated, purified, and finally

Table 13.4 Clinical applications of botulinum toxin

Focal dystonia
Blepharospasm
Lid apraxia
Oromandibular-facial-lingual dystonia
Cervical dystonia (torticollis)
Laryngeal dystonia (spasmodic dysphonia)
Task-specific dystonia (occupational cramps)
Other focal dystonias (idiopathic, secondary)

Other involuntary movements
Voice, head, and limb tremor
Palatal myoclonus
Hemifacial spasm tics

Inappropriate contractions
Strabismus
Nystagmus
Myokymia
Bruxism
Stuttering
Painful rigidity
Muscle contraction headaches
Lumbosacral strain and back spasms
Radiculopathy with secondary muscle spasm
Spasticity
Spastic bladder
Achalasia (esophageal, pelvirectal)
Other spasmic disorders

Other potential applications
Protective ptosis
Cosmetic (wrinkles, facial asymmetry)
Debarking dogs
Other

Table 13.5 Properties of different types of botulinum toxin tested in clinical trials

	Botox (botulinum toxin type A)	Dysport (abobotulinumtoxinA)	Xeomin (botulinum toxin type A)	Prosigne (botulinum toxin type A)	Neuronox (botulinum toxin type A)	Mybloc/ NeuroBloc (botulinum toxin type B)
Manufacturer	Allergan, Inc., Irvine, CA, USA	Ipsen Ltd, Slough, Berks, UK	Merz Pharmaceuticals, Frankfurt am Main, Germany	Lanzhou Institute of Biological Products, Lanzhou, China	CJ Corp/ Medy-Tox, Inc., Seoul, South Korea	Elan Plc, Dublin, Ireland
BTX serotype	A	A	A	A	A	B
Strain	Hall A	Ipsen strain	Hall A	?	?	Bean B
Site of SNARE hydrolysis	SNAP-25	SNAP-25	SNAP-25	SNAP-25	SNAP-25	VAMP
Reconstituted pH	7.4	7.4	7.4	6.0	6.8	5.6
Other constituents (per vial)	HSA 500 µg NaCl 900 µg	HSA 125 µg Lactose 2500 µg	HSA 1 mg Sucrose 5 mg	Gelatin 5 mg Dextran 25 mg Sucrose 25 mg	HS 500 µg NaCl 900 µg	?
Product-specific units/vial	100	500	100	100	100	$2.5/5.0/10.0 \times 10^9$
Protein weight/ vial (mg)	4.5	4.3	0.6			50 (5000 U vial)

crystallized with ammonium sulfate. The crystalline toxin is diluted from milligram to nanogram concentrations, freeze-dried, and dispensed as a white powder in small vials containing 100 mouse units (U) of the toxin. When isolated from bacterial cultures, BTX is noncovalently associated with nontoxic macromolecules, such as hemagglutinin. These nontoxic proteins enhance toxicity by protecting the neurotoxin from proteolytic enzymes in the gut, but they apparently have no effect on the potency of the toxin if injected parenterally. Although the efficacy and duration of benefits of BTX-B or Mybloc, formerly NeuroBloc (Elan), are thought to be generally comparable to those of BTX-A (Botox and Dysport), no head-to-head comparisons between the various products have been performed. An in-vivo study using injections into the extensor digitorum brevis in healthy volunteers suggested that the muscle paralysis from BTX-B was not as complete or long-lasting as that from BTX-A (Sloop et al., 1997). Whether M-wave amplitude is a reliable measure of clinical response and whether the doses of BTX-A (7.5–10 U) and BTX-B (320–480 U), with a B/A ratio of about 45:1, are comparable are debatable. The apparently longer duration of action of BTX-A compared to that of BTX-B could possibly be explained by the observation that VAMP that is cleaved by BTX-B cannot form stable SNARE (soluble N-ethlymaleimide sensitive factor attachment protein receptor or SNAP receptor or neuronal synaptosome-associated proteins) complex and it turns over to form new VAMP, whereas SNAP-25, the substrate for BTX-A, forms a truncated SNAP-25$_A$, which prevents degradation of SNARE, as a result of which the inhibition of exocytosis persists for 40–60 days. This correlates well with the reappearance of the original terminals (de Paiva et al., 1999). De Paiva and colleagues (1999) noted that a single intramuscular injection of BTX-A

into the sternomastoid muscles of mice caused the formation of functional neuronal sprouts that connected with the muscle fiber. The primary BTX-A-intoxicated nerve terminal was incapable of neurotransmitter exocytosis; it produced new sprouts that were capable of exocytosis with subsequent upregulation of adjacent nicotinic receptors on the muscle fiber, thus forming a functional synapse. After a certain period of time, such as 3 months, consistent with return of clinical function of the muscle and wearing-off response from the previous injection, the original BTX-A-intoxicated terminal resumed exocytosis, and the sprouts regressed to return the neuromuscular junction to its original state. Other studies have also shown that the prolonged duration of action of BTX-A is due to persistence of catalytically active enzyme in the muscle cell (Adler et al., 2001). A physiologic study in monkeys showed that BTX-B diffuses less extensively than BTX-A into adjacent and remote muscles (Arezzo et al., 2002). In contrast to Botox, Mybloc is a solution that does not require reconstitution, and it may be stored in a refrigerator rather than a freezer. The commercial preparations are complex proteins that must be dissociated from the active neurotoxin molecule to exert the paralytic effect. This dissociation, which is pH dependent, unmasks the binding site on the heavy chain.

In addition to Botox, Mybloc, and Dysport (Truong et al., 2005), a new formulation of BTX-A, NT 201, has been recently introduced (Benecke et al., 2005). This formulation of BTX-A, which is free of complexing proteins, has been reported to be equivalent, in terms of efficacy and safety, to Botox in healthy volunteers and in patients with blepharospasm (Roggenkamper et al., 2006; Jankovic, 2009b) and cervical dystonia (Benecke et al., 2005). While low antigenicity has been predicted with this new formulation of BTX, no

Table 13.6 Risk factors for development of blocking antibodies (immunoresistance)

- The dose (protein load) per treatment session
- The total cumulative dose
- Antigenicity of the botulinum toxin drug
- Frequency of exposure (inter-dose interval)
  - Booster injections
- Prior history of immunoresistance
  - Cross-reactivity
- Individual (genetic) characteristics
  - Possible: female gender, younger age

Table 13.7 Long-term effects of repeat botulinum toxin injections in cervical dystonia

- 326 were enrolled (mean age 50.1 years; 69.9% female) and 77% (251/326) completed the study
- Mean dose per session: 148.4–213.0 U
- Median 9 treatments over a mean of 2.5 years (3.2 months to 4.2 years)
- Adverse events: weakness, dysphagia, neck pain, and injection pain
- Only 4/326 subjects (1.2%) had at least one positive antibody assay result
- Conclusions: BTX-A treatment is safe and effective for the chronic treatment of cervical dystonia. The current formulation of BTX-A rarely causes neutralizing antibodies in cervical dystonia subjects treated for up to 4 years

From: Brin MF, Comella CL, Jankovic J, Lai F, Naumann M; CD-017 BoNTA Study Group. Long-term treatment with botulinum toxin type A in cervical dystonia has low immunogenicity by mouse protection assay. Mov Disord 2008;23:1353–1360.

long-term data exist, and in view of the low frequency of blocking antibodies reported with the new formulation of Botox (see later) (Jankovic et al., 2003; Brin et al., 2008; Naumann et al., 2010) (Tables 13.6 and 13.7), it is not clear what role the new NT 201 BTX will play in the future treatment of dystonia. Patients resistant to BTX-A often initially respond to BTX-B, but a recent study showed that continued treatment with Myobloc is associated with high incidence of blocking antibodies (Jankovic et al., 2006).

The primary effect of BTX is to induce paralysis of injected skeletal muscles, especially the most actively contracting muscles. BTX paralyzes not only the extrafusal fibers but also the intrafusal fibers, thus decreasing the activity of Ib muscle afferents (Filippi et al., 1993). This might explain the effect of BTX on reciprocal inhibition. In untreated patients with dystonia, the second phase of reciprocal inhibition is usually decreased. BTX "corrects" the abnormal reciprocal inhibition by increasing the second phase, possibly through its effect on the muscle afferents (Priori et al., 1995). While the effect on intrafusal fibers might contribute in part to the beneficial action of BTX in patients with dystonia, this is not its main action because BTX is effective in facial dystonia, even though the facial muscles do not have spindles.

Measuring variations in fiber diameter and using acetylcholine-esterase staining as indexes of denervation,

Borodic and colleagues (1994) showed that BTX diffuses up to 4.5 cm from the site of a single injection (10 U injected in the rabbit longissimus dorsi). Since the size of the denervation field is determined largely by the dose (and volume), multiple injections along the affected muscle rather than a single injection should therefore contain the biologic effects of the toxin in the targeted muscle (Borodic et al., 1992). Blackie and Lees (1990) also showed that frequency of dysphagia could be reduced by 50% when multiple rather than single injections are used.

A small percentage of patients receiving repeated injections develop antibodies against BTX, causing them to be completely resistant to the effects of subsequent BTX injections (Greene et al., 1994; Jankovic and Schwartz, 1995; Jankovic, 2002) (Tables 13.6 and 13.7). In one study, 24 of 559 (4.3%) patients treated for cervical dystonia developed BTX antibodies (Greene et al., 1994). The authors suggested that the true prevalence of antibodies might be more than 7%. In addition to patients with BTX antibodies, they studied 8 patients from a cohort of 76 (10.5%) who stopped responding to BTX treatments. These BTX-resistant patients had a shorter interval between injections, more booster injections, and a higher dose at the non-booster injection compared to nonresistant patients treated during the same period. As a result of this experience, clinicians are warned against using booster injections and are encouraged to extend the interval between treatments as long as possible, certainly at least 1 month, and to use the smallest possible dose. In addition to high dosages, young age is a potential risk factor for the development of immunoresistance to BTX-A (Jankovic and Schwartz, 1995; Hanna and Jankovic, 1998; Hanna et al., 1999). Some of the patients who developed BTX-A antibodies have benefited from injections by immunologically distinct preparations, such as BTX-F and BTX-B (Greene and Fahn, 1992b; Mezaki et al., 1994). After 1–3 years, some patients become antibody negative, and when reinjected with the same type of toxin, they may again experience transient benefit (Sankhla et al., 1998). The original preparation of Botox contained 25 ng of neurotoxin complex protein per 100 units, but in 1997, the Food and Drug Administration approved a new preparation that contains only 5 ng per 100 units, which should have lower antigenicity (Aoki et al., 1999). In fact, in a 3-year follow-up of patients treated with the current Botox, no evidence of blocking antibodies was found, compared to a 9.4% frequency of blocking antibodies in patients treated with the original Botox for the same period of time (Jankovic et al., 2003). The low antigenicity of the current Botox is also supported by the findings from a longitudinal, multicenter study in which de novo subjects were treated with Botox and only 4/326 (1.2%) subjects tested positive for antibodies by the mouse protective assay during the course of up to 15 cycles of treatment (Brin et al., 2008) (Table 13.7).

The preliminary data suggest that BTX-B provides clinical effects similar to those of BTX-A, but the duration of benefits is shorter (Comella et al., 2005) and Myobloc appears to have greater antigenicity than Botox, particularly in patients with prior resistance to BTX-A (Jankovic et al., 2007). To compare autonomic effects of BTX, Tintner and colleagues (2005) randomized patients with cervical dystonia to receive either BTX-A or BTX-B in a double-blind manner. Efficacy and physiologic questionnaire measures of autonomic function were assessed at baseline and 2 weeks after injection. Patients who were treated with BTX-B had significantly less saliva production ($P < 0.01$) and greater severity of constipation ($P = 0.037$) than those treated with BTX-A but did not differ with respect to other tests of autonomic function, including changes in blood pressure, heart rate, and ocular function. The autonomic effects of BTX-B were reviewed in several additional reports (Wan et al., 2005).

Many clinical studies have provided evidence not only that BTX is safe and effective, but also that this therapy leads to meaningful improvements in quality of life (Naumann and Jankovic, 2004; Jankovic et al., 2004), and the benefits are long-lasting (Mejia et al., 2005) (Video 13.1). Despite its proven therapeutic value, there are still many unresolved issues and concerns about BTX. These include lack of standardization of biologic activity of the different preparations of BTX, poor understanding of toxin antigenicity, variations in the methods of injection, and inadequate assays for BTX antibodies (Brin et al., 2008). Training guidelines for the use of botulinum toxin have been established (American Academy of Neurology, 1994). Clinicians who are interested in utilizing BTX chemodenervation in their practice must be aware of these concerns and must exercise proper precautions to minimize the potential risks associated with BTX. Most important, they should become thoroughly familiar with the movement disorders that they intend to treat and with the anatomy at the injection site. Possible contraindications to the use of BTX include the presence of myasthenia gravis (Emerson, 1994), Eaton–Lambert syndrome, motor neuron disease, aminoglycoside antibiotics, and pregnancy. Besides occasional complications, usually related to local weakness, a major limitation of BTX therapy is its high cost. Several studies analyzing the cost-effectiveness of BTX treatment, however, have demonstrated that the loss of productivity as a result of untreated dystonia and the cost of medications or surgery more than justify the financial expense of BTX treatments. It is likely that future research will result in the development of new, more effective neuromuscular blocking agents that provide therapeutic chemodenervation with long-term benefits and at lower cost.

Blepharospasm

The effectiveness of BTX in blepharospasm was first demonstrated in double-blind, placebo-controlled trials (Fahn et al., 1985b; Jankovic and Orman, 1987). In a subsequent report of experience with BTX in 477 patients with various dystonias and hemifacial spasm, Jankovic and colleagues (1990) reviewed the results in 90 patients who had been injected with BTX for blepharospasm. Moderate or marked improvement was noted in 94% of the patients. The average latency from the time of the injection to the onset of improvement was 4.2 days; the average duration of maximum benefit was 12.4 weeks, but the total benefit lasted considerably longer: an average of 15.7 weeks. While 41% of all treatment sessions were followed by some side effects (ptosis, blurring of vision or diplopia, tearing, and local hematoma), only 2% of these affected patient's functioning. Complications usually improved spontaneously in less than 2 weeks. These results are consistent with those of other studies (Elston,

1994). There is no apparent decline in benefit, and the frequency of complications actually decreases after repeat BTX treatments (Jankovic and Schwartz, 1993a).

The efficacy and safety of another type of BTX-A, NT-201 (or Xeomin), in the treatment of blepharospasm was also confirmed by a prospective, double-blind, placebo-controlled, randomized, multicenter study involving 109 patients (mean total dose of Xeomin per treatment visit was 64.8 U), in which the Jankovic Rating Scale severity subscore was significant reduced compared to placebo ($P < 0.001$). The most commonly reported adverse effects related to Xeomin versus placebo were eyelid ptosis (18.9 vs. 8.8%), dry eye (16.2 vs.11.8%), and dry mouth (16.2 vs. 2.9%) (Jankovic, 2009b; Jankovic et al., 2011). In a multicenter, clinical, fixed-dose, trial Dysport (40, 80, and 120 units/eye) or placebo (in a 3:1 randomization ratio) were administered to 119 patients with blepharospasm, 85 of whom completed the 16-week follow-up; several parameters showed robust improvement in Dysport arms compared to placebo (Truong et al., 2008).

In addition to the four different BTX-A preparations available on the market in one or more countries, Botox (Allergan Inc., Irvine, CA, USA), Dysport (Ipsen Ltd, Slough, UK), Xeomin (Merz Pharmaceuticals, Frankfurt am Main, Germany) (Albanese, 2011), and Prosigne (Lanzhou Biological Products, China), Meditoxin (Medy-Tox, Seoul, Korea; also known as Neuronox) was introduced for the treatment of blepharospasm and is currently available in Korea (Yoon et al., 2009). All these types were evaluated in blepharospasm and were found to be comparable with respect to clinical efficacy and adverse effects.

Reasons for the gradual enhancement in efficacy and reduction in the frequency of complications with repeat treatments include greater experience and improvements in the injection technique. For example, one controlled study showed that an injection into the pretarsal rather than preseptal portion of the orbicularis oculi is associated with significantly lower frequency of ptosis (Jankovic, 1996). Ptosis can be prevented also by injecting initially only the lateral and medial portions of the upper lid, thus avoiding the midline levator muscle. We usually initially inject 5 U in each site in the upper lid and 5 U in the lower lid laterally only. This finding has been confirmed by others (Cakmur et al., 2002).

The functional improvement, experienced by the vast majority of patients after BTX injection, is difficult to express numerically. Many patients could not work, drive, watch television, or read prior to the injections. As a result of reduced eyelid and eyebrow spasms, most can now function normally. In addition to the observed functional improvement, there is usually a meaningful amelioration of discomfort, and because of less embarrassment, the patients' self-esteem also frequently improves. BTX injections are now considered by many to be the treatment of choice for blepharospasm (American Academy of Ophthalmology, 1989; American Academy of Neurology, 1990). In addition to idiopathic blepharospasm, BTX injections have been used effectively in the treatment of blepharospasm induced by drugs (e.g., levodopa in parkinsonian patients or neuroleptics in patients with tardive dystonia), dystonic eyelid and facial tics in patients with Tourette syndrome, and blepharospasm associated with apraxia of eyelid opening (Jankovic, 1994;

Aramideh et al., 1995; Lepore et al., 1995; Jankovic, 1995a, 1996; Forget et al., 2002).

Oromandibular dystonia

Oromandibular dystonia is among the most challenging forms of focal dystonia to treat with BTX (Blitzer et al., 1989; Charous et al., 2011); it rarely improves with medications, there are no surgical treatments, and BTX therapy can be complicated by swallowing problems. The masseter muscles are usually injected in patients with jaw-closure dystonia; in patients with jaw-opening dystonia, either the submental muscle complex or the lateral pterygoid muscles are injected. In a total of 91 patients treated in 271 visits, the overall improvement was rated as 2.6 (0 = no response to 4 = marked improvement in spasms and function) (Jankovic and Schwartz, 1991b). A meaningful reduction in the oromandibular-lingual spasms and an improvement in chewing and speech were achieved in more than 70% of patients. The improvement was noted within an average of 5.5 days after injection and lasted an average of 11.5 weeks. Patients with dystonic jaw closure responded better than those with jaw-opening dystonia. A temporary swallowing problem, noted in fewer than one-third of patients and in only 17% of all treatment sessions, was the most frequent complication. Early treatment with BTX may prevent dental and other oral complications, including temporomandibular joint syndrome (Blitzer and Brin, 1991; Charous et al., 2011). BTX can provide lasting improvement not only in patients with primary (idiopathic) dystonia but also in orolingual-mandibular tardive dystonia. Clenching and bruxism are frequent manifestations of oromandibular dystonia, although nocturnal and diurnal bruxism can occur even without evident dystonia (Tan and Jankovic, 1999, 2000). Oromandibular involuntary movements caused by hemimasticatory spasms and other disorders such as Satoyoshi syndrome have been also successfully treated with BTX (Merello et al., 1994; Yaltho and Jankovic, 2011).

Laryngeal dystonia (spasmodic dysphonia)

Until the introduction of BTX, the therapy of spasmodic dysphonia was disappointing. The anticholinergic and benzodiazepine drugs only rarely provide meaningful improvement in voice quality. Unilateral transection of the recurrent laryngeal nerve, although effective in most patients, frequently causes unacceptable complications, and the voice symptoms often recur (Dedo and Izdebski, 1983). A surgical procedure that involves denervation of the adductor branch of the recurrent laryngeal nerve with reinnervation of the distal sumps with branches of the ansa cervicalis nerve was reported to produce marked improvement in patients with adductor spasmodic dysphonia (Berke et al., 1999), but further studies are needed to confirm this initial observation.

Several studies have established the efficacy and safety of BTX in the treatment of laryngeal dystonia, and this approach is considered by most to be the treatment of choice for spasmodic dysphonia (Brin et al., 1987; Blitzer et al., 1988; Jankovic et al., 1990; Brin et al., 1992; Ludlow, 1990; Brin et al., 1998; Blitzer et al., 2002). Before a patient can be considered a potential candidate for BTX injections, the diagnosis of spasmodic dysphonia must be confirmed by detailed neurologic, otolaryngologic, and voice assessment and documented by video and voice recordings.

Three approaches are currently used in the BTX treatment of spasmodic dysphonia: (1) unilateral EMG-guided injection of 5–30 U (Jankovic et al., 1990), (2) bilateral approach, injecting with EMG guidance 1.25–4 U in each vocal fold (Brin et al., 1992), and (3) an injection via indirect laryngoscopy without EMG (Ford et al., 1990). Irrespective of the technique, most investigators report about 75–95% improvement in voice symptoms. One controlled study, however, concluded that unilateral injections "may provide both superior and longer lasting benefits" than bilateral injections (Adams et al., 1993). The dosage can be adjusted depending on the severity of glottal spasms and the response to previous injections. Adverse experiences include transient breathy hypophonia, hoarseness, and rare dysphagia with aspiration.

Although more complicated and less effective, BTX injections into the posterior cricoarytenoid muscle with the EMG needle placed posterior to the thyroid lamina may be used in the treatment of the abductor form of spasmodic dysphonia (Brin et al., 1989, 1992). Using a multidisciplinary team approach, consisting of an otolaryngologist who is experienced in laryngeal injections and a neurologist who is knowledgeable about motor disorders of speech and voice, BTX injections can provide effective relief for most patients with spasmodic dysphonia (American Academy of Neurology, 1990; American Academy of Otolaryngology, 1990). Outcome assessments clearly show that BTX injections for spasmodic dysphonia produce measurable improvements in the quality of life of patients with this disorder (Courey et al., 2000). BTX may be useful in the treatment of voice tremor and stuttering, but the results are less predictable (Ludlow, 1990; Brin et al., 1994; Warrick et al., 2000).

Cervical dystonia

The goal of therapy of cervical dystonia is not only to improve abnormal posture of the head and associated neck pain, but also to prevent the development of secondary complications such as contractures, cervical radiculopathy, and cervical myelopathy (Treves and Korczyn, 1986; Waterston et al., 1989).

With the use of TWSTRS and other scales, the efficacy and safety of BTX in the treatment of cervical dystonia have been demonstrated in several controlled and open trials (Greene et al., 1990; Jankovic and Schwartz, 1990; Poewe et al., 1992; Jankovic et al., 1994; Tintner and Jankovic, 2001a; Jankovic, 2002, 2004c; Truong et al., 2005; Brin et al., 2008) (Videos 13.2 and 13.3). In one double-blind, placebo-controlled study of 55 patients with cervical dystonia, 61% improved after BTX-A injection (Greene et al., 1990). BTX has been found to be superior not only to placebo but also to trihexyphenidyl (Brans et al., 1996). In a study of 66 consecutive patients with idiopathic cervical dystonia, Brans and colleagues (1996) compared the effectiveness of BTX-A (Dysport) with that of trihexyphenidyl in a prospective, randomized, double-blind design. Dysport or saline was injected under EMG guidance at study entry and again after 8 weeks. Patients were assessed for efficacy at baseline and after 12 weeks by different clinical rating scales. Sixty-four patients completed the study, 32 in each group. The mean dose of BTX-A was 292 U (first session) and 262 U (second session). The mean dose of trihexyphenidyl was 16.25 mg. TWSTRS (primary outcome) and other scales showed a significant improvement in favor of BTX-A, and adverse effects were significantly less frequent than in the group of patients randomized to trihexyphenidyl. In a multicenter, double-blind, randomized, controlled trial assessing the safety and efficacy of Dysport in cervical dystonia patients, 80 patients were randomly assigned to receive one treatment with Dysport (500 U) or placebo (Truong et al., 2005). Dysport was significantly more efficacious than placebo at weeks 4, 8, and 12 as assessed by TWSTRS (10 point vs. 3.8 point reduction in total score, respectively, at week 4; $P \leq 0.013$). Of participants in the Dysport group, 38% showed positive treatment response, compared to 16% in the placebo group (95% confidence interval 0.02–0.41). The median duration of response to Dysport was 18.5 weeks. Side effects were generally similar in the two treatment groups; only blurred vision and weakness occurred significantly more often with Dysport. No participants in the Dysport group converted from negative to positive antibodies after treatment. These results confirm previous reports that Dysport (500 U) is safe, effective, and well tolerated in patients with cervical dystonia. 🎥

Open-label studies generally report a more dramatic improvement, partly because of a placebo effect and, more important, because of greater flexibility in selecting the proper dosage and site of injection. Most trials report that about 90% of patients experience improvement in function and control of the head and neck and in pain. The average latency between injection and the onset of improvement (and muscle atrophy) is 1 week, and the average duration of maximum improvement is 3–4 months. On average, the injections are repeated every 4–6 months. Patients with long-duration dystonia have been found to respond less well than those who were treated relatively early, possibly because prolonged dystonia produced contractures (Jankovic and Schwartz, 1991b). In one study, 28% of patients experienced some complication, such as swallowing difficulties, neck weakness, and nausea, sometime during the course of their treatment (some patients had up to 12 visits in 5 years). Dysphagia, the most common complication, was encountered in 14% of all 659 visits, but in only five instances was this problem severe enough to require changing to a soft or liquid diet. Complications are usually related to focal weakness, although distant and systemic subclinical and clinical effects, such as generalized weakness and malaise, rarely occur, possibly as a result of blood distribution or retrograde axonal transport to the spinal motor neurons (Garner et al., 1993). Most complications resolve spontaneously, usually within 2 weeks. An injection into one or both sternocleidomastoid muscles was most frequently associated with dysphagia (Jankovic and Schwartz, 1991b; Comella et al., 1992b). One study showed that dosages as small as 20 units administered as a single injection into the sternocleidomastoid muscle completely eliminated muscle activity and could produce neck weakness and dysphagia (Buchman et al., 1994). In an analysis of patients who received five or more injections, the beneficial response was maintained and the frequency of complications with repeat injections actually declined, presumably as a result of improving skills

(Jankovic and Schwartz, 1993a). Lindeboom and colleagues (1998) found that neurologic impairment and pain usually improve following BTX injections, but only functional status measures differentiate between patients who improve and those who have an insufficient response. There have been only a few long-term studies of BTX treatment in cervical dystonia. Brashear and colleagues (2000) showed that two-thirds of patients who received BTX reported the injections always helped. Another long-term study showed that 75% of patients continued to benefit for at least 5 years and only 7.5% developed secondary unresponsiveness; only 1.3% discontinued BTX therapy because of intolerable side effects (Hsiung et al., 2002).

Results similar to those obtained with BTX-A have been obtained in patients treated for cervical dystonia with BTX-B (Tsui et al., 1995; Lew et al., 1997; Figgitt and Noble, 2002). In a double-blind, controlled trial of 122 patients with cervical dystonia treated with BTX-B, there was a dose response effect, particularly at doses of 10 000 units (Lew et al., 1997). Using TWSTRS, 77% of the patients were found to respond at week 4. Other studies have subsequently confirmed the efficacy of BTX-B (Brashear et al., 1999), even in patients who are resistant to BTX-A (Brin et al., 1999). In a 16-week, randomized, multicenter, double-blind, placebo-controlled trial of BTX-B, 109 patients, who previously responded well to BTX-A, were randomized into one of the treatment groups: placebo, 5000 U, and 10 000 U administered into two to four cervical muscles (Brashear et al., 1999). At week 4, the total TWSTRS score improved by 4.3, 9.3 ($P = 0.01$), and 11.7 ($P = 0.0004$), respectively, when compared to baseline, and this was accompanied by significant improvements in pain, disability, and severity. The estimated median time until the total TWSTRS score returned to baseline was 63, 114, and 111 days, respectively. The most frequent side effects associated with BTX-B included dysphagia and dry mouth. An identical design was used in another study of BTX-B in cervical dystonia with one exception: the patients were resistant to BTX-A as determined by the frontalis-type A test (F-TAT) (Brin et al., 1999). A total of 77 patients were randomized to receive placebo or 10 000 U of BTX-B. At week 4, the total TWSTRS scores improved by 2 (placebo) and 11 (10 000 U) ($P = 0.0001$). There was also significant improvement in secondary and tertiary outcome measures, including global assessments and pain visual analog scores, as well as other measures of pain, disability, and severity. The estimated duration of effect, based on a Kaplan–Meier survival analysis, was 112 days (12–16 weeks). Subsequent studies have suggested that dosages as high as 45 000 U of BTX-B (Myobloc) per session may be effective and safe in patients with cervical dystonia.

The most important determinants of a favorable response to BTX treatments are a proper selection of the involved muscles and an appropriate dosage (Table 13.8). EMG may be helpful in some patients with obese necks or in whom the involved muscles are difficult to identify by palpation (Dubinsky et al., 1991; Gelb et al., 1991). One study attempted to determine the usefulness of EMG-assisted BTX injections and found that the percentage of patients who showed any improvement after BTX was similar whether the injections were assisted by EMG or not (Comella et al., 1992a). Comella et al. (1992a) also noted that "a significantly greater magnitude of improvement" was present in patients treated with the EMG-assisted method and that

Table 13.8 Examination of patients with cervical dystonia

1. Find the most uncompensated position
   - The patient is instructed to allow the head to "draw" into the maximal abnormal posture without resisting the dystonic "pulling" (with eyes open and closed)
   - Examine while standing, walking, sitting, and writing
2. Passively move the head
   - To define the dystonic posture
   - To localize the contracting muscles
   - To determine the full range of motion
   - To determine whether there are contractures
3. Palpate contracting muscles
   - To localize the involved muscles
   - To estimate the muscle mass
   - To find points of tenderness
4. EMG (needed rarely)
   - To localize involved muscles that cannot be palpated
   - To guide the injection into the muscles that are difficult to access

there was "a significantly greater number of patients with marked benefit" in the group that was randomly assigned to the EMG-assisted method of treatment. Since the majority (70–79%) of patients had previously been treated with BTX, some might have been experiencing residual effects from previous injections, making the interpretation of the results difficult. Furthermore, the patients who were treated without EMG assistance received a higher dose, indicating more severe dystonia, thus possibly explaining the lesser degree of observed improvement. The general consensus among most BTX users is that EMG is not needed in the vast majority of patients, except in rare instances when the muscles cannot be adequately palpated or the patient does not obtain adequate relief of symptoms with the conventional approach (Jankovic, 2001b). BTX treatment not only provides effective symptomatic relief in patients with cervical dystonia but has also dramatically changed the natural history of the disease as it also prevents contractures. Early introduction of BTX has been shown to prevent contractures even in patients with congenital torticollis (Collins and Jankovic, 2006).

Writer's cramp and other limb dystonias

Treatments of writer's cramp with muscle relaxation techniques, physical and occupational therapy, and medical and surgical therapies have been disappointing. Several open (Rivest et al., 1990; Jankovic and Schwartz, 1993b; Karp et al., 1994; Priori et al., 1995; Pullman et al., 1996; Quirk et al., 1996; Wissel et al., 1996) and double-blind controlled (Yoshimura et al., 1992; Tsui et al., 1993; Cole et al., 1995) trials have concluded that BTX injections into selected hand and forearm muscles probably provide the most effective relief in patients with these task-specific occupational dystonias. In some studies, fine wire electrodes were used to localize bursts of muscle activation during the task, and the toxin was injected through a hollow EMG needle into the belly of the most active muscle (Cole et al., 1995). Similar beneficial results, however, were obtained in other studies without complex EMG studies (Rivest et al., 1990). Several lines of evidence support the notion that an intramuscular injection

of BTX into the forearm muscles corrects the abnormal reciprocal inhibition (Priori et al., 1995).

Jankovic and Schwartz (1993b) studied the effects of BTX in 46 patients with hand dystonia who had injections into their forearm muscles in 130 treatment sessions. The average age was 49.4 years, and the dystonic symptoms had been present for an average of 8.6 years. After careful examination and palpation of the forearm muscles during writing, the toxin was injected into either the wrist flexors (116 injections) or the wrist extensors (52 injections). The average baseline severity of dystonia was 3.5 on a 0–4 rating scale. The average peak effect response for all treatment sessions was 2.3 (0 = no response to 4 = maximum benefit). The latency from injection to onset of effect averaged 5.6 days, and the benefit lasted an average of 9.2 weeks. Temporary hand weakness, the chief complication of this treatment, occurred in 54% of patients and in 34% of all treatment sessions. However, nearly all patients preferred the temporary weakness, which was usually mild, to the disabling writer's cramps. Although one study showed that only 14 of 38 (37%) of needle placement attempts reached the proper hand muscles in the absence of EMG guidance, this does not mean that placement with EMG guidance correlates with better results, since the selection of the muscle involved in the hand dystonia is based on clinical examination, not on EMG (Molloy et al., 2002). One study showed that voluntary activity of the hand immediately after the treatment for 30 minutes enhanced the weakness produced by the injection which may, therefore, allow reduction in dosage and optimize the benefits (Chen et al., 1999).

In addition to improving writer's cramp, BTX might provide relief in other task-specific disorders affecting typists, draftsmen, musicians, athletes, and other people who depend on skilled movements of their hands (Schuele et al., 2005). Other focal distal dystonias, besides those involving the hands, might be amenable to treatment with BTX. Patients with Parkinson disease, progressive supranuclear palsy, corticobasal degeneration, and other forms of parkinsonism or stroke-related hemiplegia occasionally develop secondary fixed dystonia of the hand (dystonic clenched fist), which might benefit in terms of pain and hygiene from local BTX injections (Cordivari et al., 2001). Patients with foot dystonia as a manifestation of primary (idiopathic) dystonia and patients with parkinsonism who experience foot dystonia as an early symptom of their disease or, more commonly, as a complication of levodopa therapy might benefit from local BTX infections (Pacchetti et al., 1995). BTX injections into the foot–toe flexors or extensors might not only alleviate the disability, pain, and discomfort that are often associated with such dystonia but also improve gait. Whether BTX injections will play an important role in the treatment of recurrent painful physiologic foot and calf cramps has yet to be determined.

Other indications for botulinum toxin

It is beyond the scope of this chapter to review the rapidly broadening indications for BTX therapy. The reader is referred to some recent reviews on this topic (Brin et al., 2002; Jankovic and Brin, 2002; Jankovic 2004a; Jankovic et al., 2009) and to Simpson et al. (2008) for evidence-based recommendations. Based on a thorough review of clinical trials with

Table 13.9 Evidence-based recommendations for the therapeutic use of botulinum toxin for treatment of movement disorders

Disorder	No. Trials/ Subjects	Botulinum toxin formulation	Recommendations
Cervical dystonia	7/584	Botox (1), Dysport (3), Myobloc (3)	Should be offered (A)
Blepharospasm	2/17	Botox	May be offered (B)
Focal limb dystonia (upper extremity)	3/47	Botox, Dysport, not specified	May be offered (B)
Laryngeal dystonia (adductor)	1/13	Botox	May be offered (B)
Essential tremor (UE)	2/158	Botox	May be offered (B)
Hemifacial spasm	2/19	Botox, Dysport	May be considered (C)
Tics	1/18		May be considered (C)

From Simpson DM, Blitzer A, Brashear A, et al. Report of the Therapeutics and Technology Assessment Subcommittee of the AAN. Neurology 2008;70:1699–1706.

BTX, the American Academy of Neurology has made the following evidence-based recommendations: "BoNT should be offered as a treatment option for the treatment of cervical dystonia (Level A), may be offered for blepharospasm, focal upper extremity dystonia, adductor laryngeal dystonia, and upper extremity essential tremor (Level B), and may be considered for hemifacial spasm, focal lower limb dystonia and motor tics (Level C)" (Simpson et al., 2008) (Table 13.9).

Surgical treatment of dystonia

Although surgery has been used in the treatment of dystonia for a long time (Cooper 1965), there has been a recent resurgence in this approach, largely because of improvements in surgical and imaging techniques and as a result of surgical benefits observed in patients with tremor and Parkinson disease (Jankovic, 1998; Lang, 1998; Ondo et al., 2001).

Central ablative procedures and deep brain stimulation

Improved understanding of the functional anatomy of the basal ganglia and physiologic mechanisms underlying movement disorders, coupled with refinements in imaging and surgical techniques, has led to a resurgence of interest in thalamotomy in patients with disabling tremors, dystonia, and other hyperkinetic movement disorders (Grossman and Hamilton, 1993; Jankovic et al., 1996; Ondo et al., 2001). The observation, supported by both physiologic and positron emission tomographic studies, that there is a disruption of pallidothalamic-cortical projections in dystonia provides some rationale for treating dystonia by interrupting the abnormal outflow from the thalamus to the overactive prefrontal motor cortex (Lenz et al., 1990; Mitchel et al., 1990; Ceballos-Baumann et al., 1995).

In a longitudinal study of 17 patients with severe dystonia, 8 (47%) had a moderate to marked improvement in their abnormal postures and functional disability following thalamotomy (Cardoso et al., 1995). Patients with primary and secondary dystonia had similar responses, but 43% of the patients with primary dystonia deteriorated during a mean follow-up of 32.9 months, whereas only 30% of patients with secondary dystonia deteriorated during a mean follow-up of 41 months. Neurologic complications were observed in 6 of 17 patients (35%) immediately after surgery, but deficits (contralateral weakness, dysarthria, pseudobulbar palsy) persisted in only one subject. Mild weakness contralateral to the surgery was the most common complication, noted in 3 patients immediately following the procedure. The one patient who underwent bilateral procedures had no detectable dysarthria. These results are consistent with other studies that have reported improvement in 34–70% of patients with dystonia following thalamotomy (Cooper, 1976; Andrew et al., 1983; Tasker et al., 1988). While most studies concluded that distal dystonia responded more favorably to thalamotomy than axial dystonia, Andrew and colleagues (1983) felt that their patients with axial dystonia, including torticollis, also improved after thalamotomy. Most investigators, however, feel that the best candidates for thalamotomy are patients who have disabling, particularly unilateral, dystonia (hemidystonia) that is unresponsive to medical therapy. Patients with preexisting dysarthria are also good candidates because they have less to lose from thalamotomy-related speech disturbance. Patients with secondary (symptomatic) dystonia seem to respond better than those with idiopathic dystonia. Thalamotomy should not be recommended for patients with facial, laryngeal, and cervical or truncal dystonia.

The role of pallidotomy in the treatment of dystonia is currently being reevaluated in view of the emerging use of deep brain stimulation (Jankovic et al., 1997; Eltahawy et al., 2004). In one study of eight patients with severe generalized dystonia, there was 59% and 62.5% improvement in the Fahn–Marsden Dystonia Scale and in the Unified Dystonia Rating Scale, respectively, following pallidotomy (Ondo et al., 1998). The experience with pallidotomy continues to show favorable long-term effects, particularly in patients with primary dystonia (Ondo et al., 2001; Yoshor et al., 2001). Although the surgery does not slow or halt the progression of the underlying disease, most patients continue to benefit. The procedure is usually well tolerated, and the benefits have persisted for more than 10 years in most patients with primary dystonia. Pallidotomy has been also reported to be effective in a 47-year-old woman with paroxysmal dystonia induced by exercise (Bhatia et al., 1998).

Although there are no data from healthy humans, microelectrode recordings from patients with generalized dystonia indicate that the mean discharge rates (about 50 Hz) in the GPi are lower than those in patients with Parkinson disease (80–85 Hz) (Lozano et al., 1997) or parkinsonian primates (70–75 Hz) (Filion and Tremblay, 1991) but higher than those in hemiballism (Vitek et al., 1998, 1999) and that the proportion of GPi cells that respond to stimulation is higher in patients with dystonia than in those with hemiballism (Lenz et al., 1998). In comparison to normal or parkinsonian primates, the GPi discharges in patients with dystonia seem to be more irregular, with more bursting and pauses, and the receptive fields to passive and active movements seem to be widened (Kumar et al., 1999). The intraoperative neurophysiologic recordings in 15 patients with dystonia were compared with those of 78 patients with Parkinson disease undergoing pallidotomy; the discharge rates were lower in frequency and more irregular in the GPi and GPe of patients with dystonia (Sanghera et al., 2003).

Physiologic studies in patients with dystonia, based on lower mean discharge rates in GPe and GPi (Vitek et al., 1998, 1999), suggest overactivity of both direct (striatum–GPi) and indirect (striatum–GPe–GPi) pathways; the dopamine receptor ligand PET studies (Perlmutter et al., 1997; Asanuma et al., 2005) suggest increased activity in the direct and decreased activity in the indirect pathway. This is compatible with FDG PET studies supportive of excessive activity in the direct pathway (Eidelberg et al., 1995). In multiple reports, pallidotomy (Lozano et al., 1997; Ondo et al., 1998; Vitek et al., 1999) and GPi DBS (Coubes et al., 2000; Tronnier and Fogel, 2000; Vercueil et al., 2001; Bereznai et al., 2002; Vidailhet et al., 2005; Diamond et al., 2006; Isaias et al., 2008, 2009; Sensi et al., 2009) appear to be effective procedures for patients with dystonia (Fig. 13.2) (Videos 13.4, 13.5, and 13.6). Both procedures may provide benefit by disrupting the abnormal GPi pattern and thus reduce cortical overactivation, characteristic of dystonia (Eidelberg et al., 1995). Primary dystonia clearly responds better than secondary dystonia to either pallidotomy or GPi DBS, although patients with pantothenate kinase-associated neurodegeneration also experience marked improvement (Coubes et al., 2000; Eltahawy et al., 2004).

DBS targeting GPi has generally replaced ablative surgery in patients with disabling dystonia (Ostrem and Starr, 2008). Since an ablative lesion or high-frequency stimulation of the GPi can both produce and improve dystonia, this suggests it is the pattern of discharge in the basal ganglia rather than the actual location or frequency of discharge that is pathophysiologically relevant to dystonia (Münchau et al., 2000). In a prospective, multicenter study

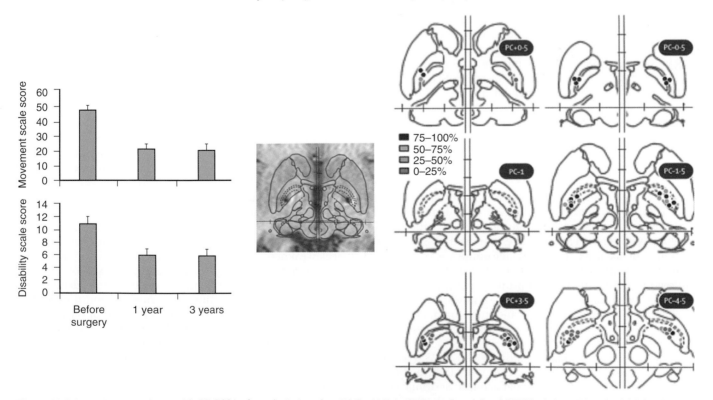

BILATERAL, PALLIDAL, DEEP BRAIN STIMULATION IN PRIMARY GENERALIZED DYSTONIA: A PROSPECTIVE 3-YEAR FOLLOW-UP STUDY

22 patients with primary generalized dystonia. Motor improvement, observed at 1 year (51%), was maintained at 3 years (58%).

75–100%
50–75%
25–50%
0–25%

Figure 13.2 Long-term experience with GPi DBS in dystonia. *Redrawn from Vidailhet M, Vercueil L, Houeto JL, et al., French SPIDY Study Group. Bilateral, pallidal, deep-brain stimulation in primary generalised dystonia: a prospective 3 year follow-up study. Lancet Neurol 2007;6:223–229.*

of 22 patients with generalized dystonia, seven of whom had a DYT1 mutation, the Fahn–Marsden Dystonia Scale score (FMDRS) improved after bilateral GPi DBS from a mean of 46.3 ± 21.3 to 21.0 ± 14.1 at 12 months (P < 0.001) (Vidailhet et al., 2005). A "blinded" review of the videos at 3 months showed improvement with stimulation from a mean of 34.63 ± 12.3 to 24.6 ± 17.7. The improvement in mean dystonia motor scores was 51%, and one-third of the patients improved more than 75% compared to preoperative scores. In addition, there was a significant improvement in health-related quality of life as measured by the SF-36, but there was no change in cognition or mood. Although the sample was rather small, the authors were not able to find any predictors of response such as DYT1 gene status, anatomic distribution of the dystonia, or location of the electrodes. Patients with the phasic form of dystonia improved more than those with tonic contractions and posturing. The maximum benefit was not achieved in some patients until 3–6 months after surgery. Vercueil and colleagues (2001) described 10 patients with bilateral GPi DBS; 5 had a major improvement, 2 had a moderated improvement, and 1 had a minor improvement after 14 months. They concluded that GPi DBS is much more effective than thalamic DBS for the treatment of dystonia. In a 2-year follow-up of 31 patients with primary generalized dystonia, Coubes and colleagues (2004) noted a mean improvement in clinical and functional FMDRS of 79% and 65%, respectively. There was no difference in response between DYT1-positive and DYT1-negative patients, but the magnitude of improvement was greater in children than in adults. Kupsch et al. (2006) compared GPi DBS with sham stimulation in a randomized, controlled clinical trial of 40 patients with primary segmental or generalized dystonia. The primary endpoint was the change from baseline to 3 months in the severity of symptoms, according to the movement subscore on the FMDRS. Two investigators who were unaware of treatment status assessed the severity of dystonia by reviewing videotaped sessions. Three months after randomization, the change from baseline in the mean (± SD) movement score was significantly greater in the neurostimulation group (−15.8 ± 14.1 points) than in the sham-stimulation group (−1.4 ± 3.8 points, P < 0.001). There was other evidence of benefit from DBS in this study. Several studies have demonstrated a gradual deterioration of dystonia over 48 hours or longer after GPi DBS is interrupted but this is rapidly reversible once the DBS is turned on (Grabli et al., 2009). In a study of 39 patients with dystonia undergoing GPi DBS, short duration of disease was identified as the only predictor of good outcome (among 32 patients with mobile dystonia the FMDRS score improved 87.8%) but the presence of fixed axial skeletal deformities was associated with poor outcome (Isaias et al., 2008). In a long-term follow-up of 30 patients with primary and generalized dystonia followed for up to 8 years, the hardware and stimulation adverse events were rare and the implantable pulse generators were replaced on the average every 24 months (Isaias et al., 2009).

In addition to primary dystonia, GPi DBS has been reported to be effective in patients with tardive dystonia (Trottenberg et al., 2005), cranial-cervical dystonia (Foote et al., 2005; Hebb et al., 2007; Ostrem et al., 2007) and other forms of segmental dystonia (Krauss et al., 2002). In addition, bilateral GPi DBS has been reported to be effective in patients with neurodegeneration with brain iron accumulation (NBIA) (Timmermann et al., 2010). Further studies are needed before surgery is recommended for these forms of dystonia. For example, blepharospasm associated with craniocervical dystonia has been reported to be exacerbated by bilateral GPi DBS (Vagefi et al., 2008). Although DBS has not been used frequently in the treatment of cranial-cervical dystonia, both GPi and STN have been targeted in the DBS treatment of this form of dystonia (Ostrem et al., 2011). GPi DBS has also been found helpful in the treatment of dystonic or parkinsonian camptocormia, an extreme flexion of the trunk (Jankovic, 2010).

Peripheral surgery

Peripheral denervation procedures were used extensively for cervical dystonia prior to the advent of BTX therapy. In one series of patients with cervical dystonia seen before 1990, 40 of 300 (13%) patients elected to have this type of surgery (Jankovic et al., 1991). While 10% of the patients noted worsening after the surgery, 38% experienced a noticeable improvement in the ability to control their head position or in reduction of the neck pain.

Three procedures have been used in the treatment of cervical dystonia: (1) extradural selective sectioning of posterior (dorsal) rami (posterior ramisectomy) with or without myotomy, (2) intradural sectioning of anterior cervical roots (anterior cervical rhizotomy), and (3) microvascular decompression of the spinal accessory nerve. Although the first procedure, championed by Bertrand (Bertrand and Molina-Negro, 1988), is considered by many clinicians to be the procedure of choice, no study has compared the different surgical approaches. Bertrand and Molina-Negro (1988) reported that 97 of 111 (87%) patients had "excellent" or "very good" results. In a smaller series, five of nine (56%) patients had moderate benefit that was sustained during up to 21 months of follow-up (Davis et al., 1991). The procedure is performed under general anesthesia without a paralyzing agent so that intraoperative nerve root stimulation can be used to identify the innervation to the dystonic muscles. This information, coupled with preoperative EMG, is used to avulse selected nerve roots, usually the branches of the spinal accessory nerve and the posterior rami of C1 through C6. Thorough avulsion of the peripheral branches is believed to be essential in preventing recurrences. Pain seems to improve more than the abnormal posture following the cervical muscle denervation, although some patients complain of stiff neck, sometimes lasting several months, after the surgery. Other complications may include local numbness, neck weakness, and rarely dysphagia. The chief disadvantage of anterior rhizotomy compared to posterior primary ramisectomy is that the former procedure causes denervation of both involved and uninvolved muscles, and it cannot be carried out at or below the C4 level because of the potential for involvement of the roots to the phrenic nerve, leading to paralysis of the diaphragm. The posterior ramisectomy (C2 to C6) allows more selective denervation of the involved muscles. Krauss and colleagues (1997) reported the effects of 70 intradural or extradural approaches in 46 patients with severe cervical dystonia. During a mean duration of follow-up of 6.5 years, 21 (46%) of the patients reported excellent or

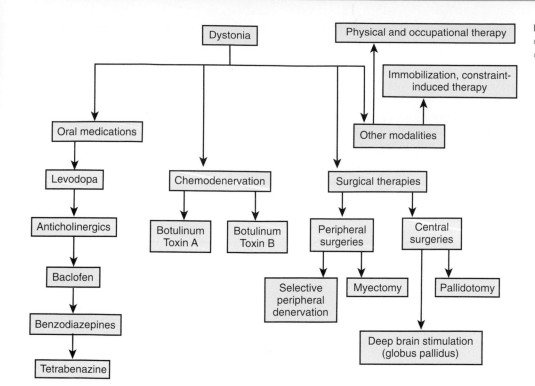

Figure 13.3 Therapeutic algorithm in dystonia. *Redrawn from Jankovic J. Treatment of dystonia. Lancet Neurol 2006;5:864–872.*

marked improvement on a global outcome scale. There was no difference in the distribution of outcome when patients who still responded to BTX were compared with the BTX nonresponders. Using a modified TWSTRS scale, there was statistically significant improvements not only in the severity of dystonia but also in occupational and domestic work as well as in various activities of daily living. The results of this study are comparable with those of Ford and colleagues (1998b), who reported on an open-label, retrospective study of selective denervation for severe cervical dystonia (torticollis) in 16 patients who were refractory to injections with BTX-A. Using functional capacity scales, they concluded that 6 (37.5%) patients had "a moderate or complete return of normal neck function." Despite some improvement in 12 of 14 (85.7%) patients on the TWSTRS dystonia rating scale applied to "blinded" ratings of videotaped examinations, the surgery failed to return patients to their occupations. On the basis of the reported experience, we conclude that surgical treatment tailored to the specific pattern of dystonic activity in the individual patient is a valuable alternative in the long-term management of cervical dystonia, particularly for patients who are anxious to avoid having the intracranial surgical procedure of DBS targeting the GPi.

Surgical treatments, such as facial nerve lysis and orbicularis oculi myectomy, once used extensively in the treatment of blepharospasm, have been essentially abolished because BTX treatment is usually very effective and because postoperative complications, such as ectropion, exposure keratitis, facial droop, and postoperative swelling and scarring, are common (Chapman et al., 1999). Similarly, recurrent laryngeal nerve section, once used in the treatment of spasmodic dysphonia (Dedo and Izdebski, 1983), is used rarely and only when BTX fails to provide a satisfactory relief. Another once popular procedure, spinal cord stimulation for cervical dystonia, has been shown to be ineffective by a controlled trial (Goetz et al., 1988).

Medical, surgical, and other therapeutic approaches to dystonia have been described in several recent reviews (Jankovic 2006; Jankovic, 2009a) (Fig. 13.3).

Other therapies

Inhibiting expression of mutant torsinA could be potentially a powerful therapeutic strategy in DYT1 dystonia. Using small interfering RNA (siRNA) to silence the expression of mutant torsinA, Gonzalez-Alegre and colleagues (2003) successfully suppressed expression of this abnormal protein in transfected cells that was allele-specific. Novel and experimental therapies are needed in order to make incremental advances in the treatment of dystonia (Jinnah and Hess, 2008).

Therapeutic guidelines

In summary, patients with segmental or generalized dystonia beginning in childhood or adolescence should be initially tried on levodopa/carbidopa up to 1000 mg of levodopa per day. If this therapy is successful, it should be maintained at a lowest possible dose. If it is ineffective after 3 months, then high-dose anticholinergic (e.g., trihexyphenidyl) therapy should be instituted, and the dosage should be increased to the highest tolerated level. If the results are poor, then baclofen, benzodiazepines, carbamazepine, and tetrabenazine should be tried. Some patients may require triple therapy consisting of an anticholinergic agent (e.g., trihexyphenidyl), a monoamine-depleting drug (e.g., tetrabenazine), and a dopamine receptor-blocking drug (e.g., fluphenazine, pimozide, risperidol, or clozapine) (Marsden et al., 1984). Tetrabenazine alone or with anticholinergic drugs is particularly useful in the treatment of tardive dystonia. In some patients, BTX injections may be helpful to control the most disabling symptom of the segmental or generalized dystonia. In most patients with adult-onset dystonia, the distribution is usually focal; therefore, BTX injections are usually considered the treatment of choice. Besides the abnormal movement and posture, pain, associated depression, anxiety, and other psychological comorbidities can have an important impact on the quality of life of patients with cervical dystonia and must be appropriately treated (Ben-Shlomo et al., 2002). In some patients, this treatment might need to be supplemented by other drugs noted previously or by surgical peripheral denervation. DBS should be reserved only for patients whose symptoms continue to be disabling despite optimal medical therapy. Any form of therapy should, of course, be preceded by a thorough evaluation designed to rule out secondary causes of dystonia. Finally, it is important to emphasize that patient education and counseling are essential components of a comprehensive therapeutic approach to all patients with dystonia (see the Appendix).

References available on Expert Consult: www.expertconsult.com

Appendix

Dystonia Medical Research Foundation
One East Wacker Drive, Suite 2810
Chicago, IL 60601-1905
Telephone: (312) 755-0198
in Canada (800) 361-8061
Fax: (312) 803-0138
Email: dystonia@dystonia-foundation.org
Website: http://www.dystonia-foundation.org

National Spasmodic Torticollis Association
9920 Talbert Avenue #233
Fountain Valley, CA 92708
Telephone: (800) 487-8385
Email: nstamail@aol.com
Website: http://www.torticollis.org

The Bachmann-Strauss Dystonia and Parkinson Foundation
Fred French Building
551 Fifth Avenue, at 45th St
Suite 520
New York, NY 10176
Telephone: (212) 682-9900
Fax: (212) 987-0662
Email: info@bsdpf.org
Website: http://www.dystonia-parkinsons.org

Spasmodic Torticollis/Dystonia
PO Box 28
Mukwonago, WI 53149
Telephone: (888) 445-4598
Email: info@spasmodictorticollis.org
Website: http://www.spasmodictorticollis.org

Care4Dystonia
440 East 78th Street
New York, NY 10021
Telephone: 212-249-2808
Email: bekadys@aol.com
Website: http://www.care4dystonia.org

Benign Essential Blepharospasm Research Foundation
PO Box 12468
Beaumont, TX 77726-2468
Telephone: (409) 832-0788
Fax: (409) 832-0890
Email: bebrf@blepharospasm.org
Website: http://blepharospasm.org

For further information about movement disorders contact:

WE MOVE: Worldwide Education and Awareness for Movement Disorders
5731 Mosholu Avenue
Bronx, New York, NY 10024
Telephone: (347) 843-6132
Fax: (718) 601-5112
Email: wemove@wemove.org
Website: http://www.wemove.org

CHAPTER **14**

Huntington disease

Chapter contents

Introduction	311		Genetics	318
Epidemiology	311		Pathogenesis	322
Clinical aspects	311		Treatment	326
Natural course	314		Experimental therapeutics	333
Neuroimaging	315		Appendix	334
Neuropathology and neurochemistry	316			

Introduction

George Huntington published his essay "On Chorea" in 1872 (Huntington, 1872), one year after graduating from Columbia College of Physicians and Surgeons while practicing general medicine with his father on Long Island. Soon afterward, the eponym Huntington's chorea was adopted in the literature to draw attention to chorea (derived from the Latin *choreus*, meaning "dance" and Greek *choros*, meaning "chorus") as the clinical hallmark of this neurodegenerative disorder. However, since many other manifestations of the disease exist and since chorea might not even be present, the term *Huntington disease* (HD) (OMIM 143100) is more appropriate (Penney and Young, 1998; Jankovic, 2006; Fahn and Jankovic, 2009). Although chorea (known as the dancing mania) has been recognized since the Middle Ages, the origin of the affected families described by Huntington was traced to the early seventeenth century in the village of Bures in southeast England. The inhabitants of this area later migrated to various parts of the world, accounting for the marked variation in the regional prevalence of HD.

This chapter will focus on HD; other diseases, such as Huntington disease-like type 1 (HDL1), HDL2, and HDL3, dentatorubral-pallidoluysian atrophy, and spinocerebellar atrophy type 17 (SCA17) that may present as HD-like phenotypes are discussed in Chapter 15 and other reviews (Toyoshima et al., 2004; Schneider et al., 2006; Schneider et al., 2007; Wild et al., 2008; Jankovic and Fahn, 2009; Fekete and Jankovic, 2010).

Epidemiology

While the estimated prevalence of HD in the United States is 2 to 10 per 100 000 population (Kokmen et al., 1994),

which translates to about 30 000 people with HD and another 200 000 at risk of developing the disease, the prevalence is geographically heterogeneous, and in certain regions of the world it is as high as 560 per 100 000 (Moray Firth, Scotland) and 700 per 100 000 (Lake Maracaibo, Venezuela) (Harper, 1992). Americo Negrette, a Venezuelan physician, first observed the dancing mania of Maracaibo in the 1950s, and his findings later led to the discovery of the gene locus and gene mutation for HD (Okun and Thommi, 2004). Because many epidemiologic studies were done before the advent of genetic testing, the true prevalence of the HD gene is not known. DNA testing has largely replaced other tests, such as magnetic resonance imaging (MRI) of the brain, in the evaluation of patients with HD.

Clinical aspects

The rich repertoire of neurologic, behavioral, and cognitive manifestations of HD makes it one of the most intriguing of all neurodegenerative disorders. In a study involving 1901 patients with HD, the following were considered the most frequent presenting symptoms, in descending order: chorea, trouble walking, unsteadiness, irritability, depression, clumsiness, speech difficulty, memory loss, dropping of objects, lack of motivation, paranoia, intellectual decline, sleep disturbance, hallucination, weight loss, and sexual problems (Foroud et al., 1999). The Unified Huntington's Disease Rating Scale (UHDRS) was developed to assess and quantify various clinical features of HD, specifically motor function, cognitive function, behavioral abnormalities, and functional capacity (Huntington Study Group, 1996; Siesling et al., 1998). A shortened version of the UHDRS has been validated (Siesling et al., 1997). In addition, assessment protocol has been developed to evaluate various neurologic and

DOI: 10.1016/B978-1-4377-2369-4.00014-7

behavioral features in HD patients who are undergoing striatal grafting (CAPIT-HD Committee, 1996). When so-called "soft signs" are identified at the initial evaluation, the cumulative relative risk of HD diagnosis at 1.5 years is 4.68 times greater than in controls (Langbehn et al., 2007).

Patients with HD often have poor insight into their chorea and are more likely to report consequences of the movement disorder, such as dropping objects, than "twitching" or other features of chorea, and there is little or no relationship between direct experience or awareness of involuntary movement and actual chorea scores (Snowden et al., 1998). This may explain why the presence and degree of chorea seem to correlate poorly with functional decline (Feigin et al., 1995). Besides chorea, other motor symptoms that typically affect patients with HD include dystonia, postural instability, ataxia, dystonia, bruxism, myoclonus, tics and tourettism, dysarthria, dysphagia, and aerophagia (Vogel et al., 1991; Carella et al., 1993; Thompson et al., 1994; Ashizawa and Jankovic, 1996; Hu and Chaudhuri, 1998; Louis et al., 1999; Tan and Jankovic, 2000; Jankovic and Ashizawa, 2003; Walker, 2007) (Videos 14.1, 14.2, 14.3, and 14.4). A characteristic feature of HD is the inability to maintain tongue protrusion, representing motor impersistence (sometimes also referred to as "negative chorea") (Videos 14.5 and 14.6).

Chorea is clearly not merely a cosmetic or embarrassing symptom, but this cardinal feature of HD may affect fine and gross motor function, activities of daily living, gait and balance, eventually impacting on the quality of life, and likely contributing to weight loss, falls, social isolation, loss of employability, and increased morbidity and dependence on others, eventually leading to institutionalization (Wheelock et al., 2003). In one study, only the change in the UHDRS chorea score correlated with the change in the complex task performance, such as peg insertion (Andrich et al., 2007). One study compared 45 HD patients with a history of at least one fall to 27 healthy controls (Grimbergen et al., 2008). The fallers had more chorea, bradykinesia, aggression and cognitive decline. The HD patients had decreased gait velocity and a decreased stride length. In one study of 24 patients with HD, 14 (58.3%) reported at least two falls within the previous 12 months and the fallers had worse scores on Berg Balance Scale (BBS) and the Timed "Up & Go" (TUG) test (Busse et al., 2009).

Hung-up and pendular reflexes are also typically present in patients with HD (Video 14.6) (Brannan, 2003). Some patients can "camouflage" their chorea by incorporating the involuntary movements into semipurposeful activities, so-called "parakinesia" (Video 14.7). Rarely, patients with HD present with tics and other features suggestive of adult-onset Tourette syndrome ("tourettism") (Jankovic and Ashizawa, 1995) (Video 14.8).

In a study of 593 members of a large kindred in Venezuela, generation of fine motor movements and of rapid eye saccades was found to be impaired in about 50% of at-risk individuals (Penney et al., 1990). Since at-risk individuals with these findings were more likely than those without them to develop overt HD within several years, these abnormalities were thought to represent the earliest clinical manifestations of the disease. If the first examination was normal, there was only a 3% risk of developing symptomatic HD within 3 years. HD patients seem to have greater defects in

initiating internally than externally generated saccades (Tian et al., 1991). In 215 individuals at risk for HD or recently diagnosed with HD, a high-resolution, video-based eye tracking system demonstrated three types of significant abnormalities while performing memory-guided and anti-saccade tasks: increased error rate, increased saccade latency, and increased variability of saccade latency (Blekher et al., 2006). In another study initiation deficits of voluntary-guided, but not reflexive saccades were found in individuals with preclinical HD (Golding et al., 2006). Voluntary-guided saccades in 25 presymptomatic HD individuals have been found to correlate with deficits in white matter tracts as determined by diffusion tensor MRI (Klöppel et al., 2008). In addition to abnormal eye saccades, patients with HD demonstrate other neuro-ophthalmologic abnormalities, such as increased blink rates (Karson et al., 1984; Xing et al., 2008), irregular elevations of eyebrows due to choreic contractions of the frontalis muscles and eye closures with irregular narrowing of palpebral fissures, rarely leading to frank blepharospasm, and apraxia of eyelid opening and closure (Bonelli and Niederwieser, 2002).

Using quantitative assessments, Siemers and colleagues (1996) found subtle but significant abnormalities in simple and choice movement time and reaction time in 103 truly presymptomatic carriers of the HD gene. These deficits correlated well with the number of cytosine-adenine-guanine (CAG) trinucleotide repeats (see later). In a follow-up longitudinal study of 43 at-risk individuals, Kirkwood and colleagues (1999) found that the following variables declined more rapidly among the presymptomatic gene carriers (n = 12) than among the noncarriers (n = 31): psychomotor speed (digit symbol subscale of the Wechsler Adult Intelligence Scale), optokinetic nystagmus, and rapid alternating movements. In contrast to UHDRS, which is not very sensitive in detecting early clinical signs of HD, careful gait and balance analysis has detected gait bradykinesia and dynamic balance impairment in presymptomatic HD gene carriers with otherwise normal neurologic examination (Rao et al., 2008). In the Predict-HD study, 505 at-risk individuals, 452 of whom had more than 39 CAG repeats, but had not yet met clinical criteria for the diagnosis of HD, the striatum MRI volume decreased from 17.06 cm^3, at diagnostic confidence level of 0, to 14.89 cm^3, at diagnostic confidence level of 3 (probable HD, with a mean CAG repeat number of 44 and mean motor UHDRS score of 16.92) (Paulsen et al., 2006). The study found that smaller striatal volume, reduced finger tapping speed and consistency, and impaired odor identification were among the best markers of "pre-clinical" HD (Paulsen et al., 2008). Additional analyses found that even subtle abnormality in finger tapping (bradykinesia), tandem gait, Luria test, saccade initiation, and chorea were associated with high probability of disease diagnosis (Biglan et al., 2009).

While hyperkinesia, usually in the form of chorea, is typically present in adult-onset HD, parkinsonism (an akinetic-rigid syndrome) is characteristic of juvenile HD, also termed Westphal variant. Bradykinesia, usually evident in patients with the rigid form of HD, when it coexists with chorea might not be fully appreciated on a routine examination (van Vugt et al., 1996; Thompson et al., 1988; Sánchez-Pernaute et al., 2000). Variability in isometric grip forces while grasping an object has been found to correlate well with UHDRS and with progressive motor deficits associated with HD (Reilmann et al., 2001). Assessing simple repetitive movements, such as tapping, correlates with UHDRS and may be used to follow progression of HD (Andrich et al., 2007). Fast simple wrist flexion movements were found to be significantly slower in 17 patients with HD compared to controls (Thompson et al., 1988). While bradykinesia was most pronounced in the rigid-akinetic patients, it was also evident in patients with the typical choreic variety of HD. When bradykinesia predominates, the patients exhibit parkinsonian findings, some of which can be subtle. Using a continuous wrist-worn monitor of motor activity, van Vugt and colleagues (1996) also provided evidence of hypokinesia in patients with HD, particularly when they were treated with neuroleptics. Micrographia may be one manifestation of underlying parkinsonism; when chorea predominates, the handwriting is characterized by macrographia (Phillips et al., 1994). Bradykinesia in HD may be an expression of postsynaptic parkinsonism as a result of involvement of both direct and indirect pathways. This might explain why a reduction in chorea with antidopaminergic drugs rarely improves overall motor functioning and indeed can cause an exacerbation of the motor impairment. In their excellent review, Berardelli and colleagues (1999) argue that "bradykinesia results from degeneration of the basal ganglia output to the supplementary motor areas concerned with the initiation and maintenance of sequential movements" and "may reflect failure of thalamocortical relay of sensory information." Although bradykinesia associated with HD usually does not respond to dopaminergic therapy, late-onset levodopa-responsive HD presenting as parkinsonism has been well documented (Reuter et al., 2000).

Besides chorea, the other two components of the HD cardinal triad include cognitive decline and various psychiatric symptoms, particularly depression (Paulsen et al., 2001a). Depression, poor impulse control, and other behavioral and socioeconomic factors associated with HD contribute to the markedly increased risk of suicide in patients with HD. Suicide rate in patients with HD is 138/100 000 person-years as compared to 12–13/100 000 person-years in the general population. Thus, the risk of suicide is ten times greater in HD than in the general population (Bird, 1999; Almqvist et al., 1999). In a study of 506 individuals with documented or suspected HD, suicide represented the third most common cause of death, accounting for 12.7% of 157 ascertained deaths, after bronchopneumonia (31.8%) and heart disease (15.3%) (Schoenfeld et al., 1984). In a review of records of 452 deceased patients diagnosed with HD, 5.7% of deaths were attributed to suicide, 4 times the expected rate for the corresponding US white population (Farrer, 1986). In a cross-sectional study of 2835 patients with "definite" diagnosis of HD, with disease onset at age 20 years or later, mean age of 49.6 years, and duration of symptoms for a mean 7.6 years, 50.3% reported seeking treatment for depression and 10.3% reported at least one suicide attempt (Paulsen et al., 2005b). Patients endorsing current symptoms of depression were twice as likely to have attempted suicide in the past as those who deny symptoms of depression (15.7% vs. 7.1%). In another study, using UHDRS in 4171 patients with HD, the frequency of suicidal ideation doubled from 9.1% in at-risk persons with normal neurologic examination to 19.8% in at-risk individuals with soft neurologic signs and increased to 23.5% in persons with "possible" HD. In

patients with diagnosed HD, the risk of suicidal ideation increased from 16.7% at stage 1 to 21.6% at stage 2, and decreased thereafter to 19.5%, 14.1%, and 9.8% in stages 3, 4, and 5, respectively (Paulsen et al., 2005a). Thus the most critical periods of suicide risk are immediately before receiving a formal diagnosis of HD and in stage 2 of the disease, when activities, such as driving and taking care of one's finances are beginning to be restricted and patients are becoming more dependent on others. While some studies (Foroud et al., 1995) showed that cognitive deficits correlated with the number of CAG repeats in asymptomatic carriers of the HD gene, other studies found no correlation between cognitive decline and CAG repeats in symptomatic patients with HD (Zappacosta et al., 1996). The neurobehavioral symptoms typically consist of personality changes, agitation, irritability, anxiety, apathy, social withdrawal, impulsiveness, depression, mania, paranoia, delusions, hostility, hallucinations, psychosis, and various sexual disorders (Fedoroff et al., 1994; Litvan et al., 1998). In a study of 52 patients with HD, Paulsen and colleagues (2001a) found the following neuropsychiatric symptoms in descending order of frequency: dysphoria, agitation, irritability, apathy, anxiety, disinhibition, euphoria, delusions, and hallucinations (Video 14.9). Affective disorders, such as depression, often preceded the onset of motor symptoms. In one study of presymptomatic individuals at risk for HD, gene carriers were 1.74 times (95% CI 1–3.07) more likely to report depression than non-carriers, and the rate of depression increased the closer the subject was to the clinical onset (Julien et al., 2007). Behaviors such as agitation, anxiety, and irritability have been related to hyperactivity of the medial and orbitofrontal cortical circuitry (Litvan et al., 1998). This is in contrast to the apathy and hypoactive behaviors that are seen in progressive supranuclear palsy, attributed to a dysfunction in the frontal cortex and associated circuitry. Progressive decline in attention and executive function, consistent with frontostriatal pathology, has been found in early HD (Ho et al., 2003). Criminal behavior, closely linked to the personality changes, depression, and alcohol abuse, has been reported to be more frequent in patients with HD than in nonaffected first-degree relatives (Jensen et al., 1998). Such behavior might be a manifestation of an impulsive disorder as part of disinhibition, seen not only in HD but also in other frontal lobe–basal ganglia disorders, particularly Tourette syndrome (Brower and Price, 2001).

Cognitive changes, manifested chiefly by loss of recent memory, poor judgment, and impaired concentration and acquisition, occur in nearly all patients with HD; but some patients with late-onset chorea never develop dementia (Britton et al., 1995). In one study, dementia was found in 66% of 35 HD patients (Pillon et al., 1991). Tasks requiring psychomotor or visuospatial processing, such as skills tested by the Trail Making B and Stroop Interference Test, are impaired early in the course of the disease and deteriorate at a more rapid rate than memory impairment (Bamford et al., 1995). In addition to deficits in visual and auditory perception, patients with HD have impaired recognition of emotional facial expression (Sprengelmeyer et al., 1996). The presence of apraxia and other "cortical" features has cast doubt on this classification (Shelton and Knopman, 1991). In one study, ideomotor apraxia was found in three of nine HD patients, and seven of nine made some apraxic errors. It could not be determined whether the apraxia was due to involvement of frontal cortex or to involvement of subcortical structures (Shelton and Knopman, 1991). Speech and language may be also affected in HD, possibly as a result of striatal degeneration (De Diego-Balaguer et al., 2008). One study showed that high levels of insulin-like growth factor I (IGFI) are associated with cognitive deficits in HD (Saleh et al., 2010).

Although neurobehavioral symptoms precede motor disturbances in some cases, de Boo and colleagues (1997) showed that motor symptoms are more evident than cognitive symptoms in early stages of HD. Symptoms of REM behavioral sleep disorders may precede the onset of chorea or other motor symptoms of HD by many years (Arnulf et al., 2008). Asymptomatic at-risk individuals who are positive for the HD gene or the marker do seem to differ in their cognitive performance from asymptomatic at-risk individuals who are negative for the HD gene or marker (Giordani et al., 1995; Foroud et al., 1995; Lawrence et al., 1998). Most studies have found that neuropsychological tests do not differentiate between presymptomatic individuals who are positive for the HD gene and those who are negative (Strauss and Brandt, 1990; de Boo et al., 1997), but some studies have found that cognitive changes might be the first symptoms of HD (Hahn-Barma et al., 1998). In a longitudinal study by the Huntington Study Group of 260 individuals who were considered to be at risk for HD, Paulsen and colleagues (2001b) found that this group had worse scores on the cognitive section of the UHDRS at baseline, an average of 2 years before the development of motor manifestations of the disease.

In addition to motor, cognitive, and behavioral abnormalities, most patients with HD lose weight during the course of their disease, despite increased appetite (Marder et al., 2009). Weight loss in HD increases with higher CAG repeats (Aziz et al., 2008). Weight loss is not unique for HD among the neurodegenerative disorders; for example, it is typically seen in patients with Parkinson disease (Jankovic et al., 1992). The pathogenesis of weight loss in HD is unknown, but one study showed that patients with HD have a 14% higher sedentary energy expenditure than that of controls and that this appears to be correlated with the severity of the movement disorder (Pratley et al., 2000). The lower body mass index in HD parallels the weight loss in transgenic mice, suggesting that it represents a clinical expression of the gene abnormality associated with HD (Djousse et al., 2002; Aziz et al., 2008). Weight loss, and alterations in sexual behavior and wake–sleep cycle, frequently found in patients with HD, have been attributed to involvement of the hypothalamus even in early stages of HD as demonstrated by positron emission tomography (PET) and postmortem studies (Politis et al., 2008). Juvenile HD is associated with higher CAG repeats; 54% have 60 or more CAG repeats (Ribai et al., 2007).

About 10% of HD cases have their onset before age 20. This juvenile HD is usually inherited from the father (father vs. mother inheritance for patients with onset before 10 years is 3:1) and it typically presents with the combination of progressive parkinsonism, dementia, ataxia, myoclonus, and seizures. Myoclonus is particularly common in patients with juvenile HD (Video 14.10) and progressive myoclonic epilepsy has been reported as the initial presentation of juvenile HD (Gambardella et al., 2001) (Videos 14.10, 14.11, and 14.12).

Natural course

The natural course of HD varies; on the average, duration of illness from onset to death is about 15 years for adult HD, but it is about 4–5 years shorter for the juvenile variant. Patients with juvenile onset (<20 years) and with late onset (>50 years) of symptoms have the shortest duration of the disease (Foroud et al., 1999) (Fig. 14.1) (Videos 14.11 and 14.12). Using the Total Functional Capacity Scale, longitudinal follow-up of patients with HD showed a 0.72 unit/year rate of decline (Marder et al., 2000). Clinical-pathologic studies have demonstrated a strong inverse correlation between the age at onset and the severity of striatal degeneration (Myers et al., 1988). Striatal degeneration as measured by immunostaining with tyrosine hydroxylase (TH) is more pronounced in HD than in Parkinson disease (Huot et al., 2007). A review of clinical and pathologic data in 163 HD patients showed that patients with juvenile or adolescent onset had much more aggressive progression of the disease than patients with onset in middle and late life. Because of lack of efficacy, the clinical trial conducted by the Huntington Study Group that compared coenzyme Q10 (CoQ10) and remacemide, known as CARE-HD and involving 347 patients with documented HD, provides the best available data on the natural history of HD (Huntington Study Group, 2001). In this study, after 20 months, the Functional Assessment score decreased by 2.51 points, Total Functional Capacity score decreased by 1.95 points, and the Independence Scale score decreased by 8.58 points. Analysis of data collected by the Huntington Study Group on 1026 patients with HD, followed for a median of 2.7 years, concluded that the rate of progression was significantly more rapid with a younger age at onset and longer CAG repeats (Mahant et al., 2003). Although chorea and dystonia were not major determinants of disability, chorea was associated with weight loss.

Progressive motor dysfunction, dementia, dysphagia, and incontinence eventually lead to institutionalization and death from aspiration, infection, and poor nutrition (Leopold and Kagel, 1985). Among 4809 HD subjects, 3070 of whom had a definite diagnosis of HD, 228 (7.4%) resided

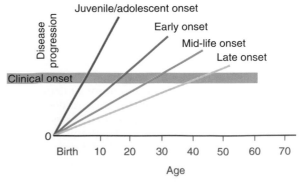

Figure 14.1 Progression of HD related to age at onset.

in a skilled nursing facility, and these residents had worse chorea, bradykinesia, gait abnormality, and imbalance, as well as more obsessions, compulsions, delusions, and auditory hallucinations, and they were more aggressive and disruptive than their counterparts living at home (Wheelock et al., 2003). In a study of 1642 patients with HD, 27.2% had some obsessive-compulsive features and nearly one-quarter received treatment for obsessive-compulsive disorder (Anderson et al., 2010). The HD patients with obsessive-compulsive disorder were older, had poorer functioning, and a longer duration of illness than those without these features, and more psychiatric comorbidities such as depression, suicidal ideation, aggression, delusions, and hallucinations. Quality of life is markedly affected by HD; the "work" and "alertness behavior" domains of the Sickness Impact Profile are affected the most (Helder et al., 2001). One study that assessed health-related quality of life (HrQoL) by SF-36 showed that depressive mood and functional disability are key factors in HrQoL for people with HD (Ho et al., 2009).

Neuroimaging

Caudate atrophy, as measured by the ratio of intercaudate to outer-table distances, has traditionally been used as an index of striatal atrophy in HD, and it has been demonstrated to correlate well with the degree of cognitive impairment in early HD (Bamford et al., 1995). Subsequent studies, however, showed that a reduction in the volume of putamen, measured by MRI, was a more sensitive index of neurologic dysfunction than caudate atrophy (Harris et al., 1992; Rosas et al., 2001). This suggests that the putamen is underdeveloped in HD or that it is one of the earliest structures to atrophy. Striatal volume loss correlates with length of CAG repeats (Rosas et al., 2001). Several MRI volumetric and single photon emission computed tomography (SPECT) blood flow studies have shown that basal ganglia volume and blood flow are reduced even before individuals become symptomatic with HD (Harris et al., 1999; Aylward et al., 2004; Paulsen et al., 2006; Leoni et al., 2008) and that widespread degeneration occurs in early and middle stages of HD (Rosas et al., 2003). Patients with the akinetic-rigid form of HD are more likely to show striatal hyperintensity on T2-weighted MRI than patients with the choreic form of HD (Oliva et al., 1993). Both neuroimaging and postmortem studies indicate that regional thinning of the cortical ribbon, particularly involving the sensorimotor region, is affected in early HD and "might provide a sensitive prospective surrogate marker for clinical trials of neuroprotective medications" (Rosas et al., 2002; Rosas et al., 2005). Altered cortex morphology with enlargement of gyral crowns and abnormally thin sulci were demonstrated using three-dimensional MRI, obtained in 24 subjects with preclinical HD and 24 matched healthy subjects (Nopoulos et al., 2007). The authors concluded that "These findings lend support to the notion that, in addition to the degenerative process, abnormal neural development may also be an important process in the pathoetiology of HD."

Using voxel-based MRI morphometry to identify differences between presymptomatic carriers and gene-negative controls, Thieben and colleagues (2002) found significant

reductions in the gray matter volume in the left striatum, bilateral insula, dorsal midbrain, and bilateral intraparietal sulcus in the gene carriers. Other techniques, such as real-time sonography, showed abnormalities not only in the caudate but also in the substantia nigra of patients with HD (Postert et al., 1999). Using tensor-based morphometry, Kipps and colleagues (2005) were able to demonstrated progression of gray matter atrophy in presymptomatic HD mutation carriers compared to controls. Certain MRI techniques focusing on the gray matter have allowed successful identification of presymptomatic HD gene mutation (Klöppel et al., 2009). Other imaging studies have suggested that myelin breakdown and changes in ferritin iron distribution underlie the regional toxicity and may be important in pathogenesis of HD (Bartzokis et al., 2007). Pre-HD individuals have been found to have lower gross gray matter and white matter volume, and voxel-wise analysis demonstrated local gray matter volume loss, most notably in regions consistent with basal ganglia-thalamocortical pathways, whereas pre-HD individuals showed widespread reductions in white matter integrity, probably due to a loss of axonal barriers (Stoffers et al., 2010). In another study, not only were the volumes of the caudate nucleus and putamen reduced in premanifest HD long before predicted onset (>10.8 years), but atrophy of the accumbens nucleus and pallidum was also apparent in premanifest HD (van den Bogaard et al., 2010). In addition, the 12-month whole-brain atrophy rates were greater in early HD individuals as well as premanifest gene-positive carriers (less than 10.8 years from predicted diagnosis compared with controls) (Tabrizi et al., 2011). All gene-positive groups also showed faster rates of caudate and putamen atrophy over 12 months compared with controls. The whole-brain and caudate atrophy rates were found to correlate with the UHDRS total functional capacity score and with cognitive and quantitative motor measures. While these studies are intriguing, it is, however, still too early to conclude that neuroimaging can be used as a surrogate marker in future trials of putative neuroprotective agents.

In addition to striatal atrophy shown by neuroimaging studies, a variety of techniques, such as ^{18}F-2-fluoro-2-deoxyglucose PET and SPECT, have been used to demonstrate hypometabolism and reduced regional cerebral blood flow in the basal ganglia and the cortex (Kuwert et al., 1990; Hasselbach et al., 1992; Harris et al., 1999). PET studies of presymptomatic HD carriers have shown initial (compensatory) thalamic hypermetabolism with subsequent decline heralding the onset of HD symptoms and signs in a setting of steady decline of striatal raclopride binding (Feigin et al., 2007).

Abnormalities in striatal metabolism measured by PET scans may precede caudate atrophy (Grafton et al., 1990). Regional cerebral metabolic rate of glucose consumption has been found to be decreased by 62% in the caudate, by 56% in the lenticular nucleus, and by 17% in the frontal cortex (Kuwert et al., 1990). Bilateral reduction in the uptake of technetium-99m HM-PAO and iodine-123 IMP in the caudate and putamen has been demonstrated by SPECT in patients with HD (Nagel et al., 1991). Using PET and [^{11}C] flumazenil binding to GABA receptors in the striatum, Künig and colleagues (2000) found marked reduction in the caudate (but not in the putamen) of HD patients compared to normal controls. The authors interpreted these findings as

Table 14.1 Huntington disease: neuropathology

Neuronal loss and gliosis in the cortex and striatum (caudate and putamen)

Early loss of medium-sized, spiny striatal neurons: SNc, GPe, SNr, GPi

Loss of large (17 to 44 μm) striatal interneurons

Loss (<40%) of neurons in SN

Intranuclear inclusions and dystrophic neurons in cortex and striatum

PATHOLOGY OF HD

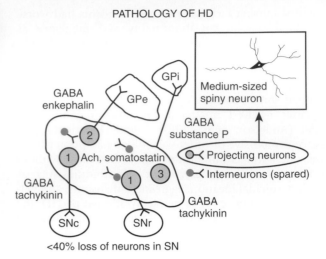

Figure 14.2 Pathologic changes associated with HD from the earliest stages (1) to more advanced stages (3). Ach, acetylcholine; GABA, gamma-aminobutyric acid.

indicative of compensatory GABA receptor upregulation in the striatal (putamen) GABAergic medium spiny neurons projecting to the pallidum. As microglial activation has been found to be correlated with neuronal degeneration, techniques designed to image microglial activation, such as [^{11}C] (R)-PK11195 (PK) PET, show that microglia activation correlates with severity of the disease (e.g., UHDRS score) and is inversely related to D2 density as demonstrated by raclopride PET studies (Pavese et al., 2006). Similar findings were reported in presymptomatic HD gene carriers who had lower striatal raclopride binding than the controls but significantly higher striatal and cortical PK binding (Tai et al., 2007). This study provided strong evidence that widespread microglial activation occurs even in preclinical stages of HD and that this early pathologic change correlates with striatal neuronal dysfunction (see below).

Neuropathology and neurochemistry

Pathologic studies have provided evidence for primary involvement of the basal ganglia–thalamocortical circuitry in HD (Joel, 2001). Postmortem changes in HD brains include neuronal loss and gliosis in the cortex and the striatum, particularly the caudate nucleus (Table 14.1). Morphometric analysis of the prefrontal cortex in HD patients reveals loss of cortical pyramidal cells, particularly in layers III, V, and VI (Sotrel et al., 1991). At the cortical level motor dysfunction seems to correlate with primary motor cortex cell loss whereas mood symptomatology is associated with cell loss in the cingulate cortex (Thu et al., 2010). Chorea seems to be related to the loss of medium spiny striatal neurons projecting to the lateral pallidum (GPe), whereas rigidakinetic symptoms correlate with the additional loss of striatal neurons projecting to the substantia nigra compacta (SNc) and medial pallidum (GPi) (Albin et al., 1990b; Albin, 1995). Pathologic studies have suggested that the earliest changes associated with HD consist of degeneration of the striato-SNc neurons followed by striato-GPe and striato-SNr neurons and finally striato-GPi neurons (Hedreen and Folstein, 1995; Albin, 1995) (Fig. 14.2). There appears to be a correlation between the number of CAG repeats and the severity of pathology; longer trinucleotide repeat length is associated with greater neuronal loss in the caudate and putamen (Furtado et al., 1996). In addition, significant association between pronounced mood dysfunction and loss of the GABA(A) receptor marker in striosomes of the striatum has been found in an autopsy study of 35 HD brains and 13 controls (Tippett et al., 2007). Increased density of oligodendrogliocytes and intranuclear inclusions was found in the tail of the caudate nucleus among presymptomatic HD gene

carriers, suggesting that pathologic changes occur long before the onset of symptoms (Gómez-Tortosa et al., 2001). In addition to neuronal loss in the basal ganglia, there is evidence of increased iron in this brain area as measured by MRI, which in part might contribute to the regional neurotoxicity (Bartzokis et al., 2007).

Using specific monoclonal antibodies against phosphorylated and nonphosphorylated neurofilaments and neuronal cell adhesion molecules, Nihei and Kowall (1992) found marked abnormalities in these cytoskeletal components in the striatal neurons of HD brains. The earliest degenerative changes, the loss of medium-sized spiny neurons containing calbindin, enkephalin, and substance P immunoreactivity, occur in the dorsomedial aspect of the caudate and putamen (Ferrante et al., 1991). The enkephalin neurons appear to die before the substance P neurons. In contrast, the spiny striatal cholinergic and somatostatin-containing interneurons are spared. As a result of these degenerative changes, the matrix zone of the striatum is reduced in size, while the patches (striosomes) remain unaltered. In one postmortem study, however, calbindin D28k mRNA in the striata of HD brains was normal, while the preproenkephalin neurons were markedly reduced in the HD caudate nucleus (Richfield et al., 1995). Another class of medium-sized (8–18 μm) striatal interneurons, characterized by intense immunostaining against calcium-binding protein calretinin, was found to be markedly increased in the striatum of brains of patients with HD compared to controls (Cicchetti and Parent, 1997). In contrast, the density of the larger, 17–44 μm, interneurons was markedly decreased. Since both populations of interneurons express calretinin, the implication of the findings of the study is that calretinin, for some as yet unknown reason, protects the medium-sized neurons but not the large neurons against HD-related degeneration.

Curtis and colleagues (2003) observed an interesting phenomenon in the brains of patients with HD. When they were compared to non-HD control brains, there was marked increase in cell proliferation in the subependymal layer, and the degree of cell proliferation increased with pathologic severity and increasing CAG repeats in the HD gene. These results suggest that progenitor cell proliferation and neurogenesis occur in the diseased adult human brain, providing further evidence for regeneration.

Huntingtin (Htt), the product of the HD gene (see below), is expressed throughout the brain in both affected and unaffected regions; therefore, its contribution to neurodegeneration in HD is unclear. Using quantitative in-situ hybridization methods, Landwehrmeyer and colleagues (1995) showed that the expression of *Htt* mRNA was not selectively increased in the neurons that were particularly susceptible to degeneration in HD. The authors suggested that this lack of correlation indicates that the gene mutation is not sufficient to produce the disease and that other factors probably also play a role in its pathogenesis. Since the mutated Htt is not limited to vulnerable neurons, other factors besides mutated Htt must play a role in the neuronal degeneration associated with HD (Gourfinkel-An et al., 1997). An immunohistochemical study showed that neuronal staining for Htt is reduced in the striatal medium-sized spiny neurons, but the large striatal neurons that are spared in HD retain normal levels of Htt (Sapp et al., 1997). Surprisingly, however, Htt staining was markedly reduced in both segments of the globus pallidus. This suggests a postsynaptic response to a reduction in striatal inputs; or it might indicate that the globus pallidus is for some yet unknown reason preferentially involved in HD.

N-terminal mutant Htt also binds to synaptic vesicles and inhibits their glutamate uptake in vitro (Li et al., 2000). Using a transgenic mouse model generated by introducing mutant polyQ tract into one of the mouse genes, Li and colleagues (2000) found aggregated Htt only in medium striatal neurons, neurons that are most susceptible to degeneration in HD. The aggregated Htt was first found in the neuronal nucleus and later in synaptic terminals. Scherzinger and colleagues (1999) found that the aggregation of Htt protein is time- and concentration-dependent, suggesting "a nucleation-dependent polymerization." Aggregation was proportional to repeat length, and no aggregation could be induced for a repeat length of 27 or fewer glutamines. This might in part explain the inverse correlation of repeat length and age at onset. Since the probability of neural death in HD with time is constant and since the age at onset is inversely dependent on the length of repeats, it has been suggested that the polyglutamine aggregates are toxic when directed to the nucleus and cause the cell death in HD (Yang et al., 2002). This is supported by the physics of protein aggregation as a result of transition to a new intramolecular configuration (Perutz and Windle, 2001).

The finding of neuronal intranuclear inclusions and dystrophic neurites in the two regions that are most affected in HD, the cortex and striatum, has revolutionized our understanding of the genetic-pathologic mechanisms of this heredodegenerative disorder (DiFiglia et al., 1997). Using an antiserum against the NH_2-terminus of Htt, DiFiglia and colleagues (1997) found intense labeling localized to neuronal intranuclear inclusions in brains of three juvenile and six adult cases of HD. These inclusions had an average diameter of 7.1 μm and were almost twice as large as the nucleolus. The neurons with these inclusions were found in all cortical layers and the medium-sized neurons of the striatum but not in the globus pallidus or the cerebellum. They were more frequent in juvenile HD, and in these cases, the

inclusions were found not only in the nuclei but also in the cytoplasm. The inclusions were not found in the cortex of one subject who had the HD gene but was still asymptomatic but were found in his striatum, thus providing evidence that these changes preceded clinical onset and might be critical in the pathogenesis of the disease. In addition, the investigators found spherical and slightly ovoid dystrophic neurites in cortical layers 5 and 6. None of the control brains demonstrated this finding, and antibodies raised against the internal site of Htt failed to differentiate the HD brains from those of controls. Subsequent studies showed that the NH_2-terminus of mutant Htt is cleaved by apopain and is ubiquitinated. Thus, ubiquitin staining can be also used to localize these inclusions. These inclusions are composed of granules, straight and tortuous filaments, and fibrils, and they are not membrane bound. Similar inclusions have been demonstrated in the HD transgenic mouse (Davies et al., 1997). Since the aggregates in the nucleus consist mostly of N-terminal fragments of the whole Htt protein, it has been postulated that the protein has to be cleaved before it enters the nucleus. Mutant Htt fragments accumulate in axon terminals and interfere with glutamate uptake (Li et al., 2000) and, as occurs in other polyglutamine disease, impair axonal transport (Szebenyi et al., 2003; Gunawardena and Goldstein, 2005). Using a yeast artificial chromosome transgenic mouse model of HD, Tang and colleagues (2005) found that repetitive application of glutamate elevates cytosolic Ca^{2+} levels in medium spiny neurons from the HD mouse but not from the wild-type or control mouse. They further found that the FDA-approved anticoagulant enoxaparin (Lovenox), a calcium blocker, the mitochondrial Ca^{2+} uniporter blocker ruthenium 360, and the dopamine depletor tetrabenazine (TBZ) (Tang et al., 2007) are neuroprotective. Thus, abnormal Ca^{2+} signaling seems to be directly linked with the degeneration of medium spiny neurons in the caudate nucleus in HD; therefore, calcium channel blockers could have a therapeutic potential for treatment of HD. Studies with the yeast artificial chromosome (YAC128) transgenic HD mouse model provide evidence for a connection between glutamate receptor activation, disturbed calcium (Ca^{2+}) signaling, and apoptosis of HD striatal neurons (Tang et al., 2005, 2007). Furthermore, glutamate and dopamine signaling pathways acting via D1 receptors induce elevation of Ca^{2+} signals and cause TBZ-induced striatal cell loss in these mice, suggesting potential neuroprotective effects of this dopamine depletor. Further support and mechanistic insight comes from studies using *Drosophila* that express expanded full-length human huntingtin and elevated intracellular Ca^{2+} levels (Romero et al., 2008). The increased Ca leads to increased neurotransmitter release, motor dysfunction, and progressive neuronal degeneration. Partially blocking Ca channel activity, or partially impairing neurotransmission, restores the Ca levels and motor dysfunction and suppresses neurodegeneration. Since the findings in *Drosophila* of altered Ca homeostasis are in agreement with the early observations by Tang et al. (2007) in mammalian systems, Ca channel blockers may be useful in HD patients.

While some studies have shown a moderate (40%) degree of neuronal degeneration in the substantia nigra, particularly noticeable in the medial and lateral thirds (Oyanagi et al., 1989), this is probably not sufficient to cause bradykinesia in either choreic or rigid-akinetic HD patients (Albin

Table 14.2 Huntington disease: neurotransmitters, peptides, and receptors

↓↓ CAT

↓↓ GABA, GAD

↓↓ enkephalin, substance-P, cholecystokinin, angiotensin, and met-enkephalin

↑ somatostatin, TRH, neurotensin, neuropeptide-Y

↓ Glutamate (↑ CSF glutamate)

↑↑ 3-hydroxyanthranilic acid oxidase, DA, GABA, cholinergic-muscarinic, and benzodiazepine receptors

↓↓ NMDA, ↓ phencyclidine and quisqualate receptors

CAT, choline acetyl transferase; DA, dopamine; GABA, gamma-aminobutyric acid; GAD, glutamic acid decarboxylase; NMDA, N-methyl-D-aspartate receptors; TRH, thyroid-releasing hormone.

et al., 1990a). Measurements of brain dopamine concentrations and cerebrospinal fluid (CSF) homovanillic acid levels have yielded conflicting results (Table 14.2). In one study, CSF homovanillic acid was normal in 51 patients with early HD, and there was no correlation between homovanillic acid levels and degree of parkinsonism (Kurlan et al., 1988). Dopamine, acetylcholine, and serotonin receptors are decreased in the striatum. Using PET imaging of dihydrotetrabenazine as a marker of striatal vesicular monoamine transporter (VMAT) type 2, Bohnen et al. (2000) found reduced binding especially in the posterior putamen, similar to Parkinson disease, particularly in patients with akinetic-rigid HD.

Postsynaptic loss of dopamine receptors might be responsible for the parkinsonian findings in some HD patients (Sánchez-Pernaute et al., 2000). Dopamine D2 receptors, imaged with iodobenzamide–SPECT, have provided evidence of D2 receptor loss in HD (Brucke et al., 1991). Using PET to measure binding of specific D1 and D2 receptor ligands in the striatum, Weeks and colleagues (1996) found that these two receptors are markedly decreased in individuals who have the HD mutation but who are still presymptomatic. In another study, Andrews and colleagues (1999) showed that loss of striatal D1 and D2 binding as determined by PET was significantly greater in the known mutation carriers than in the combined at-risk and gene-negative patients. Although some studies found that the loss of D2 receptors correlates significantly with motor and cognitive slowing (Sánchez-Pernaute et al., 2000), other studies failed to show any correlation between clinical and psychological assessments and the loss of striatal D2 receptors (Pavese et al., 2003). Turjanski and colleagues (1995) showed that HD patients with rigidity had more pronounced reduction of these receptors (also measured by PET) compared with HD patients without rigidity. Since D2 binding was normal in a patient with chorea associated with systemic lupus erythematosus, the authors concluded that the presence of chorea is not determined by alterations in striatal dopamine receptor binding.

Loss of the medium-sized spiny neurons, which normally constitute 80% of all striatal neurons, is associated with a marked decrease in GABA and enkephalin levels. After examining two brains of presymptomatic individuals carrying the HD gene, Albin and colleagues (1992) concluded that

striatal neurons projecting to the GPe and SN, but not those that project to the GPi, are preferentially involved in early stages of HD and even in the presymptomatic phase. Likewise, cannabinoid receptors are preferentially lost in the GPe (Blazquez et al., 2011). In contrast, the cholinergic and somatostatin striatal interneurons seem to be relatively spared in HD. Other neuropeptide alterations in HD include a decrease in substance P, cholecystokinin, and met-enkephalin and an increase in somatostatin, thyrotropin-releasing hormone, neurotensin, and neuropeptide Y. Prior to any clinical signs, in addition to the loss of cannabinoid receptors there is also loss of adenosine A2a receptor binding and increased GABA-A receptor binding in the GPe. As the disease progresses, there is typically loss of D1 receptors in the striatum as well as cannabinoid and D1 in the substantia nigra, eventually involving the rest of the basal ganglia. The preferential loss of enkephalinergic striatal neurons correlates with the appearance of chorea (Albin et al., 1992). Loss of substance P/dynorphin neurons correlates with the increase in dystonia in the later stages of disease (Table 14.2).

Evidence of immune activation not only of central microglia but also of the peripheral system is supported by the findings of increased levels of cytokines, such as interleukin 6 (IL-6) levels in HD gene carriers, with a mean of 16 years before the predicted onset of clinical symptoms (Björkqvist et al., 2008). The same study also found that monocytes from HD patients expressed mutant Htt. Autonomous immune activation was also noted in macrophages and microglia from HD mouse models, and in the CSF and striatum of HD patients. There are no reliable peripheral markers of HD, but 24S-hydroxycholesterol, previously found to be associated with neurodegeneration, has been found to be significantly decreased in patients in all stages of HD, although it was not different from controls among pre-manifest subjects, while caudate volume, as measured by MRI morphometry, was significantly decreased even in pre-HD subjects (Leoni et al., 2008). This is consistent with other MRI studies discussed earlier.

Although HD has been traditionally considered as a degenerative disease of the brain, mutant Htt is ubiquitously expressed throughout the body and HD is now recognized to be associated with abnormalities in peripheral tissues (van der Burg et al., 2009).

Genetics

For some time, HD has been regarded as truly an autosomal dominant disease in that homozygotes were thought to be no different from heterozygotes. However, subsequent studies have provided evidence that homozygotes (n = 8) have a more severe clinical course than that of heterozygotes (n = 75), even though the age at onset is similar (Squitieri et al., 2003). This suggests that the more rapid progression is a consequence of greater toxic effects because of doubling of mutated proteins and aggregate formation (see later). Linkage studies in HD families from various ethnic origins and countries have found that, despite the marked variability in phenotypic expression, genetic heterogeneity is unlikely. Localization of a gene marker near the tip of the short arm of chromosome 4 in 1983 by Gusella and colleagues (Gusella

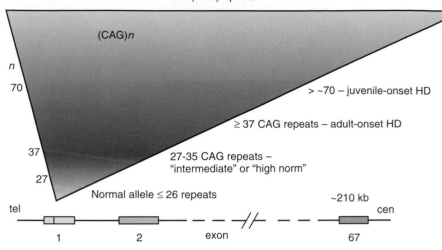

Huntingtin gene

Htt (IT15)-4p16.3

(CAG)*n*

n

70 — > ~70 – juvenile-onset HD

≥ 37 CAG repeats – adult-onset HD

37 —
27 — 27-35 CAG repeats –
"intermediate" or "high norm"

Normal allele ≤ 26 repeats

~210 kb

tel — cen

1   2   exon   67

Figure 14.3 Relationship between CAG repeats and age at onset.

et al., 1983) initiated an intensive search for the abnormal gene, which was finally cloned 10 years later (Bates et al., 1991; Pritchard et al., 1991; Wexler et al., 1991; Huntington's Disease Collaborative Research Group, 1993). The mutation that is responsible for the disease consists of an unstable enlargement of the CAG repeat sequence in the 5′ end of a large (210 kb) gene, *huntingtin (Htt)*, also called *IT15* (Huntington's Disease Collaborative Research Group, 1993). This gene, located at 4p16.3, contains 67 exons and encodes a previously unknown 348 kDa protein, named Htt, without homology to known protein sequences (Fig. 14.3). The expanded CAG repeat, located in exon 1, alters Htt by elongating a polyglutamine segment near the NH_2-terminus.

The study of HD, the prototype of trinucleotide repeat neurodegenerative diseases, has provided important insights into the pathogenesis of a growing number of disorders caused by accumulation of misfolded proteins (Everett and Wood, 2004). Whereas the number of repeats varies between 10 and 29 copies in unaffected individuals, the HD gene contains 36–121 of such repeats (Kremer et al., 1994). There are some alleles that do not cause HD in individuals carrying the allele but become unstable in the next generation. These alleles are termed *intermediate*, and their lower limit of CAG repeats might be as low as 27 (Nance, 1996). Of the 11 cases that lacked the triplet expansion, 5 had a prior history of Sydenham chorea during childhood, indicating the possibility of recurrence of autoimmune chorea. The intermediate-sized CAG repeats range from 27 to 35, but rare cases with CAG repeats in this range develop the full symptomatology of HD. One case, a 75-year-old man with 15-year history of the clinical manifestation of HD, was reported to have only 34 CAG repeats (Andrich et al., 2008). An autopsy-proven case of HD with only 29 CAG repeats has been reported (Kenney et al., 2007c; Kenney and Jankovic, 2008). We also studied a 50-year-old man with typical symptoms of HD since age 43 but without a family history of HD. His maternally derived allele had 17 CAG repeats, but his paternally derived allele had 45 CAG expands. His completely asymptomatic 80-year-old father and 76-year-old paternal uncle had 30 CAG repeats each. This patient indicates that a

relatively short expansion (of 30 CAG repeats) might be unstable, particularly if it is of paternal origin, and might spontaneously expand in successive generations resulting in so-called sporadic HD (Alford et al., 1996). Since that time several cases of HD phenotype with less than 36 CAG repeats have been described and the clinical, genetic, and prognostic implications of the "intermediate" CAG repeat range is currently being re-examined. To assist with genetic counseling in these subjects, Hendricks et al. (2009) estimated that the probability that a male with intermediate or "high normal" (27–35) CAG repeats in one allele will have an offspring with an expanded penetrant allele ranges from 1/6241 to 1/951. Besides DNA CAG length, larger somatic CAG repeat length expansions (somatic instability) is associated with earlier disease onset and probably more rapid progression (Swami et al., 2009).

Approximately 11% of patients with clinically suspected HD exhibit no family history of HD, and some of these patients might have "new" mutations (Goldberg et al., 1993; Davis et al., 1994). In a study of 28 patients with clinically probable HD, but without a family history of HD, 25 (89%) patients were confirmed by DNA testing to have HD, and 5 of 16 (31%) patients with clinically doubtful HD had expanded triplet repeats, confirming the diagnosis of HD (Davis et al., 1994).

Several studies have demonstrated that the number of repeats inversely correlates with the age at onset (anticipation) (Duyao et al., 1993; Snell et al., 1993; Ashizawa et al., 1994; Gusela and MacDonald, 1995; Furtado et al., 1996; Brinkman et al., 1997; Nance et al., 1997; Maat-Kievit et al., 2002; Marder et al., 2002; Ravina et al., 2008). Brinkman and colleagues (1997) retrospectively examined the relationship between CAG length and age at onset and found a 50% probability of developing HD symptoms by age 65 when the CAG repeat length is 39 and by age 30 when the CAG repeat length is 50. The inverse relationship between age of onset and number of CAG repeats was confirmed in a Dutch cohort of 755 affected patients (Maat-Kievit et al., 2002). The correlation was stronger for paternal inheritance than for maternal inheritance. CAG repeat length also inversely correlates with late-stage outcomes, such as nursing home admission and placement of percutaneous endoscopic gastrostomy (Marder et al., 2002). One analysis, based on the data from the CARE-HD trial, modeled progression over 30 months on UHDRS and concluded that 10 additional CAG repeats were associated with a 7.7 (63%) increase on the UHDRS total motor score and 9.2 (81%) points in progression on the Independence Scale (Ravina et al., 2008). One study showed that increasing CAG repeat size in normal *Htt* gene diminishes the association between mutant CAG repeat size and disease severity and progression in HD (Aziz et al., 2009).

The Huntington Study Group is conducting two studies to prospectively characterize the transition from health to illness (phenoconversion): (1) PHAROS (Pilot Huntington At Risk Observational Study) and (2) PREDICT (Predictors of Huntington Disease). Although some studies suggest a possible correlation between the length of CAG repeats and the rate of progression (Illarioshkin et al., 1994; Brandt et al., 1996; Antonini et al., 1998), other studies have found no correlation between the CAG repeats and progression (Ashizawa et al., 1994; Kieburtz et al., 1994; Claes et al., 1995) or between age at onset and progression of disease (Feigin et al., 1995). The rate of disease progression is generally faster in paternally transmitted HD independent of the CAG repeat length (Ashizawa et al., 1994). Because of the poor correlation between the number of CAG repeats and the rate of progression, some investigators have argued that the number of CAG repeats should not be disclosed to the patient or even to the physician. This may not, however, be practical and many patients insist on knowing the number of CAG repeats. We believe that (1) the CAG repeat size should be disclosed to appropriately informed physicians and counselors who take care of the patient, (2) appropriate training should be provided to inform physicians and counselors about the implications of the CAG repeat size in HD, and (3) information regarding the CAG repeat size should be disclosed to patients on the patient's request, given that appropriate counseling is made available to the patient (Jankovic et al., 1995). When appropriate genetic counseling and a multidisciplinary approach are used in presymptomatic testing, the risk of adverse events such as psychological distress and depression requiring hospitalization or leading to attempted suicide may be as low as 2% (no difference between carriers and noncarriers) (Goizet et al., 2002). Noninvasive prenatal diagnosis of HD was confirmed in three of four at-risk fetuses in whom the father was affected with HD by direct analysis of the cell-free fetal DNA in maternal plasma (Bustamante-Aragones et al., 2008).

There is no difference in the mean number of repeats between patients presenting with psychiatric symptoms and those with chorea and other motor disorders, although, as expected, the rigid juvenile patients have the largest number of repeats (MacMillan et al., 1993; Nance and the US Huntington Disease Genetic Testing Group, 1997). The trinucleotide repeat is relatively stable over time in lymphocyte DNA but may be unstable in sperm DNA. This appears to account for the marked increase in the number of trinucleotide repeats to offspring by affected fathers, leading to a 10:1 ratio of juvenile HD when the affected parent is the father. However, after isolating X- and Y-bearing sperm of HD transgenic mice, Kovtun and colleagues (2004) found that the

CAG distribution is the same as that in the founding fathers, suggesting that the "gender-dependent changes in CAG repeat length arise in the embryo."

Analyzing DNA for the expansion of respective trinucleotide repeats utilizing polymerase chain reaction and Southern blotting has provided the means for a reliable diagnostic test that does not require participation of other family members. Such a test is helpful not only in confirming the diagnosis in index cases, but also in clarifying the diagnosis in atypical cases and asymptomatic at-risk individuals. In one study, 4 of 15 tests on presymptomatic individuals using linkage analysis were positive for the HD gene (Meissen et al., 1988). While all the individuals with positive results experienced transient symptoms of depression, none reported suicidal ideation. One year after the results of gene testing were disclosed, both increased-risk and the decreased-risk individuals had overall no increase in depression or deterioration in psychological well-being (Wiggins et al., 1992). A high rate of suicidal ideation, however, was found in a Swedish study of 13 HD carriers and 21 noncarriers (Robins Wahlin et al., 2000). In another study of 171 presymptomatic gene carriers compared to 414 noncarriers, Kirkwood and colleagues (2000) found that the carriers performed significantly worse on the digit symbol, picture arrangement, and arithmetic subscales of the Weschler Adult Intelligence Scale–Revised and various movement and choice–time measures. Other studies have addressed the natural history and progression of HD in the early and middle stages (Kirkwood et al., 2001). An adjustment to results of testing appears to depend more on the individual's psychological makeup before the testing than on the testing itself (Meiser and Dunn, 2000). Because of potential psychological and legal implications of positive identification of a HD gene mutation in an asymptomatic, at-risk individual, predictive testing must be performed by a team of clinicians and geneticists who are not only knowledgeable about the disease and the genetic techniques, but also sensitive to the psychosocial and ethical issues associated with such testing. Although, as a result of the discovery of the HD gene, the cost of presymptomatic testing has been substantially reduced, the currently recommended extensive pretesting and posttesting counseling is still quite costly. An assessment of the cost–benefit ratio should be carried out. When the DNA test for HD became available, it was thought that demand for testing for HD in asymptomatic at-risk individuals would be high (Tyler et al., 1992), but recent studies have demonstrated a decline in the number of applicants (Maat-Kievit, et al., 2000). In one study only 3–4% of at-risk individuals have requested a presymptomatic test, and requests for prenatal diagnosis are rare (Lacone et al., 1999).

Important insights into the potential function of Htt have been gained by the study of various mouse models in which the HD homolog gene was inactivated (knock-out models) (Duyao et al., 1995) or expanded CAG repeats are introduced into the mouse hypoxanthine phosphoribosyltransferase gene (knock-in models) (Reddy et al., 1999). Homozygous inactivation resulted in embryonic death, suggesting that Htt is critical for early embryonic development. Since this model does not mimic adult HD and homozygote individuals apparently are indistinguishable from heterozygotes, it suggests that the HD gene mutation involves "gain" rather than "loss" in function. This hypothesis, however, has been challenged because the earlier studies suggesting no phenotypic difference between heterozygous and homozygous HD were based on linkage studies and focused predominantly on the age at onset (Cattaneo et al., 2001). Furthermore, homozygous transgenic mice expressing mutant Htt cDNA have a shorter lifespan than that of heterozygous mice. This suggests that either a double-dose of mutant Htt or loss of the normal allele (loss of function) contributes to the disease. Either wild-type or mutant Htt is needed for normal brain development. Huntingtin is associated with vesicle membranes and microtubules and as such probably has a role in endocytosis, intracellular trafficking, and membrane recycling. Thus, HD appears to result from a new toxic property of the mutant protein (gain of function) and loss of neuroprotective activity of the normal Htt (loss of function) (Cattaneo et al., 2001; Borrell-Pagès et al., 2006).

There are currently three types of HD transgenic mouse models: (1) mice expressing fragments, usually one or two exons of the human *huntingtin* gene that contain the polyglutamine expansion (R6/2 and N-171-82Q mice); (2) transgenic mice expressing the full-length human *huntingtin* gene with expanded polyglutamine tract (YAC128 mice); and (3) knock-in mice with pathogenic CAG repeats inserted into the existing CAG expansion (*Hdh*QIII) (Hersch and Ferrante, 2004). Interestingly, the more genetically accurate the model, the more variable and subtle is the phenotype. Thus, the fragment models are used more frequently for therapeutic research, and these studies are then confirmed in the full-length models. Full-length Htt, when expressed in transgenic mice, does not appear to produce neurologic disease, but only the shortened or truncated form of the protein appears to be toxic to neuronal cells. Except for the mouse model that expresses the full-length *Htt* gene with 72 CAG repeats and displays selective striatal pathology at 12 months of age (Hodgson et al., 1999), all transgenic-mouse cell lines develop intranuclear inclusions and neurodegeneration in widespread areas of the brain. Using viral-vector-mediated expression, several investigators have been able to produce aggregates starting within 5 days after transduction and associated with striatal degeneration in rats and even in primates (Kirik and Bjorklund, 2003). Formation of inclusions correlated with longer CAG expansions and shorter protein fragments. Overexpression of a short fragment of Htt, carrying 82 glutamine repeats, in the putamen produced progressive dyskinesia and putaminal intranuclear aggregates and striatal degeneration (Regulier et al., 2003). Although intranuclear inclusions in HD are traditionally thought to be neurotoxic, recent studies provide evidence that they are actually neuroprotective (Arrasate et al., 2004). Using a robotic microscope imaging system that can follow the survival of individual neurons over several days, the authors found that neuronal death was related to the length of polyglutamine expansions in the Htt protein, not to the increase in size or number of inclusion bodies. Therefore, this study suggests that the inclusions protect neurons by reducing the levels of toxic diffuse forms of mutant Htt. Furthermore, compounds that promote the formation of inclusions lessen the pathology of HD (Bodner et al., 2006).

The R6/2 transgenic mouse line has been studied most extensively (Mangiarini et al., 1999; Ona et al., 1999). These mice develop normally until 5–7 weeks of age, when they start manifesting irregular gait, abrupt shuddering movements, and resting tremors, followed by epileptic seizures, muscle wasting, and premature death at 14–16 weeks. Striatal neurons show ubiquitinated neuronal inclusions, similar to those seen in the brains of patients with HD. Analysis of glutamate receptors in symptomatic 12-week-old R6/2 mice revealed decreases compared with age-matched littermate controls (Cha et al., 1998). Other neurotransmitter receptors that are known to be affected in HD were also decreased in R6/2 mice, including dopamine and muscarinic cholinergic, but not gamma-aminobutyric acid (GABA) receptors. D1-like and D2-like dopamine receptor binding was drastically reduced to one-third of control in the brains of 8- and 12-week-old R6/2 mice. Altered expression of neurotransmitter receptors precedes clinical symptoms in R6/2 mice and may contribute to subsequent pathology. Biochemical analysis at 12 weeks shows a marked reduction in striatal aconitase (Tabrizi et al., 2000), indicative of damage by superoxide (O_2) and peroxynitrite ($ONOO^-$), similar to human HD (Tabrizi et al., 1999). In addition, the R6/2 transgenic mouse has a marked reduction in striatal and cortical mitochondrial complex IV activity and increased immunostaining for inducible nitric oxide synthase and nitrotyrosine (Tabrizi et al., 2000). Since these changes occur before evidence of neuronal death, the described findings suggest that mitochondrial dysfunction and free radical damage play an important role in the pathogenesis of HD. Indeed, mutant Htt has been found to attach to the outer mitochondrial membrane, causing the mitochondria permeability transition pores to open, allowing an influx of calcium and releasing cytochrome c (Choo et al., 2004). N171 mice, in which the transgene is driven by the prion promoter, have been used also as models of HD, but they have not been subjected to as rigorous examination as the R6/2 mice. In another study mice in which the *PGC-1a* gene had been knocked out developed brain lesions in the striatum and PGC-1α levels in those particular neurons were much lower among mice with the HD mutation than in normal mice (Cui et al., 2006). Since PGC-1α is involved in energy metabolism, this study shows that transcriptional repression of PGC-1α leads to mitochondrial dysfunction and supports other studies suggesting that energy deficits contribute to neurodegeneration in HD (Ross and Thompson, 2006). One study of polymorphism in *PGC-1a* gene in over 400 individuals with HD concluded that PGC-1α (which is inhibited by mutant Htt) has a small modifying effect on the progression of HD (Taherzadeh-Fard et al., 2009). In addition to the mouse models, there are several *Drosophila* models (Zoghbi and Botas, 2002). These are now being utilized to better understand the pathogenic mechanisms of HD-related neurodegeneration and for testing drugs that might have a potential for favorably modifying the disease (Agrawal et al., 2005; Imarisio et al., 2008). For example, expanded full-length Htt (128QHtt) mutant *Drosophila* exhibit behavioral, neurodegenerative, and electrophysiologic phenotypes, thought to be caused by a Ca^{2+}-dependent increase in neurotransmitter release (Romero et al., 2008). According to this study and in contrast to previous belief, the expanded protein does not have to be cleaved to be neurotoxic. Since partial loss of function in synaptic transmission (syntaxin, Snap, Rop) and voltage-gated Ca^{2+} channel genes suppresses both the electrophysiologic and the neurodegenerative phenotypes, it has been postulated that increased neurotransmission plays a key role in the neuronal degeneration caused by expanded CAG repeats in human HD.

In addition to the sub-primate models, progress is being made in developing a transgenic model of HD in a rhesus macaque monkey that expresses polyglutamine-expanded *Htt* (Yang et al., 2008; Wang et al., 2008a). The primate model was produced by injecting 130 mature rhesus oocytes with high titer of lentiviruses expressing *Htt* gene exon1 with 84 CAG repeats and green fluorescent protein (GFP) gene. After a transfer or 30 embryos into 6 surrogates, 5 liveborns were delivered at full term, including two sets of twins. Unfortunately, only one monkey survived one month and the others died at birth or shortly thereafter. The monkey that survived one month presumably demonstrated chorea and dystonia 2 days after birth, but these involuntary movements are difficult to characterize in infants. Brain autopsy showed abundant distribution of transgenic Htt in the cortex and striatum and nuclear inclusions and neuropil aggregates. Similar to the HD mouse models, which demonstrate more severe phenotypes, the transgenic monkeys expressing exon1 *Htt* with a 147-glutamine repeat (147Q) died early and showed abundant neuropil aggregates in swelling neuronal processes (Wang et al., 2008a).

Pathogenesis

Multiple processes have been postulated to relate CAG expansion to neurodegeneration, including aberrant interaction between the mutant Htt and transcriptional factors and coactivators (Anderson et al., 2008; Ross and Tabrizi, 2011) (Fig. 14.4). For example, aberrant interaction with histone acetyltransferase interferes with acetylation and deacetylation of histones. Abnormal histone deacetylation, catalyzed by histone deacetylases, leads to tightly packed chromatin structure and transcriptional repression. Histone deacetylase inhibitors have been suggested as potential treatment

strategies in HD and other neurodegenerative disorders (Chuang et al., 2009). Mutant Htt has been also shown to abnormally interact with histone acetyltransferases interfering with acetylation of histone proteins and also leading to transcriptional repression. Decreasing transcriptional activation by abnormal interaction between mutant Htt and the transcription factor cAMP-response element binding protein (CREB)-binding protein (CBP), a mediator of cell survival signals containing a short polyglutamine stretch, is another mechanism of cell death (Nucifora et al., 2001; Mantamadiotis et al., 2002). CBP is a coactivator for the transcription factor CREB linking DNA-binding proteins to RNA polymerase II transcription complex and functioning in histone acetyltransferase complex. By recruiting CREB into cellular aggregates, the mutant Htt prevents it from participating as a coactivator in CREB-mediated transcription, supporting the toxic gain-of-function mechanism of cell death in HD. The polyglutamine-containing domain of abnormal Htt protein directly binds the acetyltransferase domains of CBP and p300/CBP-associated factor (P/CAF) (Steffan et al., 2001). This reduces acetyltransferase activity and decreases acetylation of histones, proteins that package DNA. This in turn results in a decrease in gene transcription. Therefore, histone-deacetylase inhibitors could prevent HD-related neurodegeneration. Indeed, inhibition of histone deacetylase by sodium butyrate has been shown to partially protect HD R6/2 mice from neurodegeneration and against 3-nitropropionic acid neurotoxicity (Ferrante et al., 2003). According to current understanding, an inhibitor of κB kinase-mediated phosphorylation of the amino terminus of huntingtin targets mutant huntingtin into the nucleus, where it interferes with gene transcription (Krainc et al., 2010a, 2010b). When acetylated by CBP, mutant huntingtin is transported into autophagosomes for degradation, but mutant huntingtin that is not cleared accumulates in the nucleus and cytoplasm in the form of inclusions. Thus, recent neuroprotective strategies focus on increasing phosphorylation or acetylation of the mutant huntingtin to improve its clearance and reduce its neuronal toxicity. Several studies have

HD PATHOGENESIS

Figure 14.4 Possible pathogenic mechanisms of HD.

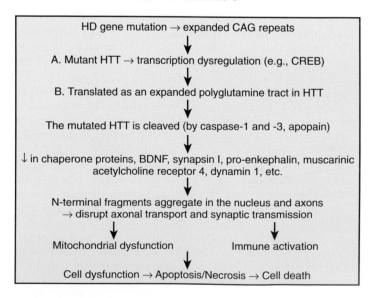

demonstrated impaired autophagy in animal models of HD, suggesting that inefficient engulfment of cytosolic components by autophagosomes may contribute to the HD-related neurodegeneration (Martinez-Vicente et al., 2010).

Transcriptional dysregulation as a pathogenic mechanism of neurodegeneration in HD has been also suggested by the study by Dunah and colleagues (2002), which showed that Htt interacts with the transcriptional activator Sp1 and coactivator TAFII130. Sp1, the first of many transcriptional activators isolated from human cells, binds to GC-box on the promoter region of DNA. It contains glutamine-rich activation domains that selectively bind to core components of the transcriptional machinery, such as the TAFII13 subunit of TFIID, which contains TATA-box-binding protein and multiple TATA-box-binding protein-associated factors. Therefore, one of the earliest steps in the development of HD may involve deregulation of specific transcriptional programs as suggested by Dunah and colleagues (2002), who demonstrated that mutant Htt inhibited Sp1 binding to DNA in postmortem brain tissues of both presymptomatic and affected HD patients. As a result, the RNA polymerase II is not able to locate the dopamine D2 receptor promoter region, and the gene cannot be transcribed (Freiman and Tjian, 2002).

It has been postulated that the common theme linking all the diseases pathogenetically with polyglutamine-tract expansion is that the various proteins (e.g., Htt, atrophin, androgen receptor, and ataxins), as a result of an increase in size of their intrinsic polyglutamine sequences, accumulate in the nucleus, forming insoluble amyloid-like fibrils and then somehow interfere with normal cellular metabolism (Davies et al., 1998). Proteolytic cleavage of a glutathione-S-transferase-Htt fusion protein results in spontaneous formation of insoluble aggregates. The aggregate formation is directly related to Htt and polyglutamine length; a polyglutamine tract of 51 glutamines or longer results in these aggregates (Scherzinger et al., 1997; Martindale et al., 1998). It has been hypothesized that after the expanded CAG repeat in the HD gene is transcribed in the Htt mRNA and then translated as an expanded polyglutamine tract in Htt, the mutated protein is cleaved (e.g., by caspase, apopain). This, the earliest step in the pathogenesis of HD, is followed by the liberation of polyglutamine-containing fragments, which are linked by transglutaminase to other proteins containing lysine residues, resulting in formation of perinuclear aggregates, eventually leading to neuronal apoptosis (Bates, 2003). The formation of inclusions, however, is not required for the initiation of cell death; in fact, neuronal intranuclear inclusions might have a protective role (Saudou et al., 1998). Kuemmerle and colleagues (1999) found that aggregate formation occurs predominantly in spared striatal interneurons rather than in the spiny neurons that are typically affected in HD. Thus, Htt aggregates do not predict neuronal death and might actually protect against polyglutamine-induced neurotoxicity. Several lines of evidence suggest that the expanded polyglutamine fragment of mutant Htt decreases protein degradation by the proteasome (Martin, 1999; Bence et al., 2001). The protein aggregates appear to be simultaneously inhibitors of the ubiquitin-proteasome system and the products that result from its inhibition. Arfaptin 2 has been shown to promote Htt protein aggregation, possibly by impairing proteasome function (Peters et al., 2002).

Aggregating proteins besides Htt, including α-synuclein, tau, mutant SOD1, and mutant ubiquitin, inhibit proteasome function (Cookson, 2004). In addition to the brain, proteasomal dysfunction has been demonstrated in the skin fibroblasts of patients with HD (Seo et al., 2004). In the striatum, however, dysfunction of the proteasomal system correlated with neuronal pathology and decreased levels of brain-derived neurotrophic factor (BDNF), which is normally upregulated by wild-type Htt; decreased mitochondrial complex II/III activity; and increased levels of ubiquitin (Seo et al., 2004).

Abnormal clearance of mutant Htt due to impaired phosphorylation, which normally tags certain amino acids with phosphates for destruction by the cellular waste handling systems, proteasomes and lysosomes, is increasingly recognized as an important mechanism of cell loss in HD and in other neurodegenerative disorders. Htt is phosphorylated by the inflammatory kinase IKK, which regulates additional posttranslational modifications, including Htt ubiquitination, sumoylation, and acetylation, and increases Htt nuclear localization, cleavage, and clearance mediated by lysosomal-associated membrane protein 2A (LAMP-2A) and Hsc70 (Thompson et al., 2009). The mutant Htt interferes with proteasome activity and lysosomal degradation becomes impaired, partly as a result of age-related reduction of the LAMP-2A. Furthermore, impaired phosphorylation on serines 13 and 16 of the N-terminal 17 amino acids of Htt has been demonstrated to impair clearance of mutated Htt, but genetic engineering to either mimic phosphorylation (phosphomimetic) or resist it (phosphoresistant) in mice prevented formation of Htt clumps (Gu et al., 2009). Thus these and other studies show that uncleared mutant Htt and Htt fragments can accumulate and become toxic by interfering with cellular function and axonal transport.

The impairment of proteasomal degradation of mutant Htt leads to caspase-mediated apoptosis (Jana et al., 2001). Jana and colleagues (2001), for example, found "massive accumulation" of polyubiquitinated mutant, but not normal, Htt after 2 days of expression in mouse neural cells, indicating lack of proteasomal processing of the mutant protein. Decline of proteasomal activity with time in the soluble fraction of the cell and an increase in the insoluble portion correlated with increased accumulation of proteasomal components in cell aggregates. The expression of mutant Htt (or inhibition of proteasomes with lactacystin) was associated with activation of caspases and release of mitochondrial cytochrome c, indicators of apoptosis. Studies have demonstrated that wild-type Htt upregulates transcription of cortically derived BDNF (Zuccato et al., 2001). Thus, a decrease in BDNF appears to play an important role in the pathology and pathogenesis of HD by causing dysfunction of striatal enkephalinergic neurons (Canals et al., 2004; Cattaneo et al., 2005). Furthermore, since wild-type Htt has been found to transport BDNF, it is not surprising that mutated Htt interferes with intracellular transport of this trophic factor (Gauthier et al., 2004). This suggests that as a result of mutated Htt in HD, there is insufficient neurotrophic support for striatal neurons and that treatment with BDNF might possibly restore or rescue the damaged striatal neurons. Rapamycin, an antibiotic that acts as a specific inhibitor of mTOR, a kinase that regulates important cellular processes, has been found to attenuate Htt accumulation and cell death in cell models of HD, possibly by enhancing the clearance of proteins that abnormally accumulate and aggregate in the cytoplasm (Ravikumar et al., 2004). Therefore, drugs such as rapamycin might play a role also in other neurodegenerative diseases that result from accumulation of unwanted protein aggregates.

Htt also interacts with chaperone proteins that unfold the expanded mutant Htt protein, preventing the aggregate formation in a cell culture model (Jana et al., 2001). Studies have shown that processing of polyglutamine-containing proteins by proteases (e.g., caspases) liberates truncated fragments with expanded polyglutamine tracts that can form aggregates through hydrogen bonding or transglutaminase activity and may be toxic to the cell. Abnormalities in proteasome function are associated with altered expression of stress-response proteins or heat-shock proteins that function as chaperones. The chaperones normally maintain proteins in an appropriate conformation and denature misfolded proteins (aggregates) (Kobayashi and Sobue, 2001). Overexpression of these chaperone proteins protects cells from toxicity induced by Htt with expanded polyglutamines (Jana et al., 2001; Kobayashi and Sobue, 2001). It has been postulated that the mutant Htt with an expanded polyglutamine tract, which is resistant to proteasome-mediated protein processing, overloads the proteasome machinery, enhancing the pathogenic effects of mutant Htt. Since truncated proteins that contain the expanded polyglutamine tract appear to be more toxic than the full-length protein, blocking proteolytic processing, aggregation, and nuclear uptake might be reasonable therapeutic strategies.

To examine the possible role of caspase-1, a cysteine protease that is important in regulating apoptosis, in the pathogenesis of cell death associated with HD, Ona and colleagues (1999) crossbred R6/2 with a transgenic mouse expressing dominant-negative mutant of caspase-1 in the brain. The inhibition of caspase-1 delayed the disease onset by 7.3 days and prolonged survival by 20.4 days. Furthermore, it significantly delayed the appearance of neuronal inclusions and neurotransmitter alterations. Although abnormal protein aggregation has been postulated to play an important role in the pathogenesis of HD, DiFiglia and colleagues (Kim et al., 1999) showed that aggregation was not intimately involved in cell death. While general inhibitors of caspases prolonged cell life, they did not alter aggregation, whereas specific caspase 3 inhibitors inhibited aggregation but had no effect on survival. Thus, continuous influx of the mutant protein is required to maintain inclusions. To determine whether caspase cleavage of Htt is a key event in the selective neurodegeneration in HD, Graham et al. (2006) found that mice expressing mutant Htt, resistant to cleavage by caspase-6 but not caspase-3, maintained normal neuronal function and did not develop striatal neurodegeneration and were protected against neurotoxicity induced by multiple stressors including NMDA, quinolinic acid, and staurosporine. These findings suggest that proteolysis of Htt at the caspase-6 cleavage site is critical for neurodegeneration in HD, which is enhanced by excitotoxicity. This and other studies provide strong evidence that caspases are important in the pathogenesis of cell death in HD and other neurodegenerative diseases.

The finding that N-methyl-D-aspartate (NMDA) receptors are markedly reduced in the putamen and cerebral cortex was the first clue that suggested an NMDA-mediated excitotoxicity as a mechanism of neuronal degeneration in HD (Young et al., 1988; Tabrizi et al., 1999). In addition to the 92% reduction in NMDA binding, phencyclidine binding was reduced by 67% and quisqualate by 55% in the same HD brains. The NMDA receptor density was decreased by 50% in the brain of a presymptomatic HD gene carrier, suggesting that the loss of the excitatory receptors occurred early in the course of the disease (Albin et al., 1990b). In contrast to the study by Young and colleagues (1988), no single excitatory amino acid receptor was selectively affected. Using quantitative in-vitro autoradiography, Dure and colleagues (1991) found a 50–60% reduction in binding sites of all the major excitatory receptors (NMDA, MK-801, glycine, kainate, and AMPA) in the caudate nucleus of HD brains. Furthermore, as was noted earlier, mutated Htt protein might interfere with vesicular glutamate uptake and thus contribute to excitotoxicity (Li et al., 2000).

In support of the excitotoxic theory is the observation that certain excitatory neurotoxins produce useful animal models of HD. Although the activity of 3-hydroxyanthranilic acid oxidase, the synthesizing enzyme for quinolinic acid, is markedly increased in the striatum of HD brains (Schwarcz et al., 1988), the concentration of quinolinic acid, an NMDA agonist, in the CSF and brains of patients with HD is normal (Heyes et al., 1991). Nevertheless, intrastriatal injections of quinolinic acid preferentially damage the medium-sized spiny neurons containing calbindin Dk28, enkephalin, and substance P, the very same neurons that degenerate in HD (Beal et al., 1991a; Ferrante et al., 1993). The striatal patch-matrix pattern closely resembles that seen in HD. Pretreatment with MK-801, a noncompetitive NMDA antagonist, protects the striatum from the quinolinic acid neurotoxicity. Despite neuronal loss and astrogliosis, the axons are spared, which might account for relatively normal dopamine, norepinephrine, and serotonin levels. GABA levels are markedly decreased in the GPe of these animals, similar to HD, indicating early loss of GABA afferents from the striatum to the GPe in both HD and the experimental model. In addition to pathologic and biochemical similarities between this animal model and HD, the animals also exhibit choreic movements. In addition to quinolinic acid, another excitotoxin that has been implicated in the pathogenesis of HD is glutamate. The observation that glutamate levels are decreased in the striatum of HD brains has been interpreted to be a result of chronic failure of the normal reuptake mechanism for glutamate released from the corticostriatal afferent terminals (Perry and Hansen, 1990). The resulting increase in concentration of glutamate at synapses might cause damage to the striatal neurons. The increased extracellular glutamate might also explain the finding of increased CSF glutamate in some patients with HD. Additional support for the excitotoxic theory of HD is provided by the observation that a lesion with the excitotoxin ibotenic acid, a glutaric acid agonist, in a striatum of the baboon produces behavioral and neuropathologic changes similar to those seen in patients with HD (Hantraye et al., 1990).

One hypothesis of mechanisms of cell death in HD is that a defect in mitochondrial energy metabolism makes certain neurons more vulnerable to the excitotoxic effects of endogenous glutamate (Beal, 1992; Bossy-Wetzel et al., 2008). It has been postulated that mutant Htt might cause mitochondrial dysfunction by either interfering with transcription of nuclear-encoded mitochondrial proteins or by causing damage directly to the mitochondria and interfering with Ca^{2+} buffering or mitochondria membrane potential (Bossy-Wetzel et al., 2008). Panov and colleagues (2002) showed that lymphoblast mitochondria from patients with HD and brain mitochondria from transgenic HD mice have a lower membrane potential and depolarize at lower calcium loads than mitochondria from controls. Since this defect preceded the onset of pathologic or behavioral abnormalities by months, the authors concluded that "mitochondrial calcium abnormalities occur early in HD pathogenesis and may be a direct effect of mutant Htt on the organelle." Intrastriatal injections of inhibitors of oxidative phosphorylation, such as amino oxyacetic acid or MPP+, or a systemic administration of 3-nitropropionic acid (3-NP), a mitochondrial poison, into animals produce even more striking resemblance to HD than when "pure" excitotoxins are used (Beal et al., 1991b; Storey et al., 1992; Brouillet et al., 1993; Beal et al., 1993). Studies have shown that 3-NP induces striatal neurodegeneration via c-Jun N-terminal kinase/c-Jun module (Garcia et al., 2002). Accidental ingestion of 3-NP has resulted in putaminal necrosis and delayed onset of dystonia and chorea in humans (Ludolph et al., 1991). The age-dependent neurotoxicity of 3-NP, demonstrated by increased striatal lactate levels in the older animals, appears to be related to the effect of 3-NP on energy metabolism. Severe defects have been demonstrated in the activities particularly of complexes II and III in the caudate nuclei of HD patients (Gu et al., 1996; Tabrizi et al., 1999). Using spectrophotometric techniques, Browne and colleagues (1997) found 29% and 67% reductions in the activity of the complex II to III in the caudate and putamen of HD brains, respectively. In addition, there was a 62% reduction in the complex IV activity. This finding provides further support for the potential role of oxidative damage in the pathogenesis of HD. The possibility that mitochondrial function is impaired in HD is supported by the observation of 5-fold to 11-fold increase in cortical mitochondrial DNA deletion in the brains of HD patients (Horton et al., 1995). Dichloroacetate, which stimulates pyruvate dehydrogenase complex, has been found to increase survival and improve motor function and prevent striatal atrophy in R6/2 and N171-82Q transgenic mouse models of HD (Andreassen et al., 2001). A "toxic-oxidation cycle" has been proposed as an important mechanism in neurodegeneration associated with HD (Kovtun et al., 2007). According to this hypothesis the accumulation of DNA oxidized bases, as a result of impaired function of the repair enzyme 7,8-dihydro-8-oxogunaine-DNA glycosylate (OGG1), overwhelms the repair machinery in the genome with generation of single-strand breaks (SSB), ultimately leading to further CAG expansion and neuronal death.

Defects in mitochondrial oxidative phosphorylation have been postulated to decrease cellular ATP production, resulting in a concomitant decrease in sodium-potassium ATPase activity and partial membrane depolarization. Under normal circumstances, the NMDA receptor-associated channels are blocked by a voltage-dependent Mg^{2+} system that pumps Mg^{2+} out of the cell. As a result of decreased ATPase activity, caused by the inhibition of oxidative phosphorylation, the normal resting potential cannot be maintained, resulting in the opening of the channel and influx of calcium. This triggers a cascade of events leading to a production of free radicals and associated oxidative damage to various cellular elements. Thus, as a result of inhibition of oxidative phosphorylation, even low levels of excitatory amino acids become toxic, a process that is referred to as slow excitotoxicity. More recent studies provide evidence that HD is associated with transcriptional dysregulation associated with interference in transcription mediated by Sp1 and CREB-binding protein (CBP) coupled with mitochondrial impairment due to reduced activity of peroxisome proliferator-activated receptor-γ coactivator 1α (PGC-1α), which regulates the expression of many nuclear-encoded mitochondrial proteins and proteins that provide protection against reactive oxygen species (ROS) (Greenamyre, 2007).

It has been suggested that in HD, as a result of prolonged excitatory neurotransmission, certain neurons become "exhausted" and switch from aerobic to anaerobic glycolytic metabolism, leading to the production and accumulation of lactate. Increased lactate concentration in the cerebral cortex of patients and animal models of HD, postulated to be due to global cerebral energy failure, has been demonstrated by proton magnetic resonance spectroscopy (Jenkins et al., 1998). Subsequently ^{1}H magnetic resonance spectroscopy was used to measure N-acetylaspartate, creatine, and choline, and a reduction in these markers correlated well with the progression of the disease and with striatal atrophy (Sánchez-Pernaute et al., 1999). Administration of agents that improve energy metabolism, such as CoQ10 and nicotinamide, might protect animals against toxicity produced by malonate, a complex II inhibitor (Beal et al., 1994). Using ^{31}P magnetic resonance spectroscopy to measure lactate in the muscle and ^{1}H magnetic resonance spectroscopy to measure lactate in the basal ganglia and the cortex, Koroshetz and colleagues (1997) showed that treatment with CoQ10 was associated with a significant decrease in cortical lactate concentrations in patients with HD. There is, however, no evidence that this biochemical change is in any way associated with clinical improvement or slowing of disease progression. Furthermore, increased lactate could not be confirmed by other studies (Hoang et al., 1998). A National Institutes of Health-sponsored multicenter study designed to evaluate the efficacy of CoQ10 and remacemide, an NMDA antagonist, is currently being conducted by the Huntington Study Group (see later).

The obvious question still to be answered is how the mutation in the HD gene leads to selective damage of certain neuronal populations. One explanation is that there are certain genes or proteins that are uniquely expressed in the striatum and cortex making these structures particularly vulnerable to neurodegeneration. For example, the *CalDAG-GEFI* gene has been found to be markedly downregulated in the brains of individuals with HD as well as in mouse models of the disease (Crittenden et al., 2010). By following mutant mice for up to 9 months, the investigators showed that this reduction occurs gradually, in parallel with the progression of the disease and when they blocked the expression of the gene using siRNA, the striatal neurons were protected from Htt-induced damage. Thus, the striking downregulation of CalDAG-GEFI in HD could be a protective mechanism against mutant Htt (mHtt), but even switching off of the gene is eventually unsuccessful, resulting in the striatal neurodegeneration.

There is a growing body of evidence to support the notion that neurodegeneration in HD is due to abnormal interaction between mutant Htt and transcription factors and other proteins interfering with normal transcriptional regulation (Paulson and Fischbeck, 1996; Roses, 1996; Anderson et al., 2008). One of the most provocative clues to the selective vulnerability of neuronal damage in HD was provided initially by Li and colleagues (1995). These investigators identified a protein, called Htt-associated protein (HAP1), that specifically binds to Htt. Subsequent studies have demonstrated that HAP1 and Htt are anterogradely transported in axons. HAP1 normally interacts with kinesin light chain, a subunit of the kinesin motor complex that drives anterograde transport along microtubules, and it links to transport proteins such as growth factor receptor tyrosine kinase (TrkA) (Rong et al., 2006). However, when mutant Htt is present HAP1 is unable to carry out its trafficking function, leading to degeneration of nerve terminals. Other Htt-interacting proteins have been identified, such as glyceraldehyde-3-phosphate dehydrogenase (GAPDH), HAP1, HIP14, apopain, α-adaptin, ubiquitin, calmodulin, and PSD95 (Reddy et al., 1999; Young, 2003; Yanai et al., 2006). The Htt protein might also interact with clathrin and adaptor protein-2, which are involved in endocytosis and other proteins (Li and Li, 2004). The small guanine nucleotide-binding protein, Rhes (Ras homolog enriched in striatum), which is localized to the striatum and to much lesser extent in the cortex, but not in the cerebellum, binds physiologically to mHtt and leads to selective cytotoxicity (Subramaniam et al., 2009). The mechanism of the cytotoxicity is not clear, but Rhes has been shown to markedly decrease aggregation of mHtt, presumably by Rhes-mediated sumoylation which involves binding of the small ubiquitin-like modifier (SUMO) to the mHtt. Thus, Rhes-elicited disaggregation of mHtt probably accounts for the localized neuropathology of HD in the striatum and to lesser extent in the cortex. Therefore, drugs that block the binding of Rhes to mHtt may exert neuroprotective effects in HD.

There are many other Htt interacting proteins, identified with high-throughput screening, that may modify polyglutatime neurotoxicity leading to neurodegeneration (Kaltenbach et al., 2007). The long tract of glutamines in mutant HD protein weakens the interaction with Htt-associated protein, which is then free to bind the protein Hippi and activate apoptosis through caspase-8 and caspase-3. The latter also cleaves Htt, producing fragments that eventually form intraneuronal inclusions (Gervais et al., 2002). Wild-type Htt has been found to partially protect cells against noxious stimuli, and removal of the caspase sites is beneficial for the cells (Young, 2003). Htt has been found to be normally palmitoylated at cysteine 214, which is essential for its trafficking and function and this process is regulated by the palmitoyl transferase Htt-interacting protein 14 (HIP14). Expansion of the polyglutamine tract of Htt results in reduced interaction between mutant Htt and HIP14 and consequently in a marked reduction in palmitoylation and increased formation of inclusions and neuronal toxicity (Yanai et al., 2006). These pathologic changes may be partly corrected by overexpression of HIP14.

The relationship of the abnormal interaction of Htt with other proteins and how this interaction contributes to the pathogenesis of HD is still unclear. It is possible that as the Htt polyglutamine tract expands and changes its tertiary configuration, it blocks the ATP-dependent import mechanisms for succinate dehydrogenase entry into the mitochondria in the striatum. This might lead to selective, localized energy depletion and pathologic changes that are typically associated with HD. As the expansion increases, the impairment of import mechanism becomes less selective, and the pathology becomes more widespread. Thus, in HD, in addition to the typical involvement of the striatum, the GPe and GPi, SNc, and cerebellum become involved, and the patient manifests additional features, such as rigidity, bradykinesia, and ataxia (Furtado et al., 1996). Morphometric analyses of structural MRI demonstrated marked cerebellar atrophy and white matter loss in patients with HD (Fennema-Notestine et al., 2004). Although activity of glyceraldehyde-3-phosphate dehydrogenase, an Htt-binding protein, is normal in the brains of patients with HD, the activity of aconitase, an Fe-S-containing tricarboxylic acid cycle enzyme, is reduced to 8% in the caudate, 27% in the putamen, and 52% in the cerebral cortex of HD brains (Tabrizi et al., 1999). Since this enzyme is particularly sensitive to inhibition by peroxynitrite $ONOO^-$ and superoxide $O_2^{\cdot-}$, it is considered be a good marker of excitotoxic cell damage.

Htt may also contribute to the apoptotic cell death in HD; it has been found to be cleaved by apopain, an apoptosis-specific cysteine protease (Goldberg et al., 1996). It has been postulated that the aggregates of mutant Htt (DiFiglia et al., 1997) cannot be properly removed from the cell and therefore might interfere with the metabolic activities of the affected neurons. Since ubiquitin is important in protein degradation and this process requires energy, the cells that are most vulnerable to the accumulation of the ubiquitin-Htt aggregates are those whose metabolic function has been already compromised, possibly as a result of toxins that interfere with oxidative phosphorylation. This concept then might link this new finding of region-selective accumulation of Htt aggregates and inclusions (DiFiglia et al., 1997) with the theories of regional impairment of energy metabolism (Beal et al., 1994). More recently, the molecular pathogenesis of HD has been considered to result from a decrease in specific chaperone proteins, such as Hdj1, Hsp70, αSGT, and βSGT, as demonstrated in R6/2 mice (Hay et al., 2004). Antigliadin antibodies have been demonstrated in 44% of patients with HD, but this probably represents an epiphenomenon and a nonspecific finding, as it has been also demonstrated in ataxia and other neurodegenerative disorders (Bushara et al., 2004).

Recent findings, based largely on studies in fruit flies, suggest that neurodegeneration in polyglutamine diseases such as HD and SCA3 may be due to RNA toxicity (Li et al., 2008).

Treatment

HD is one of few neurodegenerative diseases in which the diagnosis can be made long before the onset of clinical symptoms. This offers an opportunity to intervene in the earliest stages of the neurodegenerative cascade, perhaps even before the disease-related cell loss is initiated. Thus, HD is an excellent model for testing early neuroprotective treatments (Yamamato et al., 2000; Beal and Ferrante, 2004;

Leegwater-Kim and Cha, 2004; Ryu and Ferrante, 2005; Bodner et al., 2006; Adam and Jankovic, 2008; Imarisio et al., 2008; Hersch and Rosas, 2008; Phillips et al., 2008; Roze et al., 2008; Jankovic, 2009; Frank and Jankovic, 2010; Ross and Tabrizi, 2011). There is currently no treatment to stop or slow the progression of HD, but experimental therapeutics in transgenic mouse models promise to translate some of the pathogenesis-targeted strategies into clinical trials (Beal and Ferrante, 2004). These models, for example, have been used to demonstrate potential disease-modifying effects of caspase inhibitors (Ona et al., 1999; Chen et al., 2000; Yamamoto et al., 2000). In another study, 2% creatine has been found to increase survival from 97.7 days to 114.6 days, and this was associated with a reduction in the number of Htt-positive aggregates in the striatum of transgenic HD mice (Ferrante et al., 2000). In a pilot study, 10 g/day of creatine was well tolerated for 12 months by 13 patients with HD, except for transient nausea and diarrhea in 2 patients (Tabrizi et al., 2003). In a randomized, double-blind, placebo-controlled study of 64 patients with HD, 8 g/day of creatine administered for 16 weeks was well tolerated and was associated with an increase in serum and brain creatine and a reduction in serum 8-hydroxy-2′-deoxyguanosine, an indicator of oxidative injury to DNA (Hersch et al., 2006). In a placebo-controlled trial, using 5 g/day of creatine, Verbessem and colleagues (2003) showed no improvement in functional, neuromuscular, or cognitive status in patients with early to moderate HD. Although weight loss is very common in HD, paradoxically, food restriction (fasting) slows disease progression in transgenic mice (Duan et al., 2004). The same group also showed that paroxetine, a serotonin uptake inhibitor, improves survival in transgenic mice while preventing weight loss (Duan et al., 2004). Using the R6/1 HD mice, van Dellen and colleagues (2000) showed that the onset of neurologic deficit was significantly delayed if the mice were raised in an enriched and stimulating environment. Furthermore, environmental enrichment delayed the degenerative loss of peristriatal cerebral volume and rescued protein deficits, possibly through rescuing transcription or protein transport problems (Spires et al., 2004). Similarly, environmental stimulation was found to enhance the health and life expectancy in R6/2 mice that were transgenic for exon 1 (Carter et al., 2000). It is therefore possible that occupational therapy, based on the principle of environmental enrichment, could delay the onset of HD. These findings showing that environmental enrichment slows disease progression in HD mouse models have been confirmed by other studies (Hockly et al., 2002). In support of the role of environment in expression of HD symptoms is the observation of discordance after 7 years in monozygotic twins with HD (Friedman et al., 2005).

Knowledge of the natural history of HD is critical for the design of neuroprotective trials (Paulsen et al., 2006). Although several agents, such as CoQ10 and nicotinamide, are being tested in clinical trials to determine whether they exert a neuroprotective effect in humans, only symptomatic treatments have been found to be useful in HD patients at this time. CoQ10 (ubiquinone) carries electrons from complexes I and II to complex II of the mitochondrial electron transport chain (Jankovic and Ashizawa, 2003; Ryu and Ferrante, 2005). As such, it can act as an antioxidant or as a pro-oxidant, depending on the cell's redox potential (Shults

and Schapira, 2001). In the pilot study, CoQ10, at doses of 600 and 1200 mg/day, has been found to be well tolerated, although some patients may experience adverse effects, such as headache, heartburn, fatigue, and increased involuntary movements (Feigin et al., 1996). In a multicenter clinical trial conducted by the Huntington Study Group that compared CoQ10 and remacemide, an NMDA ion channel blocker, 347 patients with documented HD were randomized to receive CoQ10 300 mg twice daily, remacemide hydrochloride 200 mg three times daily, both, or placebo, the so-called CARE-HD study (Huntington Study Group, 2001). The patients were evaluated every 4–5 months for 30 months. Although patients who were treated with CoQ10 showed a trend toward slowing in total functional capacity decline (13%), this difference failed to reach statistical significance. Furthermore, CoQ10 was associated with higher frequency of stomach upset, and remacemide treatment was associated with higher frequency of nausea, vomiting, and dizziness. Because of these rather disappointing results, routine use of CoQ10 in patients with HD is not warranted. Likewise, remacemide, although relatively well tolerated at 200 and 600 mg/day (Kieburtz et al., 1996), cannot be recommended for the treatment of HD. In a 6-week open-label trial, another antiglutamatergic drug, riluzole (100 mg/day), was found to be well tolerated and to be associated with a 35% reduction in the chorea rating score (Rosas et al., 1999). The Huntington Study Group (2003) also found that riluzole at 200 mg/day significantly improved chorea scores but without improving functional capacity, and because of abnormalities in liver transaminase, this drug could not be recommended for routine use in HD. In a large, randomized, double-blind placebo-controlled trial, conducted by the European Huntington's Disease Initiative Study Group, 537 genetically-confirmed HD patients were randomized 2:1 to receive riluzole 100 mg/day or placebo for 3 years, and assessed periodically with the UHDRS (Landwehrmeyer et al., 2007). No concomitant use of other anti-choreic medications was allowed (wash-out period was 1 month). A total of 379 patients completed the study; the main reasons for discontinuation were the introduction of additional anti-choreic treatment and consent withdrawal. Although well tolerated, riluzole had no significant effect on chorea, behavioral, cognitive, independence, and functional scores compared to the placebo group at 3 years or at any other time point during the study. The potentially useful role of riluzole in favorably modifying the progression of HD is supported by studies in animal models of HD (Schiefer et al., 2002). Schiefer and colleagues (2002) were able to significantly increase survival time of R6/2 HD transgenic mice treated with riluzole. Furthermore, they showed that striatal neuronal intranuclear inclusions were less ubiquitinated and were surrounded by ubiquitinated microaggregates in riluzole-treated animals compared to controls. Staining with antibodies directed against the mutated Htt revealed no significant difference in this component of neuronal intranuclear inclusions. Minocycline, a second-generation antibiotic with high levels of blood–brain barrier permeability, has been shown to delay disease progression in the mouse model R6/2 of HD, possibly by inhibiting caspase-1 and caspase-3 mRNA upregulation and decreasing inducible nitric oxide synthase (Chen et al., 2000). Thirty patients (19 women and 11 men) between the ages of 21 and 66 years with symptomatic and genetically confirmed HD were treated with minocycline at the Baylor College of Medicine Huntington's Disease Center for at least 6 months (Thomas et al., 2003). Assessments included the Abnormal Involuntary Movements Scale, the UHDRS, and the Mini-Mental State Examination, performed at baseline and every 2 months throughout the study period. Laboratory studies at baseline and at 2-month intervals included complete blood and platelet counts and renal and liver function tests. In this pilot study, we showed that minocycline was well tolerated over the 6-month observation period, although no significant improvement was observed on any clinical assessment. No changes were noted in any of the laboratory tests. There was no evidence of any adverse interaction between minocycline and any of the concomitant medications. Our findings are similar to those reported by others (Bonelli et al., 2003). Future multicenter trials should focus not only on the long-term tolerability of minocycline but also, more important, on its potential disease-modifying effects. Interestingly, paroxetine, a commonly used serotonin reuptake inhibitor, has been found to slow the progression in *Htt* mutant mice (Duan et al., 2004). Early and sustained treatment with essential fatty acids has been demonstrated to protect against motor deficits in R6/1 transgenic mice expressing exon 1 and a portion of intron 2 of the *huntingin* gene (Clifford et al., 2002).

A growing body of evidence supports the notion that preformed polyglutamine aggregates are highly toxic when directed to the cell nucleus; therefore, recent research has focused on pharmacologic intervention aimed at inhibiting aggregate formation (Bates, 2003; Sanchez et al., 2003; Bossy-Wetzel et al., 2004; Hay et al., 2004). One such strategy is to use histone deacetylase inhibitors, such as valproic acid, phenylbutyrate, suberoylanilide hydroxamic acid (SAHA), pyroxamide, vorinostat, and other molecules to arrest polyglutamine-dependent neurodegeneration (Marks et al., 2001; Steffan et al., 2001; Butler and Bates, 2006; Chuang et al., 2009). In *Drosophila* flies expressing 93Q Htt, the histone deacetylase inhibitors suberoylamide hydroxamic acid and sodium butyrate suppressed neuronal degeneration (Steffan et al., 2001; Kazantsev et al., 2002; Agrawal et al., 2005). Suberoylamide hydroxamic acid also ameliorates motor deficits in the R6/2 mouse model of HD (Hockly et al., 2003). Geldanamycin, a benzoquinone ansamycin antibiotic that binds to Hsp90 and activates the stress response, has been found in some in-vitro cell culture models of HD to prevent polyQ aggregation, presumably by activating a heat-shock response (Sittler et al., 2001). Geldanamycin and radicicol have been found to delay aggregate formation in cell cultures and to increase soluble exon 1 huntingtin at concentrations that are capable of inducing Hsp40 and Hsp70 expression, indicating that chaperone induction favorably changes the biophysical properties of the aggregates (Hay et al., 2004). These drugs do not cross the blood–brain barrier, however, and therefore might not be clinically useful. Intraperitoneal injections of cystamine, an amino acid derivative that competitively inhibits transglutaminase, into transgenic HD mice ameliorated tremor and gait abnormalities and prolonged survival from 92 to 103 days (Karpuj et al., 2002). Keene and colleagues (2002) reported that treatment with tauroursodeoxycholic acid, a hydrophilic bile acid, prevented neuropathology and

associated behavioral deficits in the 3-nitropropionic acid rat model of HD and reduced striatal neuropathology in the R6/2 transgenic HD mouse. Inhibition of polyglutamine oligomerization by the azo dye Congo red interferes with the ability of expanded polyglutamine to induce cytotoxic events, thus facilitating the degradation of expanded polyglutamine by making it more accessible to proteasome (Sanchez et al., 2003). Congo red has also been found to inhibit the assembly of protofibrils into fibrils, thus preventing toxicity from mature fibrils (Poirier et al., 2002). Trehalose, a disaccharide composed of two glucose molecules, has been found to alleviate polyglutamine-mediated pathology in the R6/2 transgenic model of HD, including a 30% reduction in brain aggregates (Tanaka et al., 2004). Trehalose, which appears to bind directly to proteins with expanded polyglutamines, is highly soluble and therefore can be administered orally. Since it appears to have no toxicity, the drug is a promising therapeutic agent for various polyglutamine diseases, not just HD. Another strategy is to reduce the toxic effects of pathogenic fragment of Htt by small ubiquitin-like modifier (SUMO)-1, which at least partially prevents aggregation of Htt in vitro (Steffan et al., 2004). However, in a *Drosophila* model of HD, sumoylation of Htt fragment exacerbates neurodegeneration, whereas ubiquitination reduces HD pathology. These findings suggest that SUMO-1 blockers might delay the progression of HD. Some unorthodox attempts are under way to test various putative neuroprotective agents, such as CoQ10, creatine, cystamine, omega-3 fatty acids, trehalose, and blueberry extract (Couzin, 2004). A component of green tea polyphenol (−)–epigallocatechin-3-gallate (EGCG) has been found to potently inhibit the aggregation of mutant Htt exon 1 protein, and when fed to transgenic HD flies overexpressing a pathogenic Htt exon 1 protein, photoreceptor degeneration and motor function improved (Ehrnhoefer et al., 2006). Another approach, currently investigated in HD mouse models, is the use of an engineered virus to make an intracellular antibody or "intrabody" that will clear the cytoplasm of mutated Htt (Wang et al., 2008b). Improving clearance of the mutant protein is another strategy that is being explored in experimental models of HD. For example, increased acetylation of the mutant Htt at lysine residue 444 (K444) in a *C. elegans* model of HD facilitates trafficking of mutant Htt into autophagosomes and improves clearance of the mutant protein by macroautophagy (Jeong et al., 2009). Intrabody against the proline-rich domain of Htt (Happ1) has been found to improve motor and cognitive deficits as well as the neuropathology found in the lentiviral, R6/2, N171-82Q, YAC128, and BACHD models of HD (Southwell et al., 2009).

Transglutaminase inhibitors, such as cystamine and monodansyl cadaverine, reduce aggregate formation and, as such, might be potential therapeutic agents in diseases caused by CAG-repeat expansion (Igarashi et al., 1998). By inhibiting the HD mutant transgene with tetracycline, Yamamoto and colleagues (2000) were able to show that the neurodegeneration can be not only prevented but also reversed. Preliminary data based on pilot clinical trials suggest that minocycline is well tolerated and that it is not associated with serious adverse events or laboratory test abnormalities (Bonelli et al., 2003; Thomas et al., 2004). In a pilot safety and tolerability study of 30 patients with HD who were given minocycline over a 6-month period, minocycline was found to be well tolerated during this study period, and no serious adverse events were noted (Thomas et al., 2004). Minocycline was also found to be well tolerated in a larger, double-blind, placebo-controlled study of 60 HD patients (Huntington Study Group, 2004). It has been also found to have a potential neuroprotective role in other neurodegenerative disorders (Zemke and Majid, 2004). Smith and colleagues (2003), however, found no effect of minocycline or doxycycline on behavioral abnormalities or Htt aggregates in R6/2 mice.

Another caspase inhibitor with potential neuroprotective effects, currently being tested in patients with HD, is ethyl eicosapentaenoate (LAX-101, ethyl-EPA, Miraxion). This pure, highly unsaturated fatty acid, concentrated chiefly in fish oil, has been found to be effective in some pilot trials in HD and schizophrenia. In a small ($n = 24$) double-blind, placebo-controlled study of LAX-101, Vaddadi and colleagues (2002) showed possible improvement in both the orofacial and total components of the UHDRS after 6 months of treatment. In one double-blind, placebo-controlled study ethyl-EPA has been found to have a possible stabilizing effect on the progression of HD (Puri et al., 2005). Because of the encouraging results, a multicenter trial of ethyl-EPA, TREND-HD, was conducted in North America. A multicenter, randomized, double-blind, placebo-controlled trial of ethyl-EPA (1 g twice daily) for 6 months involving 316 HD patients, 190 of whom completed the 12-month trial, showed improvement in the Total Motor Score 4 (TMS-4) component of the UHDRS (Huntington Study Group, 2008). While ethyl-EPA has not been found to be effective for the movement symptoms of HD when taken over 6 months, after 12 months those subjects who received ethyl-EPA for 12 continuous months had no deterioration in their UHDRS Total Motor Score, while those who received active treatment for only 6 months worsened ($P = 0.02$) (Huntington Study Group, 2008). Thus, improvement in motor symptoms may require long-term treatment with ethyl-EPA. These important observations, of course, have obvious therapeutic implications and suggest that caspase inhibitors might play a role in the treatment of HD and related neurodegenerative disorders (Friedlander, 2000; Sanchez Mejia and Friedlander, 2001).

Latrepirdine (Dimebon), originally developed in Russia as an antihistamine drug, has been also found to inhibit butyrylcholinesterase and acetylcholinesterase as well as NMDA receptor, and may also act as a mitochondrial enhancer by inhibiting mitochondrial permeability transition pore opening (although the latter presumably requires higher dosages than those used in clinical trials). It has been also found to exert neuroprotective effects in HD models and in a phase II trial of Alzheimer disease. A phase II clinical trial conducted by the Huntington Study Group (HSG) showed that latrepirdine significantly improved mean MMSE scores compared with stable performance in the placebo group but there were no significant treatment effects on the UHDRS or the Alzheimer's Disease Assessment Scale-cognitive subscale (ADAS-cog) (Kieburtz et al., 2010).

Phenylbutyrate, which increases brain histone acetylation, decreases histone methylation levels, enhances the ubiquitin-proteasomal pathway, and downregulates caspases, has been found to exert significant neuroprotective effects in a transgenic mouse model of HD (Gardian et al., 2005), and is currently being investigated as a potential neuroprotective drug by the HSG. Lithium has been found to induce autophagy via inositol monophosphatase (IMPase) inhibition, a process independent of the mammalian target of rapamycin (mTOR) induced autophagy (Pan et al., 2008), but combining it with rapamycin may be particularly useful in the treatment of neurodegenerative diseases, such as HD. But, in contrast to enhancement of autophagy via IMPase inhibition, the inhibition of glycogen synthase kinase-3β (GSK-3β) by lithium has the opposite effect (Sarkar et al., 2008). Various drugs have been found to induce autophagy and as such have been proposed to be potentially useful in slowing neurodegeneration associated with HD. These included L-type Ca^{2+} channel antagonists, the K^+ATP channel opener minoxidil, and the Gi signaling activator clonidine. These drugs appear to regulate autophagy through mechanisms other than the cyclical (mTOR) pathway, in which cAMP regulates inositol trisphosphate levels, influencing calpain activity, which completes the cycle by cleaving and activating Gs alpha, which regulates cAMP levels (Williams et al., 2008).

Until effective neuroprotective therapy is found, the management of patients with HD will focus primarily on relief of symptoms designed to improve their quality of life (Handley et al., 2006; Jankovic, 2006; Bonelli and Hofmann, 2007; Adam and Jankovic, 2008; Frank and Jankovic, 2010). In a European survey of 2128 registered HD patients, 84% were prescribed symptomatic treatment, 50% were treated for depression, and 28% received anti-choreic medications (Priller et al., 2008). Psychosis, one of the most troublesome symptoms, usually improves with neuroleptics, such as haloperidol, pimozide, fluphenazine, and thioridazine. These drugs, however, can induce tardive dyskinesia and other adverse effects; therefore, they should be used only if absolutely needed to control symptoms. Clozapine (Clozaril), an atypical antipsychotic drug that does not cause tardive dyskinesia, might be a useful alternative to the typical neuroleptics, but its high cost, risk of agranulocytosis, and other potential side effects might limit its use, particularly since it has anti-choreic effects only in relatively high doses (Bonuccelli et al., 1994; van Vugt et al., 1997). It is likely that the other atypical antipsychotics, such as olanzapine (Zyprexa) (Paleacu et al., 2002) and quetiapine fumarate (Seroquel), will also provide a beneficial effect. Anxiolytics and antidepressants also might be useful in some patients with psychiatric problems. Donepezil, a procholinergic drug that is used in the treatment of Alzheimer disease, was found to be ineffective in the treatment of cognitive impairment or chorea associated with HD (Fernandez et al., 2000).

One of the most effective drugs in the treatment of hyperkinetic movement disorders, including chorea, is TBZ (Jankovic and Beach, 1997; Kenney and Jankovic, 2006). This drug, approved under the brand name Xenazine by the Food and Drug Administration in 2008 for chorea associated with HD, is also marketed in other countries as Nitoman. A potent and selective depletor of dopamine and, to a lesser degree, norepinephrine and serotonin from nerve terminals, it has been shown to be effective in the treatment of a variety of hyperkinetic movement disorders. The effects of TBZ are largely restricted to the CNS, which differentiates it from another monoamine depletor, reserpine, an old antihypertensive drug that produces both central and peripheral depletion. By inhibiting the brain synaptic VMAT, TBZ impairs uptake of monoamines and serotonin into synaptic vesicles, causing them to remain in the cytoplasm, where they are rapidly degraded by monoamine oxidases (Fig. 14.5). There are two types of VMAT: type 1 (VMAT1) and type 2 (VMAT2), which are coded by two distinct genes, 8p21.3 and 10q25, respectively. In humans, VMAT2 is nearly exclusively expressed in the CNS neurons, whereas VMAT1 is present in the peripheral nerve terminals. TBZ exhibits a 10 000-fold higher affinity for human VMAT2 than for human VMAT1, reversibly binding to the intravesicular part of VMAT2. Reserpine, on the other hand, binds irreversibly to the cytoplasmic site of both VMAT1 (peripheral) and VMAT2 (central). These pharmacologic differences probably account for the absence of hypotension and gastrointestinal side effects with TBZ compared to reserpine. Also, the

duration of action is much shorter with TBZ, about 12 hours versus several days. In contrast to reserpine, which depletes all the monoamines and serotonin equally, TBZ preferentially depletes dopamine. Finally, despite early reports of dopamine receptor inhibition, more recent studies suggest that since the affinity of TBZ for the dopamine D2 receptor is 1000-fold lower than its affinity for VMAT2, it is unlikely that the weak dopamine D2 receptor antagonism is involved in the therapeutic effects of TBZ. This might be one reason why tardive dyskinesia has never been reported to occur with TBZ, one of the chief advantages of this drug over the neuroleptic, dopamine receptor-blocking, drugs.

Although TBZ can cause or exacerbate depression, sedation, akathisia, and parkinsonism, in our experience it is clearly the most effective and safest anti-chorea drug (Jankovic and Beach, 1997; Ondo et al., 2002; Kenney and Jankovic, 2006; Kenney et al., 2007a, 2007b; Fasano and Bentivoglio, 2009; Jankovic, 2009) (Video 14.13). In one study of 15 patients who were treated for an average of 7 months at a mean dose of TBZ of 68 ± 27.1 mg/day (range: 25–150 mg/day), a "blinded" rating of videotapes showed improvement in motor scores in 12 (80%), and the mean score improved from 16 ± 3.6 to 13 ± 3.8 (Ondo et al., 2002). Adverse events included akathisia, insomnia, constipation, depression, drooling, and subjective weakness. Paradoxically, some patients with HD benefit from dopaminergic drugs, particularly when the disease is associated with parkinsonism (Racette and Perlmutter, 1998). In a multicenter, double-blind, placebo-controlled trial of TBZ involving 84 ambulatory patients with HD (TETRA-HD), TBZ treatment resulted in a reduction of 5.0 units in chorea severity compared with a reduction of 1.5 units on placebo treatment (adjusted mean effect size = −3.5 ± 0.8 UHDRS units (mean ± standard error); 95% confidence interval: −5.2 to −1.9; P < 0.0001) (Huntington Study Group, 2006) (Fig. 14.6). About 50% of TBZ-treated subjects had a 6-point or greater improvement compared with 7% of placebo-treated

TETRABENAZINE MECHANISM OF ACTION

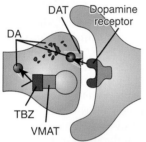

- Tetrabenazine selectively and reversibly inhibits striatal VMAT2
- Cytoplasmic dopamine rapidly degraded by monoamine oxidase (MAO) in synaptic terminal → presynaptic depletion
- Selective for dopamine >> norepinephrine and/or 5–HT
- Tetrabenazine reduces dopamine transmission selectively in the CNS

DAT = dopamine transporter
VMAT = vesicular monoamine transporter
DA = dopamine
TBZ = tetrabenazine

Figure 14.5 Mechanisms of action of tetrabenazine.

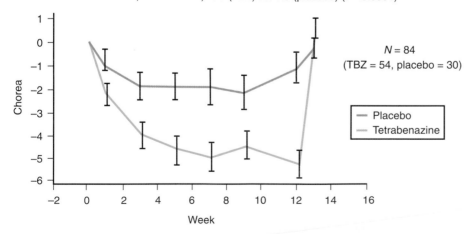

MEAN CHANGE IN UHDRS TOTAL MAXIMAL CHOREA SCORE
(Primary Study Endpoint: From Baseline to Week 12)

Mean score decline (UHDRS units): 5.0 (TBZ) vs. 1.5 (placebo) (P <0.0001)

N = 84
(TBZ = 54, placebo = 30)

— Placebo
— Tetrabenazine

There was blinded washout of study drug at week 12. Change favors tetrabenazine
(P = 0.0001; ANCOVA (ITT-LOC). Chorea scale range: 0 to 28
ANCOVA = analysis of covariance; ITT-LOC = intent-to-treat analysis

Figure 14.6 Results of placebo-controlled trial of tetrabenazine in HD. *From Huntington Study Group. A randomized, double-blind, placebo-controlled trial of tetrabenazine as antichorea therapy in Huntington disease. Neurology 2006;66:366–372.*

subjects. There was also a significant benefit on ratings of clinical global improvement. There were five study withdrawals in the TBZ group and five serious adverse events in four subjects (drowning suicide, complicated fall, restlessness/suicidal ideation, and breast cancer), compared with one withdrawal and no serious adverse events in the placebo group. This study concluded that TBZ, at adjusted dosages of up to 100 mg/day, was effective for the treatment of chorea in HD and was generally safe and well tolerated. In a retrospective study of 448 patients with hyperkinetic movement disorders (98 with chorea), treated with TBZ (mean dose at the last visit 60.4 ± 35.7 mg) for up to 21.6 years (mean 2.3 ± 3.4 years) at Baylor College of Medicine between 1997 and 2004, and evaluated with a clinical response scale (1: marked reduction in abnormal movements, 5: worsening), TBZ was found to be effective across the spectrum of the hyperactive movement disorders treated (Kenney and Jankovic, 2006). The percentage of patients with chorea that had a response of 1 or 2 at the last visit was 84.4%. The most common side effects, all dose related, were drowsiness (25%), parkinsonism (15.4%), depression (7.6%), akathisia (7.6%), with less common side effects including nausea/vomiting, nervousness/anxiety, and insomnia. Many patients are willing to tolerate side effects such as parkinsonism (sometimes effectively treated with amantadine, levodopa, dopamine agonists) because of TBZ's beneficial effects on their hyperkinetic movement disorder. Even though this study was retrospective and open-label, it provides valuable information regarding the long-term tolerability and safety of the treatment with TBZ of hyperkinetic movement disorders. These observations have been confirmed by other, albeit smaller, longitudinal studies including one in which 68 patients with HD were followed for a mean period of 34.4 ± 25.2 months (Fasano et al., 2008a). An open-label, extension study following the TETRA-HD study showed that TBZ is a safe and effective drug (Frank et al., 2009).

TBZ is not only a dopamine depletor but may also decrease the brain serotonin and norepinephrine concentrations, with a potential for causing or worsening depression. To answer the question whether TBZ is contraindicated in depression, a retrospective study examined the effects of TBZ in 518 patients treated with TBZ for hyperkinetic movement disorders, of which 52.5% had a history of depression prior to the treatment (Kenney et al., 2006). Of the patients without depression at the time of the treatment initiation, 11.4% were newly diagnosed with depression, and 18.4% of the patients with a previous diagnosis of depression at the time when the treatment with TBZ was started had a worsening of their depression. Overall 15.1% of patients experienced depression for the first time or had an exacerbation of the preexisting depression. On the other hand, there are patients whose depression improves with the TBZ treatment because of the marked benefit on the underlying hyperkinesia. Although depression is a known side effect of TBZ and may be potentially exacerbated by TBZ, a diagnosis of preexisting depression should not necessarily constitute an absolute contraindication for initiating the treatment with TBZ if the patient is otherwise a good candidate, but close monitoring of such patients is clearly warranted. There are no reports to this date of tardive dyskinesia induced by TBZ, this representing a major advantage of this medication over neuroleptics.

The clinical pharmacokinetics of TBZ was studied in an open-label observational study (Kenney et al., 2007a). Ten patients with HD were assessed with serial motor UHDRS and Beck Depression Inventory at baseline and following their morning dose of TBZ, after at least 12 hours off from the last dose. There was an average of 42.4% reduction in chorea, with effect lasting between 3.2 and 8.1 hours (mean 5.4 ± 1.3 hours). Therefore, a minimum of three times a day dosing may be required in most patients to sustain the antichorea effects without wearing off. The best tolerated dose of TBZ, necessary to provide an adequate control of symptoms, varies greatly between individuals, from as low as 12.5 mg/day to as high as 400 mg/day. Although no blood levels or other pharmacokinetic data were obtained during this study, the findings suggest that the wash-out period of TBZ is short. This is also supported by a double-blind study of 30 HD patients treated with TBZ, randomly assigned to one of three groups: the first group of 12 patients stopped TBZ (which was replaced with a placebo) on day 1 (withdrawal group), the second group followed the same protocol on day 3 (partial withdrawal), while the third group continued the treatment with TBZ (non-withdrawal group) (Frank et al., 2008). The withdrawal group experienced reemergent chorea at day 3, with a difference in the UHDRS change of 5.33 units, compared to 2.94 units in the non-withdrawal group, which was in the hypothesized direction ($P < 0.077$). Post hoc analysis of the linear trend was positive for reemergent chorea ($P = 0.0486$) and provides further support for the effectiveness of TBZ in reducing chorea. TBZ has been found to be as effective as other neuroleptics, including "atypical" neuroleptics such as aripiprazole (Brusa et al., 2009), in reducing chorea with similar adverse effect profile, but it clearly has a lower risk of tardive syndrome. The Cochrane review, which examined 22 trials (1254 subjects) (Mestre et al., 2009a), concluded that based on available evidence, only TBZ showed a clear efficacy for the control of chorea.

Several guidelines on the treatment of HD have been published (Walker, 2007; Adam and Jankovic, 2008; Phillips et al., 2008; Jankovic, 2009; Mestre et al., 2009a, 2009b; Frank and Jankovic, 2010) (Fig. 14.7). Modulation of the dopaminergic system by presynaptically depleting dopamine, postsynaptically blocking dopamine receptors, or by activation of presynaptic dopamine receptors (autoreceptors) has been also suggested as a strategy to treat symptoms of HD. Apomorphine, a dopamine agonist that presumably acts by stimulating presynaptic D2 receptors and thus inhibiting dopamine release, has been found to be effective in five patients with HD, in whom it was continuously infused subcutaneously for 5 days (Vitale et al., 2007). A novel dopaminergic modulator, OSU6162, has been reported to improve chorea in a patient with HD (Tedroff et al., 1999), but further studies on the pharmacology and clinical efficacy of the drug are needed. Pridopidine (ACR16, Huntexil), a molecule similar to OSU162, is considered a "dopaminergic stabilizer" in that it stimulates or inhibits dopaminergic signaling depending on the dopaminergic tone and as such has been also classified as a partial dopamine receptor agonist or antagonist with preferential action on dopaminergic autoreceptors resulting in functional D2 antagonism (Rung et al., 2008). The drug may also decrease glutamatergic activity. Further studies by Carlsson and colleagues (Rung et al.,

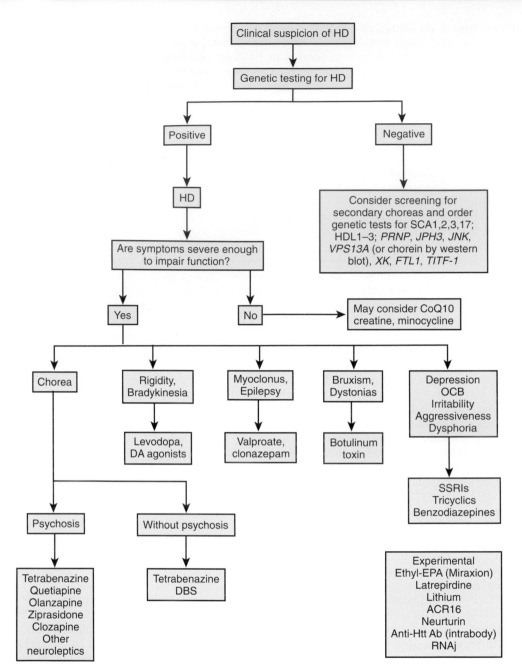

Figure 14.7 Symptomatic treatment of HD.

2008) have suggested that ACR16 has an "allosteric" effect on D2 receptors causing an enhanced response to dopamine and "orthosteric" effect, antagonizing dopamine. The plasma half-life increases from around 8 hours after a single dosing to about 15–20 hours at steady state. Although in a phase II trial in Europe the primary endpoint, the weighted cognitive score, did not significantly change and there was no significant improvement in chorea, the patients showed improvement in parkinsonian and gait scores and the drug was well tolerated (personal communication). Phase III (MermaiHD), which included 437 HD patients in 32 European centers with 92% compliance, failed to meet the primary endpoint, the modified Motor Score (mMS) (adopted from the UHDRS), after a 6-month trial of 45 mg twice daily. Further analysis showed that the significance value for the primary

study endpoint of $P = 0.042$ did not meet the prespecified level of $P < 0.025$, but with inclusion of the clinically relevant CAG number adjustment, the P value is <0.02. There were no serious adverse effects detected. The NeuroSearch press release concluded that the drug "demonstrates a superior treatment effect in patients with an elevated CAG number score (considered a surrogate marker for rate of progression and disease prognosis) and that the significant improvements observed in mMS are driven primarily by positive effects on fine motor skills, gait and balance." In contrast to the MermaiHD trial, in which about 40% of the patients were also receiving antipsychotics, the North American, phase IIb (HART) trial, involving 220 HD patients, currently under way, has excluded patients on antipsychotic or antidepressant drugs.

Baclofen, a putative GABA agonist, provides neither symptomatic nor protective effects in HD (Shoulson et al., 1989). Whether blocking glutamate release from the presynaptic terminals by drugs such as riluzole or lamotrigine (Brodie, 1992) or whether other antiglutamatergic drugs will be effective in slowing down the otherwise inexorable progression of the disease awaits further studies. In a double-blind, placebo-controlled trial, lamotrigine failed to slow HD progression but was found to improve symptoms and lessen chorea; 54% of patients on lamotrigine reported symptomatic improvement versus 15% of those on placebo, and the chorea subscale measure showed less deterioration for lamotrigine than for placebo (Kremer et al., 1999). Dystonia and bruxism, occasionally present in patients with HD, can be effectively treated with local injections of botulinum toxin (Tan et al., 2000). Pallidotomy, known to be effective in the treatment of levodopa-induced dyskinesias in patients with Parkinson disease, has been found also useful in the treatment of dystonia associated with HD (Cubo et al., 2000). Bilateral pallidal stimulation at 40 and 130 Hz improved chorea in one patient with HD (Moro et al., 2004).

Since NMDA supersensitivity might be responsible in part for chorea in patients with HD, selective NMDA antagonists might ameliorate this symptom. In a double-blind, controlled trial of 22 patients with HD, amantadine (400 mg/day) reduced extremity chorea by 36% (Verhagen Metman et al., 2002). In addition to symptomatic effect, amantadine might confer a neuroprotective effect. In another randomized placebo-controlled trial, amantadine at 300 mg/day had no effect on HD-associated chorea (O'Suilleabhain and Dewey, 2003). A 2-hour intravenous infusion of amantadine in a double-blind, randomized crossover study showed reduction in dyskinesias scores after both intravenous and oral administration (Lucetti et al., 2003). In a pilot trial of 9 patients with HD, memantine when titrated to the maximum dose of 20 mg/day, and followed for 3.8 ± 1.0 months, showed a significant decrease in total UHDRS motor scores ($P = 0.008$), mostly due to a significant ($P = 0.008$) decrease in the maximum chorea rating at their final visit (11.5 ± 6.3 to 4.8 ± 3.8) (Ondo et al., 2007). There was no significant change in their cognitive ($P = 0.625$) or behavioral ($P = 0.258$) ratings or total functional capacity ($P = 0.078$) and independence scale rating ($P = 1.000$). There were minimal adverse events, such as drowsiness and worsening of balance, speech, and social interaction.

Another group of medications used in the treatment of HD-related symptoms, such as depression, anxiety, and obsessive-compulsive disorder, are the selective serotonin uptake inhibitors (SSRIs). Fluoxetine, one of the SSRIs, has been also shown to stimulate CREB, increase production of BDNF, enhance glycogenolysis, block voltage-gated calcium and sodium channels, and decrease the conductance of mitochondrial voltage-dependent anion channels, and as such it may potentially exert neuroprotective effect in HD (Mostert et al., 2008). Nabilone, a synthetic analog of delta-9-tetrahydrocannabinol, the major psychoactive component of cannabis, has been found to exert modest symptomatic benefit in chorea associated with HD (Curtis et al., 2009).

In another Cochrane review of the literature, evaluating neuroprotective strategies, of 8 randomized, double-blind, placebo-controlled clinical trials (1366 subjects), no compounds studied thus have been found to provide disease-modifying effects although they were generally safe and well tolerated (Mestre et al., 2009b). Subjects were treated for a mean of 52 weeks (range 30–144 weeks) with one of the following compounds: vitamin E, idebenone, baclofen, lamotrigine, creatine, CoQ10 + remacemide, ethyl-eicosapentaenoic acid, and riluzole. All studies to date have used clinical scales to measure progression of disease, and future studies will likely need to use a more sensitive biomarker for disease onset and progression.

Palliative surgery, including pallidotomy and deep brain stimulation (DBS), has been tried in a few patients with severe chorea associated with HD but despite some improvement in chorea, the disease has continued to progress (Kang et al., 2011). When targeting the globus pallidus interna, DBS at a frequency of 40 Hz has been able to reduce chorea without producing parkinsonian features although the overall motor function and quality of life may not improve (Fasano et al., 2008b).

Experimental therapeutics

Following up on some encouraging results from animal studies, the delivery of trophic factors, such as nerve growth factor and ciliary neutrophic factor by genetically modified cells, into the striatum of patients with HD has become a reachable goal (Kordower et al., 1999; Mittoux et al., 2000; McBride et al., 2004). Implantation of nerve growth factor-producing fibroblasts into the rat striatum appeared to protect these animals against neurotoxic effects of the excitatory amino acids quinolate and quisqualate (Schumacher et al., 1991). Whether intrastriatal implantations of genetically engineered cells designed to produce trophic factors, such as ciliary neutrophic factor (Emerich et al., 1997; Kordower et al., 1999), or fetal cells will be useful in the treatment of HD awaits the results of further animal and clinical studies (Freeman et al., 2000; Bachoud-Levi et al., 2002; Peschanski et al., 2004; Reuter et al., 2008). The observation that implanted fetal neuronal cells survive in the HD brain and reconstitute damaged neuronal connections suggests that the host HD disease process does not affect the grafted tissue. No change in functional status or hyperkinetic movements was observed in 12 HD patients who were treated with transplantation of fetal porcine striatal cells (St Hillaire et al., 1998), but in another study (Bachoud-Levi et al., 2000), motor and cognitive improvement was noted in three of five patients after staged grafting of both striatal areas with human fetal neuroblasts. In their subsequent study, the investigators showed that the three patients who received fetal striatal allografts and demonstrated clinical improvement had a reduction of striatal and cortical hypometabolism as measured by F-deoxyglucose PET, whereas in the two patients who did not show clinical improvement, the striatal and cortical metabolism progressed (Gaura et al., 2004). Hauser and colleagues (2002) reported the results of an uncontrolled pilot study of transplantation of fetal striatal cells into the postcommissural putamen of seven patients with HD. There was no change in the primary outcome variable, the motor component of UHDRS, and three subjects suffered four subdural hemorrhages. Furthermore, the placebo effect, which was the same as the treatment effect (>20% improvement), lasted 18 months. Although the authors conclude that transplantation of human fetal striatal cells is feasible and that "a lack of significant worsening might reflect clinical benefit in a progressive neurodegenerative disease," this study should be viewed as a negative study. It should, however, also provide a stimulus for future randomized, blind, and adequately controlled studies (Greenamyre and Shoulson, 2002). In five patients with HD followed for up to 6 years, the subjects were found to improve during the first 2 years and then their function again deteriorated (Bachoud-Levi et al., 2006). Autopsy studies, however, show that despite prolonged survival of the graft for up to 6 years or longer, there is poor integration with the host striatum, which probably accounts for the poor efficacy of this approach (Keene et al., 2007). Although fetal grafting in the treatment of HD is still being pursued in some, chiefly European, centers (Peschanski et al., 2004), it is unlikely that this approach will become an acceptable therapeutic

strategy, especially with a recent report of symptomatic mass as a result of the graft overgrowth (Keene et al., 2009). The mechanisms of graft degeneration in HD are not well understood, but have been attributed to allograft immunoreactivity, microglial responses targeted to grafted cells and, similar to grafts in PD, cell-to-cell neurotoxicity (Cicchetti et al., 2011). Similarly, although adipose tissue stem cells implanted in the striata of R6/2 mice transgenic for HD showed some benefits, it is unlikely that this will translate into a clinically useful therapeutic strategy (Lee et al., 2009).

In addition, an initiative, Systemic Evaluation of Treatment for Huntington's Disease, has been developed to systematically evaluate various strategies as potential treatments for HD (http://www.huntingtonproject.org; Walker and Raymond, 2004). One of the most promising approaches to the treatment of HD is neurturin, delivered via adeno-associated virus type 2 (AAV2) vector. Support for this statement is provided by an encouraging report using this approach in rats that received the neurotoxin 3NP (Ramaswamy et al., 2007).

Finally, RNA interference (RNAi) has been suggested as a promising therapeutic strategy, but further work is needed to determine whether this method can suppress the expression of only the mutated, but not the normal, *Htt* gene, for how long the suppression is required, and what the potential negative effects of knocking down mutated and wild-type *Htt* are (Harper, 2009). Furthermore, silencing of the wild-type and mutant *Htt* using small hairpin RNA administered via lentiform vectors and an amelioration of HD pathology was demonstrated in a rodent model of HD (Drouet et al., 2009).

A listing of available and experimental therapies for HD is provided in Table 14.3. In an evidence-based review of 218 publications on pharmacologic interventions in HD since 1965, Bonelli and Wenning (2006) found 20 level I, 55 level II, 54 level III trials, and 89 case reports. Chorea, the primary endpoint in nearly all studies, showed some improvement with haloperidol and fluphenazine, with less evidence for olanzapine. The analysis failed to result in any treatment recommendation of clinical relevance.

Table 14.3 Treatment of Huntington disease

Adequate nutrition

Physical, speech, and occupational therapy

Treat/prevent aspiration, fecal impaction, incontinence

Support: life-planning, disability benefits, household help, home equipment, supervise smoking, child care, day care, institutional care, hospice

Caregiver support

Anxiolytics: benzodiazepines, propranolol, clonidine

Antidepressants: tricyclics (nortriptyline, amitriptyline, imipramine); SSRIs (fluoxetine, sertraline, fluvoxamine, paroxetine, venlafaxine, citalopram)

DA receptor-blocking drugs or DA-depleting drugs for severe chorea, psychosis: quetiapine, olanzapine, ziprasidone, clozapine, fluphenazine, risperidone, haloperidol, tetrabenazine (TBZ)

Glutamate release inhibitors and receptor blockers (remacemide, riluzole)

Mitochondrial electron transport enhancers and free radical scavengers (CoQ10, nicotinamide, creatine)

Caspase and iNOS inhibitors (minocycline, ethyl eicosapentaenoate or ethyl-EPA, LAX-101)

Histone deacetylase inhibitors

Trophic factors

Fetal transplants

References available on Expert Consult: www.expertconsult.com

Appendix

Hereditary Disease Foundation
3960 Broadway, 6th Floor
New York, NY 10032
Telephone: (212) 928-2121
Fax: (212) 928-2172
Email: cures@hdfoundation.org
Website: http://www.hdfoundation.org

Huntington's Disease Society of America
505 Eighth Avenue
Suite 902
New York, NY 10018
Telephone: (800) 345-HDSA (4372)
Fax: (212) 239-3430
Email: hdsainfo@hdsa.org
Website: http://www.hdsa.org/

Huntington Study Group
University of Rochester
HSG Administrative Office
1351 Mt. Hope Avenue, Suite 223
Rochester, NY 14620
Telephone: (800) 487-7671
Website: http://www.huntington-study-group.org

International Huntington Association
Gerrit Dommerholt
Callunahof 8, 7217 ST Harfsen
The Netherlands
Telephone: (31) 573-431-595
Email: iha@huntington-assoc.com
Website: http://www.huntington-assoc.com

Other related websites

http://www.wemove.org

CHAPTER 15

Chorea, ballism, and athetosis

Chapter contents

Introduction	335
Dentatorubral-pallidoluysian atrophy and HD-like disorders	335
Other Huntington disease-like disorders	337
Neuroacanthocytosis	339
Neurodegeneration with brain iron accumulation	341
Other familial choreas	342
Infectious chorea	343
Postinfectious and autoimmune choreas	343
Other autoimmune choreas	344
Other choreas	345
Treatment of chorea	346
Ballism	346
Treatment of ballism	347
Athetosis	347
Treatment of athetosis	348
Appendix	349

Introduction

Chorea consists of involuntary, continual, abrupt, rapid, brief, unsustained, irregular movements that flow randomly from one body part to another. Patients can partially and temporarily suppress the chorea and frequently camouflage some of the movements by incorporating them into semi-purposeful activities (parakinesia). The inability to maintain voluntary contraction (motor impersistence), such as manual grip (milkmaid grip) or tongue protrusion, is a characteristic feature of chorea and results in dropping of objects and clumsiness. Chorea should be differentiated from "pseudo-choreoathetosis," a movement disorder that is phenomeno-logically similar to chorea or athetosis (slow chorea) due to loss of proprioception (Sharp et al., 1994). Muscle stretch reflexes are often "hung-up" and "pendular." Affected patients typically have a peculiar, irregular, and dance-like gait. The pathophysiology of chorea is poorly understood, but in contrast to parkinsonism, dystonia, and other movement disorders, intracortical inhibition of the motor cortex is normal in chorea (Hanajima et al., 1999). In addition, semiquantitative analysis of single photon emission computed tomography in patients with hemichorea due to various causes suggests that there is an increase in activity in the contralateral thalamus, possibly due to disinhibition as a result of loss of normal pallidal inhibitory input (Kim et al., 2002).

Chorea may be a manifestation of a primary neurologic genetic disorder, such as Huntington disease (HD), or it may occur as a neurologic complication of systemic, toxic, or other disorders (Rosenblatt et al., 1998; Cardoso, 2004;

Cardoso et al., 2006; Jankovic and Fahn, 2009) (Tables 15.1 and 15.2, Fig. 15.1). Chorea may be seen in normal infants, but these movements usually disappear by age 8 months, and some of these movements may be purposeful (Van der Meer et al., 1995).

In this chapter we will briefly mention HD, but the focus will be on non-HD causes of chorea, as HD-like phenotypes without the HD genotype are increasingly being described and must be recognized. Several neurodegenerative disorders, some with expanded trinucleotide repeats, have been reported as phenocopies of HD, including spinocerebellar atrophy, particularly SCA2 and SCA3 (Kawaguchi et al., 1994), pure cerebello-olivary degeneration (Fox et al., 2003), and dentatorubral-pallidoluysian atrophy (DRPLA) (see below) (La Spada et al., 1994; Ikeuchi et al., 1995; Komure et al., 1995; Warner et al., 1995; Ross et al., 1997; Rosenblatt et al., 1998; Wild et al., 2008). In a study of 285 patients with clinical features consistent with HD, but who tested negative for HD by a DNA analysis, the following diagnoses were identified: five cases had Huntington disease-like type 4 (HDL4), one had HDL1, one had HDL2, and one patient had Friedreich ataxia (Wild et al., 2008).

Dentatorubral-pallidoluysian atrophy and HD-like disorders

Dentatorubral-pallidoluysian atrophy (DRPLA) is an autosomal dominant neurodegenerative disorder that is particularly prevalent in Japan, but it has been also identified in Europe and in African-American families ("Haw River

DOI: 10.1016/B978-1-4377-2369-4.00015-9

Table 15.1 Differential diagnosis of chorea

Developmental choreas

Physiologic chorea of infancy

Chorea minima

Idiopathic choreas

Buccal-oral-lingual dyskinesia and edentulous orodyskinesia

In older adults, senile chorea (probably several causes)

Hereditary choreas

Huntington disease

Benign hereditary chorea (*TITF1* gene)

Neuroacanthocytosis (*VPS13A* gene)

Other heredodegenerations: Huntington disease-like (HDL) disorders (e.g., prion protein *PRNP*, *junctophilin* or *JPH3* genes), dentatorubral-pallidoluysian atrophy (*c-Jun NH-terminal kinase*, *JNK* gene), spinocerebellar ataxias (SCA2, SCA17), ataxia telangiectasia, ataxia with oculomotor apraxia type 1 (*aprataxin* gene), ataxia with oculomotor apraxia type 2 (due to mutations in the *senataxin* gene), tuberous sclerosis of basal ganglia, pantothenate kinase associated neurodegeneration, other neurodegenerations with brain iron accumulation (Hallervorden–Spatz disease), Wilson disease, neuroferritinopathy, infantile bilateral striatal necrosis (IBSN)

Neurometabolic disorders

Lesch–Nyhan syndrome, lysosomal storage disorders, amino acid disorders, Leigh disease, porphyria; glucose transporter type 1 deficiency syndrome (Pérez-Dueñas et al., 2009)

Drugs

Neuroleptics (tardive dyskinesia, withdrawal emergent syndrome), dopaminergic drugs, anticholinergics, amphetamines, cocaine, tricyclics, oral contraceptives

Toxins

Alcohol intoxication and withdrawal, anoxia, carbon monoxide, manganese, mercury, thallium, toluene

Metabolic and endocrine disorders

Hypernatremia, hyponatremia, hypomagnesemia, hypocalcemia, hypoglycemia, hyperglycemia (nonketotic)

Hyperthyroidism, hypoparathyroidism

Pregnancy (chorea gravidarum)

Acquired hepatocerebral degeneration

Renal failure

Nutritional (e.g., ketogenic diet, beriberi, pellagra, vitamin B1 and B12 deficiency, particularly in infants)

Infectious and postinfectious

Sydenham chorea

Encephalitis lethargica

Various other infectious and postinfectious encephalitis, Creutzfeldt–Jakob disease, Lyme disease, mycoplasma

Immunological

Systemic lupus erythematosus

Henoch–Schönlein purpura

Acquired immunodeficiency disease

Acute disseminated encephalomyelitis (ADEM)

Vascular

Infarction or hemorrhage

Arteriovenous malformation, moyamoya disease

Polycythemia rubra vera

Antiphospholipid syndrome

Migraine

Following cardiac surgery with hypothermia and extracorporeal circulation in children (choreathetosis and orofacial dyskinesia, hypotonia, and pseudobulbar signs or CHAP syndrome)

Tumors

Trauma

Other secondary choreas

Cerebral palsy (anoxic), kernicterus, sarcoidosis, multiple sclerosis, disease, Behçet disease, polyarteritis nodosa, mitochondrial disorders

Miscellaneous

Paroxysmal dyskinesias (choreoathetosis), familial dyskinesia, and facial myokymia

---

syndrome") (Burke et al., 1994; Thomas and Jankovic, 2001; Wardle et al., 2009) (Table 15.3). Usually beginning in the fourth decade, the disorder may occur as an early-onset DRPLA (before 20 years of age), manifested by a variable combination of myoclonus, epilepsy, and mental retardation, or late-onset DRPLA (after 20 years of age), manifested by cerebellar ataxia, choreoathetosis, dystonia, rest and postural tremor, parkinsonism, and dementia (Video 15.1).

Unstable CAG expansion has been identified as the mutation in the *DRPLA* (or *ATN1*) gene on chromosome 12p13.31 (Koide et al., 1994; Komure et al., 1995; Warner et al., 1995; Becher et al., 1997; Ross et al., 1997). The *DRPLA* gene codes for protein that has been identified as a phosphoprotein, c-Jun NH(2)-terminal kinase, one of the major factors involved in its phosphorylation. In DRPLA, this protein appears to be slowly phosphorylated; thus, it may delay a process that is essential in keeping neurons alive

(Okamura-Oho et al., 2003). Similar to HD, there is an inverse correlation between the age at onset and the number of CAG repeats (Ikeuchi et al., 1995). The early onset of DRPLA is associated with greater number of CAG repeats (62–79) as compared to the late-onset type (54–67 repeats) (Ikeuchi et al., 1995). Testing for the various gene mutations will undoubtedly lead to better recognition and appreciation of the spectrum of clinical and pathologic changes associated with these disorders. For example, a family with spastic paraplegia, truncal ataxia, and dysarthria, but without other clinical features of DRPLA, has been found to show homozygosity for an allele that carries intermediate CAG repeats in the *DRPLA* gene (Kuroharas et al., 1997). The *DRPLA* gene is expressed predominantly in neurons, but neurons that are vulnerable to degeneration in DRPLA do not selectively express the gene (Nishiyama et al., 1997).

Neuroimaging studies in patients with DRPLA often show evidence of cortical, brainstem, and cerebellar atrophy and

Table 15.2 Differential diagnosis of inherited and sporadic choreas

Inherited disorders	Sporadic disorders
• HD	• Static encephalopathy (CP)
• HDL1, HDL2, HDL3	• Essential (senile) chorea
• DRPLA	• Sydenham chorea
• Neuroacanthocytosis	• Vascular chorea
• SCA2, 3, 17	• Polycythemia vera
• NBIA	• Sporadic Creutzfeldt–Jakob disease
– Pantothenate kinase associated neurodegeneration (PKAN), neuroferritinopathy, aceruloplasminemia, infantile neuroaxonal dystrophy	• Systemic lupus erythematosus
	• Antiphospholipid syndrome
	• Hyperthyroidism
	• AIDS
• Benign hereditary chorea	• Tardive dyskinesia
• Wilson disease	• Metabolic encephalopathy
• Mitochondrial disorders	– Hepatolenticular degeneration
• Ataxia with oculomotor apraxia (types 1 and 2)	– Nonketotic hyperglycemia
• Ataxia telangiectasia	– Hypoglycemia
	– Renal failure
	– Ketogenic diet

Table 15.3 Clinical features of dentatorubral-pallidoluysion atrophy (DRPLA)

Early onset	Late onset
<20 years	>20 years
Mild–moderate	Moderate–severe
Myoclonus	Ataxia (severe)
Epilepsy	Choreoathetosis
Mental retardation	Dystonia
62–79 CAG repeats	Rest and postural tremor
	Parkinsonism
	Dementia
	MRI – white matter changes
	54–67 CAG repeats

widespread white matter changes (Koide et al., 1997; Muñoz et al., 1999, 2004). Neuropathologic findings consist chiefly of degeneration of the dentatorubral system, globus pallidus externa (GPe), subthalamic nucleus, and, to a lesser extent, striatum, substantia nigra, inferior olive, and thalamus (Warner et al., 1994) as well as demyelination and reactive astrogliosis in the cerebral white matter (Muñoz et al., 2004). Involvement of oligodendrocytes in autopsied brains and an increased number of affected glia, as well as larger expansions in CAG in these glia, in transgenic mice might explain the widespread demyelination (Yamada et al., 2002). Several pathologic reports have noted widespread deposition of lipofuscin. Similar to HD and other diseases associated with CAG repeat expansions, DRPLA has also been associated with the formation of perinuclear aggregates that can be prevented by the use of transglutaminase inhibitors such as cystamine and monodansyl cadaverine (Igarashi et al., 1998). These intranuclear inclusions stain intensely with

ubiquitin (Becher and Ross, 1998). Subsequent studies have demonstrated accumulation of mutant atrophin-1 in the neuronal nuclei, rather than neuronal intranuclear inclusions, as the predominant pathologic feature in this neurodegenerative disorder (Yamada et al., 2001).

Other Huntington disease-like disorders

An autosomal dominant HD-like neurodegenerative disorder, now classified as HDL1 and mapped to chromosome 20p (Xiang et al., 1998), is a familial prion disease with an expanded PrP. A 192-nucleotide insertion in the region of the prion protein gene (*PRNP*) encoding an octapeptide repeat in the prion protein, was found in a single family with HD phenotype, suggesting that *PRNP* mutations can result in HD phenocopies (Moore et al., 2001).

Another disorder, termed HDL2, is characterized by onset in the fourth decade, involuntary movements such as chorea and dystonia as well as other movement disorders (bradykinesia, rigidity, tremor), dysarthria, hyperreflexia, gait abnormality, psychiatric symptoms, weight loss, and dementia with progression from onset to death in about 20 years (Margolis et al., 2001, 2004; Walker et al., 2003a). The disorder appears to be present exclusively or predominantly in individuals of African origin. The neuroimaging and neuropathologic findings are very similar to those in HD, except that there appears to be more severe involvement of the occipital cortex (Greenstein et al., 2007), and the intranuclear inclusions stain with 1C2 but not with anti-huntingtin antibodies. Unlike the family linked to chromosome 20p, seizures are not present in the HDL2 family. All 10 affected family members had a CAG repeat expansion of 50–60 triplets. The gene was later mapped to chromosome 16q24.3 and was found to encode junctophilin-3, a protein of the junctional complex linking the plasma membrane and the endoplasmic reticulum (Holmes et al., 2001). Although acanthocytosis was emphasized by Walker and colleagues (2002, 2003b) in their initial report and in one of three patients reported subsequently (Walker et al., 2003b), we have not been able to confirm the presence of acanthocytes in one member of the original family or in the other members when we carefully examined the peripheral smear.

The mutation associated with HDL2 has been identified as a CTG/CAG trinucleotide repeat expansion within the junctophilin-3 (*JPH3*) gene. In the normal population, the repeat length ranges from 6 to 27 CTG triplets, whereas affected individuals have 41–58 triplets. One family, previously described as "autosomal dominant chorea–acanthocytosis with polyglutamine-containing neuronal inclusions" (see later) (Walker et al., 2002), was subsequently found to have the triple nucleotide expansion of HDL2 (Stevanin et al., 2003; Walker et al., 2003b). The CTG repeat expansion at the HDL2 locus has been found to be responsible for 2% of patients with typical features of HD but without expanded CAG repeats in the *IT15* gene and 0.2% of all HD families, again providing evidence that HD is clinically and genetically heterogeneous (Stevanin et al., 2002). This group later analyzed 252 patients with an HDL phenotype, including 60 with typical HD, who had tested negative for pathologic expansion in the *IT15* gene and found two patients that had an abnormal CTG expansion in

DIAGNOSTIC EVALUATION OF CHOREA

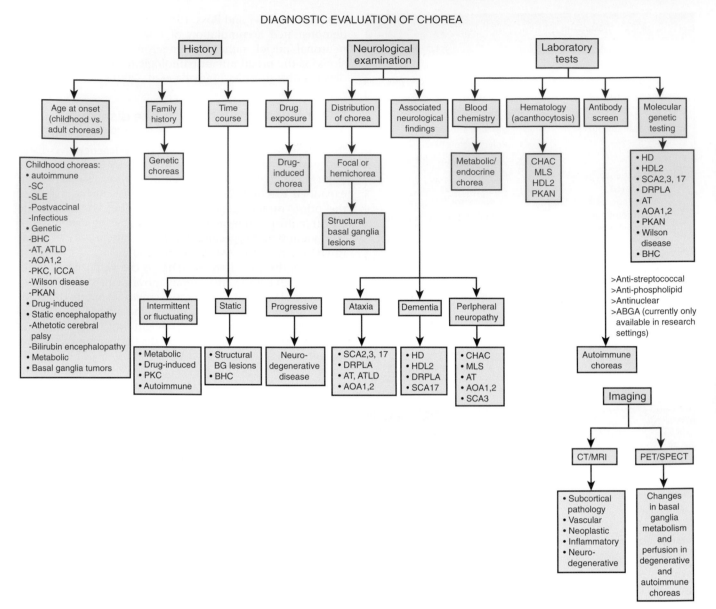

Figure 15.1 Evaluation of chorea.

the *JPH3* gene and two other patients with abnormal CAG expansion in the gene coding for TATA-binding protein (TBP/SCA17), important in initiation of transcription (Stevanin et al., 2003; Toyoshima et al., 2004; Schneider et al., 2006). SCA17, categorized as HDL4, has many clinical features that overlap with HD (Schneider et al., 2007; Bech et al., 2010). Thus, the frequency of mutation in either the *JPH3* gene or *TBP* gene among patients with HDL phenotype is about 3%. Initially, the TBP expansion was found in the family with SCA17, characterized clinically by intellectual deterioration, cerebellar ataxia, epilepsy, and chorea. CUG repeat-containing RNA foci, resembling myotonic dystrophy type 1, were detected in neurons of HDL2 brains, suggesting that RNA toxicity may play a role in the pathogenesis of this neurodegenerative disorder (Rudnicki et al., 2007). HLD2 resembles HD clinically and pathologically more than any other disease (Rudnicki et al., 2008).

While the majority of genetic forms of chorea are inherited in an autosomal dominant pattern, a novel autosomal recessive neurodegenerative HDL disorder has been described (Kambouris et al., 2000). Beginning at 3–4 years of age and manifested by chorea, dystonia, ataxia, gait disorder, spasticity, seizures, mutism, intellectual impairment, and bilateral frontal and caudate atrophy, this neurodegenerative disorder has been linked to 4p15.3, different from the 4p16.3 HD locus, but confirmation of this finding is lacking. Although classified as HDL3, because of its AR inheritance and clinical features atypical for HD, it should not be categorized as HDL. In fact the HDL terminology should be replaced with specific disorders in which genetic mutation has been identified.

Some cases of neuronal intranuclear inclusion disease, caused by expanded CAG repeats and characterized by the combination of extrapyramidal signs, lower motor neuron

Table 15.4 Clinical and genetic features of neuroacanthocytosis

- "Neuroacanthocytosis" coined to replace Levine–Critchley syndrome and choreoacanthocytosis and to draw attention to the heterogeneous presentation with a variety of hyperkinetic and hypokinetic movement disorders in addition to other neurologic deficits and abnormal laboratory findings
- Chorea–acanthocytosis (ChAc, MIM 200150)
  - Autosomal recessive
  - *VPS13A* gene (9q21, 73 exons); ~100 different mutations
  - Encodes a large protein, chorein (3174 amino acids)
  - Chorein required for trafficking of proteins between cell organelles; interferes with membrane functions
  - It is widely expressed in various tissues, but its expression is absent or severely reduced in ChAc
  - Absence of expression of chorein (Western blot) in RBC membrane is strongly suggestive of a diagnosis of ChAc (www.naadvocacy.org)

Table 15.5 Classification of neuroacanthocytosis

I. Normal lipids
1. Autosomal dominant
   a. Without inclusions
   b. With polyglutamine-containing neuronal inclusions (Walker et al., 2002)
2. Autosomal recessive: 9q21 (73 exons)
   a. Multiple mutations in the chorea acanthocytosis gene coding for chorein (Rampoldi et al., 2001; Ueno et al., 2001)
3. Sporadic

II. Hypobetalipoproteinemia (Mars et al., 1969)

III. Abetalipoproteinemia (Bassen and Kornzweig, 1950)

IV. Aprebetalipoproteinemia (Bohlega et al., 1998)

V. Hypoprebetalipoproteinemia
1. HARP syndrome: Hypoprebetalipoproteinemia, acanthocytosis, retinitis pigmentosa, and pallidal degeneration: similar to NBIA-1 (HSD)

VI. X-linked (McLeod syndrome) (Allen et al., 1961) Xp21
1. Neuroacanthocytosis: http://www.naadvocacy.org

signs, and cognitive and behavioral abnormalities resulting in death by the third decade, also show intranuclear aggregates, similar to the other CAG disorders (Lieberman et al., 1998).

Neuroacanthocytosis

After HD, neuroacanthocytosis is perhaps the most common form of hereditary chorea (Table 15.4). Previously also referred to as chorea–acanthocytosis, it is now recognized that this multisystem, neurodegenerative disorder can be expressed by a wide variety of clinical and laboratory abnormalities, hence the term *neuroacanthocytosis* (Spitz et al., 1985; Danek et al., 2005; Walker et al., 2006, 2007; Thomas and Jankovic, 2006) (Table 15.5). The term was coined by Jankovic et al. (1985) to replace the old term Levine–Critchley syndrome choreoacanthocytosis to draw attention to the heterogeneous presentation with a variety of hyperkinetic (chorea, dystonia, tics) and hypokinetic (parkinsonism) movement disorders in addition to other neurologic deficits and abnormal laboratory findings. Symptoms usually first begin in the third and fourth decades of life (range: 8–62 years) with lip and tongue biting followed by orolingual (eating) dystonia, motor and phonic tics, generalized chorea, and stereotypies (Video 15.2). Other features include cognitive and personality changes, seizures, dysphagia, dysarthria, vertical ophthalmoparesis, parkinsonism, amyotrophy, areflexia, evidence of axonal neuropathy, and elevated serum creatine kinase without evidence of myopathy. Hardie and colleagues (1991) reviewed the clinical, hematologic, and pathologic findings in 19 patients (10 males and 9 females) with a mean age of 32 years (range: 8–62 years) with more than 3% acanthocytes on peripheral blood smear. Twelve of these patients with neuroacanthocytosis were familial, and seven were sporadic; two had the McLeod phenotype (see later). In their series, Hardie and colleagues (1991) found a variety of movement disorders, including chorea (58%), orofacial dyskinesia (53%), dystonia (47%), vocalizations (47%), tics (42%), and parkinsonism (34%). Although lip and tongue biting was observed in only 16%

of the patients, this is a characteristic feature of neuroacanthocytosis and when present, it strongly suggests the diagnosis. The use of a mouth guard has been reported to be effective in the treatment of oral self-mutilation associated with neuroacanthocytosis (Fontenelle and Leite, 2008). Besides movement disorders other associated features included dysarthria (74%); absent or reduced reflexes (68%); dementia (63%); psychiatric problems such as depression, anxiety, and obsessive-compulsive disorder (58%); dysphagia (47%); seizures (42%); muscle weakness and wasting (16%); and elevated creatine phosphokinase (CK) in 58%. Magnetic resonance volumetry and fluorodeoxyglucose positron emission tomography (PET) show striatal atrophy in patients with neuroacanthocytosis (Jung et al., 2001).

Although autosomal dominant, X-linked recessive, and sporadic forms of neuroacanthocytosis have been reported, the majority of the reported families indicate autosomal recessive inheritance. Genome-wide scan for linkage in 11 families with autosomal recessive inheritance showed a linkage to a marker on chromosome 9q21, indicating a single locus for the disease (Rubio et al., 1997). Ueno and colleagues (2001) carried out a linkage-free analysis in the region of chromosome 9q21 in the Japanese population and identified a 260 bp deletion in the EST (expressed sequence tags) region K1AA0986 in exon 60, 61 that was homozygous in patients with neuroacanthocytosis and heterozygous in their parents. Further sequencing has identified a polyadenylation site with a protein with 3096 amino acid residues that has been named "chorein" by the authors. This deletion is not found in normal Japanese and European populations (Ueno et al., 2001). In another study by Rampoldi and colleagues (2001) in European patients, a novel gene encoding a 3174-amino-acid protein on chromosome 9q21 with 73 exons was identified. They identified 16 mutations in the chorea acanthocytosis (ChAc) gene, later renamed *VPS13A* gene. These mutations were identified in various exons. They suggested that chorea acanthocytosis encodes an evolutionarily conserved protein that is involved in protein sorting (Rampoldi et al., 2002). Other single heterozygous mutations have been identified in this gene (Saiki et al., 2003). Molecular analysis by screening all 73 exons of the *VPS13A* gene showed marked genotype–phenotype heterogeneity (Lossos et al., 2005). The function of the protein product, chorein, is not yet fully understood, but it is probably involved in intracellular protein trafficking. Using anti-chorein antisera, the expression of chorein in peripheral red blood cells has been found to be absent or markedly reduced in patients with neuroacanthocytosis, but not with McLeod syndrome or with HD (Dobson-Stone et al., 2004). Loss of chorein expression, measured by Western blot analysis has been found to be a reliable diagnostic test for neuroacanthocytosis.

Walker and colleagues (2002) described a family with chorea or parkinsonism as well as cognitive changes, inherited in an autosomal dominant pattern. At autopsy, there was marked degeneration of the striatum and intranuclear inclusion bodies immunoreactive for ubiquitin, expanded polyglutamine CGG repeats, and torsinA. Interestingly, one of the patients had fragile X syndrome, and two had expanded trinucleotide repeats at permutation range, previously associated with postural/kinetic tremor, parkinsonism, ataxia, and cognitive decline (Hagerman et al., 2001). The family reported by Walker and colleagues (2002) turned out to have the trinucleotide repeat expansion associated with HDL2, but subsequent analysis of the family shed doubt on the presence of acanthocytes as a feature of the HDL2 syndrome (Walker et al., 2003a).

Two patients from the original study by Rubio and colleagues (1997) were found to have the McLeod phenotype, an X-linked (Xp21) recessive form of acanthocytosis associated with depression, bipolar and personality disorder, and neurologic manifestations, including chorea, involuntary vocalizations, seizures, motor axonopathy, hemolysis, liver disease, and high creatine kinase levels (Witt et al., 1992; Danek et al., 2001a, 2001b). Neuroimaging usually reveals caudate and occasionally cerebellar atrophy with a rim of increased T2-intensity in the lateral putamen. Functional neuroimaging studies show evidence of downregulation of D2 dopamine receptors. In contrast to the autosomal recessive form of neuroacanthocytosis linked to mutations in *VPS13A* gene on chromosome 9, patients with McLeod syndrome usually do not exhibit lip-biting or dysphagia. This multisystem disorder is associated with low reactivity of Kell erythrocyte antigens (weak antigenicity of red cells) due to absence of XK, a 37 kDa, 444-amino-acid, membrane protein that forms a complex with the Kell protein. The disorder is caused by different mutations in the *XK* gene encoding for the XK protein (Ho et al., 1996; Danek et al., 2001a; Jung et al., 2001). Mutations identified by various authors include frame shift mutations in exon 2 at codon 151, deletion at codon 90 in exon 2 and at codon 408 in exon 3, and splicing mutations in intron 2 of the *XK* gene (Dotti et al., 2000; Ueyama et al., 2000; Danek et al., 2001a; Jung et al., 2001). Rarely, neuroacanthocytosis may be associated with abetalipoproteinemia due to mutations in the microsomal triglyceride transfer protein (Sharp et al., 1993).

In addition to acanthocytosis, the patients exhibit retinopathy; malabsorption, including that of vitamin E; low serum cholesterol levels; and abnormal serum lipoprotein electrophoresis. Aprebetalipoproteinemia can also cause movement disorders and acanthocytosis (Bohlega et al., 1998).

An examination of wet blood or Wright-stained, fast dry, blood smear usually reveals over 15% of red blood cells as acanthocytes. In mild forms of acanthocytosis, scanning electron microscopy might be required to demonstrate the red blood cell abnormalities (Feinberg et al., 1991). In a recent study of two patients with pathologically proven neuroacanthocytosis, Feinberg and colleagues (1991) noted that the yield in demonstrating acanthocytosis may be increased by using a coverslip because the contact with glass causes the fragile cells to undergo morphologic changes. Diluting the blood with normal saline, incubating the Wright-stained smear with EDTA, using a scanning electron microscope, and other techniques designed to increase "echinocytotic stress" are also helpful (Feinberg et al., 1991; Orrell et al., 1995). The characteristic acanthocytic appearance of red blood cells has been attributed to abnormalities in transmembrane glycoprotein band 3 that can be demonstrated on gel electrophoresis. It is not yet clear how the gene mutation leads to the abnormal morphology of the red cells.

By using high-performance liquid chromatography, fatty acids of erythrocyte membrane proteins were analyzed in six patients with neuroacanthocytosis (Sakai et al., 1991). In comparison with normal controls and patients with HD, erythrocytes of patients with neuroacanthocytosis showed a marked abnormality in the composition of covalently bound fatty acids: an increase in palmitic acid (C16:0) and a decrease in stearic acid (C18:0).

Brain magnetic resonance imaging (MRI) in patients with neuroacanthocytosis usually shows caudate and more generalized brain atrophy, but some cases also show extensive white matter abnormalities (Nicholl et al., 2004). Caudate hypometabolism and atrophy have been demonstrated by PET studies and by neuroimaging. Similar to the findings in Parkinson disease, PET scans in six patients with neuroacanthocytosis showed a reduction to 42% of normal in [^{18}F]dopa uptake in the posterior putamen; in contrast to Parkinson disease, however, there was a marked reduction in the striatal [^{11}C]raclopride (D2) receptor binding (Brooks et al., 1991).

Neuronal loss and gliosis were particularly prominent in the striatum and pallidum but may also affect the thalamus, substantia nigra, and anterior horns of the spinal cord (Rinne et al., 1994b). The neuronal loss in the substantia nigra is most evident in the ventrolateral region, similar to Parkinson disease, but the nigral neuronal loss is more widespread in neuroacanthocytosis (Rinne et al., 1994a). The preservation of the cerebral cortex, cerebellum, subthalamic nucleus, pons, and medulla may serve to differentiate pathologically between neuroacanthocytosis, HD, and DRPLA. Brain biochemical analyses showed low substance P in the substantia nigra and striatum and increased levels of norepinephrine in the putamen and pallidum (DeYebenes et al., 1988).

Unfortunately, there is no effective treatment for patients with neuroacanthocytosis. The associated parkinsonism rarely improves with dopaminergic therapy, probably because there is loss of postsynaptic dopamine receptors. We have seen some patients whose condition remained static for several years, followed by further progression and an eventual demise as a result of aspiration pneumonia or other complications of chronic illness.

Neurodegeneration with brain iron accumulation

A group of neurodegenerative disorders, formerly known as Hallervorden–Spatz disease, has been receiving increasing attention as the genetic and pathogenic mechanisms of the various subtypes become elucidated. Because of Hallervorden's terrible past and his shameless involvement in active euthanasia (Shevell, 2003), this group of disorders has been renamed neurodegeneration with brain iron accumulation (NBIA). The prototype form of NBIA consists of an autosomal recessive disorder characterized by childhood-onset progressive rigidity, dystonia, choreoathetosis, spasticity, optic nerve atrophy, and dementia, and has been associated with acanthocytosis (Malandrini et al., 1996; Racette et al., 2001; Thomas et al., 2004). Although chorea is not a typical feature of NBIA, "senile chorea" has been described in a patient with pathologically proven NBIA type1 (NBIA-1) (Grimes et al., 2000).

The most classic NBIA, NBIA-1, is the pantothenate kinase-associated neurodegeneration (PKAN). Linkage analyses initially localized the NBIA-1 gene on 20p12.3–p13; subsequently, a 7 bp deletion and various missense mutations were identified in the coding sequence of the *PANK2* gene, which codes for pantothenate kinase (Zhou et al., 2001; Hayflick et al., 2003). Pantothenate kinase is an essential regulatory enzyme in coenzyme A biosynthesis. It has been postulated that as a result of phosphopantothenate deficiency, cysteine accumulates in the globus pallidus of brains of patients with NBIA-1. It undergoes rapid auto-oxidation in the presence of nonheme iron that normally accumulates in the globus pallidus interna (GPi) and substantia nigra, generating free radicals that are locally neurotoxic. Interestingly, atypical subjects were found to be compound heterozygotes for certain mutations for which classic subjects were homozygous. The disorder with the clinical phenotype of NBIA associated with mutations in the *PANK2* gene is now referred to as pantothenate kinase-associated neurodegeneration or PKAN (Thomas et al., 2004). On the basis of an analysis of 123 patients from 98 families with NBIA-1, Hayflick and colleagues (2003) found that "classic Hallervorden–Spatz syndrome" was associated with *PANK2* mutation in all cases and that one-third of "atypical" cases had the mutations within the *PANK2* gene. Those who had the *PANK2* mutation were more likely to have dysarthria and psychiatric symptoms, and all had the typical "eye-of-the-tiger" abnormality on MRI with a specific pattern of hyperintensity within the hypointense GPi (McNeill et al., 2008).

Neuroacanthocytosis and NBIA may overlap in some clinical features. While PKAN may be associated with acanthocytosis, another neuroacanthocytosis syndrome, linked to PKAN, is the hypoprebetalipoproteinemia, acanthocytosis, retinitis pigmentosa, and pallidal degeneration (HARP) syndrome (Orrell et al., 1995). This disorder is associated with dystonia, particularly involving the oromandibular region,

Table 15.6 Differential diagnosis of neurodegeneration with brain iron accumulation (NBIA)

- Pantothenate kinase-associated neurodegeneration
- Neuroferritinopathy
- Aceruloplasminemia
- Infantile neuroaxonal dystrophy (NBIA-2)
  - Karak syndrome
  - PLAN (PLA2G6-associated neurodegeneration). The *PLA2G6* gene encodes a calcium-independent phospholipase A2 enzyme that catalyzes the hydrolysis of glycerophospholipids; early-childhood-onset axial hypotonia, spasticity, bulbar dysfunction, ataxia, and dystonia
  - PLAN without iron deposition; adult-onset, levodopa-responsive dystonia–parkinsonism

rather than chorea and self-mutilation. Indeed, a homozygous nonsense mutation in exon 5 of the *PANK2* gene that creates a stop codon at amino acid 371, found in the original HARP patient, establishes that HARP is part of the pantothenate kinase-associated neurodegeneration disease spectrum (Ching et al., 2002; Houlden et al., 2003).

The classification of NBIA is continuously being revised as our understanding of this group of disorders is improving. In addition to PKAN, other forms of NBIA include neuroferritinopathy, infantile neuroaxonal dystrophy, and aceruloplasminemia, and PLA2G6-associated neurodegeneration (PLAN), with mutations in the *PLA2G6* gene, on chromosome 22q13.1 (Schneider et al., 2009) (Table 15.6, Fig. 15.2). These disorders are chiefly manifested by childhood-onset axial hypotonia, spasticity, bulbar dysfunction, ataxia, dystonia, and choreoathetosis, as well as MRI changes indicative of iron deposition in the globus pallidus and substantia nigra (Kurian et al., 2008). Previously diagnosed as infantile neuroaxonal dystrophy, now classified as NBIA-2, PLAN may also present as adult-onset, levodopa-responsive dystonia–parkinsonism without iron on brain imaging (McNeill et al., 2008; Paisan-Ruiz et al., 2008; Schneider et al., 2009). Another gene, *FA2H*, when mutated, has been found to cause not only leukodystrophy and hereditary spastic paraplegia, but also NBIA (Kruer et al., 2010). The *FA2H*-associated neurodegeneration (FAHN) is characterized by childhood-onset gait impairment, spastic paraparesis, ataxia, and dystonia (Kruer et al., 2010; Schneider and Bhatia, 2010). FA2H is involved in lipid and ceramide metabolism. Another form of NBIA was highlighted by a report of 11 children with a biochemical profile suggestive of dopamine transporter deficiency syndrome (Kurian et al., 2011). Presenting in infancy, this disorder is usually characterized by severe parkinsonism-dystonia syndrome, but chorea, oculomotor deviations, and spasticity may also dominate the clinical phenotype. The CSF ratio of homovanillic acid to 5-hydroxyindoleacetic acid is usually increased. This autosomal recessive disorder has been attributed to homozygous or compound heterozygous *SLC6A3* mutations and complete loss of dopamine transporter activity in the basal nuclei (indicated by abnormal DAT Scan SPECT). Regression of symptoms after 6 months of iron chelation with deferiprone has been reported in some patients with NBIA (Forni et al., 2008).

BRAIN IRON HOMEOSTASIS AND NEURODEGENERATIVE DISEASE

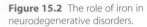

Figure 15.2 The role of iron in neurodegenerative disorders.

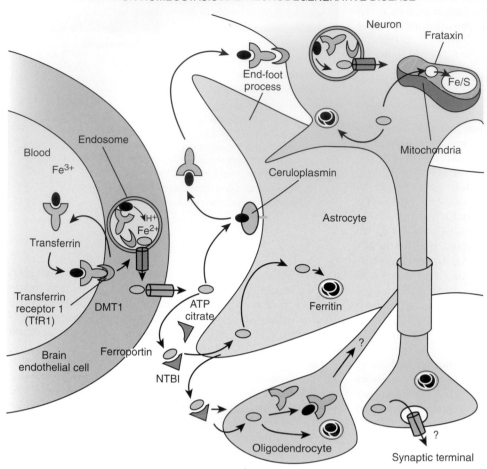

Table 15.7 Clinical features of benign hereditary chorea

- Onset in early childhood
- Progresses until second decade → static or spontaneously improves (may persist >60)
- No dementia or other abnormalities
- MRI normal, but may show hypoplastic pallidum, lack of differentiation of medial and lateral components, and bilateral signal hyperintensities on T2-weighted images
- No pathologic changes, but may have reduced number of striatal and neocortical interneurons
- Autosomal dominant associated with mutation in *TITF1* gene on chromosome 14q13–q21.1
- *TITF1* gene mutation should be considered in patients with chorea, mental retardation, chronic lung disease and congenital hypothyroidism, hence the term brain–lung–thyroid (BLT) syndrome
- May improve markedly with levodopa

Other familial choreas

Besides HD and neuroacanthocytosis, genetically transmitted choreas include benign hereditary chorea (BHC), a nonprogressive chorea of childhood onset (Wheeler et al., 1993; Kleiner-Fisman and Lang, 2007; Adam and Jankovic, 2010) (Table 15.7). BHC usually starts in early childhood and progresses until the second decade, after which time it remains static or even spontaneously improves. The patients may have a slight motor delay because of chorea, slight gait ataxia, and their handwriting may be impaired, but the disorder is self-limiting after adolescence in most cases, although it may persist as a mild chorea beyond age 60 years. Inherited as an autosomal dominant disorder, BHC has been linked to a marker on chromosome 14q13.1–q21.1 (de Vries et al., 2000; Fernandez et al., 2001; Breedveld et al., 2002) and a novel single nucleotide substitution in the *TITF1* gene (also referred to as *TTF*, *Nkx2.1*, and *T/ebp*), coding for a transcription essential for the organogenesis of the lung, thyroid, and basal ganglia, has been identified in one Canadian family (Kleiner-Fisman et al., 2003; Kleiner-Fisman and Lang, 2007; Ferrara et al., 2008) (http://www.ncbi.nlm.nih.gov/sites/GeneTests/). This syndrome has been also described in patients with deletion of not only the *TITF1* gene but also the contiguous *PAX9* gene (Devos et al., 2006). These mutations should be considered in children and adults with chorea, mental retardation, congenital hypothyroidism, and chronic lung disease, hence the term brain–lung–thyroid syndrome proposed for this disease (Willemsen et al., 2005; Devos et al., 2006). MRI has been generally reported to be unremarkable but some cases showed hypoplastic pallidum, lack of differentiation of medial and lateral components, and bilateral signal hyperintensities on T2-weighted MRI images (Kleiner-Fisman and Lang, 2007).

Two autopsied brains from patients with BHC due to *TITF1* showed no pathologic abnormalities (Asmus et al., 2005), but specific immunochemical investigations suggested reduced number of striatal and neocortical interneurons, consistent with a defect in migration normally mediated by the *TITF1* gene (Kleiner-Fisman et al., 2005).

Adult-onset, autosomal dominant, benign chorea without dementia, initially reported in Japan, in which HD, HDL1, HDL2, DRPLA, SCA17, and mutations in the *TITF1* gene were excluded, revealed linkage to a novel locus on chromosome 8q21.3–q23.3 in two Japanese families with "benign hereditary chorea type 2" (BHC2) (Shimohata et al., 2007). Surprisingly, BHC may improve markedly with levodopa (Asmus et al., 2005). The existence of BHC has been questioned because many patients who were initially diagnosed with the disorder were later found to have some other diagnosis, such as myoclonic dystonia, hereditary essential myoclonus, tics, and HD (Schrag et al., 2000).

Essential chorea is a form of adult-onset, nonprogressive chorea without family history of chorea or other symptoms suggestive of HD and without evidence of striatal atrophy on neuroimaging studies. Sometimes referred to as senile chorea, essential chorea usually has its onset after age 60, and in contrast to HD, it is not associated with dementia or positive family history. Some cases of senile chorea, however, have been reported to have pathologic changes identical to HD; others have had predominant degeneration of the putamen rather than the caudate (Friedman and Ambler, 1990). The CAG repeat length should, by definition, be normal, but Ruiz and colleagues (1997) found abnormal CAG expansion in three of six clinically diagnosed cases of senile chorea. Although the authors suggest that some patients with senile chorea have a sporadic form of HD, the term *essential* (or *senile*) *chorea* should be reserved for those patients with late-onset chorea without family history, without dementia, without psychiatric problems, and without CAG expansion. These criteria are necessary in order to separate senile or essential chorea from HD. Hereditary chorea without dementia and with a benign course has been also described (Behan and Bone, 1977).

Choreoathetosis, along with developmental regression, mental retardation, pendular nystagmus, optic atrophy, dysphagia, dystonia, spasticity, and severe bilateral striatal atrophy with response to biotin, is a feature of familial infantile bilateral striatal necrosis (IBSN) (Straussberg et al., 2002; Basel-Vanagaite et al., 2006). IBSN, an autosomal recessive neurodegenerative disorder, was found to be associated with mutation of *nup62* on chromosome 19q13.32–13.41 (Basel-Vanagaite et al., 2006).

Ataxia telangiectasia, an autosomal recessive multisystem disease, is another disorder often associated with chorea. In a retrospective analysis of the clinical characteristics in 18 adult patients with ataxia telangiectasia from 9 families and 6 unrelated adults documented with elevated alphafetoprotein, chromosomal instability, and mutations in the *A-T mutated* (*ATM*) gene and measurements of ATM protein expression and kinase activity, chorea–athetosis was present in 14/18 (78%) cases (Verhagen et al., 2009). Other common abnormalities included dysarthria, oculomotor apraxia, dystonia, rest tremor, neuropathy, immunodeficiency, restricted respiratory function, and malignancies. Not all affected individuals have telangiectasia.

Another disorder, rarely considered in the differential diagnosis of chorea, is familial dyskinesia and facial myokymia (FDFM), characterized by childhood-onset adventitious movements and perioral or periorbital myokymia. These movements may be paroxysmal in early stages, increase in frequency and severity, and become constant in the third decade, without intellectual impairment or shortening of lifespan. Frontotemporal dementia, particularly associated with TAR-DNA binding protein (TDP)-43 abnormalities due to *TARDBP* mutations, may be associated not only with amyotrophic lateral sclerosis, but also supranuclear gaze palsy and chorea (Kovacs et al., 2009).

Infectious chorea

A variety of infections that affect the central nervous system have been associated with chorea. Acute manifestations of bacterial meningitis, encephalitis, tuberculous meningitis, and aseptic meningitis include movement disorders such as chorea, athetosis, dystonia, or hemiballismus (Alarcon et al., 2000). Human immunodeficiency virus (HIV) has also been reported to cause chorea and other features of HD, either as the result of human immunodeficiency virus encephalitis (Sevigny et al., 2005) or as the result of focal opportunistic infections such as toxoplasmosis (Nath et al., 1987; Gallo et al., 1996; Pardo et al., 1998; Piccolo et al., 1999).

Postinfectious and autoimmune choreas

Sydenham disease

Occasionally still referred to as St Vitus' chorea or St Vitus' dance (Krack, 1999), Sydenham chorea was described originally by Thomas Sydenham, an English physician, in 1686. Considered an autoimmune disorder, a consequence of infection with group A β-hemolytic streptococcus (GABHS), the phenomenology has broadened to include not only chorea but also a variety of other neurologic, psychiatric, cardiac, rheumatologic, and other disorders (Swedo, 1994; Cardoso et al., 1997; Cardoso, 2004) (Videos 15.3 and 15.4). Since chorea is only one of many neurologic and nonneurologic manifestations, the term *Sydenham disease* is preferred, rather than *Sydenham chorea*, but the latter is used so frequently in the literature that its usage will be difficult to change. Osler, in his seminal paper "On Chorea and Choreiform Affections," published in 1894, drew attention to the distinction between Sydenham disease and HD (Goetz, 2000). Although the majority of the patients have bilateral involvement, the distribution of chorea is usually asymmetrical, and pure hemichorea can be seen in 20% of all Sydenham disease patients. The individual contractions are slightly longer in Sydenham disease (>100 ms) compared to those in HD (50–100 ms) (Hallett and Kaufman, 1981). Other features of Sydenham disease include dysarthria and decreased verbal output, hypometric saccades, oculogyric crisis, papilledema, central retinal artery occlusion, and seizures. Similar to Tourette syndrome (Kwak et al., 2003b), migraine is more common in children with Sydenham disease than in controls (Teixeira et al., 2005). Unlike arthritis and carditis, which occur soon after streptococcal infection, chorea and various neurobehavioral symptoms may be delayed for 6 months or longer and may be the sole manifestation of rheumatic fever (Stollerman, 1997). In 50 consecutive patients with rheumatic fever, 26% developed chorea, but arthritis was more frequent in patients without chorea (84%) than in those with chorea (31%) (Cardoso et al., 1997). 📷

Some features of Sydenham disease overlap with those of Tourette syndrome. Although tics are often differentiated from chorea by the presence of premonitory sensation, reported by more than 90% of patients with Tourette syndrome (Kwak et al., 2003a), some patients with chorea also report sensory symptoms (Rodopman-Arman et al., 2004). There is controversy as to whether pediatric autoimmune neuropsychiatric disorders associated with streptococcal infections (PANDAS), discussed in more detail in Chapter 16, which may be associated with motor and phonic tics, is a variant of Sydenham disease or a separate entity (Kurlan, 2004; Kurlan et al., 2008; Singer et al., 2008).

Behavioral problems associated with Sydenham disease include irritability, emotional lability, obsessive-compulsive disorder, hyperactivity, learning disorders, and other behavioral problems that are typically observed in patients with Tourette syndrome. One study compared 56 patients with Sydenham disease with 50 rheumatic fever patients and 50 healthy subjects and found that obsessive-compulsive behavior was present in 19%, obsessive-compulsive disorder in 23.2%, and attention deficit-hyperactivity disorder in 30.4%, all significantly more frequently than in the rheumatic fever or healthy controls (Maia et al., 2005). The neurobehavioral symptoms usually begin within 2–4 weeks after the onset of the choreic movements. The disorder tends to resolve spontaneously in 3–4 months but may persist in half of the patients during a 3-year follow-up (Cardoso et al., 1999). Female gender and the presence of carditis might be risk factors for persistent disease. In some cases of Sydenham disease, the chorea recurs during pregnancy (chorea gravidarum) or when the patient is exposed to estrogen. Sydenham disease, once relatively common, is now encountered relatively rarely in developed countries (Eshel et al., 1993). Recurrences of Sydenham disease are not associated with anti-basal ganglia antibodies (Harrison et al., 2004).

In addition to occasionally elevated titers of antistreptolysin O (ASO), which is not specific for GABHS infection as it can also reflect group G, the majority of patients with Sydenham disease have been found to have IgG antibodies reacting with neurons in the caudate and subthalamic nuclei (Kiessling et al., 1993; Swedo et al., 1993). These antineuronal antibodies are found in nearly all patients with Sydenham disease (Swedo, 1994; Abraham et al., 1997; Mittleman, 1997). The rheumatic B-cell alloantigen D8/17 is also frequently found in patients with rheumatic chorea, but it is not clear whether this could be used as a diagnostic test (Feldman et al., 1993). Anti-basal ganglia antibodies have been identified in patients with acute and persistent Sydenham disease, providing further evidence that the disease is an antibody-mediated disorder (Church et al., 2002).

MRI is usually normal in patients with Sydenham disease except for selective enlargement of the caudate, putamen, and globus pallidus (Giedd et al., 1995). In contrast to other choreic disorders, PET scans in patients with Sydenham disease indicate increased rather than decreased striatal glucose consumption (Weindl et al., 1993).

The standard of care for all children diagnosed with Sydenham disease, even in cases of isolated chorea, is secondary prevention with penicillin to reduce the risk of recurrences of chorea but especially to reduce the likelihood that future GABHS infections could cause carditis and permanent valvular damage (Panamonta et al., 2007; Cardoso, 2008). Current recommendations in the United States are for treatment until age 21 years with either monthly intramuscular or daily oral penicillin. Although cephalosporins are equally effective, penicillin, 500–1000 mg of penicillin G four times per day or one intramuscular injection of 600 000 to 1.2 million units of benzathine penicillin, is considered the drug of choice for pharyngitis caused by GABHS infection (Garvey and Swedo, 1997). Despite an adequate (10-day) course, the bacteriologic failure rate is as high as 15%, and some patients develop rheumatic fever. Therefore, oral rifampin 20 mg/kg every 24 hours for four doses is recommended during the last 4 days of the 10-day course of penicillin therapy. Alternatively, oral rifampin 10 mg/kg can be given every 12 hours for eight doses with one dose of intramuscular benzathine penicillin G. Another alternative is oral clindamycin 20 mg/kg/day in three doses for 10 days. The best prevention of rheumatic fever is accurate diagnosis and adequate treatment of the initial acute pharyngitis. Penicillin prophylaxis is advisable in all patients for at least 10 years after rheumatic fever. Symptomatic treatment usually consists of anti-dopaminergic drugs such as tetrabenazine, valproic acid, and carbamazepine until the condition resolves spontaneously. A double-blind, placebo-controlled study of prednisone showed beneficial effects on Sydenham disease (Paz et al., 2006).

Other autoimmune choreas

Besides Sydenham disease, another poststreptococcal disorder which may include chorea, but more commonly is characterized by parkinsonism and dystonia is poststreptococcal acute disseminated encephalomyelitis (PSADEM), associated with the anti-basal ganglia antibodies (Dale et al., 2001). Although both Sydenham disease and PSADEM are associated with MRI T2 hyperintensities, the lesions described in PSADEM had normal T1 sequences and the white matter and brainstem are additionally involved. Chorea has been also recognized in a variety of other autoimmune processes, such as systemic lupus erythematosus (SLE). Chorea occurs in 2% of patients with SLE, and choreic movements precede the diagnosis of SLE in 22% of these cases. Choreic movements associated with pregnancy (chorea gravidarum) and with birth control pills probably result from a common pathogenesis, and chorea gravidarum may be the first manifestation of SLE or may represent as a variant of Sydenham disease. Chorea in SLE has been associated with the presence of antiphospholipid antibodies, a heterogeneous group of antibodies that produce platelet endothelial dysfunction and promote thrombogenesis. The primary antiphospholipid syndrome is characterized by the presence of antiphospholipid antibodies in patients who have autoimmune phenomena but insufficient clinical or serologic features to be classified as having SLE. Antiphospholipid antibody syndrome is defined by a clinical event of thrombosis or miscarriage in the setting of persistently present and sufficiently high titers of antibodies, either anticardiolipin IgG or IgM, lupus anticoagulant, or anti-B2-glycoprotein 1 ("Sapporo" criteria) (Orzechowski et al., 2008). In a cohort of 1000 patients who met the Sapporo criteria for definite antiphospholipid syndrome, chorea occurred in 13 (1.3%) patients. In addition to a hypercoagulable state, a variety of neurologic and movement disorders, such as chorea, ballism, dystonia, parkinsonism and paroxysmal dyskinesias have been associated with the antiphospholipid syndrome (Gutrecht et al., 1991; Lang et al., 1991; Cervera et al., 1997; Martino et al., 2006; Wu et al., 2007; Huang et al., 2008; Orzechowski et al., 2008). Other clinical features include spontaneous abortions, arthralgias, Raynaud phenomenon, digital infarctions, transient ischemic attacks, and stroke (Sanna et al., 2006). Antiphospholipid antibodies present in patients with this syndrome include lupus anticoagulant, anticardiolipin antibody, and anti-β2-glycoprotein-I antibodies. Anticardiolipin antibodies, frequently found in SLE, are absent in patients with Sydenham disease. Contralateral striatal hypermetabolism was documented by an ^{18}F-fluorodeoxyglucose PET scan in a 23-year-old woman with alternating hemichorea and antiphospholipid syndrome (Furie et al., 1994). The striatal D1 and D2 receptor binding, measured by PET scans, was normal in one patient with SLE (Turjanski et al., 1995).

Other choreas

One of the most common forms of chorea encountered in a movement disorder clinic is drug-induced chorea associated with the use of dopaminergic or antidopaminergic drugs, anticonvulsants, and other drugs (Hyde et al., 1991; Jankovic, 1995). Levodopa-induced dyskinesia is often manifested by stereotypies, dystonia, and myclonus as well as chorea (Jankovic, 2005) (Video 15.5). Although the dominant hyperkinetic movement disorder seen in patients with tardive dyskinesia is stereotypy, some patients have associated chorea, and chorea is the chief manifestation in children with withdrawal emergent syndrome. Chorea, often accompanied by ataxia and deafness, has also been associated with mitochondrial DNA mutations (Nelson et al., 1995) and other evidence of mitochondrial cytopathies, including mutations in the *POLG* gene (Caer et al., 2005; Wong et al., 2008). The disorder of early-onset ataxia with oculomotor apraxia and hypoalbuminemia due to mutations in the *aprataxin* gene on chromosome 19p13 has also been associated with chorea (Shimazaki et al., 2002).

Besides vasculitis, chorea has been associated with a variety of other vascular etiologies, but few have been documented pathologically. The topic of vascular chorea has been reviewed in a report of an 85-year-old woman who developed progressive dementia and chorea at age 70 (Bhatia et al., 1994). At autopsy, her brain showed neostriatal neuronal loss and gliosis associated with congophilic angiopathy and atherosclerosis. Hemichorea has been also reported following endarterectomy for carotid stenosis (Galea et al., 2008).

During the 1980s, there was an increase in the number of children with chorea as sequelae to cardiac surgery, but with modification of treatment strategies during the perioperative period, the incidence of this complication has subsequently decreased (Robinson et al., 1988). This post-pump chorea appears to be associated with prolonged time on pump, deep hypothermia, and circulatory arrest (Medlock et al., 1993; Newburger et al., 1993; du Plessis et al., 2002) (Videos 15.6 and 15.7). Others have suggested that hypoxia rather than hypothermia is critical in the development of CHAP syndrome (choreathetosis and orofacial dyskinesia, hypotonia, and pseudobulbar signs) after surgery for congenital heart disease. In most patients, the chorea persists, and fewer than 25% improve with antidopaminergic therapy such as haloperidol. Steroid-responsive chorea was described in a patient after heart transplant (Blunt et al., 1994). Although the chorea may improve, long-term studies have shown that these children have persistent deficits in memory, attention, and language (du Plessis et al., 2002).

A variety of systemic (Janavs and Aminoff, 1998), metabolic, and neurodegenerative disorders can be associated with chorea, such as hypocalcemia or hypercalcemia, hyperglycemia (Ahlskog et al., 2001; Chu et al., 2002; Oh et al., 2002; Pisani et al., 2005; Sitburana and Ondo, 2006), hyperthyroidism (Pozzan et al., 1992), B12 deficiency (Pacchetti et al., 2002), Lesch–Nyhan syndrome (Jankovic et al., 1988; Jinnah et al., 1994; Ernst et al., 1996), propionic acidemia (Nyhan et al., 1999), and other metabolic disorders such as glutaric aciduria, gluscose transporter type 1 deficiency (Pérez-Dueñas et al., 2009), and GM1 gangliosidosis (Shulman et al., 1995; Stacy and Jankovic, 1995).

Chorea (with or without associated ballism) has been reported as the presenting feature of renal failure (Kujawa et al., 2001) and paraneoplastic striatal encephalitis (Tani et al., 2000; Vernino et al., 2002; Kinirons et al., 2003; Grant and Graus, 2009; Kleinig et al., 2009). In a series of 16 patients with paraneoplastic chorea, 11 had small-cell carcinoma, all had CRMP-5 IgG, and 6 had ANNA-1 (anti-Hu) antibodies (Vernino et al., 2002). Another metabolic cause of chorea is liver disease, particularly chronic acquired hepatocerebral degeneration (Thobois et al., 2002) (Video 15.8). Many of the metabolic choreas are associated with abnormalities on MRI scans. For example, hepatocerebral degeneration and hyperglycemic chorea are often associated with high signal intensity on T1-weighted MRI, involving the striatum and pallidum (Ahlskog et al., 2001; Thobois et al., 2002; Sitburana and Ondo, 2006). In a report of two patients with hyperglycemic hemichorea–hemiballism, Chu and colleagues (2002) found high signal intensities on T1- and T2-weighted images as well as on diffusion-weighted MRI accompanied by a reduction in diffusion coefficient, suggestive of hyperviscosity, rather than petechial hemorrhages, as the mechanism of edema in the striatum. This is also supported by another study of seven patients with hyperglycemic choreoathetosis using MRI and MR spectroscopy (Kandiah et al., 2009). Interestingly, the presence of high acanthocyte count may predispose patients with diabetes to develop hyperglycemic chorea (Pisani et al., 2005). Other disorders frequently associated with this MRI abnormality include manganese toxicity, Wilson disease, abnormal calcium metabolism, neurofibromatosis, hypoxia, and hemorrhage. Chorea has been associated with a variety of other causes, including cerebrospinal fluid leak (Mokri et al., 2006).

Another disorder associated with chorea and frequently misdiagnosed as Huntington disease is neuroferritinopathy, a progressive but potentially treatable disorder caused by mutations in the ferritin light chain gene (*FTL1*), located on 19q13.3–q13.4. Patients may be initially diagnosed as "idiopathic dystonia," "Parkinson disease," "Huntington disease," and a variety of other disorders. In a study of 41 genetically homogeneous subjects with the 460InsA mutation in *FTL1*, the mean age at onset was 39.4 ± 13.3 years (range: 13–63), beginning with chorea in 50%, focal lower limb dystonia in 42.5%, and parkinsonism in 7.5% (Chinnery et al., 2007). The disease progressed over a 5–10-year period, eventually leading to aphonia, dysphagia and severe, often asymmetrical, motor disability, and finally dementia in the advanced stages. A characteristic action-specific facial dystonia was present in 65%. Serum ferritin levels were low in the majority of males and postmenopausal females, but may be normal, particularly in premenopausal females. MRI typically shows gradient echo T2* hypointensity in red nuclei, substantia nigra, and globus pallidus; brain imaging was abnormal in all affected individuals and one presymptomatic carrier, with T1 hyperintensity in the globus pallidus and posterior putamen (Chinnery et al., 2007).

Treatment of chorea

The first step in the treatment of chorea is the identification of a specific etiology. Chorea has been treated successfully with drugs that interfere with central dopaminergic function, such as the dopamine receptor-blocking drugs (neuroleptics), reserpine, and tetrabenazine (Jankovic and Beach, 1997; Chatterjee and Frucht, 2003; Kenney and Jankovic, 2006; Sitburana and Ondo, 2006; Fasano and Bentivoglio, 2009; Jankovic, 2009). Indeed, tetrabenazine provides the most effective relief of chorea with only minimal, dose-related side effects, such as drowsiness, insomnia, depression, and parkinsonism. Tetrabenazine is effective not only for the treatment of chorea associated with HD (Ondo et al., 2002; Huntington Study Group, 2006), but also for choreatic disorders associated with tardive dyskinesia (Ondo et al., 1999), cerebral palsy (CP), and post-pump encephalopathy (Chatterjee and Frucht, 2003) (Video 15.6). While some studies have suggested that sodium valproate may be effective in the treatment of chorea (Daoud et al., 1990; Hoffman and Feinberg, 1990), other reports have been less conclusive (Sethi and Patel, 1990). Levetiracetam has been reported to markedly improve a patient with CP and postinfectious chorea (Recio et al., 2005).

There is no consensus as to the optimal management of autoimmune chorea. Patients with Sydenham disease should be treated with penicillin prophylactically to prevent rheumatic fever. Symptomatic suppression of chorea with dopamine antagonists may lessen disability. Anticoagulation, immunosuppressants, and plasmapheresis have been utilized with variable success, and the frequent occurrence of spontaneous remissions makes the results of treatment difficult to interpret. Until prospective therapeutic trials can be designed, careful selection of treatment that best seems to suit the severity of the patient's illness might be indicated. The presence of true vasculitis might require more aggressive management. Steroids are sometimes recommended for the treatment of autoimmune chorea, and this treatment was found effective also in chorea associated with heart

transplant (Blunt et al., 1994). Stereotactic surgery is occasionally needed in very severe and disabling cases of hemichorea/hemiballism (Krauss and Mundinger, 2000).

Ballism

Chorea, athetosis, and ballism represent a continuum of involuntary, hyperkinetic movement disorders. Ballism is a form of forceful, flinging, high-amplitude, coarse, chorea (Videos 15.9 and 15.10). Ballism and chorea are often interrelated and may occur in the same patient (Harbord and Kobayashi, 1991). The involuntary movement usually affects only one side of the body; the term *hemiballism* is used to describe unilateral ballism. Although various structural lesions have been associated with ballism (Rossetti et al., 2003), damage to the subthalamic nucleus and the pallido-subthalamic pathways appears to play a critical role in the expression of this hyperkinetic movement disorder (Guridi and Obeso, 2001). Subthalamotomy has been found to ameliorate the motor disturbances in human and experimental parkinsonism, but the procedure can produce transient or permanent hemiballism (Bergman et al., 1990; Aziz et al., 1991; Guridi and Obeso, 2001; Chen et al., 2002).

When caused by a hemorrhagic or ischemic stroke, the movement disorder is often preceded by hemiparesis. Anterior parietal artery stroke, without any evidence of involvement of the basal ganglia, thalamus, or subthalamic nucleus, has been associated with contralateral hemiballism and neurogenic pain (Rossetti et al., 2003). This and other similar cases suggest that the lesion associated with hemiballism may extend beyond the contralateral subthalamic nucleus and connecting structures into the adjacent internal capsule. Less common causes of hemiballism include abscess, arteriovenous malformation, cerebral trauma, hyperosmotic hyperglycemia (Ahlskog et al., 2001), multiple sclerosis, and tumor (Glass et al., 1984). Rarely, ballism occurs bilaterally (paraballism), usually due to bilateral basal ganglia strokes or calcification (Inbody and Jankovic, 1986; Vidakovic et al., 1994). In a series of 21 patients with hemiballism, hemichorea, or both, an identifiable cause was found in all (Dewey and Jankovic, 1989). Stroke was the most common cause, followed by tumors, abscesses, encephalitis, vasculitis, and other causes. In a series of 23 patients with hemiballism and 2 with biballism, Vidakovic and colleagues (1994) found ischemic and hemorrhagic strokes to be the most common causes of hemiballism. Only two patients had "pure" hemiballism, and only six showed a lesion in the subthalamic nucleus on neuroimaging studies. The prognosis for spontaneous remission was good; nine patients completely recovered, and in seven additional patients, there was complete recovery of the ballism, but mild chorea had persisted. While hemichorea–hemiballism is usually contralateral to a basal ganglia lesion, ipsilateral hemichorea–hemiballism has been described in patients with contralateral hemiparesis (Krauss et al., 1999). The mechanism of this peculiar phenomenon is unknown. Survival rates following vascular hemiballismus are similar to those of vascular disease, with only 32% survival and 27% stroke-free survival 150 months following the onset of the movement disorder (Ristic et al., 2002).

Other causes of ballism include encephalitis, Sydenham disease, SLE, basal ganglia calcifications, tuberous sclerosis, and overlap between Fisher syndrome and Guillain–Barré syndrome (Odaka et al., 1999; Postuma and Lang, 2003). In addition to structural lesions, metabolic disorders, such as hyperglycemia (Sitburana and Ondo, 2006), nutritional vitamin D deficiency (Fernandez et al., 2007), and certain drugs, such as phenytoin and lamotrigine (Yetimalar et al., 2007), have been associated with ballism.

Treatment of ballism

The frequent occurrence of spontaneous remission makes the assessment of therapy difficult. Dopamine receptor-blocking drugs such as haloperidol, chlorpromazine, pimozide, and atypical neuroleptics have been used most frequently (Dewey and Jankovic, 1989; Bashir and Manyam, 1994; Shannon, 2005). Dopamine-depleting drugs, such as reserpine and tetrabenazine, have also been used successfully (Jankovic and Beach, 1997). Tetrabenazine is our preferred drug for its rapid onset of action and its effectiveness, without the danger of inducing tardive dyskinesia if chronic antidopaminergic treatment is needed (Sitburana and Ondo, 2006). Other drugs that are sometimes beneficial in the treatment of ballism include sodium valproate and clonazepam. Finally, ventrolateral thalamotomy and other stereotactic surgeries may be needed to control violent and disabling contralateral hemiballism (Cardoso et al., 1995; Krauss and Mundinger, 2000). Although effective and relatively safe, this procedure should be used only as a last resort in patients with disabling and medically intractable movement disorder.

Athetosis

Athetosis is a slow form of chorea that consists of writhing movements resembling dystonia, but in contrast to dystonia, these movements are not sustained, patterned, repetitive, or painful. Originally described by Hammond in acquired hemidystonia and by Shaw in CP, athetosis should be viewed as a movement disorder separate from dystonia (Morris et al., 2002a). The relationship of athetosis to chorea is highlighted not only by the continuously changing direction of movement but also by the observation that chorea often evolves into athetosis or vice versa. In some patients, particularly children, chorea and athetosis often coexist, hence the term choreoathetosis. Dystonia, particularly involving the trunk causing opisthotonic posturing, also frequently accompanies athetosis, particularly in children with CP (Video 15.11). In contrast to idiopathic dystonia, athetosis associated with perinatal brain injury often causes facial grimacing and spasms, particularly during speaking and eating, and the bulbar function is usually impaired. 🎥

Athetosis is typically present in children with CP, but may be caused by many various etiologies (Kyllerman, 1982; Kyllerman et al., 1982; Foley, 1983; Murphy et al., 1995; Goddard-Finegold, 1998; Morris et al., 2002b; Cowan et al., 2003; Ashwal et al., 2004; Koman et al., 2004; Bax et al., 2006; Keogh and Badawi, 2006). In a study of 431 children diagnosed with CP, 26.2% had hemiplegia, 34.4% had diplegia, 18.6% had quadriplegia, 14.4% had dyskinesia, and 3.9% had ataxia (Bax et al., 2006). In a study of 1817

of the 2357 (77%) children born preterm (22–32 weeks of gestation) who survived at least 5 years, CP was diagnosed in 9%, and 5% had severe, 9% moderate, and 25% minor disability; cognitive and motor disability was most common in children born at 24–28 weeks of gestation (49%) (Larroque et al., 2008). In addition to motor disorders manifested chiefly by weakness and hypertonia (i.e., spasticity, rigidity, athetosis, dystonia), patients with CP may also have cognitive impairment, epilepsy, visual and hearing problems, and other neurologic deficits. Although many patients with dyskinetic CP have well-preserved intellectual function, most of them have a variety of comorbidities. In one study the following comorbidities were documented: nonverbal 22.2% (54/243), active afebrile seizure disorder 16.9% (41/243), severe auditory impairment 11.5% (28/243), cortical blindness 9.5% (23/243), and gavage feeding requirement 7.8% (19/243) (Shevell et al., 2009). Children with ataxic-hypotonic, spastic quadriplegic, and dyskinetic CP subtypes experienced about five times the numerical burden (i.e., frequency) of comorbidities compared to children with the spastic diplegic or hemiplegic variants; dyskinetic children had a particularly high frequency of nonverbal skills (8/16, 50%) and auditory impairment (6/16, 38%).

As a result of hypertonia, many patients with untreated CP develop fixed contractures. With the advent of botulinum toxin treatment, intrathecal baclofen infusion, and selective dorsal rhizotomy, coupled with aggressive physical therapy and antispastic drugs, these sequelae can be largely prevented.

Although there has been a steady decline in infant mortality, the incidence of CP has remained unchanged. Because of the higher frequency of premature births, the frequency of certain types of CP, such as spastic diplegia, has been increasing. In one study of children born at 25 or fewer completed weeks of gestation, half of the patients at 30 months of age were considered disabled, 18% were diagnosed with CP, and 24% had gait difficulties (Wood et al., 2000).

Kernicterus, once a common cause of CP due to bilirubin encephalopathy associated with neonatal jaundice, is now quite rare, although still an important cause of childhood disabilities in developing countries (Maisels, 2009). Besides delayed developmental milestones and athetotic or dystonic movements, patients with kernicterus often exhibit vertical ophthalmoparesis, deafness, and dysplasia of the dental enamel. Hearing abnormalities, very common in chronic bilirubin encephalopathy, can be present as the only finding of kernicterus. The high-frequency sensory neural hearing loss has been attributed to damage to the cochlear nuclei and auditory nerves, possibly as a result of bilirubin's interference with intracellular calcium homeostasis (Shapiro and Nakamura, 2001). Unconjugated bilirubin can also cause damage to endoplasmic reticulum membranes leading to neuronal excitotoxicity and mitochondrial energy failure.

Although improved perinatal care has reduced the frequency of birth-related injuries, birth asphyxia with anoxia is still a relatively common cause of CP (Kuban and Leviton, 1994; Cowan et al., 2003). Expression of tyrosine hydroxylase was reduced in the putamen in cases of acute kernicterus and in the globus pallidus of acute and chronic postkernicterus (Hachiya and Hayashi, 2008).

The cause of CP is multifactorial. Intrauterine insults, particularly chorioamnionitis and prolonged rupture of membranes (Murphy et al., 1995), might be responsible for many of the cases of CP. In one study of 351 full-term infants with neonatal encephalopathy, early seizures or both, excluding infants with congenital malformations and obvious chromosomal disorders, MRI showed evidence of an acute insult in 69–80% (Cowan et al., 2003). The higher figure correlated with evidence of perinatal asphyxia. The vast majority of children with neurologic deficits associated with perinatal asphyxia show abnormalities within the basal ganglia with shrinkage of the striatum. In addition, defects in myelination are often associated with a marbled gross appearance (hypermyelination-status marmoratus) or dysmyelination.

The border zones between the major cerebral arteries ("watershed") is most vulnerable to asphyxia (Folkerth, 2005). In the striatum, the excitatory glutamate receptors and GABAergic neurons are particularly sensitive to asphyxia. Striatal neurons also die by glutamate-mediated excitotoxicity in which apoptosis may be delayed over days to weeks. Leukomalacia was the most common MRI abnormality, found in 42.5%, followed by basal ganglia lesions in 12.8%, cortical/subcortical lesions in 9.4%, malformations in 9.1%, and infarcts in 7.4%. Although athetosis is usually associated with perinatal brain injury, the neuroimaging studies often fail to show basal ganglia pathology.

Both above-normal and below-normal weight at birth are also significant risk factors for CP (Jarvis et al., 2003). These data strongly suggest that events in the immediate perinatal period are most important in the neonatal brain injury. An analysis of 58 brains of patients with clinical diagnosis of CP showed wide morphologic variation, but the authors were able to classify the brains into three major categories: thinned cerebral mantle ($n = 10$), hydrocephalus ($n = 3$), and microgyria–pachygyria ($n = 45$) (Tsusi et al., 1999). Of the 19 brains that were examined microscopically, four showed heterotopic gray matter, three showed cortical folding (cortical dysplasia), and three showed neuronal cytomegaly. The majority of the examined brains showed a variable degree of laminar disorganization in the cortex and disorientation of neurons, suggesting impaired neuronal migration during cortical development. Because 5–10% of patients with athetoid CP have a family history, genetic factors are considered important in the pathogenesis of this disorder (Fletcher and Foley, 1993). In a study based on a Swedish registry, 40% of cases of CP were thought to have a genetic basis (Costeff, 2004).

A growing number of studies also draw attention to inflammation and coagulation abnormalities in children with CP. The increased concentrations of interleukins, tumor necrosis factor, reactive antibodies to lupus anticoagulant, anticardiolipin, antiphospholipid, antithrombin III, epidermal growth factor, and other abnormal cytokine patterns may play an important role in the etiology of CP (Nelson et al., 1998; Kaukola et al., 2004). Kadhim and colleagues (2001) suggest that an early macrophage reaction and associated cytokine production and coagulation necrosis, coupled with intrinsic vulnerability of the immature oligodendrocyte, lead to periventricular leukomalacia, the most common neuropathologic changes found in premature infants who develop CP. Although infection and inflammation, along with free radicals, can activate the process that leads to periventricular leukomalacia and even to delayed progression (Scott and

Jankovic, 1996), the cause or pathogenesis of CP is still not well understood.

Often referred to as static encephalopathy, the neurologic deficit associated with CP may progress with time. Motor development curves derived by assessing patients with the Gross Motor Function Measure, used to prognosticate gross motor function in patients with CP, indicate that, depending on their level of impairment (levels I to V) 3–10 years after birth, the natural course becomes static (Rosenbaum et al., 2002). We and others, however, found that some patients continue to progress, and others may progress after a period of static course. In about half of the patients with CP, the abnormal movements become apparent within the first year of life, but in some cases, they might not appear until the fifth decade or even later. The mechanism by which such "delayed-onset" movement disorder becomes progressive after decades of a static course is unknown, but aberrant regeneration and sprouting of nerve fibers has been considered (Scott and Jankovic, 1996). In contrast to the other forms of CP (e.g., diplegic or spastic and hemiplegic), the athetoid variety, which constitutes only about a quarter of all cases, is usually not associated with significant cognitive impairment or epilepsy. Although here we emphasize athetosis, the most common movement disorder in patients with CP is spasticity (Albright, 1995).

Many other disorders associated with developmental delay and intellectual disability can cause athetosis. Chromosomal microarray has been recommended for genetic testing of individuals with unexplained developmental delay/intellectual disability, autism spectrum disorders, or multiple congenital anomalies (Miller et al., 2010). Some are due to errors in metabolism and include acidurias, lipidoses, and Lesch–Nyhan syndrome (Jankovic et al., 1988; Stacy and Jankovic, 1995) (Table 15.1). Finally, athetotic movements, or "pseudoathetosis," can be seen in patients with severe proprioceptive deficit (Sharp et al., 1994).

Treatment of athetosis

Athetosis usually does not respond well to pharmacologic therapy. Because dopa-responsive dystonia is sometimes confused with athetoid CP, it is prudent to treat all these patients with levodopa. If levodopa fails to provide any meaningful benefit, then anticholinergic drugs should be tried in the same manner as when treating dystonia. Although generally recommended, physical therapy might or might not prevent contractures, and its role in altering the eventual outcome is uncertain (Palmer et al., 1988). Other complications of CP, such as carpal tunnel syndrome, cervical spondylosis with radiculopathy, and myelopathy, require independent assessment and treatment (Hirose and Kadoya, 1984; Treves and Korczyn, 1986). Bilateral GPi deep brain stimulation has been reported to produce about 24.4% improvement in the Burke–Fahn–Marsden scale in adult patients with dystonia–choreoathetosis associated with CP (Vidailhet et al., 2009).

References available on Expert Consult: www.expertconsult.com

Appendix

Testing for various causes of chorea is available at the following:

http://www.ncbi.nlm.nih.gov/sites/
  entrez?db=omim
http://www.athenadiagnostics.com/content/
  diagnostic-ed/genetic_testing
http://www.genome.gov
http://www.mayomedicallaboratories.com/
  testcatalog/index.html
http://www.geneticalliance.org.uk/
http://www.genetests.org
http://www.massgeneral.org/neurology/
  research/resourcelab.aspx?id=43/
http://www.kumc.edu/gec/
http://www.pdgene.org
http://www.familytreedna.com/default.aspx
http://www.horizonmedicine.com/
http://www.diagenic.com/
http://www.23andme.com
http://ccr.coriell.org/

HDL1 – Lab of Pierluigi Gambetti, MD

National Prion Disease Pathology
Surveillance Center
Institute of Pathology
Case Western Reserve University
2085 Adelbert Road, Room 418
Cleveland, Ohio 44106
Telephone: (216) 368-0587
Fax: (216) 368-4090
Email: cjdsurv@case.edu

HDL2 – Lab of Russell Margolis, MD

Neurogenetic Testing Laboratory
Johns Hopkins University
600 North Wolfe Street
Meyer 2-181
Baltimore, MD 21287
Telephone: (410) 955-1349

Neuroacanthocytosis

Loss of chorein expression has been found to be a reliable diagnostic test and the analysis by Western blot test is available without charge by sending 20–30 mL of EDTA blood to Dr B. Baker, Munich, Germany (Benedikt. Bader@med.uni-muenchen.de) through the support of the Advocacy for Neuroacanthocytosis patients (http://www.naadvocacy.org).

Western blot for chorein

Prof. Dr Adrian Danek
Neurologische Klinik
und Poliklinik
Klinikum der Universität München,
Campus Großhadern
Marchioninistraße 15
81377 Munich
Germany
Telephone: ++ 49 89 7095 6676
Fax: ++ 49 89 7095 6671
Email: adrien.danek@med.uni-muenchen.de/

VPS13A gene testing

Koichiro Sakai, MD, PhD
Ishikawa, Japan
Email: ksakai@kanazawa-med.ac.jp

CHAPTER 16

Tics and Tourette syndrome

Chapter contents

Introduction	350	Etiology of tics (secondary tourettism)	368
Phenomenology of tics	351	Epidemiology	369
Clinical features of Tourette syndrome	353	Treatment	369
Pathogenesis	359	Appendix	379
Genetics	366		

Introduction

Tourette syndrome (TS), which should be more appropriately called Gilles de la Tourette syndrome, is a neurologic disorder manifested by motor and vocal or phonic tics usually starting during childhood and often accompanied by obsessive-compulsive disorder (OCD), attention-deficit hyperactivity disorder (ADHD), poor impulse control, and other comorbid behavioral problems (Shapiro and Shapiro, 1992; Cohen and Leckman, 1994; Hyde and Weinberger, 1995; Feigin and Clarke, 1998; Leckman and Cohen, 1999; Freeman et al., 2000; Robertson, 2000; Jankovic, 2001a; Leckman et al., 2001; Leckman, 2002; Stein, 2002; Singer, 2005; Albin and Mink, 2006; Leckman et al., 2006; Bloch et al., 2011; Jankovic and Kurlan, 2011). Once considered a rare psychiatric curiosity, TS is now recognized as a relatively common and complex neurobehavioral disorder (Table 16.1). There has been speculation that many notable historical figures, including Dr Samuel Johnson and possibly Wolfgang Amadeus Mozart (Simkin, 1992; Ashoori and Jankovic, 2007), were afflicted with TS.

One of the earliest reports of TS dates to 1825, when Itard (1825) described a French noblewoman with body tics, barking sounds, and uncontrollable utterances of obscenities. Sixty years later, the French neurologist and a student of Charcot, Georges Gilles de la Tourette (1885) reviewed Itard's original case and added eight more patients. He noted that all nine patients shared one feature: they all exhibited brief involuntary movements or tics; additionally, six made noises, five shouted obscenities (coprolalia), five repeated the words of others (echolalia), and two mimicked others' gestures (echopraxia) (Goetz and Klawans, 1982; Kushner, 1999). Although Tourette considered the disorder he described to be hereditary, the etiology was ascribed

to psychogenic causes for nearly a century following the original report. The perception of TS began to change in the 1960s, when the beneficial effects of neuroleptic drugs on the symptoms of TS began to be recognized (Shapiro and Shapiro, 1968). This observation helped to refocus attention from psychogenic etiology to central nervous system (CNS) etiology. Despite these advances TS is still often misunderstood and wrongly labeled as a mental or psychiatric disorder. For example, insurance compensation for patients with TS is often compromised because the TS-related diagnostic codes (307.22 = Tic Disorder, 307.23 = Tourette Syndrome) are currently included in the ICD-9 series for mental disorders (290–319). Therefore, the code 333.3 = Tics of Organic Origin or 349.9 = Unspecified Nervous System Disorder may result in more appropriate compensation. If payment is denied, an appeal letter to the insurance company specifying that TS is a neurologic disorder along with some literature and links to a credible website may be required.

The cause of TS is yet unknown, but the disorder appears to be inherited in the majority of patients (Pauls et al., 1988, 1991; Tolosa and Jankovic, 1998; Jankovic, 2001a; Leckman, 2002; Paschou et al., 2004; Singer, 2005). The clinical expression of this genetic defect varies from one individual to another, fluctuations in symptoms are seen within the same individual, and different manifestations occur in various family members (Kurlan, 1994). This variable expression from one individual to another, even within members of the same family, contributes to diagnostic confusion. Without a specific biologic marker, the diagnosis depends on a careful evaluation of the patient's symptoms and signs by an experienced clinician. Educational efforts directed to physicians, educators, and to the general public have increased awareness about TS. In addition, the media have drawn increasing public attention to this condition. As a result of this improved awareness, the self-referral rate of patients has increased, and

DOI: 10.1016/B978-1-4377-2369-4.00016-0

Table 16.1 Summary of epidemiologic studies in Tourette syndrome (TS)

- 0.7% (1142 children, 2nd, 5th, 8th grades – Houston, TX)
- 0.6% (3034 children, 1/95 M and 1/759 F – Los Angeles)
- 6.1% (135/553 children, K–6th grade) had persistent tics (TS); 24% observed to have motor tics during at least one month of the 8-month study
- 3.8% (339/1596, 9–17 years old – Rochester, NY) had TS; 21% had tics after 60–150 minutes of observation, M > F, higher frequency of OCD, ADHD, oppositional defiant behavior, separation anxiety, overanxious disorder, simple and social phobia, agoraphobia, and depression
- Worldwide prevalence of TS in children has been reported to range from 0.3% to 0.8%

the correct diagnosis is made earlier than was the case in the past. Many patients, however, still remain undiagnosed, or their symptoms are wrongly attributed to habits, allergies, asthma, dermatitis, hyperactivity, nervousness, and many other conditions (Jankovic et al., 1998; Hogan and Wilson, 1999).

Phenomenology of tics

Tics, the clinical hallmark of TS, are relatively brief and intermittent movements (motor tics) or sounds (vocal or phonic tics). Recognition of the full spectrum of phenomenology of tics is critical to the diagnosis of TS (Jankovic, 2008). Motor tics typically consist of sudden, abrupt, transient, often repetitive and coordinated (stereotypical) movements that may resemble gestures and mimic fragments of normal behavior, vary in intensity, and are repeated at irregular intervals (Videos 16.1 to 16.8). Currently accepted criteria for the diagnosis of TS require both types of tics to be present (Robertson, 1989; Golden, 1990; Tourette Syndrome Classification Study Group, 1993; Jankovic, 1997; Singer, 2000). This division into motor and vocal/phonic tics, however, is artificial, because vocal/phonic tics are actually motor tics that involve respiratory, laryngeal, pharyngeal, oral, and nasal musculature. Contractions of these muscles may produce sounds by moving air through the nose, mouth, or throat. The term *phonic tic* is preferable, since not all sounds produced by TS patients involve the vocal cords.

To better understand the categorization of tics and how they fit in the general schema of movement disorders, it might be helpful to provide a simple classification of movements (Jankovic, 1992). All movements can be categorized into one of four classes:

1. Voluntary
   a. Intentional (planned, self-initiated, internally generated)
   b. Externally triggered in response to some stimulus (e.g., turning the head toward a loud noise or withdrawing the hand from a hot plate)
2. Semivoluntary (unvoluntary)
   a. Induced by an inner sensory stimulus (e.g., the need to "stretch" a body part)
   b. Induced by an unwanted feeling or compulsion (e.g., compulsive touching or smelling)
3. Involuntary
   a. Nonsuppressible (e.g., reflexes. seizures, myoclonus)
   b. Suppressible (e.g., tics, tremor, dystonia, chorea, stereotypy)
4. Automatic
   a. Learned motor behaviors performed without conscious effort (e.g., the act of walking or speaking).

Recent studies have shown that automatic, learned behaviors appear to be encoded in the sensorimotor portion of the striatum (Jog et al., 1999). Some support for the proposed classification is provided by the findings of Papa and colleagues (1991). They recorded normal premovement (readiness) electroencephalographic, slow, negative potential (the Bereitschaftspotential) 1–1.5 seconds prior to self-induced, internally generated (voluntary) movement in normal individuals but not before externally triggered movement induced by electrical stimulation (Colebatch, 2007). Most tics can be categorized as either semivoluntary (unvoluntary) or involuntary (suppressible). In some cases, learned voluntary motor skills are incorporated into the tic repertoire. This is exemplified by a case of a woman with TS who incorporated sign language into her tic behavior, suggesting that semantics is more important than phonology in the generation of tics (Lang et al., 1993).

Tics may be simple or complex. Simple motor tics involve only one group of muscles, causing a brief, jerk-like movement. They are usually abrupt in onset and rapid (clonic tics), but they may be slower, causing a briefly sustained abnormal posture (dystonic tics) or an isometric contraction (tonic tics) (Jankovic and Fahn, 1986; Jankovic, 1992). Examples of simple clonic motor tics include blinking, nose twitching, and head jerking. Rhythmical clonic tics may rarely resemble tremor or rhythmical myoclonus, such as palatal myoclonus (Schwingenschuh et al., 2007; Adam et al., 2009). Simple dystonic tics include blepharospasm, oculogyric movements, bruxism, sustained mouth opening, torticollis, and shoulder rotation (Videos 16.3 and 16.9). Tensing of abdominal or limb muscles is an example of a tonic tic (Video 16.10). To characterize clonic and dystonic tics further, 156 patients with TS were studied; 89 (57%) exhibited dystonic tics, including oculogyric deviations (28%), blepharospasm (15%), and dystonic neck movements (7%) (Jankovic and Stone, 1991). Since patients with dystonic tics did not differ significantly on any clinical variables from those with only clonic tics, we concluded that despite previous reports (Feinberg et al., 1986), the presence of dystonic tics should not be considered atypical or unusual. In fact, on subsequent observation, the patient in Feinberg and colleagues' case report was shown to be a case of TS with typical dystonic tics (Fahn, 1987). Dystonic tics should be distinguished from persistent dystonia, which is typically seen in patients with primary dystonia (Jankovic and Fahn, 2002). Dystonic (and tonic) muscle contraction might be responsible for so-called blocking tics (Video 16.11). These blocking tics are due to either prolonged tonic or dystonic tics that interrupt ongoing motor activity such as speech (intrusions) or a sudden inhibition of ongoing motor activity (negative tic). Clonic and dystonic tics may occasionally occur in patients with primary dystonia more frequently than in the general population. In nine patients with coexistent TS and persistent primary dystonia, the onset of tics was at a mean age of 9 years, while dystonia followed the onset of tics by a mean of 22 (10–38) years (Stone and Jankovic, 1991). Other reports have drawn attention to the possible association of tics and dystonia, although the two disorders may coexist by chance alone (Pringsheim et al., 2007). The occasional co-occurrence of tics and dystonia in the same family, however, provides additional evidence for a possible etiologic relationship between the two disorders (Németh et al., 1999; Yaltho et al., 2010). Dopa-responsive dystonia with mutations in the *GCH1* gene and TS was found in various members of a large Danish family (Romstad et al., 2003).

Motor (particularly dystonic) and phonic tics are preceded by premonitory sensations in over 80% of patients (Cohen and Leckman, 1992; Banaschewski et al., 2003; Kwak et al., 2003a; Woods et al., 2005; Prado et al., 2008). This premonitory phenomenon consists of localizable sensations or discomforts, such as a burning feeling in the eye before an eye blink, tension or a crick in the neck that is relieved by stretching of the neck or jerking of the head, a feeling of tightness or constriction that is relieved by arm or leg extension, nasal stuffiness before a sniff, a dry or sore throat before throat clearing or grunting, and itching before a rotatory movement of the scapula. Rarely, these premonitory sensations, termed in one report *extracorporeal phantom tics*, involve sensations in other people and objects and are temporarily relieved by touching or scratching them (Karp and Hallett, 1996). In one study, premonitory sensations were experienced by 92% of 135 patients with TS, and these were localized chiefly to the shoulder girdle, palms, midline abdominal region, posterior thighs, feet, and eyes (Cohen and Leckman, 1992). We administered a questionnaire regarding various aspects of premonitory sensations associated with their motor tics to 50 TS patients with a mean age of 23.6 ± 16.7 years (Kwak et al., 2003a). Forty-six of 50 (92%) subjects reported some premonitory sensations, the most common of which was an urge to move and an impulse to tic ("had to do it"). Other premonitory sensations included an itch, tingling/burning, numbness, and coldness. Thirty-seven (74%) also reported intensification of premonitory sensations if the patient was prevented from performing a motor tic; 36 (72%) reported relief of premonitory sensations after performing the tic; and 24 (48%) stated that their motor tic would not have occurred if they had had no premonitory sensation. Twenty-seven of 40 patients (68%) described a motor tic as a voluntary motor response to an involuntary sensation rather than as a completely involuntary movement. Besides the local or regional premonitory sensations, this premonitory phenomenon may be a nonlocalizable, less specific, and poorly described feeling, such as an urge, anxiety, anger, and other psychic sensations. The observed movement or sound sometimes occurs in response to these premonitory phenomena, and these movements or sounds have been previously referred to as sensory tics (Kurlan et al., 1989; Chee and Sachdev, 1997). In a study of 60 patients with tic disorders, 41 (68%) thought that all their tics were intentionally produced, and 15 (25%) additional patients had both voluntary and involuntary movements; thus, 93% of the tics were perceived to be "irresistibly but purposefully executed" (Lang, 1991). This "intentional" component of the movement may be a useful feature in differentiating tics from other hyperkinetic movement disorders, such as myoclonus and chorea. The sensations or feelings that often precede motor tics usually occur out of a background of relative normalcy and are clearly involuntary, even though the movements (motor tics) or noises (phonic tics) that occur in response to these premonitory symptoms may be regarded as semivoluntary or unvoluntary. Chee and Sachdev (1997) suggest that sensory tics, which we and others refer to as premonitory sensations, "represent the subjectively experienced component of neural dysfunction below the threshold for motor and phonic tic production." Many patients report that they have to repeat a particular movement to relieve the uncomfortable urge until "it feels good." The "just right" feeling has been associated with compulsive behavior, and as such, the "unvoluntary" movement may be regarded as a compulsive tic (Leckman et al., 1994). While many patients describe a gradually increasing inner tension as tic suppression is maintained and a rebound effect of a flurry of tics when the tics are finally expressed, formal objective studies of tic frequency during and after voluntary suppression have failed to detect a rebound increase (Meidinger et al 2005; Himle and Woods 2005) and, when reinforced, tic suppression may last at least 40 consecutive minutes (Woods et al., 2008).

Complex motor tics consist of coordinated, sequenced movements resembling normal motor acts or gestures that are inappropriately intense and timed (Videos 16.6, 16.12, and 16.13). They may be seemingly nonpurposeful, such as head shaking or trunk bending, or they may seem purposeful, such as touching, throwing, hitting, jumping, and kicking. Additional examples of complex motor tics include gesturing "the finger" and grabbing or exposing one's genitalia (copropraxia) or imitating gestures (echopraxia). Burping, vomiting, and retching have been described as part of the clinical picture of TS, but it is not clear whether this phenomenon represents a complex tic or some other behavioral manifestation of TS (Rickards and Robertson, 1997). Air swallowing is another unusual tic described in TS (Weil et al., 2008). Another unusual tic is ear dyskinesia, which consists of anterior-posterior displacement of the external ear (Cardoso and Faleiro, 1999). Complex motor tics may be difficult to differentiate from compulsions, which frequently accompany tics, particularly in TS. A complex, repetitive movement may be considered a compulsion when it is preceded by, or associated with, a feeling of anxiety or panic, as well as an irresistible urge to perform the movement or sound because of fear that if it is not promptly or properly executed, "something bad" will happen. However, this distinction is not always possible, particularly when the patient is unable to verbalize such feelings. Some coordinated movements resemble complex motor tics but may actually represent pseudovoluntary movements (parakinesias) that are designed to camouflage the tics by incorporating them into seemingly purposeful acts, such as adjusting one's hair during a head jerk.

Simple phonic tics typically consist of sniffing, throat clearing, grunting, squeaking, screaming, coughing, blowing, and sucking sounds. Complex phonic tics include linguistically meaningful utterances and verbalizations, such as shouting of obscenities or profanities (coprolalia), repetition of someone else's words or phrases (echolalia), and repetition of one's own utterances, particularly the last

Table 16.2 Classification of tics

A. Primary

1. Sporadic
   a. Transient motor or phonic tics (<1 year)
   b. Chronic motor or phonic tics (>1 year)
   c. Adult-onset (recurrent) tics
   d. TS
2. Inherited
   a. TS

B. Secondary

1. Inherited
   a. Huntington disease
   b. Primary dystonia
   c. Neuroacanthocytosis
   d. NBIA1 (neurodegeneration with brain iron accumulation type 1)
   e. Tuberous sclerosis
   f. Wilson disease
   g. Duchenne muscular dystrophy
2. Infections: encephalitis, Creutzfeldt–Jakob disease, neurosyphilis, Sydenham disease
3. Drugs: amphetamines, methylphenidate, pemoline, levodopa, cocaine, carbamazepine, phenytoin, phenobarbital, lamotrigine, antipsychotics, and other dopamine receptor-blocking drugs (tardive tics, tardive tourettism)
4. Toxins: carbon monoxide
5. Developmental: static encephalopathy, mental retardation syndromes, chromosomal abnormalities, autistic spectrum disorders (Asperger syndrome)
6. Chromosomal disorders: Down syndrome, Kleinfelter syndrome, XYY karyotype, fragile X syndrome, triple X and 9p mosaicism, partial trisomy 16, 9p monosomy, citrullinemia, Beckwith–Wiedemann syndrome
7. Other: head trauma, stroke, neurocutaneous syndromes, schizophrenia, neurodegenerative diseases

C. Related manifestations and disorders

1. Stereotypies/habits/mannerisms/rituals
2. Self-injurious behaviors
3. Motor restlessness
4. Akathisia
5. Compulsions
6. Excessive startle
7. Jumping Frenchman

syllable, word, or phrase in a sentence (palilalia). Some TS patients also manifest sudden and transient cessation of all motor activity (blocking tics) without alteration of consciousness.

In contrast to other hyperkinetic movement disorders, tics are usually intermittent and may be repetitive and stereotypic (Table 16.2). Tics may occur as short-term bouts or bursting or long-term waxing and waning (Peterson and Leckman, 1998). They vary in frequency and intensity and often change distribution. Typically, tics can be volitionally suppressed, although this might require intense mental effort (Banaschewski et al., 2003). Suppressibility, although characteristic and common in tics, is not unique or specific for tics, and this phenomenon has been well documented in

other hyperkinetic movement disorders (Walters et al., 1990). Using functional magnetic resonance imaging (MRI), Peterson and colleagues (1998a) showed decreased neuronal activity during periods of suppression in the ventral globus pallidus, putamen, and thalamus. There was increased activity in the right caudate nucleus, right frontal cortex, and other cortical areas that are normally involved in the inhibition of unwanted impulses (prefrontal, parietal, temporal, and cingulate cortices). Using event-related functional magnetic resonance imaging in 26 children with bipolar disorder, deficits in the ability to engage striatal structures and the right ventral prefrontal cortex were found during unsuccessful inhibition, thus suggesting that deficits in motor inhibition contribute to impulsivity and irritability in children with bipolar disorder and possibly also with TS (Leibenluft et al., 2007).

Besides temporary suppressibility, tics are characterized by suggestibility and exacerbation with stress, excitement, boredom, fatigue, and exposure to heat (Lombroso et al., 1991). Emotional stress associated with life events or other stresses have been documented to potentially markedly exacerbate tics, but onset of TS is not necessarily related to stressful life events (Wood et al., 2003; Hoekstra et al., 2004; Horesh et al., 2008). Tics may also increase during relaxation after a period of stress.

In contrast to other hyperkinetic movement disorders that are usually completely suppressed during sleep, motor and phonic tics may persist during all stages of sleep (Cohrs et al., 2001; Jankovic et al., 1984; Silvestri et al., 1990; Fish et al., 1991; Hanna and Jankovic, 2003; Rothenberger et al., 2001). In addition, patients with TS often have disturbances of sleep, such as increased sleep fragmentation, higher frequency of arousals, decreased rapid eye movement (REM) sleep, and enuresis (Hanna and Jankovic, 2003). Many patients note a reduction in their tics when they are distracted while concentrating on mental or physical tasks (such as when playing a video game or during an orgasm). Other patients experience increased frequency and intensity of their tics when distracted, especially when they no longer have the need to suppress the tics. Tics are also typically exacerbated by dopaminergic drugs and by CNS stimulants, including methylphenidate and cocaine (Cardoso and Jankovic, 1993). Finally, it should be noted that there is a broad spectrum of movements that may be present in patients with TS that can be confused with tics, such as akathisia, chorea, dystonia, compulsive movements, and fidgeting as part of hyperactivity associated with ADHD (Jankovic, 1997; Kompoliti and Goetz, 1998; Wilens et al., 2004).

Clinical features of Tourette syndrome

Motor symptoms

TS, the most common cause of tics, is manifested by a broad spectrum of motor and behavioral disturbances (Table 16.3). This clinical heterogeneity often causes diagnostic difficulties and presents a major challenge in genetic linkage studies. To aid in the diagnosis of TS, the Tourette Syndrome Classification Study Group (1993) formulated the following criteria for definite TS: (1) Both multiple motor and one or more phonic tics have to be present at some time during the

Table 16.3 Demographic and clinical features in a large database of patients with TS (Tourette International Consortium) (Freeman et al., 2009)

Number (80 sites; 60% North America; 66% Psychiatry: 27% Neurology)	6805
Male:Female ratio	4.4:1
Mean age at onset of tics	6.4 years
Mean age at diagnosis of TS	13.2 years
Delay in diagnosis	6.4 years
Family history	51.7%
TS only, no comorbidity	14.2%
Attention-deficit hyperactivity disorder	55.6%
Obsessive-compulsive disorder/behavior	54.9%
Conduct/oppositional defiant disorder	12.3%
Anger control problems	27.6%
Learning disability	22.0%
Mood disorder	16.9%
Anxiety disorder	16.8%
Pervasive developmental disorder	4.6%

illness, although not necessarily concurrently. (2) Tics must occur many times a day, nearly every day, or intermittently throughout a period of more than 1 year. (3) The anatomic location, number, frequency, type, complexity, or severity of tics must change over time. (4) Onset must be before age 21. (5) Involuntary movements and noises cannot be explained by other medical conditions. (6) Motor and/or phonic tics must be directly witnessed by a reliable examiner at some point during the illness or must be recorded by videotape or cinematography. Probable TS type 1 meets all the criteria except for number 3 and/or number 4, and probable TS type 2 meets all the criteria except for number 1; it includes either a single motor tic with phonic tics or multiple motor tics with possible phonic tics. In contrast to the criteria outlined by the Diagnostic and Statistical Manual of Mental Disorders, Fourth Edition (DSM-IV) (1994), the Tourette Syndrome Classification Study Group criteria do not include a statement about "impairment." There is considerable controversy about the DSM-IV criteria, which require that "marked distress or significant impairment in social, occupational or other important areas of functioning" be present. Therefore, patients with mild tics that do not produce an impairment would not satisfy the diagnostic criteria for TS, according to DMS-IV. This criterion will be deleted from the fifth edition of the DSM. Kurlan (1997) suggested another set of diagnostic criteria for genetic studies and introduced the term *Tourette disorder* for patients who have "functional impairment." This, however, does not take into account the marked fluctuation in symptoms and severity; some patients may be relatively asymptomatic at one time and clearly functionally impaired at another time. The TSA International Genetic Collaboration developed the Diagnostic Confidence Index, which consists of 26 confidence factors, with weightings given to each of them and a total maximum score of 100. The most highly weighted diagnostic confidence factors

include history of coprolalia, complex motor or vocal tics, a waxing and waning course, echophenomenon, premonitory sensations, an orchestrated sequence, and age at onset. The Diagnostic Confidence Index was found to be a useful instrument in assessing the lifetime likelihood of TS (Robertson et al., 1999). Several instruments, some based on ratings of videotapes, have been developed to measure and quantitate tics, but they all have some limitations (Goetz and Kompoliti, 2001; Goetz et al., 2001). The most widely used instrument to assess tics is the Yale Global Tic Severity Scale (YGTSS), which consists of two broad domains: Total Tic Severity (with two sub-domains: Motor and Phonic Tics) and Impairment. Within each category there are five dimensions, score 0–5: number of tics, frequency, intensity, complexity, and interference. The total tic score ranges from 0 to 50; the usual ranges in most studies is 15 to 30. A health-related quality of life scale (HR-QOL) has been developed and validated for internal consistency, test–retest reliability and against other clinical scales (Cavanna et al., 2008). Utilization of the HR-QOL scale showed that comorbidities such as ADHD and OCD rather than tic severity are more predictive of the long-term outcome.

The clinical criteria are designed to assist in accurate diagnosis, in genetic linkage studies and in differentiating TS from other tic disorders (Jankovic, 1993b) (Table 16.2). There is a body of evidence to support the notion that many, if not all, patients with other forms of idiopathic tic disorders represent one end of the spectrum in a continuum of TS (Kurlan et al., 1988). The most common and mildest of the idiopathic tic disorders is the transient tic disorder (TTD) of childhood. This disorder is essentially identical to TS except the symptoms last less than 1 year and therefore the diagnosis can be made only in retrospect. Transient tic disorder has been estimated to occur in up to 24% of schoolchildren (Shapiro et al., 1988). Chronic multiple tic disorder is also similar to TS, but the patients have either only motor or, less commonly, only phonic tics lasting at least 1 year. Chronic single tic disorder is the same as chronic multiple tic disorder, but the patients have only a single motor or phonic tic. This separation into transient tic disorder, chronic multiple tic disorder, and chronic single tic disorder seems artificial because all can occur in the same family and probably represent a variable expression of the same genetic defect (Kurlan et al., 1988).

Although the diagnostic criteria require that the onset is present before the age of 21, in 96% of patients the disorder is manifested by age 11 (Robertson, 1989). In 36–48% of patients, the initial symptom is eye blinking, followed by tics involving the face and head. Blink rate in TS is about double of that of normal, age-matched controls (Tulen et al., 1999). During the course of the disease, nearly all patients exhibit tics involving the face or head, two-thirds have tics in the arms, and half have tics involving the trunk or legs. According to one study, the average age at onset of tics is 5.6 years, and the tics usually become most severe at age 10; by 18 years of age, half of the patients are tic-free (Leckman et al., 1998). In a study of 58 adults who had been diagnosed with TS during childhood, Goetz and colleagues (1992) found that tics persisted in all patients but were moderate or severe in only 24%, although 60% had moderate or severe tics during the course of the disease. Tic severity during childhood had no predictive value for the future course, but patients with mild tics during the preadult period had mild tics during adulthood. In a longitudinal study that involved structured interviews of 976 children aged 1–10 years, 776 of whom were reassessed 8, 10, and 15 years later, tics and ADHD symptoms were associated with OCD symptoms in late adolescence and early adulthood (Peterson et al., 2001). Furthermore, ADHD was associated with lower IQ and lower social status, whereas OCD was associated with higher IQ. These findings are similar to those of another study designed to address the long-term prognosis of children with TS as they reach adulthood (Bloch et al., 2006). In this study 46 children with TS underwent a structured interview at a mean age of 11.4 years, and again at 19.0 years. The mean worst-ever tic severity score was 31.6 out of a possible 50 on the YGTSS, and occurred at a mean age of 10.6 years. By the time of the second interview, mean YGTSS score decreased to 10. This first prospective longitudinal study also showed that only 22% continued to experience mild or greater tic symptoms (YGTSS scores, ≥10) at follow-up, while nearly one-third were in complete remission of tic symptoms at follow-up. In contrast to the study by Goetz et al. (1992), the severity of childhood tics was predictive of increased tic severity at follow-up. The peak OCD severity occurred 2 years after peak tic severity. Interestingly, a 10-point increase in baseline IQ increased the risk of OCD symptoms at follow-up by 2.8-fold. The authors point out that the later average onset of OCD symptoms indicates the importance of counseling parents about the possibility of OCD development in children recently diagnosed with tics. Although the long-term prognosis for TS is generally favorable for most patients, a minority of cases may have persistent, severe tic symptoms which may be resistant to medications (Eapen et al., 2002). In another study, the investigators reviewed videotapes of 31 patients, with an average age of 24.2 ± 3.5 years, approximately 12 years after their initial video and found that 90% of the adults still had tics, even though they often considered themselves tic-free (Pappert et al., 2003). There was, however, a significant improvement in tic disability and tic severity. When 40 children and 31 adults with TS were compared no difference in tic phenomenology or severity was found, but children were more frequently managed without medications, and sedation was more common in adults but weight gain was more common in children (Cubo et al., 2008).

Although the vast majority of tics in adults represent recurrences of childhood-onset tics, rare patients may have their first tic occurrence during adulthood (Chouinard and Ford, 2000). In adults with new-onset tics, it is important to search for secondary causes, such as infection, trauma, stroke (Kwak and Jankovic, 2002; Gomis et al., 2008), multiple sclerosis (Nociti et al., 2009), cocaine use, neuroleptic exposure, and peripheral injury (Video 16.14) (Chouinard and Ford, 2000; Jankovic, 2001b; Jankovic and Mejia, 2006). One study of eight patients with adult-onset tics (three of whom had childhood-onset OCD and three of whom had a family history of tics and OCD) found that in comparison to the patients with more typical childhood-onset tics, the former group had more severe symptoms, greater social morbidity, and less favorable response to medications (Eapen et al., 2002). Poor motor control, which can lead to poor penmanship and, at times, almost illegible handwriting, can contribute to the academic difficulties faced by many patients with TS.

Table 16.4 Clinical features of severe ("malignant") TS

- Malignant TS defined as ≥2 emergency room visits or ≥1 hospitalizations for TS symptoms or its associated behavioral comorbidities
- Of 332 TS patients evaluated during the 3-year period, 17 (5.1%) met criteria for malignant TS
- Compared to patients with nonmalignant TS, those with malignant TS were significantly more likely to have a personal history of obsessive-compulsive behavior/disorder, complex phonic tics, coprolalia, copropraxia, self-injurious behavior, mood disorder, suicidal ideation, and poor response to medications

Tics, although rarely disabling, can be quite troublesome for TS patients because they cause embarrassment, interfere with social interactions, and at times can be quite painful or uncomfortable. Rarely, cervical tics may be so forceful and violent, the so-called "whiplash tics," that they may cause secondary neurologic deficits, such as cervical artery dissection (Norris et al., 2000), and noncompressive (Isaacs et al., 2010) or compressive cervical myelopathy (Krauss and Jankovic, 1996) (Video 16.2). The truncal bending tics, which resemble intermittent, repetitive camptocormia, may cause secondary degenerative changes in the thoracic spine (Azher and Jankovic, 2005) (Video 16.5). These disabling tics and other severe symptoms of TS draw attention to the subset of patients with TS so severe that they may be life-threatening, hence labeled as "malignant" TS (Table 16.4). Of 332 TS patients evaluated at Baylor College of Medicine Movement Disorders Clinic during a 3-year period, 17 (5.1%) met criteria for malignant TS, defined as ≥2 emergency room (ER) visits or ≥1 hospitalizations for TS symptoms or its associated behavioral comorbidities (Cheung et al., 2007). The patients exhibited tic-related injuries, self-injurious behavior (SIB), uncontrollable violence and temper, and suicidal ideation/attempts. Compared to patients with nonmalignant TS, those with malignant TS were significantly more likely to have a personal history of obsessive-compulsive behavior/disorder (OCB/OCD), complex phonic tics, coprolalia, copropraxia, SIB, mood disorder, suicidal ideation, and poor response to medications. Severe or malignant TS, associated with SIB and other disabling features, has been also reported in families, including consanguineous kindreds (Motlagh et al., 2008).

Vocalizations have been reported as the initial symptom in 12–37% of patients, throat clearing being the most common (Robertson, 1989). Phonic tics can be quite troublesome for patients and those around them. In addition to involuntary noises, some patients have speech dysfluencies that resemble developmental stuttering, and up to half of all patients with developmental stuttering have been thought to have undiagnosed TS (Abwender et al., 1998). Coprolalia, perhaps the most recognizable and certainly one of the most distressing symptoms of TS, is actually present in only half of patients (Videos 16.8 and 16.15). When describing the distress caused by his severe coprolalia, one of our patients remarked that immediately after shouting an obscenity, he reaches out with his hand in an attempt to "catch the word and bring it back before others can hear it." Coprolalia appears to be markedly influenced by cultural background.

Although in one retrospective analysis of 112 children with TS, only 8% exhibited coprolalia (Goldenberg et al., 1994), the true prevalence of coprolalia in TS children and adults is about 50% in the US population, when mental coprolalia (without actual utterance) is included. In a study of 597 individuals with TS from seven countries, coprolalia occurred at some point in the course of the disease in 19.3% of males and 14.6% of females, and copropraxia in 5.9% of males and 4.9% of females (Freeman et al., 2009). Coprolalia has been reported to occur in only 26% of Danish patients and 4% of Japanese patients (Robertson, 1989). Copropraxia has been found in about 20% of patients, echolalia in 30%, echopraxia in 25%, and palilalia in 15%. Although coprolalia is a characteristic feature of TS and, based on functional MRI studies, attributed to abnormal activation particularly in the left middle frontal gyrus and right precentral gyrus, and possibly the caudate nucleus, cingulate gyrus, cuneus, left angular gyrus, left inferior parietal gyrus, and occipital gyri (Gates et al., 2004), this language abnormality is not universally present or specific for TS.

Except for tics, the neurologic examination in patients with TS is usually normal. In one case-control study, TS patients were found to have a shorter duration of saccades, but the saccades were performed with a greater mean velocity than in normal controls, and the TS patients had fewer correct antisaccade responses, suggesting a mild oculomotor disturbance in TS (Farber et al., 1999). Although the ability to inhibit reflexive saccades is normal, TS patients make more timing errors, indicating an inability to appropriately inhibit or delay planned motor programs (LeVasseur et al., 2001).

Behavioral symptoms

Patients with TS generally have normal intelligence and may even perform better and faster than age-matched controls on certain tasks that require grammar skills that depend on procedural, rather than declarative memory (Walenski et al., 2007). While TS patients have no cognitive deficits, they often exhibit a variety of behavioral symptoms, particularly ADHD and OCD (Figs 16.1 and 16.2) (Gaze et al., 2006). In the Tourette International Consortium (TIC) database, which includes information on 3500 patients with TS evaluated by neurologists or psychiatrists, only 12% had tics only, without other comorbidities (Freeman et al., 2000). Kurlan and colleagues (2002) interviewed 1596 children, aged 9–17, in schools in Rochester and Monroe Counties, New York, and identified tics in 339 children (21%) after 60–150 minutes of observation. They found the following behavioral problems more frequently (*P* < 0.05) in children with tics than in those without tics: OCD, ADHD, separation anxiety, overanxious disorder, simple phobia, social phobia, agoraphobia, mania, major depression, and oppositional defiant behavior. Also, children with tics were younger (mean age: 12.5 vs. 13.3 years) and were more likely to require special education services (27% vs. 19.8%).

A thorough discussion of the pathogenesis of comorbid disorders and their relationship to TS is beyond the scope of this review, and the reader is referred to some recent reviews on these topics (Tannock, 1998; Stein, 2002). The diagnosis of ADHD and OCD is based on clinical history; there are no laboratory or other tests that reliably diagnose these

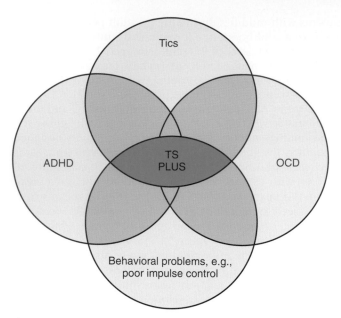

Figure 16.1 An overlap of disorders typically coexisting in patients with TS. *Redrawn from Jankovic J: Tourette's syndrome. N Engl J Med 2001;345:1184–1192.*

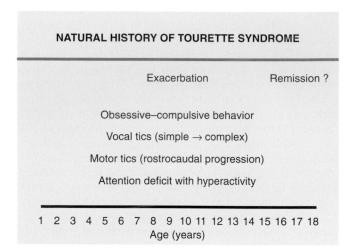

Figure 16.2 Typical progression of symptoms associated with TS. *Redrawn from Jankovic J: Tourette's syndrome. N Engl J Med 2001;345:1184–1192.*

neurobehavioral disorders (Dulcan and AACAP Works Group on Quality Issues, 1997; Goldman et al., 1998; Swanson et al., 1998). These comorbid behavioral conditions often interfere with learning and with academic and work performance (Singer et al., 1995b). In contrast to tics, ADHD and obsessional symptom severity are significantly associated with impaired social and emotional adjustment (Carter et al., 2000). The clinician should be skilled not only in the recognition and treatment of ADHD but also in documenting the ADHD-related deficits (Richard et al., 1998). Such documentation is essential for the parents and educators in order to provide the optimal educational setting for the affected individual.

Since nearly all studies on the frequency of associated features have been based on a population of TS patients who have been referred to physicians, usually specialists, there is a certain selection bias; therefore, accurate figures on the prevalence of these behavioral disorders in TS patients are not available. It has been estimated, however, that 3–6% of the school-aged population suffers from ADHD (Goldman et al., 1998), and probably a majority of patients with TS have had symptoms of ADHD, OCD, or both at some time during the course of their illness (Coffey and Park, 1997). In a review of 1500 patients with TS, 48% were diagnosed as having ADHD, a figure that is consistent with the results of other studies (Comings and Comings, 1988b). The symptoms of ADHD may be the initial manifestations of TS and may precede the onset of motor and phonic tics by about 3 years. During this time, therapy with stimulant drugs may trigger the onset of tics and may precipitate the emergence of other TS symptoms (Price et al., 1986).

There are three types of ADHD: predominantly inattentive, predominantly hyperactive-impulsive, and combined (Dulcan AACAP Works Group on Quality Issues, 1997) (Table 16.5). ADHD is one of the most common neurobehavioral disorders, affecting 3–10% of children and 4% of adults (Wilens et al., 2004; Rappley, 2005). Adults with ADHD often have childhood histories of educational and discipline problems; and during adulthood, they usually have lower socioeconomic status, lower rates of professional employment, and higher rates of marital problems, driving violations, and other life failures. In a genome scan of 106 families, including 128 affected sib-pairs with estimated heritability of 60–80%, evidence of a gene locus was found on chromosomes 4, 9, 10, 11, 12, 16, and 17 (Smalley et al., 2001). Although attention deficit is certainly one of the most common and disabling symptoms of TS, in many patients the inability to pay attention is due to not only a coexistent ADHD but also uncontrollable intrusions of thoughts. Some patients are unable to pay attention because of a compulsive fixation of gaze. For example, while they are sitting in a classroom or a theater or during a conversation, their gaze becomes fixated on a particular object, and despite concentrated effort, they are unable to break the fixation. As a result, they miss the teacher's lesson or a particular action in a play. Another reason for impaired attention in some TS patients is mental concentration exerted in an effort to suppress tics. Yet another cause for inattention is the sedative effect of anti-TS medications. It is therefore important to determine which mechanism or mechanisms are most likely to be responsible for the patient's attention deficit. This is particularly important in selecting the best therapeutic approach. Despite growing publicity about ADHD, there is little evidence of widespread overdiagnosis or overtreatment of ADHD (Goldman et al., 1998). One study showed that children and adolescents with ADHD as compared to those without ADHD are more likely to have major injuries and asthma, and their 9-year medical costs are double (Leibson et al., 2001). The mechanism of ADHD with or without TS is not well understood, and there are no specific pathologic abnormalities identified. However, by using high-resolution MRI, abnormal morphology was observed in the frontal cortices, reduction in the anterior temporal cortices, and increased gray matter in the posterior and inferior parietal cortices in children and adolescents with ADHD (Sowell et al., 2003).

That OCD is a part of the spectrum of neurobehavioral manifestations in TS is now well accepted (Rapoport, 1988; Towbin, 1988; Black, 1992; Stein, 2002). OCD, with an estimated lifetime prevalence of 2–3% (Sasson et al., 1997; Snider and Swedo, 2000) and an incidence of 0.55 per 1000 person-years (Nestadt et al., 1998), is one of the most frequent causes of disability (Jenike, 2004). It may occur alone without other features of TS (Micallef and Blin, 2001). The instrument used most frequently to measure the severity of OCD is the Yale-Brown Obsessive Compulsive Scale (Scahill et al., 1997). A distinction should be made between obsessive-compulsive symptoms or traits, obsessive-compulsive personality disorder, and OCD. Obsessions are characterized by intense, intrusive thoughts, such as concerns about bodily wastes and secretions; unfounded fears; need for exactness, symmetry, evenness, and neatness; excessive religious concerns; perverse sexual thoughts; and intrusions of words, phrases, or music. Compulsions consist of subjective urges to perform meaningless and irrational rituals, such as checking, counting, cleaning, washing, touching, smelling, hoarding, and rearranging. Leckman and colleagues (1994) have drawn attention to the frequent occurrence of the "just right" perception in patients with

Table 16.5 Attention-deficit hyperactivity disorder/hyperkinetic disorder (HKD) (ICD-10, DSM-IV)

Inattention (IN)

Fails to attend to details
Difficulty sustaining attention
Does not seem to listen
Fails to finish
Difficulty organizing tasks
Avoids sustained effort
Loses things
Distracted by external stimuli
Forgetful

Hyperactivity (H)

Fidgets with hands or feet
Leaves seat in classroom
Runs about or climbs
Difficulty playing quietly
Motor excess ("on the go")
Talks excessively

Impulsivity (IMP)

Talks excessively
Blurts out answers
Difficulty waiting turn
Interrupts or intrudes on others

Attention-Deficit Hyperactivity Disorder Diagnostic Subtypes (DSM-IV)

Combined: six or more from the IN domain and six or more from the H/IMP domain
Inattentive: six or more from the IN domain and less than six from the H/IMP domain
Hyperactive/impulsive: six or more from the H/IMP domain and fewer than six from the IN domain

HKD (ICD-10)

Six or more from the IN domain, three or more from the H domain, and one or more from the IMP domain

OCD and TS. While obsessional slowness accounts for some of the school problems experienced by TS patients, cognitive slowing (bradyphrenia) is also a contributing factor (Singer et al., 1995b). Patients with OCD can usually be divided into those with a predominantly cognitive form (in which an idea is followed by a ritual) and those with a sensorimotor type (in which a physical sensation is followed by a movement). In contrast to primary OCD, in which the symptoms relate chiefly to hygiene and cleanliness, the obsessive symptoms that are associated with TS usually involve concerns with symmetry, violent aggressive thoughts, forced touching, fear of harming self or others, and need for saying or doing things "just right" (Eapen et al., 1997b). A principal-components factor analysis of 13 categories that are used to group types of obsessions and compulsions in the Yale-Brown Obsessive Compulsive Scale symptom checklist identified the obsessions and checking and the symmetry and ordering factors as particularly common in patients with tic disorders (Leckman et al., 1997a). Miguel and colleagues (2000) showed that patients who have OCD associated with TS tend to have more bodily sensations occurring either before or during the patient's performance of the repetitive behaviors as well as mental sensations including urge only, energy release (mental energy that builds up and needs to be discharged), and "just right" perceptions. Cognitive inflexibility manifested by impaired task-switch ability in patients with OCD has been suggested to be due to "imbalance in brain activation between dorsal and ventral striatal circuits (Gu et al., 2008).

In addition to an idiopathic sporadic or familial disorder and TS, OCD has been reported to occur as a result of a variety of lesions in the frontal-limbic-subcortical circuits (Berthier et al., 1996; Kwak and Jankovic, 2002; Voon, 2004). Although both ADHD and OCD are regarded as integral findings of the syndrome, only OCD has been shown to be genetically linked to TS (Alsobrook and Pauls, 1997). A pathogenic link between TS and OCD is also suggested by the finding in one study that 59% of 54 patients with OCD had a lifetime history of tics, and 14% fulfilled the criteria for TS during the 2–7-year follow-up (Leonard, 1992). Alsobrook and Pauls (2002) identified four significant factors: (1) aggressive phenomena (e.g., kicking, temper fits, argumentativeness), (2) purely motor and phonic tic symptoms, (3) compulsive phenomena (e.g., touching of others or objects, repetitive speech, throat clearing), and (4) tapping and absence of grunting, which accounted for 61% of the phenotypic symptom variance in TS probands and their first-degree relatives.

An important link between motor and behavioral manifestations of TS is the loss of impulse control. Many TS patients suffer from poor impulse control, disinhibition of aggression and emotions, and obsessive thoughts that may dictate their actions. Indeed, many behavioral symptoms of TS, including some complex tics, coprolalia, copropraxia, and many behavioral problems, can be explained by loss of normal inhibitory mechanisms (disinhibition) manifested by poor impulse control. It is as though the TS patients have lost their ability to suppress vestiges of primitive behavior. Poor impulse control might also explain the inability to control anger, as a result of which many patients have frequent and sometimes violent, temper outbursts, and rages. Rarely, TS patients exhibit inappropriate sexual aggressiveness and antisocial, oppositional, and even violent, unlawful, or criminal behavior. TS, indeed, serves as a model medical disorder that can predispose one to engage in uncontrollable and offensive behaviors that are misunderstood by the law-abiding community and the legal justice system (Jankovic et al., 2006). The social and legal aspects of TS patients have yet to be investigated, but there is growing concern regarding media misrepresentation that attributes violent criminal behavior in certain individuals to TS. Although TS should not be used as an excuse to justify unlawful or criminal behaviors, studies are needed to determine whether TS-related symptoms and neurobehavioral comorbidities predispose TS patients to engage in such behaviors. Often, the avolitional nature of behaviors in response to involuntary internal thought and emotional patterns is supported by the subsequent remorse and lack of secondary gain. This suggests that the preponderance of unlawful acts committed by TS patients are not premeditated but may result from a variety of TS-related mechanisms such as poor impulse control, OCD associated with addictive behavior (e.g., drugs, alcohol, gambling), attention-deficit disorder (ADD), and distractibility (e.g., motor vehicle accidents). A previous study (Comings and Comings, 1987) compared conduct in 246 TS patients to that of controls for behaviors such as lying, stealing, fighting or inability to stop fighting, violence against animals, physically attacking peers or parents, vandalism, running away from home, starting fires, poor temper control, alcohol and drug abuse, and other misdemeanors. Thirty-five percent of TS patients had a conduct score higher than 13, significantly greater than the 2.1% of controls with high scores ($P < 0.0005$). All behaviors with the exception of running away from home and trouble with the law occurred at a significantly greater rate in TS patients. Although no difference was found for the law variable, TS patients were significantly more likely to vandalize ($P < 0.0005$), fight ($P < 0.0005$), abuse drugs or alcohol ($P < 0.003$), and steal ($P < 0.015$). An interesting finding in this study was that certain behaviors, such as starting fires, shouting, and physically attacking, were significantly greater only in TS patients with comorbid ADD, supporting the well-established association of ADD in conduct disorder. It was estimated from this study that 10–30% of conduct disorder cases in non-economically disadvantaged children may be attributed to a possible TS gene. In a more recent study, however, TS accounted for only 2% of all cases that were referred for forensic psychiatric investigation in Stockholm, Sweden, between 1990 and 1995; 15% of the subjects had ADHD, 15% had PDD, and 3% had Asperger syndrome (Siponmaa et al., 2001).

Focal frontal lobe dysfunction, demonstrated in TS by various functional and imaging studies, has been associated with an impulsive subtype of aggressive behavior (Brower and Price, 2001). It has been postulated that impulse disorders stem from exaggerated reward-, pleasure-, or arousal-seeking brain centers, resulting in failure of inhibition. Animal studies of rats with lesions of the nucleus accumbens core, the brain region that is noted for reward and reinforcement, showed that the lesioned rats preferred small, immediate rewards over larger, delayed rewards (Cardinal et al., 2001). In addition to the ventromedial prefrontal cortices, lesions in the amygdala have also been known to result in altered decision-making processes and a disregard for future consequences (Bechara et al., 2000).

One of the most distressing symptoms of TS is a self-injurious behavior (SIB), which has been reported in up to 53% of all patients (Robertson, 1989; Robertson et al., 1990). A common form of SIB is damage of skin by biting, scratching, cutting, engraving, or hitting, particularly in the eye and throat (compulsions), often accompanied by an irresistible urge (obsession) (Jankovic et al., 1998) (Videos 16.16 and 16.17). In some patients SIB can be life-threatening, hence the term "malignant" TS (Cheung et al., 2007). The mechanism of self-injurious behavior is not well understood, but the recently described animal model may shed some light on this very important behavioral disorder that may accompany TS. A mouse with genetic deletion of *Sapap3*, a gene that codes for postsynaptic scaffolding protein at excitatory striatal synapses, has been proposed as a possible model of OCD as its phenotype is characterized by excessive compulsive grooming resulting in self-injurious behavior, such as facial hair loss and skin lesions (Welch et al., 2007). The similarity of this behavior to OCD is further supported by the observation that the mice markedly improved after treatment with a selective serotonin reuptake inhibitor. Thus, SIB appears to be related to OCD, which has treatment implications. Besides OCD, SIB also correlates with impulsivity and impulse control (Mathews et al., 2004). Conduct disorders and problems with discipline at home and in school are recurrent themes during discussions of behavioral problems with TS families. The inability to suppress or "edit" intentions due to a "dysfunctional intention editor" has been proposed as one of the chief reasons for poor impulse control in patients with TS (Baron-Cohen et al., 1994).

The TS gene(s) may, in addition to tics, ADHD, and OCD, express itself in a variety of behavioral manifestations, including learning and conduct disorders, schizoid and affective disorders, antisocial behaviors, oppositional defiant disorder, anxiety, depression, conduct disorder, severe temper outbursts, rage attacks, impulse control problems, inappropriate sexual behavior, and other psychiatric problems (Comings, 1987; Robertson, 2000). Personality disorder and depression have been reported in 64% of patients with TS (Robertson et al., 1997). Whether these behavioral problems indeed occur with higher frequency in TS patients and whether they are pathogenically linked to TS are debatable (Comings and Comings, 1988a; Pauls et al., 1988).

Besides comorbid behavioral conditions, TS has been reported to be frequently associated with migraine headaches. In one study, 26.6% of TS patients, with a mean age of 11.9 years, exhibited migraine headaches (Barabas et al., 1984). We found migraine headaches in 25 carefully screened TS patients at a significantly greater rate than the estimated 11–13% in the general adult population ($P < 0.0001$) and the general pediatric population ($P < 0.04$) (Kwak et al., 2003b). This compares to 4.0–7.4% in the general population of school-aged children. The Tourette International Consortium Database (Freeman et al., 2000), which at the time of publication included information on 3500 patients with TS collected from 64 centers from around the world, showed that only 12% of patients with TS had no other disorders; ADHD was seen in 60%, symptoms of OCD in 59%, anger control problems in 37%, sleep disorder in 25%, learning disability in 23%, mood disorders in 20%, anxiety disorders in 18%, and SIB in 14%.

Pathogenesis

Neurophysiology

Although the pathogenic mechanisms of TS are still unknown, the weight of evidence supports an organic rather than psychogenic origin, probably involving the basal ganglia circuitry (Leckman et al., 1997b; Palumbo et al., 1997; Jankovic, 2001a; Leckman, 2002; Berardelli et al., 2003; Albin and Mink, 2006) (Fig. 16.3). Despite the observation that some tics may be voluntary, at least in part, physiologic studies suggest that tics are not mediated through normal motor pathways utilized for willed movements (Obeso et al., 1982). Using back-averaging techniques, Obeso and colleagues (1982) observed normal Bereitschaftspotential in six subjects who voluntarily simulated tic-like movements, but no such premovement potential was noted in association with an actual tic. The common absence of premotor potentials in simple motor tics suggests that tics are truly involuntary or that they occur in response to some external cue (Papa et al., 1991). Karp and colleagues (1996), however, documented premotor negativity in two of five patients with simple motor tics. Although the investigators could not correlate the presence of Bereitschaftspotential with the premonitory sensation, the physiology of the premovement phenomenon requires further studies. Transmagnetic stimulation used to study cortical excitability in 11 TS patients found evidence of motor-cortical disinhibition at rest (Heise et al., 2010).

Conventional neurophysiologic investigations have found that TS patients have defective inhibitory mechanisms, as is suggested by the increased duration of the late response of the blink reflex and reduced inhibition at paired pulse testing (Smith and Lees, 1989; Berardelli et al., 2003). TS patients also have exaggerated audiogenic startle response (Gironell et al., 2000). About 20% patients with TS have exaggerated startle responses, which may fail to habituate with repetition (Stell et al., 1995).

As was noted before, functional MRI showed decreased neuronal activity during periods of suppression in the ventral globus pallidus, putamen, and thalamus and increased activity in the right caudate nucleus, right frontal cortex, and other cortical areas that are normally involved in the inhibition of unwanted impulses (prefrontal, parietal, temporal, and cingulate cortices) (Peterson et al., 1998a). In another study of three patients with TS, functional MRI showed marked reduction or absence of activity in secondary motor areas while the patient attempted to maintain a stable grip-load force control (Serrien et al., 2002). The authors interpreted the findings as an ongoing activation of the secondary motor reflecting patients' involuntary urges to move. In a study of children with ADHD, functional MRI showed increased frontal activation and reduced striatal activation on various tasks and an enhancement of striatal function after treatment with methylphenidate (Vaidya et al., 1998). Functional MRI studies show decreased neuronal activity during periods of suppression in the ventral globus pallidus, putamen, and thalamus and increased activity in the caudate,

HYPOTHETICAL BASAL GANGLIA CIRCUITRY MODEL OF TICS

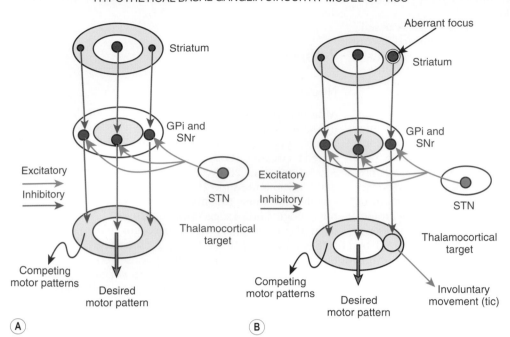

Figure 16.3 Basal ganglia circuitry relevant to pathophysiology of tics. GPi, globus pallidus interna; STN, subthalamic nucleus; SNr, substantia nigra pars reticulata.

frontal cortex, and other cortical areas that are normally involved in the inhibition of unwanted impulses (prefrontal, parietal, temporal, and cingulated cortical areas) (Peterson, 2001). By using event-related functional MRI (fMRI) in 10 patients with TS, a brain network of paralimbic areas such as anterior cingulate and insular cortex, supplementary motor area (SMA), and parietal operculum (PO) was identified that predominantly activated before tic onset, whereas at the beginning of tic action, significant fMRI activities were found in sensorimotor areas including superior parietal lobule bilaterally and cerebellum (Bohlhalter et al., 2006). Using resting-state functional connectivity MRI (rs-fcMRI) in 33 adolescents with TS, Church et al. (2009) found anomalous connections primarily in the frontoparietal network, suggesting widespread immature functional connectivity, particularly in regions related to adaptive online control.

Transcranial magnetic stimulation studies have demonstrated a shortened cortical silent period and defective intracortical inhibition (determined in a conditioning test paired-stimulus paradigm) in patients with TS (Orth et al., 2005) and OCD (Greenberg et al., 1998), thus providing a possible explanation for intrusive phenomena. Subsequent studies utilizing the same technique have demonstrated that patients with tic-related OCD have more abnormal motor cortex excitability than OCD patients without tics (Greenberg et al., 2000). Transcranial magnetic stimulation studies have also demonstrated that TS children have a shorter cortical silent period but that their intracortical inhibition was not different from that of controls, although intracortical inhibition is reduced in children with ADHD (Moll et al., 2001). There is evidence of additive inhibitory deficits, as demonstrated by reduced intracortical inhibition and a shortened cortical silent period in children with TS and comorbid ADHD. In another study, ADHD more than tics were associated with short-interval intracortical

inhibition (Gilbert et al., 2004). Both short-interval intracortical inhibition and short-interval afferent inhibition, modulated by nicotinic receptors, were reduced in eight patients with TS (ages 24–38 years) as compared to ten matched healthy controls (Orth et al., 2005). Comprehensive discussion of the neuroscience of ADHD is beyond the scope of this chapter, but the reader is referred to some recent reviews of this topic (Castellanos and Tannock, 2002).

Sleep studies have provided additional evidence that some tics are truly involuntary. Polysomnographic studies in 34 TS patients recorded motor tics in various stages of sleep in 23 patients and phonic tics in 4 patients (Glaze et al., 1983; Jankovic and Rohaidy, 1987). Additional sleep studies have suggested that some patients with TS have alterations of arousal, decreased percentage (up to 30%) of stage 3/4 (slow wave) sleep, decreased percentage of REM sleep, paroxysmal events in stage 4 sleep with sudden intense arousal, disorientation and agitation, restless legs syndrome, and periodic leg movement in sleep (Voderholzer et al., 1997; Chokroverty and Jankovic, 1999; Picchietti et al., 1999). Restless legs syndrome has been reported to be present in about 10% of patients with TS and in 23% of parents (Lesperance et al., 2004). In this regard, it is of interest that in a study in which 14 single-nucleotide polymorphisms were typed spanning the three genomic loci in 298 TS trios, 322 TS cases (including 298 probands from the cohort of TS trios), and 290 control subjects, it was found that the same variant of the gene *BTBD9* that increases the risk of restless legs syndrome also increases the risk of TS without obsessive-compulsive disorder or attention-deficit disorder ("pure" TS) (Rivière et al., 2009). Other sleep-related disorders that are associated with TS include sleep apnea, enuresis, sleepwalking and sleep talking, nightmares, myoclonus, bruxism, and other disturbances (Rothenberger et al., 2001; Hanna and Jankovic, 2003).

Neuroimaging

Although standard anatomic neuroimaging studies in TS are unremarkable, by using special volumetric, metabolic, blood flow, ligand, and functional imaging techniques, several interesting findings have been reported that have strong implications for the pathophysiology of TS (Peterson, 2001; Albin and Mink, 2006; Frey and Albin, 2006) (Fig. 16.3). Careful volumetric MRI studies have suggested that the normal asymmetry of the basal ganglia is lost in TS (Peterson et al., 1993; Singer et al., 1993; Peterson, 2001). In one study, the normal left > right asymmetry (Singer et al., 1993) in the volume in the right anterior brain, right caudate, and right pallidum was reversed in TS subjects (Castellanos et al., 1996). Caudate volumes have been reported to correlate significantly and inversely with the severity of tic and OCD in early adulthood (Bloch et al., 2005). The volumetric studies, however, have not always produced consistent results (Moriarty et al., 1997). In another volumetric MRI study, Frederickson and colleagues (2002) found evidence of smaller gray matter volumes in the left frontal lobes of patients with TS, further supporting the findings of loss of normal left > right asymmetry. Quantitative MRI studies have found a subtle, but possibly important, reduction in the volume of caudate nuclei in patients with TS. In 10 pairs of monozygotic twins, the right caudate was smaller in the more severely affected individuals, providing evidence for the role of environmental events in the pathogenesis of TS (Hyde et al., 1995). In contrast, the corpus callosum has been found to be larger in children with TS than in normal controls (Baumgardner et al., 1996). Subsequent study showed that this finding was gender-related and was present only in boys with TS (Mostofsky et al., 1999). An MRI-DTI study of monozygotic twins showed that the mean fractional anisotropy values were significantly lower, particularly in the posterior portion of the corpus callosum, in the twin affected with TS (Cavanna et al., 2010). Using voxel-based morphometry and high-resolution MRI in 31 TS patients, increased gray matter was found in the left mesencephalon compared to 31 controls (Garraux et al., 2006). This finding, however, could not be replicated in a smaller study of 14 boys with TS using the same technique (Ludolph et al., 2006). This latter study found increased gray matter volumes in bilateral ventral putamen and regional decreases in gray matter volumes in the left hippocampus gyrus. The difference was attributed to younger mean age in the latter study compared to the previous study (12.5 vs. 32 years). Diffusion-tensor MRI (DT-MRI) used to investigate the structural integrity of basal ganglia and thalamus in 23 children with TS found increased mean water diffusivity bilaterally in the putamen and decreased anisotropy in the right thalamus, indicating impairment of white matter integrity in the fronto-striatal-thalamic circuit at a microstructural level (Makki et al., 2008). Using tractography of the fronto-striato-thalamic circuit, the same group showed that TS patients had significantly lower probability of connection between caudate nucleus and anterior-dorsolateral-frontal cortex on the left and that OCB was negatively associated with connectivity score of the left caudate and anterior dorsolateral-frontal cortex, and was positively associated with connectivity score for the subcallosal gyrus and for the lentiform nucleus (Makki et al., 2009). Additional imaging studies have identified frontal and parietal cortical thinning, most prominent in ventral portions of the sensory and motor homunculi in patients with TS (Sowell et al., 2008). Dopaminergic hyperfunction (Albin et al., 2003), possibly as a result of overproduction of synapses in mid-childhood (Giedd et al., 1999), might be associated with increased striatal volume in childhood which may be lost in adulthood.

Positron emission tomography (PET) scanning has shown variable rates of glucose utilization in basal ganglia as compared to controls. In one study, [^{18}F]fluorodeoxyglucose PET has shown evidence of increased metabolic activity in the lateral premotor and supplementary motor association cortices and in the midbrain (pattern 1), and decreased metabolic activity in the caudate and thalamic areas (limbic basal ganglia–thalamocortical projection system) (pattern 2) (Eidelberg et al., 1997). Pattern 1 is reportedly associated with tics, and pattern 2 correlates with the overall severity of TS. In a follow-up study, involving 12 TS adult patients (untreated for >2 years) and 12 controls, the investigators found a TS-related metabolic pattern which was characterized by increased premotor cortex and cerebellum activity, and reduced resting activity of the striatum and orbitofrontal cortex (Pourfar et al., 2011). They also provided evidence for an OCD-related pattern which was characterized by reduced activity of the anterior cingulate and dorsolateral prefrontal cortical regions associated with relative increases in primary motor cortex and precuneus. This pattern significantly correlated with the severity of the OCD symptoms.

In contrast to dystonia, which is characterized by lentiform nucleus-thalamic metabolic dissociation, attributed to overactivity of the direct striatopallidal inhibitory pathway, the pattern of TS is characterized by concomitant metabolic reduction in striatal and thalamic function. The authors suggested that this pattern can be explained by a reduction in the indirect pathway, resulting in reduction in subthalamic nucleus (STN) activity. This is in part consistent with another study that found evidence of increased activation in the direct pathway, but the activity in the prefrontal cortex and STN has been found to be increased presumably as a result of compensatory activation (Baym et al., 2008). Using event-related [^{15}O]H$_2$O PET combined with time-synchronized audiotaping and videotaping of six patients with TS, Stern and colleagues (2000) found increased activity in the sensorimotor, language, executive, paralimbic, and frontal-subcortical areas that was temporarily related to the motor and phonic tics and the irresistible urge that precedes these behaviors. Using a similar technique Lerner et al. (2007) found robust activation of cerebellum, insula, thalamus, and putamen during tic release. Rauch and colleagues (1997) showed bilateral medial temporal (hippocampal/parahippocampal) activation on PET in patients with OCD as compared to normal controls and absence of activation of inferior striatum, seen in normal controls. Various neuroimaging studies have also demonstrated moderate reduction in the size of the corpus callosum, basal ganglia (particularly caudate and globus pallidus), and frontal lobes (Filipek et al., 1997) and striatal hypoperfusion (Vaidya et al., 1998) in patients with ADHD.

An autopsy study of three TS brains found consistent increases in dopamine transporter (DAT) and D2 receptor as well as D1 and α-2A density, suggesting that dopaminergic hyperfunction in the frontal lobe may play a role in the pathophysiology of TS (Yoon et al., 2007). Another pathological study showed a marked increase in total number of neurons in the globus pallidus interna (GPi) and decreased number in the globus pallidus externa (GPe) and in the caudate nucleus of brains of patients with TS (Kalanithi et al., 2005). Furthermore, an increased number and proportion of the GPi neurons were positive for the calcium-binding protein parvalbumin in tissue from TS subjects, whereas lower densities of parvalbumin-positive interneurons were observed in both the caudate and putamen of TS subjects. These abnormalities have been interpreted as indicating a developmental defect in the migration of some GABAergic neurons.

Neurochemistry

An alteration in the central neurotransmitters has been suggested chiefly because of relatively consistent responses to modulation of the dopaminergic system (Harris and Singer, 2006). Dopamine antagonists and depletors generally have an ameliorating effect on tics, whereas drugs that enhance central dopaminergic activity exacerbate tics (Jankovic and Rohaidy, 1987; Jankovic and Orman, 1988). Low cerebrospinal fluid homovanillic acid, coupled with a favorable response to dopamine receptor-blocking drugs, has been interpreted as evidence in support of the notion that tics and TS are due to supersensitive dopamine receptors (Singer, 2000). Postmortem binding studies of dopamine receptors, however, have failed to provide support for this hypothesis (Singer, 2000).

Neurochemical studies of TS have been hampered by the lack of available postmortem brain tissue. Biochemical abnormalities in the few postmortem brains that have been studied include low serotonin, low glutamate in the medial globus pallidus, and low cyclic AMP in the cortex (Singer, 2000). Haber and Wolfer (1992) reported that in a blind rating of five TS brains, three had low dynorphin immunoreactivity in the ventral portion of the medial globus pallidus. A defect in tryptophan oxygenase in TS has been proposed by Comings (1990), who analyzed 1400 blood samples from patients with TS or ADHD and their relatives and controls; he found decreased platelet serotonin and low blood tryptophan levels in TS patients and their parents. In support of the "tryptophan hypothesis" is a study that used alpha-[^{11}C]methyl-L-tryptophan (AMT) positron emission tomography (PET) to assess global and focal brain abnormalities of tryptophan metabolism in 26 children with TS and nine controls. The findings indicate that tryptophan uptake is significantly decreased in the dorsolateral prefrontal cortex and increased in the thalamus of TS patients (Behen et al., 2007).

One intriguing hypothesis, supported partly by the increased ^{3}H-mazindol binding to the presynaptic dopamine uptake carrier sites, suggests that TS represents a developmental disorder resulting in dopaminergic hyperinnervation of the ventral striatum and the associated limbic system (nucleus accumbens) (Singer et al., 1991). Using [^{11}C]raclopride PET and amphetamine stimulation, Singer and colleagues (2002) found evidence for increased dopamine release in the putamen of patients with TS. They postulate that in TS, there is increased activity of the dopamine transporter leading to increased dopamine concentration in the

dopamine terminals and stimulus-dependent increase in dopaminergic transmission. Support for this hypothesis has been provided by the imaging studies of Albin and colleagues (2003). The authors used PET with the vesicular monoamine transporter type 2 ligand [^{11}C]dihydrotetrabenazine that binds to type 2 vesicular monoamine transporter (VMAT2) to quantify striatal monoaminergic innervation in patients with TS ($n = 19$) and control subjects ($n = 27$). With voxel-by-voxel analysis, the investigators found increased [^{11}C]dihydrotetrabenazine binding in the ventral striatum (right > left) in patients with TS as compared to age-matched controls. However, a subsequent PET study involving 33 adults with TS and utilizing not only [^{11}C]dihydrotetrabenazine but also [^{11}C]methylphenidate, a ligand for DAT, binding, found no differences between subjects with TS and controls (Albin et al., 2009). In a study of 8 patients with TS and 8 controls [^{11}C]FLB 457 PET in conjunction with an amphetamine challenge used to evaluate extrastriatal D2/D3 receptor binding and DA release, TS patients showed decreased [^{11}C]FLB 457 binding potentials bilaterally in cortical and subcortical regions outside the striatum, including the cingulate gyrus, middle and superior temporal gyrus, occipital cortex, insula, and thalamus (Steeves et al., 2010). Furthermore, amphetamine challenge induced widespread increased DA release in TS patients, which extended more anteriorly to involve anterior cingulate and medial frontal gyri. The authors suggested that "reductions in D2/D3 receptor binding in both frontal cortex and thalamus are consistent with recently published preliminary data demonstrating similar abnormalities of D2/D3 binding in TS patients using a different PET ligand." A postmortem examination of two brains of patients with typical childhood-onset TS and one with adult-onset tics showed that the prefrontal cortex rather than the striatum showed most abnormalities, including increased D2 receptor protein, as well as increases in dopamine transporter, VAMP2, and α-2A (Minzer et al., 2004).

Although this idea is highly speculative, it is possible that the genetic defect in TS somehow interferes with the normal regulation of the neuronal progenitor cells during development, thus resulting in the increased innervation of the ventral striatum (Ikonomidou et al., 1999; Itoh et al., 2001; Hanashima et al., 2004). This implies that the genetic defect somehow interferes with the programmed cell suicide that is needed to control cell proliferation in normal development and growth. The ventral striatum is the portion of the basal ganglia that is anatomically and functionally linked to the limbic system. The link between the basal ganglia and the limbic system might explain the frequent association of tics and complex behavioral problems, and a dysfunction in the basal ganglia and the limbic system seems to provide the best explanation for the most fundamental behavioral disturbance in TS, namely, loss of impulse control and a state of apparent "disinhibition." The notion that deficits in inhibitory functions are at the core of the clinical phenotype associated with TS is supported by studies by Baron-Cohen and colleagues (1994) showing that patients with TS are not able to appropriately edit their intentions and by Swerdlow and colleagues (1996) showing that TS patients demonstrate deficits on the visuospatial priming tasks.

Functional neuroimaging studies have been used to aid in the understanding of neurotransmitter and receptor alterations in TS. Using [^{123}I]β-carboxymethoxy-3β-(4-iodophenyl) tropane (CIT) single photon emission computed tomography scans, Malison and colleagues (1995) demonstrated a mean 37% increase in binding of this dopamine transporter ligand in the striatum in five adult patients with TS as compared to age-matched controls. In contrast, Heinz and colleagues (1998) found no difference in [^{123}I] β-CIT binding in the midbrain, thalamus, or basal ganglia between 10 TS patients and normal control subjects. There was, however, a significant negative correlation between the severity of phonic tics and β-CIT binding in the midbrain and thalamus. In another study involving 12 TS adult patients, β-CIT scans showed evidence of increased dopamine transporter binding (Müller-Vahl et al., 2000). Combining single photon emission computed tomography and MRI, Wolf and colleagues (1996) found 17% greater binding of IBZM, a D2 receptor ligand, in the caudate (but not putamen) nucleus in five of the more affected monozygotic twins who were discordant for TS. It is important to note, however, that two of the five subjects were taking neuroleptics for up to 6 weeks prior to the single photon emission computed tomography studies. These findings, if confirmed by other studies of neuroleptic-naive patients, support the notion that the presynaptic dopamine function is enhanced in TS. This might, in turn, lead to a reduced inhibitory pallidal output to the mediodorsal thalamus. The observation that in patients with Parkinson disease the severity of childhood-onset tics was not influenced by the development of parkinsonism or by its treatment with levodopa, however, argues against the role of dopamine in the pathogenesis of TS symptoms (Kumar and Lang, 1997a). This is supported by the results of PET ligand studies showing normal D2 receptor density (Turjanski et al., 1994). Furthermore, Meyer and colleagues (1999) used PET imaging of (+)-α-[^{11}C]dihydrotetrabenazine to determine the density of vesicular monoamine transporter type 2, a cytoplasm-to-vesicle transporter that is linearly related to monoaminergic nerve terminal density unaffected by medications, in 8 TS patients and 22 controls. This study showed no significant difference in terminal density between patients and controls, thus failing to provide support for the concept of increased striatal innervation. However, these studies do not exclude the possibility of abnormal regulation of dopamine release and uptake. Subsequent study involving 19 adult patients with TS showed that the [^{11}C]dihydrotetrabenazine-binding potential is significantly increased, thus supporting the notion that striatal monoaminergic innervation is increased in the ventral striatum (right > left) of TS patients (Albin et al., 2003). The results of this study contrasted with previous findings of 30–40% increase in dopamine transporter (Müller-Vahl et al., 2000; Singer et al., 2001). Furthermore, in a small sample of TS patients, PET studies, have demonstrated a 25% increase in accumulation of fluorodopa in the left caudate ($P = 0.03$) and a 53% increase in the right midbrain ($P = 0.08$) (Ernst et al., 1999). These findings indicate possible dopaminergic dysfunction in the cells of origin and in the dopaminergic terminals, suggesting increased activity of dopa decarboxylase.

Functional imaging has provided insights into the mechanisms not only of TS but also of ADHD. In 53 adults with ADHD (without tics) when compared to 44 healthy controls, a reduction in dopamine markers was demonstrated, using ^{11}C-cocaine as a marker for dopamine transporter and ^{11}C-raclopride, a ligand for D2/D3 receptors (Volkow et al., 2009).

Despite some limitations and inconsistencies, the imaging, ligand, and biochemical studies provide support for the hypothesis that the corticostriatal-thalamic-cortical circuit plays an important role in the pathogenesis of TS and related disorders (Witelson, 1993; Peterson, 2001). The dorsolateral prefrontal circuit, which links Brodmann's area 9 and 10 with the dorsolateral head of the caudate, appears to be involved with executive functions (manipulation of previously learned knowledge, abstract reasoning, organization, verbal fluency, and problem solving; it is closely related to intelligence, education, and social exposure) and motor planning. An abnormality in this circuit has been implicated in ADHD. The lateral orbitofrontal circuit originates in the inferior lateral prefrontal cortex (area 10) and projects to the ventral medial caudate. An abnormality to this circuit is associated with personality changes, mania, disinhibition, and irritability. Last, the anterior cingulate circuit arises in the cingulate gyrus (area 24) and projects to the ventral striatum, which also receives input from the amygdala, hippocampus, medial orbitofrontal cortex, and entorhinal and perirhinal cortex. A variety of behavioral problems, including OCD, may be linked to an abnormality in this circuit.

Reduced metabolism or blood flow to the basal ganglia, particularly in the ventral striatum, most often in the left hemisphere, has been demonstrated in the majority of the studies involving TS subjects. These limbic areas are thought to be involved in impulse control, reward contingencies, and executive functions, and these behavioral functions appear to be abnormal in most patients with TS. The radioligand studies have been less consistent, but they provide some support for increased D2 receptor density in the caudate nucleus. Imaging studies of presynaptic markers such as dopa decarboxylase, dopamine, and dopamine transporter have produced results that are even less consistent. Future imaging and ligand studies should include children, since this population has been largely excluded because of ethical considerations. The studies should also rigorously characterize comorbid disorders and should take into consideration potential confounding variables, such as the secondary effects of chronic illness and medications.

Immunology

The potential role of immunologic mechanisms and specifically antineuronal antibodies is currently being explored in a variety of neurologic disorders, including TS (Allen, 1997; Hallett and Kiessling, 1997; Hallett et al., 2000; Morshed et al., 2001; Church et al., 2003; Harris and Singer, 2006; Singer et al., 2008; Martino et al., 2009). Several studies have suggested that exacerbations of TS symptoms correlated with an antecedent group A β-hemolytic streptococcus (GABHS) infection (demonstrated by elevated antistreptococcal titers) and the presence of serum antineuronal antibodies (Kiessling et al., 1993). Epitopes of streptococcal M proteins have been found to cross-react with the human brain, particularly the basal ganglia, and may be pathogenetically important in various neurologic disorders, such as Sydenham disease, TS-like syndrome, dystonia, and parkinsonism (Bronze and Dale, 1993; Dale et al., 2001). In 10 patients with poststreptococcal acute disseminated encephalomyelitis (PSADEM) following exposure to GABHS, Dale and colleagues (2001) showed antibasal ganglia antibodies in all with three (60, 67, and 80 kDa) dominant bands. Furthermore, MRI showed hyperintense basal ganglia in 80% of the patients. The B-lymphocyte antigen D8/17 is considered to be a marker for rheumatic fever but is also frequently overexpressed in patients with tics, OCD, and autism (Murphy et al., 1997; Swedo et al., 1997; Hoekstra et al., 2001). In one study, children and adults with TS had significantly higher serum levels of antineuronal antibodies against the putamen, but not the caudate or globus pallidus, as compared to controls (Singer et al., 1998). The potential relevance of this finding has been questioned, however, since there is no relationship between the presence of the antineuronal antibodies and age at onset, severity of tics, or the presence of comorbid disorders. Trifiletti and Packard (1999) have confirmed the presence of a specific brain protein at an apparent molecular weight of 83 kDa that is recognized by antibodies in the serum of 80–90% of patients with TS or OCD (Trifiletti and Packard 1999). They concluded that there may be a subset of patients with TS and OCD, perhaps up to 10% of all cases, in whom a streptococcal infection triggers the onset of symptoms (Trifiletti and Packard, 1999). In a large case-control study of 150 patients with tics compared to 150 controls, Cardona and Orefici (2001) found a correlation between the occurrence of tics and prior exposure to streptococcal antigens and that the severity of tic disorder correlates with the magnitude of the serologic response to streptococcal antigens measured by antistreptolysin O (ASO) titers (38% of the children with tics compared with 2% of the control subjects had ASO titers $\geq$500 IU, ($P < 0.001$)). In another study involving 25 adult patients with TS and 25 healthy controls, increased antibody titers against streptococcal M12 and M19 proteins were found in the TS group as compared to the healthy controls (Müller et al., 2001). In yet another study involving 81 patients with TS, 27 with Sydenham disease, 52 with autoimmune disorders, and 67 normal controls, Morshed and colleagues (2001) found elevated titers of IgG antineuronal antibodies in diseased individuals compared to controls, but there was no relationship between the antibody titers and the age, severity of TS, or comorbid disorders. Church and colleagues (2003) studied 100 patients with TS, 50 children with neurologic disease, 40 with recent uncomplicated streptococcal infection, and 50 healthy adults. They found elevated ASO titers in 64% of TS children compared with 15% of pediatric controls ($P < 0.0001$) and in 68% of adults with TS compared with 12% of adult neurologic controls and 8% of adult healthy controls ($P < 0.05$). Evidence of basal ganglia antibodies were found in 20–27% of TS patients, compared to 2–4% of controls. Similar to the proposed antigen in Sydenham disease, the most common antigen in TS was 60 kDa protein. Furthermore, 91% of patients with positive basal ganglia antibodies were found to have elevated ASO titers, whereas only 57% of those without such antibodies had high ASO titers. The authors concluded that these findings "suggest a pathogenic similarity between Sydenham disease and some patients with TS." In another study, 65% of 65 patients with atypical movement disorders, including dystonia and tics, had antibasal ganglia antibodies (Edwards et al., 2004b). Edwards and colleagues (2004a) also reported four adult cases of tic disorder and stereotypies associated with the presence of antibasal ganglia antibodies. There was no difference when clinical features of TS patients (53 children and 75 adults) with and without antinuclear antibodies, determined by Western immunoblot showing bands for at least 1 of 3 reported striatal antigens (40, 45, and 60 kDa), were compared (Martino et al., 2009). When brain MRI T1 and diffusion tensor (DTI) imaging was compared in 9 adults with TS who had antibasal ganglia antibodies with 13 without detectable antibodies, the voxel-based morphometry analysis failed to detect any significant difference in gray matter density between the two groups, again suggesting lack of relevance of the antibasal ganglia antibodies to the pathogenesis of TS. Although there are many inconsistencies in the reported results related to autoantibodies in TS, and increased activation of immune responses in TS has been suggested by some investigators, further studies are needed before it can be concluded that TS is an autoimmune disorder (Martino et al., 2009).

Development of dyskinesias (paw and floor licking, head and paw shaking) and phonic utterances has been reported in rodents after the microinfusion of dilute IgG from TS subjects into their striatum (Hallett et al., 2000). They extended their initial observations by demonstrating that intrastriatal microinfusion of TS sera or gamma immunoglobulins (IgG) in rats produced stereotypies and episodic utterances, analogous to involuntary movements seen in TS, and confirmed the presence of IgG selectively bound to striatal neurons (Hallett et al., 2000). Peterson and colleagues (2000) found that ADHD was associated significantly with titers of two distinct antistreptococcal antibodies, ASO and antideoxyribonuclease B, but no significant association was seen between antibody titers and a diagnosis of either chronic tic disorder or OCD. When basal ganglia volumes were included in these analyses, the relationships between antibody titers and basal ganglia volumes were significantly different in OCD and ADHD subjects compared with other diagnostic groups. Higher antibody titers in these subjects were associated with larger volumes of the putamen and globus pallidus nuclei.

Variably referred to as pediatric autoimmune neuropsychiatric disorders associated with streptococcal infections (PANDAS) or pediatric infection-triggered autoimmune neuropsychiatric disorders (PITANDS), this area is one of the most controversial topics in pediatric neurologic and psychiatric literature (Kurlan, 1998b; Trifiletti and Packard, 1999; Hoekstra et al., 2002; Murphy and Pichichero, 2002; Church et al., 2003; Snider and Swedo, 2003; Kurlan, 2004; Gabbay et al., 2008; Gilbert and Kurlan, 2009; Schrag et al., 2009). The following are the diagnostic criteria for pediatric infection-triggered autoimmune neuropsychiatric disorders, which are similar to those for PANDAS except that they define an episode of illness more specifically:

1. The patient must have met diagnostic criteria for a tic disorder or OCD at some point in life.
2. Symptom onset must have occurred between 3 years of age and puberty.
3. Symptom onset must be clinically sudden or demonstrate a pattern of sudden, recurrent clinically significant symptom exacerbations and remissions.

4. Increased symptoms must be pervasive and severe enough to warrant consideration of a treatment intervention or, if untreated, last for at least 4 weeks. Symptom exacerbations should not occur exclusively during a period of stress or illness.

5. There must be evidence of an antecedent or concomitant infection. This evidence might include a positive throat culture; positive GABHS serologic findings (antistreptolysin O antibodies with a peak at 3–6 weeks or anti-DNAase B antibodies with highest titers at 6–8 weeks); or a history of illness such as pharyngitis, sinusitis, or flu-like symptoms (Allen, 1997). Since GABHS infections are quite common (an average of three episodes during childhood), it is difficult to make the association between such infections and the subsequent development or exacerbation of tics or OCD.

The PANDAS concept has some other shortcomings: (1) The streptococcal infection may cause stress, which can exacerbate tics; (2) some patients with PANDAS may simply have a variant of Sydenham disease; and (3) there is no established temporal link between antecedent streptococcal infection and the exacerbation of tics. One piece of evidence supporting the notion that PANDAS simply represents one spectrum of Sydenham disease is the frequent occurrence of TS comorbidities in patients with Sydenham disease. One study compared 56 patients with Sydenham disease with 50 rheumatic fever patients and 50 healthy subjects; it found that obsessive-compulsive behavior (OCB) was present in 19%, OCD in 23.2%, and ADHD in 30.4% of Sydenham disease patients, all significantly more frequent than in the rheumatic fever or healthy controls (Maia et al., 2005). Nevertheless, the concept of postinfectious OCD is gradually seeping into the literature, even though definite proof is still lacking (Leonard et al., 1999). One observation, yet to be confirmed, that has been used in support of the autoimmune hypothesis of TS is that infusion of sera from patients with TS who have high titers of antibodies against nuclear or neural protein into ventrolateral striata of rats was associated with a higher rate of oral stereotypies as recorded by "blinded" raters (Taylor et al., 2002). This observation, however, could not be reproduced by other investigators who infused sera from patients with TS who had antiputaminal antibodies ($n = 9$) and from patients with PANDAS ($n = 8$) into the striatum of rats (Loiselle et al., 2004). No stereotypic behavior or abnormal movements were observed. Furthermore, there was no difference in antibasal ganglia antibodies between patients with PANDAS and patients with TS as measured by enzyme-linked immunosorbent assay (Singer et al., 2004). In a study of 40 subjects prospectively evaluated with intensive laboratory testing for GABHS for an average of 2 years with additional testing at the time of any clinical exacerbations, Kurlan et al. (2008) found that 5 of 64 exacerbations were temporally associated (within 4 weeks) with a GABHS infection, which was significantly higher than the number that would be expected by chance alone (1.6). In another study no correlation between a variety of immune markers and clinical exacerbations in children with PANDAS was found, arguing against autoimmunity as a pathophysiologic mechanism in this disorder (Singer et al., 2008). In a study that involved consecutive ratings of tics and behavioral symptoms in 45 cases and 41 matched control subjects over a 2-year period, only a small minority of children with TS and early-onset OCD were found to be sensitive to antecedent GABHS infections (Lin et al., 2010). In a case-control study of a large primary care database of 678 862 patients with an average follow-up of 5.08 years, no support was found for a strong relationship between streptococcal infections, neuropsychiatric syndromes such as OCD or TS, or PANDAS (Schrag et al., 2009). Although, in contrast to the Schrag et al. (2009), similar health services database studies in the United States found modest statistical associations between streptococcal infections and tic or OCD diagnoses, "current evidence indicates that for the ordinary TS/OCD phenotype of waxing and waning symptoms, GABHS infection does not seem to be an important etiologic factor and therefore not an appropriate target for assessment or therapy" (Gilbert and Kurlan, 2009).

Untreated GABHS infection is often complicated by rheumatic fever within 10–14 weeks and by Sydenham disease within several months. Several studies have provided evidence for an overlap between TS and Sydenham disease, tics and OCD being manifested in both disorders (Church et al., 2003). It is therefore not clear whether TS and OCD are independent sequelae of GABHS or whether the observed symptoms of TS and OCD are manifestations of Sydenham disease. In a 3-year prospective study of 12 children, 5 to 11 years old, with documented acute GABHS tonsillopharyngitis, Murphy and Pichichero (2002) noted a sudden onset of OCD symptoms in all patients and tics in 3 patients concurrently with the acute infection or within 4 weeks. These symptoms resolved in all patients within 2 weeks of initiation of antibiotic therapy. Although this intriguing hypothesis requires further studies, plasmapheresis, intravenous IgG, and immunosuppressant therapies are currently being investigated in the treatment of TS (Allen, 1997). In a study of 30 children in whom OCD or tics were presumably triggered or exacerbated by GABHS, there were striking improvements in various measures of OCD after intravenous immunoglobulin (IVIg) and in tics after plasma exchange (Perlmutter et al., 1999). Twenty-nine children with PANDAS were randomized in a partially double-blind fashion (no sham plasmapheresis) to an IVIg, IVIg placebo (saline), and plasmapheresis (PEX) group. One month after treatment, the severity of obsessive-compulsive symptoms (OCS) was improved by 58% and 45% in the PEX and IVIg groups, respectively, compared to only 3% in the IVIg control group. In contrast, tic scores were only improved after PEX treatment (i.e., reductions of 49% (PEX), 19% (IVIg), and 12% (IVIg placebo)). Improvements in both tics and OCS were sustained for 1 year. However, there was no control PEX group, and the control comparisons were limited to the 1-month visit. Furthermore, there was no relationship between rate of antibody removal and therapeutic response. Until the results of this study are confirmed, these treatment modalities are not justified in patients with TS. Furthermore, because of uncertainties about the possible cause-and-effect relationship between GABHS and tics and OCD, an antibiotic treatment for acute exacerbations of these symptoms is currently considered unwarranted (Kurlan, 1998b). Some studies have suggested that encephalitis lethargica is also part of the spectrum of poststreptococcal autoimmune diseases (Dale et al., 2004; Vincent, 2004).

Other hypotheses

Although direct evidence is still lacking, TS is currently viewed as a disorder of synaptic transmission involving disinhibition of the corticostriatal-thalamic-cortical circuitry. Several studies have provided evidence in support of the notion that the basal ganglia, particularly the caudate nucleus, and the inferior prefrontal cortex play an important role in the pathogenesis of not only TS but also comorbid disorders, particularly OCD (Baxter et al., 1992; McGuire, 1995; Swoboda and Jenike, 1995). For example, Laplane and colleagues (1989) described eight patients with bilateral basal ganglia lesions (anoxic or toxic encephalopathy) who showed stereotyped activities and OCB; extrapyramidal signs were mild or absent. Several imaging studies (reviewed earlier in the chapter) have implicated the ventral striatum–limbic system complex as playing an important role in the primitive reproductive behavior. A disturbance in sex hormones and certain excitatory neurotransmitters that normally influence the development of these structures may be ultimately expressed as TS (Kurlan, 1992). This hypothesis may explain the remarkable gender difference in TS, with males outnumbering females by 3 to 1; the exacerbation of symptoms at puberty and during the estrogenic phase of the menstrual cycle (Schwabe and Konkol, 1992); the characteristic occurrence of sexually related complex motor and phonic tics; and a variety of behavioral manifestations with sexual content. According to this hypothesis, the gene defect in TS results in an abnormal production of gonadal steroid hormones and increased trophic influence exerted by the excitatory amino acids, causing disordered development and increased innervation of the striatum and the limbic system. This is consistent with the finding of increased presynaptic dopamine uptake sites in brains of patients with TS (Singer et al., 1991).

Although there are no animal models of TS, studies of stereotypies in animals may provide insight into the pathogenesis of habits, rituals, tic-like, and impulsive behaviors in humans (Graybiel, 2008; Cools, 2008). These studies have shown that a broad spectrum of repetitive behaviors and rituals can become habitual and stereotyped through learning, partly as a result of experience-dependent neuroplasticity. Several families of horses with equine self-mutilation syndrome have been described with features that resemble human TS (Dodman et al., 1994). These horses exhibit a variety of stereotypic behaviors, such as glancing, biting at the flank or pectoral areas, bucking, kicking, rubbing, spinning, rolling, and vocalizing (squealing). Similar to TS, this condition is much more common in young males, is typically exacerbated by stress and during restful nonvigilance or boredom, and may be triggered by head trauma and relieved by castration. Genetic factors, however, seem to be most important.

Genetics

Finding a genetic marker and, ultimately, the gene has been the highest priority in TS research during the past decade (Keen-Kim and Freimer, 2006). Unfortunately, despite concentrated effort by many investigators, the TS gene has thus far eluded this intensive search. A systematic genome scan using 76 affected sib-pair families with a total of 110 sib-pairs showed two regions, 4q and 8p, with a LOD score of 2.38 and 2.09, respectively; four additional regions, on chromosomes 1, 10, 13, and 19, had a LOD score over 1.0 (Tourette Syndrome Association International Consortium on Genetics, 1999). An analysis of 91 Afrikaner nuclear families with one or more affected children provided evidence of linkage to loci on chromosomes 2p11, 8q22, and 11q23–q24, respectively (Simonic et al., 2001). This provides support for the finding in a previous study of a large French Canadian family of a LOD score of 3.24 for association with chromosome 11q23 (Merette et al., 2000). Other gene loci that are of interest in TS include 17q25 (Paschou et al., 2004) and 18q22 (Cuker et al., 2004). Assuming that genetic heterogeneity is not an important factor in TS, over 95% of the genome has been already excluded (Pakstis et al., 1991; Heutink et al., 1992). A linkage of TS with a known gene defect may help in the search for the TS gene. In this regard, a 16-year-old boy with typical TS was found to have a deletion of the terminal portion of the short arm of chromosome 9 (Taylor et al., 1991). A 7;18 translocation was identified in a patient with the sporadic form of TS, and the relevant regions in chromosome 18q22.3 and 7q22–q31 will be searched for possible markers (Boghosian-Sell et al., 1996; Patel, 1996). The identification of balanced reciprocal translocation near 18q22.1 in families with TS and a deletion in the same locus in one patient with tics and OCD (and dysmorphic facial features) led to the tentative assignment of the TS gene in this region (Alsobrook and Pauls, 1997). Two families with translocations involving the 8q13 have been identified (Crawford et al., 2003). Linkage disequilibrium has been demonstrated between a D4 receptor locus (on chromosome 11) and TS (Grice et al., 1996). It is possible that the clue to the TS gene(s) will come from genetic studies of ADHD. In this regard, it is of interest that a genome-wide scan in patients with ADHD identified five "hot spots": 17p11 (MLS = 2.98) and four nominal regions with MLS values greater than 1.0, including 5p13, 6q14, 11q25, and 20q13 (Ogdie et al., 2003). On the basis of analysis of several genomic regions, 17q25 appears to be of special interest, having the highest LOD score of 2.61 ($P = 0.002$) (Paschou et al., 2004). Intronic variants in BTBD9, which has been associated with restless legs syndrome and periodic limb movements, have been also associated with TS (Rivière et al., 2009). A genome-wide screening of single nucleotide polymorphism (SNP) genotyping microarray identified five exon-affecting rare variants on 1q21.1, 2p16.3, and 10q21.3 loci, not found in 73 ethnically matched controls (Sundaram et al., 2010). Some of these copy number variants have been implicated previously by other studies in schizophrenia, autism, and ADHD. Although potentially important, this study has many limitations and the data have to be interpreted cautiously (Scharf and Mathews, 2010).

A major advance in the search for the elusive TS gene or genes has been made by the discovery of a frameshift mutation in the Slit and Trk-like 1 (*SLITRK1*) gene on chromosome 13q31.1 (Abelson et al., 2005). These variants were absent in 172 other TS and in 3600 control chromosomes. *SLITRK1* gene mutation, however, is a rare cause of TS (Deng et al., 2006; Fabbrini et al., 2007; Scharf et al., 2008). One parent of a TS patient carried the *SLITRK1* mutation but displayed only symptoms of trichotillomania. In a study of

44 families with one or more members who had trichotillomania, two mutations in the *SLITRK1* gene were found among some individuals with trichotillomania but not in their unaffected family members (Zuchner et al., 2006). *SLITRK1* mutations have been estimated to account for 5% of trichotillomania cases. The *SLITRK1* gene has been found to be expressed in brain regions previously implicated in TS, such as the cortex, hippocampus, thalamic, subthalamic, and globus pallidus nuclei, striatum, and cerebellum and it appears to play a role in dendritic growth. Analysis of 988 parents of children with TS estimated the prevalence of *SLITRK1* variants as 0.1% (Sharf, personal communication). Another gene mutation implicated in TS is the L-histidine decarboxylase gene (*HDC*) mutation W317X, located on 15q21.1–15q21.3, inherited in an autosomal dominant fashion in a two-generation family (Ercan-Sencicek et al., 2010). L-histidine decarboxylase is the rate-limiting enzyme that catalyzes the biosynthesis of histamine from histidine. Histaminergic neurons are located chiefly in the posterior hypothalamus but have widespread axonal connections. Although these findings suggest the possibility of using pharmacologic manipulation of histaminergic neurotransmission to treat TS, it is unknown how histamine abnormalities might cause or contribute to TS symptoms. Although potentially an important finding, it is unlikely that the W317X mutation is relevant to the pathogenesis of TS in most cases as the mutation was not found in 720 other patients with TS. Intriguingly, however, chromosomal inv(15) (q13;q22.3), which includes the 15q21.1–15q21.3 region, was identified in one of our patients, a 10-year-old boy with tics (Jankovic and Deng, 2007). Although mutations in *HDC* and *SLITRK1* are only rarely associated with TS, careful studies of monogenic cases may provide insights into the pathogenesis of this complex neurobehavioral disorder. Another potential candidate gene mutation is *Gln20X* mutation in the 5-hydroxytryptamine receptor 2B gene (*HTR2B*, MIM 601122), reported to be associated with impulsivity in a Finnish population of violent criminals, but none of the 252 samples of patients with TS showed the *Gln20X* mutation (Guo et al., 2011).

Current concepts of the genetics of TS support a sex-influenced autosomal dominant mode of inheritance with a nearly complete penetrance for males and 56% penetrance for females when only tics are considered and 70% when OCD is included (Robertson, 1989; Pauls et al., 1991). Comings and Comings (1992), however, have proposed that TS is a semidominant, semirecessive disorder. This model takes into account the common observation that both parents of a TS child often exhibit TS or a forme fruste of TS and that the full and more severe motor-behavioral syndrome in the offspring represents a homozygous state (Fig. 16.4). Indeed, bilineal transmission was noted in 33% (considering tics) and 41% (considering tics or OCB) of TS families (Kurlan et al., 1994). In another study, McMahon and colleagues (1996) examined 175 members of a large, four-generation, TS family as well as 16 spouses who married into this family. Interestingly, they found evidence of TS in 36% of the family members and in 31% of the married-in spouses (some form of a tic was found in 67% and 44%, respectively). Multivariate analysis showed that tics were more severe in the offspring of both parents with tics. This study raises the possibility of assortative mating (like marrying

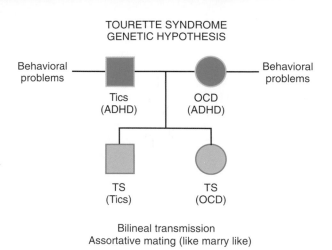

TOURETTE SYNDROME
GENETIC HYPOTHESIS

Figure 16.4 Bimodal distribution typically present in TS nuclear families.

like) in TS, in contrast to random, nonassortative mating, which is presumed in the general population. Thus, bilineal transmission may lead to frequent homozygosity and high density of TS in some families. Walkup and colleagues (1996) failed to find TS in both parents, but when the broader definition was allowed, 19% of families had both parents affected. Using rigorous diagnostic criteria, we found that 25% of our TS cases had both parents with some features of TS: tics, 8%; OCB, 4%; and ADD, 12% (Hanna et al., 1999) (Fig. 16.4). The TS patients were compared with a control population of 1142 students who were observed in second-, fifth-, and eighth-grade classrooms. In contrast to the 5% frequency of ADD in one parent of controls, the occurrence of tics was 31% in at least one parent of TS cases, 45% in at least one parent of ADD cases, and 41% in at least one parent of OCB cases. Among all the parents of TS cases, tics were present in 24%, OCB in 25%, and ADD in 34%, whereas only 3% of parents of controls exhibited ADD. Bilineal transmission violates the standard principle of one-trait-one-locus, and it might explain why a gene marker has not yet been identified in TS despite intense collaborative research effort. These results are similar to those of Lichter and colleagues (1999), who found bilineal transmission in 6% of patients; tics or OCB were represented bilineally in 22% of patients. In a large family study and segregation analysis, Walkup and colleagues (1996) provided evidence for a mixed model of inheritance rather than a simple autosomal mode of inheritance. This complex model of inheritance suggests that the majority of TS patients have two copies of the gene, one from each parent. This is consistent with the observation that many TS patients have both parents affected.

Based on various epidemiological-genetic studies, the rate of TS in the parents of a proband ranges from 6.5% to 16%, with fathers demonstrating a much higher risk (11.9–23.1%) compared to mothers (1–9.6%) (Pauls et al., 1991; Walkup et al., 1996). A Japanese population study, however, found the rate of TS for both parents was 1.9% and the rate of tics for both parents was approximately 11.5% (Kano et al., 2001). Siblings have approximately an 8% risk of TS and a 9.7–22% risk of OCD. The empiric risk to offspring of a proband with TS was reported as 22% for TS and greater than 50% for a tic disorder (McMahon et al., 2003). In bilineal families the risk of TS for offspring increased to 42.8% compared to 15% for unilineal families. Additionally, rates of any tic diagnosis, OCD, and ADHD were increased (McMahon et al., 2003).

Twin studies, showing 89% concordance for TS and 100% concordance for either TS or chronic multiple tic disorder, provide strong support for the genetic etiology of TS (Alsobrook and Pauls, 1997; Singer, 2000). How much influence environmental factors have on the phenotypic expression of this disorder is not known. In searching for nongenetic factors in the pathogenesis of TS, Leckman and colleagues (1990) found that maternal life stress, nausea, and vomiting during the first trimester of pregnancy were some of the perinatal factors that influenced the expression of the TS gene. In a study of 16 pairs of monozygotic twins, 94% of whom were concordant for tics, low birth weight was a strong predictor of tic severity, supporting a relationship between birth weight and phenotypic expression of TS (Hyde et al., 1992). Kurlan (1994) hypothesized that the clinical features associated with TS may occur to a variable degree in the course of normal childhood development and that genetic influences determine the severity of clinical symptoms in a given individual with TS. Eapen and colleagues (1997a) found evidence for earlier age at onset in maternally transmitted cases, suggesting genomic imprinting. The evidence for genomic imprinting in TS is, however, quite weak, and the genetic mechanism of TS remains elusive (Sadovnick and Kurlan, 1997). Because of phenotypic overlap between TS and Rett syndrome and myoclonus–dystonia, we have examined the genes for the latter disorders and found no mutations in our TS population (De Carvalho Aguiar et al., 2004).

One of the major concerns with the genetic linkage studies has been the lack of specificity of the current clinical criteria for diagnosis of TS. The boundaries of neurologic and behavioral manifestations of TS have not been clearly defined. While some investigators believe that the spectrum of behavioral expression of TS gene is quite broad, encompassing, in addition to ADHD and OCD, such diverse symptoms as conduct disorders, stuttering, dyslexia, panic attacks, phobias, depression, mania, and severe anxiety (Comings, 1987; Comings and Comings 1988a), others argue that more restrictive criteria for TS are needed, particularly for genetic linkage studies (Pauls et al., 1991). Pauls and colleagues (1991) studied 338 biological relatives of 86 TS probands and compared them to 21 biologically unrelated relatives of adopted TS probands. They confirmed their earlier observations and concluded that TS and OCD are etiologically related. The debate as to whether TS, OCD, and ADHD are genetically related or whether they merely represent comorbid neurobehavioral disorders will not be resolved until a TS-specific genetic marker is found.

Discovering the gene or genes for OCD would have important implications for TS and would help to clarify the relationship between the two disorders. One study showed that men with OCD are significantly more likely to have both alleles of the gene for catechol-O-methyltransferase in a low activity form (L/L) than in the L/H form (Karayiorgou et al., 1997). As was noted earlier, the B-lymphocyte antigen D8/17 has been suggested to be a possible peripheral marker for childhood-onset OCD and TS (Murphy et al., 1997).

Etiology of tics (secondary tourettism)

While TS is probably the most common cause of tics, there are many other neurologic disorders that are manifested by tics and other symptoms of TS, supporting the notion of a multifactorial genesis of TS (Table 16.2) (Jankovic, 2001a; Jankovic and Mejia, 2006). Of these, tics associated with static encephalopathy, autistic spectrum disorders, neuroacanthocytosis (Spitz et al., 1985; Saiki et al., 2004), Huntington disease (Jankovic and Ashizawa, 1995), pantothenate kinase-associated neurodegeneration (Pellecchia et al., 2005), fragile X syndrome (Schneider et al., 2008), beta-mannosidase deficiency (Sedel et al., 2006) and certain drugs such as dopamine receptor-blocking drugs, cocaine, and antiepileptics (Cardoso and Jankovic, 1993; Bharucha and Sethi, 1995; Kumar and Lang, 1997b; Lombroso, 1999) are particularly important to consider, especially in patients who do not fulfill the clinical criteria of TS. In one report, lamotrigine, a phenyltriazine drug that is structurally unrelated to other antiepileptic medications, was associated with dose-related motor and phonic tics in three children and features of OCD in one (Lombroso, 1999). The author speculated that in these rare cases, lamotrigine in high doses inhibited the presynaptic release of excitatory amino acids and resulted in an abnormal regulation of dopamine uptake in the striatum, leading to the production of tics and related TS symptoms. Rarely, "tourettism" can follow head trauma (Krauss and Jankovic, 1997; Kumar and Lang, 1997b); nonspecific cerebral insults, such as ischemia, hypoxia, and hypothermia (Singer et al., 1997); or striatal encephalitis due to varicella zoster (Dale et al., 2003). The study of the mechanisms of the secondary tourettism could provide insights into the pathogenesis of TS. For example, while TS symptoms have been reported to be exacerbated by various structural lesions involving the basal ganglia and the limbic system (Jankovic, 2001a), one patient with TS had complete resolution of tics after an MRI-proven midbrain lesion due to Wernicke encephalopathy (Pantoni et al., 1997). This suggests that an intact midbrain tegmentum is required for the expression of motor tics.

Autistic spectrum disorders (or pervasive developmental disorders) represent one of the largest groups of pediatric disorders in which features of TS, such as tics, ADHD, and OCD, may be present. In a study of 7288 participants enrolled in the Tourette Syndrome International Database Consortium Registry, 334 (4.6%; 1 of every 22 participants) had a comorbid pervasive developmental disorder, 13 times the expected rate (Burd et al., 2009). Autism is a behaviorally defined syndrome manifested by poor social interaction; disordered language; and atypical responses to people, objects, and events (Volkmar and Pauls, 2003). The syndrome is typically associated with severe disturbances in cognition, language, and behavior that appear before the age of 30 months. Stereotypic movements include body rocking, repeated touching and sniffing of objects, ritualistic ordering, and insistence on precisely following routines. Similar to TS, there is about 3 : 1 male : female preponderance. A study of children 3–10 years old found a 0.34% prevalence of autism with cognitive impairment in 68% (Yeargin-Allsopp et al., 2003). A review of home videos during early development in 17 autistic children found evidence of abnormal movement at the age of 4–6 months and sometimes even at birth, long before the diagnosis of autism (Teitelbaum et al., 1998). The authors suggest that their findings support the view that movement disturbances play an intrinsic part in the phenomenon of autism, that movement disturbances in autistic children are present at birth, and that such movement disturbances can be used to diagnose the presence of autism in the first few months of life. Other studies have suggested that TS symptoms are more common than expected in patients with autism, with an estimated frequency of 6.5% (Baron-Cohen et al., 1999). Asperger syndrome is a form of pervasive developmental disorder in which language and self-help skills are relatively intact. It is often considered a mild form of autism, but its relationship to other autistic disorders has not been well defined. Asperger syndrome patients frequently exhibit repetitive movements (stereotypies) and may have motor and phonic tics in addition to other behavioral abnormalities (Ringman and Jankovic, 2000). Other childhood behavioral disorders that may overlap in symptomatology with autism and TS include Williams syndrome, characterized by remarkable conversational skills and excessive empathy; Prader–Willi syndrome, associated with temper tantrums and obsessive-compulsive behavior; Angelman syndrome, characterized by hyperactivity and a constantly happy disposition (Cassidy and Morris, 2002); and Rett syndrome, an X-linked autistic disorder associated with stereotypies and other movement disorders. However, we excluded mutations in *MECP2* gene on chromosome X28, responsible for Rett syndrome (Rosa et al., 2003). We also excluded mutations in the *SGCE* gene, responsible for the dystonia–myoclonus syndrome, which shares some clinical features with TS, in a population of well-defined TS (De Carvalho Aguiar et al., 2004).

Other related conditions that may have resemblance to tics and TS are the jumping Frenchmen of Maine, "ragin' Cajuns" of Louisiana, latah of the Malays, and myriachit of Siberia (Lees, 2001). First described in 1878, these culture-bound conditions are characterized by an excessive startle response, sometimes with echolalia, echopraxia, or forced obedience. It is considered by some as an operant conditioned behavior rather than a neurologic or even hysteric disorder (Saint-Hilaire et al., 1986). The rare late-onset startle-induced tics may resemble these culture-bound syndromes and other startle responses (Tijssen et al., 1999). Rarely, psychogenic tics are present in patients with TS, but this very rare occurrence is difficult to confirm clinically (Kurlan et al., 1992).

The discussion of the numerous causes of tics and other manifestations of TS is beyond the scope of this review, and the reader is referred to other reviews of secondary causes of tics (Kumar and Lang, 1997b; Jankovic 2001b; Jankovic and Mejia, 2006).

Epidemiology

Discovery of a disease-specific marker would be helpful not only in improving our understanding of this complex neurobehavioral disorder but also in clarifying the epidemiology of TS (Kadesjo and Gillberg, 2000; Scahill et al., 2001).

Up to 24% of children may have tics sometime during their childhood (Robertson, 2008a, 2008b). The prevalence rates have varied markedly and have been estimated to be as high as 4.2% when all types of tic disorders are included (Costello et al., 1996) and 1/83 (1.2%) (Comings and Comings, 1988b) or as low as 28.7/100 000 (0.03%) (Caine et al., 1988) and 1/10 000 (0.01%) (Singer, 2000). There are many reasons for this wide variation, the most important of which are different ascertainment methods, different study populations, and different clinical criteria. Since about one-third of patients with tics do not even recognize their presence, it is difficult to derive more accurate prevalence figures for TS without a well-designed door-to-door survey (Kurlan et al., 1987). In one study, 3034 students in three schools in Los Angeles were monitored over a 2-year period by a school psychologist; the frequency of definite TS was 1 in 95 males and 1 in 759 females (Comings et al., 1990). Because the observed population included special education children, the authors adjusted the final prevalence figure to 0.63%. This figure is similar to that derived from our own observational study of 1142 children in second, fifth, and eighth grades of a general school population, among whom 8 children (0.7%) had some evidence of TS (Hanna et al., 1999). In another school-based study involving 167 randomly selected 13- and 14-year-olds in English high schools, the prevalence of TS based on DSM III-R was estimated at 3%, but 18% screened positive for tics (Mason et al., 1998). A follow-up study with improved methods found a TS prevalence of 0.76–1.85% (Hornsey et al., 2001). Snider and colleagues (2002) observed 553 schoolchildren (kindergarten to sixth grade) monthly over an 8-month period and found tics in 135 (24%); 34 children had persistent tics (6.1%). Those with persistent tics were more likely to be males and had more behavioral problems than those without persistent tics. Kurlan and colleagues (2001) found that 27% of 341 special education students had tics compared to 19.7% of 1255 students in regular classroom programs; the frequency of TS was 7% and 3.8%, respectively. In another study, based on an interview of 1596 children, Kurlan and colleagues (2002) found that 339 (21%) had tics. Children with tics were younger, were more likely to be male and attend special education classes, and had a lower mean IQ. The prevalence of tics was studied in 867 children attending two schools in the Basque country and was estimated to be 6.5% (Linazasoro et al., 2006). Thus, epidemiologic studies have shown that 20–30% of children exhibit tics sometime during childhood and 2–3% of children develop some features of TS, although the worldwide prevalence of TS in children has been reported to range from 0.3% to 0.8% (Scahill et al., 2009).

It is not known why tics disappear in the majority of children and further studies are needed to understand mechanisms of conversion from pre-TS state to TS.

Treatment

The first step in the management of patients with TS is proper education of the patient, relatives, teachers, and other individuals who frequently interact with the patient about the nature of the disorder (Scahill et al., 2006; Jankovic, 2009; Shprecher and Kurlan, 2009). School principals, teachers, and students can be helpful in implementing the therapeutic strategies. In addition, the parents and the physician should work as partners in advocating the best possible school environment for the child. This might include extra break periods and a refuge area to allow release of tics, waiving time limitations on tests or adjusting timing of tests to the morning, and other measures designed to relieve stress. National and local support groups can provide additional information and can serve as a valuable resource for the patient and his or her family (see the Appendix at the end of the chapter).

Before deciding *how* to treat TS-related symptoms, it is important to decide *whether* to treat them. Even in our referrals, and presumably in more severely affected populations of patients, about 20% do not need pharmacologic therapy. Counseling and behavioral modification might be sufficient for those with mild symptoms. Medications, however, may be considered when symptoms begin to interfere with peer relationships, social interactions, academic or job performance, or activities of daily living. Because of the broad range of neurologic and behavioral manifestation and varying severity, therapy of TS must be tailored specifically to the needs of the individual patient (Jimenez-Jimenez and Garcia-Ruiz, 2001; Lang, 2001; Silay and Jankovic, 2005; Gilbert, 2006; Jankovic and Kurlan, 2011) (Table 16.6). The most troublesome symptoms should be targeted first. Medications should be instituted at low doses, titrated gradually to the lowest effective dosage, and tapered during nonstressful periods (e.g., summer vacations). Another important principle of therapy in TS is to give each medication and dosage regimen an adequate trial. This approach will avoid needless changes made in response to variations in symptoms during the natural course of the disease. While an evidence-based approach, based on double-blind, placebo-controlled studies, is desirable to objectively evaluate the efficacy of a drug, long-term observational studies provide useful information about not only the efficacy of the drug but also its safety (Mesulam and Petersen, 1987).

Before discussing pharmacologic therapy of TS symptoms, it is appropriate to make a few remarks about behavioral therapy (Piacentini and Chang, 2001; Piacentini et al., 2010). Different forms of behavioral modification have been recommended since the disorder was first described, but until recently, very few studies of behavioral treatments have been subjected to rigorous scientific scrutiny. Most of the reported studies suffer from poor or unreliable assessments, small sample size, short follow-up, lack of controls, no validation of compliance, and other methodologic flaws. Given these limitations, the following behavioral techniques have been reported to provide at least some benefit: (1) massed (negative) practice (voluntary and effortful repetition of the tic leads to a build-up of a state termed *reactive inhibition*, at which point the subject is forced to rest and not perform the tic due to a build-up of a negative habit), (2) operant techniques/contingency management (tic-free intervals are positively reinforced, and tic behaviors are punished), (3) anxiety management techniques (relaxation training), (4) exposure-based treatment (desensitization to address tic triggering phenomena such as premonitory sensory urges), (5) awareness training (direct visual feedback, self-monitoring, and awareness-enhancing techniques, such as saying the letter "T" after each tic), and (6) habit-reversal training (HRT),

Table 16.6 Treatment strategies in Tourette syndrome

Tics
Clonazepam
Fluphenazine
Pimozide
Haloperidol
Thiothixene
Trifluoperazine
Molindone
Sulpiride
Tiapride
Flunarizine
Olanzapine
Risperidone
Quetiapine
Clozapine
Tetrabenazine
Pergolide
Nicotine
Naltrexone
Flutamide
Cannabinoid
Botulinum toxin

Obsessive-compulsive disorder
Imipramine
Clomipramine
Fluoxetine
Sertraline
Nefazodone
Fluvoxamine
Paroxetine
Venlafaxine
Citalopram
Lithium
Buspirone
Clonazepam
Trazodone
Clonazepam

Attention-deficit disorder/attention-deficit hyperactivity disorder
Clonidine
Imipramine
Nortriptyline
Desipramine
Deprenyl
Bupropion
Guanfacine
Carbamazepine
Dextroamphetamine
Methylphenidate
Adderal
Pemoline
Modafinil
Atomoxetine
Mecamylamine
Neurosurgery

consisting of competing response training with reenactment of tic movements while looking in a mirror, training to detect and increase awareness of one's tics, identification of high-risk situations, training to isometrically contract the tic-opposing muscles, and training to recognize and resist tic urges (Piacentini and Chang, 2001; Deckersbach et al., 2006; Himle et al., 2006; Piacentini et al., 2010). Wilhelm and colleagues (2003) studied 32 patients with TS who were randomly assigned to 14 sessions of either HRT (awareness training, self-monitoring, relaxation training, competing response training, and contingency management) or supportive psychotherapy. The 16 patients who were assigned to the HRT group "improved significantly" and "remained significantly improved over pretreatment at 10-month follow-up." This approach has been also found useful in the management of phonic tics (Woods et al., 2003). Another behavioral therapeutic approach is the so-called exposure plus response prevention, already found useful in the treatment of OCD. The behavioral intervention, called Comprehensive Behavioral Intervention for Tic Disorders (CBIT), is primarily based on HRT which employs competing-response training, which is different from deliberate tic suppression in that it teaches the patient to initiate a voluntary behavior to manage the premonitory urge. CBIT also includes relaxation training and a functional intervention. In a multicenter study designed to test the efficacy of CBIT, 126 children aged 9–17 with moderate to severe TS were randomly assigned to receive either CBIT or supportive counseling and education about TS (Piacentini et al., 2010). About one-third of the children in the study were on a stable dose of anti-tic medication. Behavioral intervention led to a significantly greater decrease on the YGTSS (24.7 vs. 17.1) from baseline to endpoint compared with very minimal change in the control treatment group (24.6 vs. 21.1), with the overall effect size of 0.68. Furthermore, 52.5% of children receiving CBIT were rated as significantly improved, compared to 18.5% of those in the control group. The decrease of 7.6 points (31% from baseline) on the Total Tic score of the YGTSS in the CBIT group is less than the decrease reported in clinical trials of antipsychotic medications or topiramate (Jankovic et al., 2010). Although the attrition rate was only 9.5% and 87% of available responders apparently exhibited continued benefit for 6 months following treatment, there are some limitations to the CBIT that were not fully acknowledged in the study. The success of this behavioral management is critically dependent on active involvement by the parents and the therapist, both of whom must be well trained and skilled in the various CBIT techniques (Woods et al., 2008). Given the demands on time and effort on the part of the patient, the therapist, and parents, it is unlikely that all parties will be able to maintain the needed compliance with the training program to provide sustained benefit. There is also some concern as to whether the mental effort required to fully comply with the various components of CBIT could actually interfere with patient's attention and learning. While there has been a great deal of effort exerted over the last several decades making the scientific, clinical, and lay community understand the biological basis of TS, the reported response to behavioral therapy may be misinterpreted by some as evidence that tics and TS are of psychological etiology. This is one reason why behavioral therapies are often not covered by insurance or other third party payers. Thus, only a limited number of patients will be able to access this behavioral therapy as compared to pharmacologic treatment, which actually may be more effective. Nevertheless, behavioral therapies are useful ancillary techniques in patients whose response to other therapies, including pharmacotherapy, is not entirely satisfactory.

Management of tics

The goal of treatment should be not to completely eliminate all the tics, but to achieve a tolerable suppression of the tics (Jankovic, 2009). Because of the variability of tics in terms of severity, frequency, and distribution, the assessment of efficacy of a therapeutic intervention on tics is often quite problematic. A number of tic-rating scales have been utilized, but none of them are ideal. Although at-home videotapes can be used to capture tics that are not appreciated by patients or when patients are examined in the clinic, video-based tic rating scales have many shortcomings (Goetz et al., 1999, 2001).

Despite these limitations, controlled and open trials have found that of the pharmacologic agents that are used for tic suppression, the dopamine receptor-blocking drugs (neuroleptics) are clearly most effective (Robertson, 2000; Jimenez-Jimenez and Garcia-Ruiz, 2001) (Tables 16.5 and 16.6). Haloperidol (Haldol) and pimozide (Orap) are the only neuroleptics that have actually been approved by the Food and Drug Administration (FDA) for the treatment of TS. In one randomized, double-blind, controlled study, pimozide was found to be superior to haloperidol with respect to efficacy and side effects (Sallee et al., 1997). We prefer fluphenazine (Prolixin) as the first-line anti-tic pharmacotherapy, since it appears to have a lower incidence of sedation and other side effects. If fluphenazine fails to adequately control tics, we substitute risperidone (Risperdal) or pimozide. We usually start with fluphenazine, risperidone, and pimozide at 1 mg at bedtime and increase by 1 mg every 5–7 days. If these drugs fail to control tics adequately, then we try haloperidol, thioridazine (Mellaril), trifluoperazine (Stelazine), molindone (Moban), or thiothixene (Navane). Risperidone, a neuroleptic with both dopamine- and serotonin-blocking properties, has been shown to be effective in reducing tic frequency and intensity in most (Bruun and Budman, 1996; Bruggeman et al., 2001), but not all studies (Robertson et al., 1996). A double-blind, placebo-controlled, 8-week, trial in which 24 patients were randomly assigned risperidone in doses of 0.5–6.0 mg/day (median dose of 2.5 mg/day) and 24 were assigned to placebo, risperidone was found to be significantly ($P < 0.05$) superior to placebo on the Global Severity Rating of the Tourette Syndrome Severity Scale (Dion et al., 2002). The proportion of patients who improved by at least one point on this seven-point scale was 60.8% in the risperidone group and 26.1% in the placebo group. Hypokinesia and tremor increased in the risperidone group, but there were no other extrapyramidal side effects. Fatigue and somnolence were the most common adverse events associated with risperidone. In another placebo-controlled study, 12 patients who were randomized to risperidone had a 36% reduction in tic symptoms compared to 11% reduction in the 14 patients receiving placebo (Scahill et al., 2003). One randomized, double-blind study found risperidone to be more effective than clonidine in the treatment of TS-associated OCD (Gaffney et al., 2002). Risperidone has been also found to be effective in the treatment of tantrums, aggression, and SIB in children with autism (Research Units on Pediatric Psychopharmacology Autism Network, 2002). Some atypical, second-generation neuroleptics have been found to increase the risk of obesity and type 2 diabetes, but risperidone and ziprasidone appear to be associated with a lower risk of these complications (Gianfrancesco et al., 2002; Stahl and Shayegan, 2003).

It is not clear whether the atypical neuroleptics, such as clozapine (Clozaril), olanzapine (Zyprexa), or quetiapine (Seroquel), will be effective in the treatment of tics and other manifestations of TS. Quetiapine (Seroquel), a dibenzothiazepine that blocks not only D1 and D2 receptors but also $5HT_{1A}$ and $5 HT_2$ receptors, has been reported to provide beneficial effects in some patients with TS, but the clinical improvement might not be sustained. Ziprasidone (Geodon), a potent blocker of 5-HT_{2A}, 5-HT_{2C}, 5-HT_{1A}, 5-HT_{1D}, and α_1 receptors more than D2 or D3 receptors, was found to decrease tic severity by 35% compared to a 7% change in the placebo group (Sallee et al., 2000). Because of its relatively high D2 receptor occupancy, ziprasidone is pharmacologically more similar to risperidone and olanzapine than to clozapine and quetiapine (Mamo et al., 2004). Since TS patients may have increased cortical 5-HT_2 density, it is possible that the beneficial effects of some of the atypical drugs is mediated by their 5-HT_2 and 5-HT_3 blocking effects (Haugbol et al., 2007). A few small studies have indeed shown some benefit in patients with TS treated with serotonin antagonists such as ketanserin and ondansetron (Bonnier et al., 1999; Toren et al., 2005). Similar to pimozide, ziprasidone may prolong the QT interval (Blair et al., 2005) but has the advantage over other atypical neuroleptics in that it is less likely to cause weight gain and sexual side effects. It also appears to have strong antiapathy, promotivational, and antidepressant effects. The clinical significance of a prolonged QT interval is controversial, but it may be associated with *torsades de pointes*, which can potentially degenerate into ventricular fibrillation and sudden death. Besides pimozide and ziprasidone, other drugs that can prolong the QT interval include haloperidol, risperidone, thioridazine, and desipramine. However, according to experts, the low rate of QTc prolongation in *torsades de pointes* is not likely to be a serious problem (Glassman and Bigger, 2001). Aripiprazole (Abilify), another atypical antipsychotic medication (Goodnick and Jerry, 2002; Seo et al., 2008), acts as an antagonist of D2 receptors in the mesolimbic pathway, but also as a partial D2 agonist. It displays strong 5-HT_{2A} receptor antagonism and is similar to ziprasidone in also having agonistic activity at the 5-HT_{1A} receptor. As a partial dopamine agonist it reduces dopamine synthesis and release through an agonist action at the dopamine autoreceptor. Among the atypical antipsychotics, aripiprazole displays the lowest affinity for α1-adrenergic (α1), histamine (H1), and muscarinic (M1) receptors and, as such, has a relatively low incidence of side effects, including orthostatic hypotension, weight gain, sedation, dry mouth, and constipation. In one study 10 of 11 patients with TS were reported to improve with 10–20 mg daily dose of aripiprazole (Davies et al., 2006). The role of antipsychotic drugs, such as paliperidone and bifeprunox, atypical neuroleptics that also act as mood stabilizers in the treatment of tics and TS, is unknown (Nasrallah, 2008).

Tetrabenazine, a monoamine-depleting drug that acts by inhibiting VMAT2, is a powerful anti-tic drug, approved in 2008 for the treatment of chorea associated with Huntington disease (Jankovic and Beach, 1997; Kenney and Jankovic, 2006; Kenney et al., 2007) (Fig. 16.5). This drug has been found very effective in the treatment of TS. In 92 patients with TS treated with tetrabenazine at Baylor College of Medicine, for a mean of 1.6 years (up to 20.4 years) at a maintenance dose of 53.3 mg/day (range: 6.25–150 mg), 77.8% reported complete or nearly complete abolishment of tics (Silay and Jankovic, 2005). Tetrabenazine was generally well tolerated, although some patients experienced drowsiness (32.6%), nausea/vomiting (8.7%), depression (7.6%), insomnia (6.5%), akathisia (5.4%), and other less frequent, dose-related side effects. The drug has the advantage over the conventional neuroleptics in that it does not cause tardive dyskinesias. Furthermore, it appears to be associated with less weight gain than the typical neuroleptics (Ondo et al., 2008).

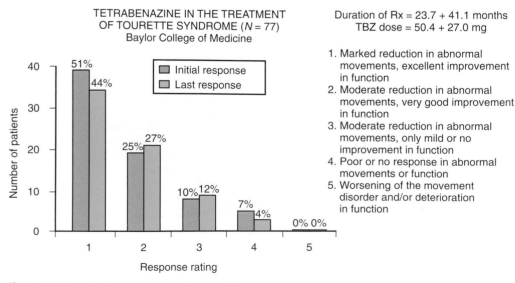

Figure 16.5 Results of tetrabenazine treatment in TS.

The side effects associated with neuroleptics, such as sedation, depression, weight gain, and school phobia, seem to be somewhat less frequent with fluphenazine than with haloperidol and the other neuroleptics (Bruun and Budman, 1996). The most feared side effects of chronic neuroleptic therapy include tardive dyskinesia and hepatotoxicity. In addition, pimozide may prolong the QT interval; therefore, patients who are treated with the drug must have an electrocardiogram before starting therapy. We repeat the electrocardiogram about 3 months later and once a year thereafter. It is important to note that certain antibiotics, such as clarithromycin, can raise the blood levels of pimozide and indirectly contribute to the drug's cardiotoxicity. Tardive dyskinesia, usually manifested by stereotypic involuntary movements, is only rarely persistent in children. However, tardive dystonia, a variant of tardive dyskinesias that is most frequently encountered in young adults, may persist and occasionally progresses to a generalized and disabling dystonic disorder (Singh and Jankovic, 1988; Silva et al., 1993) (Video 16.18). Other movement disorders that are associated with neuroleptics include bradykinesia, akathisia, and acute dystonic reactions (Jankovic, 1995). Therefore, careful monitoring of the patients is absolutely essential, and whenever possible, the dosage should be reduced or even discontinued during periods of remission or during vacations.

Several non-neuroleptic treatments have been reported to be effective in the treatment of tics. The dopamine agonist pergolide has been found to be useful in an open-label trial in 32 patients with TS, particularly if the TS is associated with restless legs syndrome (Lipinski et al., 1997). In another study, 24 patients with TS (ages 7–17 years) who were medication-free for 4 weeks prior to treatment were randomized to receive either placebo or pergolide (150–300 μg daily) for 6 weeks, followed by a 2-week washout, and then crossed over to the other treatment arm (Gilbert et al., 2000). Nineteen patients completed the study. Tic severity, as determined by the main outcome measure, the YGTSS, fell by 50% on pergolide versus 42% on placebo ($P < 0.0011$). There was no significant difference between the two treatments on the Clinical Global Impression-Severity scale or on the parent-rated Tic Severity Self Report. In a follow-up, randomized, placebo-controlled trial, the researchers concluded that "pergolide appeared to be an efficacious and safe medication for tic reduction in children, and may also improve attention deficit hyperactivity disorder symptoms" (Gilbert et al., 2003). Ropinirole, another dopamine agonist, has been also found to be effective in the treatment of TS (Anca et al., 2004). These findings seem paradoxical in view of the well-known beneficial effects of dopamine receptor blockers. It is possible, however, that the observed effects of dopamine agonists could be mediated by their action on dopamine D2 autoreceptors, thus reducing endogenous dopamine turnover. A single-blind levodopa challenge in six adult patients with TS resulted in a decrease in self-rated tic severity (Black and Mink, 2000), but this preliminary study needs to be confirmed by a larger and well-designed clinical trial. Pramipexole, a D3 and D2 receptor agonist, is currently being studied in a double-blind, placebo-controlled trial.

Clonazepam is another drug that is sometimes useful in treating patients with TS, particularly in the treatment of clonic tics. Since some of the premonitory sensations resemble obsessions and the tics may be viewed as "compulsive" movements, anti-OCD medications can be also helpful. Treatment of the premonitory sensations may lead to improvement of these tics. Since sex steroids affect the expression of TS gene and also modulate multiple neurotransmitter systems, antiandrogens have been tried in the treatment of TS. Flutamide, an acetanilid nonsteroidal androgen antagonist, has been found in one double-blind, placebo-controlled study to modestly and transiently reduce motor, but not phonic, tics, with a mild improvement in associated symptoms of OCD (Peterson et al., 1998b). Because of potentially serious side effects, such as diarrhea and fulminant hepatic necrosis, this drug should be reserved only for those patients in whom tics remain a disabling problem despite optimal anti-tic therapy. Baclofen, a $GABA_B$ autoreceptor agonist, has been found to markedly decrease the severity of motor and phonic tics in 95% of 264 patients with TS (Awaad, 1999), but a double-blind, placebo-controlled, crossover trial of nine patients with TS showed that the beneficial response to baclofen was due to improvement in the overall impairment score rather than a reduction of tic activity (Singer et al., 2001). Donepezil, a noncompetitive inhibitor of acetylcholinesterase, has been reported anecdotally to suppress tics (Hoopes, 1999).

Ever since the discovery that cannabinoids markedly potentiate neuroleptic-induced hypokinesis in rats and that their effects on the extrapyramidal motor system may be mediated through nicotinic cholinergic receptors, there has been growing interest in nicotine as a treatment of various movement disorders, including TS (Sanberg et al., 1993). Several of our patients in fact have reported that herbal cannabinoid helped them control their tics more than prescribed medications and some have reported benefits from the synthetic cannabinoid dronabinol (Marinol) (2.5–5 mg 2–3 times per day), used to control nausea, although this treatment is not considered practical or safe because chronic use may lead to addiction and other potential adverse events. Delta9-tetrahydrocannabinol (THC) was reported to reduce tics in a single-dose, cross-over study in 12 patients and in a 6-week, randomized trial in 24 patients with TS (Müller-Vahl, 2003). Based on the available evidence the Cochrane review concluded that there was "not enough evidence to support the use of cannabinoids in treating tics and obsessive compulsive behaviour in people with Tourette's syndrome" (Curtis et al., 2009). Nicotine gum (e.g., Nicorette, 2 mg) and transdermal nicotine patch (e.g., Nicoderm, 7 mg) have been reported to potentiate the anti-tic effects of neuroleptics, but this observation needs to be confirmed by a placebo-controlled study (Silver et al., 1996; Sanberg et al., 1998; Hughes et al., 1999). Open trials indicate that nicotine may suppress tics even in patients who have not been treated with D2 receptor-blocking drugs. The onset of anti-tic effect is quite rapid (0.5–3 hours) and the effects appear to persist for about 10 days after a 24-hour application of the patch (to the deltoid area). Side effects of the nicotine patch include local irritation and itching, nausea (in up to 70% lasting 4–6 hours), and transient headache with or without dizziness. There was apparently no evidence of nicotine dependence in these open trials. Although nicotine is a potent agonist of nicotinic acetylcholine receptors, when used chronically it causes desensitization of these receptors, thus exerting an antagonist effect. This is consistent with the observation that mecamylamine (Inversine, approved by the FDA as an antihypertensive and antismoking drug at 2.5 mg twice a day), an antihypertensive agent that acts as a peripheral ganglionic blocker with central antinicotinic, anticholinergic properties, improved tics as well as behavioral problems in 11 of 13 patients with TS at doses up to 5 mg/day (Sanberg et al., 1998). A subsequent double-blind, placebo-controlled study, however, failed to demonstrate a significant benefit on the symptoms associated with TS (Silver et al., 2001). Nicotine also causes the presynaptic release of acetylcholine, GABA, norepinephrine, dopamine, serotonin, vasopressin, and β-endorphins (Toth et al., 1992). Although the mechanism of action of nicotine in TS is unknown, it is interesting that nicotine initially activates midbrain dopamine neurons, but after longer exposure to nicotine, these neurons become desensitized, thus possibly accounting for the antidopaminergic (and anti-tic) effect of the drug (Pidoplichko et al., 1997). Recent studies suggest that nicotine inhibits some (e.g., α4β2), but not other (e.g., α3β4), striatal nicotinic receptors and that this inhibition could persist for several days (Lindstrom, 1997). Finally, there have been several anecdotal reports of marijuana helping various symptoms of TS. This is consistent with the finding that cannabinoid receptors are densely located in the output nuclei of the basal ganglia and that activation of these receptors increases GABAergic transmission and inhibition of glutamate release (Müller-Vahl et al., 1999). Some patients clearly benefit from taking the cannabinoid dronabinol (Marinol) at doses of 2.5–10 mg twice a day. Although levetiracetam has been found to be effective in the treatment of tics in an open-label trial involving 60 patients with TS (Awaad et al., 2005), it is not clear whether this will be useful in the treatment of TS. Topiramate has been found to be effective in some open-label studies (Abuzzahab and Brown, 2001) as well as in a multicenter, placebo-controlled trial (Jankovic et al., 2010) (Fig. 16.6). Other drugs that are used in the treatment of tics include sulpiride, tiapride, metoclopramide, and piquindone (Jimenez-Jimenez and Garcia-Ruiz, 2001; Scahill et al., 2006).

Motor tics may be successfully treated with botulinum toxin (BTX) injections in the affected muscles (Videos 16.15 and 16.19) (Kwak et al., 2000; Aguirregomozcorta et al., 2008). Such focal chemodenervation ameliorates not only the involuntary movements but also the premonitory sensory component. We initially treated 10 TS patients with BTX injections into the involved muscles, and all experienced moderate to marked improvement in the intensity and frequency of their tics (Jankovic, 1994). Subsequent experience with a large number of patients has confirmed the beneficial effects of BTX injections in the treatment of motor and phonic tics (Vincent, 2008), including severe coprolalia (Scott et al., 1996). Furthermore, those patients in whom premonitory sensations preceded the onset of tics noted lessening of these sensory symptoms. The benefits last 3–4 months, on the average, and there are usually no serious complications. In a follow-up study of 35 patients treated for troublesome or disabling tics in 115 sessions, the mean peak effect response was 2.8 (range: 0–4) (Kwak et al., 2000). The mean duration of benefit was 14.4 weeks (up to 45 weeks). The latency to onset of benefit was 3.8 days (up to 10 days). The mean duration of tics prior to initial injections was 15.3 years (range: 1–62 years), and the mean duration of follow-up was 21.2 months (range: 1.5–84 months). Twenty-one of 25 (84%) patients with notable premonitory sensory symptoms derived marked relief of these symptoms from BTX (mean benefit: 70.6%). Patients reported an overall global response of 62.7%. The total mean dose (units) was 502.1 (range: 15–3550), the number of visits was 3.3 (range: 1–16), and the mean dose per visit was 119.9 (range: 15–273). The sites of injections in descending order were as follows: cervical or upper thoracic (17), upper face (14), lower face (7), voice (4), upper back and shoulder (3), scalp (1), forearm (1), leg (1), and rectus abdominis (1). Complications included mild, transient neck weakness (4); mild, transient dysphagia (2); ptosis (2); nausea, 1 day (1); hypophonia (1); fatigue (1); and generalized weakness, 7 days (1). We concluded that BTX is effective and well tolerated in the treatment of tics. An additional and consistent finding was the relief of disturbing premonitory sensations. In a placebo-controlled study of 18 patients with simple motor tics, Marras and colleagues (2001) found a 39% reduction in the number of tics per minute within 2

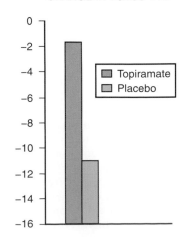

A RANDOMIZED, DOUBLE-BLIND, PLACEBO-CONTROLLED STUDY OF TOPIRAMATE IN THE TREATMENT OF TOURETTE SYNDROME

- *N* = 29 (26 males)

- Mean age 16.5 ± 9.89 years

- The Total Tic Score (TTS), the primary endpoint, improved by 14.29 ± 10.47 points from baseline to visit 5 (Day 70) compared to 5.00 ± 9.88 point change in the placebo group (*P* = 0.0259)

- There were also improvements in the other components of the YGTSS and various secondary measures

- No differences were observed in the frequency of adverse events between the two treatment groups

CHANGE IN YGTSS-TTS

Figure 16.6 Topiramate in TS. YGTSS, Yale Global Tic Severity Scale. *Data from Jankovic J, Jimenez-Shahed J, Brown LW. A randomised, double-blind, placebo-controlled study of topiramate in the treatment of Tourette syndrome. J Neurol Neurosurg Psychiatry 2010;81:70–73.*

weeks after injection with BTX compared to a 6% increase in the placebo group ($P = 0.004$). In addition, there was a 0.46 reduction in urge scores with BTX compared to a 0.49 increase in the placebo group ($P = 0.02$). This preliminary study, however, lacked the power to show significant differences in other measured variables, such as severity score, tic suppression, pain, and patient global impression. Furthermore, the full effect of BTX might not have been appreciated at only 2 weeks; a single treatment protocol does not reflect the clinical practice of evaluating patients after several adjustments in doses and sites of injections; and the patients' symptoms were relatively mild, since the patients "did not rate themselves as significantly compromised by their treated tics" at baseline (Kurlan, 2001). A larger sample and a longer follow-up will be needed to further evaluate the efficacy of BTX in the treatment of tics and to demonstrate that this treatment offers clinically meaningful benefit. BTX, however, not only improves motor and phonic tics and the associated premonitory sensations, but also life-threatening tics, such as dystonic cervical tics that otherwise would cause compressive myelopathy or radiculopathy (Cheung et al., 2007; Aguirregomozcorta et al., 2008).

A single-blind, placebo-controlled trial of two 20-minute applications of repetitive transcranial magnetic stimulation on two consecutive days provided no evidence that repetitive transcranial magnetic stimulation is of any benefit for patients with TS (Munchau et al., 2002), Improvement lasting up to 3 months with 1 Hz repetitive transcranial magnetic stimulation to bilateral supplementary motor area has been reported in patients with adult TS (Mantovani et al., 2007).

Management of behavioral symptoms

Attention-deficit hyperactivity disorder

Behavioral modification, school and classroom adjustments, and other techniques described previously may be useful in the management of behavioral problems associated with TS for some selected patients, but in our experience, these approaches are rarely effective and at best play an ancillary role. Such behavioral strategies, however, may provide important emotional support for the patient and the family members and may be helpful in raising self-esteem and improve motivation (Peterson and Cohen, 1998).

Pharmacologic therapy is usually required when behavioral measures do not allow for a satisfactory adaptation and the symptoms of ADHD impair interpersonal relationships and interfere with academic or occupational performance (Elia et al., 1999; Zametkin and Ernst, 1999; Riddle and Carlson, 2001; Silay and Jankovic, 2005). It is estimated that there are more than 4 million children in the United States diagnosed with ADHD and compared to their non-ADHD peers, children with ADHD suffer lower grades and achievement scores, and higher dropout rates. While only half of the patients used anti-ADHD medications, several studies have found that such medications improve math and reading grades and overall have a favorable impact on academic performance (Scheffler et al., 2009).

CNS stimulants, such as methylphenidate (Ritalin, Ritalin SR, and Ritalin LA), controlled-release methylphenidate (Concerta), controlled-delivery methylphenidate (Metadate CD), methylphenidate oral solution or chewable tablets (Methylin), transdermal methylphenidate, once-a-day patch (Daytrana), dexmethylphenidate (Focalin and Focalin XR), methamphetamine (Desoxyn), dextroamphetamine (Dexedrine), a mixture of amphetamine salts with a 75:25 ratio of dextroamphetamine and levoamphetamine (Adderall), and pemoline (Cylert) are clearly the most effective agents in the treatment of ADHD. The National Institute of Mental Health (NIMH) Collaborative Multimodal Treatment Study of Children with Attention Deficit Hyperactivity Disorder, the most comprehensive study of treatment strategies for ADHD, found medication to be superior to behavioral treatment (MTA Cooperative Group, 1999). The initial dose for methylphenidate is 5 mg in the morning and the dose can be gradually advanced up to 20–60 mg/day (0.3–0.7 mg/kg/dose). Methylphenidate has been found useful not only in the treatment of attention deficit but also as a short-term therapy for conduct disorders (Klein et al., 1997). Dextroamphetamine doses are usually one-half of those of methylphenidate. Pemoline dose should be given as a single morning dose that is approximately 6 times the daily dose of methylphenidate. These drugs usually have a rapid onset of action but also have a relatively short half-life. The long-acting preparations, such as Ritalin-SR (20 mg), are less reliable and less effective than two doses of standard preparation. Dexedrine Spansule has the advantage of greater range of available doses (5, 10, and 15 mg). Some studies (Manos et al., 1999; Pliszka et al., 2000), supported by our own experience, suggest that Adderall is better tolerated, produces less anorexia and sedation, and may be longer lasting than methylphenidate, and it can be used as a one-time morning dose. Only future studies will determine the utility of the new formulation of methylphenidate using a novel controlled-release delivery system designed for once-daily oral dosing (Concerta: 18–36 mg methylphenidate; Metadate CD: 20 mg methylphenidate; Adderall XR: 5–30 mg/day). Metadate CD is formulated to release 6 mg of methylphenidate from immediate-release and 14 mg from extended-release beads. Tolerance, while rare, is more likely to occur with the long-acting formulations, but this has not been demonstrated in patients with ADHD. Besides the possible development of tolerance, potential side effects of these stimulant drugs include nervousness, irritability, insomnia, anorexia, abdominal pain, and headaches. In one study, dextroamphetamine was found to cause more insomnia and negative emotional symptoms than methylphenidate (Efron et al., 1997). Pemoline can rarely produce chemical hepatitis and even fulminant liver failure. Liver enzymes should be assessed before administration, but because the onset of hepatitis is unpredictable, routine laboratory studies are not useful. The parents should be instructed to notify the physician if nausea, vomiting, lethargy, malaise, or jaundice appears. Although some studies have suggested growth retardation, this effect, if present at all, is very minimal and probably clinically insignificant. Whether other CNS stimulants such those used as appetite suppressants (e.g., sibutramine, Meridia, and Reductil) would be useful in the treatment of ADD or tics is not known (Arterburn et al., 2004). Lisdexamfetamine dimesylate (LDX, Vyvanse), a therapeutically inactive amphetamine prodrug that was developed with the goal of providing an extended duration of effect with pharmacologically active d-amphetamine molecule gradually released by rate-limited hydrolysis, has been approved by the FDA in 2007 for the treatment of ADHD. In a phase III, multicenter, randomized, double-blind, forced-dose, parallel-group study that was conducted at 40 centers across the United States, children aged 6–12 years with ADHD were randomly assigned to receive LDX 30, 50, or 70 mg with forced-dose titration, or placebo (Biederman et al., 2007). Efficacy was assessed using the ADHD Rating Scale Version IV (ADHD-RS-IV), the Conners Parent Rating Scale (CPRS), and the Clinical Global Impression of Improvement scale. Of the 290 randomized patients, 230 completed the trial. Significant improvements in ADHD-RS-IV scores were seen with all doses (30–70 mg) of LDX compared with placebo (all, $P < 0.001$), and in CPRS scores with all LDX doses versus placebo throughout the day (all, $P < 0.001$ for all comparisons). The most frequently reported adverse events among patients receiving LDX were typical of amphetamine products: decreased appetite (39% with active treatment vs. 4% with placebo), insomnia (19% vs. 3%), upper abdominal pain (12% vs. 6%), headache (12% vs. 10%), irritability (10% vs. 0%), vomiting (9% vs. 4%), weight decrease (9% vs. 1%), and nausea (6% vs. 3%); most were mild to moderate and occurred in the first week.

CNS stimulants may exacerbate or precipitate tics in up to 25% of patients (Robertson and Eapen, 1992). If the symptoms of ADHD are troublesome and interfere with a patient's functioning, however, it is reasonable to use these CNS stimulants and titrate the dosage to the lowest effective level (Wilens et al., 1995) (Tables 16.5 and 16.6). More recent studies suggest that while CNS stimulants may exacerbate tics when they are introduced into the anti-TS treatment regimen, with continued use these drugs can be well tolerated without tic exacerbation (Gadow et al., 1999; Law and Schachtar, 1999; Kurlan, 2002; Tourette's Syndrome Study Group, 2002). The dopamine receptor-blocking drugs can be combined with the CNS stimulants if the latter produce unacceptable exacerbation of tics. If one stimulant is ineffective or poorly tolerated, another stimulant should be tried.

While methylphenidate was initially thought to work by raising brain levels of dopamine, more recent studies have suggested that its beneficial effects on ADHD are mediated via the serotonin system (Gainetdinov et al., 1999). A strain of mice with an inactivated gene for dopamine transporter has been described to have behavioral symptoms similar to those in children with ADHD. The hyperactivity of the mice was markedly ameliorated by methylphenidate, and this improvement correlated with an increase in brain serotonin. Other investigators have provided evidence that ADHD is a noradrenergic disorder (Biederman and Spencer, 1999). Although it has been suggested that long-term use of CNS stimulants might lead to substance abuse, some studies have demonstrated that untreated ADHD is a significant risk factor for substance abuse and that treatment of ADHD with CNS stimulants significantly reduces the risk for substance use disorder (Biederman et al., 1999).

α_2-Adrenergic agonists and tricyclic antidepressants are also useful in the treatment of ADHD, particularly if CNS stimulants are not well tolerated or are contraindicated. Clonidine (Catapres), a presynaptic α_2-adrenergic agonist that is used as an antihypertensive because it decreases plasma norepinephrine, improves symptoms of ADHD and impulse control problems. Although initially found to be marginally effective in controlling motor tics (Leckman et al., 1991), clonidine has not been found to be an effective anti-tic agent in other studies. Singer and colleagues (1995a) reported a double-blind, placebo-controlled study involving children with ADHD ($n = 37$) randomized to 6-week medication cycles with clonidine (0.05 mg four times a day), desipramine (25 mg four times a day), or placebo. Desipramine, but not clonidine, was significantly more effective than placebo. The usual starting dose is 0.1 mg at bedtime, and the dosage is gradually increased up to 0.5 mg/day in three divided doses. Although a multicenter controlled clinical trial showed that clonidine alone or in combination with methylphenidate is an effective anti-tic drug (Tourette's Syndrome Study Group, 2002), our experience has suggested that the perceived benefit might not be due to a specific anti-tic efficacy, but rather might be a nonspecific anxiolytic effect or due to its benefit for comorbid disorders (see later). The drug is also available as a transdermal patch (Catapres TTS-1, TTS-2, TTS-3, corresponding to 0.1, 0.2, and 0.3 mg, respectively) that should be changed once a week, using a different skin location. Side effects include sedation, lightheadedness, headache, dry mouth, and insomnia. Because of its sedative effects, some clinicians use clonidine as a nighttime soporific agent. Although the patch can cause local irritation, it seems to cause fewer side effects than oral clonidine.

Another drug that is increasingly used in the treatment of ADHD and impulse control problems is guanfacine (Tenex, Intuniv), which is available as 1 mg or 2 mg tablets. The initial dose is 0.5 mg at bedtime with gradual increases, as needed, to final doses up to 4–6 mg/day. Pharmacologically similar to clonidine, guanfacine may be effective in patients in whom clonidine has failed to control the behavioral symptoms. Guanfacine may have some advantages over clonidine in that it has a longer half-life, it appears to be less sedating, and it produces less hypotension. It also seems to be a more selective α_2-noradrenergic receptor agonist and binds more selectively to the postsynaptic α_{2A}-adrenergic receptors located in the prefrontal cortex. While both clonidine and guanfacine appear to be effective in the treatment of attention deficit with and without hyperactivity, they appear to be particularly useful in the management of oppositional, argumentative, impulsive, and aggressive behavior. Although less effective than methylphenidate (Ritalin) (see later), the drugs have an advantage over methylphenidate in that they do not increase tics (Horrigan and Barnhill, 1995). The efficacy of this drug is supported by a pilot study of 13 patients with ADHD (but without TS) (Hunt et al., 1995). Another study, a 4-week, double-blind, placebo-controlled study of mild TS patients, however, failed to show significant neuropsychiatric or tic benefits (Cummings et al., 2002). The most frequently encountered side effects of the two drugs include sedation, dry mouth, itchy eyes, dizziness, headaches, fatigability, and postural hypotension. The beneficial effects might not be appreciated for several weeks after initiation of therapy, and the symptoms might markedly intensify if the medications are withdrawn abruptly. We have found deprenyl or selegiline (Eldepryl), a monoamine oxidase-B inhibitor, to be effective in controlling the symptoms of ADHD without exacerbating tics (Jankovic, 1993a). Using the DuPaul Attention Deficit Hyperactivity Scale, the efficacy of this drug in ADHD has been confirmed by a double-blind placebo-controlled study (Feigin et al., 1996).

It is not clear how deprenyl improves symptoms of ADHD, but the drug is known to metabolize into amphetamines. Other drugs that are frequently used in relatively mild cases of ADHD include imipramine (Tofranil), nortriptyline (Pamelor), and desipramine (Norpramin). Because of potential cardiotoxicity, an electrocardiogram or cardiologic evaluation might be needed before initiation of desipramine therapy, and follow-up electrocardiograms should be performed every 3–6 months. Bupropion (Wellbutrin), an atypical antidepressant with stimulant properties, may be also useful in the management of ADHD, although like the other CNS stimulants, it may possibly exacerbate tics (Spencer et al., 1993). Some nonstimulant drugs such as modafinil and atomoxetine (inhibitor of presynaptic norepinephrine transporter) (Michelson et al., 2001; Kratochvil et al., 2002) have been reported to be useful in the treatment of ADHD associated with TS. Atomoxetine (Strattera), not a controlled substance, which was approved by the FDA in 2002, is the first anti-ADHD medication to be approved for adults as well as children. Metabolized primarily through the CYP2D6 enzymatic pathway and excreted in the urine, atomoxetine has a mean half-life of 5.2 hours. The usual starting dose is 0.5 mg/kg of body weight or 25 mg/day, and the dose can be gradually increased up to 40–50 mg twice a day. Anorexia, insomnia, sedation, tremor, and sexual dysfunction are the most frequent side effects. In one study (Kelsey et al., 2004), the efficacy of atomoxetine administered once daily among children with ADHD was assessed throughout the day, including the evening and early morning. This study was a randomized, multicenter, double-blind, placebo-controlled trial conducted at 12 outpatient sites in the United States. A total of 197 children, 6–12 years of age, who had been diagnosed as having ADHD on the basis of the criteria of the Diagnostic and Statistical Manual of Mental Disorders, fourth edition, were randomized to receive 8 weeks of treatment with atomoxetine or placebo, dosed once daily in the mornings. ADHD symptoms were assessed with parent and investigator rating scales. Among children 6–12 years of age who had been diagnosed as having ADHD, once-daily administration of atomoxetine in the morning provided safe, rapid, continuous, symptom relief that lasted beyond the evening hours, into the morning hours. Overall, atomoxetine treatment was safe and well tolerated. Another prospective, multicenter open-label assessment of atomoxetine in non-North American children and adolescents with ADHD supported the efficacy and safety of atomoxetine (Buitelaar et al., 2004). In another study, TS patients were randomly assigned to double-blind treatment with placebo ($n = 56$) or atomoxetine (0.5–1.5 mg/kg/day, $n = 61$) for approximately 18 weeks. Subjects receiving atomoxetine showed significantly greater improvement on ADHD symptom measures, but significant increases were seen in mean pulse rate and rates of treatment-emergent nausea, decreased appetite, and decreased body weight (Spencer et al., 2008). Comparative studies assessing the relative efficacy and safety of atomoxetine versus CNS stimulants in patients with TS and comorbid ADHD are needed.

Modafinil, a nonschedule stimulant, α_1 receptor agonist that also acts on GABA and glutamate, has been found to be ineffective in a double-blind, placebo-controlled study of ADHD (Pliszka, 2003). Desmopressin, either as a nasal spray or in tablet form, with or without imipramine, can be used in the treatment of enuresis, which is frequently associated with ADHD.

Obsessive-compulsive disorder

The role of cognitive-behavioral therapy in the treatment of OCD has not been well defined, although some investigators argue that when used alone or in combination with pharmacotherapy, it is the psychotherapeutic treatment of choice (March et al., 2001; Micallef and Blin, 2001; Jenike, 2004). This therapy utilizes repeated exposure to provocative stimuli in an attempt to prevent the rituals and other compulsions. The Pediatric OCD Treatment Study showed that cognitive-behavioral therapy alone or in combination with a selective serotonin uptake inhibitor (SSRI) provides the best results in children and adolescents with OCD (Pediatric OCD Treatment Study Team, 2004). In a study of 10 OCD patients and 12 control subjects, PET scans showed significant decreases in glucose metabolism in the thalamus bilaterally and an increase in activity in the right dorsal anterior cingulate cortex, a region involved in reappraisal and suppression of negative emotions after cognitive-behavioral therapy (Saxena et al., 2009).

Although imipramine and desipramine have been reported to be useful in the treatment of OCD, the most effective drugs are the SSRIs (Dolberg et al., 1996; Flament and Bisserbe, 1997; Grados and Riddle, 2001; Hensiek and Trimble, 2002; Silay and Jankovic, 2005). These include fluoxetine (Prozac), fluvoxamine (Luvox), clomipramine (Anafranil), paroxetine (Paxil), sertraline (Zoloft), venlafaxine (Effexor), citalopram (Celexa), and escitalopram (Lexapro), the S-enantiomer of citalopram. Controlled trials have found all these agents, except for escitalopram, to be effective in the treatment of OCD. Only a few comparative studies have been performed of the various agents in patients with TS and OCD, but clomipramine (Anafranil), fluvoxamine (Luvox), fluoxetine (Prozac), and sertraline (Zoloft) are particularly effective. Sertraline, particularly when combined with cognitive-behavioral therapy, has been found to significantly reduce anxiety in a randomized, controlled trial involving 488 children with anxiety disorder (Walkup et al., 2008). The initial dosage of clomipramine is 25 mg at bedtime, and the dosage can be gradually increased up to 250 mg/day, using 25 mg, 50 mg, or 75 mg capsules after meals or at bedtime. Fluoxetine, paroxetine, and citalopram should be started at 20 mg after breakfast, and the dosage can be increased up to 80 mg/day. In contrast to clomipramine and fluvoxamine, the other SSRIs should be started as a morning, after-breakfast dose.

Although comparative trials have been lacking, meta-analyses have provided some useful information. A comprehensive meta-analysis found venlafaxine particularly effective in the treatment of depression and inducing remission compared to the other SSRIs, possibly because of its dual effect by inhibiting both serotonin and noradrenaline (Nemeroff et al., 2008). Long-term clinical trials indicate that fluoxetine and sertraline are the best tolerated of the SSRIs (Flament and Bisserbe, 1997). A double-blind comparison of fluvoxamine and clomipramine showed equal efficacy, although clomipramine had a more rapid onset of effect, but fluvoxamine was better tolerated (Milanfranchi et al., 1997). In addition to its antidepressant and anti-OCD effects, fluvoxamine has been found to be an effective treatment for children and adolescents with social phobia and anxiety (Research Unit on Pediatric Psychopharmacology Anxiety Study Group, 2001). There is some evidence that fluvoxamine sensitizes sigma receptors, which may lead to potentiation of dystonia in animals (Stahl, 1998). In a multicenter, randomized controlled study of 187 children and adolescents, sertraline was found to be safe and effective in the treatment of OCD (March et al., 1998). Up to 25% of patients with OCD show no meaningful improvement with the SSRIs and may therefore require polypharmacy (Laird, 1996). Certain drugs, such as lithium and buspirone, have been reported to augment the SSRIs. There is little information about the potential synergistic effects of different SSRIs, although some patients clearly feel that the combination of two SSRIs is more effective than when they are used as monotherapy. In some treatment-refractory cases, SSRIs might need to be combined with buspirone, clonazepam, lithium, and even neuroleptics (Goodman et al., 1998). When a combination or polypharmacy is used, it is prudent practice to discuss with the patients potential adverse reactions, including the serotonin syndrome (confusion, hypomania, agitation, myoclonus, hyperreflexia, sweating, tremor, diarrhea, and fever), withdrawal phenomenon, and possible extrapyramidal side effects. Acute parkinsonism was reported in adult patients with TS who were treated with the combination of serotonin reuptake inhibitors and neuroleptics (Kurlan, 1998a). Despite unsubstantiated evidence about an increased risk of suicide, some regulatory agencies, including the British Medicines and Health Care Products Regulatory Agency, found in December 2003 that the "balance of risks and benefits for the treatment of major depressive disorder in under 18s is judged to be unfavorable for sertraline, citalopram and escitalopram"; fluoxetine has been exempt because of its favorable "balance of risks and benefits" (see www.mhra.gov.uk). Systematic review of published and unpublished data on SSRIs in the treatment of childhood depression raised some questions about the safety and efficacy of these drugs in this population of depressed patients (Whittington et al., 2004). In addition to the SSRIs, anxiolytics, such as alprazolam and clonazepam, have been used with modest success. Similarly, monoamine oxidase (MAO) inhibitors, trazodone, and buspirone have limited efficacy in the treatment of OCD. Finally, surgical treatment such as deep brain stimulation of the subthalamic nucleus and other subcortical areas, may be used as a last resort in patients with disabling, medically intractable OCD (Mallet et al., 2008; Greenberg et al., 2010).

Other behavioral problems

There are many other behavioral problems that may be even more troublesome for patients with TS than ADHD or OCD. As was noted, treatment of ADHD often improves impulse control problems that are frequently associated with TS. Sudden, explosive attacks of rage, which occur in a considerable proportion of patients with TS, have been found to respond to SSRIs, such as paroxetine (Bruun and Budman, 1998).

It can be only speculated at this time whether antagonists of excitatory amino acids or antiadrenergic agents, such as flutamide, will exert a protective effect in TS. However, future therapeutic interventions should include strategies that are designed not only to control symptoms but also to alter the natural course of the disease.

Surgical treatments

Surgical treatment of TS is controversial. While the overall experience of stereotactic ablative surgery in the treatment of tics has been rather disappointing, an increasing number of reports have provided evidence that deep brain stimulation (DBS) involving thalamus, globus pallidus and other targets may be a very effective strategy to treat uncontrollable tics (Temel and Visser-Vandewalle, 2004; Diederich et al., 2005; Houeto et al., 2005; Ackermans et al., 2006; Shahed et al., 2007; Ackermans et al., 2008 and 2011; Porta et al., 2009). Experience with 17 patients, median age 23 years (range 11–40), who were treated with ablative procedures between 1970 and 1998 was reviewed by Babel et al (2001). Unilateral zona incerta and ventrolateral/ventromedial lesioning was used and occasional second surgery on the contralateral side was performed. The authors concluded that the procedure(s) "sufficiently" reduced both motor and phonic tics. Transient complications were reported in 68% of patients and only one patient suffered permanent complication. Medial thalamus has long been considered a target not only in ablative procedures but also in DBS treatment of tics and OCD (Vandewalle et al., 1999; Nuttin et al., 1999; Diederich et al., 2005). Nuttin et al. (2003) noted beneficial effects in OCD with bilateral anterior capsular stimulation after one year of stimulation, but all six patients remained defective in several domains of health-related quality of life. A report of a 42-year-old man with severe motor and phonic tics controlled by high-frequency deep brain stimulation (DBS) of thalamus is quite encouraging (Vandewalle et al., 1999). In another report, a 36-year-old woman with a childhood history of tics, severe coprolalia, and SIB, stimulation of either the thalamus (centromedian-parafascicular complex) or the anteromedial part of the internal globus pallidus markedly improved the three components of her TS (Houeto et al., 2005). The GPi has been increasingly used as the target in patients with disabling tics because of its extensive connections to the prefrontal cortex, an area that influences cognition and mood (Diederich et al., 2005; Shahed et al., 2007; Dehning et al., 2008). This selection is supported by previous reports of successful treatment with bilateral GPi DBS in two TS patients. In one study, a comparison of bilateral GPi to bilateral medial thalamic stimulation in the same patient found greater tic reduction (95% vs. 80%) at lower settings with GPi stimulation (Diederich et al., 2005), but another report described similar degrees of improvement using either site (Ackermans et al., 2006). In a 16-year-old boy with disabling, medically intractable TS, bilateral GPi DBS resulted in 63% improvement in Yale Global Tourette Syndrome Scale, 85% improvement in Tic Symptom Self Report, and 51% improvement in SF-36, a quality of life measure (Shahed et al., 2007). Furthermore, the patient was able to return to school. Although these observations must be confirmed by a controlled trial before DBS can be recommended even to severely affected patients, it suggests that stimulation of certain targets involved in the limbic striatopallidal-thalamocortical system could be beneficial in the treatment of various aspects of TS. STN DBS has been reported to be effective in a patient with PD and coexistent TS (Martinez-Torres et al., 2009), but it should be noted that DBS targeting STN may occasionally lead to increased impulsivity, similar to pathologic gambling seen in patients treated with dopamine agonists, which may possibly be due to impaired ability to self-modulate decision processes and cognitive control (Frank et al., 2007). Although DBS may be associated with behavioral and cognitive complications, neuropsychological and psychiatric comorbidities in TS should not necessarily be a contraindication to DBS, as these conditions may in fact improve after GPi stimulation.

Careful selection of patients, experience with DBS procedure, and comprehensive assessments at baseline and at follow-up visits are essential for successful outcome of DBS in TS (Mink et al., 2006). DBS of the median part of the thalamus also resulted in a marked improvement in tics (Bajwa et al., 2007). DBS of ventral capsule and ventral striatum has been also reported to be effective in patients with severe OCD (Greenberg et al., 2006). Based on a double-blind assessment of five patients with TS undergoing bilateral thalamic DBS, there was a significant ($P < 0.03$) reduction in the modified Rush Video-Based Rating Scale score (primary outcome measure) and improvement was also noted in motor and phonic tic counts as well as on the YGTSS and TS Symptom List scores (secondary outcome measures) (Maciunas et al., 2007). In addition, there was evidence of improvement in the quality of life indices and three of five patients had marked improvement according to all primary and secondary outcome measures. In another double-blind clinical trial, involving 6 TS patients with DBS targeting the centromedian nucleus–substantia periventricularis–nucleus ventrooralis internus crosspoint, the tic severity during "on" stimulation was significantly lower than during "off" stimulation, with substantial improvement (37%) on the YFTS (mean 41.1 ± 5.4 vs. 25.6 ± 12.8, $P = 0.046$) (Ackermans et al., 2011). The benefits were sustained one year after surgery with significant improvement (49%) on the YGTS (mean 42.2 ± 3.1 vs. 21.5 ± 11.1, $P = 0.028$) when compared with preoperative assessments. There were no improvements in secondary outcome measures and there was some deterioration in attention. Serious adverse events included one small hemorrhage ventral to the tip of the electrode, one infection of the pulse generator, subjective gaze disturbances

and reduction of energy levels in all patients. In the largest reported series, 18 TS patients underwent bilateral DBS of the centromedian parafascicular (CM-Pfc) and ventralis oralis (Vo) complex of the thalamus (Servello et al., 2008). Followed up to 18 months, most patients apparently showed improvement in tics as well as OCD, self-injurious behavior, and other comorbidities. In a prospective 24-month follow-up of 15 of the original 18 patients, there continued to be marked improvement in tics, OCD, anxiety, and depression with subjective perception of improved social functioning and quality of life (Porta et al., 2009). It would be helpful to know what happened to the 3 patients not included in this open-label, observational study. Also a blinded review of videos before and after treatment would provide more objective measure of efficacy (Black, 2009). Finally, the observation that vagal nerve stimulation also favorably modifies the frequency and intensity of facial tics suggests that the brainstem plays a role in generation of modulation of tics (Diamond et al., 2006).

References available on Expert Consult: www.expertconsult.com

Appendix

Tourette Syndrome Association (TSA)
42–40 Bell Boulevard, Suite 205
Bayside, NY 11361-2820
Telephone: (718) 224-2999
Email: mark.levine@tsa-usa.org
Website: http://www.tsa-usa.org/

Other relevant websites
http://www.ed.gov
http://www.nih.gov
http://www.wemove.org

Obsessive Compulsive Foundation
http://www.ocfoundation.org/

Children and adults with attention-deficit disorder
http://www.chadd.org/
http://www.ets.org/disabilities/documentation/documenting_adhd/

CHAPTER **17**

Stereotypies

Chapter contents

Pathophysiology of stereotypies	380		Obsessive-compulsive disorder and tic disorders	386
Physiologic stereotypies	382		Other stereotypies	387
Developmental disorders	382		Treatment	388
Schizophrenia and catatonia	386			

Stereotypies may be defined as involuntary or unvoluntary (in response to or induced by inner sensory stimulus or unwanted feeling), coordinated, patterned, repetitive, rhythmic, seemingly purposeless movements or utterances (Jankovic, 1994, 2005; Singer, 2009; Sanger et al., 2010; Singer et al., 2010). Although stereotypies typically occur in children with autism or other pervasive developmental disorders, they can also occur in adults. Each child tends to have his or her own repertoire of movements, but typical motor stereotypies encountered in children with autism include body rocking, head nodding, head banging, hand waving, covering ears, fluttering of fingers or hands in front of the face, repetitive and sequential finger movements, eye deviations, lip smacking, and chewing movements, pacing, object fixation, and skin picking. Phonic stereotypies include grunting, moaning, and humming. Stereotypies are usually either continuous, such as those seen in patients with tardive dyskinesias and Rett syndrome, or intermittent, as seen in autism (see Chapter 1). Tics in Tourette syndrome (TS), although mostly intermittent movements, are usually stereotypic in that the movements repeat themselves. In their classic monograph on tics, Meige and Feindel (1907) distinguished between stereotypies and motor tics by describing the latter as acts that are impelling but not impossible to resist, whereas the former, while illogical, are without an irresistible urge. The word "stereotypic," however, has been removed from the description of tics in the *Diagnostic and Statistical Manual of Mental Disorders*, Fifth Edition (DSM-V), expected to be published in 2013. Mannerisms, which are gestures that are peculiar or unique to the individual, may at times seem stereotypic (patterned), but they are usually not continuous. Automatisms in patients with seizures can be viewed as paroxysmal stereotypies (Sadleir et al., 2009). There is often an overlap between stereotypies and self-injurious behavior, such as biting, scratching, and hitting (Jankovic et al., 1998; Schroeder et al., 2001; Lutz et al., 2003).

In addition to motor and phonic types, stereotypies can be classified as either simple (e.g., foot tapping, body rocking) or complex (e.g., complicated rituals, repeatedly sitting down and rising from a chair). Stereotypies can also be described according to the distribution of the predominant site of involvement (orolingual, hand, leg, truncal). The term stereotypy should be used to describe a phenomenologic, not an etiologic, category of hyperkinetic movement disorders. However, recognition of stereotypy as a distinct movement disorder can logically lead from a phenomenologic to an etiologic diagnosis (Table 17.1). Thus, stereotypy is a motor-behavioral disorder that is found most frequently in patients who are in the borderland between neurology and psychiatry.

Pathophysiology of stereotypies

There is no clear anatomic-clinical correlation for stereotypies, although it is believed that both cortical and subcortical structures are involved. While dysfunction in the basal ganglia has been implicated in the pathogenesis of certain stereotypies, some studies have also provided evidence for the role of the mesolimbic system, particularly the nucleus accumbens–amygdala pathway, in the pathogenesis of stereotypic movements. Stereotypies with or without associated obsessive-compulsive behavior (OCB) have been observed in patients with structural lesions in different anatomic areas, including bilateral lesions of the medial frontoparietal cortices (Sato et al., 2001; Kwak and Jankovic, 2002) and cerebellum (Hottinger-Blanc et al., 2002). Studies of stereotypies in animals may provide insight into the pathogenesis of habits, rituals, and other repetitive behaviors in humans (Graybiel, 2008).

Stereotypic behavior is common in animals in lower species up to and including the primates and are particularly common in farm and zoo animals that are housed in

© 2011 Elsevier Ltd, Inc, BV

DOI: 10.1016/B978-1-4377-2369-4.00017-2

Table 17.1 Classification of stereotypies

Physiologic

- Mannerisms or habits
- Normal developmental stereotypies
- Spasmus nutans
- Shuddering attacks
- Gratification (masturbatory) behavior

Pathologic

- Mental retardation
- Pervasive developmental disorders (autism)
- Schizophrenia
- Catatonia
- Obsessive-compulsive disorder
- Frontotemporal degeneration
- Tourette syndrome
- Neuroacanthocytosis
- Restless leg syndrome
- Epileptic automatism
- Structural lesions (medial-frontoparietal cortex, cerebellum)
- Tardive (dopamine receptor-blocking drugs) and other dyskinesias (levodopa)
- Akathisia
- Psychogenic

restraining environments with low stimulation (Garner et al., 2003; Lutz et al., 2003) (Video 17.1). Self-injurious behavior, observed in 14% of housed monkeys, may be viewed as a form of stereotypy (Novak, 2003). Therefore, stereotypy has been viewed as either a self-generating sensory stimulus or a motor expression of underlying tension and anxiety. The repetitive and ritualistic behavior that some animals display has been used as an experimental model of obsessive-compulsive disorder (OCD). Indeed, studies of animal and human stereotypies have provided important insights into relationships between motor function and behavior. Some veterinarian scientists have even suggested changing the nomenclature of stereotypies to OCB, but there is little evidence to indicate that the stereotypic behavior that is observed in animals is driven by underlying obsessions and represents compulsive behavior (Garner et al., 2003; Low, 2003). A study of 136 Romanian children with a history of early institutional care showed that in comparison to those placed in foster care, institutional care was associated with much higher frequency of stereotypies, again highlighting the importance of restrained environment in the pathogenesis of stereotypies (Bos et al., 2010).

Most studies of stereotypic behavior in experimental animals have focused on the role of dopaminergic systems in the basal ganglia and limbic structures. Intrastriatal injection of dopamine and systemic administration of both presynaptically active dopaminergic drugs, such as amphetamine, and postsynaptically active dopamine agonists, such as apomorphine, in rats produce dose-related repetitive sniffing, gnawing, licking, biting, rearing, head bobbing, grooming, and other stereotyped learned activities.

The observation that self-biting behavior induced by dopaminergic drugs in 6-hydroxydopamine rats and monkeys with a unilateral lesion in the ventral medial tegmentum can be blocked by a selective D1 antagonist SCH 23390 suggests that self-injurious behavior is mediated primarily by the D1 receptors (Schroeder et al., 2001). Selective dopamine receptor agonists and antagonists have been used in experimental models to study different effects of D1 and D2 receptors on stereotypic behavior. SKF 38393, a D1 agonist, produced no stereotypic behavior in normal rats, but it did enhance stereotypy induced by apomorphine, a mixed D1 and D2 agonist (Koller and Herbster, 1988). This suggests that the D2 dopamine receptors mediate stereotypic behavior and that activation of the D1 receptors potentiates these D2-mediated effects. Additional evidence for the role of D2 dopamine receptors in the pathogenesis of stereotypies is the observation that upregulation of D2 receptors (e.g., with haloperidol, a selective D2 antagonist) but not of D1 receptors (e.g., with SCH 23390, a selective D1 antagonist), enhanced apomorphine-induced stereotypies (Chipkin et al., 1987). Drug-induced models of stereotypy, however, might not accurately reflect spontaneous or disease-related repetitive behaviors. Using several selective dopaminergic agonists (apomorphine, SKF81297, and quinpirole) as well as intrastriatal administration of the D2 receptor antagonist raclopride to study stereotypic behaviors in the deer mouse model of spontaneous and persistent stereotypy showed that spontaneously emitted and drug-induced stereotypies may have different mechanisms (Presti et al., 2004). Nevertheless, these studies suggest that the striatal dopaminergic system is significantly involved in stereotypic behaviors. Oral and forelimb stereotypies can be induced in the rat with injections of amphetamine into the ventrolateral striatum (Canales et al., 2000), and certain genes can be activated in the striosomes with these drugs when they are administered orally (Canales and Graybiel, 2000). These studies provide further support for basal ganglia involvement in stereotypies. Although there is experimental evidence from rodent and primate studies to support the notion that differential activation of striosomes in the basal ganglia plays an important role in pathophysiology of stereotypies (Saka and Graybiel, 2003), some recent studies found that motor stereotypies do not require enhanced activation of striosomes (Glickstein and Schmauss, 2004). In addition to the basal ganglia, the pontine tegmentum has been implicated in certain stereotypies, particularly repetitive involuntary leg movements that are somewhat similar to the leg movements in patients with restless legs syndrome (Lee et al., 2005). Indeed, bilateral 6-hydroxydopamine (6-OHDA) lesioning in the A11 nucleus of C57BL/6 mice has been associated with an increase in motor, stereotypic, behavior resembling restless legs syndrome activity (Qu et al., 2007).

Besides the classic neurotransmitters, evidence is accumulating in support of involvement of neuropeptides as modulators of stereotypic behavior. For example, microinjection of cholecystokinin and neurotensin into the medial nucleus accumbens markedly potentiated apomorphine-induced stereotypy (Blumstein et al., 1987). Since injection of these peptides into the striatum had no effect on the apomorphine-induced stereotypy, these studies provide additional evidence for the involvement of the limbic system in the pathogenesis of this movement disorder. Improvement in self-injurious behavior observed in autistic children after administration of the opiate blockers naloxone and naltrexone has been interpreted as evidence for the role of endogenous opiates (e.g., β-endorphins) in this abnormal behavior (Sandman, 1988). Additional support for the role of endorphins in self-injurious and stereotypic behavior is the finding of elevated plasma and cerebrospinal fluid levels of β-endorphins in autistic patients with these behavioral abnormalities (Sandman, 1988). More recently, the emphasis has shifted to the serotonin system, supported by the observation that certain animal behaviors improve with serotonin uptake inhibitors (Hugo et al., 2003; Andersen et al., 2010).

Physiologic stereotypies

Certain stereotypies, such as hair twisting, drumming with fingers, tapping of the feet, adduction–abduction, and crossing–uncrossing and other repetitive movements of the legs, may be part of a repertoire of movements, also referred to as mannerisms or habits, seen in otherwise healthy individuals (Bonnet et al., 2010). Developmental and benign movement disorders in childhood include: benign jitteriness or myoclonus of newborn, sleep-related rhythmic movements, spasmus nutans, paroxysmal tonic gaze, benign paroxysmal torticollis, shuddering attacks, transient dystonia of infancy, gratification (masturbatory) behavior, mirror movements, Sandifer syndrome and a variety of normal stereotypies (Bonnet et al., 2010). In infants and children, there seems to be a progression of normal stereotypies (Castellanos et al., 1996). For example, thumb sucking and hand sucking in infancy are later replaced by body rocking, head rolling, and head banging. Some infants demonstrate head stereotypies that resemble bobble-head doll syndrome, sometimes associated with ataxia but without any other neurologic deficit and normal subsequent development (Hottinger-Blanc et al., 2002). A review of 40 "normal" children, aged 9 months to 17 years, with complex hand and arm stereotypies, such as flapping, shaking, clenching, posturing, and other "ritual" movements, showed that the movements can be temporarily suppressed in nearly all when cued (Mahone et al., 2004). Although the children were classified as "normal," 25% had comorbid attention-deficit hyperactivity disorder (ADHD), and 20% had learning disability, probably due to referral bias, since this group is also known for their work in TS. This referral bias was supported by a relatively high family history of sterereotypies (25%) and tics (33%). A variety of stereotypies can be observed in children (Castellanos et al., 1996; Tan et al., 1997) and young adults (Niehaus et al., 2000) without any other neurologic deficits. We have observed otherwise normal children with persistent head stereotypies similar to the bobble-head syndrome but without abnormal neuroimaging studies. Stereotypies may also occur during development of otherwise normal children who are congenitally blind (Troster et al., 1991) or deaf (Bachara and Phelan, 1980).

Head banging is seen in up to 15% of normal children (Sallustro and Atwell, 1978). Some girls exhibit stereotypic crossing and extending of legs, which actually represents a self-gratifying or masturbatory behavior (Mink and Neil, 1995; Yang et al., 2005; Bonnet et al., 2010) (Video 17.2). Otherwise normal children can also develop bruxism, nail biting, trichotillomania, and other stereotypic behaviors.

These behaviors have been often attributed to underlying generalized anxiety disorder or OCD. While motor stereotypies most frequently occur in a setting of mental retardation or autism, in a clinical cohort of 100 normally developing children with motor stereotypies, some involuntary or unvoluntary movements were continued in 62% of the children followed for over 5 years (Harris et al., 2008). Nearly half the children with continuing stereotypies exhibit other comorbidities, including ADHD (30%), tics (18%), and OCB or OCD (10%). It is possible, however, that many of these children had TS, as suggested by the comorbidities typically associated with TS and positive family histories of involuntary movements in 25%. The study also suggested that the clinical course of children who exhibit head nodding may be more favorable than that of children whose motor stereotypy predominantly involves the hands and arms. In another study designed to better characterize stereotypic movements and differentiate them from tics, Freeman and colleagues (2010) evaluated 40 children (31 males), with mean age at onset of stereotypies at 17 months, without self-injurious behavior, intellectual disability, sensory impairment, or an autistic spectrum disorder and found neuropsychiatric comorbidity in 30 (ADHD in 16, tics in 18, developmental coordination disorder in 16, and OCD in 2). In contrast to their parents, children liked their movements, which were usually associated with excitement or imaginative play. Of the 39 children followed for longer than 6 months, the behavior stopped or occurred primarily privately in 25.

Thus, while stereotypies can occur in otherwise normal individuals, when accompanied by other behavioral and neurologic findings, this form of hyperkinesia usually indicates the presence of an underlying neurologic and/or psychiatric disorder.

Developmental disorders

It is beyond the scope of this chapter to review the current notions about the clinical features and pathogenesis of mental retardation, but the reader is referred to a review of this topic (Nokelainen and Flint, 2002). In one study of 102 institutionalized mentally retarded people, with a mean age of 35 years (range: 21–68 years), 34% exhibited at least one type of stereotypy (rhythmic movement, 26%; bizarre posturing, 13%; object manipulation, 7%; and others) (Dura et al., 1987). In another study, 100 individuals with severe or profound intellectual disability were randomly selected and followed for 26 years (Thompson and Reid, 2002). Their behavior was recorded through carer and psychiatrist ratings using the Modified Manifest Abnormality Scale of the Clinical Interview Schedule. The follow-up evaluations found that stereotypies, emotional abnormalities, eye avoidance, and other behavioral symptoms persist. Although there seems to be an inverse correlation between stereotypies and IQ, stereotypic behavior may be seen even in those who are mildly retarded. In some mental retardation disorders, typically Lesch–Nyhan syndrome, stereotypies are associated with self-injurious behavior (Videos 17.3 and 17.4). Supersensitivity of D1 receptors, possibly in response to abnormal arborization of dopamine neurons in the striatum, has been postulated as a possible mechanism of

Table 17.2 Clinical features associated with autism

- Insistence on sameness; resistance to change
- Difficulty in expressing needs; uses gestures or pointing instead of words
- Aggressive and self-injurious behavior
- Repeating words or phrases in place of normal, responsive language
- Laughing, crying, showing distress for reasons not apparent to others
- Prefers to be alone; aloof manner
- Tantrums
- Difficulty in mixing with others
- May not want to cuddle or be cuddled
- Little or no eye contact
- Unresponsive to normal teaching methods
- Sustained odd play
- Spins objects
- Inappropriate attachments to objects
- Apparent over-sensitivity or under-sensitivity to pain
- No real fears of danger
- Noticeable physical over-activity or extreme under-activity
- Uneven gross/fine motor skills
- Not responsive to verbal cues; acts as if deaf although hearing tests in normal range

self-injurious behavior in Lesch–Nyhan syndrome (Jankovic et al., 1988).

Autism

Autism is a type of pervasive developmental disorder (PDD), sometimes referred to as autistic spectrum disorders, with onset during infancy or childhood, characterized by impairment in reciprocal social and interpersonal interactions, impairment in verbal and nonverbal communication, markedly restricted repertoire of activities and interests, and stereotyped movements (Bodfish et al., 2001; Gritti et al., 2003; Lam et al., 2008) (Table 17.2). Many autistic patients also exhibit other abnormal behaviors, such as preoccupations, circumscribed interest patterns, abnormal object attachments, cognitive rigidity, and exaggerated sensory responses. Earlier studies have suggested that about 0.1% of all children are autistic (Sugiyama and Abe, 1989), but more recent epidemiologic studies have estimated that the prevalence of autistic disorders and related pervasive developmental disorders ranges between 0.3% (Yeargin-Allsopp et al., 2003) and 0.6% (Chakrabarti and Fombonne, 2001). In children and adults with autism of any cause, stereotypies and other self-stimulatory activities constitute the most recognizable symptoms. Typical stereotypies that are seen in autistic individuals include facial grimacing, staring at flickering light, waving objects in front of the eyes, producing repetitive sounds, arm flapping, rhythmic body rocking, repetitive touching, feeling and smelling of objects, jumping, walking on toes, and unusual hand and body postures. In a study of motor stereotypies recorded during 15 minutes of videos of standardized play sessions in 277 children (209 males, 68 females), 129 with autistic disorder and 148 cognitively-matched

non-autistic developmentally disordered children, hand/finger repetitive movements and pacing, jumping, and spinning movements during gait were two types of stereotypies that were especially suggestive of autism (Goldman et al., 2009).

The motor manifestations are often associated with insensitivity or excessive sensitivity to sensory stimuli including pain and extremes of temperature, preoccupations with perceptual sensations such as lights or odors, insistence on preservation of sameness, and absence of fear or other emotional reactions. Self-stimulatory and self-injurious behaviors, such as self-biting and head banging, are also common. In addition to these and other behavioral and developmental abnormalities, some autistic individuals have isolated areas of remarkable and sometimes spectacular mental skills, the so-called savant syndrome (Miller, 1999; Treffert, 1999). The mechanism of the savant phenotype in the setting of autism is not well understood but studies of one genetic model of autism, the Shank1 knock out mice, may provide some insight (Hung et al., 2008). The Shank family of post-synaptic scaffold proteins has been found to be abundantly present in the postsynaptic density of central excitatory synapses. When these postsynaptic proteins are altered as in Shank1 knock-out mice, surprisingly the mice displayed enhanced performance in a spatial learning task, although their long-term memory retention in this task was impaired (Hung et al., 2008). The authors suggested that the superior learning ability of these mutant mice was similar to what has been observed human autistic savants.

There are many causes of autism, including fragile X syndrome and a variety of eponymically classified types such as Kanner, Heller, Asperger, Down, and Rett syndromes (Ringman and Jankovic, 2000). Asperger syndrome is one of the most common forms of autism, found in 1 to 3 children in 1000 (Gillberg, 1989). Characterized by social isolation in combination with odd and eccentric behavior, Asperger syndrome shares many features with infantile autism. Several studies have indeed noted an overlap in various clinical and demographic characteristics between Asperger syndrome and infantile autism (Szatmari et al., 1989). In one study of 23 patients, the children with Asperger syndrome seemed to have relatively poor motor skills and had a stiff and awkward gait (without armswing), and their speech development was delayed, although they acquired better expressive speech than the children with infantile autism. In contrast to infantile autism, Asperger syndrome usually does not become fully manifest until 30–36 months of age, but some children may have their first symptoms in infancy. A study of seven patients with the combination of Asperger syndrome and TS showed magnetic resonance imaging (MRI) evidence of cortical and subcortical abnormalities in five of these patients (Berther et al., 1993). Because children with Asperger syndrome are generally brighter than those with other forms of autism, it has been suggested that Asperger syndrome merely represents a mild variant of autism. In a study of eight patients with Asperger syndrome and an additional four with other forms of pervasive developmental disorder who were referred to the Baylor College of Medicine movement disorders clinic for evaluation of tics, all patients exhibited stereotypic movements; in addition, seven had tics, and six of these met inclusion diagnostic criteria for TS (Ringman and Jankovic, 2000). Of the six patients with clinical features of both Asperger syndrome and TS, three had severe congenital sensory deficits, suggesting that sensory deprivation contributes to the development of adventitious movements in this population. Other autistic children also showed features of TS (Rapin, 2001).

In patients with mental retardation and autism, irrespective of etiology, stereotypies are often associated with self-injurious behavior. This is particularly true for patients with body-rocking movements, a stereotypy that is most often associated with self-hitting (Rojahn, 1986). While head banging and other self-injurious behavior may occur in normal children, this type of behavior is usually abnormal and is particularly common in patients who also exhibit stereotypic behavior.

Some studies in autistic children reported that stereotypy interfered with learning, suggesting that treatment of stereotypies in patients with autism facilitates learning (Koegel and Covert, 1972) and implied that controlling stereotypic behavior was a necessary precondition for learning. Drugs that block postsynaptic dopamine and serotonin receptors, such as risperidone, have been found to be effective in the treatment of tantrums, aggression, self-injurious behaviors, and stereotypies in patients with autistic disorders (Research Units on Pediatric Psychopharmacology Autism Network, 2002; Gagliano et al., 2004). These benefits, however, must be weighed against potential side effects, such as sedation, weight gain, and parkinsonism. Other agents that are used in the treatment of autistic disorders include central nervous system stimulants, anticonvulsants, naltrexone, lithium, anxiolytics, and other treatments, but well-controlled, double-blind studies are lacking (Owley, 2002). The pathogenesis of autism is still unknown; one hypothesis suggests that in autistic children, the normal high brain serotonin synthesis capacity is somehow disrupted during early development (Chugani and Chugani, 2000), which might explain the beneficial effects of selective serotonin uptake inhibitors in some patients with autism (DeLong, 1999).

Although the cause of autism is not yet clear, genetic studies, including high concordance in monozygotic twins, strongly argue for the role of genetic abnormalities in the pathogenesis of this developmental disorder. One potential candidate gene involved in autism is the *CNTNAP2* gene on chromosome 7q35 that codes for contactin associated protein-like 2, a neurexin family member involved in myelination of axons (Alarcón et al., 2008; Arking et al., 2008; Bakkaloglu et al., 2008). Another locus implicated in the genetics of autism is on chromosome 16p13.1 (Ullmann et al., 2007).

Dysfunction of the frontal-parietal cortex, neostriatum, thalamus, and cerebellum in autistic patients has been suggested by various cerebral metabolic and imaging studies. MRI studies have found left frontal and brainstem atrophy in some autistic patients (Hashimoto et al., 1989), but other studies have failed to find any characteristic abnormalities on MRI scans of autistic children (Kleiman et al., 1992). More recent MRI studies have found white matter enlargement in patients with autism (Herbert et al., 2004). Other imaging studies have shown that autistic children have a reversal of asymmetry in frontal language-related cortex (De Fosse et al., 2004). Neuropathologic studies have not found consistent abnormalities, but most have found increased cell density and smaller neuronal size in the limbic system, decreased number of Purkinje cells in the cerebellum, and cerebellar cortical dysgenesis, but additional studies utilizing new techniques are needed before a consistent picture will emerge (Palmen et al., 2004).

Rett syndrome

Although the genes for most autistic disorders have yet to be identified, many researchers investigating the cause of autism believe that most of the "idiopathic" forms of autism are genetic in origin (Muhle et al., 2004; Chahrour and Zoghbi, 2007). Rett syndrome is an autistic disorder that occurs almost exclusively in girls and is manifested clinically by stereotypic movements and other movement disorders (Fitzgerald et al., 1990a; Percy, 2002; Roze et al., 2007; Temudo et al., 2008) (Videos 17.5 and 17.6). The prevalence of Rett syndrome has been reported to range between 1 in 10 000 and 1 in 28 000 (Kozinetz et al., 1993). In contrast to infantile autism and mental retardation, patients with Rett syndrome tend to have normal development until 6–18 months of age; this is then followed by gradual regression of both motor and language skills. Usually between the ages of 9 months and 3 years, there is a gradual social withdrawal and psychomotor regression with loss of acquired communication skills. Acquired finger and hand skills are gradually replaced by stereotypic hand movements, including hand clapping, wringing, clenching, washing, patting, rubbing, picking, and mouthing (Fitzgerald et al., 1990a; Temudo et al., 2008) (Figs 17.1 and 17.2). In an analysis of 83 patients with Rett syndrome, 53 with *MECP2* gene mutation, 62% had hand stereotypies, and in combination with bruxism, these features seemed to differentiate between Rett patients with and without mutation (Temudo et al., 2008). Among 12 girls with confirmed Rett syndrome 14 years old or older, the mean age at onset of stereotypies was 19.4 months consisting chiefly of hand repetitive movements, pill-rolling, mouthing, and twisting and these can persist into middle age (Vignoli et al., 2009),

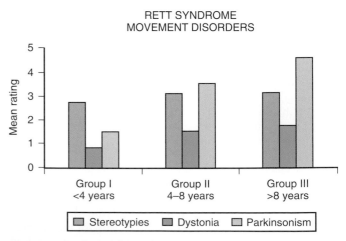

Figure 17.1 Diagnostic features associated with Rett syndrome. *From Fitzgerald PM, Jankovic J, Glaze DG, et al: Extrapyramidal involvement in Rett's syndrome. Neurology 1990;40:293–295.*

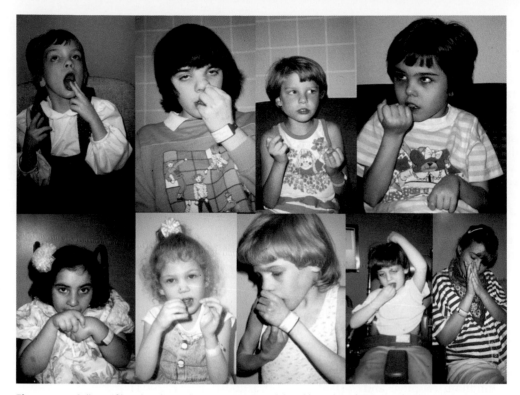

Figure 17.2 Collage of hand and mouthing stereotypies exhibited by girls with Rett syndrome.

but may evolve into parkinsonism in older age (Roze et al., 2007). Boys with *MECP2* duplication, in addition to autism, also manifested streotypies and choreic movements (Ramocki et al., 2009).

Besides hand stereotypies, girls with Rett syndrome often exhibit body-rocking movements and shifting of weight from one leg to the other. Although most girls with Rett syndrome are able to walk, they tend to walk on their toes; their gait is usually broad-based and apraxic and associated with retropulsion and loss of balance. Other motor disturbances include respiratory dysregulation with episodic hyperventilation and breath holding, bruxism, ocular deviations, dystonia, myoclonus, athetosis, tremor, jerky truncal and gait ataxia, and parkinsonian findings. In a study of 32 patients with Rett syndrome, aged 30 months to 28 years, Fitzgerald and colleagues (1990b) suggested that the occurrence of the different motor disorders seem to be age-related. The hyperkinetic disorders were more common in younger girls, while bradykinetic disorders seemed more prominent in the older ones. Although typically diagnosed in young girls, the diagnosis of Rett syndrome should be also considered in adult women with stereotypies and psychomotor retardation (Roze et al., 2007).

The pathophysiologic basis of the motor disturbances in Rett syndrome has not been fully elucidated (Akbarian, 2003). MRI studies have shown generalized brain and bilateral caudate atrophy (Reiss et al., 1993). Electroencephalographic recordings show age-related progressive deterioration characterized by slowing, loss of normal sleep characteristics, and the appearance of epileptiform activity. In a few postmortem examinations of brains of people with Rett syndrome, besides marked reduction in both gray and white matter volume, particularly involving the caudate nucleus (Subramaniam et al., 1997), some studies also found spongy degeneration of cerebral and cerebellar white matter, deposition of lipofuscin, and depigmentation of the substantia nigra and locus coeruleus (Hagberg, 1989). The various neuropathologic findings have been interpreted as a failure in the proper development or maintenance of synaptic connections. Since there is no evidence of a neurodegenerative process, there is a possibility of a therapeutic intervention that might not only alter the symptoms but also favorably modify the natural course of the disease.

The major advance in understanding the biology of Rett syndrome has come with the discovery of a gene that is responsible for most, but not all, cases of the Rett phenotype. Since the initial discovery of the gene in 1999 (Amir et al., 1999), loss-of-function mutations of the X-linked gene encoding methyl-CpG binding protein 2 (MECP2) have been found to be responsible for more than 80% of Rett cases (Akbarian, 2003). The phenotypic spectrum of *MECP2* mutations is broadening, and it includes not only the classic Rett syndrome but also Rett variants, mentally retarded males, and autistic children (Neul and Zoghbi, 2004). The function of the MECP2 protein is still unknown, but it is expressed ubiquitously in neurons and binds primarily, but not exclusively, to methylated DNA; it is thought to regulate gene expression, chromatin composition, and chromosomal architecture and might be important for maintenance of neuronal chromatin during late development and in adulthood. The MECP2 protein is expressed exclusively in neurons at the time when they are starting to form synapses. In the cerebellum, the Purkinje cells, which are born early, strongly express MECP2 soon after birth, but granule cells, which mature later, do not express the protein until several weeks after birth. Thus, the protein is not turned on until it is needed for the formation of synapses. Furthermore, selective knock-out of the gene in mice results in a Rett-like phenotype, including a reduction in brain atrophy and neuronal dystrophy. Rett syndrome appears to be a disorder of synapse formation and proliferation.

A broad range of mutations associated with MECP2 have been described involving not only girls and women but also males; they include a variety of autistic spectrum disorders, such as Angelman syndrome, learning disability, and fatal encephalopathy (Percy, 2002). Some *MECP2* mutations, such as p.R133C or p.R294X, are associated with milder symptoms and relatively late onset of neurologic manifestations, including stereotypies (Temudo et al., 2008, 2010; Fehr et al., 2010). Although stereotypies are sometimes present in patients with TS, Rosa and colleagues (2003) excluded mutations in the *MECP2* gene in a population of patients with TS.

Using a mouse heterozygous for a conditionally silenced *MECP2* gene, containing a stop cassette flanked by *loxP* sites, researchers are exploring potential therapeutic strategies in Rett syndrome. The animal model shares some clinical characteristics of Rett syndrome, including inertia, breathing abnormalities, gait abnormalities, hindlimb clasping, and weight gain between 4 and 12 months, which then stabilizes. Mice also expressed a Cre-recombinase enzyme linked to a tamoxifen receptor. When *MECP2* gene is activated in mice, symptoms such as breathing and mobility difficulties ceased. Over a 7-week period, the mice often became indistinguishable from healthy counterparts. When exposed to tamoxifen, Cre targeted the *loxP* sequences and removed the stop cassette, restoring expression of MECP2 (Guy et al., 2007). Tamoxifen appeared to reverse or prevent these symptoms. These findings suggest that gene therapy is a reachable goal in the treatment of Rett syndrome.

Other developmental genetic disorders

Patients with Williams syndrome, a hypersociable behavior associated with hemizygous 1.5 Mb deletion in chromosome band 7q11.23 that includes about 24–28 genes, such as elastin (*ELN*), *LIM kinase-1*, *RFC2*, *LIMK1*, and *CYLN2* genes, also can present with slow, complex, persistent head stereotypies (Doyle et al., 2004; Meyer-Lindenberg et al., 2006) (Video 17.7). There is also a suggestion that some of the stereotypic behavior in patients with Williams syndrome may be due to associated restless legs syndrome as many patients with Williams syndrome seem to have a frequent coexistence of periodic limb movement in sleep (Arens et al., 1998). Other developmental disorders associated with repetitive, stereotypic behaviors include Angelman, Cornelia de Lange, fragile X, Lowe, Prader–Willi, cri-du-chat, Smith–Magenis syndromes, and Primrose syndrome (Moss et al., 2009). Primrose syndrome consists of cognitive and motor delay, facial dysmorphism with enlarged and calcified external ears, cataracts, hearing impairment, spastic paraparesis with joint contractures, and distal muscle wasting in addition to motor tics, hand stereotypies, and self-flagellating behaviors (Dalal et al., 2010).

Schizophrenia and catatonia

Various stereotypies were described in schizophrenic patients long before neuroleptics were first introduced for the treatment of psychotic disorders. Since stereotypies in untreated childhood schizophrenia have not been well studied, the discussion of this topic is beyond the scope of this review (Ihara et al., 2002). In a study of 200 antipsychotic-naive patients with schizophrenia spectrum disorders a variety of abnormal involuntary movements, such as grimacing, stereotypies and abnormal blinking, were observed along with catatonia, echo-phenomena, catalepsy, and parkinsonism (Peralta et al., 2010).

Obsessive-compulsive disorder and tic disorders

Stereotypies can be encountered in various tic disorders, including TS and neuroacanthocytosis, both of which can be also associated with OCD. Neuroacanthocytosis and TS are discussed in Chapters 15 and 16, respectively; therefore, only a brief discussion of other tic disorders and OCD follows. Also, the reader is referred to recent reviews on this topic (Jankovic, 2001a, 2001b; Jenike, 2004).

Progression from a hyperkinetic to a bradykinetic movement disorder, as seen in Rett syndrome, may be also encountered in neuroacanthocytosis, another disorder that is manifested by stereotypic and self-injurious (e.g., lip and tongue biting) behavior. Symptoms usually first begin in the third and fourth decades but may start during childhood, with lip and tongue biting followed by orolingual ("eating") dystonia, motor and phonic tics, generalized chorea, distal and body stereotypies, parkinsonism, vertical ophthalmoparesis, and seizures. Other features include cognitive and personality changes, dysphagia, dysarthria, amyotrophy, areflexia, evidence of axonal neuropathy, and elevated serum creatine kinase without evidence of myopathy. Besides movement disorders, other associated features included dysarthria; absent or reduced reflexes; dementia; psychiatric problems, such as depression, anxiety, and OCD; dysphagia; seizures; muscle weakness and wasting; and elevated creatine phosphokinase. Magnetic resonance volumetry and fluorodeoxyglucose PET show striatal atrophy in patients with neuroacanthocytosis (Jung et al., 2001).

Although autosomal dominant, X-linked-recessive, and sporadic forms of neuroacanthocytosis have been reported, the majority of the reported families indicate autosomal recessive inheritance. Genome-wide scan for linkage in 11 families with autosomal recessive inheritance showed a linkage to a marker on chromosome 9q21, indicating a single locus for the disease. Sequencing has identified a polyadenylation site with a protein with 3096 amino acid residues, which has been named chorein, and subsequent studies have identified multiple mutations in the *CHAC* gene (Rampoldi et al., 2001).

OCD is a psychiatric disorder that is frequently accompanied by stereotypic movements (Jenike, 2004). Foot tapping, crossing and uncrossing the legs, tapping fingers on a chair arm, and similar stereotypic behaviors may be associated with obsessive-compulsive symptoms (Niehaus et al., 2000).

OCD was once considered a rare psychiatric disorder, but recent epidemiologic studies indicate that the lifetime prevalence of OCD is approximately 2.5% (Snider and Swedo, 2000). Compulsions might be difficult to differentiate from stereotypies. In contrast to stereotypies, compulsions are usually preceded by or associated with feelings of inner tension or anxiety and a need to perform the same act repeatedly in the same manner. Examples of compulsions are ritualistic hand washing; repetitively touching the same place; evening up; and arranging and checking doors, locks, and appliances. Reports of focal striatal lesions giving rise to severe OCD and the frequent association of OCD with basal ganglia disorders such as TS, Parkinson disease, and Sydenham disease (Church et al., 2002; Kwak and Jankovic, 2002) provide additional support for the link between abnormal behavior, such as OCD, and extrapyramidal dysfunction (Cummings, 1993; Rosario-Campos et al., 2001).

Other stereotypies

It is well known that stereotypies often accompany a variety of behavioral disorders, such as anxiety, obsessive-compulsive disorders (OCD), TS, schizophrenia, autism, mental retardation, akathisia, restless legs syndrome, and a variety of neurodegenerative disorders, including frontotemporal dementia (Nyatsanza et al., 2003; Mateen and Josephs, 2009; Singer, 2009), neuroferritinopathy (Ondo et al., 2010), and postinfectious disorders such as subacute sclerosing panencephalitis (SSPE) (Jankovic et al., 1998) (Video 17.8).

Akathisia – a combination of restless movements that resemble complex stereotypies, such as hair and face rubbing, picking at clothes, crossing and uncrossing legs, adduction-abduction and up-and-down leg pumping, sitting down and standing up, marching in place, pacing and shifting weight, and feelings of restlessness – is typically a manifestation of tardive dyskinesia but may be also seen in patients with Parkinson disease, in patients with various forms of mental retardation and autism (Bodfish et al., 1997), and as part of tardive dyskinesia (see below) (Video 17.9).

In some individuals, particularly those who abuse amphetamines or cocaine and in patients with Parkinson disease taking levodopa and particularly dopamine agonists, certain stereotypic behaviors, called punding, are seen (Fernandez and Friedman, 1999; Evans et al., 2004; Stamey and Jankovic, 2008; Voon et al., 2009; Brust, 2010). These include compulsive sorting of objects, nail polishing, shoe shining, hair dressing, and intense fascination with repetitive handling and examining of mechanical objects, such as picking at oneself or taking apart watches and radios, or sorting and arranging of common objects, such as lining up pebbles, rocks, or other small objects. This stereotypic behavior has not been previously described in children, even in those taking central nervous system stimulants for ADHD, although no studies specifically designed to study punding in children have been reported.

Tardive dyskinesia

Repetitive and patterned movements, phenomenologically identical to stereotypy, are characteristically seen in patients with tardive dyskinesia (Jankovic, 1995; Mejia and Jankovic, 2010). All types of movement disorders, including parkinsonism, tremor, chorea, dystonia, tics, myoclonus, and stereotypy, can result from the use of dopamine receptor-blocking drugs (neuroleptics) both acutely and chronically (tardive). See Chapter 19 in this volume for a detailed review. The most typical form of tardive dyskinesia, the orofacial-lingual-masticatory movement, is one of the best examples of a stereotypic movement disorder (Miller and Jankovic, 1990). Tardive dystonia tends to occur more frequently in younger patients, although it is quite rare in children. Tardive stereotypy is more typically observed in middle-aged or elderly patients, particularly women, and this is a very rare complication in children. However, there is a report of a 1-year-old girl who developed orofacial-lingual stereotypy at age 2 months after a 17-day treatment with metoclopramide for gastroesophageal reflux (Mejia and Jankovic, 2005; Pasricha et al., 2006; Kenney et al., 2008). The stereotypy, documented by sequential videos, persisted for at least 9 months after the drug was discontinued. This patient, perhaps the first documented case of tardive dyskinesia in an infant, draws attention to the possibility that this disorder is frequently unrecognized in young children.

Although with the advent of atypical neuroleptics, the incidence of tardive dyskinesia was thought to markedly decrease, there are a growing number of reports of tardive dyskinesia in patients, including children, treated with atypical (second and third generation) neuroleptics (Mejia and Jankovic, 2010; Peña et al., 2011). Campbell and colleagues (1997), in their 15-year-long prospective double-blind, placebo-controlled study of autistic children exposed to haloperidol reported that tardive dyskinesia developed in 9 of 118 children (7.6%) (Campbell et al., 1997).

In a comprehensive review of 702 patients reported in 17 studies of children exposed to dopamine receptor blocking drugs, 69 (9.8%) patients, 60% of whom were female, had tardive dyskinesia (Mejia and Jankovic, 2010). The children were treated with the neuroleptics for various psychiatric conditions ($n = 463$, 65.9%), autism ($n = 118$, 16.8%), mental retardation ($n = 116$, 16.5%), TS ($n = 5$, 0.7%), and gastro-esophageal reflux disease (GERD; $n = 2$, 0.3%). The phenomenology of tardive dyskinesia consisted chiefly of orofacial stereotypies with or without dystonic or choreic movements of the trunk and limbs.

The most important step in the management of tardive dyskinesia is prevention. Dopamine receptor-blocking drugs, particularly the typical neuroleptics, should be used only if other drugs do not adequately control the behavior or neurologic disorder, such as TS. Although the risk of tardive dyskinesia is highest in the elderly population, the causative drugs should be avoided whenever possible, even in children. Atypical antipsychotics might be better alternative medications with less risk of causing tardive dyskinesia, but even the atypicals have been reported to cause tardive dyskinesia (Peña et al., 2011). Drugs that have been found to be useful in the treatment of tardive dyskinesia include clonazepam and other benzodiazepines and dopamine depletors such as tetrabenazine (Jankovic and Beach, 1997; Vuong et al., 2004; Kenney and Jankovic, 2006). Beta-blockers and opioids have also been found effective in some patients with akathisia. Antidepressant citalopram was not found to be effective in children with repetitive behaviors associated with autism (King et al., 2009).

Treatment

Treatment of stereotypies is quite challenging . In addition to behavioral therapy (Miller et al., 2006), some patients benefit from pharmacologic therapy targeted to relieve associated comorbidities, such as anxiety, OCD, and impulse control problems. In addition, tetrabenazine has been found to be very effective in the treatment of the involuntary repetitive movements (Kenney and Jankovic, 2006). Pharmacologic treatment of tardive stereotypies is covered in more detail in Chapter 19.

References available on Expert Consult: www.expertconsult.com

CHAPTER **18**

Tremors

Chapter contents

Introduction	389	Kinetic tremors	407
Assessment of tremors	391	Pathophysiologic mechanisms of rest and action tremors	408
Rest tremors	391	Other tremors	412
Postural tremors	394	Appendix	414

Introduction

Tremor is a rhythmic, oscillatory movement produced by alternating or synchronous contractions of antagonist muscles. It is the most common form of involuntary movement, but only a small fraction of those who shake will seek medical attention. Indeed, in one epidemiologic study of normal controls, 96% were found to have clinically detectable postural tremor, and 28% had a postural tremor of "moderate amplitude" (Louis et al., 1998e).

Tremors can be classified according to their phenomenology, distribution, frequency, or etiology (Hallett, 1991; Lou and Jankovic, 1991a; Bain, 1993; Findley, 1993; Deuschl et al., 1998a; Jankovic, 2000; Deuschl et al., 2001; Jankovic and Lang, 2008; Deuschl and Elble, 2009). Phenomenologically, tremors are divided into two major categories: rest tremors and action tremors (Table 18.1). Rest tremor is present when the affected body part is fully supported against gravity and not actively contracting; rest tremor is diminished or absent during voluntary muscle contraction and during movement. Action tremors occur with voluntary contraction of muscles, and they can be subdivided into postural, kinetic, task-specific or position-specific, and isometric tremors. Postural tremor is evident during maintenance of an antigravity posture, such as holding the arms in an outstretched horizontal position in front of the body. Some parkinsonian patients exhibit postural tremor that emerges after a latency of a few seconds. This tremor, referred to here as reemergent tremor, probably represents a rest tremor that has been "reset" during posture holding (Jankovic et al., 1999) (Fig. 18.1). The relationship of this reemergent tremor to the typical rest tremor is supported by the observation that this reemergent repose tremor shares many characteristics with the typical rest tremor; it has the same 3–6 Hz frequency, and it also responds to dopaminergic therapy

(Video 18.1). Kinetic tremor can be seen when the voluntary movement starts (initial tremor), during the course of the movement (dynamic tremor), and as the affected body part approaches the target, such as while performing the finger-to-nose or the toe-to-finger maneuver (terminal tremor, also called intention tremor). Task-specific tremors occur only during, or are markedly exacerbated by, a certain task, such as while writing (primary handwriting tremor) (Video 18.2), while speaking or singing (voice tremor) (Rosenbaum and Jankovic, 1988; Soland et al., 1996b), or while smiling (Schwingenschuh et al., 2009). Besides writing, task specific tremors may be triggered during other activities, such as while playing golf, particularly when putting (Video 18.3). Position-specific tremors occur while holding a certain posture (e.g., the "wing-beating" position or holding a spoon or a cup close to the mouth). One example of a task- or position-specific tremor is the tremor that occurs in performing the dot test ("dot approximation test"), during which the subject, seated at the desk with elbow elevated to a 90° shoulder abduction, is asked to hold the tip of the pen as close as possible to a dot on a horizontal paper without touching the dot. Patients with essential tremor (ET), to be discussed later, or other action tremors usually exhibit exacerbation of the tremor during this specific task. A variant of this tremor occurs in performing the modified finger–nose–finger test, during which the subject stands in front of a paper mounted on a wall and is asked to mark the center of the drawn target and to make a mark with a felt-tipped pen five times (Louis et al., 2005a). Isometric tremor occurs during a voluntary contraction of muscles that is not accompanied by a change in position of the body part, such as maintaining of a tightly squeezed fist or while standing (e.g., orthostatic tremor; see later). 📹

Tremors can be also classified according to their anatomic distribution – for example, head, tongue, voice, and trunk. Orolingual tremors include physiologic, essential, task- and

Table 18.1 Classification and differential diagnosis of tremors

A. Rest tremors

1. Parkinson disease (PD)

2. Other parkinsonian syndromes

a. Multiple system atrophies (SND, SDS, OPCA)

b. Progressive supranuclear palsy

c. Cortical-basal-ganglionic degeneration

d. Parkinsonism–dementia–ALS of Guam

e. Diffuse Lewy body disease

f. Progressive pallidal atrophy

3. Heredodegenerative disorders

a. Huntington disease

b. Wilson disease

c. Neuroacanthocytosis

d. NBIA1 (Neurodegeneration with brain iron accumulation 1)

e. Gerstmann–Sträussler–Scheinker disease

f. Ceroid lipofuscinosis

4. Secondary parkinsonism

a. Toxic: MPTP, CO, Mn, methanol, cyanide, CS_2

b. Drug-induced: dopamine receptor blocking drugs neuroleptics ("rabbit syndrome"), dopamine-depleting drugs (reserpine, tetrabenazine), lithium, valproate, amiodarone, flunarizine, cinnarizine

c. Vascular: multi-infarct, Binswanger disease, "lower body parkinsonism"

d. Trauma: pugilistic encephalopathy, midbrain injury

e. Tumor and paraneoplastic

f. Infectious: postencephalitic, fungal, AIDS, subacute sclerosing panencephalitis, Creutzfeldt–Jakob disease

g. Metabolic: hypoparathyroidism, chronic hepatic degeneration, mitochondrial cytopathies

h. Normal pressure hydrocephalus

5. Severe essential tremor (ET)

6. Midbrain (rubral) tremor

7. Tardive tremor

8. Myorhythmia

9. Spasmus nutans

B. Action tremors

1. Postural tremors

a. Physiologic tremor

b. Enhanced physiologic tremor:

(1) Stress-induced: emotion, exercise, fatigue, anxiety, fever

(2) Endocrine: hypoglycemia, thyrotoxicosis, pheochromocytoma, adrenocorticosteroids

(3) Drugs: β-agonists (e.g., theophylline, terbutaline, epinephrine), dopaminergic drugs (levodopa, dopamine agonists), stimulants (amphetamines), psychiatric drugs (lithium, neuroleptics, tricyclics), methylxanthines (coffee, tea), valproate, amiodarone, cyclosporine, interferon

(4) Toxins: Hg, Pb, As, Bi, Br, alcohol withdrawal

c. Essential tremor

(1) Autosomal dominant

(2) Sporadic

d. Postural tremor associated with

(1) Dystonia

(2) Parkinsonism

(3) Myoclonus

(4) Hereditary motor-sensory neuropathy (Roussy–Levy)

(5) Kennedy syndrome (X-linked spinobulbar atrophy)

e. PD and other parkinsonian syndromes

f. Tardive tremor

g. Midbrain (rubral) tremor

h. Cerebellar hypotonic tremor (titubation)

i. Neuropathic tremor: motor neuron disease, peripheral neuropathy, peripheral nerve injury, reflex sympathetic dystrophy

2. Kinetic (intention, dynamic, termination) tremors

a. Cerebellar disorders (cerebellar outflow): multiple sclerosis, trauma, stroke, Wilson disease, drugs and toxins

b. Midbrain lesions

3. Task- or position-specific tremors

a. Handwriting

b. Orthostatic

c. Other (e.g., occupational) task-specific tremors

4. Isometric

a. Muscular contraction during sustained exertion

C. Miscellaneous tremors and other rhythmic movements

1. Myoclonus: rhythmical segmental myoclonus (e.g., palatal), oscillatory myoclonus, asterixis, mini-polymyoclonus

2. Dystonic tremors

3. Cortical tremors

4. Epilepsia partialis continua

5. Nystagmus

6. Clonus

7. Fasciculation

8. Shivering

9. Shuddering attacks

10. Head bobbing (third ventricular cysts)

11. Aortic insufficiency with head titubation

position-specific, dystonic, orthostatic, parkinsonian, palatal (also termed palatal myoclonus), drug-induced, hereditary, and psychogenic (Erer and Jankovic, 2007; Silverdale et al., 2008). Because of the complexity of limb tremors, it is best to describe them according to the joint about which the oscillation is most evident – for example, metacarpal-phalangeal joints, wrist, elbow, and ankle tremor. In most tremors, the frequency ranges between 4 and 10 Hz, but the cerebellar tremors may be slower, with a frequency of 2–3 Hz. The "slow" tremors (frequency: 1–3 Hz) are sometimes referred to as myorhythmia and are usually associated with brainstem pathology (Masucci et al., 1984; Cardoso and Jankovic, 1996; Tan et al., 2007a). The "fast" tremors (frequency: 11–20 Hz) may be distinct tremor disorders,

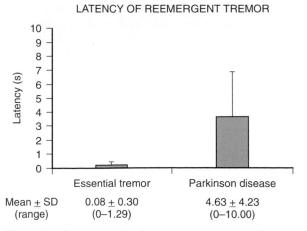

LATENCY OF REEMERGENT TREMOR

	Essential tremor	Parkinson disease
Mean ± SD	0.08 ± 0.30	4.63 ± 4.23
(range)	(0–1.29)	(0–10.00)

Figure 18.1 Rest tremor of Parkinson disease reemerges after a latency when arms are outstretched or in a wing-beating position.

such as orthostatic tremor, or may represent harmonics of other tremors. The clinical characteristics of tremors provide the most important clues to their etiology (Table 18.1).

Assessment of tremors

There have been many attempts to quantitate tremor, but it is not apparent whether electromyographic (EMG), accelerometric, or other methods of measuring tremor correlate with clinical rating scales. Indeed, one study suggested that assessments of spirography and handwriting correlate better with overall functional tremor-related disability than electrophysiologic methods (Bain et al., 1993). However, because the physiologic measurements and the clinical ratings were not performed simultaneously and because of other technical problems, interpretation of the study is difficult. Elble and colleagues (1996) described the use of a digitizing tablet in quantification of tremor during writing and drawing. Although relatively good inter-trial correlations were obtained with this method, the tablet does not capture the speed of writing or the amount of effort exerted by the patient in an attempt to control the tremor while writing. One study found high inter-observer reliability using a diagnostic protocol for ET (Louis et al., 1998a). The investigators also found high specificity and sensitivity of a screening questionnaire when compared to the physician's examination in patients with definite and probable ET, but actual examination of the subjects is necessary to detect mild ET (Louis et al., 1998b). In another study, the authors concluded that when a limited number of tests are available in large epidemiologic surveys, a test such as the finger–nose maneuver may be used to screen populations for ET, whereas to exclude normal subjects, the spiral drawing test, water pouring test, or arm extension test may be utilized (Louis et al., 1999a). A performance-based test for ET has been validated and compared to other measures of tremor (Louis et al., 1999b). Although this performance-based test was thought to objectively assess functional capacity in patients with ET, the test seems somewhat cumbersome to perform because it requires a variety of props, such as a milk carton, a glass, a soup spoon, a bowl, a saucer, a wallet, coins, an

electrical socket, a thread and needle, a strip of buttons, and a telephone. Using other instruments, the modified Klove–Matthews Motor Steadiness Battery and the Nine-Hole Steadiness Tester, Louis and colleagues (2000c) showed that these portable instruments provide a reliable and valid means of collecting objective quantitative data on tremor severity. A Tremor Disability Questionnaire has been developed and found to reliably correlate with multiple measures of tremor severity (Louis et al., 2000a). Another screening instrument for ET, consisting of seven items and a spiral drawing, has been found to have 70.5% sensitivity, 68.2% specificity, and 64.9% positive predictive value (Lorenz et al., 2008). A simple, user-friendly clinical tool, with even higher sensitivity, specificity and predictive value, is needed to assess tremors in the clinic and in the field. A teaching videotape for assessment of ET was developed to improve the uniform application of the Washington Heights–Inwood Genetic Study of Essential Tremor (Louis et al., 2001a). Using a clinical evaluation (interview and videotaped examination) and an electrophysiologic evaluation (quantitative computerized tremor analysis using accelerometry and EMG), Louis and Pullman (2001) found a very high concordance rate between the two methods in 51 of 54 (94%) subjects, suggesting that using either technique would arrive at a similar diagnosis. Although not yet validated, the Unified Tremor Rating Assessment developed by the Tremor Research Group has been used in a number of clinical, therapeutic trials (Bain, 1993; Jankovic et al., 1996). The other scale that has been used in several tremor studies is the Fahn–Tolosa–Marin Tremor Rating Scale (TRS) (Fahn et al., 1993). While the inter-rater reliability of this scale is relatively poor, there is a good consistency, with average Spearman correlation of 0.87, when the same rater repeatedly assesses the tremor (Stacy et al., 2007). Using the TRS, Putzke et al. (2006) showed that the total score increased by about 2 points during prospective follow-up of patients with ET over a mean of 3.6 years and that older age, longer duration of disease, and asymmetric onset of tremor were associated with increased tremor severity. Another tremor rating scale, the Tremor Research Group (TRG) Essential Tremor Rating Scale (TETRAS), is currently being validated against the TRS (Elble et al., 2008). The TETRAS has been found to correlate well with quantitative assessments using the Kinesia™ (CleveMed) system (Mostile et al., 2010). Any assessment of tremor must take into account minute-to-minute and hour-to-hour amplitude variability (Koller and Royse, 1985), and potential provocations, such as voluntary isometric contraction in the case of action tremors and walking and counting backwards in the case of rest tremor (Raethjen et al., 2008).

Rest tremors

Diagnosis

Rest tremor is most typically present in patients with Parkinson disease (PD). In one study, all 34 patients with pathologically proven cases of idiopathic (Lewy body) parkinsonism demonstrated typical rest tremor sometime during the course of their illness (Rajput et al., 1991). Although this study suggests that parkinsonian patients who do not exhibit rest tremor probably do not have idiopathic parkinsonism (PD), another study, involving 100 pathologically proven cases of PD, found that 32% of all patients apparently never manifested tremor during the course of their disease (Hughes et al., 1993).

Several studies have suggested that the natural course of PD is in part related to the presence or absence of tremor (Hughes et al., 1993). The tremor-dominant PD may be associated with earlier age at onset, less cognitive decline, and slower progression than the type of PD that is dominated by postural instability and gait difficulty (PIGD) (Jankovic et al., 1990). Clinical-pathologic correlations are needed to answer the question as to whether the tremor-dominant form and the PIGD-dominant form represent different diseases or merely variants of one disease, namely, PD. In support of the former is the finding that only 27% of patients with the PIGD form of idiopathic parkinsonism had Lewy bodies at autopsy (Rajput et al., 1993). In another clinical-pathologic study, Hirsch and colleagues (1992) demonstrated that patients with PD and prominent tremor have degeneration of a subgroup of midbrain (A8) neurons, whereas this area is spared in PD patients without tremor. This observation supports the hypothesis that differential damage of subpopulations of neuronal systems is responsible for the diversity of phenotypes seen in PD and other parkinsonian disorders. It is unclear whether the occasional patients with long-standing unilateral tremor and minimal or no other parkinsonian findings have a benign form of PD, as is suggested by positron emission tomography (PET) scans showing low fluorodopa uptake in the contralateral putamen (Brooks et al., 1992), or whether this condition represents a separate disease entity. In contrast to patients with the PIGD form of PD, patients with tremor-dominant PD have increased metabolic activity in the pons, thalamus, and motor association cortices (Antonini et al., 1998). When rest tremors involve the fingers, hands, lips, jaw, and tongue in the same individual, they share a common frequency, suggesting that they are of central origin (Hunker and Abbs, 1990). This pattern, however, changes during sleep in that non-rapid eye movement sleep transforms the alternating tremor that is typically seen in the awake patient into subclinical repetitive muscle contractions of variable frequency and duration during sleep stages I to IV, and the tremor disappears during rapid eye movement sleep (Askenasy and Yahr, 1990).

Rest tremor has other causes besides PD and related parkinsonian disorders (see Table 18.1). Patients with severe ET may have tremor at rest and prominent kinetic tremor. It is not known whether the ET patients with rest tremor have associated PD, whether they later develop other features of PD, or whether the rest tremor is a feature of ET (Jankovic, 1989; Shahed and Jankovic, 2007). Some patients with lesions in the cerebellar outflow pathways, particularly in the superior cerebellar peduncle near the red nucleus (cerebellar outflow, midbrain or "rubral" tremor, also referred to as Holmes tremor), also have tremor at rest, probably due to an interruption of the nigrostriatal pathway (Remy et al., 1995). This irregular, slow (2–5 Hz), predominantly unilateral tremor may be associated with other neurologic signs, such as ataxia, bradykinesia, and ophthalmoplegia. It is often associated with midbrain pathology, such as multiple sclerosis, stroke, tumor, or arteriovenous malformation (Lee et al., 2008). It rarely responds to any medical therapy, but

wrist weights, levodopa, dopamine agonists, amantadine, propranolol, clonazepam, isoniazid, and levetiracetam (Ferlazzo et al., 2008) may be effective in reducing the amplitude of this, often disabling, tremor. The affected arm or leg may be also ataxic and may be associated with third nerve palsy (Benedikt syndrome) (Video 18.4). The cerebellar outflow tremor is most often caused by trauma, stroke, multiple sclerosis, and Wilson disease (Lou and Jankovic, 1993; Krauss et al., 1995; Miwa et al., 1996; Alarcon et al., 2004). Strokes involving the posterior circulation may involve the thalamus, producing slow (1–3 Hz) rest and postural tremors, sometimes referred to as myorhythmia (Masucci et al., 1984; Cardoso and Jankovic, 1996; Miwa et al., 1996).

Myorhythmia is a slow (1–3 Hz) frequency, continuous or intermittent, relatively rhythmic movement that is present at rest but may persist during activity (Masucci et al., 1984; Cardoso and Jankovic, 1996). It may be associated with palatal myoclonus, and it disappears with sleep. Except for the slower frequency, the presence of flexion–extension rather than the typical supination–pronation pattern, and the absence of associated parkinsonian findings, myorhythmia resembles a parkinsonian tremor. In the cases that were examined at autopsy, the sites of maximum pathology involved chiefly the brainstem (particularly the substantia nigra and the inferior olive) and the cerebellum. The etiology for myorhythmia includes brainstem stroke, cerebellar degeneration, Wilson disease, and Whipple disease (Masucci et al., 1984; Tison et al., 1992; Cardoso and Jankovic, 1996).

Palatal myoclonus, sometimes referred to as palatal tremor, has some features of tremor, but in contrast to tremor which is produced by alternating or synchronous contractions of antagonist muscles, the palatal movement is produced by rhythmical contractions of agonist muscles, hence the term myoclonus is preferred despite the arguments raised against this nosology (Zadikoff et al., 2006). Palatal myoclonus, a form of segmental myoclonus, is manifested by rhythmical contractions of the soft palate resulting from acute or chronic lesions involving the Guillain–Mollaret triangle linking dentate nucleus with the red nucleus via the central tegmental tract to the inferior olivary nucleus. Symptomatic palatal myoclonus (SPM) usually persists during sleep, while essential palatal myoclonus (EPM), frequently associated with an ear-clicking sound, disappears with sleep. In EPM the muscle agonist is the tensor veli palatini, which opens the eustachian tube and is innervated by the trigeminal nerve. In SPM the palatal movement is due to contractions of the levator veli palatini, innervated by the facial nucleus and nucleus ambiguus. When the tensor muscle contracts, as in EPM, the entire soft palate moves, whereas only the edges of the soft palate move when the levator muscle contracts in SPM. Symptomatic, but not essential, palatal myoclonus is often associated with hypertrophy of the inferior olive (Goyal et al., 2000). SPM has been associated with a variety of lesions involving the brainstem as well as some neurodegenerative disorders such as Alexander disease (Pareyson et al., 2008).

Treatment with neuroleptics can also cause persistent tremor, referred to as tardive tremor (Stacy and Jankovic, 1992). This rest, postural, and kinetic tremor, with a frequency of 3–5 Hz, is aggravated by, and persists after, neuroleptic withdrawal and improves after treatment with the dopamine-depleting drug tetrabenazine. The tremor may be accompanied by other tardive movement disorders, including akathisia, chorea, dystonia, myoclonus, and stereotypy. There is usually no family history or other explanation for the tremor.

Spasmus nutans is characterized by the triad of nystagmus, abnormal head position, and irregular, multidirectional head nodding that disappears during sleep. This self-limited and often familial condition is first noted between the ages of 4 and 12 months, and it usually disappears within a year or two. Another oculomotor cause of head tremor is "head-shaking nystagmus" seen in patients with lateral medullary infarction (Choi et al., 2007). The 2–3 Hz horizontal head shaking has been postulated to be caused by unilateral impairment of nodulo-uvular inhibition of the velocity storage.

Treatment

The treatment of rest tremors is similar to that of parkinsonism (Jankovic and Marsden, 1998; also see Chapter 6). Secondary and potentially curable causes should be excluded, particularly when there are associated features to suggest disorders other than PD (see Table 18.1). Anticholinergic and dopaminergic drugs provide the most effective relief of rest tremors. Clozapine, an atypical neuroleptic that does not significantly exacerbate parkinsonism but can cause potentially serious side effects such as agranulocytosis, has been shown to be effective in the treatment of parkinsonian tremor (and ET) (Bonuccelli et al., 1997; Friedman et al., 1997; Ceravolo et al., 1999). Ethosuximide, an anticonvulsant that blocks low-threshold Ca^{2+} conductance in the thalamus, has been shown to reduce tremor in MPTP monkeys and to potentiate the effects of a D2 agonist (Gomez-Mancilla et al., 1992). However, ethosuximide was found ineffective in a pilot study of six PD patients with drug-resistant tremor (Pourcher et al., 1992). Mirtazapine (Remeron), a novel antidepressant that enhances noradrenergic and serotonergic transmission and acts as a presynaptic alpha-2, 5-HT$_2$, and 5-HT$_3$ receptor antagonist, has been reported to improve rest tremor (Pact and Giduz, 1999). Other drugs reported to have a possible beneficial effect in patients with ET include mirtazapine, clozapine, sodium oxybate, dimethoxymethyl-diphenyl-barbituric acid (T-2000), and carisbamate (Lyons and Pahwa, 2008). High-amplitude parkinsonian tremors and rest tremors caused by disorders other than PD usually do not improve with pharmacologic therapy. In some cases, botulinum toxin (BTX) injections in the involved muscles produce a satisfactory reduction in the tremor amplitude (Jankovic and Schwartz, 1991; Jankovic et al., 1996; Hou and Jankovic, 2002). A multicenter, randomized, double-blind, controlled trial confirmed the results of an earlier study (Jankovic et al., 1996) that BTX injections produce significant reduction in the postural hand tremor of ET and modest functional improvement (Brin et al., 2001). By avoiding injections of the forearm extensor muscles we prevent finger extensor weakness, a relatively frequent complication reported in the earlier studies (Pacchetti et al., 2000).

Ventral lateral thalamotomy, particularly involving the ventral intermediate nucleus of the thalamus (VIM), was considered the neurosurgical treatment of choice for

disabling, drug-resistant tremors until the later 1980s when the ablative procedure was replaced by high-frequency deep brain (thalamic) stimulation (DBS) (Benabid et al., 1991; Fox et al., 1991; Jankovic et al., 1995b). Although effective in a majority of cases, the tremor recurs in about 20% of patients, and there is a considerable risk of contralateral hemiparesis, hemianesthesia, ataxia, speech disturbance, and other potential complications. These are compounded when the procedure is performed bilaterally. Thalamic DBS is now the surgical treatment of choice for patients with disabling tremors (Deiber et al., 1993; Benabid et al., 1996; Pahwa and Koller, 2001; Ondo et al., 2001a, 2001b; Pahwa et al., 2006) (see also Chapter 7). This technique has been proposed for chronic treatment of parkinsonian, essential, and other tremors. Using high-frequency (100 Hz) stimulation, with the tip of a monopolar electrode implanted stereotactically in the VIM contralateral to the disabling tremor, Benabid and colleagues (1991) noted "complete relief" of contralateral tremor in 27 of 43 (63%) thalami that were stimulated and "major improvement" in 11 (23%). The series included 26 patients with PD and 6 with ET, 7 of whom had previously been treated with thalamotomy. The benefit of thalamic stimulation was maintained for up to 29 months (mean follow-up: 13 months). The results were similar in their subsequent report of long-term effects of chronic VIM stimulation in 117 patients, 74 of whom had bilateral implantation (Benabid et al., 1996). The most robust tremor suppression was noted in patients with PD (n = 80); but patients with ET (n = 20) also benefited, although 18.5% deteriorated with time. Dysarthria and ataxia still occurred, but the patients were able to adjust the intensity of stimulation to ameliorate these side effects, though at the expense of increased tremor. Nevertheless, the investigators felt that the reversible nature of the side effects was the chief advantage of DBS over the permanent lesion produced by thalamotomy. To compare thalamic DBS with thalamotomy, Schuurman and colleagues (2000) conducted a prospective, randomized study of 68 patients with PD, 13 with ET, and 10 with multiple sclerosis. They found that the functional status improved more in the DBS group than in the thalamotomy group, and tremor was suppressed completely or almost completely in 30 of 33 (90.9%) patients in the DBS group and in 27 of 34 (79.4%) patients in the thalamotomy group. Although one patient in the DBS group died after an intracerebral hemorrhage, DBS was associated with significantly fewer complications than was thalamotomy. This procedure may be also advantageous in elderly patients and when bilateral effects are desirable (Blond et al., 1992). We found that bilateral thalamic DBS is more effective than unilateral DBS in controlling bilateral appendicular and midline tremors of ET and PD, and thalamic DBS does not seem to improve meaningfully any parkinsonian symptoms other than tremor (Ondo et al., 2001a). In addition, we found that VIM DBS produces modest improvement, rather than tremor augmentation as previously suggested, in ipsilateral tremor in patients with ET (Ondo et al., 2001b). A review of long-term efficacy of VIM DBS in 39 patients (20 with PD and 19 with ET) showed that the benefits may be maintained for at least 6 months (Rehncrona et al., 2003). In one of our patients, minimal foreign body reaction and gliosis around the electrodes was found 12 years after implantation, the longest reported follow-up with autopsy examination after DBS, supporting the long-term safety of DBS (DiLorenzo et al., 2010).

In addition to improving distal tremor associated with PD and ET, VIM DBS can effectively control ET head tremor, which usually does not respond to conventional therapy (Koller et al., 1999). Other midline tremors, such as voice, tongue, and face tremor, also may improve with unilateral VIM DBS, although additional benefit can be achieved with contralateral surgery (Obwegeser et al., 2000). The risk of local gliosis with chronic stimulation of the thalamus is minimal (Caparros-Lefebvre et al., 1994). Unfortunately, thalamic stimulation does not appear to be as effective in patients with predominantly kinetic and axial tremors, and it does not improve other parkinsonian features such as bradykinesia, rigidity, and levodopa-related motor complications. Furthermore, while VIM DBS is very effective in improving PD tremor, when performed bilaterally it is often associated with dysarthria and postural and gait abnormality (Pahwa et al., 2006) as a result of which the subthalamic nucleus (STN) has been suggested as a more appropriate target in PD patients with severe tremor (Limousin et al., 1998; Benabid et al., 2000; Diamond et al., 2007; Fishman, 2008). The mechanism of action of DBS is unknown, but "jamming" of low-frequency oscillatory inputs has been suggested as a possible mechanism for the antitremor effects of DBS. Regional cerebral blood flow, measured by PET scan, demonstrated that tremor suppression was associated with decreased cerebellar blood flow and, presumably, decreased synaptic activity in the cerebellum (Deiber et al., 1993).

In 1992, Laitinen of Stockholm, Sweden, reported the results of 90 pallidotomies in 86 patients with severe PD (Laitinen et al., 1992). The external, posteroventral portion of the medial globus pallidus interna (GPi) was the intended target for the stereotactically placed lesion. Nearly all patients had "marked improvement in tremor and akinesia." In addition, some patients apparently also noted improvement in their gait, speech, and pain. Only two patients suffered permanent visual field defect, and one had "minor stroke with hemiparesis." Several pallidotomy series have since confirmed the beneficial effects of pallidotomy on various parkinsonian symptoms, including tremor (Jankovic and Marsden, 1998). These results provide support for the notion that the GPi is "hyperactive" in PD and that surgical or chemical lesions of these structures may have a therapeutic value not only in controlling tremor but also in improving bradykinesia (Bergman et al., 1990; Aziz et al., 1991). Although some investigators (Subramanian et al., 1995) have suggested that posteroventral pallidotomy is as effective as thalamotomy in controlling parkinsonian tremor, others (Dogali et al., 1995) feel that pallidotomy provides only partial relief of tremor.

Postural tremors

Diagnosis and clinical features

Physiologic tremor

Normal and enhanced physiologic tremors are the most common forms of postural tremor, but they rarely require medical attention. Postural tremors are clinically similar despite different etiologies. In contrast to ET, the frequency of physiologic tremor can be slowed by mass loading (Elble and Koller, 1990). Indeed, there appear to be two components to physiologic tremor: variable frequency (peak: 8 Hz), which is dependent on loading, and consistent frequency (peak: 10 Hz), which is independent of peripheral influence. The latter suggests central origin of the tremor, as is presumed the case in ET. Thus the amplitude of ET is less dependent on the position of the tested limb than is the amplitude of other postural tremors, including physiologic tremors (Sanes and Hallett, 1990).

Essential tremor

Although the term "essential" implies necessary or desirable, it actually means that there is no known cause and the term is synonymous with "idiopathic." The term "essential tremor" did not gain regular and widespread currency until a century or so after its initial use in 1874 by Pietro Burresi, a professor of medicine at the University of Siena, Italy (Louis et al., 2008b). He coined the term "tremore semplice essenziale" or "simple essential tremor" when he described the case of an 18-year-old man suffering from severe tremor of the arms when engaged in voluntary movement as well as head tremor. While the amplitude of ET tends to increase with age, the tremor frequency decreases with age (Elble et al.,1994; Elble, 2000b). The tremor of ET is typically a postural or kinetic tremor with frequency varying between 4 and 10 Hz. Although the frequency of the tremor is relatively constant in a particular individual, the amplitude may vary and in some cases may be even suppressed by mental concentration and distraction (Koller and Biary, 1989; Kenney et al., 2007).

Epidemiology of ET

In the past the modifier "benign" was used ("benign ET") to indicate favorable prognosis of ET, even though it is now well accepted that ET can produce marked physical and psychosocial disability (Busenbark et al., 1991; Jankovic, 2000; Sullivan et al., 2004; Louis, 2005; Benito-León and Louis, 2006; Elble et al., 2006). Furthermore, in a longitudinal, prospective, population-based study, ET has been found to be associated with increased mortality at an estimated risk ratio of 1.59 (95% CI 1.11–2.27, $P = 0.01$) (Louis et al., 2007a). Meta-analysis of epidemiologic studies has found the prevalence of ET to range between 0.01% and 20.5%, but the pooled prevalence is 0.9%; the prevalence in people ≥65 years old is 4.6% and may be as high as 21.7% in people ≥95 years old; the prevalence is higher in males than females (Louis and Ferreira, 2010). There are many other estimates (Haerer et al., 1982; Louis et al., 1995, 1998d; Dogu et al., 2003) such as 5.5% in people over the age of 40 years (Rautakorpi et al., 1982) and 14% in people 65 years old or older (Moghal et al., 1994) (Table 18.2). In one epidemiologic study, 108 of 1056 (10%) nondemented individuals in upper Manhattan, aged 65 years or older, reported "shaking" (Louis et al., 1996). Neurologic examination confirmed rest tremor in 8.3% and action tremor in 17.6%, and the prevalence of PD and ET was estimated to be 3.2% and 10.2%, respectively. In a door-to-door survey of people aged 40 years or older in Mersin Province, Turkey, the prevalence of ET was found to be 4% (Dogu et al., 2003). In another population-based survey, involving 5278 subjects aged 65 years or older

Table 18.2 Prevalence and incidence of essential tremor

Prevalence

- 0.4%–5.5% – community-based studies
- 14% in people ≥65 years
- 4% – a door-to-door survey of people ≥40 years in Mersin Province, Turkey

Incidence

- 616/100 000 person-years – a population-based study of 5278 subjects ≥65 years in central Spain followed for a median of 3.3 years
  - 64/83 (77.1%) incident cases had not been previously diagnosed, and only 4 (4.8%) were taking antitremor medications

Table 18.3 Proposed classification of essential tremor

A. Definite essential tremor

1. Inclusions

a. Bilateral postural tremor with or without kinetic tremor involving hands or forearms, which is visible and persistent and is long-standing in duration (>5 years)

b. Tremor involving body parts other than the upper limbs may be present, the tremor may be asymmetrical, amplitude may fluctuate, and the tremor might or might not produce disability

2. Exclusions

a. Neurologic signs, except for Froment sign

b. Causes of enhanced physiologic tremor

c. Concurrent or recent exposure to tremorgenic drugs

d. Direct or indirect trauma to the central and peripheral nervous systems

e. Historical or clinical evidence of psychogenic origins of tremor

f. Convincing evidence of sudden onset or evidence of stepwise deterioration

B. Probable essential tremor

1. Inclusions

The same as for definite ET, but the tremor may be confined to body parts other than hands and the duration is greater than 3 years

2. Exclusions

a. Primary orthostatic tremor, which is an isolated, high-frequency (14–18 Hz), bilaterally synchronous leg tremor on standing or voluntary contraction of leg muscles

b. Isolated voice, tongue, or chin tremors

c. Position- and task-specific tremors

C. Possible essential tremor

1. Inclusions

a. Type 1. Satisfy criteria for definite or probable ET but exhibit other recognizable neurologic disorders, such as:

(1) Parkinsonism, dystonia, myoclonus, peripheral neuropathy, or restless legs syndrome

(2) Other neurologic signs of uncertain significance not sufficient to make a diagnosis of a recognizable neurologic disorder, such as mild extrapyramidal signs (hypomimia, decreased armswing, and mild bradykinesia)

b. Type 2. Monosymptomatic and isolated tremors of uncertain relationship to ET. This includes position- and task-specific tremors, such as occupational tremors (primary writing tremors); primary orthostatic tremor; isolated voice, chin, tongue, and leg tremor; and unilateral postural hand tremor

2. Exclusions

Same as points 2a–f for definite ET

Members of the Tremor Research and Investigation Group: M. Brin, C. Contant, R. Elble, L. Findley, J. Jankovic, W. Koller, P. LeWitt, A. Rajput.
From Findley LJ, Koller WC. Definitions and behavioural classifications. In Findley LJ, Koller WC (eds): *Handbook of Tremor Disorders*. New York, Marcel Dekker, 1995, pp 1–5.

in central Spain who were followed for a median of 3.3 years, the adjusted annual incidence was determined to be 616 per 100 000 person-years; 64 of the 83 (77.1%) incident cases had not been previously diagnosed, and only 4 (4.8%) were taking antitremor medications (Benito-León et al., 2005). In yet another population-based study of northern Italian adults in which all participants were examined and classified by movement specialists using rigorous diagnostic criteria, tremors comprised the most common category of movement disorders, followed by restless legs syndrome (Wenning et al., 2005). These epidemiologic studies provide strong evidence that the prevalence and incidence of ET are higher than was previously recognized.

Diagnosis of ET

Although ET was described as early as the nineteenth century (Dana, 1887; Louis, 2010), there is still considerable controversy about the diagnostic criteria for ET (Chouinard et al., 1997; Louis et al., 1998c; Jankovic, 2000; Louis, 2010; Quinn et al., 2011). In one study of 71 patients, 37% diagnosed with ET based on the criteria for ET adapted from the consensus statement of the Movement Disorders Society (Deuschl et al., 1998a) were misdiagnosed, usually either as PD or dystonia (Jain et al., 2006). This is partly due to a lack of a disease-specific marker for ET. No specific pathologic changes indicative of PD were noted in 20 brains of ET patients that were examined at autopsy (Rajput et al., 2004). However, this study is fundamentally flawed, since all patients who were selected for the study had a diagnosis of ET at the time of death and patients who started with ET and later developed PD would have been excluded (Jankovic, 2004). It is of interest that one patient with severe ET that began at age 45 and no parkinsonian features, at the time of her death at age 91 years had Lewy bodies localized to the locus coeruleus, providing further evidence of a connection between ET and Lewy body disease (Louis et al., 2005b). The controversy about the possible association of ET and PD should be clarified once the genetic basis and pathophysiology of ET are understood. Until then, the operational diagnostic criteria must rely on the presence of typical clinical characteristics. The presence or absence of certain clinical characteristics may be used to categorize ET into "definite," "probable," and "possible" (Table 18.3). The diagnostic criteria may be used or modified according to specific needs. For example, for

genetic linkage studies, only "definite" ET may be acceptable, whereas in studies that are designed to explore the clinical spectrum of ET, including associated features, the "possible" ET category might be more appropriate (Table 18.4). Family history, alcohol sensitivity, and propranolol responsiveness, while characteristic of ET, should not be considered necessary for the diagnosis. More recently, core and secondary

Definite

1. Bilateral arm tremor with 2+ amplitude rating in at least one arm and 1+ in the other arm

or

2. Predominant cranial-cervical tremor with 2+ amplitude rating and 1+ rating in at least one arm. The head tremor is rhythmic, without directional preponderance, and without asymmetry of cervical muscles

3. Exclude obvious secondary causes of tremor: for example, physiologic, drug-induced, Charcot–Marie–Tooth (CMT), chronic inflammatory demyelinating polyradiculoneuropathy (CIPD), PD

(Coexistent dystonia is allowed, but coexistent PD is not)

Probable

1. 1+ arm tremor bilaterally

or

2. Isolated cranial-cervical tremor with 2+ amplitude rating

or

3. Convincing history of ET

4. Exclude obvious secondary causes of tremor: for example, physiologic, drug-induced, CMT

(Coexistent dystonia is allowed; coexistent PD is allowed if there is a convincing history of preexisting ET)

Possible

1. Isolated 1+ cranial-cervical tremor
2. Task/position specific hand/arm tremor
3. Unilateral arm tremor
4. Orthostatic tremor

Tremor rating: 0, none perceived; 1, slight (barely noticeable); 2, moderate, noticeable, probably not disabling (<2 cm excursions); 3, marked, probably partially disabling (2–4 cm excursions); 4, severe, coarse, disabling (>4 cm excursions). Participants in the July 1996 NIH meeting: J. Beach, S.B. Bressman, M.F. Brin, D. De Leon, L. Goldfarb, M. Hallett, J. Jankovic, W. Koller, D. Mirel, K. Wilhemsen. From Brin MF, Koller W. Epidemiology and genetics of essential tremor. Mov Disord 1998;13(Suppl. 3),55–63.

criteria were proposed to facilitate a practical approach to the diagnosis of ET (Elble, 2000a). Core criteria include bilateral action tremor of the hands and forearms (but not rest tremor), absence of other neurologic signs, except for the Froment sign (a "cogwheel" phenomenon on passive movement of the affected limb with voluntary movement of the contralateral limb), and isolated head tremor without signs of dystonia, although the latter is rare. A recent analysis of ET patients from two large population-based studies and one large clinic-based cohort revealed no cases of pure head tremor in 583 patients (Louis and Dogu 2009). Therefore, patients with pure head tremor probably should not be regarded as definite ET. Head tremor is seen in about 18% of population-based cases of ET and in 37% of clinical samples of ET (Louis and Dogu, 2009). Secondary criteria include long duration (>3 years), a positive family history, and a beneficial response to alcohol (Mostile and Jankovic, 2010). Another feature, seen in about a third of patients with ET, is mirror movements (Louis et al., 2009d), more typically observed in patients with focal dystonia (Sitburana et al., 2009). There are red flags that indicate a diagnosis other than ET, such as unilateral tremor, present in only

4.4% of cases of ET (Phibbs et al., 2009), leg tremor, rigidity, bradykinesia, rest tremor, gait disturbance, focal tremor, isolated head tremor with abnormal posture (head tilt or turning), sudden or rapid onset, and drug treatment that may cause or exacerbate tremor. Thus head tremor is usually a manifestation of ET or cervical dystonia; it is almost never seen in PD unless there is coexistent ET (Roze et al., 2006; Gan et al., 2009).

A review of the clinical features in 350 consecutive patients who were referred to the Movement Disorders Clinic at Baylor College of Medicine and diagnosed with ET has shown that although tremor is clearly the most troublesome symptom, it is not necessarily the only symptom in patients with ET (Lou and Jankovic, 1991b) (Tables 18.1 and 18.3). This is supported by the reports of well-studied families in which some members have typical ET, while others have dystonia, parkinsonism, or a combination of all three disorders (Jankovic et al., 1997; Farrer et al., 1999; Bertoli-Avella et al., 2003; Yahr et al., 2003; Spanaki and Plaitakis, 2009). One multigenerational family, 36 members in five generations, had an admixture of ET, PD, and dystonia (Yahr et al., 2003). Two twin brothers with ET and PD had the classic pathologic features of PD at autopsy. The authors concluded, "This unusual set of clinical and pathologic circumstances can hardly be attributed to chance occurrence and raises the question of a specific genetic mutation and/or clustering, which may link ET with PD." In a study of the first-degree relatives of 303 PD probands and 249 controls from Crete, ET was present in the relatives of PD patients more often than in those of controls (OR: 3.64, $P < 0.001$) and the risk was even greater (OR: 4.48) when the affected proband had tremor-dominant or mixed PD (Spanaki and Plaitakis, 2009). Twelve subjects had both ET and PD phenotypes. The authors concluded that "in certain families ET and PD are genetically related probably sharing common hereditary predisposition." Retrospective chart review at the Neurological Institute (NI) of New York showed that 56.7% of 210 PD patients versus 33.3% of 210 Parkinson-plus syndrome patients ($P < 0.001$) had kinetic tremor on examination and patients with PD were more likely to have a diagnosis of ET assigned by an NI neurologist (5.3% vs. 0.0%, OR 12.85, 95% CI 1.66–99.8, $P = 0.001$) (Louis and Frucht, 2007). Patients with PD were three to thirteen times more likely to have diagnoses of ET than patients with Parkinson-plus syndromes, thus confirming "the link between ET and PD, and possibly, between ET and Lewy body disease." In another large family, originally from Cuba, manifested by parkinsonism and ET, the parkinsonism was linked to a marker on chromosome 19p13.3–q12, but it did not cosegregate with ET (Bertoli-Avella et al., 2003). Other gene mutations associated with PD have not been found in patients with ET alone (Deng et al., 2006a). Some, but not all (Adler et al., 2011) studies have suggested that there is an association between ET and dystonia and between ET and parkinsonism (Jankovic et al., 1997; Yahr et al., 2003; Shahed and Jankovic, 2007; Fekete and Jankovic, 2011) (Fig. 18.2). In addition to dystonic tremor, patients with dystonia frequently have postural ET-like tremor present in body parts distal to the dystonia, and they have a higher-than-expected family history of postural tremor (Chan et al., 1991; Jankovic et al., 1991; Deuschl et al., 1997; Jankovic and Mejia, 2005; Schneider et al., 2007). Asymmetric dystonic hand tremor may be initially

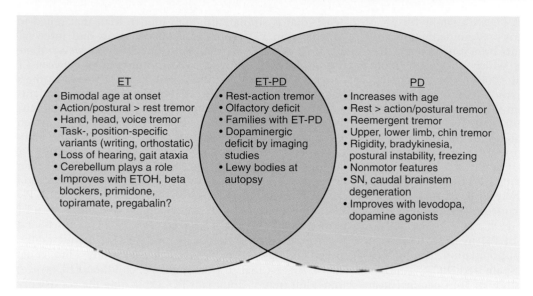

Figure 18.2 Overlap between and differentiation of essential tremor and Parkinson disease. ETOH, ethanol. SN, substantia nigra.

misdiagnosed as PD-related tremor and, along with rest tremor associated with ET, may be responsible for scans without evidence of dopamine deficiency (SWEDDs) (Schneider et al., 2007; Bain, 2009; Schwingenschuh et al., 2010; Stoessl, 2010). When 25 tremulous SWEDDs patients were compared to 25 tremor-dominant PD patients, the former group lacked true bradykinesia, they had evidence of dystonia, and head tremor, whereas reemergent tremor, true fatiguing or decrement, good response to dopaminergic drugs, and presence of nonmotor symptoms favored PD (Schwingenschuh et al., 2010). Whether the hand tremor that is seen in about 25% (10–85%) of patients with cervical dystonia represents an enhanced physiologic tremor, ET, dystonic tremor, or some other form of postural tremor is unknown (Jankovic et al., 1991; Deuschl et al., 1997). Although the frequency of ET and the limb tremor in patients with cervical dystonia are similar, the tremor amplitude in patients with dystonia is smaller and the tremor is more irregular, suggesting that the two types of tremors, while similar, arise from different types of oscillators (Shaikh et al., 2008). The observation of significant overlap in association between variants in *LINGO1* and ET and PD (see below) provides support for the genetic association between the two common movement disorders (Vilariño-Güell et al., 2010a).

The clinical heterogeneity of ET suggests that there may be different subtypes. Indeed, Louis and colleagues (2000b) found that patients with older onset (>60 years) and those without head tremor progressed more rapidly than did patients with young-onset tremor and those with head tremor. They also later found that head tremor was present four times more frequently in women than in men (Louis et al., 2003; Hardesty et al., 2004). Using the medical records linkage system of the Rochester Epidemiology Project, the authors identified ET patients who also had an autopsy report and found that women with ET were six times more likely to develop head tremor than men (Hardesty et al., 2004). The presence of jaw tremor, seen in 7.5–18.0% of patients with ET, has been found to be associated with older age at onset, more severe action tremor in arms, and the presence of head and voice tremor (Louis et al., 2006a). In

a study of 34 patients with voice tremor, 93% were female and the voice tremor typically began in the seventh decade (62.9 ± 15.0 years) (Sulica and Louis, 2010). More than a third had a first-degree relative with tremor and more than a quarter reported a beneficial effect of ethanol. In this study only 11 (32.3%) were aware of an arm tremor and 10 (29.4%) had been misdiagnosed as spasmodic dysphonia. Only 56% of treated patients found botulinum toxin helpful and the response was often incomplete. Jaw tremor was also significantly associated with rest tremor, suggesting that some patients with ET and jaw tremor may convert to PD. Besides ET and PD, jaw tremor may be a manifestation of dystonia (Schneider and Bhatia, 2007). Lower extremity tremor is usually mild or asymptomatic (Poston et al., 2009).

The ongoing debate as to whether ET is a monosymptomatic or heterogeneous disorder or phenotypic manifestation of multiple entities will probably not be resolved until disease-specific physiologic, genetic, or other biologic markers are identified (Schrag et al., 2000; Elble, 2002; Jankovic, 2002; Elble and Tremor Research Group, 2006; Louis, 2009; Deuschl and Elble, 2009). One hypothesis is that the various nonmotor signs linked to ET could be secondary to "abnormal neuronal oscillation" (Deuschl and Elble, 2009), but his would not explain the heterogeneous presentation of ET. Also, the proposed classification of ET into "hereditary" (unequivocal family history), "sporadic" (no immediate family member with ET), and "senile" (onset after age 65) is too artificial and not easily applicable. Some studies have suggested that there is an association between ET and parkinsonism (Jankovic et al., 1997; Yahr et al., 2003; Shahed and Jankovic, 2007; Fekete and Jankovic, 2011), but other studies have not found a link (Adler et al., 2011) (Fig. 18.2). Differentiation between ET and PD is critical particularly in early stages since ET has been found to be erroneously treated with anti-PD drugs in 12.4% of 402 community cases re-evaluated by a movement disorder specialist (Meara et al., 1999). Postural tremor, similar to ET, has been reported to occur in as many as 93% of patients with PD and to correlate with the ipsilateral rest tremor but not with age at onset or disease duration (Louis et al., 2001e).

Furthermore, in 22 patients with PD with family history of ET, 90% (20 of 22) had a tremor-predominant subtype of PD, suggesting that "these patients have inherited a genetic susceptibility factor for tremor, which affects the motor phenotype of PD" (Hedera et al., 2009). Phenomenologically similar to ET, the postural tremor of PD has been linked by some investigators to coexistent ET (Geraghty et al., 1985; Jankovic, 1989; Jankovic et al., 1997; Jankovic 2000). Others, however, believe that the coexistence of the two disorders simply "represents a chance occurrence of two common diseases" (Pahwa and Koller, 1993). On the basis of an analysis of 678 patients diagnosed as having ET, some by movement disorder specialists and others by private practice neurologists, 6.1% were found to have concomitant PD, and 6.9% had coexisting dystonia (Koller et al., 1994). The authors concluded that "the frequency of PD in ET is more than would be reported in the general population." In the Neurological Disorders in Central Spain (NEDICES) study, a longitudinal, population-based study of 3813 people (mean age 73.4 ± 6.6 years), after a median of 3.3 years, 12 (5.8%) of 207 ET cases developed parkinsonism compared with 56 (1.6%) of 3606 controls, with adjusted relative risk (RR) of 3.47 (95% confidence interval 1.82–6.59; $P < 0.001$) (Benito-León et al., 2009b). Six (3.0%) of 201 ET cases developed incident PD versus 24 (0.7%) of 3574 controls, with adjusted RR of 4.27 (95% confidence interval 1.72–10.61; $P = 0.002$). The authors concluded that "Patients with ET were four times more likely than controls to develop incident PD during prospective follow-up."

The coexistence of ET and PD may be difficult to recognize because once a patient develops PD, the postural tremor is usually attributed to the disease, and it is therefore difficult to diagnose ET in a patient who already has symptoms of PD (Shahed and Jankovic, 2007; Louis, 2009; Fekete and Jankovic, 2011) (Fig. 18.2). While rest tremor may be observed in patients with advanced ET, it may also be the initial manifestation of coexistent PD (Shahed and Jankovic, 2007; Fekete and Jankovic, 2010). The "postural tremor" that is seen in many patients with PD may represent an enhanced physiologic tremor (Forssberg et al., 2000), coexistent ET (Geraghty et al., 1985; Jankovic, 1995), or a reemergent classical rest tremor (Jankovic et al., 1999) with the same frequency and clinical characteristics as the typical rest tremor. This reemergent tremor is also often exacerbated during walking. In contrast to ET, which is seen immediately when patients outstretch their arms, the reemergent tremor of PD usually appears after a latency of several seconds (Jankovic et al., 1999). Furthermore, this PD-related tremor often responds to levodopa, whereas the postural tremor of ET does not (Kulisevsky et al., 1995). It is actually this action tremor that seems to correlate with motor disability rather than the typical rest tremor, which correlates chiefly with social handicap (Zimmermann et al., 1994). The clinical characteristics, however, may not always reliably differentiate between the two types of postural tremor (Henderson et al., 1995). We found a higher frequency of the 263 bp allele of the NACP-Rep1 polymorphism not only in patients with PD (odds ratio: 3.86) but also in patients with ET (odds ratio: 6.42), but not in patients with Huntington disease, supporting a genetic link between PD and ET (Tan et al., 2000). Further evidence that ET and PD may be related is the observation that patients with ET have an olfactory deficit that is similar, although milder, than that noted in patients with PD (Louis et al., 2002; Louis and Jurewicz, 2003; Djaldetti et al., 2008). In one study, however, there was no difference in results of olfactory testing between ET patients and controls (Shah et al., 2008). We and others (Gimenez-Roldan and Mateo, 1991) have noted that patients with ET seem to have a higher propensity toward neuroleptic-induced parkinsonism than do patients without ET, although a formal epidemiologic study is needed to confirm this clinical observation. To examine an ET–PD relationship, we described 22 patients with childhood-onset ET who later developed PD (Shahed and Jankovic, 2007; Fekete and Jankovic, 2011). Of 11 patients reporting asymmetric ET, PD symptoms began on the same side as the more severe ET tremor in 10 (90.9%, $\chi^2 = 0.66$, $P = 0.024$), with 68.2% reporting change in tremor as their first PD manifestation. These findings, supported by another study (Tan et al., 2006), suggest that in some patients, childhood ET evolves into adult tremor-dominant PD, explaining the coexistence of ET and PD within the same patient and family. It has been postulated that ET-related gene mutations may predispose some patients to subsequent development of PD. In a study of 53 patients with ET–PD combination, compared to 53 PD and 150 ET patients, the side of the greatest initial ET severity corresponded to the side of the greatest PD severity (Minen et al., 2008). In another study involving 13 patients who presented originally with asymmetrical postural tremor and no rest tremor for at least 10 years (mean: 19.2 years) and were initially diagnosed with ET, all patients subsequently developed evidence of PD (Chaudhuri et al., 2005). The onset of levodopa-responsive PD was manifested by rest tremor for a mean of 2.5 years before final presentation in the clinic. Furthermore, five patients who had β-CIT single photon emission computed tomography (SPECT) all showed reduced uptake in the contralateral striatum. It is not clear whether these patients with a long-standing history of asymmetrical postural tremor have PD at onset, whether patients with unilateral postural tremor (isolated tremor) or asymmetrical postural tremor (atypical ET) who later develop PD represent an overlap between ET and PD, or whether this type of postural tremor is an early marker for PD (Grosset and Lees, 2005).

In a population-based study (981 first-degree relatives of 162 patients with PD and of 838 first-degree relatives of 147 controls), the risk of ET was significantly increased for relatives of patients with onset of PD ($P = 0.006$) (Rocca et al., 2007). Also, in a referral-based sample (981 first-degree relatives of 162 patients with PD and of 838 first-degree relatives of 147 controls), the risk of ET among relatives increased with younger onset of PD in patients ($P = 0.001$) and was higher in relatives of PD patients with the tremor-predominant or mixed form when compared with relatives of patients with the akinetic-rigid form, and in men compared with women. The authors concluded that "These findings suggest that PD and ET may share familial susceptibility factors." In a case-control study of 600 subjects evaluated for tremor, ET was significantly more frequent in patients with PD (12/204, 5.9%) compared to diseased controls (2/206, 1%) and healthy controls (1/190, 0.5%) (Tan et al., 2008). The authors concluded that "PD patients were 5–10 times more likely to have ET compared diseased and healthy controls."

In addition to genetic factors, there may be environmental factors that determine the occurrence of ET and its relationship to PD. For example, heavy cigarette smoking has been associated with lower risk of PD and ET (Louis et al., 2008a). Although some studies have concluded dementia is more frequent in patients with ET than in controls (Bermejo-Pareja et al., 2007), and one study reported the adjusted odds ratios to vary between 1.64 and 1.84 (Thawani et al., 2009), a relationship between ET and Alzheimer disease has not been established (Elble et al., 2007a).

The possibility of additional cochlear involvement in ET is supported by the observation of high occurrence of partial or complete deafness in patients with ET (Ondo et al., 2003). Among 250 patients with ET, 42 (16.8%) patients wore hearing aids, compared to only 2 of 127 (1.6%) PD patients and 1 of 127 (0.8%) controls ($P < 0.0001$). Pure tone audiometry demonstrated age-dependent higher-frequency loss among patients with ET as compared to the general population. High risk of hearing loss among patients with ET has been confirmed by other studies (Benito-León et al., 2007). The combination of ET, sensorineuronal hearing loss, and early graying has been suggested to be a unique disorder, separate from Waardenburg syndrome (Karmody et al., 2005). Although mental functioning is usually intact in patients with ET, detailed testing of cognitive performance has found some subtle abnormalities on tests of verbal fluency, naming, mental set-shifting, verbal working memory, and other tests of cognitive function (Benito-León et al., 2006a) and elderly patients with ET may possibly have an increased risk of dementia compared with those without ET (Benito-León et al., 2006b). Furthermore, depression has been found to occur in about a third of the patients with ET, almost as frequently as in PD (Lombardi et al., 2001; Miller et al., 2007). These deficits have been interpreted as suggesting involvement of frontocerebellar circuits. In a cross-sectional study of personality, patients with ET were found to have a tendency to have increased levels of pessimism, fearfulness, shyness, anxiety, and easy fatigability, but none of these traits correlated with the severity of the tremor (Chatterjee et al., 2004).

ET appears to be a heterogeneous disorder, as is suggested by the multiple gene loci that have so far been identified and by the frequent association with other disorders, such as parkinsonism, dystonia, and myoclonus (Jankovic et al., 1997; Jankovic, 2002; Yahr et al., 2003; Deng et al., 2006b; Shahed and Jankovic, 2007) (Fig. 18.2). Postmortem studies of patients with ET have not provided evidence for nigrostriatal pathology in ET, but patients who had a diagnosis of PD at time of death (even though ET might have preceded the onset of PD) would have been excluded from these clinical-pathologic studies (Jankovic, 2004; Rajput et al., 2004). Furthermore, there is indirect evidence suggesting nigrostriatal impairment in some patients with ET. We found that relatives of patients with PD have at least a 2.5 times higher (those with the combination of ET–PD: 10 times higher) frequency of tremor than normal controls, providing additional support for the association of ET and PD (Jankovic et al., 1995a). Furthermore, about 20% of patients with ET have a rest tremor that has the clinical and physiologic characteristics of PD tremor (Cohen et al., 2003). However, when 9 brains of patients who exhibited advanced ET and upper extremity rest tremor (without any other

evidence of parkinsonism) were examined with alpha-synclein staining, only two had Lewy bodies in the dorsal vagus nucleus and locus ceruleus, but none had Lewy body-containing neurons and/or Lewy neurites in the basal ganglia (Louis et al., 2011). Although this pathological study suggests that rest tremor in patients with ET is not associated with PD pathology, 19 of 24 (80%) patients with ET and rest tremor without other parkinsonian features had abnormal DAT uptake on DaTscan, particularly in the putamen (deVerdal et al., 2011). Similarly, a fourfold increase in prevalence of isolated tremor among relatives of patients with PD as compared to controls was found by Payami and colleagues (1994). Interestingly, among 196 twins with postural or kinetic tremors, Tanner and colleagues (2001) found that 137 had PD or had a twin with PD.

Imaging studies have been helpful in providing insight into the relationship between ET and PD. A 10–13% reduction in ^{18}F-dopa uptake in the striatum of patients with ET as compared to controls (Brooks et al., 1992) suggests a physiologically important compromise of the dopaminergic system in patients with ET (Jankovic et al., 1993). Furthermore, ^{18}F-dopa uptake constants (Ki) in 5 of 32 asymptomatic relatives of patients with PD who had isolated postural tremor were reduced on average by 23% ($P < 0.001$) (Piccini et al., 1997). The mean Ki for the other 27 asymptomatic relatives was decreased by 17% ($P < 0.001$). Using ^{123}I-IPT SPECT to image the striatal dopamine transporter, Lee and colleagues (1999) found the mean bilateral uptake in nine patients with isolated postural tremor (ET) to be slightly lower than that in normal control subjects (3.60 vs. 3.80), but this did not reach statistical significance. Six other patients in whom rest tremor developed 4–18 years (mean: 11.5 ± 6.7) after the onset of postural tremor without other parkinsonian features, however, had a significant reduction in the dopamine transporter compared to normal controls (2.61 vs. 3.83, $P < 0.05$) but lower than PD patients (1.97 contralateral and 2.35 ipsilateral). They concluded that some patients with postural tremor may acquire rest tremor in association with mild substantia nigra neuronal loss. Although the majority of ET patients have normal dopamine transporter (DAT) SPECT, some cases may start with isolated postural tremor, phenomenologically identical to ET, and later develop PD. In one study the mean latency between the onset of asymmetrical postural tremor and PD was 19.2 years whereas the mean latency between onset of rest tremor and PD was 2.5 years (Chaudhuri et al., 2005). In one study of 61 subjects presenting with "isolated atypical tremors defined as unilateral either postural, resting or mixed" followed at baseline and at mean 28.4 ± 7.2 months with ^{123}I-FPCIT SPECT, those ($n = 25$) with normal baseline scan had only tremor at follow-up, and of the 36 with abnormal baseline scan, 23 (64%) developed PD, while the remaining patients had only tremor (presumably ET) (Ceravolo et al., 2008). They suggested that term "isolated tremor with dopaminergic presynaptic dysfunction" is used for the patients with unilateral or asymmetrical tremor with abnormal DAT SPECT. Whether the use of ^{123}I-FPCIT SPECT in differentiating ET from PD is cost-effective is not clear, although one Italian study suggested some cost savings when using this diagnostic tool (Antonini et al., 2008). In one study FP-CIT SPECT showed that the pattern of dopaminergic loss over time is different between ET and PD, but both disorders exhibit impairment of DAT in the caudate nucleus (Isaias et al., 2010). Although this and other imaging studies reported by the same group (Isaias et al., 2008) provide important insights into the selective caudate dopaminergic deficit as a possible link between the two common disorders, some studies have reported that DAT SPECT remains normal over time in patients with mixed tremor (a combination of postural and rest tremor) (Arabia et al., 2010). Since medial substantia nigra (that predominantly projects to the caudate nucleus) is particularly involved in the tremor-dominant PD and is associated with more caudate loss of DAT, it is possible that tremor-dominant PD and ET share a selective dopaminergic loss in the caudate nucleus. This, in turn, may lead to a dysfunction of the caudate-thalamic pathway and disinhibition of the thalamic autorhythmic pacemakers, clinically expressed as tremor. Indeed, β-CIT SPECT, which mainly reflects serotonin transporters, is lower in the thalamus of patients with tremor-dominant PD as compared to those with non-tremor PD (Caretti et al., 2008). In addition to thalamus, the caudate also projects to the inferior olive and cerebellum, both implicated in the pathophysiology of ET, and supported by growing evidence or cerebellar pathology in ET. The clinical overlap between the two disorders undoubtedly contributes to the 10–15% frequency of patients diagnosed with mild PD who have SWEDDs (Schneider et al., 2007; Bain, 2009; Schwingenschuh et al., 2010; Stoessl, 2010).

A relationship between ET and nigral degeneration is supported by the finding of hyperechogenicity of substantia nigra on midbrain sonography in 16% of 44 ET patients as compared to 3% of 100 controls and 75% of 100 patients with PD (Stockner et al., 2007). Although not demonstrated by all studies (Doepp et al., 2008; Budisic et al., 2009), the slightly increased hyperechogenicity of the substantia nigra on midbrain sonography provides further support for the notion that some ET patients may later develop parkinsonism.

Although the relatively frequent coexistence of ET and dystonia supports the notions that there is a pathogenetic link between the two disorders, linkage analysis has excluded the dystonia (DYT1) gene on chromosome 9 in hereditary ET (Conway et al., 1993; Dürr et al., 1993). This suggests that the genes for these two disorders are on separate loci or that the relationship between the two disorders is physiologic rather than genetic. Münchau and colleagues (2001) studied 11 patients with classic ET and compared them to 19 patients with cervical dystonia and arm tremor. They found that the latency of the second agonist burst during ballistic wrist flexion movements was later in ET patients than in those with arm tremor associated with cervical dystonia. Furthermore, the latter group had a greater variability in reciprocal inhibition than the ET group. Patients with normal presynaptic inhibition had simultaneous onset of their arm tremor with onset of their cervical dystonia (mean age: 40 years), whereas patients with reduced or absent presynaptic inhibition had an earlier age at onset (mean 14 years), and the interval between the onset of the tremor and the onset of cervical dystonia was longer (mean: 21 years). This suggests that the mechanisms of arm tremor in patients with ET and cervical dystonia are different. The association between ET, dystonia, and PD is suggested by reports of families with manifestations of these three disorders in different or same members of the families (Jankovic et al., 1997; Yahr et al., 2003).

ET-like tremor has been described in patients with hereditary myoclonus and with hereditary motor-sensory neuropathy (sometimes referred to as Roussy–Levy syndrome) (Cardoso and Jankovic, 1993). ET-like tremor occurs in other genetic diseases, the study of which may provide important insights into possible genetic heterogeneity in families with clinically similar tremor. For example, postural tremor similar to that seen in ET has been reported in patients with Kennedy disease, also called X-linked recessive spinal and bulbar muscular atrophy, which is caused by a mutation characterized by expansion of CAG repeats in the gene on the X chromosome (Sperfeld et al., 2002). ET may also be associated with higher-than-expected frequency with restless legs syndrome (Ondo and Lai, 2006). The validity and meaning of such associations, however, are disputed, and the controversies are not likely to be resolved until a disease-specific marker (e.g., an ET-linked genetic locus) is identified. A diagnostic marker for ET would also help to resolve the question as to whether site-, position-, and task-specific tremors, such as primary handwriting tremor and orthostatic tremor, are distinct entities or whether these tremors represent clinical variants of ET (Rosenbaum and Jankovic, 1988; FitzGerald and Jankovic, 1991; Britton et al., 1992b; Danek, 1993; Soland et al., 1996b; Sander et al., 1998) (Table 18.5). It is still not clear whether primary writing tremor is a variant of ET, a type of focal dystonia such as writer's cramp, or a separate nosological entity (Hai et al., 2010; Quinn et al., 2011).

Orthostatic tremor, first described by Heilman in 1984, is a fast (14–16 Hz) tremor, involving mainly the legs and trunk, but cranial muscles may be also involved (Koster et al., 1999) (Video 18.5). The latter observation suggests that supraspinal mechanisms play a role in the pathophysiology of orthostatic tremor. This is further supported by the finding of high intermuscular coherence between the two sides, providing evidence that the tremor originates from a common site (Lauk et al., 1999), and a high degree of EMG coherence between right and left muscle groups. This is in contrast to ET or PD tremors, in which there is no such left/right coherence, and these tremors are probably generated by more than one oscillator (Raethjen et al., 2000). Some authors have suggested that coherent high-frequency tremor in the legs may be a normal response to perceived unsteadiness when standing still and that orthostatic tremor may be an exaggeration of this response (Sharott et al., 2003). Others have postulated that orthostatic tremor merely unmasks 16 Hz central oscillators involved in postural tremor (McAuley et al., 2000). While there is robust evidence for a supraspinal origin of orthostatic tremor, the spinal cord may also serve as the generator of the tremor as suggested by the presence of a 16 Hz tremor in a man with complete paraplegia (Norton et al., 2004). Present chiefly on standing, orthostatic tremor may be precipitated also by isometric contraction of the upper limbs as well as facial and jaw muscles (Boroojerdi et al., 1999; Koster et al., 1999). This suggests that the generation of orthostatic tremor is more likely related to isometric force control rather than to regulation of stance. Orthostatic tremor is often associated with a feeling of unsteadiness and calf cramps, relieved by sitting or a supine position. Fung and colleagues (2001)

Table 18.5 Categorization of tremors

Rest	Action		Kinetic	Miscellaneous
	Postural			
• Parkinsonian	• Physiologic		• Cerebellar	• Idiopathic
– PD	• Enhanced physiologic		– Multiple sclerosis	• Psychogenic
– Secondary	– Stress		– Stroke	• Other involuntary
– P-plus	– Endocrine		– Degenerative	rhythmic movements
• ET variants	– Drugs, toxins		– Wilson disease	– Convulsions
• Midbrain	• Essential tremor		– Drugs, toxins	– Myoclonus
• Myorhythmia	• Orthostatic		• Midbrain	– Asterixis
	• Other position-specific tremors		• Task-specific	– Nystagmus
	• PD (reemergent)		• Cortical	– Fasciculations
	• Dystonic			– Clonus
	• Cerebellar			
	• Myorhythmia			
	• Cortical			
	• Neuropathic			
	• Fragile X-associated tremor/ataxia syndrome (FXTAS)			

postulated that "the sensation of unsteadiness arises from a tremulous disruption of proprioceptive afferent activity from the legs". The leg cramps are presumably due to a high-frequency (tetanic) contraction of the calf muscles. The muscle contraction can be "heard" by auscultating over the thigh or calf and listening for the characteristic thumping sound (Brown, 1995).

The pathophysiology of orthostatic tremor is not well understood, but some have suggested that it is a variant of ET. In support of the association between ET and orthostatic tremor is the relatively high occurrence of postural tremor, phenomenologically identical to ET, and the presence of family history of tremor in the majority of patients with orthostatic tremor (FitzGerald and Jankovic, 1991). Furthermore PET findings indicative of bilateral cerebellar (and contralateral lentiform and thalamic) dysfunction, similar to those observed in ET, have been also reported in patients with orthostatic tremor (Wills et al., 1996). Some studies have also suggested that there is a dopaminergic deficit in orthostatic tremor. Leg tremor, phenomenologically similar to orthostatic tremor, may be the initial manifestation of PD, particularly due to *parkin* mutation (Kim and Lee, 1993; Deng et al., 2006b). Some patients with orthostatic tremor respond to levodopa (Wills et al., 1999) and dopamine agonists (Finkel, 2000). Furthermore, [^{123}I]-FP-CIT SPECT showed evidence of marked reduction of dopamine transporter in patients with orthostatic tremor (Katzenschlager et al., 2003).

Tremor that is present predominantly or only on standing, but usually of much lower frequency than the classic orthostatic tremor, can be also seen in other conditions, including parkinsonism, ET, head trauma, pontine lesions, and other disorders (Gabellini et al., 1990; Benito-León et al., 1997). In contrast to ET, orthostatic tremor does not respond to the conventional anti-ET medications, but usually improves with clonazepam and gabapentin (Rodrigues et al., 2006). In one study, five of nine patients with orthostatic tremor benefited from levodopa (Wills et al., 1999). In a review of 41 patients with orthostatic tremor, Gerschlager and

colleagues (2004) found that 24 (58%) patients had associated postural arm tremor, and 10 (25%) had "orthostatic tremor plus"; 6 (15%) patients had parkinsonism. The response to medications was generally poor, but some, particularly those with associated parkinsonism, responded to dopaminergic therapy. Whether dopamine agonists and other antiparkinsonian treatments, including thalamotomy and VIM or STN/GPi DBS, will provide benefit to patients with orthostatic tremor remains to be determined. VIM DBS may be an effective treatment for patients with medically resistant orthostatic tremor (Guridi et al., 2008; Espay et al., 2008). Chronic spinal cord stimulation has been reported to be effective in two patients with medically intractable orthostatic tremor (Krauss et al., 2006).

The age at onset for ET showed a bimodal distribution with peaks in the second and sixth decades (Lou and Jankovic, 1991b). This was evident in both genders and in patients with and without dystonia and parkinsonism. Patients with early-onset (<30 years) ET had significantly more hand involvement, were more likely to have associated dystonia, and were more likely to improve with alcohol than were those with later onset (>40 years) ET ($P < 0.05$). There were no significant differences in any clinical variables between patients with and without a family history of tremor. Patients with older-onset ET, sometimes also referred to as "senile tremor," tend to have more rapid progression and more degenerative pathology than the younger-onset patients (Louis et al., 2009b). The relative lack of important differences between subgroups (early versus late onset, familial versus sporadic, mild versus severe, low versus high frequency) suggests that ET represents a single disease entity with a variable clinical expression. This conclusion is supported by a recent study by Koller and colleagues (1992). In their clinical and physiologic study of 61 patients, they found a frequency below 7 Hz in 79% of the patients, a positive family history in 72%, an amelioration with alcohol in 75%, an amelioration with primidone in 71%, and an amelioration with propranolol in 46%. Since no significant correlations could be found to suggest any particular grouping, they concluded that "essential tremor cannot be classified into subtypes."

Epidemiologic studies indicate that up to 5% of the adult population has ET, and 5–30% of adults with ET report symptom onset during childhood (Ferrara and Jankovic, 2009). Childhood-onset ET is usually hereditary, begins at a mean age of 6 years, and affects boys three times as often as girls. In a study of 39 patients with childhood-onset ET, a mean age at onset of 8.8 ± 5.0 years, and a mean age at evaluation of 20.3 ± 14.4 years, we found that some had their initial symptoms as early as infancy (Jankovic et al., 2004). A family history of tremor was noted for 79.5% of the patients. Eighteen (46.2%) patients had some neurologic comorbidity, such as dystonia, which was noted in 11 (28.2%) patients. Only 24 (61.5%) patients were treated with a specific antitremor medication; 5 of the 12 patients who were treated with propranolol experienced improvement. Other studies of childhood-onset ET also found male preponderance and paucity of head tremor (Louis et al., 2001b; Tan et al., 2006). Some investigators have suggested that "shuddering attacks" of infancy might be the initial manifestation of ET (Vanasse et al., 1976; Kanazawa, 2000).

Some isolated site-specific tremors, such as those involving the head and trunk (Rivest and Marsden, 1990) and some task- or position-specific tremors, might actually represent forms of dystonic tremor (Elble et al., 1990; Jedynak et al., 1991; Bain et al., 1995). Dystonic tremor is typically irregular and position-sensitive and when the patient is allowed to move the affected body part into the position of the maximal "pull", the tremor often ceases, the so-called "null point" (Videos 18.6 and 18.7). Some patients with dystonic tremor present with asymmetric rest hand tremor and decreased armswing which may lead to initial misdiagnosis of PD (Jankovic and Mejia, 2005; Schneider et al., 2007; Bain, 2009). Although there is some overlap between primary writing tremor and dystonic writer's cramp, the former is not usually associated with an excessive overflow of EMG activity into the proximal musculature, and the reciprocal inhibition of the median nerve H-reflex on radial nerve stimulation is normal (Bain et al., 1995; Modugno et al., 2002). The latter two features are typical of dystonia, and their presence in patients with task-specific tremors suggests that despite the absence of overt dystonia, these tremors represent forms of focal dystonia (Rosenbaum and Jankovic, 1988; Soland et al., 1996b). The overlap with primary handwriting tremor is supported by the observed activation of brain areas on functional magnetic resonance imaging (MRI) that are commonly activated in ET and dystonic writer's cramp. Other causes of postural tremor include midbrain (rubral) lesions. In a study of six patients with midbrain tremors, PET studies indicated dopaminergic striatal denervation, supported by markedly decreased fluorodopa uptake in the ipsilateral striatum (Remy et al., 1995). This nigrostriatal denervation, however, was not accompanied by striatal dopamine receptor supersensitivity, and the density of striatal D2 receptors did not change. Furthermore, the density of dopamine transporter is the same as that in normal controls (Antonini et al., 2001). Another form of postural tremor with bilateral high-frequency (14 Hz) synchronous discharges was reported in a patient with sporadic olivopontocerebellar atrophy (Manto et al., 2003).

Genetics

A family history of tremor has been reported in 17–100% of patients with ET (Busenbark et al., 1996; Louis and Ottman, 1996). The reason for such a large discrepancy is that unless all the symptomatic and asymptomatic members of the family are examined, the number of affected relatives will be under-ascertained (Jankovic et al., 1997; Louis et al., 1999b). Tremor in relatives is often wrongly attributed to aging, stress, nervousness, PD, alcoholism, or an associated illness or medications. In a study of 169 relatives of 46 ET patients, 12 (7.5%) were diagnosed as having probable or definite ET, but only 2 were reported by probands to have tremor (sensitivity: 16.7%); only 1 of 136 normal relatives were reported to have tremor (specificity: 99.3%) (Louis et al., 1999b). In other studies, the investigators found that 23% of elderly individuals had ET, and relatives of ET patients were five times more likely to develop the disease than a control population (Louis et al., 2001c), and first-degree relatives were more likely to have tremor compared to relatives of controls than were second-degree relatives (Louis et al., 2001d). Factors that were associated with more accurate reporting were female informant, increased tremor severity, sibling relationship, and higher level of education. In a comprehensive study of 20 index patients with hereditary ET and their 93 first-degree relatives and 38 more distant relatives, Bain and colleagues (1994) examined 53 definite and 18 possible cases. Similar to the findings of Lou and Jankovic (1991a), the investigators found a bimodal distribution and autosomal dominant inheritance with nearly complete penetrance by the age of 65 years. In contrast to some previous studies, they found no cases of dystonia, PD, task-specific tremors, or primary orthostatic tremors, but migraine headaches occurred with a higher-than-expected frequency of 26%. About 50% were alcohol-responsive, but there was marked heterogeneity of responsiveness between and within families (Mostile and Jankovic, 2010). In contrast, in a study of 252 members in four large kindreds with ET, three of the kindreds had a total of 41 members with the combination of ET and dystonia, and two had associated parkinsonism (Jankovic et al., 1997). Besides the one kindred with "pure" ET without any associated disorders (Jankovic et al., 1997), we subsequently studied 216 individuals of another large kindred with "pure" ET. The observation of earlier age at onset in successive generations suggests the phenomenon of anticipation, although the relatively small number of subjects and the possibility of ascertainment bias preclude any definite conclusions. Since ET is so common in the general population, bilineal transmission is not rare, and the amplitude of tremor appears to be greater in the children than in either affected parent (Rajput and Rajput, 2006). The younger the age at onset of ET, the higher the frequency of positive family history. In one study, 91% of cases with onset before the age of 20 years had a family history of tremor (Louis and Ottman, 2006).

Although the genetic origin of ET is widely recognized, the gene or genes responsible for ET have eluded intensive search by several groups of investigators (Deng et al., 2007) (Table 18.6). A genome scan of 16 ET Icelandic families containing 75 affected relatives with "definite" ET identified a marker for the familial ET gene, *FET1* or *ETM1*, on chromosome 3q13.1 (Gulcher et al., 1997). An analysis of a large

Table 18.6 A review of genetic studies in essential tremor

- *ETM1* – 3q13.1
  - A genome scan of 16 ET Icelandic families containing 75 affected relatives with "definite" ET (and in Tajikistan)
- *ETM2* – 2p24.1
  - Linkage established in 3 "pure" ET families and in 1 family with ET-parkinsonism, dystonia
- 6p22.3–24.1
  - Linkage in two ET families
- D3 receptor gene (*DRD3*) – 3q13.3
  - Ser9Gly variant associated with increased risk and younger age at onset of ET
- *Lingo 1* and *2*

Czech-American family established linkage to a locus *ETM2* on chromosome 2p22–p25 (Higgins et al., 1997). Two of our families with "pure" ET and one with ET–parkinsonism–dystonia also mapped to the same locus (Higgins et al., 1998). On the basis of studies of genetically diverse populations of ET, the locus has been narrowed to 2p24.1 with a candidate interval to a 192-kilobase interval between the loci *etm1231* and *APOB* (Higgins et al., 2004). More recently, a missense mutation ($828C{\rightarrow}G$) in the *HS1-BP3* gene was identified in two American families with ET and was absent in 150 control samples (300 chromosomes) (Higgins et al., 2005, 2006). The $828C{\rightarrow}G$ mutation causes a substitution of a glycine for an alanine residue in the HS1-BP3 protein (A265G), which is normally highly expressed in motor neurons and Purkinje cells and regulates the Ca^{2+}/calmodulin-dependent protein kinase activation of tyrosine and tryptophan hydroxylase. Studies in our own population of patients with ET and suitable controls, however, have led us to conclude that the variant might not be pathogenic for ET and might simply represent a polymorphism in the *HS1-BP3* gene (Deng et al., 2005). A linkage to 6p23 with a LOD score ranging from 1.265 to 2.983 was identified in two ET families, but further studies are needed to determine whether this merely represents a susceptibility locus or whether this gene region contains a causative gene (Shatunov et al., 2006). Variants in the coding region of the D3 receptor gene (*DRD3*), localized on 3q13.3, have been found to be associated with ET in some families and in a case-control study (Lucotte et al., 2006). In a genome-wide scan involving families from France and North America, Ser9Gly variant in the *DRD3* gene was found to increase dopamine affinity 4–5-fold and produce a gain-of-function abnormality as demonstrated by increased cAMP dopamine-mediated response and prolonged mitogen-associated protein kinase (MAPK) signal (Jeanneteau et al., 2006). The *DRD3Gly* was found to be associated with an increased risk for and age at onset of ET in Spanish (García-Martín et al., 2009) and French populations (Lorenz et al., 2009). This variant, however, has not been found in the majority of Asian (Tan et al., 2007b) or Italian (Vitale et al., 2008) patients with ET, and some have argued against the role of *DRD3* gene in the pathogenesis of ET (Blair et al., 2008).

When the genome-wide scan of 452 ET patients was compared to that of 14 378 controls, a marker in intron 3 of *LINGO1* gene on chromosome 15q24.3 was found to be significantly associated with ET (Stefansson et al., 2009). In several large European and American populations, the odds ratios for carriers of one G allele averaged 1.55, with $P = 10^{-9}$. Odds increased to 2.4 for carrying two G alleles. Based on this and the prevalence of the allele, the population attributable risk of the variant was 20%. Another study involving a North American population demonstrated a significant association between *LINGO1* rs9652490 and essential tremor ($P = 0.014$) and PD ($P = 0.0003$), again suggesting that variations in *LINGO1* can increase risk of ET and provide the first evidence of a genetic link between ET and PD (Vilariño-Güell et al., 2010a, 2010b). Furthermore, a slightly higher frequency of the allele G of *LINGO1* marker rs9652490 was found in ET patients of Asian origin (Tan et al., 2009). *LINGO1* may be potentially pathogenic as it has been implicated in axon regeneration, and when mutated it may be responsible for fusiform swellings of Purkinje cell axons, similar to those found in autopsied brains of patients with ET.

Another marker for ET has been mapped to chromosome 4p14–p16.3 (MIM 168601) in a family with autosomal dominant PD (Farrer et al., 1999, 2004). This family, however, was later found to have α-synuclein gene (SNCA) triplication, and this SNCA triplication segregated with parkinsonism but not the postural tremor (Singleton et al., 2003). This suggests that the postural tremor is a coincidental finding. Since not all families map to the three known loci (ETM1, ETM2, or the 4p locus) (Kovach et al., 2001), it is likely that familial tremor has not only marked phenotypic but also genetic heterogeneity and that additional gene loci will be identified in the near future. Furthermore, models other than autosomal dominant, including interaction between susceptibility genes and environmental risk factors, should be considered (Ma et al., 2006).

In 1935, Minor (1935), a Russian neurologist, not only stated that "the older one is, the more likely one displays tremor (ET)," but also suggested "that a factor for longevity was also contained in the tremor gamete." In support of the latter hypothesis, he offered the description of 51 cases of "hereditary tremor" associated with longevity. The longevity was based on patients' parents and grandparents usually being older than 70 years. His "control group" consisted of 11 cases of parkinsonism in which "no example of longevity was found out." However, the author did not state who in the ET families had tremor, and he did not provide any details on his parkinsonian patients (clinical features, ages of the subjects and relatives), and normal controls were not examined. Supporting the clinical observation that patients with ET live longer than a controlled population, Jankovic, Beach and colleagues (Jankovic, 1995) found that parents of patients with ET who had tremor (presumably ET) lived on the average 9.2 years longer than did parents without tremor. The association of familial tremor with significantly increased longevity suggests that familial tremor confers some anti-aging influence. Alternatively, patients with ET might have an underlying personality trait that encourages dietary, occupational, and physical habits that promote longevity. Furthermore, the small amounts of alcohol to calm the tremor might prolong life; and finally, the tremor itself might be viewed as a form of exercise that would have long-standing beneficial effects on general health (Mostile and Jankovic, 2010). Despite the overwhelming evidence that ET is of genetic origin, some researchers have suggested that environmental factors might also play a role, particularly since concordance among monozygotic twins is only 60% (Louis, 2001; Tanner et al., 2001). However, in another study involving 92 twins with ET from the Danish twin registry, the concordance rate was 93% among monozygotic twins and 29% among dizygotic twins when the Tremor Research and Investigation Group consensus criteria were used (Lorenz et al., 2004).

Treatment

In designing protocols to study the effects of a therapeutic intervention on tremor-related functional impairment and on the mean amplitude (and frequency) of tremor, it is important to take into account the marked intraindividual and interindividual and diurnal variations in physiologic and pathologic tremors (van Hilten et al., 1991; Deuschl et al., 2011). Factors such as anxiety, caffeine, or alcohol intake, drugs, and even temperature (Lakie et al., 1994) can affect hour-to-hour variations in the amplitude of tremor. Caffeine, a nonselective adenosine receptor antagonist, can trigger or exacerbate tremor and the observed marked increase in the DBS-induced release of ATP from local astrocytes, which metabolizes to adenosine, has been suggested as one possible mechanism of DBS in suppression of tremor (Bekar et al., 2008).

Even without specific triggers or exacerbating factors, the ET amplitude may vary by 30–50% from hour to hour (Koller and Royse, 1985). The antitremor drugs exert their ameliorating effects by reducing tremor amplitude without any effect on tremor frequency. Reduction of tremor amplitude, however, does not always translate into improvement in function. There are currently no uniformly accepted ET rating scales, but the Unified Tremor Rating Assessment developed by the Tremor Research and Investigation Group

(Jankovic et al., 1996; Ondo et al., 2000) and the Tremor Rating Scale developed by the Tremor Research Group (Tintner and Tremor Research Group, 2004) have been used in several studies.

The treatment of postural tremor depends largely on its severity; many patients require nothing more than simple reassurance. Most patients who are referred to a neurologist, however, have troublesome tremors that require pharmacologic or surgical treatments (Ondo and Jankovic, 1996; Bain, 1997; Lyons et al., 2003) (Fig. 18.3). The large-amplitude and slow-frequency postural tremors usually do not respond to any pharmacologic therapy. Since alcohol reduces the amplitude of ET in about two-thirds of patients, some use it regularly for its calming effect, and some use it prophylactically – for example, before an important engagement at which the presence of tremor could be a source of embarrassment. Although evidence concerning the risk of alcoholism among ET patients is contradictory, regular use of alcohol to treat ET is inadvisable (Mostile and Jankovic, 2010). One epidemiologic, prospective, population-based study in central Spain involving 3285 elderly participants, 76 of whom developed incident ET, concluded that baseline alcohol consumption was associated with substantially higher risk of developing ET (Louis et al., 2009a). They suggested that the alcohol may be in part responsible for the cerebellar toxicity associated with ET. Although the authors dismiss the possibility that the participants who developed incident ET between the baseline and follow-up evaluations had preclinical ET at baseline, because they answered "no" when asked at baseline whether their arms or legs shook, many patients deny having tremor before the onset of alcohol consumption but validation by other family members often confirms that they had tremor prior to alcohol. Furthermore, family members of ET patients sometimes consume alcohol without being aware that it "calms" their tremor. Arguing against alcohol as contributing to the

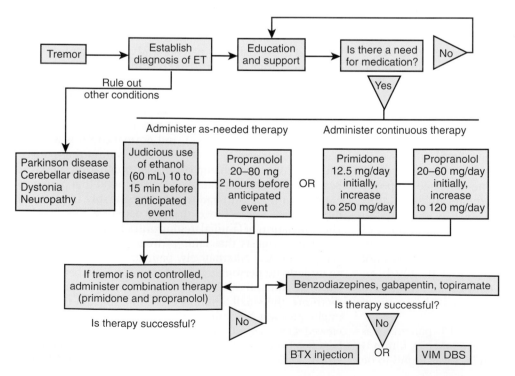

Figure 18.3 Therapeutic algorithm in essential tremor.

cause of ET is also the observation that many patients with ET never drink alcohol (Mostile and Jankovic, 2010).

The mechanism by which alcohol reduces tremor (effective blood level is only 300 mg/L (0.03%)) is unknown, but it is thought to act centrally, since infusion of alcohol into the brachial artery of a tremulous arm is ineffective (Growdon et al., 1975). Furthermore, the amplitude of the central but not peripheral components of ET is decreased after alcohol consumption (Zeuner et al., 2003a). Alcohol is known to affect multiple neurotransmitters, and it might stabilize neuronal membranes by potentiating gamma-aminobutyric acid (GABA) receptor-mediated chloride influx. A pilot trial (n = 12) of 1-octanol, a food additive approved by the Food and Drug Administration that was previously demonstrated to suppress harmaline tremor (see below), found that it significantly decreased amplitude of ET for about 90 minutes after oral dose of 1 mg/kg (Bushara et al., 2004). The benefits and tolerance (except for unusual taste) of this drug were demonstrated in an open-label trial at doses up to 64 mg/kg (Shill et al., 2004).

Treatment of ET and other action tremors is not optimal. In a survey of 261 patients with ET about a third who had been prescribed medication for tremor had discontinued the therapy and another third of cases with severe tremor had stopped medication (Louis et al., 2010). Propranolol, a β-adrenergic blocker, remains the most effective drug for the treatment of ET and enhanced physiologic tremors, but other beta-blockers may also ameliorate postural tremor (Caccia et al., 1989; Calzetti et al., 1990; Koller et al., 2000) (Table 18.7). Propranolol is less effective in head tremor than hand tremor (Calzetti et al., 1992). Although a central mechanism of action has been suggested for this group of drugs, some beta-blockers exert potent antitremor activity even though they are not lipid soluble and hence do not cross the blood–brain barrier. This suggests that the therapeutic effect of beta-blockers may be mediated, at least in part, by the peripheral β-adrenergic receptors (Guan and Peroutka, 1990). The major side effects of propranolol and, to a lesser degree, other beta-blockers include fatigability, sedation, depression, and sexual impotence. A critical review of 42 articles, based on controlled trials, concluded that despite the conventional wisdom, "there is no significant increased risk of depressive symptoms and only small increased risk of fatigue and sexual dysfunction" associated with beta-blocker therapy (Ko et al., 2002). These drugs are contraindicated in the presence of asthma, second-degree atrioventricular block, and insulin-dependent diabetes. Contrary to traditional

recommendations, they may be used safely in patients with stable congestive heart failure due to left ventricular systolic dysfunction (Packer et al., 1999). The efficacy of sotalol, a nonselective β-antagonist, in reducing ET is comparable to that of propranolol and atenolol, even though both atenolol and sotalol have very low lipid solubility and therefore act mainly through peripheral mechanisms (Leigh et al., 1983). Arotinolol, an alpha- and beta-blocker that is used as an antiobesity drug, was found to be as effective as propranolol in a randomized crossover study (Lee et al., 2003).

The antitremor effect of primidone has been confirmed by several open trials and placebo-controlled studies (Koller and Royse, 1986). By starting primidone at a very low dose (25 mg at bedtime), the occasional idiosyncratic acute, toxic side effects (nausea, vomiting, sedation, confusion, and ataxia) can be prevented. Since there is little or no correlation between blood levels and tremolytic effects, the daily dosage should be gradually increased over a period of several weeks until the optimal therapeutic response is achieved. Dosages above 250 mg/day are only rarely necessary. The antitremor effect of primidone is largely attributed to the parent compound rather than to its metabolites, phenylethylmalonamide (PEMA) or phenobarbital (Sasso et al., 1991). In one study (Koller and Royse, 1986), primidone alone was found to decrease tremor more than propranolol alone, but a combination of the two drugs might be more efficacious than either drug alone. In a double-blind, placebo-controlled, crossover study, Gorman and colleagues (1986) found that both propranolol and primidone significantly reduced tremor compared to placebo. There is no evidence that either one of these primary anti-ET drugs is more efficacious than the other, but acute adverse effects with primidone and chronic side effects of propranolol limit therapy. The combination of the two drugs might be more efficacious than monotherapy (Koller and Royse, 1986). Although the benefits are usually maintained, the dosages might have to be increased after the first year to sustain the antitremor effectiveness. A double-blind study of 87 patients with ET, however, showed that low doses of primidone (250 mg/day) were as effective as, or more effective than, high doses (750 mg/day) (Serrano-Duenas, 2003).

In addition to beta-blockers and primidone, the benzodiazepine drugs, such as diazepam, lorazepam, clonazepam, and alprazolam (Gunal et al., 2000), as well as barbiturates, also may have some ameliorating effects on ET or its variants (Ondo and Jankovic, 1996). In a double-blind, crossover, placebo-controlled study, 22 patients with ET received in random order alprazolam, acetazolamide, primidone, and placebo for 4 weeks, each separated by a 2-week washout period. The study demonstrated that alprazolam was superior to placebo and equipotent to primidone, whereas there was no statistically significant difference between acetazolamide and placebo (Gunal et al., 2000). The mean effective daily dose of alprazolam was 0.75 mg, and no troublesome side effects were reported by the patients who took alprazolam. Clonazepam was shown to be ineffective in controlling ET in one double-blind study, but at a mean dose of 2.2 mg/day, it improved kinetic tremor (Biary and Koller, 1987). Methazolamide (Neptazane), a sulfonamide that is used in the treatment of glaucoma, was reported to be effective in the treatment of ET (Muenter et al., 1991). Ten of 28 patients apparently achieved moderate to complete relief of

---

Table 18.7 Evidence-based recommendations for treatment of ET (Quality Standards Subcommittee of the AAN)

- Propranolol and primidone reduce limb tremor (Level A)
- Alprazolam, atenolol, gabapentin (monotherapy), sotalol, and topiramate (Level B)
- Propranolol reduces head tremor (Level B)
- Clonazepam, clozapine, nadolol, and nimodipine (Level C)
- Botulinum toxin A in limb, head and voice tremor (Level C)
- Chronic DBS and thalamotomy (Level C)
- Surgical treatment of head and voice tremor and the use of gamma knife thalamotomy (Level U)

their tremor. The average maintenance dose was 129 mg/day, and reported side effects included sedation, nausea, epigastric discomfort, and parasthesias. Aplastic anemia, the most feared complication, did not occur during the 6-month (10 weeks to 29 months) follow-up. The beneficial effects of methazolamide suggested by this open trial, however, could not be confirmed by a double-blind controlled study (Busenbark et al., 1993). Although our personal experience with this drug has been disappointing, we have found that up to 10–20% of patients who were previously unresponsive to other antitremor treatments note a marked improvement in their tremor with methazolamide. Flunarizine, a calcium channel blocker, was reported to improve ET in 13 of 15 patients (Biary and Deeb, 1991). This drug, however, is not available for use in the United States, and it can produce parkinsonism and tardive dyskinesia. Another calcium channel blocker, nimodipine at 120 mg/day, was found to improve ET in 8 of 15 patients who completed a double-blind, placebo-controlled trial (Biary et al., 1995). Anecdotally, fenofibric acid (Trilipix), a lipid regulating agent, has been reported to also improve ET.

Despite some encouraging results with gabapentin based on pilot studies, subsequent double-blind controlled studies showed mixed results (Louis, 1999), ranging from no benefit (Pahwa et al., 1998) to modest improvement (Ondo et al., 2000) to a marked benefit comparable to that obtained with propranolol (Gironell et al., 1999). Topiramate, a broad-spectrum anticonvulsant, has been also reported to reduce ET in a double-blind, placebo-controlled trial at 400 mg/day dose (Connor, 2002). Although well tolerated, topiramate may cause parasthesias and weight loss and may adversely affect cognition (Thompson et al., 2000). Some patients who are unresponsive to conventional treatments do improve even with low-dose (50 mg/day) topiramate (Gatto et al., 2003). In a multicenter, double-blind, placebo-controlled trial involving 208 patients (topiramate, 108; placebo, 100) the final visit score (last observation carried forward) was lower in the topiramate group than with placebo ($P < 0.001$) (Ondo et al., 2006). Mean percentage improvement in overall TRS scores was 29% with topiramate at a mean final dose of 292 mg/day and 16% with placebo ($P < 0.001$) and topiramate was associated with greater improvement in function and disability ($P = 0.001$). The most common adverse effects were parasthesias (28%), weight loss (22%), and taste perversion (19%), but only the following adverse effects resulted in discontinuation of the drug: paresthesia (5%), nausea (3%), concentration/attention difficulty (3%), and somnolence (3%). Overall, adverse events were treatment limiting in 31.9% of topiramate patients and 9.5% of placebo patients. Thus, this multicenter study showed that topiramate was effective in the treatment of ET with acceptable tolerability profile. In a pilot, open-label, crossover trial designed to compare zonisamide and arotinolol in 14 patients with ET using the Fahn–Tolosa–Marin clinical rating scale at baseline and 2 weeks after administration of each drug, both drugs were found to have significant and equal antitremor effect, but zonisamide was more effective for voice, face, tongue, and head tremors (Morita et al., 2005). In a subsequent double-blind, placebo-controlled trial involving 20 patients with ET, zonisamide failed to provide any improvement in clinical rating scales, although it reduced tremor by accelerometry (Zesiewicz et al., 2007a).

Zonisamide was, however, found to be more effective than propranolol in the treatment of isolated head tremor (Song et al., 2008). One study showed that 200 mg/day seemed to the optimal dose for zonisamide in the treatment of ET (Handforth et al., 2009). Levetiracetam, another antiepileptic, was shown to have a significant antitremor effect in one double-blind, placebo-controlled trial at 1000 mg as a single dose (Bushara et al., 2005), but not in other studies (Handforth and Martin, 2004; Ondo et al., 2004; Elble et al., 2007b). Pregabalin has been found effective in a pilot, double-blind, placebo-controlled trial (Zesiewicz et al., 2007b), but not in a double-blind, placebo-controlled trial (Ferrara et al., 2009b).

Mirtazapine has been reported to improve rest tremor (Pact and Giduz, 1999), but in a double-blind, placebo-controlled trial, the drug was not found to exert a significant benefit in ET (Pahwa and Lyons, 2003). Finally, clozapine has been found to effective in selected drug-resistant patients with ET (Ceravolo et al., 1999). Gabapentin (Onofrj et al., 1998), levodopa (Wills et al., 1999), primidone, clonazepam, and phenobarbital seem to be particularly useful in patients with orthostatic tremor (Cabrera-Valdivia et al., 1991; FitzGerald and Jankovic, 1991). Despite earlier reports, amantadine has not been found effective in patients with ET in a randomized, placebo-controlled trial, and in some patients actually exacerbated the postural tremor (Gironell et al., 2006). Sodium oxybate, a salt of gamma-hydroxybutyrate (GHB), may suppress tremor in a manner similar to alcohol (Frucht et al., 2005).

Other treatment modalities for postural tremors include injections of BTX into muscles that are involved in the production of the oscillatory movement and various surgical approaches. In one open trial of BTX treatment, 67% of 51 patients with various disabling tremors noted at least some improvement (Jankovic and Schwartz, 1991). The average duration of improvement was 10.5 weeks, and side effects were chiefly related to local muscle weakness; 40% of 42 patients who were injected in the neck muscles to control head tremor and 60% of 10 patients who were injected in the forearm muscles to control hand tremor improved. Other studies have demonstrated the usefulness of BTX in the treatment of hand tremor (Trosch and Pullman, 1994). A double-blind, placebo-controlled trial has demonstrated a mild to moderate efficacy of BTX injections in patients with severe hand ET (Jankovic et al., 1996) and in patients with ET involving the head (Pahwa et al., 1995; Wissel et al., 1997). Although in one study, only 20–30% of patients with voice tremor were found to benefit from vocal cord injections of BTX, the majority of patients benefited from a subjective reduction in vocal effort that might have been attributable to reduced laryngeal airway resistance (Warrick et al., 2000). In another study involving 27 patients with adductor spasmodic dysphonia and vocal tremor and in four patients with severe vocal tremor alone, a significant improvement in various acoustic measures was observed after thyroarytenoid and interarytenoid BTX injections and less tremor was demonstrated in 73% of the paired comparisons (Kendall and Leonard, 2010). Although 67% of the patients with spasmodic dysphonia and vocal tremor wished to continue to receive BTX injections, only one patient with severe vocal tremor wished to continue with injections. BTX may also be effective in primary writing tremor, although a specially designed writing device might be a simpler and at least as effective treatment (Espay et al., 2005).

Peripheral deafferentation with anesthetic is currently being re-explored as a potential treatment of focal dystonia and tremor (Rondot et al., 1968; Pozos and Iaizzo, 1992; Kaji et al., 1995). An injection of 5–10 mL of 0.5% lidocaine into the target muscle not only improved focal dystonia, but also reduced the amplitude of the postural tremor. This short effect (<24 hours) can be extended for up to several weeks if ethanol is injected simultaneously (Kaji, personal communication). In a study of 10 patients with ET, Gironell and colleagues (2002) reported a transient (<1 hour) improvement in tremor after transient magnetic stimulation of the cerebellum.

The neurosurgical treatments, including DBS, that were discussed in the section on rest tremors may be also efficacious in patients with action hand tremors (Benabid et al., 1991; Blond et al., 1992; Deiber et al., 1993; Jankovic et al., 1995b; Koller et al., 1997), head tremors (Koller et al., 1999), and even task-specific tremors (Racette et al., 2001). It is of interest that cerebellar lesions can abolish ET, but it is unlikely that this observation will lead to surgically induced cerebellar lesions as a therapeutic modality in patients with ET (Dupuis et al., 1989). On the other hand, chronic cortical stimulation has been reported to improve contralateral action tremor (Nguyen et al., 1998). The observation that injection of muscimol, a GABA$_A$ agonist, into the VIM thalamus improved tremor in patients with ET suggests that GABA agonists might be useful in the treatment of ET (Pahapill et al., 1999). On the basis of the observation that vagus nerve stimulation has a nonspecific calming effect in treated epileptic patients and that it suppresses harmaline-induced tremor (see below) in rats (Handforth and Krahl, 2001), a multicenter trial was conducted to study the effects of vagus nerve stimulation in patients with essential and parkinsonian tremor, but no meaningful benefit was demonstrated (Handforth et al., 2003).

Kinetic tremors

Diagnosis

Kinetic tremor is typically associated with lesions or diseases that involve the cerebellum or its outflow pathways. The term *kinetic tremor* more accurately describes the oscillation occurring with limb movement than the classic term *intention tremor*, which is ambiguous because it implies tremors that are present when "contemplating, initiating, performing, or completing a movement" (Lou and Jankovic, 1993). It is important to recognize that kinetic tremor is not simply a consequence of cerebellar ataxia (Diener and Dichgans, 1992), hypotonia, dysmetria, or dysdiadochokinesia but that the different motor disorders may coexist, often causing severe functional disability (Sabra and Hallett, 1984). Although kinetic tremor was traditionally considered a predominantly proximal tremor, using wrist (distal) or whole-arm (proximal) visually guided tracking in patients with multiple sclerosis showed a major frequency component at 4–5 Hz, most of the action tremor being distal rather than proximal (Liu et al., 1999).

In addition to this action, kinetic tremor patients with cerebellar lesions often exhibit postural tremors and titubation. The term *titubation* simply refers to a rhythmic oscillation of the head or trunk, presumably caused by hypotonia of the axial muscles. Kinetic cerebellar outflow tremor might be a component of the thalamic ataxia syndrome characterized in addition to the tremor by contralateral ataxia, hemisensory loss, and transient hemiparesis caused by a lesion in the mid to posterior thalamus involving the dentatorubrothalamic and ascending sensory pathways (Solomon et al., 1994). Kinetic terminal and postural tremors have been reported to result from repetitive transcranial magnetic stimulation, possibly by interfering with cerebellar inflow to the motor cortex (Topka et al., 1999). Although kinetic tremors are more difficult to assess than ET or PD tremors, by using handwriting, spirals, and other tests, objective assessments of kinetic tremors, such as those seen in multiple sclerosis, can be reliably obtained (Alusi et al., 2000). In a study of 100 patients with definite multiple sclerosis, Alusi and colleagues (2001b) found 58 with tremor, but it was symptomatic in only 38 and incapacitating in 10. The authors concluded that multiple sclerosis tremors are usually related to involvement of the cerebellum.

Treatment

Some causes of tremor, such as alcohol withdrawal, phenytoin, lithium, amiodarone, and valproate toxicity (Nouzeilles et al., 1999) and cerebellar tumors and abscesses are specifically treatable. Tremor and ataxia in such cases can resolve after the underlying cause is removed. Some kinetic tremors can be reduced by attaching weights to the wrist, but this method provides only limited improvement in function (Aisen et al., 1993).

No drugs have been shown to reduce cerebellar tremor satisfactorily and reproducibly, but the application of wrist weights before eating may enable to patient feed himself. Isoniazid was initially thought to improve cerebellar, postural tremor more than kinetic tremor (Sabra and Hallett, 1984), but the results of a double-blind trial were disappointing (Hallett et al., 1991). Sechi and colleagues (1989) reported that carbamazepine was effective in the treatment of cerebellar tremor, possibly by reducing hyperactivity in thalamic neurons. Ten patients, seven with multiple sclerosis and three with cerebrovascular disease, were followed for 2–24 months. All patients improved on a clinical rating scale and by accelerometric recording when given carbamazepine, 400–600 mg daily. There was no improvement with placebo. Trelles and colleagues (1984) reported that cerebellar kinetic tremor secondary to multiple sclerosis and to olivopontocerebellar degeneration responded to clonazepam treatment at a daily dose of 8–15 mg. Alcohol not only improves ET but also may improve tremor associated with multiple sclerosis (Hammond and Kerr, 2008). Glutethimide, a piperidinedione derivative with sedative and anticholinergic effects, has recently been reported to be effective at doses of 750–1250 mg/day in action tremors, including ET, cerebellar tremors, and midbrain tremors (Aisen et al., 1991). The encouraging results from this open trial await confirmation by properly designed controlled studies. Even if it is found to be effective, however, the potential side effects of glutethimide, including respiratory depression, aplastic anemia, and physical and psychological dependence, will limit its usefulness. Buspirone, a serotonin (5-HT$_{1A}$) agonist was reported to be useful in some patients with mild cerebellar ataxia, but placebo-controlled study is needed before it can be concluded that this drug is effective in cerebellar ataxia or tremor (Lou et al., 1995). Baker and colleagues (2000) found that cannabinoids control tremor in a mouse model of multiple sclerosis, but the effects of tetrahydrocannabinol in patients with cerebellar outflow tremor are unknown. Levetiracetam has been also found to be effective in rare cases (Ferlazzo et al., 2008).

Stereotactic thalamotomy has been reported to successfully relieve kinetic tremor in patients with multiple sclerosis and other etiologies (Andrew, 1984). Radiofrequency lesions in the VIM seem to provide the best control of tremor with the lowest risk of neurologic deficit (Speelman and Manen, 1984; Nagaseki et al., 1986; Alusi et al., 2001a), although thalamic DBS has been also reported to be useful in selected patients with cerebellar-outflow tremor due to multiple sclerosis or other causes (Whittle et al., 1998; Montgomery et al., 1999). A recent report of the Quality Standards Subcommittee of the American Academy of Neurology, based on a review of evidence-based publications, published the following practice parameters related to therapies for ET. Propranolol and primidone reduce limb tremor (Level A); alprazolam, atenolol, gabapentin (monotherapy), sotalol, and topiramate are probably effective in reducing limb tremor (Level B); propranolol reduces head tremor (Level B); clonazepam, clozapine, nadolol, and nimodipine possibly reduce limb tremor (Level C); BTX type A may reduce limb, head, and voice tremor, but this treatment is limited by potential adverse effects (Level C); chronic DBS and thalamotomy are highly efficacious but potentially risky procedures (Level C); and there is insufficient evidence regarding surgical treatment of head and voice tremor and the use of gamma knife thalamotomy (Level U) (Zesiewicz et al., 2005) (Table 18.7).

Pathophysiologic mechanisms of rest and action tremors

Our understanding of mechanisms that are involved in generation of tremors has been facilitated by the development of neurophysiologic and other quantitative techniques such as EMG recordings and uniaxial and triaxial accelerometers and by the application of computer technology to analyze the frequency spectra and other tremor-related physiologic variables (Elble and Koller, 1990; Gresty and Buckwell, 1990; Elble et al., 1994; Louis et al., 2001b). A frequency of 6 Hz is usually the maximum rate of oscillation produced by a voluntary effort. During a voluntary contraction, motor units usually start firing at 8 Hz, and tetanic fusion frequency is reached at 15–20 Hz. Different parts of the human limb have mechanical characteristics (inertia and stiffness) that determine its natural resonant frequency. Such frequency is inversely related to the mass of the body part: finger, 25 Hz; wrist, 9 Hz; and elbow, 2 Hz.

There is a growing body of evidence supporting the notion that central oscillators are important in the generation of physiologic and pathologic tremors (Pare et al., 1990; Plenz and Kitai, 1999; McAuley and Marsden, 2000; Brown, 2003;

Gatev et al., 2006). Using microelectrode recordings in awake or decerebrate monkeys who have been curarized and whose limbs were deafferented by sectioning C2 to T4 dorsal roots, Lamarre (1984) demonstrated spontaneous 3–6 Hz rhythmic discharges in the ventral thalamus and 7–12 Hz activity in the olivocerebellar system. Deafferenting the thalamus by a lesion in the ventromedial tegmentum of the midbrain facilitates synchronization of thalamic neurons, which is ultimately expressed as a spontaneous, 3–6 Hz, parkinsonian rest tremor. The amplitude of these discharges and associated tremors is markedly enhanced by the tremorgenic drug harmaline. Harmaline-induced tremor is currently considered the most reliable animal model of ET as it generates both postural and kinetic tremors. It has been postulated that harmaline induces release of glutamate and acts as a potent reversible monoamine oxidase inhibitor. These and possibly other pharmacologic effects of harmaline result in facilitating low-threshold calcium conductance with resultant oscillatory activity of the olivocerebellar system, and eventual coupling and synchrony in the inferior olivary nucleus. Ethanol reduced harmaline-induced tremor, and possibly ET, by desynchronizing the olivary discharges, in part by decreasing glutamate (Manto and Laute, 2008). There are two types of harmaline-induced tremors, both of which appear to originate in the inferior olivary nucleus: an 8–12 Hz tremor in normal animals (analogous to physiologic tremor) and a 6–8 Hz tremor in monkeys with lesions in the dentate nucleus. Single-unit recordings from patients with parkinsonian tremors showed that neurons in the thalamic ventral nuclear group show rhythmic activity that correlated with EMG activity. Some, but not all, of these cells responded to somatosensory activity, indicating the importance of peripheral modulation (Lenz et al., 1994). In addition to the thalamus, there are other subcortical nuclei – particularly the subthalamic nucleus (STN) and external globus pallidus (GPe) – that contain neuronal populations that produce synchronized oscillating bursts at 0.4, 0.8, and 1.8 Hz in a cell-culture environment (Plenz and Kitai, 1999). In addition to the low-frequency (<10 Hz) oscillations, there are 11–30 Hz and >60 Hz oscillatory activities within the subthalamopallidal-thalamocortical circuit (Brown, 2003). In PD, synchronized oscillatory activity in the 10–50 Hz band (often termed "β-band") prevalent in the basal ganglia thalamocortical circuit may be important in mediating certain parkinsonian features, including bradykinesia and tremor, and can be reduced by dopaminergic treatments (Gatev et al., 2006). Furthermore, there is evidence that as a result of dopaminergic deficiency, the normal independent firing of pallidal neurons changes to both low-frequency (4–7 Hz) and high-frequency (10–16 Hz) oscillatory activity, which can be also recorded from the STN, and these oscillations often correlate with arm tremor (Bergman et al., 1998). This pacemaker could be responsible for the generation of tremor under pathologic conditions such as dopaminergic deficiency in PD. Therefore, surgical treatments of PD, such as lesion or stimulation of the GPi or STN, might act by desynchronizing the oscillatory basal ganglia–thalamocortical network activity. Such microelectrode-guided stereotactic operations in PD allow for single-cell recordings in the globus pallidus, thalamic nuclei, and other subcortical structures, leading to hypotheses about the normal and abnormal function of the basal ganglia. One such study, for example, found tremor-locked cells in the center median-parafascicular complex of the thalamus with low-threshold calcium spike type bursts in central lateral nucleus and the paralamellar division of mediodorsal nucleus of the thalamus (Magnin et al., 2000).

Intracellular recordings from brainstem sections have demonstrated that neurons in the inferior olive have spontaneous oscillatory activity (Llinas, 1988; Kepler et al., 1990; Bevan et al., 2002). The autorhythmic properties of these neurons make this brainstem nucleus a prime candidate as a neuronal generator for tremor. In the olivary neurons, low-threshold Ca^{2+} conductance at the somatic membrane enables these neurons to generate action potentials (low-threshold spike) even at subthreshold depolarization. A fast-action potential, generated by Na^+ current into the cell body, is followed by a slow, high-threshold Ca^{2+} spike that activates prolonged (80–100 ms), K^+-mediated hyperpolarization. This is followed by an abrupt rebound response, generated by low-threshold Ca^{2+} conductance, often large enough to generate a second, Na^+-dependent, action potential, and the cycle repeats itself. In addition to the olivary nucleus, there are other areas of the brain, particularly the STN and globus pallidus, that display spontaneous rhythmic activities. In the STN neurons, voltage-gated Na^+ channels inactivate slowly during the depolarizing phase of the oscillation. In addition, Ca^{2+}-dependent K^+ current is activated by Ca^{2+} entry through high-voltage Ca^{2+} channels that open briefly during each Na^+ action potential (Bevan et al., 2002). Harmaline enhances normal hyperpolarization, which is terminated by Ca^{2+} influx and rebound excitation, leading to rhythmic activation of the neurons. Besides harmaline, there are many toxins that can produce tremors in animals and provide useful models for the study of tremors (Wilms et al., 1999). Microelectrode-guided single-cell recordings in patients with PD showed that the average firing rate in the GPi was 91 ± 52 Hz, and that in the globus pallidus externa was 60 ± 21 Hz (Magnin et al., 2000). In addition, rhythmic, low-threshold calcium spike bursts are often recorded in the pallidum and medial thalamus; some, but not all, are synchronous (in phase) with the typical rest tremor. It has been postulated that the low-threshold calcium spike bursts contribute to rigidity and dystonia by activating the supplementary motor area.

Physiologic tremor is present in all humans. It is an asymptomatic oscillation of a body part, resulting from a complex interaction between local mechanical-reflex mechanisms and central oscillators (McAuley and Marsden, 2000) (Fig. 18.4). The mechanical-reflex component is determined partly by the ballistocardiogram, mechanical properties of the muscle, motor neuron firing characteristics, stretch reflex and muscle spindle feedback, supraspinal influences, and state of activation of the muscle beta receptors (Marsden, 1984). The frequency of this component is inversely proportional to the mass and stiffness of the limb; thus, increasing the external mass load decreases the tremor frequency (Elble and Koller, 1990). Besides this variable frequency component, which is determined largely by the mechanical properties of the oscillating body part, spectral analyses of normal physiologic tremor show another, generally smaller, component with a relatively consistent frequency peak at about 10 (8–12) Hz. This 10 Hz frequency component is independent of peripheral influence, and it persists even after

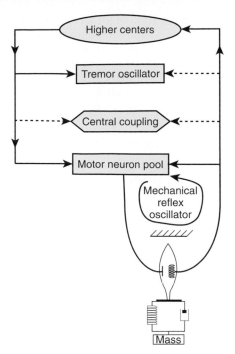

Figure 18.4 Central and peripheral mechanisms of tremors.

deafferentation, suggesting that this component of physiologic tremor is centrally generated. Supraspinal influence on physiologic tremor is supported by the observation that the loss of visual input when the eyes are closed reduces or abolishes this tremor. The amplitude of physiologic tremor is determined largely by the degree of synchronization of motor unit discharges, modulated by muscle spindle Ia afferents. This process is exaggerated during anxiety, exercise, fatigue, and other conditions that are known to enhance peripheral β-adrenergic activity, and it may result in a visible tremor called enhanced physiologic tremor (Table 18.1).

In most pathologic tremors, such as the rest or reemergent tremor of PD (Jankovic et al., 1999), the central oscillators are thought to drive the tremor, and the peripheral mechanisms are thought to merely modify or modulate its amplitude (Marsden, 1984; Britton et al., 1992a). Magnetic brain stimulation can also modify certain pathologic tremors, providing further evidence that these tremors are centrally generated (Britton et al., 1993). The motor pathways that are involved in transmission of signals from these central generators are not well understood. Inhibition of tremor by lesions in the basal ganglia outflow nuclei and in the thalamus suggests that these subcortical nuclei are involved in the pathophysiology of tremors. In parkinsonian states, as a result of nigrostriatal dopamine depletion, excessive GABA-mediated inhibition of the GPe within the indirect striatopallidal pathway leads to a disinhibition of the STN and enhanced glutamate-mediated excitatory drive to the basal ganglia output nucleus (GPi) (DeLong, 1990). This increased drive from the output nuclei is reinforced by reduced inhibitory input to the GPi through the direct pathway. The typical 3–6 Hz rest tremor of PD possibly results from increased inhibition of the thalamic neurons that normally suppress the oscillators or from hyperpolarization of the oscillator neurons. In PD, the increased inhibitory output from the GPi leads to deafferentation of the thalamus, particularly the reticular nucleus, and synchronization of local neuronal networks with intrinsic properties to spontaneously discharge (Lamarre, 1984; Huntsman et al., 1999). This spontaneous bursting is transmitted via the thalamocortical-spinal circuitry to the motor neurons in the spinal cord, causing synchronization of motor unit discharges, ultimately expressed as an oscillatory movement.

Pathophysiology of Parkinsonian tremor

In support of the role of the thalamus in the generation of parkinsonian rest tremor is the observation that the ventral thalamus of patients with PD contains a population of neurons that fire spontaneously and rhythmically and that their firing frequency correlates relatively well with the frequency of tremor, recorded by EMG in the contralateral limb (Lenz et al., 1988). Furthermore, a lesion in the nucleus ventralis intermedius (VIM) or electrical stimulation of the nucleus, so-called deep brain stimulation (DBS), abolishes contralateral rest tremor (Kelly et al., 1987; Benabid et al., 1991, 1996; Hubble et al., 1997; Koller et al., 1997; Ondo et al., 1998; Limousin et al., 1999). That parkinsonian tremor is centrally driven is supported by the observation that complete paralysis of extensor forearm muscles as a result of radial nerve palsy actually increased the amplitude of the tremor without changing its frequency (Pullman et al., 1994). Volkmann and colleagues (1996) used magnetoencephalography to study parkinsonian resting tremor, and on the basis of these studies, they concluded that the typical 3–6 Hz parkinsonian tremor is generated by the same central mechanisms that are involved in voluntary rapid alternating movements. They proposed the following sequence of events for typical parkinsonian rest tremor: increased inhibitory output from GPi → hyperpolarization and activation of low-threshold calcium conductance in anterior ventrolateral nucleus (VLa) → 5–10 ms → activation of lateral premotor and motor cortex → 25–30 ms → EMG activity → 100 ms → activation of the central sulcus (reafferent input from muscle spindle to area 3a) → second activation of the somatosensory cortex by the antagonist contraction. The study of pacemaker neuronal networks as well as fast and slow oscillations within the basal ganglia circuitry will undoubtedly provide important insights into the pathophysiology of rhythmic involuntary movements such as tremors (Plenz and Kitai, 1999; Ruskin et al., 1999).

Pathophysiology of essential tremor

It has been suggested that the postural tremor of ET arises from spontaneous firing of the inferior olivary nucleus, which drives the cerebellum and its outflow pathways via the thalamus to the cerebral cortex and then to the spinal cord (Deuschl and Elble, 2000). In contrast to physiologic tremor, the frequency of ET does not decrease with mass loading, indicating a primary role of central mechanisms in ET (Elble and Koller, 1990). On the other hand, local cooling may significantly reduce the amplitude of ET, without changing its frequency (Lakie et al., 1994). Abnormal triphasic pattern with a delayed second agonist burst and other kinematic problems in response to a ballistic movement further support impaired cerebellar function in patients with ET (Koster et al., 2002). In addition, impaired eyeblink conditioning in

patients with ET has been used as evidence of functional disturbance in the olivocerebellar circuits (Kronenbuerger et al., 2007). MRI scans, including diffusion-weighted imaging, have found no abnormalities associated with ET (Martinelli et al., 2007). Using a 3-tesla MRI in 19 ET patients (mean age 69.8 ± 9.4 years) and 20 age- and gender-matched controls, Benito-León et al. (2009a) found that ET patients with severe tremor had significantly more white matter changes in the midbrain, both occipital lobes, and right frontal lobe, and gray matter changes bilaterally in the cerebellum. Diffusion tensor imaging (DTI) MRI showed microstructural abnormalities in the dentate nucleus and superior cerebellar peduncle in patients with ET, providing further support for neurodegenerative pathology of cerebellar structures in ET (Nicoletti et al., 2010).

The involvement of the olivocerebellar-thalamocortical circuitry in ET is supported by changes in the cerebellar blood flow as measured by PET during inhalation of C15-labeled O_2 (Jenkins et al., 1993). Using this technique, the authors compared the cerebellar and cerebral blood flow in patients with ET and normal controls. They found that when the control subjects were holding one arm outstretched (in the absence of tremor), there was increased blood flow in the contralateral sensorimotor cortex and the supplementary motor area. In contrast, unilateral postural arm tremor in patients with ET was associated with markedly increased blood flow to *both cerebellar hemispheres*; in both premotor cortices; and to the contralateral striatal, thalamic, and sensorimotor cortex (but not the supplementary motor area). Passive and voluntary flexion–extension movements of the wrist significantly increased the blood flow only in the ipsilateral cerebellum. The investigators suggested that the increased flow in the cerebellum reflected increased activity of neurons involved in generation of tremor and that ET was due to oscillation within the olivocerebellar pathways, relayed by way of the thalamus and motor cortex to the spinal cord. Using a higher-resolution camera, the investigators were additionally able to demonstrate bilateral midbrain activation in the region of the red nuclei during tremor, but there was no change in the activity of the inferior olive either at rest or during postural tremor (Wills et al., 1994). Additional evidence of increased activation of the cerebellum and red nucleus in ET has been provided by functional MRI studies (Bucher et al., 1997). The preponderance of evidence, based on PET and functional MRI studies, indicates that the inferior olive probably does not play an important role in the generation of ET. This is in contrast to one previous study that indicated the involvement of the inferior olive in ET, suggested by the finding of glucose hypermetabolism during activation (finger-to-nose) of tremor in patients with ET (Dubinsky and Hallett, 1987). The absence of activity in the inferior olive and the bilateral overactivity of cerebellar-rubral-thalamic connections suggest that the tremor generator for ET is located in the cerebellum rather than the inferior olive. This conclusion is further supported by the finding of abnormal bilateral overactivity of cerebellar connections, as measured by regional cerebral blood flow determined by PET with ^{15}O-labeled water, in patients with primary writing tremor and primary orthostatic tremor (Wills et al., 1995, 1996). Furthermore, alcohol has been found to suppress cerebellar synaptic overactivity in patients with ET, which in turn increases afferent input to the inferior olive (Boecker et al., 1996). In one study, 25% of ET patients were found to have moderate or severe kinetic tremor and other elements of cerebellar dysfunction (Deuschl et al., 2000). The demonstration by magnetic resonance spectroscopy of reduced N-acetyl-L-aspartate/creatine and N-acetyl-L-aspartate/choline ratios in the cerebellum of patients with ET compared to controls provides additional evidence for cerebellar dysfunction in ET (Pagan et al., 2003).

Cerebellar pathology, including loss of Purkinje cells, has been also described in some brains of patients with ET (Louis et al., 2006b; Axelrad et al., 2008; Louis and Vonsattel, 2008) but this finding has not been replicated by others (Rajput et al., 2011). In one of the largest clinical-pathologic studies, involving 33 ET and 21 control brains, 8 (24.2%) brains were found to have Lewy bodies in the brainstem, mainly in the locus coeruleus, and these patients were older than those ET cases without Lewy bodies (Louis et al., 2007b). The major pathologic changes, however, were observed in the cerebellum, particularly marked reduction in the number of Purkinje cells and 7-fold increase in Purkinje cell torpedoes (Louis et al., 2009c). Other findings included degeneration of the dentate nucleus, Purkinje cell heterotopias and dendrite swellings. Lewy body ET cases were older than ET cases without Lewy bodies. Increased cerebellar gliosis and depletion of pigmented neurons in the locus coeruleus and substantia nigra (of which 3 had Lewy bodies) were found in a prospective study of 24 subjects enrolled in the Sun Health Research Institute and Body Donation Program (Shill et al., 2008). In a subsequent study, presumably based on the same pathologic cases, they found no difference in the putaminal tyrosine hydroxylase concentration between the ET cases (91.7 ± 113.2 ng/mg) and controls (96.4 ± 102.7 ng/mg) and concluded that "This study provides neurochemical support that ET does not appear to be pre-clinical PD." The data, however, do not support the conclusion for several reasons. First, the mean age in the pathologic series was 86.2 years and mean duration of tremor was 11.1 years; and 19/24 (79%) had a duration of ≤8 years. Although the authors do not provide the mean age at onset, based on their demographic data, the mean age at onset of ET in their population was about 81 years, which is 50 years later than the usual mean age at onset of ET of 31 years. It is, therefore, likely that most of the patients in the Shill et al. (2008) pathologic series had "senile tremor" rather than typical ET. Furthermore, patients with prior history of a movement disorder, including those with parkinsonian features, were excluded; thus, by definition, clinical, pathologic, or biochemical evidence of PD could not be demonstrated in this selected ET population.

Cerebellar dysfunction in ET is also suggested by abnormalities in tandem gait, noted in 50% of ET patients (Singer et al., 1994; Stolze et al., 2001), and by mild postural instability (Henderson et al., 1996; Overby et al., 1996). Although ataxic gait is rare, some ET patients exhibit a slightly slow or cautious pattern of walking (Kronenbuerger et al., 2009). This gait ataxia improves with alcohol at blood level of 0.45% (Klebe et al., 2005). Posturographic analysis in patients with ET showed that balance control is only minimally impaired in ET, but patients with head tremor and longer disease duration may have slightly reduced postural stability (Bove et al., 2006). ET patients also show eye

movement abnormalities indicative of cerebellar dysfunction, such as impaired smooth pursuit initiation and pathologic suppression of the vestibular-ocular reflex time constant by head tilts (otolith dumping) (Helmchen et al., 2003). Further evidence of cerebellar involvement in ET is suggested by a delay in second agonist EMG burst during rapid wrist movements (Britton et al., 1994). That the cerebellum might be involved in ET is also supported by the report of a 71-year-old man with ET in whom postural tremor disappeared on the right side after an ipsilateral cerebellar infarct (Dupuis et al., 1989). Since the amplitude of ET can be substantially reduced by thalamic lesions or thalamic stimulation (Benabid et al., 1991) and close correlation has been demonstrated between thalamic neuronal activity and forearm EMG in patients with ET (Hua et al., 1998), it is likely that the thalamus also plays an important role in the generation or transmission of ET. Despite the reported evidence of cerebellar dysfunction in patients with ET, voxel-based morphometry, however, shows no reduction in cerebellar gray matter volume (Daniels et al., 2006).

In addition to proposed cerebellar involvement in ET, there is some evidence that cerebral cortex plays a role in the generation of ET (McAuley, 2001). Using simultaneous electroencephalogram (EEG)-EMG recordings, Hellwig and colleagues (2001) showed significant corticomuscular coherences in five of nine patients with ET. This is in contrast to a previous study that used magnetoencephalography (Halliday et al., 2000). That study found that in contrast to PD rest tremor, which is associated with marked disruption to the organization of the descending motor signals, there was no coherence between the magnetoencephalogram and EMG in patients with ET. However, the interpretation of the study that primary motor cortex does not contribute to the generation or maintenance of ET has been challenged because of possible insensitivity of the method (Elble, 2000c). The limitations of the various methods that were used in these studies have been pointed out by McAuley (2001), who also noted that EEG-EMG coherence does not necessarily establish cortical origin of the tremor (McAuley, 2001). Some patients with ET have abnormal vibration-induced illusion of movement, suggesting abnormal sensorimotor processing (Frima and Grunewald, 2005).

Rarely, postural tremor that occurs during sustained isometric muscle contraction can be a manifestation of cortical reflex myoclonus (Toro et al., 1993). This "cortical tremor," with or without seizures, usually starts between 19 and 30 years of age as tremulous finger movements, with a benign course and marked response to anticonvulsants, possibly cognitive decline, and a family history suggestive of ET (Okuma et al., 1998; van Rootselaar et al., 2005). It is characterized physiologically by an 8–15 Hz, synchronous, agonist-antagonist, EMG burst lasting less than 50 ms (10–50 ms). The condition shares neurophysiologic features with myoclonus, including giant somatosensory evoked responses and C-reflexes, and it responds well to anticonvulsants such as clonazepam, primidone, and valproate but not to beta-blockers (Okuma et al., 1998). Since the EMG pattern can be influenced by transcranial magnetic and electrical stimulation but not by peripheral nerve stimulation, the rhythmic movement is thought to arise from central, possibly cortical, generators. Jerk-locked back-averaging revealed a positive EEG wave 15 ms preceding the EMG burst of the wrist extensor muscle (Okuma et al., 1998). In contrast to ET, strong cortico- and intermuscular coherence in the 8–30 Hz range was demonstrated in patients with familial cortical myoclonic tremor with epilepsy (van Rootselaar et al., 2006). The syndrome of autosomal dominant cortical tremor, myoclonus, and epilepsy has been linked to three genetic markers, on 8q24 and 2p11.1–q12.2 (Striano et al., 2005) and 5p15.31–p15 (Depienne et al., 2010). The term *familial cortical myoclonic tremor* with epilepsy has been suggested for this disorder, which has been reported in over 50 Japanese and European families (van Rootselaar et al., 2005) and in patients with spinocerebellar ataxia type 6 (Bour et al., 2008).

Other abnormalities that are found in patients with ET include high blood levels of β-carboline alkaloids. Interestingly, these endogenous compounds, also found in plant-derived foods, increase the synchrony of neuronal firing in the inferior olive and cause tremor in experimental animals and humans. Some investigators have suggested that a loss of $GABA_A$ receptors may impair signaling by cerebellar Purkinje cells and cause tremor, as has been demonstrated in mice in which the gene coding for the $GABA_A$ receptor α1 subunit has been knocked out (Jankovic and Noebels, 2005; Kralic et al., 2005). Mutations in the coding region of the *GABRA1* gene, however, do not seem to be a major genetic cause of ET (Deng et al., 2006c).

Clinical-anatomic correlations indicate that kinetic tremor is usually associated with lesions in the cerebellar outflow pathways (Lou and Jankovic, 1993). Lesions of the dentate nucleus or the superior cerebellar peduncle proximal to the decussation correlate with kinetic tremor ipsilateral to the side of the lesion, whereas lesions that are distal to the decussation result in kinetic tremor contralateral to the side of the lesion (Carrea and Mettler, 1955). Lesions in the cerebellar hemisphere tend to produce kinetic tremors with a variable frequency ranging from 5 to 11 Hz; high brainstem lesions are usually associated with tremor frequency in the range of 5–7 Hz; and lower brainstem lesions produce faster tremors, ranging from 8 to 11 Hz (Cole et al., 1988). In contrast, the frequency of classical midbrain (red nucleus) tremor is relatively slow, at 2–3 Hz. In one study of patients with multiple sclerosis, two types of action tremors were identified. One group of patients had pure kinetic tremor with a frequency of 5–8 Hz and an EMG burst duration of 75–100 ms; the other group had coexisting kinetic and postural tremor. In contrast to kinetic tremor, postural tremor had a slower (2.5–4 Hz) frequency and a higher amplitude with a longer burst duration (125–200 ms) (Sabra and Hallett, 1984). The postural tremor was thought to result from a lesion in the cerebellar outflow pathway. Cerebellar kinetic tremor is associated with errors in timing and amplitude of the EMG activities of agonists and antagonists (Flament and Hore, 1986; Hore and Flament, 1986). The important role of peripheral reflex mechanisms in the pathogenesis of cerebellar kinetic tremor is supported by the observation that the character of the tremor can be altered by mechanical loading to the tremulous limb (Sanes et al., 1988) and by improvement in writing after 3–5 min of compressive ischemia of the affected arm (Dash, 1995). Lakie and colleagues (2004) showed that reduction of tremor by ischemia may be due to an accumulation of interstitial potassium in the muscle. The frequency of the tremor can be increased by increasing the spring stiffness and by decreasing the mass.

Other tremors

Fragile X-associated tremor/ataxia syndrome

Other causes of kinetic tremor, phenomenologically similar to ET, include premutation in the fragile X gene (*FMR1*) (Hagerman et al., 2001; Berry-Kravis et al., 2003; Jacquemont et al., 2003, 2004; Leehey et al., 2003; Hagerman and Hagerman, 2004, 2008; Amiri et al., 2008). While healthy individuals have about 30 CGG repeats in the *FMR1* gene, the carriers of this premutation syndrome have 55–200 repeats. The *FMR1* CGG repeat length has been found to predict motor dysfunction in premutation carriers (Leehey et al., 2008). In addition to the ET-like tremor, frequently affecting the head, and ataxia, this fragile X-associated tremor/ataxia syndrome (FXTAS) is also associated with mild cognitive impairment with frontal executive deficit, dementia, parkinsonism, dysautonomia, erectile dysfunction, peripheral neuropathy, and generalized brain atrophy, regardless of family history (Berry-Kravis et al., 2007) (Table 18.8). FXTAS may also, rarely, occur in females with a similar phenotype but in early menopause due to ovarian failure. One of our patients with severe FXTAS-associated tremor improved markedly with thalamic DBS (Ferrara et al., 2009a). Unusual bilateral T2 middle cerebellar hyperintensities have been identified on magnetic resonance imaging in some cases (Leehey et al., 2003). Overexpression and CNS toxicity of the *FMR1* mRNA has been thought to cause this fragile-X-associated tremor/ataxia syndrome (Berry-Kravis et al., 2007; Jacquemont et al., 2007; Hagerman and Hagerman, 2008).

Although some features overlap with those of multiple system atrophy, FXTAS is a rare cause of multiple system atrophy (Biancalana et al., 2005). Patients with FXTAS and parkinsonism have been found to have normal dopamine transporter as determined by CIT-SPECT, indicating a postsynaptic dopaminergic deficit (Ceravolo et al., 2005). Postmortem studies on brains of four elderly premutation carriers showed eosinophilic intranuclear inclusions in both neuronal and astrocytic nuclei throughout the brain, particularly involving the hippocampus (Greco et al., 2002). Subsequent neuropathologic studies of patients with FXTAS showed:

Table 18.8 Clinical features of fragile X-associated tremor/ataxia syndrome (FXTAS)

- 55–200 CGG repeats (*FMR1* premutation)
- ET-like postural tremor
- Kinetic tremor
- Mild cognitive impairment with frontal executive deficit
- Ataxia
- Parkinsonism (MSA)
- Erectile dysfunction
- Peripheral neuropathy
- Premature ovarian failure
- MRI: Bilateral T2 middle cerebellar peduncle hyperintensities

(1) cerebral and cerebellar white matter disease with spongiosis in the middle cerebellar peduncles, (2) astrocytic pathology with enlarged inclusion-bearing astrocytes, and (3) intranuclear inclusions in the brain and spinal cord, including the cranial nerve nucleus XII (Greco et al., 2006). The number of inclusions seem to correlate with the number of CGG repeats (Cohen et al., 2006). The inclusions contain a variety of proteins, such as RNA binding proteins, but ubiquinated proteins represent only a small portion of all the proteins, suggesting that breakdown of proteasomal degradation is not the main mechanism of the inclusions (Iwahashi et al., 2006).It has been postulated that premutation RNA is responsible for the observed neurodegeneration (Orr, 2004). Marked loss of Purkinje cells in the cerebellum, Purkinje axonal torpedoes, and Bergmann gliosis were also found. SCA12, a rare autosomal-dominant ataxia, may also present with ET-like tremor before other signs of ataxia become evident. This form of ataxia has been associated with CAG repeat expansion in the *PPP2R2B* gene (5q31–q33) coding for protein phosphatase PP2A (Fujigasaki et al., 2001). The frequency of fragile X premutation, even in patients with tremor, parkinsonism, and ataxia, is so low that it is not cost-effective to routinely test for it even in an enriched movement disorders population (Arocena et al., 2004; Deng et al., 2004; Tan et al., 2004). Interestingly, the location of the CAG repeat expansion in the 5′ region is similar to that of the CGG repeat in *FMR1*, in which an expansion results in CpG hypermethylation and disruption of transcription, resulting in the fragile X phenotype.

Neuropathic tremors

Tremor has been described in patients with various types of peripheral neuropathy (Said et al., 1982; Shahani, 1984). Distal postural tremor was noted in patients with chronic relapsing and dysgammaglobulinemic polyneuropathies (Bain et al., 1996). The amplitude was not related to the severity of weakness or proprioceptive sensory loss, and propranolol improved the tremor in some patients. Hereditary motor and sensory neuropathy is associated with tremor, clinically similar to ET, in nearly half of cases (Cardoso and Jankovic, 1993). The frequent association between tremor caused by peripheral nerve injury and reflex sympathetic dystrophy suggests that the sympathetic nervous system contributes to the pathogenesis of peripherally induced tremor (Jankovic and Van der Linden, 1988; Deuschl et al., 1991; Cardoso and Jankovic, 1995; Jankovic, 1994; van Rooijen et al., 2011).

Tremors caused by trauma or stroke

Tremor can also occur after severe or even minimal head trauma (Biary et al., 1989; Goetz and Pappert, 1992; Jankovic, 1994; Krauss et al., 1995). Biary and colleagues (1989) described seven patients who developed postural and kinetic tremors involving various body parts up to several weeks after mild head injury without loss of consciousness. Ipsilateral predecussational dentatothalamic lesion was involved in the majority (56%) of 25 instances of severe post-traumatic tremor in 19 patients, followed by involvement of the contralateral predecussational dentatothalamic pathway (28%), dentate nucleus (4%), and thalamus (4%);

no lesion was identified by neuroimaging in 2 (8%) patients (Krauss et al., 1995). Clonazepam was effective in reducing tremor in 3 patients, and propranolol was effective in 1. Post-traumatic midbrain tremor may improve with anticholinergic and dopaminergic drugs (Samie et al., 1990), but in general, this tremor only rarely responds satisfactorily to drug therapy. Many of our patients with post-traumatic tremors have benefited from VIM thalamotomy; additional patients may benefit from thalamic stimulation (Broggi et al., 1993). In addition to trauma, a variety of tremors can occur following ischemic or hemorrhagic strokes (Ferbert and Gerwig, 1993; Miwa et al., 1996).

Trauma can also cause injury to the peripheral nerves, producing a form of neuropathic tremor, which was discussed earlier. Traumatic neck injury may cause cervical radiculopathy, which may be associated with a postural tremor in the ipsilateral arm (Hashimoto et al., 2002). Loading and ischemic nerve block reduced the frequency of the tremor, suggesting a role of the mechanical reflex mechanism and stretch reflex loop in this peripherally induced tremor.

Psychogenic tremor

One of the most challenging tasks in the diagnosis of tremors is differentiating between psychogenic and neurogenic tremors (Kenney et al., 2007) (Table 18.9). Koller and colleagues (1989) provided the following diagnostic criteria useful in the diagnosis of psychogenic tremors: (1) abrupt onset, (2) static course, (3) spontaneous remission, (4) difficulty in classifying (various combinations of rest, postural, and kinetic tremors), (5) selective disability, (6) changing amplitude and frequency, (7) unresponsiveness to antitremor drugs, (8) increasing of tremor with attention, (9) lessening of tremor with distractibility, (10) responsiveness to placebo, (11) absence of other neurologic signs, and (12) remission with psychotherapy (Video 18.8). Deuschl and colleagues (1998b) found the following features particularly characteristic of psychogenic tremor: sudden onset and

Table 18.9 Distinguishing psychogenic from essential tremor
• A "blinded" rater evaluated video segments of subjects using a standardized protocol
• $N = 33$ subjects with ET (56.8 ± 17.0 years) and 12 with psychogenic tremor (42.5 ± 11.0 years)
• Patients with psychogenic tremor were significantly more likely to have a history of sudden onset ($P = 0.03$), spontaneous remissions ($P = 0.03$), and shorter duration of tremor ($P = 0.001$)
• Family history of tremor was significantly more common in the ET group ($P = 0.001$)
• A moderate to marked degree of distraction with alternate finger tapping ($P = 0.01$) and mental concentration on serial 7 s ($P = 0.01$) was more common in psychogenic tremor
• Suggestibility with a tuning fork ($P = 0.04$) and exacerbation with hyperventilation ($P = 0.06$) seemed predictive of psychogenic tremor
• Entrainment was not different in the two groups
Data from Kenney C, Diamond A, Mejia N, et al. Distinguishing psychogenic and essential tremor. J Neurol Sci 2007;263:94–99.

variable (rarely remitting) course, coactivation sign (fluctuations in muscle tone and in tremor during passive movements), and absent finger tremor. Although overt signs of hysteria were often lacking, evidence of depression and psychosomatic conditions were common. In another study of 70 patients with psychogenic tremor, 73% had an abrupt onset, and 46% had their maximal disability at onset (Kim et al., 1999). Additional features that were found helpful in confirming the diagnosis of psychogenic tremor included spread from a focal onset to generalized tremor, variability, and entrainment. Electrophysiologic studies are rarely helpful in differentiating organic tremor from psychogenic tremor (McAuley et al., 1998). Using accelerometry, Zeuner and colleagues (2003b) demonstrated that in contrast to essential and parkinsonian tremor, patients with PT showed larger tremor frequency changes and higher individual variability while tapping. Longitudinal studies are needed to determine the natural history of psychogenic tremors. In one study, a 6-year follow-up of 64 patients with unexplained motor disorders, only 3 were later found to have an organic diagnosis (Crimlisk et al., 1998). In the Parkinson's Disease Center and Movement Disorders Clinic at the Baylor College of Medicine, psychogenic tremor is the most common of all psychogenic movement disorders, accounting for 4.1% of all patients (Jankovic and Thomas, 2006). Clinical information was obtained on 228 of 517 (44.1%) patients, who were followed for a mean of 3.4 ± 2.8 years. Among the 127 patients who were diagnosed with psychogenic tremor, 92 (72.4%) were female, the mean age at initial evaluation was 43.7 ± 14.1 years, and the mean duration of symptoms was 4.6 ± 7.6 years. The following clinical features were considered to be characteristic of psychogenic tremor: abrupt onset (78.7%), distractibility (72.4%), variable amplitude and frequency (62.2%), intermittent occurrence (35.4%), inconsistent movement (29.9%), and variable direction (17.3%). In the majority of patients, some precipitating event could be identified prior to the onset of tremor, including personal life stress (33.9%), physical trauma (23.6%), major illness (13.4%), surgery (9.4%), or reaction to a medical treatment or procedure (8.7%). Coexistent organic neurologic disorder was present in 37% of patients with psychogenic tremor; psychiatric comorbidities included depression in 50.7% and anxiety in 30.7%. Evidence of secondary gain was present in 32.3%, including maintenance of a disability status in 21.3%, pending compensation in 10.2%, and litigation in 9.4%. Improvement in tremor, reported on a global rating scale at last follow-up by 55.1%, was attributed chiefly to "effective treatment by physician" and "elimination of stressors." On the basis of the analysis of data in this largest longitudinal study of patients with psychogenic tremor, we have concluded that accurate diagnosis is not only based on exclusion of other causes but also dependent on positive clinical criteria, the presence of which should avoid unnecessary investigation. 🎥

Miscellaneous tremors

There are many other causes of tremors. One of the most common causes of tremors are certain drugs, such as antipsychotics, amiodarone, cyclosporine, lamotrigine, lithium, tricyclic antidepressants, selective serotonin reuptake inhibitors (SSRIs), valproate, and other drugs (Morgan and Sethi, 2005). In one study of 707 patients treated with amiodarone, 2.8% had some neurotoxic effects, including de novo tremor and exacerbation of essential tremor, gait ataxia, peripheral neuropathy, and cognitive impairment (Orr and Ahlskog, 2009). These side effects correlated with duration of exposure and were not always reversible. The bobble-head doll syndrome is a form of slow (2–30 Hz) oscillatory movement that is usually associated with cystic enlargement of the third ventricle, suprasellar arachnoid cysts, aqueductal stenosis, and other lesions involving the third ventricle (Goikhman et al., 1998; Bhattacharyya et al., 2003). Hereditary chin tremor, or hereditary geniospasm, is an autosomal dominant disorder characterized by recurrent episodes of chin tremor (Soland et al., 1996a; Erer and Jankovic, 2007) (Video 18.9). Usually a benign condition with a peak in the mid-twenties (although it may be persistent in men), this condition has been mapped to a marker on chromosome 9q13–q21 (Jarman et al., 1997). Some investigators have suggested that "isolated generalized polymyoclonus" may present as "whole body tremulousness" and that some of the cases are drug-induced (e.g., SSRI) or due to an autoimmune disorder (McKeon et al., 2007). Genetic phenocopies of ET include FXTAS, Kennedy syndrome, SCA12, hereditary neuropathies, Klinefelter (XXY) syndrome (Harlow et al., 2008), and the 48,XXYY syndrome, which is also associated with gait ataxia, dysarthria, and nystagmus (Tartaglia et al., 2009). 🎥

References available on Expert Consult: www.expertconsult.com

Appendix

International Essential Tremor Foundation (IETF)
PO Box 14005
Lenexa, KS 66285-4005
Telephone: (888) 387-3667
Fax: (913) 341-1296
Email: info@essentialtremor.org
Website: http://www.essentialtremor.org

CHAPTER **19**

The tardive syndromes
Phenomenology, concepts on pathophysiology and treatment, and other neuroleptic-induced syndromes

Chapter contents

Overview	415	Neurologic side effects of dopamine D2 receptor antagonists	424
Fundamentals and definitions	416		
Dopamine receptors and their antagonists	418	Tardive syndromes	430
"Atypical" antipsychotics	420	Treatment of tardive syndromes	440

Overview

The topic of tardive dyskinesia syndromes is very broad, covering different phenomenologies. This is also the appropriate chapter in which to cover nontardive neuroleptic-induced movement disorders, further extending the scope of material to review. Because of the volume of material to cover, the essential features of the tardive dyskinesia syndromes are highlighted in this summary section to allow the reader to understand the most pertinent material in a simple fashion.

1. The term "neuroleptic" was coined for reserpine when it was recognized to induce parkinsonism. Reserpine was subsequently discovered to deplete monoamines, including dopamine, and the drug-induced parkinsonian state was reversed by levodopa (Carlsson et al., 1957). When antipsychotic drugs were later found to induce parkinsonism also, they too were labeled as neuroleptics. These antipsychotic drugs were shown to block dopamine receptors, especially the D2 receptors, and this action was recognized as the pathogenic mechanism to induce parkinsonism. Drug-induced parkinsonism correlates with the dosage of the neuroleptic and disappears when the drug is withdrawn.

2. The tardive dyskinesia syndromes are the result of treatment with dopamine receptor-blocking agents (DRBAs). These disorders tend to appear late in the course of treatment, hence the term *tardive*. Syndromes with similar clinical phenomenology in the absence of a reliable history of having received such medications exclude this diagnosis. Tardive syndromes have not been caused by dopamine depletors and only rarely by the "true atypical" antipsychotics, such as clozapine. Some DRBAs are marketed for gastrointestinal problems (e.g., metoclopramide – Reglan), for depression (e.g., amoxapine (Asendin); perphenazine/amitriptyline (Triavil)), and for cough (e.g., promethazine (Phenergan)).

3. The tardive dyskinesia syndromes tend to persist and can remain permanently. It is generally believed that the sooner the offending drugs are withdrawn, the more likely it is that the syndrome will fade away with time. But evidence is lacking that prolonging the use of the drugs will increase the severity of the dyskinesia.

4. The tardive dyskinesia syndromes can occur when the patient is taking these drugs or within a period of time after stopping the drugs. The criterion should be set for the longest acceptable time after stopping the drugs that the disorder can still be considered to be due to the drugs.

5. Withdrawing the offending drugs often exacerbates the severity of the movements because of removal of dopamine receptor blockade. Increasing the dosage of these drugs often ameliorates the movements because of increasing the blockade.

6. The tardive dyskinesia syndromes present in a variety of phenomenologies. The most common is the pattern of repetitive, almost rhythmic, movements that can be labeled as stereotypic. This pattern often occurs in the oral-buccal-lingual (O-B-L) region, usually presenting as complex chewing movements with occasional popping out of the tongue and with writhing movements of the tongue when it should be at rest in the mouth. Other parts of the body may also express rhythmic movements, such as the hands, feet, and trunk. Respirations may also be affected with an altered rhythmical pattern. This pattern of dyskinesia goes by the name *classic tardive dyskinesia*, or *tardive*

DOI: 10.1016/B978-1-4377-2369-4.00019-6

dyskinesia (TD). Because the individual movements may have the speed and brevity of choreoathetosis, the name chorea has been attached by some clinicians, but this only serves to confuse because the movements of classic chorea and athetosis are random or flowing and not rhythmic. Other names that have been used are *tardive stereotypy* and *rhythmical chorea*. In this chapter the strikingly characteristic movement pattern is simply called classic tardive dyskinesia or TD. It is exceedingly rare for such a pattern to be caused by any condition besides DRBA; it can sometimes be seen with levodopa, with brainstem strokes, and as an idiopathic disorder. There are other patterns of oral dyskinesias; they should not be confused with the pattern that is seen in TD. The most common idiopathic and spontaneous oral dyskinesia is oromandibular dystonia.

7. TD is often accompanied by a feeling of inner restlessness (akathisia), which can be whole-body restlessness or uncomfortable sensations in a specific part of the body. Such focal akathisia is extremely uncomfortable and is often expressed by the patient as a burning sensation; the mouth and vaginal regions are the most common sites of such focal akathisias. Generalized akathisia is often accompanied by a pattern of movement that appears to be executed in an attempt to relieve the abnormal uncomfortable sensations. These movements are often rhythmic, repetitive, and stereotypical, such as body rocking, crossing and uncrossing of the legs, and caressing of the scalp. Sometimes these characteristic movement patterns are present without the patient's being able to express the presence of a feeling of restlessness. The discomfort of generalized akathisia can lead to constant moaning by the patient.

8. Akathisia can also occur in the early phase of treatment with DRBAs; this is called "acute akathisia" in contrast to the "tardive akathisia" described above. Acute akathisia is not persistent and will disappear on discontinuing the DRBA.

9. The third most common phenomenology in the tardive dyskinesia syndromes is dystonia, which can mimic idiopathic torsion dystonia, usually focal or segmental. Some differences include an increased tendency for tardive dystonia to cause retrocollis and opisthotonic posturing, accompanied by internal rotation of the shoulders, extension of the elbows, and flexion of the wrists. Focal tardive dystonias are usually cranial in location, particularly affecting the jaw, tongue, and facial muscles. Tardive dystonia may also be accompanied by tardive akathisia and by classic TD. The presence of classic TD or akathisia in a patient with dystonia who has had exposure to DRBA makes the diagnosis of tardive dystonia extremely likely. Tardive dystonia can occur at all ages, whereas classic TD is more common in the elderly.

10. In addition to tardive dystonia, which is usually persistent, children tend to get classic chorea, called withdrawal emergent syndrome, which is self-limiting, eventually disappearing over several weeks if the offending drugs are withdrawn.

11. Other clinical phenomenology has been described in the spectrum of the tardive dyskinesia syndromes. These include myoclonus, tremor, oculogyric crisis, and tics. Some cases that have been reported as tardive tics might have actually been the movements of tardive akathisia that were mistaken for tic-like movements.

12. The "atypical" antipsychotic agents, ranked in order of clozapine, quetiapine, and olanzapine, are less tightly bound to the D2 receptor than the typical antipsychotic agents. This pharmacologic characteristic probably accounts for these "atypicals" being much less likely to cause drug-induced parkinsonism, acute dystonic reactions, acute akathisia, neuroleptic malignant syndrome (NMS), or the tardive syndromes, but there are some case reports of these complications from these drugs.

13. At the present time, clozapine is the gold standard for the atypical antipsychotics, with quetiapine being a close second in terms of not inducing parkinsonism or worsening existing Parkinson disease. The third-ranking drug is olanzapine. Newer so-called "atypical" antipsychotics need to be in use clinically before their full side effect profile can be known, and, except for clozapine and quetiapine, they all worsen Parkinson disease and can cause TD. For example, although risperidone had been labeled an atypical antipsychotic, it readily induces and worsens parkinsonism and can induce TD; it should be removed from this classification. It therefore resembles classic antipsychotic agents. Today, the designation of first- and second-generation antipsychotics is being used, rather than typical and atypical.

14. Clozapine and quetiapine in high doses have been reported to be successful in some patients in reducing the severity of tardive dyskinesia and tardive dystonia, but there remains uncertainty whether symptoms are reduced (1) because of D2-blocking activity with high doses, (2) because there is no such activity, and tincture of time has resolved the tardive symptoms, or (3) because these drugs have some other action that can reduce TD. By and large, these two drugs are ineffective in reducing tardive symptoms at low doses, and it is likely the D2-blocking activity of their high doses that reduces symptoms. Drugs that deplete dopamine or block D2 receptors have been the most effective medications in reducing tardive disorders.

Fundamentals and definitions

A variety of neurologic adverse effects are seen with drugs that block dopamine D2 receptors. Because these complications are mainly movement disorders and likely relate to the D2 receptors in the striatum and limbic system, they are usually called extrapyramidal reactions. These are listed in Table 19.1 and are covered in the clinical sections that follow.

The term *tardive syndromes* refers to a group of disorders that fit all of the following essential criteria: (1) Phenomenologically, the clinical features are that of a movement disorder – i.e., abnormal involuntary movements or a sensation of restlessness that often causes "unvoluntary" movements;

Table 19.1 Neurological adverse effects of dopamine receptor antagonists

1. Acute reactions
   a. Acute dystonia
   b. Acute (subacute) akathisia
2. Toxicity state (overdosage)
   a. Drug-induced parkinsonism
3. Neuroleptic malignant syndrome (NMS)
4. Tardive syndromes
   a. Withdrawal emergent syndrome
   b. Classic tardive dyskinesia (TD)
   c. Tardive dystonia
   d. Tardive akathisia
   e. Tardive myoclonus
   f. Tardive tremor
   g. Tardive tics
   h. Tardive chorea
   i. Tardive parkinsonism?

Adapted from Fahn S: The tardive dyskinesias. In Matthews WB, Glaser GH (eds): Recent Advances in Clinical Neurology, vol. 4. Edinburgh: Churchill Livingstone, 1984, pp. 229–260.

Table 19.2 Terminology of the tardive syndromes

Descriptions	Equivalent common names
Tardive syndromes as a group	Tardive syndrome Tardive dyskinesia
Repetitive, rhythmic movements, usually in the oral-buccal-lingual region	Classic tardive dyskinesia (TD) Oral-buccal-lingual (O-B-L) dyskinesias Tardive stereotypy Rhythmic chorea
Dystonic movements and postures	Tardive dystonia
Restlessness and the movements that occur as a result	Tardive akathisia
Myoclonus	Tardive myoclonus
Tremor	Tardive tremor
Tics	Tardive tics Tardive tourettism
Chorea	Withdrawal emergent syndrome Tardive chorea
Oculogyria	Tardive oculogyric crisis
Parkinsonism	Tardive parkinsonism (if it exists)

(2) the disorder is caused by the patient's having been exposed to at least one DRBA within 6 months of the onset of symptoms (in exceptional cases, exposure could be up to 12 months); and (3) the disorder persists for at least 1 month after stopping the offending drug (Fahn, 1984a; Stacy and Jankovic, 1991). The question arises as to what to call persistent dyskinesias that are induced by drugs other than DRBAs. For example, Miller and Jankovic (1992) described such a patient who had been exposed to flecainide, a drug not known to be a DRBA. Another drug, buspirone, an azospirone compound, is an anxiolytic that is not known to have any dopamine receptor-blocking activity. Yet there is a report of two patients who had persistent movement disorders after prolonged treatment with this drug (LeWitt et al., 1993). One patient had cervical-cranial dystonia, and the other had an exacerbation of preexisting spasmodic torticollis and TD. It is possible, however, that future laboratory investigation will reveal flecainide and buspirone or one of their metabolites actually to be a DRBA.

Although there are several phenomenologically distinct types of tardive disorders, the collective group is referred to as *tardive dyskinesia* for historical reasons. Unfortunately, the term tardive dyskinesia is often used also to refer to a phenomenologically specific type of tardive syndrome, so the literature is often confusing; this note of caution is particularly important in trying to understand whether the author of a paper is referring to the tardive syndromes collectively or to a specific tardive syndrome. Since there could be different pathophysiologic mechanisms and treatments for the different forms of tardive syndromes, it is best that they be divided phenomenologically (Table 19.2). In this review, the tardive syndromes as a whole are referred to as tardive dyskinesia, and the specific type that was historically and initially labeled as tardive dyskinesia is referred to as classic tardive dyskinesia. Other names have been used for classic tardive dyskinesia (see Table 19.2). The phenomenologically

essential component of classic tardive dyskinesia is the presence of repetitive, almost rhythmic, movements. These are almost always present in the mouth region, and therefore are also called O-B-L dyskinesias.

Thus, tardive dyskinesia is an iatrogenic syndrome of persistent abnormal involuntary movements that occur as a complication of drugs that competitively block dopamine receptors, particularly the D2 receptor, but possibly also the D3 receptor, which is in the D2 family of receptors.

Tardive dyskinesia was first described in patients who were treated for schizophrenic psychosis with antipsychotics (Schonecker, 1957; Sigwald et al., 1959). These abnormal movements appeared late in the course of treatment, in contrast to acute dystonic reactions and drug-induced parkinsonism, which had previously been recognized as complications from antipsychotics, hence the term *tardive*. The offending antipsychotics are now known to block the D2 dopamine receptor; i.e., these drugs are DRBAs. Since the first descriptions, TD has also been noted in patients without psychiatric disorders who had other indications for using dopamine receptor antagonists, such as those with gastrointestinal complaints (Casey, 1983), with Gilles de la Tourette syndrome (Riddle et al., 1987), or with dystonia (Greene and Fahn, 1988).

Dopamine receptor antagonists produce many undesirable side effects, most of which occur relatively early in the course of treatment and are reversible on discontinuation of the medication. However, disfiguring and disabling abnormal involuntary movements were also noted to often occur late in the course of treatment and these were often noted to persist, even after discontinuation of the medication. Hence, the term "tardive" was coined, referring to the late and insidious onset (Faurbye et al., 1964). Initially the term tardive dyskinesia was equated with stereotypic repetitive movements of oral, buccal, and lingual distribution (Schonecker, 1957), but subsequently other types of movements have been recognized (Burke et al., 1982; Fahn, 1984a). As such, the concept of tardive dyskinesia has evolved and has been modified considerably since the initial recognition of the syndrome.

The prevalences of drug-induced parkinsonism and the various tardive syndromes have been compared by van Harten and colleagues (1996b) on the island of Curaçao, which has only one psychiatric facility. In 194 inpatients, the prevalence for classic tardive dyskinesia (TD) was 39.7%, that for parkinsonism was 36.1%, that for tardive dystonia was 13.4%, and that for akathisia was 9.3%. Combinations of two or more of these phenomenologies occurred in 30% of patients (van Harten et al., 1997). van Harten and colleagues (2006) continued to follow their patients over 9 years (mean duration of 18 years exposure to first-generation antipsychotic drugs); they found the annual incidence rate for classic TD to be 10.2% and for tardive dystonia to be 0.7%. Severity was associated with age and akathisia but not with drug-induced parkinsonism.

Dopamine receptors and their antagonists

Since TD is an iatrogenic disorder and the most constant feature of the syndrome is the pharmacologic class of the responsible etiologic agent, it is important to understand the nature of the drugs that produce TD (Table 19.3). Although models of abnormal basal ganglia circuitry have been proposed to explain the mechanism of TD (Marchand and Dilda, 2006), the pathophysiology is still poorly understood. Dopamine receptors are classified into five subtypes, based on the genetics of the receptors; they are labeled D1, D2, D3, D4, and D5 (Kebabian and Calne, 1979; Sokoloff et al., 1990). Table 19.4 characterizes the five dopamine receptors. It is the dopamine D2 receptor-blocking action of drugs that has been linked to the tardive syndromes and other neuroleptic drug-induced movement disorders (described later and listed in Table 19.5).

Recently introduced drugs in Table 19.3, e.g., iloperidone (Jain, 2000), ziprasidone (Hirsch et al., 2002), amisulpride (Curran and Perry, 2002), aripiprazole (Tamminga and Carlsson, 2002), paliperidone ER (Chwieduk and Keating, 2010), levosulpiride (Shin et al., 2009), and asenapine (Kane et al., 2010), need to be in clinical use for several years before their full potential in causing tardive dyskinesia syndromes can be known. The earlier ones in the above sentence have already been found to induce the acute and delayed movement disorders described in this chapter. In Table 10.3, the calcium channel blockers deserve comment. Cinnarizine (1-diphenylmethyl-4-(3-phenyl-2-propenyl) piperazine) and its difluorinated derivative flunarizine can induce parkinsonism (Teive et al., 2004). They are antagonists at the D2 receptors (Belforte et al., 2001), and they also inhibit the MgATP-dependent generation of a transmembrane proton electrochemical gradient and dopamine vesicular uptake (Terland and Flatmark, 1999). Whether either of these latter mechanisms, rather than a proposed DRBA action, is responsible for the neuroleptic activity is uncertain. In regard to

Table 19.3 Drugs that can produce tardive syndromes

Class of drug	Examples of drugs in each class
1. Phenothiazines a. Aliphatic	Chlorpromazine (Thorazine) Triflupromazine (Vesprin)
b. Piperidine	Thioridazine (Mellaril) Mesoridazine (Serentil)
c. Piperazine	Trifluoperazine (Stelazine) Prochlorperazine (Compazine) Perphenazine (Trilafon) Fluphenazine (Prolixin) Perazine
2. Thioxanthenes a. Aliphatic b. Piperazine	Chlorprothixene (Tarctan) Thiothixene (Navane)
3. Butyrophenones	Haloperidol (Haldol) Droperidol (Inapsine)
4. Diphenylbutylpiperidine	Pimozide (Orap)
5. Dibenzazepine	Loxapine (Loxitane) Asenapine (Saphris)
6. Dibenzodiazepine	Clozapine (Clozaril) Quetiapine (Seroquel)
7. Thienobenzodiazepine	Olanzapine (Zyprexa)
8. Pyrimidinone	Risperidone (Risperidal) Paliperidone ER (9-hydroxyrisperidone)
9. Benzisothiazole	Ziprasidone (Geodon)
10. Benzisoxazole	Iloperidone (Zomaril)
11. Substituted benzamides	Metoclopramide (Reglan) Tiapride (Tiapridex) Sulpiride (Meresa) Clebopride Remoxipride Veralipride (Agreal, Agradil) Amisulpride (Solian) Levosulpiride
12. Indolones	Molindone (Moban)
13. Quinolinone	Aripiprazole (Abilify)
14. Tricyclic	Amoxapine (Asendin)
15. Calcium channel blockers	Flunarizine (Sibelium) Cinnarizine (Stugeron)
16. N-acetyl-4-methoxytryptamine	Melatonin
17. Interferon-alpha	Pegylated interferon alpha 2b (IFN-α) (Pegylated = polyethylene glycol (PEG) attached to proteins)

melatonin, there is a case report of withdrawal-emergent O-B-L dyskinesias associated with akathisia that occurred with sudden discontinuation of chronic melatonin use (Giladi and Shabtai, 1999). Such withdrawal syndromes are typical of drugs that block dopamine receptors. On resumption of melatonin, the patient's O-B-L dyskinesia and

Table 19.4 Characteristics of dopamine receptors

Feature	D1	D2	D3	D4	D5
Chromosome	5q31–34	11q22–23	3q13.3	11p	4p16.3
Region	Striatum	Striatum	Accumbens	Frontal cortex	Hippocampus
DA affinity	μmolar	μmolar	nmolar	Subμmolar	Subμmolar
Agonist	SKF-82526	Bromocriptine	7-OH-DPAT	?	SKF-82526
Antagonist	SCH-23390	Haloperidol	UH 232	Clozapine	SCH-23390
Adenyl cyclase	Stimulates	Inhibits	?	Inhibits	Stimulates

Table 19.5 A brief listing of receptor binding profiles of second-generation antipsychotic agents

Drug	D1	D2	5-HT$_{2A}$	M$_2$	α_1	H$_1$
Clozapine	85	125	2	1.9	7	6
Quetiapine	455	160	220	120	7	11
Olanzapine	31	11	4	1.9	19	7
Risperidone	75	3	0.6	>10 000	2	155

Data are Ki (nM). The lower the number, the greater the affinity of the drug for the receptor. D1, dopamine D1; D2, dopamine D2; 5-HT$_{2A}$, serotonin 2A; M$_2$, muscarinic type 2; α_1, alpha NE type 1; H$_1$, histamine type 1 receptors.
Data from Worrel JA, Marken PA, Beckman SE, Ruehter VL. Atypical antipsychotic agents: A critical review. Am J Health Syst Pharm 2000;57:238–255; and Schmidt AW, Lebel LA, Howard HR Jr, Zorn SH. Ziprasidone: a novel antipsychotic agent with a unique human receptor binding profile. Eur J Pharmacol 2001;425:197–201.

akathisia cleared. Sudden cessation of the drug again brought on the symptoms; slow taper over 2 months was effective without incident. This case suggests that either the melatonin product the patient was taking was impure and was contaminated with a DRBA or melatonin itself has dopamine receptor antagonist properties. In support of the latter is the result of a blinded crossover study showing some suppression of the tardive dyskinesia with melatonin (Shamir et al., 2001). Pegylated interferon alpha-2b (IFN-α), used in the treatment of hepatitis C virus infection, has been reported to cause parkinsonism, akathisia, and acute dystonic reaction (Quarantini et al., 2007). IFN-α has been shown to decrease dopaminergic activity in mice (Shuto et al., 1997).

Some drugs that block dopamine D2 receptors are promoted for medical problems other than psychosis, but these drugs can cause drug-induced parkinsonism, acute dystonic reactions, tardive syndromes, and NMS, just like the drugs that are promoted for the treatment of psychosis. Metoclopramide (Ganzini et al., 1993) and clebopride (Sempere et al., 1994) are used mainly for dyspepsia and as antiemetic agents. Amoxapine has a tricyclic structure and is marketed as an antidepressant drug, but a metabolite has dopamine receptor-blocking activity and has been implicated in producing TD (Kang et al., 1986; Sa et al., 2001). Veralipride is a substituted benzamide that is used for the treatment of menopausal hot flushes (Masmoudi et al., 1995). Pimozide is marketed for the treatment of Tourette syndrome. Some commercial preparations contain dopamine receptor

antagonists in combination with other drugs, and this can lead to inadvertent use of these drugs. A popular combination is that of perphenazine and amitriptyline, marketed as Triavil and Etrafon. Risperidone is commercially promoted with the suggestion that it might have less risk of drug-induced complications, but this appears not to be the case. Parkinsonism and TD have been noted in association with the calcium channel antagonists flunarizine and cinnarizine (Micheli et al., 1987). Both of these medications have mild dopamine receptor antagonist activity, which is thought be the mechanism for their complications (Micheli et al., 1989). Recognition of these drugs is essential not only in making the diagnosis of TD but also in preventing the occurrence of TD by being able to avoid using them.

Clozapine is a special drug that is discussed more thoroughly later in the chapter; it has greater affinity for blocking the D4 receptor than the D2 receptor, and deserves the classification as an "atypical antipsychotic" because it rarely causes parkinsonism or worsens Parkinson disease (PD). The newer antipsychotic, quetiapine also qualifies as an atypical antipsychotic with just slightly more propensity to induce parkinsonism than clozapine. Olanzapine has more propensity to induce parkinsonism and worsen PD. Many agents that are promoted as atypical antipsychotics should not be classified as such.

The D1 and D5 receptors were both previously known as D1 receptors; both are distinct in activating adenyl cyclase. The D2, D3, and D4 receptors were all previously lumped together as the D2 receptor and are still considered in the D2 family of receptors.

The D1 and D2 receptors are found mainly in the striatum and nucleus accumbens, as well as in the substantia nigra, amygdala, cingulate cortex, and entorhinal area. The anterior lobe of the pituitary gland has only D2 receptors, and the thalamus and cerebral cortex outside of the cingulate and entorhinal area contain D1 receptors only (De Keyser et al., 1988). D2 receptor affinities of dopamine receptor antagonists correlate closely with antipsychotic and antiemetic properties of the drugs (Creese et al., 1976). Dopamine receptor antagonists are often referred to as neuroleptics or antipsychotics; the former term indicates the effect of drugs in producing parkinsonism, and the latter indicates the effect of controlling psychosis.

The D3 receptor, another target of neuroleptics, is found chiefly in the mesolimbic areas. Because it is involved in emotional behaviors, it may be involved in tardive akathisia. Clozapine, an atypical antipsychotic, which has a low potential to induce parkinsonism or tardive syndromes, is primarily a D4 receptor antagonist. However, it has some D2-blocking action, which increases with higher doses.

"Atypical" antipsychotics

The label "atypical" refers to a lower propensity of the antipsychotic agent to induce parkinsonism or a variety of other movement disorders described later (and listed in Table 19.5), that is these agents have a lower propensity to be neuroleptics. A number of epidemiologic studies have found that the atypicals are less likely to induce tardive dyskinesia and other movement disorder problems (Tarsy and Baldessarini, 2006). Dolder and Jeste (2003) found that the atypicals reduced the incidence of tardive dyskinesia by half.

Dopamine and serotonin (5-HT) receptor antagonism

Although drugs that are labeled as atypical antipsychotic agents block dopamine D2 receptors, they also block serotonin 5-HT$_{2A}$ receptors, and some investigators attribute their antipsychotic effect to this mechanism and recommend research and drug development on newer agents that block other 5-HT receptors (Meltzer, 1999).

How tightly drugs to bind to the D2 receptor (their occupancy rate) is currently considered to be important in the drug having neuroleptic potential in direct proportion. Seeman and Tallerico (1998) found that the atypical antipsychotic drugs bind more loosely than classic antipsychotic drugs (neuroleptics) to the D2 receptors. Kapur and colleagues (1999) measured D2 and 5-HT$_2$ receptor

occupancies by positron emission tomography (PET) scan for patients receiving clozapine, risperidone, or olanzapine. Clozapine showed a much lower D2 occupancy (16–68%) than risperidone (63–89%) and olanzapine (43–89%); all three showed greater 5-HT$_2$ occupancy than D2 occupancy at all doses, although the difference was greatest for clozapine. In their PET study, Moresco and colleagues (2004) found that striatal D2 receptor occupancy was significantly higher with olanzapine than with clozapine. All these studies support the relationship between receptor occupancy and the clinical observations that clozapine and quetiapine are the most "atypical," with the least propensity to cause parkinsonism, tardive syndromes, or other neuroleptic drug reactions.

Despite interest in the 5-HT$_{2A}$ receptor, it is the D2 receptor that is associated with the antipsychotic effect (Seeman, 2010). Antipsychotic clinical doses correlate with their affinities for this receptor. The receptor has high- and low-affinity states. Clozapine and quetiapine do not elicit parkinsonism and rarely result in tardive dyskinesia because they are released from D2 within 12–24 hours. Traditional antipsychotics remain attached to D2 receptors for days, preventing relapse, but allowing accumulation that can lead to tardive dyskinesia. Glutamate agonists that treat schizophrenia have affinity for the dopamine D2(High) receptor and the D3 receptor (Seeman and Guan, 2009).

A comparison of the receptor-binding profile of quetiapine, clozapine, olanzapine, and risperidone is presented in Table 19.5. Both quetiapine and clozapine have poor affinity for the dopamine D2 receptor, which probably accounts for the low incidence of inducing parkinsonism and tardive syndromes. Risperidone has the highest affinity for the D2 receptor, resembling haloperidol (see Table 19.6),

Table 19.6 A more complete listing of affinities for human receptors and rat transporters by antipsychotic drugs

Receptor	Haloperidol	Clozapine	Quetiapine	Olanzapine	Risperidone	Ziprasidone
Dopamine D1	15	53	390	10	21	9.5
Dopamine D2	0.82	36	39	2.1	0.44	2.8
Dopamine D3	2.5	22	>500	17	13	28
5-HT$_{1A}$	2600	710	>830	7100	21	37
5-HT$_{1B/1D}$						
5-HT$_{2A}$	28	4.0	82	1.9	0.39	0.25
5-HT$_{2C}$	1500	5.0	1500	2.8	6.4	0.55
5-HT$_{2D}$						
5-HT$_6$	6600	9.5	33	10	2400	n.t.
5-HT$_7$	80	21	290	120	1.6	4.9
α_1-Adrenoceptor	7.3	3.7	4.5	7.3	0.69	1.9
α_2-Adrenoceptor	1600	51	1100	140	1.8	390
Histamine H$_1$	>730	17	21	5.6	88	510
Muscarinic M$_1$	570	0.98	56	2.1	>5000	>10000

Receptor bindings are presented as Ki values (nmol/L).
Data from Horacek J. Novel antipsychotics and extrapyramidal side effects. Theory and reality. Pharmacopsychiatry 2000;33:34–42; and Schmidt AW, Lebel LA, Howard HR Jr, Zorn SH. Ziprasidone: a novel antipsychotic agent with a unique human receptor binding profile. Eur J Pharmacol 2001;425:197–201.

and is therefore more of a "typical" than an "atypical" antipsychotic.

In one PET study striatal D1 and D2 receptor occupancies were evaluated (Tauscher et al., 2004). D1 occupancy ranged from 55% with clozapine to 12% with quetiapine (rank order: clozapine > olanzapine > risperidone > quetiapine). The striatal D2 occupancy ranged from 81% with risperidone to 30% with quetiapine (rank order: risperidone > olanzapine > clozapine > quetiapine). The ratio of striatal D1/D2 occupancy was significantly higher for clozapine (0.88) relative to olanzapine (0.54), quetiapine (0.41), or risperidone (0.31). In an [^{123}I]epidepride single photon emission computed tomography (SPECT) study involving clozapine-, olanzapine-, and haloperidol-treated schizophrenia patients, as well as drug-naive patients and healthy controls, midbrain D(2/3) receptor occupancy was studied. Of those on medication, occupancy was least for those on clozapine (5%), next for those on olanzapine (28%), and greatest for those on haloperidol (40%); no significant differences were observed in the temporal poles (Tuppurainen et al., 2009). All imaging studies are compatible with the clinical results in that clozapine and quetiapine, with the least neuroleptic features, have the lowest D2 receptor occupancy rate.

Clozapine

Clozapine was the first agent to be labeled as an atypical antipsychotic and deservedly so, although rare case reports do exist of drug-induced parkinsonism (Kurz et al., 1995), but it has been reported not to induce rigidity, and it rarely induces parkinsonian tremor (Gerlach and Peacock, 1994). It has also caused rare cases of acute akathisia (Friedman, 1993; Safferman et al., 1993), acute dystonic reaction (Kastrup et al., 1994; Thomas et al., 1994), tardive syndromes (Dave, 1994), tardive dystonia (Bruneau and Stip, 1998; Molho and Factor, 1999a, van Harten et al., 2008b), tardive akathisia (Kyriakos et al., 2005), tardive oculogyria (Uzun and Doruk, 2007), and NMS (Sachdev et al., 1995; Benazzi, 1999; Lara et al., 1999; Gambassi et al., 2006). There are also parkinsonian features that are seen with clozapine. In a prospective study, seven out of 25 patients on clozapine developed TD (Bunker et al., 1996). In a retrospective study, comparison of clozapine and typical antipsychotics showed no lower prevalence of tardive dyskinesia in the clozapine group (Modestin et al., 2000). But it is not clear that the patients in the clozapine group had not been previously exposed to typical antipsychotics and had not developed TD while receiving them. What is clear from this study is that the conversion to using clozapine has not markedly reduced the prevalence of extrapyramidal syndromes; this finding supports the realization that clozapine does not effectively treat TD once it has developed. How effective its use would be in preventing TD in the first place still needs to be verified. For patients with PD, the low propensity to augment existing parkinsonism makes clozapine very useful in treating patients who have dopaminergic drug-induced psychosis (Factor and Friedman, 1997; Friedman et al., 1999).

A SPECT study measuring dopamine D2 receptor binding reveals lower binding with clozapine than with typical neuroleptics (Broich et al., 1998). In animal studies, rats that have been pretreated with haloperidol for 4 weeks develop vacuous chewing movements (VCMs) after treatment with a dopaminergic, whereas rats that have been pretreated with clozapine do not (Ikeda et al., 1999).

A problem with clozapine is that weekly blood counts are required because there is a 1% to 2% incidence of leukopenia, which is reversible if the drug is withdrawn within 1–2 weeks. Granulocyte colony-stimulating factor can be an effective means to treat the agranulocytosis (Sperner-Unterweger et al., 1998). Other common adverse effects are drowsiness, drooling, weight gain, and seizures. An unusual adverse effect with clozapine was a case of myokymia (David and Sharif, 1998). Myocarditis associated with clozapine has been reported (Hill and Harrison-Woolrych, 2008).

Quetiapine

After clozapine, quetiapine is the most favorable in being least likely to induce parkinsonism, NMS (Stanley and Hunter, 2000), or tardive syndromes. In a prospective, head-to-head comparison with risperidone treatment in schizophrenia, quetiapine had far fewer extrapyramidal adverse effects, but more orthostasis (Perez et al., 2008). D2 receptor antagonism is relatively selective for limbic than striatal receptors for clozapine and sertindole, followed by quetiapine, ziprasidone, olanzapine, and remoxipride, whereas risperidone in many respects has a profile that resembles that of haloperidol (Arnt and Skarsfeldt, 1998). In primates, quetiapine and clozapine were equally less likely to induce oral dyskinesias compared to standard antipsychotics (Peacock and Gerlach, 1999). Like clozapine, quetiapine easily induces drowsiness, so when it is used to treat dopa-induced psychosis, it should be taken at bedtime. The major advantage over clozapine is that it does not require blood tests because it does not induce agranulocytosis. However, there may be a rare risk that quetiapine can cause agranulocytosis (Ruhe et al., 2001). Since its introduction, there have been reports of acute dystonic reactions (Jonnalagada and Norton, 2000; Desarker and Sinha, 2006), acute akathisia (Prueter et al., 2003), neuroleptic malignant syndrome (El-Gaaly et al., 2009; Gortney et al., 2009), and also TD (Ghaemi and Ko, 2001). In 367 patients treated for 12 months with quetiapine (mean dose 720 mg/day), parkinsonism was seen in 10%, akathisia in 3%, dystonia in 1.4%, and "hyperkinesia" in 1.7% (Perez et al., 2008).

In a SPECT study using the D2/D3 ligand [I-123]-epidepride the percent occupancy of receptors in the limbic system (temporal lobe) and striatal receptors while patients were receiving quetiapine was 60% and 32%, respectively, which is similar to clozapine (Stephenson et al., 2000). In another SPECT study, quetiapine was shown to occupy 5-HT$_{2A}$ receptors in the frontal and temporal cortex (Jones et al., 2001). A PET study using [18F]fallypride showed similar results (Vernaleken et al., 2010).

A patient with oculogyric crisis, who failed to improve after withdrawal of antipsychotic medication, was successfully treated with quetiapine (Gourzis et al., 2007). Drug-induced parkinsonism and acute akathisia due to other neuroleptics can be reduced by switching patients to quetiapine (Cortese et al., 2008). Drowsiness and weight gain are common; postural hypotension is not infrequent. A rare complication of quetiapine is hepatotoxicity (Shpaner et al., 2008).

Olanzapine

In contrast to clozapine and quetiapine, olanzapine more readily increases parkinsonian symptoms in patients with PD (Jimenez-Jimenez et al., 1998; Molho and Factor, 1999b; Granger and Hanger, 1999), but does so less readily than risperidone and conventional antipsychotics. Drug-induced parkinsonism, including the rabbit syndrome, is seen with olanzapine (Durst et al., 2000), but less than with haloperidol (Peuskens et al., 2009). It can induce acute akathisia (Kurzthaler et al., 1997; Jauss et al., 1998) and TD but less so than haloperidol (Tollefson et al., 1997; Wood 1998). It can also induce NMS (Filice et al., 1998; Moltz and Coeytaux, 1998; Burkhard et al., 1999; Levenson, 1999; Margolese and Chouinard, 1999; Sierra-Biddle et al., 2000; Abu-Kishk et al., 2004; Zaragoza Fernandez et al., 2006), tardive dyskinesia (Herran and Vazquez-Barquero, 1999), and tardive dystonia (Dunayevich and Strakowski, 1999). Acute dystonic reactions also occur (Beasley et al., 1997; Landry and Cournoyer, 1998; Vena et al., 2006).

A direct comparison with chlorpromazine showed similar parkinsonism and acute akathisia for the two drugs (Conley et al., 1998). A double-blind comparison with haloperidol by Beasley and colleagues (1999) showed a much lower risk of developing tardive dyskinesia with olanzapine. After 1 year of exposure, 0.52% of patients developed TD with olanzapine and 7.45% developed TD with haloperidol. An open-label comparison with conventional antipsychotics after a 9-month follow-up after discharge from the hospital favored olanzapine, with TD being present in 2.3% for olanzapine (2/87), and 16.7% (12/72) for the conventional treatment (Mari et al., 2004). There are case reports of agranulocytosis induced by olanzapine (Meissner et al., 1999; Naumann et al., 1999; Tolosa-Vilella et al. 2002), including in a patient who had previously had agranulocytosis with clozapine (Benedetti et al., 1999). This has been attributed to some similar structural and pharmacologic properties of clozapine. A case of restless legs syndrome with periodic movements in sleep has been attributed to olanzapine (Kraus et al., 1999).

Olanzapine has relative regional mesolimbic dopaminergic selectivity and a broad-based binding affinity for serotonin (all 5-HT$_2$ receptor subtypes and the 5-HT$_6$ receptor), dopamine (D2, D3, and D4 receptors), muscarinic, and α_1-adrenergic receptors (Bymaster et al., 1999). A PET study in schizophrenic patients being treated with olanzapine revealed that this drug is a potent 5-HT$_2$ blocker, but also a blocker of D2 dopamine receptors similar to risperidone and less so than clozapine (Kapur et al., 1998). Patients on olanzapine were also studied with [^{123}I]iodobenzamide (IBZM) SPECT; the D2 receptor was occupied 60% and 83% of the time at doses of 5 mg/day and 10 mg/day, respectively (Raedler et al., 1999). Such high rates of occupancy probably account for olanzapine's tendency to worsen parkinsonism and induce DRBA complications, because, as was noted above, D2 receptor occupancy rates are directly related to neuroleptic potential.

Risperidone

With the success of clozapine, there is a commercial advantage for pharmaceutical companies to tout other antipsychotics as "atypical." Such has been claimed for risperidone, but this drug can readily induce parkinsonism including the rabbit syndrome (Levin and Heresco-Levy, 1999), tardive syndromes (Haberfellner 1997; Silberbauer 1998; Hong et al., 1999; Ananth et al., 2000), and NMS (Newman et al., 1997; Norris et al., 2006). The prevalence of parkinsonism from risperidone is usually considered to be less than that with conventional neuroleptics, but it was observed in 42% compared to 29% in those on haloperidol (Knable et al., 1997). Tardive dyskinesia and tardive dystonia occurred in a patient who was exposed only to risperidone (Bassitt and Garcia, 2000). The annual incidence of TD in patients taking risperidone has been estimated to be 0.3%, compared to an annual incidence in patients taking conventional neuroleptics of 5–10% (Gutierrez-Esteinou and Grebb, 1997). However, in an open-label prospective study of 255 institutionalized patients with dementia who were treated with risperidone, the 1-year cumulative incidence of TD was 2.6% (Jeste et al., 2000).

Like conventional neuroleptics, risperidone induces acute dystonic reactions in marmosets, in contrast to clozapine, which does not (Fukuoka et al., 1997). In a report of an open-label comparison with haloperidol, Rosebush and Mazurek (1999) found the two drugs to have a similar side effect profile. In a prospective follow-up of first-episode schizophrenic patients treated with risperidone, movement disorders developed in more than one-third of these patients, who had previously never been exposed to antipsychotic drugs (Lang et al., 2001). When risperidone is compared with low-potency antipsychotics, such as thioridazine, no difference was discerned in the rates of developing movement disorders (Schillevoort et al., 2001).

In a SPECT study dopamine receptor binding with IBZM showed risperidone to have effects between those of haloperidol and clozapine, with a dose–response curve for risperidone showing greater similarity to that of haloperidol (Dresel et al., 1998). A PET study showed dopamine D2 receptors occupancies of about 70% and 60% in the striatum and extrastriatum, respectively (Ito et al., 2009). Clearly, risperidone is not an "atypical" antipsychotic agent. Risperidone's occupancy of the 5-HT$_2$ receptors is about 90%, and its occupancy of the D2 receptors is between 50% and 80%, but the latter correlates with the extrapyramidal side effects (Yamada et al., 2002).

Ziprasidone

This benzisothiazole was approved by the Food and Drug Administration in 2001. There are already case reports of acute dystonic reactions (Weinstein et al., 2006; Yumru et al., 2006, Rosenfield et al., 2007), NMS, rhabdomyolysis, and pancreatitis (Murty et al., 2002; Yang and McNeely, 2002; Gray 2004). It has been reported to cause tardive dyskinesia (Mendhekar, 2005) and tardive dystonia (Papapetropoulos et al., 2005; Tsai et al., 2008). Although it is a potent 5-HT$_{2A}$ antagonist (like risperidone, olanzapine, and clozapine), it is also a D2 antagonist in humans as detected by PET scan (Bench et al., 1993, 1996). But in-vitro studies reveal much lower affinity for the D2 receptor than for the 5-HT$_{2A}$ receptor (Seeger et al., 1995), and ziprasidone also binds less tightly to the D2 receptor than dopamine (Seeman, 2002). Ziprasidone has two other unique features

Table 19.7 Adverse effect profile of "atypical" neuroleptics

Adverse effect	Haloperidol	Clozapine	Quetiapine	Olanzapine	Risperidone
Sedation	+	+++	++	+	+
Seizures	+	+++	+	+	+
Hypotension	+	+++	++	++	++
Incrased prolactin	+++	0	0	++	+
Weight gain	+	+++	++	+++	++

0, none; +, mild; ++, moderate; +++, severe.
Data from Worrel JA, Marken PA, Beckman SE, Ruehter VL. Atypical antipsychotic agents: A critical review. Am J Health Syst Pharm 2000;57:238–255.

compared to other antipsychotic agents: (1) it is a potent 5-HT$_{1A}$ agonist and thus inhibits dorsal raphe serotonergic cell firing (Sprouse et al., 1999) and increases cortical dopamine release (Rollema et al., 2000), and (2) it inhibits neuronal uptake of 5-HT and norepinephrine in a manner comparable to the antidepressant imipramine (Schmidt et al., 2001). What these unique actions might contribute to antipsychotic activity or to propensity for or against extrapyramidal reactions is unclear. Ziprasidone has been reported to induce a case of oculogyric crisis in an adult (Viana Bde et al., 2009).

Aripiprazole

This quinolinone has a novel mechanism of action. Like a number of other "atypical" antipsychotics, it is an antagonist at the 5-HT$_{2A}$ receptors. It is also a 5-HT$_{1A}$ partial agonist (Jordan et al., 2002). What is novel is that it is a partial agonist at the dopamine D2 receptor. It has a higher affinity for the presynaptic autoreceptor than for the postsynaptic receptor. Hence, it reduces dopamine synthesis and release through an agonist action at the dopamine autoreceptor (Tamminga and Carlsson, 2002). Because of its novel action as a partial D2 agonist, it was anticipated that it might cause fewer extrapyramidal adverse effects, and clinical trials reported favorable results (Kane et al., 2002). However, D2 ligand binding PET revealed a dose-related high occupancy state of 71.6% at 2 mg/day to 96.8% at 40 mg/day (Kegeles et al., 2008). With wider use, it has been shown to worsen PD (Friedman et al., 2006; Wickremaratchi et al., 2006), and there are already reports of it causing parkinsonism (López-Torres et al., 2008), NMS (Chakraborty and Johnston, 2004; Hammerman et al., 2006; Palakurthi et al., 2007), acute dystonic reactions (Desarkar et al., 2006; Fountoulakis et al., 2006), and tardive dyskinesia (Zaidi and Faruqui, 2008; Abbasian and Power, 2009; Friedman, 2010).

Amisulpride

Amisulpride, a substituted benzamide, is a highly selective antagonist for dopamine D2 and D3 receptors in the limbic region, which would predict potent antipsychotic activity with a low potential to cause extrapyramidal symptoms (Lecrubier, 2000). It binds less tightly to the D2 receptor than do the typical antipsychotics (Seeman, 2002). Using the full range of recommended amisulpride dosage, striatal occupancies up to 90% can be measured (Vernaleken et al.,

2004). It is not yet commercially available in the United States. It has already been reported to induce tardive oculogyric crisis (Mendhekar et al., 2010).

Adverse effects from second-generation antipsychotics

Aside from the D2-blocking effects described above, the five drugs in Table 19.7 have a number of other adverse effects. Sedation is a particular problem seen with each of them, but particularly clozapine and quetiapine. Metabolic side effects are now widely recognized with the second-generation antipsychotics, with weight gain a common problem (Leucht et al., 2009; Patel et al., 2009). Table 19.7 lists the common adverse effects of these drugs, along with haloperidol, for comparison.

It is not likely that drug-induced tardive syndromes will disappear because use of both typical and atypical agents continues. In a survey in Lombardy (Italy), 35 363 individuals over the age of 65 were prescribed an antipsychotic prescription (2.18 subjects per 100 inhabitants, with two-thirds receiving first-generation agents) (Percudani et al., 2004). Although there may be a lower risk of developing these disorders with "atypicals," these drugs can induce them (Table 19.8). It is even possible that if physicians consider "atypicals" safe to use, their use will increase, even in situations in which the risk from typicals might have precluded their use. In the United States, the prevalence of atypical antipsychotic use was found to be 267.1 per 100 000 subjects aged 19 years and younger and was more than twice as high for male patients as for female patients (Curtis et al., 2005).

In a large US randomized controlled trial (the CATIE study) comparing second-generation antipsychotics (olanzapine, quetiapine, risperidone, perphenazine, or ziprasidone) with the first-generation perphenazine, only olanzapine had a slightly more favorable outcome of both the patients' ability to stay on this drug for a longer duration and with slightly less drug-induced parkinsonism, akathisia, and tardive dyskinesia than all other drugs including perphenazine (Table 19.9); perphenazine fared as well as the other so-called 'atypicals' (Lieberman et al., 2005). A similar outcome was seen in a smaller British study (CUtLASS) (Jones et al., 2006). This was a randomized controlled clinical trial involving 57 centers, with flexible dosing up to 4 capsules/day in 1460 schizophrenic subjects (after excluding 33 from one center, integrity concern). The primary outcome was time to discontinuation, with a maximum observation

Table 19.8 Extrapyramidal adverse effects reported with "atypical" neuroleptics

Adverse effect	Haloperidol	Clozapine	Quetiapine	Olanzapine	Risperidone
Parkinsonism	Yes	Yes	Not yet	Yes	Yes
Acute akathisia	Yes	Yes	Yes	Yes	Yes
Acute dystonia	Yes	Yes	Yes	Yes	Yes
Neuroleptic malignant syndrome	Yes	Yes	Yes	Yes	Yes
Tardive syndrome	Yes	Yes	Yes	Yes	Yes

Table 19.9 Clinical Antipsychotic Trial of Intervention Effectiveness (CATIE) study

Drug	Dose/capsule	Mean dose	No.	Duration* (hazard ratio vs. others; $P =$)	AIMs (%)	Akathisia (%)	DIP (%)
Olanzapine	7.5 mg	20.1 mg	336	Longest duration and used as comparator	14	5	8
Quetiapine	200 mg	543.4 mg	337	0.63; 0.0001	13	5	4
Risperidone	1.5 mg	3.8 mg	341	0.75; 0.002	16	7	8
Perphenazine	8 mg	20.8 mg	261	0.78; 0.021	17	7	6
Ziprasidone	40 mg	112.8 mg	185	0.78; 0.028	14	9	4

*Duration is the amount of time on a drug before it was discontinued for any reason. Olanzapine had the longest duration, and the hazard ratios for the other drugs are based on their comparison to olanzapine.
AIMs, abnormal involuntary movements; DIP, drug-induced parkinsonism.
From Lieberman JA, Stroup TS, McEvoy JP, et al.; Clinical Antipsychotic Trials of Intervention Effectiveness (CATIE) Investigators. Effectiveness of antipsychotic drugs in patients with chronic schizophrenia. N Engl J Med 2005;353(12):1209–1223. © 2005 Massachusetts Medical Society. All rights reserved.

of 18 months. TD was present in 231 subjects at baseline, and these subjects were excluded from the perphenazine arm. The outcome had multiple comparison, requiring a P value ≤0.017 to be significant.

In a more detailed assessment of extrapyramidal side effects in the CATIE study, there were no significant differences in incidence or change in rating scales for parkinsonism, dystonia, akathisia, or tardive dyskinesia when comparing the second-generation antipsychotics with perphenazine or comparing between second-generation antipsychotics (Miller et al., 2008). Secondary analyses revealed greater rates of concomitant antiparkinsonism medication among individuals on risperidone and lower rates among individuals on quetiapine.

Metoclopramide

After the introduction of metoclopramide for gastrointestinal disorders, reports of acute dystonic reactions in children and tardive dyskinesia in adults began to appear (Cochlin, 1974; Kataria et al., 1978; Lavy et al., 1978). Today, metoclopramide has become a common cause of TD, and the legal profession has found such cases ripe for lawsuits. The annual incidence of TD from metoclopramide has been reported to be between 4.5% and 23% per year (Grimes, 1981; Ganzini et al., 1993), about the same as that for haloperidol ~5.7%/year (Tollefson et al., 1997; Beasley et al., 1999; Csernansky et al., 2002), but higher than those

for risperidone ~1.8%/year (Lemmens et al., 1999; Davidson et al., 2000; Jeste et al., 2000; Csernansky et al., 2002) and olanzapine ~1.2%/year (Tollefson et al., 1997; Beasley et al., 1999). Because antipsychotic drugs have an affinity for brain neuromelanin (Seeman, 1988), Chen and colleagues (2010) examined the amount of metoclopramide and antipsychotic drugs binding to postmortem human substantia nigra. They found that in clinical conditions the amount of metoclopramide that would bind to nigra is much higher than the amount of raclopride, haloperidol, or olanzapine that would be expected to be bound and they suggest that this binding might explain the higher annual incidence of TD induced by metoclopramide.

Neurologic side effects of dopamine D2 receptor antagonists

To better understand the tardive syndromes, it is important to recognize the variety of other movement disorders that are induced by the dopamine receptor antagonists at different points in the course of treatment. These movement disorders are often lumped together as extrapyramidal syndromes, but the lumping often hinders the effort to sort out the clinical characteristics and pathophysiology of separate syndromes. It is better to subdivide them into their phenomenologic types (see Table 19.1). Movements that may be seen include acute dystonia, acute akathisia, parkinsonism, tardive syndromes, and NMS. Both dystonia and akathisia also occur as subtypes of tardive syndromes and both subtypes are discussed in more detail in the section on tardive syndromes.

Acute dystonia

The earliest abnormal involuntary movement to appear after initiation of dopamine receptor antagonist therapy is an acute dystonic reaction. In about half of the cases, this reaction occurs within 48 hours, and in 90% of cases, it occurs by 5 days after starting the therapy (Ayd, 1961; Garver et al., 1976). The reaction may occur after the first dose (Marsden et al., 1975).

Dystonic movements are sustained muscle contractions, frequently causing twisting and repetitive movements, or abnormal postures (Fahn, 1988). In a series of 3775 patients, Ayd (1961) found that acute dystonia is the least frequent side effect, affecting about 2–3% of patients, with young males being most susceptible. The incidence rate increases to beyond 50% with highly potent dopamine receptor blockers such as haloperidol (Boyer et al., 1987). In one prospective study, Aguilar and colleagues (1994) reported that 23 of 62 patients developed acute dystonia after haloperidol was introduced, that anticholinergic pretreatment significantly prevented this, and that younger age and severity of psychosis were risk factors. In the prospective study by Kondo and colleagues (1999), 20 (51.3%) of 39 patients placed on nemonapride had dystonic reactions, onset occurring within 3 days after the initiation of treatment in 90%. As in other series, the incidence of acute dystonia was significantly higher in males than in females (77.8% vs. 28.6%, $P < 0.05$), and younger males ($\leq$30 years) had an extremely high incidence (91.7%). The incidence is much lower with the so-called atypical antipsychotics; Raja and Azzoni (2001) observed only 41 cases out of 1337 newly admitted patients treated with antipsychotics, which included 8 treated with risperidone, 1 with olanzapine, and 1 with quetiapine. A meta-analysis compared intramuscular injections of second generation antipsychotics (SGAs) to haloperidol injections (Satterthwaite et al., 2008). SGAs were associated with a significantly lower risk of acute dystonia (relative risk = 0.19) and acute akathisia (relative risk = 0.25), compared with haloperidol alone.

All agents that block D2 receptors can induce acute dystonic reactions, including risperidone (Brody, 1996; Simpson and Lindenmayer, 1997) and clozapine (Kastrup et al., 1994). One child developed an acute dystonic reaction after ingestion of a dextromethorphan-containing cough syrup (Graudins and Fern, 1996). Dextromethorphan has several different known pharmacologic actions, but D2 receptor blockade is not one of them. A case of acute dystonia following abrupt withdrawal of bupropion (DA reuptake blocker) was reported (Wang et al., 2007). A case of acute dystonia following abrupt withdrawal of dexamphetamine in a patient taking risperidone was also reported (Keshen and Carandang, 2007). Serotonergic agents have also been reported to induce acute dystonic reactions (Lopez-Alemany et al., 1997; Madhusoodanan and Brenner, 1997; Olivera, 1997). The mechanism could relate to inadequate release of dopamine from the nerve terminals in the striatum owing to the inhibitory effect of serotonin on dopamine neurons

in the substantia nigra pars compacta. The opioid σ_1 and σ_2 receptors have also been implicated (Matsumoto and Pouw, 2000).

Acute dystonic reactions most often affect the ocular muscles (oculogyric crisis), face, jaw, tongue, neck, and trunk, and less often the limbs. Oculogyric crisis has previously been noted to occur as a common feature of postencephalitic parkinsonism (Duvoisin and Yahr, 1965). A typical acute dystonic reaction may consist of head tilt backward or sideways with tongue protrusion and forced opening of the mouth, often with arching of trunk and ocular deviation upward or laterally (Rupniak et al., 1986). The forcefulness of the muscle contractions can be extremely severe and led to auto-amputation of the tongue in one patient (Pantanowitz and Berk, 1999).

Mazurek and Rosebush (1996) studied the timing in the development of an acute dystonic reaction in 200 patients who were taking a neuroleptic medication for the first time. The neuroleptic was given twice daily, and over 80% of the episodes of acute dystonia occurred between 12 noon and 11 p.m.

Reserpine and α-methylparatyrosine, which deplete presynaptic monoamines, have not been associated with acute dystonic reactions (Duvoisin, 1972; Marsden et al., 1975; Walinder et al., 1976). However, another dopamine depletor, tetrabenazine (TBZ), has been reported to induce acute dystonic reactions (Burke et al., 1985). One possible explanation for this difference is that in addition to depleting dopamine, TBZ blocks dopamine receptors (Reches et al., 1983).

It is important to mention the case described by Wolf (1973) of a patient who developed an oral dyskinesia while taking reserpine. Figure 1 in his paper clearly shows a dystonic phenomenon and not the complex, rapid, stereotypic movements of classic tardive dyskinesia. This development appeared too late after initiation of reserpine to be considered an acute dystonic reaction, however. Whether this could be an example of tardive dystonia is not clear, since the phenomenology of tardive dystonia is identical to that of naturally occurring primary dystonia; therefore, the patient could have had a coincidental case of spontaneous, idiopathic oromandibular dystonia (Fahn, 1984b). Thus, there is no absolute evidence that reserpine induces acute dystonic reactions, classic tardive dyskinesia, or tardive dystonia. In fact, symptoms of these three tardive syndromes can be suppressed by reserpine, and eventually reserpine can be withdrawn successfully in many patients without exacerbation of the symptoms (Fahn, 1983). Furthermore, the long time that reserpine has been available without a clear-cut case of tardive syndromes can be compared to the much shorter duration of use of metoclopramide, in which there are already cases of acute dystonic reactions, classic tardive dyskinesia, and tardive dystonia as a consequence of its use (Casteels-Van Daele et al., 1970; Gatrad, 1976; Pinder et al., 1976; Reasbeck and Hossenbocus, 1979; Miller and Jankovic, 1989; Lang, 1990).

Of 452 patients given high-dosage oral metoclopramide to control emesis, Kris and colleagues (1983) observed 14 who developed acute dystonic reactions. However, there was a distinct preponderance of the reactions occurring in children (6/22) compared to adults (8/430). Intravenous metoclopramide is more likely to induce it than oral administration (Pinder et al., 1976). In a study at a Veterans Administration hospital, comparing patients treated with metoclopramide and controls, the relative risk for TD was 1.67, and the relative risk for drug-induced parkinsonism was 4.0 (Ganzini et al., 1993).

The available biochemical explanations for the acute dystonic reaction are unsatisfactory, but several observations contribute to the understanding of the phenomena, relating it to dopamine, muscarinic, and sigma receptors. Acute neuroleptic administration produces sudden increase of dopamine release and increased turnover lasting for 24–48 hours after a single dose (O'Keefe et al., 1970; Marsden and Jenner, 1980). This effect is blocked by anticholinergics consistent with their efficacy in treatment of acute dystonic reactions (O'Keefe et al., 1970). Moreover, in baboons that were pretreated with reserpine and α-methylparatyrosine, which markedly reduces presynaptic dopamine concentration, haloperidol-induced acute dystonic reaction is abolished or greatly reduced (Meldrum et al., 1977). On the other hand, blockade of the postsynaptic receptor fades in about 12 hours after a single dose of antipsychotics, and supersensitivity of receptors begins to develop. Therefore, presynaptic dopaminergic excess in combination with the emerging supersensitive postsynaptic dopamine receptors could result in markedly increased striatal dopaminergic activity at about 20–40 hours after a neuroleptic dose. This period corresponds to the critical time for acute dystonic reactions in human subjects who were given a single dose of butaperazine (Garver et al., 1976). However, extrapolating the data from experimental animals to the clinical situation has its limitations including the fact that rats do not develop acute dystonic reactions. Further data on human cerebrospinal fluid (CSF) dopamine metabolites as an indicator of presynaptic function might prove to be of value in pursuing the hypothesis. Jeanjean and colleagues (1997) suggested that the σ_2 receptors could be involved in the acute dystonic reaction. They found a correlation between the clinical incidence of neuroleptic-induced acute dystonia and binding affinity of drugs for the sigma receptor.

Another animal model of acute dystonia is the common marmoset that is treated with haloperidol (Fukuoka et al., 1997). But it takes at least 6 weeks of such treatment to develop this reaction. The dystonia subsides only to reappear when haloperidol treatment is restarted; other neuroleptics, including risperidone, can also make the dystonia reappear, but clozapine was without such an effect. In this animal model, the anticholinergic agent trihexyphenidyl inhibited the induction of acute dystonia.

In patients with acute dystonic reactions, symptoms can be relieved within minutes after parenteral anticholinergics or antihistaminics (Paulson, 1960; Waugh and Metts, 1960; Smith and Miller, 1961). Diphenhydramine 50 mg, benztropine mesylate or biperiden 1–2 mg is given intravenously and can be repeated if the effect is not seen in 30 minutes. Intravenous diazepam has also been shown to be effective and can be used as an alternative therapy (Korczyn and Goldberg, 1972; Gagrat et al., 1978; Rainer-Pope, 1979). If untreated, the majority of cases still resolve spontaneously in 12–48 hours after the last dose of the dopamine receptor antagonists. Dopamine receptor antagonists with high anticholinergic activities have low incidence rates of acute dystonic reactions (Swett, 1975). Therefore, prophylactic use of

anticholinergics (Arana et al., 1988) and benztropine (Goff et al., 1991) has been studied and reported to be helpful in reducing the risk of acute dystonic reactions, especially in young patients on high-potency drugs. Three cases of recurrent episodes of acute dystonia and oculogyric crises despite withdrawal of the offending DRBAs (haloperidol in two cases, metoclopramide in one) have been reported, responding to anticholinergics each time (Schneider et al., 2009). The response of acute dystonic reactions to anticholinergics is so characteristic that it is difficult to explain the report of a few cases apparently due to amitriptyline, which has considerable anticholinergic activity and no known DRBA activity (Ornadel et al., 1992).

A case of an acute dystonic reaction occurring in an elderly person with bipolar disorder taking the serotonin uptake inhibitor paroxetine has been reported (Arnone et al., 2002). Speculation about the risk due to previous exposure to neuroleptics was raised. This class of drug can reduce firing rate of nigral dopaminergic neurons owing to their inhibition by serotonin.

Acute akathisia

The term akathisia, from the Greek, meaning unable to sit down, was coined by Haskovec in 1901 (cited by Mohr and Volavka, 2002), long before antipsychotic drugs were introduced. Akathisia was seen in some patients with advanced parkinsonism, and in others, it was frequently thought to be functional. Akathisia refers to an abnormal state of excessive restlessness, a feeling of the need to move about, with relief of this symptom on actually moving. Today, it is most frequently encountered as a side effect of neuroleptic drugs.

Two major issues of akathisia remain in confusion. First, there is no consensus about diagnostic criteria. Some authors consider akathisia to be an abnormal subjective state and regard the movements as an expression of the subjective state but not a necessary feature for the diagnosis (Van Putten, 1975). Others recognize the characteristic patterns of restless movements and consider presence of movements to be sufficient for the diagnosis (Munetz and Cornes, 1982; Barnes et al., 1983; Gibb and Lees, 1986). A second point of confusion is that akathisia occurs not only in an early-onset, self-limited form (acute akathisia), but also as a late-onset, persistent form (tardive akathisia). Much of the literature on akathisia does not distinguish between acute and tardive akathisia, which makes the interpretation of the literature difficult. The recognition of tardive akathisia as a distinct subsyndrome of tardive syndromes has been more recent (Fahn, 1978, 1983; Braude and Barnes, 1983; Weiner and Luby, 1983). For the discussion of the clinical features of akathisia, acute and tardive akathisia are lumped together, since they are similar, but their treatments and most likely their pathophysiologies are distinct.

The subjective aspect of akathisia is characterized by inner tension and aversion to remaining still. Patients complain of vague inner tension, emotional unease, or anxiety with vivid phrases such as "jumping out of my skin" or "about to explode." Subjective descriptions, however, can be nonspecific. Inner restlessness and inability to remain still can be present in a significant number of psychiatric patients without akathisia and in control subjects without psychiatric problems (Braude et al., 1983). In an attempt to clarify the issue, Braude et al. (1983) systematically surveyed the frequency of various complaints and found that inability to keep the legs still was the most characteristic complaint and was present in over 90% of patients with akathisia in contrast to about 20% of those with other psychiatric disturbances. Others noted more conservative estimation of the frequency of complaints related to the legs from 27% (Gibb and Lees, 1986) to 57% (Burke et al., 1989). Various authors also described atypical features such as "acting out," suicidal ideation, disruptive behaviors, homicidal violence, sexual torment, terror, and exacerbation of psychosis as akathitic phenomena (Van Putten and Marder, 1987). Evaluation of the subjective aspect also depends on patients' ability to describe their feelings. Those with psychosis, dementia, or learning disability are often unable to provide useful descriptions for diagnosis. Although akathisia may manifest itself as subjective feeling alone, lack of specific subjective feeling and variable expression by patients pose a diagnostic dilemma. Therefore, the presence of the motor phenomenon is very helpful for the diagnosis.

Akathisia can present as focal pain or burning, usually in the oral or genital region (Ford et al., 1994). The symptom of moaning may be a verbal expression of the subjective feeling of akathisia. Some patients may moan as part of a generalized akathitic state and have other motor evidence of akathisia, such as marching in place, inability to sit still accompanied by associated walking about, inability to lie quietly with writhing and rolling movements, and making stereotypic caressing or rocking movements. The differential diagnosis of moaning includes parkinsonism, akathisia, levodopa usage (Fahn et al., 1996), dementia, pain, and other syndromes of phonations, such as tics, oromandibular dystonia, and Huntington disease, as discussed by Fahn (1991).

The motor aspect of akathisia (akathitic movements) is generally described as excessive movements that are complex, semipurposeful, stereotypic, and repetitive. Braude and colleagues (1983) found that rocking from foot to foot, walking on the spot, and coarse tremor and myoclonic jerks of the feet were characteristic of akathitic movements. Others agree that various leg and feet movements are more common in patients with akathisia than in those with TD (Gibb and Lees, 1986; Burke et al., 1989). However, they also noted that these did not distinguish akathisia from the group that did not meet criteria for akathisia (Gibb and Lees, 1986), and movements involving other parts of the body such as trunk rocking, respiratory grunting, face rubbing, and shifting weight while sitting were also frequent (Burke et al., 1989). Although there are not enough data and consensus on the diagnostic movements of akathisia, these movements seem to be characteristic enough to be recognized by different authors who have independently documented similar phenomena.

Akathisia is seen in patients with Parkinson disease (Lang and Johnson, 1987), in patients abusing cocaine (Daras et al., 1994), and as an adverse effect of selective serotonin uptake inhibitors (Poyurovsky et al., 1995). Acute akathisia occurs not only as an adverse effect of DRBAs but also fairly commonly as an acute adverse effect of the dopamine depletors – reserpine, TBZ, and α-methyl tyrosine (Marsden and Jenner, 1980).

In Ayd's review (1961), half of the cases of acute akathisia occurred within 25 days of drug treatment and 90% occurred within 73 days. Acute akathisia was the most common side effect of DRBAs, occurring in 21.2% of patients in that study (Ayd, 1961). In a more recent study by Sachdev and Kruk (1994) of 100 consecutive patients placed on neuroleptics, mild akathisia developed in 41% and moderate to severe akathisia in 21%. In a literature review, Sachdev (1995b) reported that incidence rates for acute akathisia with conventional neuroleptics vary from 8% to 76%, with 20% to 30% being a conservative estimate. Sachdev stated that preliminary evidence suggests that the newer atypical antipsychotic drugs are less likely to produce acute akathisia. Using the criterion that both subjective and objective phenomena are required for the diagnosis of acute akathisia, Miller and colleagues (1997) found an incidence rate of 22.4%, 75% of which occurred within the first 3 days of exposure to a neuroleptic. Muscettola and colleagues (1999) found a prevalence rate of 9.4%.

The potency of neuroleptics has been associated with incidence of akathisia, ranging from 0.5% for reserpine (Marsden and Jenner, 1980) to 75% for haloperidol (Van Putten et al., 1984). Other risk factors are neuroleptic dose, the rate of dosage increase, and the development of drug-induced parkinsonism (Sachdev and Kruk, 1994). Akathisia has occurred with all second-generation antipsychotics as well as first-generation ones (Kane et al., 2009).

As with acute dystonic reactions, akathisia has also been induced by serotonergic agents (Chong, 1996; Lopez-Alemany et al., 1997). The mechanism was discussed in the above section on acute dystonia.

As was noted previously, akathisia needs to be distinguished from other conditions such as agitated depression; restless legs syndrome, in which similar subjective sensations may be described by patients but are mainly localized to legs and are present particularly at night (Blom and Ekbom, 1961); or complex motor tics with preceding aura, which show more variety of abnormal movements; and complex vocal tics (Jankovic and Fahn, 1986). Akathisia can also be obscured by other psychiatric disorders, or it could be mistaken for a psychiatric disease. For example, when patients with psychosis develop akathisia after withdrawal from antipsychotic drugs, it may be mistaken for recurrence of psychosis. Paradoxical dystonia (see Chapter 12) in which dystonic movements are relieved by movement can be mistaken for akathisia.

The pathophysiology of acute akathisia remains poorly understood. On the basis of the observation in rats that show increased locomotor activity after blockade of the mesocortical dopamine system (Carter and Pycock, 1978), reduction of this dopaminergic projection was suggested to be responsible for akathisia (Marsden and Jenner, 1980). However, tardive akathisia cannot be explained by this hypothesis because dopamine depletors can ameliorate those symptoms. The observation that acute akathisia can occur with a serotonin uptake inhibitor (Altshuler et al., 1994) indicates that inhibiting dopamine neurons in the substantia nigra by such drugs could link the dopamine system with akathisia. These types of drugs have been reported to increase parkinsonism in patients with PD (Meco et al., 1994). One attractive possibility is that akathisia might reflect an alteration of the dopaminergic mesolimbic system.

Because propranolol has been reported to be beneficial in treating acute akathisia, another suggestion is that acute akathisia results from alterations in the cingulate cortex, the piriform cortex, or area 1 of the parietal cortex based on effects of propranolol in these regions in haloperidol-treated rats (Ohashi et al., 1998).

Ayd (1961) noted that acute akathisia is self-limited, disappearing on discontinuation of neuroleptics, and is well controlled by anticholinergics despite continuation of neuroleptics. Others have noted that only patients with concomitant parkinsonism improve significantly with anticholinergics (Kruse, 1960; Braude et al., 1983). Amantadine may also help, but patients can develop a tolerance (Zubenko et al., 1984a). Beta-blockers at relatively low doses below 80 mg of propranolol per day have been noted to be effective in many studies including one with a double-blind design (Lipinski et al., 1984; Zubenko et al., 1984b; Adler et al., 1986; Dupuis et al., 1987). Nonlipophilic beta-blockers that have poor penetration to the central nervous system (CNS) are not as effective (Lipinski et al., 1984; Dupuis et al., 1987). Selective beta-blockers might not be as effective as nonselective ones (Zubenko et al., 1984b); however, when two equally lipophilic beta-blockers, propranolol and betaxolol, were compared, they were equally effective in treating acute akathisia (Dumon et al., 1992) although the former is a beta-2-blocker and the latter is a beta-1-blocker. In a rat model of acute akathisia (neuroleptic-induced defecation), a lipophilic beta-1-blocker was found to be effective in reducing the phenomenon (Sachdev and Saharov, 1997).

Clonidine also reduces central noradrenergic activity by stimulating central alpha-2 receptors and has been noted to be effective in a small number of studies. The sedating effect is pronounced, however (Adler et al., 1987). Nicotine patches have been reported to reduce akathisia (Anfang and Pope, 1997). Weiss and colleagues (1995) found cyproheptadine, an antiserotonergic agent, to be effective in ameliorating akathisia. In a small placebo-controlled trial, mianserin, a 5-HT$_2$ antagonist, was found to reduce the severity of acute akathisia (Poyurovsky et al., 1999). Trazadone has also been reported to be beneficial (Stryjer et al., 2003). Poyurovsky and Weizman (2001) discuss the potential of serotonin agents in akathisia. A literature search revealed mirtazapine to be effective and superior to propranolol (43.3% vs. 30.0%) (Hieber et al., 2008).

Parkinsonism

Neuroleptic-induced parkinsonism (usually referred to as extrapyramidal syndrome or EPS by psychiatrists and as drug-induced parkinsonism by neurologists) is a dose-related side effect and is indistinguishable phenomenologically from idiopathic PD, including high frequency of tremor and asymmetric signs (Hardie and Lees 1988). SPECT imaging of the dopamine transporter, however, may be helpful in determining whether the neuroleptic-induced parkinsonism is entirely drug-induced or an exacerbation of subclinical PD (Lorberboym et al. 2006). It develops with use of both DRBAs and dopamine-depleting drugs such as reserpine and TBZ. Some authors have noted perioral tremor and termed this rabbit syndrome, which is a localized form of parkinsonian tremor (Decina et al., 1990). The incidence of parkinsonism varies. Korczyn and Goldberg (1976) found

61%, and Muscettola and colleagues (1999) found 19.4%. Women are affected almost twice as frequently as men, which is the reverse of the ratio in idiopathic PD. Neuroleptic-induced parkinsonism also occurs increasingly with advanced age (Ayd, 1961; Hardie and Lees 1988) in parallel with the incidence of idiopathic PD.

Blockade of dopamine receptors by antagonists or depletion of presynaptic monoamines by drugs such as reserpine mimics the deficient dopamine state in PD. All DRBAs can induce parkinsonism, except clozapine (there are only rare reports with clozapine) (Factor and Friedman, 1997). Risperidone can do so (Gwinn and Caviness, 1997; Simpson and Lindenmayer, 1997), as well as olanzapine and only rarely quetiapine. Parkinsonism from neuroleptics is typically reversible when the medication is reduced or discontinued. Sometimes, the reversal can take many months; an interval of up to 18 months has been noted in the literature (Fleming et al., 1970).

Some patients show persisting parkinsonism despite prolonged discontinuation of neuroleptics (Stephen and Williamson, 1984; Hardie and Lees, 1988), giving rise to consideration of a proposed condition of tardive parkinsonism. A study of 8-week exposure of rats to haloperidol found a highly significant 32–46% loss of tyrosine hydroxylase (TH) immunoreactive neurons in the substantia nigra, and 20% contraction of the TH-stained dendritic arbor (Mazurek et al., 1998). Perhaps such pathologic changes account for some cases of prolonged drug-induced parkinsonism in humans. Several cases in the literature had initial resolution of parkinsonism and later reappearance of the symptoms without re-exposure to neuroleptics (Hardie and Lees, 1988). Two cases that had complete resolution of drug-induced parkinsonism after withdrawal of neuroleptics showed evidence of mild PD at autopsy (Rajput et al., 1982). Although one assumes that these patients had subclinical PD, the effect of neuroleptics on the disease progression is unknown. The use of the term "tardive parkinsonism" to refer to cases of persistent parkinsonism remains an enigma. Some are due to concurrent development of progressive PD, and there are no autopsied proven examples of non-PD in any example. Therefore, this suggests that there is as yet no evidence of tardive parkinsonism.

With the introduction of selective serotonin reuptake inhibitors (SSRIs) to treat depression, it has been noticed that these drugs can sometimes worsen parkinsonism in patients with PD (Meco et al., 1994) and occasionally can induce parkinsonism in patients who never had symptoms of PD (Coulter and Pillans, 1995; DiRocco et al., 1998). In an intensive monitoring program in New Zealand of the SSRI drug fluoxetine over a 4-year period, there were 15 reports of parkinsonism in 5555 patients who were exposed to the drug (Coulter and Pillans, 1995). Four of these 15 patients were also on a neuroleptic and one was on metoclopramide. In a literature search, parkinsonism was found with different classes of antidepressants, is not dose related, and can develop with short-term or long-term use (Madhusoodanan et al., 2010). The explanation for inducing or enhancing parkinsonism is that increased serotonergic activity in the substantia nigra will inhibit dopamine-containing neurons, thus causing functional dopamine deficiency in the nigrostriatal pathway (Baldessarini and Marsh, 1992).

The possibility of the existence of tardive parkinsonism comes up from time to time because some patients have continued parkinsonism despite long-term discontinuation of the DRBA (Melamed et al., 1991). However, there is always the possibility that the patient had preclinical Parkinson disease prior to developing drug-induced parkinsonism. Then, when the DRBA is withdrawn, the parkinsonism persists because of progressively worsening PD. One would need to show that there are no Lewy bodies or that the PET scan shows no loss of fluorodopa uptake in patients believed to have tardive parkinsonism.

Anticholinergics can be effective in reducing the severity of the parkinsonism induced by DRBAs, whereas dopaminergic drugs (that activate the dopamine receptors) are ineffective, probably because they are not able to displace the DRBA from its binding to the receptor. Levodopa up to 1000 mg in combination with a peripheral dopa decarboxylase inhibitor had no significant effect (Hardie and Lees, 1988), nor did apomorphine, a dopamine receptor agonist (Merello et al., 1996). On the other hand, levodopa can effectively reverse parkinsonism induced by dopamine depletors, such as reserpine. In fact, the discovery of the dopamine hypothesis for parkinsonism was based on this observation (Carlsson et al., 1957; Carlsson 1959). Treatment is usually initiated with anticholinergics or amantadine (Mindham et al., 1972; Johnson, 1978; Konig et al., 1996).

Neuroleptic malignant syndrome

NMS is an idiosyncratic reaction that can sometimes be life-threatening. The clinical triad consists of (1) *hyperthermia*, usually with other autonomic dysfunctions such as tachycardia, diaphoresis, and labile blood pressure; (2) *extrapyramidal signs*, usually increased muscle tone of rigidity or dystonia, often with accompanying elevation of muscle enzymes; and (3) *alteration of mental status*, such as agitation, inattention, and confusion. Fever is not an essential symptom (Peiris et al., 2000), and it can be delayed (Norris et al., 2006). The syndrome begins abruptly while the patient is on therapeutic, not toxic, dosages of medication. In a review of 340 clinical reports of NMS in the literature (Velamoor et al., 1994), changes in either mental status or rigidity were the initial manifestations of NMS in 82.3% of cases with a single presenting sign. All the symptoms are fully manifest within 24 hours and reach a maximum within 72 hours. There does not seem to be any relationship with the duration of therapy. NMS can develop soon after the first dose or at any time after prolonged treatment. Recovery usually occurs within 1 to several weeks, but can be fatal in 20–30% of cases (Henderson and Wooten, 1981; Gute and Baxter, 1985). Even with awareness of the potential of fatality in modern medicine, death still occurs (van Maidegem et al., 2002). Muscle biopsies have shown swelling and edema, with 10–50% of fibers involved with vacuoles but scanty mononuclear infiltration (Behan et al., 2000).

All agents that block D2 receptors can induce NMS, including risperidone (Raitasuo et al., 1994; Webster and Wijeratne, 1994; Dave, 1995; Singer et al., 1995; Levin et al., 1996), clozapine (Miller et al., 1991; Amore et al., 1997; Dalkilic and Grosch, 1997), amisulpride (Bottlender et al., 2002), olanzapine (Kontaxakis et al., 2002; Kogoj and Velikonja, 2003), and phenothiazines with antihistaminic activity, such as alimemazine (van Maidegem et al., 2002). A case of NMS associated with bupropion has been reported (Kasantikul and Kanchanatawan, 2006). TBZ has been reported to cause NMS; this seems likely to be due to its D2-blocking activity (Reches et al., 1983) rather than to its dopamine-depleting action (by blocking the vesicular dopamine transporter). Reserpine has no known dopamine receptor antagonism, only dopamine-depleting activity (also by blocking the vesicular dopamine transporter), and has not been reported to cause NMS.

In a Japanese study, 10 of 564 (1.8%) patients who received antipsychotics developed NMS (Naganuma and Fujii, 1994), many more than the 12 of 9792 patients (0.1%) reported previously (Deng et al., 1990). Risk factors that were found were psychomotor excitement, refusal of food, weight loss, and oral administration of haloperidol at 15 mg/day or above (Naganuma and Fujii, 1994). Young males appear to be more predisposed to NMS (Gratz and Simpson, 1994), but the reason for this is uncertain. In a case control study searching for risk factors, Sachdev et al. (1997) found that patients with NMS were more likely to be agitated or dehydrated, often needed restraint or seclusion, had received larger doses of neuroleptics, and more often had previous treatment with electroconvulsive therapy (ECT) before the development of the syndrome.

The pathophysiologic mechanism of NMS is not well understood. Autopsies failed to show any consistent findings (Itoh et al., 1977). A similar syndrome has been reported following abrupt withdrawal of levodopa (Friedman et al., 1985; Hirschorn and Greenberg, 1988; Keyser and Rodnitzky, 1991), suggesting a common mechanism of acute dopamine deficiency (Henderson and Wooten, 1981). IBZM SPECT in one patient showed the dopamine receptor to be blocked in the acute phase of NMS, but the patient had been receiving a D2 blocker, which would be expected to result in this finding (Jauss et al., 1996). There is a report of a patient who developed the NMS syndrome following abrupt withdrawal of the combination of a long-acting neuroleptic and an anticholinergic agent (Spivak et al., 1996). Because it responded to procyclidine administration, it implicates a muscarinic overactivity. There are also reports of an NMS-like syndrome following the sudden withdrawal of amantadine (has dopaminergic and antimuscarinic activity) (Ito et al., 2001), and following withdrawal of baclofen, with recovery after reintroduction of baclofen (Turner and Gainsborough, 2001).

The idiosyncratic nature and rarity of the syndrome remain unexplained. Ram and colleagues (1995) evaluated the structure of the D2 receptor gene in 12 patients who had a history of NMS. One patient was found to have a nucleotide substitution of an exon of the D2 gene. The A1 allele of the TaqI A polymorphism of the dopamine D2 receptor gene appears to occur more commonly in patients who developed NMS (Suzuki et al., 2001). Kishida et al. (2004) found that patients with NMS had a higher association with a polymorphism in the D2 receptor gene.

Treatment of NMS consists of discontinuing the antipsychotic drugs and providing supportive measures. Rapid relief of symptoms has been reported with the use of dantrolene, bromocriptine, or levodopa (Granato et al., 1982; Gute and Baxter, 1985). Nisijima and colleagues (1997) found levodopa to be more effective than dantrolene, but Tsujimoto and colleagues (1998) found intravenous dantrolene plus hemodialysis to be effective. Subcutaneous apomorphine has been found to be effective as a solo treatment (Wang and Hsieh, 2001). Gratz and Simpson (1994) recommended using anticholinergics in an attempt to reverse rigidity prior to utilizing bromocriptine. Carbamazepine was dramatically effective in two patients (with recurrence on withdrawal of the drug) (Thomas et al., 1998). Steroids added to standard therapy have been reported to speed recovery time (Sato et al., 2003). Re-exposure to dopamine receptor antagonists does not necessarily lead to recurrence of NMS (Singh and Albaranzanchi, 1995; Singh and Hambidge, 1998). Residual catatonia that can last weeks to months has been reported, with some patients responding to ECT (Caroff et al., 2000). Hyponatremia can sometimes occur; it has been attributed to inappropriate secretion of antidiuretic hormone and also to cerebral salt-wasting syndrome associated with the NMS (Lenhard et al., 2007). When present, salt replacement is necessary.

Tardive syndromes

The first use of dopamine receptor antagonists for psychiatric disorders was in the early 1950s, and credit for the first report of TD is given to Schonecker (1957), who reported four patients with TD induced by chlorpromazine. Sigwald and colleagues (1959) provided the first detailed descriptions of the syndrome and divided it into acute, subacute, and chronic subtypes. Uhrbrand and Faurbye (1960) published the first systematic review of the complication among 500 psychiatric patients and noted 29 patients with the disorder. Faurbye and colleagues (1964) later coined the term tardive dyskinesia and emphasized the increased incidence of the syndrome with chronic exposure. Despite numerous reports of the classic O-B-L repetitive stereotypic movements, establishment of this disorder as a distinct clinical entity took decades of epidemiologic studies (American Psychiatric Association, 1980; Jeste and Wyatt, 1982a; Kane and Smith, 1982). Confusion arose in part from the difficulty of characterizing and communicating the exact type of movements these patients develop and distinguishing these from the ones that occur spontaneously. It should be noted that these drug-induced movements can be variable in duration; they may be short-lasting and fade slowly after discontinuation of the medication, suppressed by the medication itself, or persistent.

Rigorous epidemiologic data are available only for classic tardive dyskinesia (Jeste and Wyatt, 1982a; Kane and Smith, 1982), but tardive dystonia and tardive akathisia warrant separate recognition beyond their differences in clinical phenomenology because prognosis, at-risk population, and treatment are different. Some authors have noted chronic vocal and motor tics resembling Tourette syndrome (Klawans et al., 1978; Bharucha and Sethi, 1995), and others noted myoclonic movements (Little and Jankovic, 1987; Tominaga et al., 1987) as a chronic persistent problem of neuroleptic therapy, but further studies are necessary to establish them as distinct entities. More recently, a combination of resting, postural, and action tremor has been reported in five patients that persisted despite withdrawal of the offending DRBAs and that improved with treatment with the antidopaminergic TBZ (Stacy and Jankovic, 1992). The tremor was accompanied by other tardive phenomenology, and the authors suggested that this is another tardive syndrome, calling it tardive tremor. Tardive tremor has been reported with metoclopramide (Tarsy and Indorf, 2002).

Withdrawal emergent syndrome

Withdrawal emergent syndrome was first described in children who had been on antipsychotic drugs for a long period of time and then were withdrawn abruptly from their medication (Polizos et al., 1973). The movements are choreic and resemble those of Sydenham disease (Videos 19.1 and 19.2). The abnormal movements are brief and flow from one muscle to another in a seemingly random way. They differ from the movements of classic tardive dyskinesia, which are brief, but stereotypical and repetitive. The movements in withdrawal emergent syndrome involve mainly the limbs, trunk, and neck, and rarely the oral region, which is the most prevalent site in classic tardive dyskinesia. The dyskinetic movements disappear spontaneously within several weeks after withdrawal of the DRBA. For immediate suppression of movements, dopamine receptor antagonists can be reinstituted and withdrawn gradually without recurrence of the withdrawal emergent syndrome (Fahn, 1984a). A withdrawal reaction from melatonin with O-B-L dyskinesia and akathisia was reported by Giladi and Shabtai (1999) and was described earlier in the chapter.

Withdrawal emergent syndrome is analogous to the classic tardive dyskinesia seen in adults, except that the course is more benign and movements are more generalized, resembling the choreic movements of Sydenham disease. In fact, most cases of tardive dyskinesia that have been reported in children have a benign course and the phenomenology has been reported to be more generalized choreic movements rather than stereotypic repetitive movements of oral, buccal, and lingual distribution. Acute withdrawal of chronic antipsychotic drugs in adults can also lead to transient tardive dyskinesia, which disappears within 3 months. These types of movements have been labeled withdrawal dyskinesia (Gardos et al., 1978; Schooler and Kane, 1982).

On the other hand, acute withdrawal of DRBA can precipitate a persistent akathisia (Poyurovsky et al., 1996; Rosebush et al., 1997) or dyskinesia, i.e., tardive akathisia and other tardive syndromes. Acute withdrawal should be avoided because of the propensity to induce TD, and a slow taper and withdrawal should be substituted. Abrupt withdrawal of risperidone therapy in one elderly person resulted in a near-fatal development of respiratory dyskinesia (Komatsu et al., 2005).

Classic tardive dyskinesia

Dyskinesia is a general term referring to abnormal involuntary movements. The term tardive dyskinesia has been used to refer to abnormal movements that are seen as a complication of long-term dopamine receptor antagonist therapy, mainly the type that presents with rapid, repetitive, stereotypic movements involving the oral, buccal, and lingual areas. However, over the years, other types of movements have been noted as complications of dopamine receptor antagonist therapy. These movements have more specific terminologies, such as dystonia and akathisia. Therefore, some authors refer to the type of movements that were originally described as "classic tardive dyskinesia" for lack of a more specific and distinct name for the movements (Fahn, 1989). Some have called them tardive stereotypy (Stacy and Jankovic, 1991; Jankovic, 1994) because of their repetitive, rather than random, nature. However, the stereotypical movements in classic tardive dyskinesia are so characteristic and resemble those seen in almost all patients with this disorder, in contrast to other types of stereotypies that are seen in patients with learning disability, autism, and psychosis, that the term tardive stereotypy does not convey this uniqueness and therefore seems unsatisfactory. Stereotyped hand clasping appears to be a rare form for the presentation of classic tardive dyskinesia (Kaneko et al., 1993).

On the other hand, some have used the term tardive dyskinesia as equivalent to any oral dyskinesia. It therefore needs to be emphasized that the term "tardive" has become synonymous with chronic neuroleptic complications and should be reserved for these disorders. Sustained dystonic movements of the lower face must be distinguished from classic tardive dyskinesia. Frequently, patients on anticholinergics or other medications develop oral dyskinesia with dryness of mouth. Other movements such as myokymia, myoclonus, and tics must be distinguished. The differential diagnosis of oral dyskinesia is summarized in Table 19.10, whereas Table 19.11 compares clinical features of tardive dyskinesia, Huntington disease, and oromandibular dystonia, the three most common forms of oral dyskinesias.

Clinical features of classic tardive dyskinesia

The clinical features of classic TD are quite distinct from the features of other movement disorders (Fahn, 1984a). The principal site is the face, particularly around the mouth, typically called oral-buccal-facial (O-B-L) dyskinesias. The limbs and trunk are affected less often than the mouth. Even when they are involved, it is usually in addition to involvement of the mouth. The forehead and eyebrows are seldom involved unless tardive dystonia is also present; this is in contrast to Huntington disease, in which chorea of the forehead and eyebrows is more common than choreic movements of the oral musculature. In TD, the mouth tends to show a pattern of repetitive, complex chewing motions (Video 19.3; see also Video 1.73), occasionally with smacking and opening of the mouth, tongue protrusion (flycatcher tongue) (Video 19.4), lip pursing, sucking movements, and fishlike lip puckering movements. The rhythmicity and coordinated pattern of movement are striking. This stereotypic pattern is in contrast to the dyskinesias that are seen in Huntington disease, in which the movements are without a predictable pattern. Usually, the limb involvement is limited to the distal part. Like the mouth region, the movements of the distal limbs show a repetitive pattern, earning the label of piano-playing fingers and toes. When the patient is sitting, the legs often move repeatedly, with flexion and extension movements of the toes and foot tapping. When the patient is lying down, flexion and extension of thighs may be seen. Rhythmic truncal rocking can be seen when the patient is lying, sitting, or standing (Video 19.5). The respiratory pattern can be involved with dyskinesia, causing hyperventilation at times and hypoventilation at other times (Yassa and Lai, 1986). In a study of the breathing pattern in patients with TD, patients

Table 19.10 Differential diagnosis of oral dyskinesias

1. Chorea, rhythmical, stereotypical (see also Kurlan and Shoulson, 1988)

a. Encephalitis lethargica: postencephalitic
b. Drug-induced
  i. Dopamine receptor antagonists (classic tardive dyskinesia)
  ii. Levodopa
  iii. Anticholinergic drugs
  iv. Phenytoin intoxication
  v. Antihistamines
  vi. Tricyclic antidepressants
  vii. Lithium
c. Huntington disease
d. Hepatocerebral degeneration
e. Cerebellar infarction
f. Edentulous malocclusion
g. Brainstem infarcts
h. Idiopathic

2. Dystonia

a. Idiopathic cranial dystonia (Meige syndrome)
b. Symptomatic dystonias
  i. Dopamine receptor antagonists (acute dystonia, tardive dystonia)
  ii. Other secondary dystonias (see Calne and Lang, 1988)

3. Tics

4. Tremor

a. Parkinsonian tremor of jaw, tongue, and lips
b. Essential tremor of neck and jaw
c. Cerebellar tremor of neck and jaw
d. Idiopathic tremor of neck, jaw, tongue, or lips

5. Myoclonus

a. Facial myoclonus of central origin

6. Others

a. Hemifacial spasm
b. Myokymia
c. Facial nerve synkinesis
d. Bruxism
e. Epilepsia partialis continua

Adapted from Fahn S. The tardive dyskinesias. In Matthews WB, Glaser GH, eds: Recent Advances in Clinical Neurology, vol. 4. Edinburgh: Churchill Livingstone, 1984; pp. 229–260.

had an irregular tidal breathing pattern, with a greater variability in both tidal volume and time of the total respiratory cycle (Wilcox et al., 1994). The presence of respiratory dyskinesia never causes a medical problem, although it might look alarming. Esophageal (associated with lingual) dyskinesias have also been reported, resulting in increased intraesophageal pressure and death due to asphyxiation in one patient (Horiguchi et al., 1999).

The involuntary movements of the mouth in classic tardive dyskinesia are readily suppressed by patients when asked to do so. Furthermore, the movements cease as the patient is putting food in the mouth, when talking, or when a finger is placed on the lips. Since the movements do not interfere with basic functions, patients are often unaware of their

Table 19.11 Clinical features of classic tardive dyskinesia (TD), oromandibular dystonia (OMD) and Huntington disease (HD)

Clinical signs	TD	OMD	HD
Type of involuntary movements	Stereotypic	Dystonic	Choreic
Flowing movements	0	0	+++
Repetitive movements	+++	+	±
Sustained contractions	+	+++	±
Movements of mouth	+++	+++	+
Blepharospasm	+	+++	±
Forehead chorea	±	±	++
Masticatory muscles	+++	+++	±
Nuchal muscles	+	++	±
Trunk, legs	++	0	+++
Akathisia	++	0	0
Marching in place	++	0	0
Truncal rocking	++	0	+
Motor impersistence (tongue, grip)	0	0	+++
Stuttering-ataxic gait	±	0	+++
Postural instability	0	0	+++
Effect of: antidopaminergics anticholinergics	Decrease Increase	Decrease Decrease	Decrease ±
Effect on: talking, chewing swallowing	± 0	+++ ++	+ +++

0, not seen; ±, may be seen; +, occasionally seen; ++, usually seen; +++, almost always seen.
From Fahn S, Burke RE. Tardive dyskinesia and other neuroleptic-induced syndromes. In Rowland LP, Pedley TA (eds) Merritt's Textbook of Neurology, 12th edn. Philadelphia: Lippincott Williams & Wilkins, 2010; pp. 778–781.

movements. When the patient is asked to keep the tongue at rest inside the mouth, the tongue tends to assume a continual writhing motion of athetoid side-to-side and coiling movements. The constant lingual movements might lead to tongue hypertrophy, and macroglossia is a common clinical sign. On command, however, most patients with TD can keep the tongue protruded out without darting back into the mouth for more than half a minute; patients with the chorea of Huntington disease typically cannot maintain a protruded tongue. This inability to sustain a voluntary contraction is called motor impersistence, which is not seen in TD.

Abnormal movements in schizophrenia in the absence of exposure to DRBAs

Tardive dyskinesia as an entity induced by dopamine receptor blockers has been challenged by reports claiming that spontaneous movements are sometimes encountered in patients with schizophrenia who have never been exposed to neuroleptic agents (see the review by Boeti et al., 2003). McCreadie and colleagues (2002) evaluated 37 schizophrenic patients never treated with antipsychotics and followed for 18 months. Nine (24%) had dyskinesia on both occasions, 12 (33%) on one occasion, and 16 (43%) on neither occasion. Twenty-one (57%) had dyskinesia on at least one occasion. Thirteen patients (35%) had parkinsonism on at least one occasion. It is critical that the quality of the dyskinesia be reported, because the classic O-B-L dyskinesias are very distinct and almost specific for tardive dyskinesia, whereas many other types of movements could represent a different disorder. The presence of parkinsonism, though, suggests that the patients had been exposed to neuroleptics, but that the investigators were clueless as to the exposure.

Many authors noted the existence of spontaneous oral dyskinesia occurring in untreated populations and in untreated schizophrenics. McCreadie and colleagues (1996) examined 308 elderly individuals in Madras, India, looking for abnormal movements and found them in 15%. The prevalence of spontaneous dyskinesia has been reported to be as high as 20% in psychiatric or nursing home patients (Brandon et al., 1971), but the average rate is about 5% (Jeste and Wyatt, 1982a; Kane and Smith, 1982). Others noted increasing prevalence of spontaneous dyskinesia with age (Klawans and Barr, 1982). Some studies looking at healthy elderly populations estimate the prevalence rate to be about 1% (Lieberman et al., 1984; D'Alessandro et al., 1986). Blanchet and colleagues (2004) evaluated 1018 (69.3% women) noninstitutionalized, frail elderly subjects attending day care centers to document the prevalence and phenomenology of spontaneous oral dyskinesia. The prevalence rate for spontaneous oral dyskinesia was 3.7% (4.1% for women and 2.9% for men). They reported more frequent ill-fitting dental devices, oral pain, and a lower rate of perception of good oral health compared to nondyskinetic subjects.

The true prevalence rate of spontaneous oral dyskinesia that can mimic TD may be even lower, considering the fact that many other identifiable oral dyskinesias listed in Table 19.10 such as oromandibular dystonia can be difficult to distinguish from classic tardive dyskinesia and may be counted as spontaneous dyskinesia in epidemiologic studies. On the other hand, spontaneous oral dyskinesia resembling the stereotypical O-B-L dyskinesia of classic tardive dyskinesia has been reported in an aged cynomologus monkey (Rupniak et al., 1990). Some patients with oral dyskinesias resembling those of TD and unexposed to DRBAs would seemingly be idiopathic in origin, but careful workup might reveal other etiologies (Table 19.10), including treatment with lithium (Meyer-Lindenberg and Krausnick, 1997) and brainstem infarcts (Fahn et al., 1986).

Reports of oral dyskinesias occurring in schizophrenic patients who have never been exposed to neuroleptics raise the question as to how specifically the O-B-L movements should be attributed to DRBAs and whether or not they could be due to the schizophrenia. Fenn and colleagues (1996) examined 22 never-medicated schizophrenics in Casablanca, Morocco. Three had abnormal movements that are said to be characteristic of TD. Fenton and colleagues

(1997) compared the prevalence of spontaneous oral dyskinesias among drug-naive schizophrenics and patients with other psychiatric disorders. They found that dyskinetic movements were more common in the former group. Gervin and colleagues (1998) reported 6 (7.6%) out of 79 first-episode schizophrenics to have spontaneous dyskinesias. Until movement disorder experts can evaluate the movement phenomenology, it is possible that these individuals have some disorder other than TD. Moreover, it is possible that the history of nondrug exposure is faulty. The overwhelming evidence is that the abnormal movements that are seen with DRBAs are due to these drugs.

As was mentioned earlier, a major concern in diagnosing spontaneous oral dyskinesias is the distinction between the stereotypic movements of TD and the movements of oromandibular dystonia. Authors should publish the videotape demonstrations of the abnormal movements so that the medical community can judge whether the movements do indeed fit the phenomenologic criteria of movements seen in TD.

Epidemiology, risk factors, and natural history

Epidemiologic studies looking into the prevalence of TD have been confounded by the factors that affect the detection of the abnormal involuntary movements as well as the variables that affect the prognosis of the movements. Therefore, it is not surprising to find a wide range of prevalence estimations from 0.5% to 65% in the literature (Jeste and Wyatt, 1982a; Kane and Smith, 1982). The prevalence of TD has been noted to have increased from 5% before 1965 to 25% in the late 1970s (Jeste and Wyatt, 1982a; Kane and Smith, 1982). Mean prevalence rates calculated by two different reviewers, however, agree well at around 20% (Jeste and Wyatt, 1982a; Kane and Smith, 1982).

The prevalence rates of spontaneous dyskinesias and dyskinesias in people who have been exposed to neuroleptics have been compared. In the study by Woerner and colleagues (1991) the overall prevalence of spontaneous dyskinesias was 1.3% in 400 healthy elderly people and 4.8% in elderly inpatients, with a range of 0–2% among psychiatric patients who had never been exposed to neuroleptics. These investigators reported prevalence of TD of 13.3% and 36.1% in voluntary and state psychiatric hospitals, respectively. There was an interplay between age and gender. Among younger patients, men had higher rates; among subjects over age 40 years, rates were higher in women. Van Os and colleagues (1999) also found an increased risk for men in the younger population.

In one prospective study examining development of TD with low-dose haloperidol, the 12-month incidence of probable or persistent tardive dyskinesia was 12.3% (Oosthuizen et al., 2003). In a much larger study, the annual incidence rates range from 5% in a younger population (mean age 28) (Kane et al., 1986) to 12% in an older group (mean age 56) (Barnes et al., 1983). Kane and colleagues' data (1986) also show that the cumulative incidence of TD increases linearly with increasing duration of neuroleptic exposure at least for the first 4–5 years of such exposure. In a subsequent study by these authors, Chakos and colleagues (1996) studied prospectively 118 patients in their first episode of psychosis who were treatment-naive and were then followed for up to 8.5 years while they were on neuroleptics. The cumulative incidence of presumptive TD was 6.3% after 1 year of follow-up, 11.5% after 2 years, 13.7% after 3 years, and 17.5% after 4 years. Persistent TD had a cumulative incidence of 4.8% after 1 year, 7.2% after 2 years, and 15.6% after 4 years. Thus, the earlier findings of Kane and colleagues (1986) of about 5% a year cumulative incidence seem to have been confirmed.

Jeste et al. (1999) looked at the cumulative incidence of tardive dyskinesia after exposure to neuroleptics in patients over the age of 45 years. The mean cumulative incidence was 3.4%, 5.9%, and 22.3% at 1, 3, and 12 months, respectively. Woerner and his colleagues (1998) studied patients over the age of 54 when first exposed to neuroleptics. The cumulative rates of tardive dyskinesia were 25%, 34%, and 53% after 1, 2, and 3 years of cumulative antipsychotic treatment. A greater risk of tardive dyskinesia was associated with a history of ECT treatment, higher mean daily and cumulative antipsychotic doses, and the presence of extrapyramidal signs early in treatment. From both these studies, the incidence rates for patients beginning treatment with conventional antipsychotics in their fifth decade or later are three to five times what has been found for younger patients, despite treatment with lower doses.

Studies have been carried out in other countries. A prospective study of 11 psychiatric facilities in Japan found the prevalence of TD to be 7.6%, the annual incidence rate to be 3.7%, and an annual remission rate to be 28.7% (Inada et al., 1991). On the other hand, Hayashi and colleagues (1996) reported a prevalence of 22.1% in 258 patients receiving neuroleptics. A study in Austria reported the follow-up of the 270 patients still in a psychiatric hospital after 10 years out of an original population of 861 patients; the prevalence rate of TD was 3.7% in 1982 and 12.7% in 1992; the major risk factor for TD was advanced age (Miller et al., 1995). Jeste and colleagues (1995) followed 266 patients over the age of 45 years to determine incidence and prevalence rates of tardive dyskinesia following exposure to neuroleptics, using electromechanical sensors to detect the presence of movements. Cumulative incidence of TD was 26%, 52%, and 60% after 1, 2, and 3 years, respectively. These rates, which are higher than those found by Kane and his colleagues, might reflect the sensitive sensors used, and these could possibly give false-positive findings. The same group compared the development of abnormal movements in the orofacial and limb-truncal areas in these 266 middle-aged and elderly patients treated with neuroleptics and found that the cumulative incidence of orofacial TD was 38.5% and 65.7% after 1 and 2 years, respectively, whereas that of limb-truncal TD was 18.6% and 32.6% after 1 and 2 years, respectively (Paulsen et al., 1996).

Host and treatment factors affect the development, severity, and persistence of TD, thereby resulting in different prevalence rates. Age of the patient has been the most consistent factor that adversely affects the incidence, prognosis, and severity of tardive dyskinesia (Smith and Baldessarini, 1980; Jeste and Wyatt, 1982a; Kane and Smith, 1982; Kane et al., 1986). Possibly the youngest individual who developed O-B-L tardive dyskinesia was a 2-month-old girl after a 17-day treatment with metoclopramide for gastroesophageal reflux (Mejia and Jankovic, 2005). The movements persisted for at least 9 months after the drug was discontinued.

This patient is the first documented case of tardive dyskinesia in an infant.

Female sex has been associated with increased prevalence of TD, especially in the older population (Jeste and Wyatt, 1982a; Kane and Smith, 1982; Kane et al., 1988). Several authors noted increased incidence and prevalence among patients with affective disorders compared to schizophrenia or schizoaffective disorders (Gardos and Casey, 1983). Other host factors such as presence of previous brain damage as noted by increased ventricular size remain controversial (Jeste and Wyatt, 1982a; Kane and Smith, 1982). Some noted poor treatment response of schizophrenia to drug treatment as a risk factor for development of tardive dyskinesia (Chouinard et al., 1986). The parameters of drug exposures such as dose, duration, type of neuroleptics, and drug-free intervals have been very difficult to correlate with risk of TD partly because accurate history concerning the drug treatment is usually not available and the drug itself can affect the detection of TD by masking or uncovering it.

Ethnicity has been found to be an important risk factor in both the development and prognosis of tardive dyskinesia, African-Americans being more susceptible than European-Americans (Wonodi et al., 2004a). In a meta-analysis of the literature, the only statistically significant risk factors for TD were non-white ethnicity and having developed drug-induced parkinsonism; the association with older age was suggestive but inconclusive (Tenback et al., 2009).

Prospective studies have noted that the total cumulative drug exposure correlates with incidence of withdrawal tardive dyskinesia (Kane et al., 1985), and development of TD 5 years later in patients who did not have TD initially (Chouinard et al., 1986). Continued use of DRBAs after the appearance of TD also adversely affects subsequent prognosis (Kane et al., 1986). Drug holidays were once advocated to decrease the risk of TD, but an increased number of drug-free intervals was found to worsen the prognosis after withdrawal (Jeste et al., 1979). The risk of developing TD is three times as great for patients with more than two neuroleptic interruptions as for patients with two or fewer interruptions (van Harten et al., 1998). Other than reduced risk with clozapine, olanzapine, and quetiapine, no other particular type of neuroleptic, including depot preparations, has been clearly identified as a risk factor (Yassa et al., 1988). The effect of other drugs such as anticholinergics on the incidence and prevalence of TD is controversial, although anticholinergics may increase its severity (Yassa, 1988). Lithium may decrease the chance of TD development (Kane et al., 1986; van Harten et al., 2008a). Development of parkinsonism tends to predispose patients to TD (Chouinard et al., 1986; Kane et al., 1986). Substance abuse has also been reported to be a risk factor (Bailey et al., 1997). Lacking the cytochrome P450 enzyme required for metabolism exogenous toxins because of nonfunctional alleles of the *CYP2D6* gene appears to be a risk factor for developing both TD and drug-induced parkinsonism (Andreassen et al., 1997). Another genetic risk factor is polymorphism in the ATP13A gene, especially for drug-induced parkinsonism (Kasten et al., 2011).

A review of the literature by Correll and colleagues (2004) found a lower incidence with the newer generation of antipsychotics (Table 19.12). A European consortium of

Table 19.12 Annual incidence of tardive dyskinesia comparing the second generation antipsychotics with haloperidol

Population	Second-generation antipsychotics	Haloperidol
Children	0%	
Adults	0.8%	5.4%
Mixture of adults and elderly	6.8%	
Older than 53 years	5.3%	

Data from Correll CU, Leucht S, Kane JM. Lower risk for tardive dyskinesia associated with second-generation antipsychotics: a systematic review of 1-year studies. Am J Psychiatry 2004;161(3):414–425.

investigators looking at 6-month results came to a similar conclusion (Tenback et al., 2005). In their review of the literature, Tarsy and Baldessarini (2006) also suggest that there may be a declining incidence of TD as the second-generation antipsychotics are being more regularly used. On the other hand, in a survey on elderly patients with dementia treated with older or newer generation antipsychotics, no statistical difference was found in the development of nonparkinsonian movement disorders in relation to treatment class (Lee et al., 2005). Children appear to be increasingly treated with "atypical" antipsychotics and in one study, 9% developed TD (Wonodi et al., 2007).

Although the majority of TD occurs while patients are on chronic treatment with DRBAs or shortly after discontinuing them, many cases have been reported in which the TD occurred after only a short interval of treatment and persisted. Some authors define TD arbitrarily as dyskinesias that occur after a minimum of 3 months of dopamine receptor antagonist therapy (Schooler and Kane, 1982), but it appears that there is no safe low-incidence period right after the initiation of treatment with DRBAs nor is there any particularly high-risk period. The overall risk appears to accumulate as time goes on, although whether it continues to increase linearly even after the first several years of exposure is not clear from available data. Kang and colleagues' (1986) retrospective data also show that the cumulative number of patients who developed tardive dystonia increased almost linearly from the first few months.

Probably most patients with TD have mild cases that could improve and disappear over time if the offending DRBAs were withdrawn. In an attempt to look at risk factors for the severe forms of TD, Caligiuri and colleagues (1997) conducted a longitudinal prospective study to determine the incidence of severe TD in middle-aged and elderly psychiatric patients. The cumulative incidence of severe TD was 2.5% after 1 year, 12.1% after 2 years, and 22.9% after 3 years. Risk factors for severe TD were higher daily doses of neuroleptics at study entry, greater cumulative amounts of prescribed neuroleptic, and greater severity of worsening negative psychiatric symptoms.

Once established, TD does not frequently become more severe even though the DRBA is continued (Labbate et al., 1997). Fernandez and colleagues (2001) evaluated the dyskinesia of TD and the clinical features of parkinsonism in 53 patients residing in a state psychiatric hospital over a 14-year period. TD improved and parkinsonism worsened in patients who continued to receive neuroleptic drugs. But the natural history of TD is not easy to determine because the DRBAs that cause the movement disorders also tend to suppress the movements, while they can cause drug-induced parkinsonism.

Movements that disappear with increasing dose or resumption of DRBAs have been called masked TD (Schooler and Kane, 1982). Conversely, movements of TD typically increase after discontinuation of the DRBAs. Transient dyskinesias that appear after withdrawal of DRBAs have been called withdrawal dyskinesias (Gardos et al., 1978). The term covert dyskinesia has also been used for dyskinesia that is not detectable during drug administration and is first noted during drug reduction or withdrawal and becomes permanent (Gardos et al., 1978). Therefore, the difference between withdrawal and covert dyskinesia is in duration. In fact, the spectrum of TD ranges from mild transient withdrawal dyskinesia to severe irreversible TD, which can occur during or after discontinuation of the antipsychotic drugs. These examples illustrate the complexity in the detection of TD in the presence of DRBAs. In an attempt to estimate the false-negative rate of detection for TD in patients taking DRBAs, Kane and colleagues (1988) withdrew the drug from patients who showed no evidence of TD while taking DRBAs. Withdrawal TD was seen in 34% of 70 subjects, with persistence beyond 3 months in 7 of them.

Pathophysiology

Although tardive dyskinesia is an iatrogenic condition with an established etiologic connection to dopamine receptor antagonism, the pathophysiology is not well understood. Any proposed mechanism for tardive dyskinesia will have to explain (1) the cumulative increase of risk with increasing duration of treatment, (2) frequent persistence of the condition despite discontinuation of the treatment, (3) increasing risk with age and other individual dispositions that leave only a portion of the population affected, (4) increased risk with intermittent exposure to DRBAs, and (5) clinical pharmacology of tardive dyskinesia (i.e., improvement of the condition by drugs that depress dopaminergic activity and worsening by increasing dopaminergic activity with levodopa or amphetamine).

Anatomical pathology – human and animal models

Postmortem pathologic studies are few and show nonspecific findings in the striatonigral system, which might be due to aging or other uncontrolled factors (Christensen et al., 1970). Jellinger (1977) found swollen large (i.e., cholinergic) neurons in the rostral caudate nucleus in 46% of neuroleptic-treated patients. In a review of the literature Harrison (1999) notes other studies in which cholinergic neurons are affected by these drugs. In a magnetic resonance imaging (MRI) study, 2-year exposure to neuroleptics in schizophrenic patients resulted in an increase in caudate and lenticular nucleus volume, while in those who were similarly exposed to atypical antipsychotics, there was a decrease in volume (Corson et al., 1999).

Since TD is etiologically related to DRBAs and since the clinical pharmacology is most consistent with dopaminergic

hyperactivity, many studies have been directed to the dopamine system (Klawans, 1973). Chronic dopamine receptor antagonist treatment in rats shows evidence of cell loss in ventrolateral striatum (Nielson and Lyon, 1978), changes in synaptic patterns in the striatum at the electron microscopic level (Benes et al., 1985), and increases in glutamatergic synapses in the striatum (Meshul et al., 1994). In the accumbens in rats who developed vacuous chewing movements (VCMs), the dendritic surface area is reduced, and dynorphin-positive terminals contact more spines and form more asymmetric specializations than those in animals without the syndrome (Meredith et al., 2000). Andreassen and colleagues (2001) found electron microscopic changes in rats who developed haloperidol-induced VCMs. The nerve terminal area in the striatum was increased but with a lower density of glutamate immunoreactivity. These results suggest that striatal glutamatergic transmission is affected in association with haloperidol-induced VCMs.

Anatomical pathology – in-vitro models

Galili-Mosberg and colleagues (2000) exposed neuronal and PC-12 cultures to haloperidol and its three metabolites. These induced cell death by apoptosis, which was protected by the antioxidants vitamin E and N-acetylcysteine. Marchese and colleagues (2002) found a shrinkage of TH-immunostaining (TH-IM) cell bodies in the substantia nigra pars compacta and reticulata and a reduction of TH-immunostaining in the striatum of haloperidol-treated rats with the arising of VCMs. No differences were observed in TH-IM neurons of the ventral tegmental area and nucleus accumbens versus control rats.

Rodent models – dopamine and other neurotransmitter biochemistry

In experimental animals, a short-term treatment of dopamine receptor antagonist can increase striatal dopamine synthesis and turnover that revert to normal levels within a few days despite continuing treatment (Asper et al., 1973). Receptor binding increases in 2 days and persists for up to a week (Asper et al., 1973; Klawans, 1973; Muller and Seeman, 1977). The change in receptor state correlates well with stereotypic gnawing movements by rats that are induced by a dopamine agonist such as apomorphine (Clow et al., 1980). Chronic treatment for a year in rats produces an increase in receptor binding sites by the sixth month of treatment, overcoming the initial effects of receptor blockade. The increase of receptor binding and functional hypersensitivity takes about 6 months to return to baseline after withdrawal of drug treatment. Increased response of striatal adenylate cyclase to dopamine still persists at 6 months (Clow et al., 1980). The significance of this finding is not clear. Extrapolating from this rodent model of dopaminergic supersensitivity to patients with TD has limitations. Rats do not usually develop spontaneous movements such as tardive dyskinesia, but they do demonstrate increased sensitivity to exogenously administered dopamine agonists and can develop VCMs.

The receptor supersensitivity in rodents develops in all the animals treated relatively early in the course of dopamine antagonist treatment and is completely reversible in 100% of animals shortly after withdrawal. This is clearly at odds with human TD, in which large individual variations and susceptibility factors are important and the disorder often starts late in the course of treatment and becomes persistent. Nonetheless, this model has been most useful for quick screening of potential neuroleptics that are likely to cause TD from those that are not. Calabresi and colleagues (1992) suggested that hypersensitivity of the D2 presynaptic receptors located on terminals of glutamatergic corticostriatal fibers in animals with chronic treatment with haloperidol would inhibit glutamate release in the striatum, thereby reducing the gamma-aminobutyric acid (GABA) output from postsynaptic striatal neurons. Dopamine D2 receptor occupancy appears to be a contributing factor in the development of the rodent model (Turrone et al., 2002). Andreassen and Jorgensen (2000) review the possible role of increased striatal glutamatergic activity in the rat model as an etiologic factor and suggest that excitoxicity is a possible cause of TD. Anatomic changes found by these authors were presented in the previous section.

Rodent models – behavioral changes

A common rodent model is that based on the increased rate of VCMs in rats, which develop after several months of dopamine receptor antagonist treatment (Gunne et al., 1982). The movements persist for several months after neuroleptic withdrawal. The behavioral syndrome is spontaneous in contrast to the stereotypic gnawing movement that requires apomorphine to induce. The pharmacologic response is similar to that seen with TD in that acute haloperidol alleviates the behavioral syndrome. In these aspects, this model is closer to the characteristics of human TD than models that are based on dopamine receptor supersensitivity.

The VCMs that persist after withdrawal of dopamine receptor antagonist do so at the time when the receptor-binding studies show no supersensitivity (Waddington et al., 1983). Blocking N-methyl-D-aspartate (NMDA) receptors with memantine while the rats are receiving treatment with haloperidol allowed these rats to lose the VCMs sooner than those animals who did not receive memantine (Andreassen et al., 1996). This result supports the concept that excessive NMDA receptor stimulation might be a mechanism underlying the development of persistent dyskinesias in humans. Opioid receptor antagonists were also shown to block VCMs in rats, suggesting that increases in dynorphin in the direct striatonigral pathway and enkephalin in the indirect striatopallidal pathway following chronic neuroleptic administration are both likely to contribute to tardive dyskinesia (McCormick and Stoessl, 2002).

In one study of chronic haloperidol treatment in the rat, the animals that developed VCMs were compared with those that did not develop the movements (Shirakawa and Tamminga, 1994). Whereas all animals showed an increase in the dopamine D2 family receptor binding in the striatum and in the nucleus accumbens, and an increase in GABA-A receptors in the substantia nigra pars reticulata (SNr), only those with VCMs had a significant decrease in dopamine D1 receptor density in the SNr. One explanation is that increased dopamine release from dendrites in the SNr downregulates the D1 receptor. But how this would produce dyskinesias is not clear. In dorsal striatal neurons, however, there was no change in D1 receptor mRNA nor was there a change in cell

counts in rats with neuroleptic-induced VCMs (Petersen et al., 2000).

Stereotyped behavior was evaluated in rats treated chronically with haloperidol, followed by D1 and D2 agonists. Somatostatin levels were then measured. The results suggested that somatostatin – but not enkephalin-containing striatal neurons – contribute to the expression of haloperidol-induced stereotypies (Marin et al., 1996).

Other neurotransmitters in the striatum may also be involved. Chronic haloperidol treatment in rats increases preproenkephalin messenger RNA in striatal neurons, but fail to do so in rats that develop VCMs (Andreassen et al., 1999a). Some authors noted that decreases of glutamic acid decarboxylase (GAD) and GABA in substantia nigra correlate with increased VCM rates (Gunne and Haggstrom, 1983). Others noted no consistent change in GAD and choline acetyltransferase levels (Mithani et al., 1987). However, Delfs and colleagues (1995) reported that rats treated with haloperidol for up to 12 months showed a decrease of GAD mRNA in the external globus pallidus. This result suggests that there is reduced GABAergic transmission in the projection neurons of the external pallidum. Blocking NMDA receptors with memantine while the rats are receiving treatment with haloperidol allowed these rats to lose the VCMs sooner than animals that did not receive memantine (Andreassen et al., 1996). This result supports the concept that excessive NMDA receptor stimulation could be a mechanism underlying the development of persistent dyskinesias in humans. Lesioning the subthalamic nuclei (and thus its glutamatergic efferents) eliminates VCMs after 1–3 weeks (Stoessl and Rajakumar, 1996). The 5-HT$_3$ receptor antagonist ondansetron reverses haloperidol-induced VCMs in rats (Naidu and Kulkarni, 2001).

As a test for the oxidative stress hypothesis in causing TD, rats were cotreated with coenzyme Q10 (CoQ10) along with haloperidol. Cotreatment with CoQ10 did not attenuate the development of the VCMs (Andreassen et al., 1999b). CoQ10 was absorbed, as detected in the serum, but there was no increase of CoQ10 in the brain.

Primate models with behavioral changes

The model that best resembles human tardive dyskinesia is that induced in nonhuman primates by DRBAs (Klintenberg et al., 2002). Primates show delayed onset of dyskinesia during the course of treatment and only a fraction of the population that is treated is affected by dyskinesia. The behavioral effect is spontaneous and bears resemblance to human TD. The dyskinesia also persists after withdrawal of the DRBAs. Unfortunately, neuropathologic and biochemical data from this model are limited. One group suggested that the best neurochemical correlate of dyskinesia induced by DRBAs has been a decrease in GABA and GAD activity in the substantia nigra, subthalamic nucleus, and medial globus pallidus compared to control animals without drug treatment or animals with drug treatment but without dyskinesia (Gunne et al., 1984). This finding correlates with postmortem biochemical studies on humans with TD (see the next section) and with a recent 2-deoxyglucose study in primates with TD. In the latter study, Mitchell and colleagues (1992) reported that primates with TD had a reduced glucose metabolism in the medial globus pallidus and in the ventral anterior and ventral lateral nuclei of the thalamus. These findings correlate with other similar studies of chorea and ballism and suggest a reduced subthalamopallidal output, so that the medial pallidum is not activated. Such a finding would be seen in the hemiballistic animal.

In a 5-year study of fluphenazine treatment of *Cebus apella* monkeys, re-exposure following 91 weeks of withdrawal increased dyskinesias and dystonias by 300% (Linn et al., 2001). This observation correlates with earlier clinical studies that found that intermittent treatment with neuroleptics can dramatically increase the incidence of dystonias and dyskinesias.

In a study looking for a proposed mitochondrial dysfunction in TD, baboons were treated for 41 weeks with haloperidol, producing TD; the animals were followed for another 17 weeks following withdrawal of haloperidol, during which the TD persisted (Eyles et al., 2000). Striatal mitochondria were examined by electron microscopy and showed no difference in either size or number between treated and control animals.

Human biochemistry

Postmortem analysis

In a study that was well controlled for the premortem state of patients, a significant decrease in GAD activity was found in the subthalamic nucleus of five tardive dyskinesia patients compared to age-matched controls (Andersson et al., 1989). Dopamine receptor binding is not increased in postmortem brains of tardive dyskinesia patients (Crow et al., 1982; Cross et al., 1985; Kornhuber et al., 1989). One study noted increased homovanillic acid levels in the putamen and nucleus accumbens of the postmortem brain (Cross et al., 1985).

Cerebrospinal fluid

CSF GABA concentration was found to be significantly lower in five patients with chronic schizophrenia and TD than in five patients with chronic schizophrenia without TD who were matched for age, duration of schizophrenia, and duration of neuroleptic therapy (Thaker et al., 1987). CSF cyclic-AMP is thought to reflect the dopamine receptor function, and is not significantly elevated in patients with TD. CSF dopamine metabolite studies do not show significant elevation of homovanillic acid (HVA) (Bowers et al., 1979; Nagao et al., 1979). CSF studies also showed a higher concentration of excitatory amino acid neurotransmitters and markers of oxidative stress in patients with TD, supporting the hypothesis of oxidative stress due to enhanced striatal glutamatergic neurotransmission by blocking presynaptic dopamine receptors (Tsai et al., 1998).

PET and SPECT

PET data on the postsynaptic receptor status have failed to show an elevation of striatal receptor density compared to normal controls, but there was a positive correlation with severity of TD (Blin et al., 1989). No increase in dopamine transporter binding in striatum was found in a SPECT study, indicating no loss on dopaminergic nerve terminals (Lavalaye et al., 2001). A prospective study was carried out by using FDG PET in patients receiving antipsychotic drugs. Those who later developed TD had a relative hypermetabolism in temporolimbic, brainstem, and cerebellar regions and hypometabolism in parietal and cingulate gyrus (Szymanski et al., 1996).

Dopamine release studies using amphetamine following raclopride binding of the D2 receptor showed no differences between subjects with and without TD, indicating that dopamine release does not seem to be a factor (Adler et al., 2002).

Genetics

Steen and colleagues (1997) reported that a specific allelic variation of the dopamine D3 receptor (DRD3) gene is found at a higher frequency (22–24%) of homozygosity among patients with TD compared with the relative underrepresentation (4–6%) of this genotype in patients with no TD. Subsequent studies (Segman et al., 1999; Liao et al., 2001) supported and extended an association between D3 receptor gene and TD in schizophrenia patients. A serine to glycine polymorphism in the first exon of the DRD3 gene appears to be a risk factor for developing TD (Liao et al., 2001, Ozdemir et al., 2001). Lerer and colleagues (2002) also found the presence of the glycine allele carries a higher risk for developing TD. On the other hand, Chong et al. (2003) found the serine allele to have a higher risk. A meta-analysis of genetic studies supports the view that a serine to glycine polymorphism in the D3 receptor gene has a higher risk (odds ratio = 1.17) for developing TD (Bakker et al., 2006). Other polymorphisms in *DRD3* have also been associated with TD (Zai et al., 2009).

Beta-arrestin 2 (*ARRB2*) is an important mediator between DRD2 and serine-threonine protein kinase (AKT) signal cascade. A case-control study to evaluate the association between a polymorphism (Ser280Ser) and antipsychotic-induced TD was performed amongst 381 patients (TD/non-TD = 228/153) in a Chinese population. This polymorphism was significantly more common in those with TD ($P = 0.025$) (Liou et al., 2008).

A meta-analysis of genetic studies reported that there appears to be a protective effect against developing TD by being (1) a Val-Met heterozygote or a Met carrier for *COMT* and (2) Ala-Val and Val carriers for *MnSOD*, while there is a greater risk for TD by having an A2 variant or being an A2-A2 homozygote for *DRD2* (Bakker et al., 2008).

Polymorphisms of the *CYP2D6* gene, which encodes the cytochrome P450 enzyme debrisoquine/spartein hydroxylase, has been reported to possibly be associated with an increased susceptibility to developing TD (Kapitany et al., 1998; Ohmori et al., 1998; Vandel et al., 1999).

Searches for polymorphisms in the HTR_{2A} receptor gene did not find any significant difference among patients with or without TD (Basile et al., 2001, Segman et al., 2001), but this has been inconsistent (Tan et al., 2001).

Neuroendocrine

Assessment of tuberoinfundibular dopaminergic sensitivity as a general indicator of dopamine supersensitivity shows lack of hyperresponsiveness of growth hormone and prolactin to dopamine agonist (Tamminga et al., 1977). Although these data on human TD are preliminary and indirect, the evidence for dopaminergic hypersensitivity has not been confirmed in human studies (Jeste and Wyatt, 1981; Fibiger and Lloyd, 1984).

Phenylalanine loading

In a double-blind study, 100 mg/kg of phenylalanine or placebo was given orally to 10 patients with TD (Mosnik et al., 1997); the dyskinesia was exacerbated after ingestion of phenylalanine, confirming earlier reports. Impaired phenylalanine metabolism was found in men but not in women (Richardson et al., 1999)

Human imaging

Results of imaging studies are inconsistent. In one MRI study Buchanan and colleagues (1994) found no difference between schizophrenic patients who had tardive dyskinesia and those who did not when measuring volumes of the caudate, putamen and pallidum. In contrast, Brown and colleagues (1996) reported larger caudate nuclei, particularly the right, in schizophrenic patients with TD compared to those without TD. To confuse this subject more, a computed tomographic (CT) study using special statistical methods found that the left caudate nucleus was smaller and the temporal sulci were enlarged (Dalgalarrondo and Gattaz, 1994). Brain iron was found to be normal in the basal ganglia in an MRI study (Elkashef et al., 1994).

Hoffman and Casey (1991) reviewed the literature on reports on CT evaluation of patients with tardive dyskinesia. They found that there is a trend toward larger cerebral ventricles in TD patients but that the overall difference with controls is small. Mion and colleagues (1991) compared MRI scans in young TD patients versus controls and found that the volumes of the caudate nuclei were significantly smaller in the TD patients than in normal controls and in patients on neuroleptics without TD. But covariate analysis failed to show a significant difference.

Oxidative stress and excitotoxicity

Maurer and Moller (1997) studied the effect on mitochondria of neuroleptics added to normal human brain cortex in vitro. Complex I activity was inhibited by all neuroleptics in the following order: haloperidol > chlorpromazine > risperidone >> clozapine. Haloperidol increases reactive oxygen species (generated from mitochondria) in rat cortical cell lines (Sagara, 1998). Erythrocyte Cu,Zn-superoxide dismutase activity was found to be reduced in patients on neuroleptics with TD compared to those without TD (Yamada et al., 1997). There were no differences in plasma vitamin E levels between TD and non-TD schizophrenic patients treated with neuroleptics (Brown et al., 1998). The CSF results mentioned earlier support the notion that by blocking presynaptic dopamine receptors, antipsychotics increase striatal glutamatergic transmission and subsequently excitotoxic stress (Tsai et al., 1998). Finding striatal changes in glutamate terminals in a rodent model lends support to the concept of excitotoxicity as a possible mechanism for developing TD (Andreassen et al., 2001) (see section entitled "Anatomical pathology – human and animal models").

Developing TD in the presence of dopamine deficiency states

If dopamine receptor supersensitivity plus active dopamine release from nerve terminals with activation of these supersensitive receptors plays any role in the pathogenesis of TD, then one might anticipate that a state of deficiency of dopamine storage would be incompatible with the development of TD. There appears to be some merit to this concept. Fahn and Mayeux (1980) presented the first report of a patient with PD who developed TD. Their patient had unilateral PD, was treated with a dopamine receptor blocker, and subsequently developed classic TD on the contralateral side of the body. There was no TD on the side with the parkinsonism. In essence, this case supports the notion that a marked deficiency of dopamine release renders the development of TD unlikely, as is seen in the parkinsonian half of the body. The other side probably had partial reduction of dopamine stores and reduced release of dopamine, but it was still capable of developing TD. So perhaps this suggests a quantitative requirement (i.e., a threshold of dopamine availability before an individual could develop TD). This concept is compatible with observations that patients with TD who are treated with dopamine-depleting agents, such as reserpine, can substitute the excessive movements with a parkinsonian state.

The second case was a patient with dopa-responsive dystonia (DRD) who developed TD on long-term haloperidol therapy (de la Fuente-Fernandez, 1998). In DRD, there is a reduction of dopamine stores, but not a complete depletion. So again, if the quantity of dopamine available is the critical factor, a state of DRD seems to be quantitatively sufficient with dopamine.

Pathophysiology – summary

The biochemical basis of TD is still unclear, and the explanation involving dopamine receptor supersensitivity alone does not seem to be sufficient. There is little dispute that the primary and early effect of dopamine receptor antagonist is on the dopaminergic system with presynaptic and postsynaptic hypersensitivity. However, the changes do not seem to distinguish patients who develop TD from those who do not. Gerlach (1991) suggested that TD might be due to an increased ratio of D1/D2 receptor activity. The typical neuroleptics block pre- and postsynaptic D2 receptors, leaving D1 receptors spared. Thus, it is proposed that an increased D1 receptor activation would lead to the dyskinesias.

The effect of DRBAs is not restricted to the dopaminergic system, and the influence on other interconnected systems such as cholinergic, GABAergic, and peptidergic system needs to be studied. Clinical response to antidopaminergic drugs does not necessarily indicate a central pathophysiologic process in that system either. A good example is treatment of PD with anticholinergics, which does not directly reflect the dopaminergic deficiency of the disease. Moreover, changes may occur at the ultrastructural level such as altered synaptic patterns between subsets of dopaminergic neurons and other interconnected neurons. Findings similar in humans and primate models of TD of decreased GABA activity in the subthalamic nucleus lend support to involvement of this nucleus in TD.

Oxyradicals have been implicated in the pathogenetic mechanism for the tardive syndromes (Lohr, 1991). This is based on the concept that DRBAs cause an increase in dopamine turnover, resulting in an increased synthesis of hydrogen peroxide, a metabolite of oxidative deamination of dopamine. Hydrogen peroxide, if not rapidly metabolized, will form oxyradicals, which can damage cell membranes and other cellular components. This hypothesis has received support from a study in which simultaneous administration of tocopherol to chronic haloperidol treatment in rats prevented the development of behavioral supersensitivity to apomorphine (Gattaz et al., 1993).

Additional studies and new approaches are needed to understand the pathophysiology of classic tardive dyskinesia.

Tardive dystonia

Dystonia is most often an idiopathic disorder and can occur at all ages. Persistent dystonic movement as a complication of DRBA therapy has long been noted (Druckman et al., 1962). However, it had not been studied systematically to show that this represents a distinct syndrome until reported by Burke and colleagues (1982). Tardive dystonia has a different epidemiology and pharmacologic response from those of classic tardive dyskinesia. Although secondary dystonia can be caused by many neurologic disorders (Calne and Lang, 1988), tardive dystonia is one of the most common causes (Kang et al., 1986). A rigorous epidemiologic study is not available for tardive dystonia, but the prevalence of tardive dystonia in chronic psychiatric inpatients has been estimated to be 1.5–2% (Friedman et al., 1986; Yassa et al., 1986). When mild forms of dystonia were evaluated, 27 out of 125 patients on chronic antipsychotic medications had some form of dystonia (Sethi et al., 1990), indicating that the prevalence could be higher than was initially realized. Idiopathic torsion dystonia is a much less common condition, with one of the most generous estimations of prevalence at around 1 per 3000 population (Nutt et al., 1988). Therefore, dystonic movements seem to be much more frequent in patients who have been exposed to DRBAs.

In primary dystonia, patients at younger age of onset tend to develop generalized dystonia and those with onset in adulthood are more likely to have craniocervical focal or segmental dystonia. Kang and colleagues (1986) and Kiriakakis and colleagues (1998) have reviewed large series of cases of tardive dystonia and found a similar correlation between distribution of dystonia and age at onset. They found a correlation between the site and age of onset; the site of onset ascended from the lower limbs to the face as the mean age of onset increased. But tardive dystonia rarely affects legs alone even in youngsters (Kang et al., 1986). Regardless of age at onset, tardive dystonia usually progresses over months or years from a focal onset to become more widespread; only 17% remain focal at the time of maximum severity (Kiriakakis et al., 1998). As in primary dystonia, tardive dystonia in adults tends to remain focal or segmental and tends to involve the craniocervical region.

The onset of tardive dystonia can be from days to years after exposure to a DRBA (Kang et al., 1986). Kiriakakis and colleagues (1998) found the range to extend from 4 days to 23 years of exposure (median 5, mean 6.2 ± 5.1 years) in their series of 107 patients, with a mean (±SD) age at onset of 38.3 ± 13.7 years (range 13–68 years). There is no period that is safe from development of tardive dystonia; one patient in the series by Burke et al. (1982) developed it after a one-day exposure. Men are significantly younger than women at onset of dystonia, and it develops after shorter exposure in men (Kiriakakis et al., 1998). Yassa and colleagues (1989) found that severe tardive dystonia was more common in young men while severe classic tardive dyskinesia was more common in older women.

The phenomenology of tardive dystonia can be indistinguishable from that of idiopathic dystonia, including the improvement with sensory tricks (geste antagoniste), which can be used to advantage in creating mechanical devices to reduce the severity of the dystonia (Krack et al., 1998). Focal dystonias, such as tardive cervical dystonia (Molho et al., 1998) and tardive blepharospasm (Sachdev, 1998), can resemble primary focal dystonias (Video 19.6). Retrocollis is more likely to be due to tardive dystonia (Video 19.7), and less likely head or neck trauma, while primary dystonia is uncommon (Papapetropoulos et al., 2007). A comparison of tardive and primary oromandibular dystonia (OMD) showed similar demographics, both occurring predominantly in women with jaw-closing dystonia being the most common form (Tan and Jankovic, 2000). Primary OMD patients were more likely to have coexistent cervical dystonia, and the two types of dystonia responded equally well to botulinum toxin injections. Limb stereotypies, akathisia, and respiratory dyskinesia were seen only in the tardive OMD.

One clinical presentation of tardive dystonia is particularly more characteristic of tardive dystonia, the combination of retrocollis, trunk arching backward, internal rotation of the arms, extension of the elbows and flexion of the wrists (Video 19.8) (Kang et al., 1986), whereas patients with idiopathic dystonia more often have lateral torticollis and twisting of the trunk laterally. The presence of lightning-like (myoclonic) movements in association with dystonia may be more common in tardive dystonia than in primary dystonia (Video 19.9). Reduction of dystonic movements with voluntary action such as walking is often seen in tardive dystonia. This is distinctly unusual in idiopathic dystonia in which the dystonic movements are usually exacerbated by voluntary action. It can be severe enough to jeopardize patients by causing life-threatening dysphagia (Hayashi et al., 1997; Samie et al., 1987).

Tardive dystonia tends to occur in all ages without predilection for any particular age range. The mean age of onset in the literature is about 40 years. This is in contrast to idiopathic dystonia, which shows a bimodal distribution with one early peak in childhood and another later peak in adulthood (Fahn, 1988). Tardive dystonia affects both sexes equally, and men have a younger age of onset than women. Duration of exposure to dopamine receptor antagonists at the onset of tardive dystonia can range from as short as 3 weeks to close to 40 years. The mean duration is 7 years, and as many as 20% of cases develop within a year of the therapy. If the cumulative percentage of patients is plotted against the duration of exposure, the data show a linear line extrapolated to the origin of the graph at zero. This suggests that the risk of developing tardive dystonia starts at the initiation of therapy without any safe minimum period of exposure (Kang et al., 1986).

Wojcik and colleagues (1991) reviewed 32 patients with tardive dystonia and found that most were men, but that women had a shorter exposure time to DRBAs. None of their patients had a complete remission, and the condition causes notable disability. On the other hand, van Harten and colleagues (2008b) reported a remission rate of 80% in mild cases of tardive dystonia; the patients remained on antipsychotic medications, so one cannot be certain that the underlying symptoms would not reappear after withdrawal of the DRBAs.

Many patients with tardive dystonia also have classic tardive dyskinesia at some point in their course (Kang et al., 1986; van Harten et al., 1997). It is not clear why some develop dystonia whereas others develop classic tardive dyskinesia or why some develop both. When patients have both types, dystonic symptoms are usually much more pronounced and disabling (Kang et al., 1986; Gardos et al., 1987).

The dystonia can be so severe that complications can occur. One patient with powerful retrocollis fractured the odontoid process (Konrad et al., 2004).

Tardive akathisia

Originally, akathisia was mainly thought of as an acute to subacute side effect of dopamine receptor antagonists. Various authors, however, noted different variants of akathisia that occurred late in the course of the neuroleptic therapy and/or persisted despite discontinuation of neuroleptic therapy (Braude and Barnes, 1983; Fahn, 1983; Weiner and Luby, 1983). Concomitant or subsequent development of TD was also noted (Munetz and Cornes, 1982; Burke et al., 1989). Barnes and Braude (1985) made a systematic attempt to classify the complex variety of akathisia syndromes. They defined the disorder by the presence of both the subjective and objective features and confirmed that there are acute and chronic variants of akathisia. They also distinguished two types of chronic akathisia; one that occurred early in the course at the time of increasing neuroleptic dose and persisted (acute persistent akathisia) and one that occurred during long-term therapy, sometimes during reduction of their neuroleptic dose (tardive akathisia). Burke and colleagues (1989) reviewed experience with 30 patients with persistent akathisia who met both subjective and objective criteria. They found it difficult to distinguish between acute persistent and tardive akathisia in many cases owing to imprecise information about the onset of the disorder relative to initiation of therapy. It is not clear whether these are distinct syndromes or simply two ends of a continuum. Therefore, some researchers prefer to lump them together as tardive akathisia in line with other persistent movement disorders from dopamine receptor antagonists (Burke et al., 1989). Some attempts to classify akathisia syndromes are complex (Lang, 1994; Sachdev, 1995a); a simple method is to consider persistent neuroleptic-induced akathisia to be the tardive akathisia, and withdrawal, transient akathisia to be acute akathisia, as is done here.

The clinical phenomenology of tardive akathisia is thought to be the same as that of acute akathisia. Moaning (Video 19.10; see also Video 1.36) and focal pain are more common in tardive akathisia than in acute akathisia. In Burke and colleagues' study (1989), the mean age at onset of tardive akathisia was 58 years with a range from 21 to 82 years, similar to the age range of classic tardive dyskinesia. The mean duration of dopamine receptor antagonist exposure before the onset was 4.5 years with a range from 2 weeks to 22 years. Over half of the patients had onset within 2 years. In tardive akathisia, there is a strong likelihood that there will be accompanying tardive dyskinesia (Video 19.11), or

tardive dystonia (Video 19.12) movements. All of the patients with tardive akathisia in the study by Burke and colleagues (1989) also had either tardive dyskinesia (93%) or tardive dystonia (33%) or both (27%) at the same time. But isolated tardive akathisia can exist as well. The pathophysiology of akathisia is not understood.

Treatment of tardive syndromes

The most important point to remember in the management of tardive syndromes is that they are iatrogenic disorders. One should avoid using a DRBA if possible. Patients should be forewarned of the risk of a tardive dyskinesia syndrome before being placed on the drug. In a survey of 520 psychiatrists, only 54% of them disclose this risk (Kennedy and Sanborn, 1992). A study of the impact of informed consent based on questionnaires showed that patients did retain the information both at 4 weeks and at 2 years (Kleinman et al., 1996). Another study comparing patients' knowledge of TD by a questionnaire revealed that those who were educated about the disorder had more knowledge about it 6 months later (Chaplin and Kent, 1998).

Once a tardive syndrome has been encountered, removal of the etiologic agent must be seriously considered as the first consideration. If it is to be discontinued, a slow taper appears to be safer than sudden withdrawal; the latter might exacerbate the severity of the syndrome. In classic tardive dyskinesia, prospective data show 33% remission in 2 years following elimination of the DRBA (Kane et al., 1986). In retrospective studies, the remission rates were 12% for tardive dystonia and 8% for tardive akathisia (Kang et al., 1986; Burke et al., 1989). Some of these patients remitted only after at least 5 years of abstinence from DRBAs (Klawans et al. 1984; Kang et al., 1986). Younger age is associated with better chance of remission (Smith and Baldessarini, 1980) and earlier detection and discontinuation of dopamine receptor antagonists were more favorable for remission (Quitkin et al., 1977). In a study involving chronic schizophrenics, only 1 of 49 patients who discontinued the antipsychotic drugs had a lasting recovery, but 10 others had some improvement 1 year later (Glazer et al., 1990).

There are necessary indications for long-term use of DRBAs, such as chronic psychotic disorders (American Psychiatric Association, 1980). When patients are not able to discontinue antipsychotic medications, the concern is whether their TD will inexorably get worse requiring higher and higher doses of antipsychotics to suppress the symptoms, but there are no data to indicate a worsening in most patients (Labbate et al., 1997), and the majority of patients show improvement over time (Gardos et al., 1988). Casey and colleagues (1986) noted that those with decreased neuroleptic doses showed no change in their dyskinesia score, and those with stable doses and increased doses showed a mean decrease in their dyskinesia scores at 3- to 11-year follow-up. Although these data do not answer whether the symptoms were simply masked or whether the disease itself has improved in its natural course, at least it appears that continuing antipsychotics does not necessarily aggravate the symptoms.

Therefore, a prudent approach is to keep the patients at the minimum dose of the drug necessary for their control of psychosis and add other forms of therapy for tardive dyskinesia. Many patients who are withdrawn from DRBAs still require symptomatic suppression of their movements when remission is not achieved or while waiting for remission. Since the clinical pharmacology is different in each subsyndrome, they are discussed separately.

Treatment of classic tardive dyskinesia (TD)

Dopamine depletors

The concept of employing dopamine-depleting drugs, such as reserpine and TBZ (a synthetic benzoquinolizine), is that these agents effectively reduce dopaminergic synaptic activity, thereby reducing the TD symptoms without exposing the brain to an offending DRBA. This allows the possibility that over time, the brain will heal itself and completely eliminate the TD. In contrast, DRBAs can effectively decrease TD symptoms, but the brain continues to be exposed to the same pathogenetic mechanism that caused the TD in the first place, so the brain cannot recover. Both reserpine and TBZ inhibit the vesicular monoamine transporter. By preventing monoamines from being sequestered in the nerve terminal's vesicles, they allow the monoamines to be exposed to monoamine oxidase and catabolized, thus being markedly depleted in the nerve terminals.

Dopamine-depleting drugs have rarely, if ever, been noted to produce TD. In fact, among 17 patients with TD who were treated with reserpine by Fahn (1985), 4 remitted eventually while taking reserpine and were able to come off all treatment. Reserpine depletes catecholamine stores in sympathetic nerve terminals as well as in the CNS. Side effects include parkinsonism, apathy, depression, lethargy, and orthostatic hypotension. Some patients might require fairly high doses; significant improvement was reported with up to 5–8 mg/day (Sato et al., 1971; Fahn, 1985), whereas others who used lower doses reported less dramatic responses. Reserpine has a slow onset and a prolonged duration of action, and this must be taken into consideration when doses are changed. Once control of dyskinesia has been obtained, the dosage might need readjustment because of delayed onset of the catecholamine-depleting effect of reserpine with the induction of drug-induced parkinsonism. It is usually a question of balancing benefit and this adverse effect. Sixty-four percent of 96 patients in the literature had at least 50% improvement (Jeste and Wyatt, 1982b). One of the most notable results was that of a double-blind placebo-controlled study by Huang and colleagues (1980) that showed 50% improvement on reserpine 0.75–1.5 mg/day. Fahn's long-term study (1985) showed that 13 of 17 patients had moderate to marked benefit on higher doses up to 8 mg/day. Nine of the patients who improved also took alpha-methylparatyrosine. Alpha-methylparatyrosine is a competitive inhibitor of TH, the rate-limiting step in catecholamine synthesis. It is not very effective when used alone, but can be a very powerful antidopaminergic drug when used with other presynaptically acting drugs.

TBZ has a quicker onset and shorter duration of action and has fewer peripheral catecholamine-depleting effects than reserpine. TBZ selectively inhibits vesicular monoamine transporter 2 (VMAT2), which is present in the CNS, whereas reserpine also inhibits VMAT1, found peripherally

Table 19.13 Pharmacology provile of tetrabenazine versus reserpine

Pharmacological property	Tetrabenazine	Reserpine
Mechanism of action	Selectively binds hVMAT2 *Reversibly* binds VMAT2 Binds intravesicular site	Binds hVMAT1 and hVMAT2 *Irreversibly* binds VMAT Binds cytoplasmic site
Peripheral monoamine depletion	No	Yes
Duration of action in humans	Short (approx. 12 hours)	Several days
Hypotension in humans	No	Yes
Gastrointestinal effects in humans	No	Yes

(Table 19.13). Like reserpine, TBZ has not been implicated in causing TD. However, in contrast to reserpine, TBZ does have some dopamine-receptor blocking activity (Reches et al., 1983), which probably accounts for the few reported cases of acute dystonic reaction that have been encountered clinically (Burke et al., 1985). In contrast to reserpine, remission of TD has not been reported during the treatment of TD with TBZ, although it has been seen in one of our patients (Fahn, personal observation). It would seem, therefore, that reserpine has the theoretical advantage of being more likely to allow for a remission of the TD, compared to TBZ. TBZ's major advantage is the quicker onset and fewer side effects compared to reserpine. TBZ is rapidly absorbed after oral administration and extensively metabolized during the first pass through the liver and/or the gut. One of the major metabolites, dihydrotetrabenazine, has pharmacologic actions similar to those of TBZ, although its ability to pass through the blood–brain barrier is unclear. Large individual variations are noted, and patients with hepatic dysfunction might expect alteration of pharmacokinetics (Mehvar et al., 1987). The dose has to be clinically titrated for each patient.

TBZ, clinically available in many countries, is now considered the treatment of choice for TD (Kenney and Jankovic, 2006). Improvement with TBZ was noted in 68% of 38 patients in the literature at a mean daily dose of 138 mg (Jeste and Wyatt, 1982a). Fahn (1985) reported improvement in five of six patients at doses of 75–300 mg/day in a long-term study. Kazamatsuri and colleagues (1972) noted that 54% of patients improved by at least 50% in a 6-week trial of TBZ compared to placebo treatment. Jankovic and Beach (1997) reported that 90% of patients had a marked improvement. Ondo and colleagues (1999) blindly rated videotapes taken of patients before and after TBZ treatment (mean duration of 20 weeks) and showed improvement in their dyskinesias. A major problem with TBZ therapy is with long-duration exposure. Most patients initially improve dramatically; then while maintained on the original dose some begin to develop features of parkinsonism. Lowering the dose reduces this unwanted effect, but the TD then is less well controlled. Both reserpine and TBZ can induce acute akathisia and depression, so one needs to monitor for these adverse effects and treat them if they should occur. In some cases, however, depression actually improves after the introduction of TBZ, possibly as a result of abolishment of the involuntary movements (Kenney et al., 2006). Antidepressants, including monoamine oxidase inhibitors, can be used effectively to treat the depression. The selective norepinephrine reuptake inhibitor reboxetine has been found to rapidly reverse TBZ-induced depression (Schreiber et al., 1999).

Atypical antipsychotics

By definition the atypical antipsychotics have a reduced propensity to induce extrapyramidal adverse effects, tardive dyskinesia included. However, a range of adverse effects are encountered from the variety of drugs that have at one time or another been labeled as atypical neuroleptics. Today, the dibenzodiazepines (clozapine and quetiapine) are strong candidates for this labeling, and the thienobenzodiazepine olanzapine is less so. But originally, the "atypical" label was applied to the benzamine derivatives, such as sulpiride, metoclopramide, and tiapride. However, all three compounds have been reported to induce tardive dyskinesia or NMS (Casey, 1983; Achiron et al., 1990; Miller and Jankovic, 1990; Duarte et al., 1996). Similarly, risperidone has been touted as "atypical," but it more resembles a typical antipsychotic, causing parkinsonism and inducing tardive dyskinesia (Buzan, 1996). The typical antipsychotics, including sulpiride, tiapride, and risperidone, by blocking and occupying dopamine D2 receptors, are effective in reducing the severity of tardive dyskinesia (Chouinard, 1995). But so do even stronger DRBAs, such as phenothiazines and haloperidol. The problem with using typical antipsychotics to treat TD is that they are in the class of the offending drugs and hence will prolong the exposure of the patient to the drugs that cause TD.

The question is whether the true "atypical" antipsychotics, such as clozapine and quetiapine, can reduce the symptoms of TD and still allow the healing process in the brain to proceed to eventually eliminate the pathophysiologic causation of the symptoms. There are reports of clozapine successfully reducing the abnormal movements of tardive dyskinesia and tardive akathisia (Huang et al., 1980; Wirshing et al., 1990; Bassitt and Neto, 1998) and in some patients with tardive dystonia (Lieberman et al., 1989, 1991; Van Putten et al., 1990; Friedman, 1994; Trugman et al., 1994; Wolf and Mosnaim, 1994; Raja et al., 1996; van Harten et al., 1996a; Bassitt and Neto, 1998). But the response rate is lower than that with typical antipsychotics, such as haloperidol. Clozapine permits the dyskinesia to disappear in about half the cases in one report (Gerlach and Peacock, 1994). In another, 8 of the 20 patients with TD improved after an average time of 261 ± 188 days of treatment (Bunker et al., 1996). With an average dose of approximately 400 mg/day, Bassitt and Neto (1998) obtained a 50% lessening of dyskinesia. It is still not clear whether the reduction of dyskinesia is due to the small amount of D2-blocking effect or whether actual healing of the TD can take place in the presence of clozapine.

The proof of the latter and preferred category would be the lack of reappearance when clozapine is withdrawn. There has not been a report of such a case. Without that evidence, it is likely that the reductions of tardive dyskinesia and tardive dystonia are due to the small amount of D2-blocking activity by clozapine.

There is a case report of TD improving on quetiapine 600 mg/day (Vesely et al., 2000). The patient was not withdrawn from the drug. A large randomized study on high-dose quetiapine also found quetiapine to be effective (Emsley et al., 2004), but high dosages of the atypical antipsychotics become typical by blocking D2 receptors, so the reduction of TD can be due solely to further D2 receptor blockade.

The questions that were raised from clozapine apply here as well. Is the reduction of dyskinesias due to its D2-blocking effect that would occur at high doses? If so, then withdrawal of the drug would be associated with a return of the dyskinesias. Is the reduction of dyskinesias due to a natural healing process, as has been demonstrated mainly with reserpine and somewhat with TBZ? If so, then withdrawal of the drug would not be associated with a return of the dyskinesias. The advantage of dopamine depletors, such as reserpine and TBZ, is that they allow symptomatic benefit and still allow the brain to heal spontaneously so withdrawal of medication might be possible some day.

However, clozapine and quetiapine could substitute for a typical antipsychotic in a patient with a tardive syndrome who also has psychosis, thereby controlling the psychosis and possibly still allowing a chance for a complete remission to occur. Such a remission would not take place in the presence of the typical antipsychotic. Like clozapine, quetiapine needs to be tested. Olanzapine has successfully reduced the symptoms of TD (Littrell et al., 1998). But olanzapine is not a true atypical antipsychotic, and the reduction of the symptoms and signs is probably obtained by blockading D2 receptors. This would convey no advantage over using the more classic and conventional typical antipsychotics.

Dopamine agonists

Some investigators have tried to activate the presynaptic dopamine receptors by using low doses of a dopamine agonist, which in turn would reduce the biosynthesis and release of dopamine. Another approach by Alpert and Friedhoff (1980) was the use of levodopa in an attempt to desensitize the postsynaptic dopamine receptors. This can cause initial worsening of symptoms before eventual improvement is expected after discontinuation of levodopa. Unfortunately, dopaminergic drugs can also lead to overt recurrence of underlying psychosis (Fahn, 1983). This approach has theoretical merit, but is very difficult to carry out in many patients and has not been widely used since the initial reports.

Amantadine has been reported to have some benefit (Angus et al., 1997), but it may be due to its glutamate receptor blocking effect rather than its dopaminergic effect.

Nondopaminergic medications

Although neuroleptics are most effective in controlling the abnormal movements, some patients do not respond to the treatment. Numerous investigators (Jeste and Wyatt, 1982b; Jeste et al., 1988) have attempted nondopaminergic treatments. Agents that enhance GABA transmission have been tried because of GABA's inhibitory effect on the dopaminergic system and experimental data indicating changes in the GABA system in patients and animals that have been treated with chronic neuroleptics. Use of benzodiazepines, baclofen, valproate, and γ-vinyl GABA has met with limited success, partly owing to tolerance and side effects such as worsening of psychosis. Some improvement was found with clonazepam (Thaker et al., 1990). Propranolol, fusaric acid, and clonidine decrease the noradrenergic activity and have been reported to be useful but require further study to clarify their role in treating tardive dyskinesia. Use of cholinergic drugs was based on the reciprocal dopamine–acetylcholine balance in the basal ganglia. Despite a flurry of reports in the 1970s, this modality has been quite limited, and should be reconsidered now that some adequate cholinergic drugs are available. Anticholinergics, pyridoxine, tryptophan, cyproheptadine, vasopressin, naloxone, morphine, and estrogen were reported to be of no benefit. But in a controlled clinical trial involving 15 patients, pyridoxine was found to reduce the severity of TD (Lerner et al., 2001). Buspirone has been reported to be beneficial (Moss et al., 1993), but it is not clear that this drug does not have dopamine-receptor blocking activity. Calcium channel blockers have been reported to reduce the severity of tardive dyskinesia (Kushnir and Ratner, 1989; Duncan et al., 1990; Suddath et al., 1991), but not in all studies (Loonen et al., 1992). A combination of acetazolamide and thiamine was found to reduce both TD and drug-induced parkinsonism (Cowen et al., 1997). Lithium not only may decrease the chance of TD development (Kane et al., 1986; van Harten et al., 2008a), but also may reduce its severity if applied as a treatment (van Harten et al., 2008a).

A review of randomized clinical trials was presented by Soares and McGrath (1999) with a meta-analysis when more than one randomized clinical trial had been carried out. Meta-analysis showed that baclofen, deanol, and diazepam were no more effective than a placebo. Single randomized clinical trials demonstrated a lack of evidence of any effect for bromocriptine, ceruletide, clonidine, estrogen, gamma-linolenic acid, hydergine, lecithin, lithium, progabide, selegiline, and tetrahydroisoxazolopyridinol. Meta-analysis found that five interventions were effective: levodopa, oxypertine, sodium valproate, tiapride and vitamin E; neuroleptic reduction was marginally significant. Vitamin E is more thoroughly discussed in the next paragraph. Data from single randomized clinical trials revealed that insulin, α-methyldopa, and reserpine were more effective than a placebo. Meta-analysis found that 37.3% of placebo-treated subjects improved.

A role for antioxidants has been raised (Cadet and Lohr, 1989; Behl et al., 1995). Treatment with vitamin E has been found to reduce the severity of tardive dyskinesia (Elkashef et al., 1990; Dabiri et al., 1994; Adler et al., 1998; Sajjad, 1998) or have no effect (Lam et al., 1994). The meta-analysis mentioned earlier showed effectiveness. A small clinical trial of 41 subjects comparing 1200 IU/day of vitamin E and placebo found the former to better reduce severity of abnormal involuntary movements (45.9% vs. 4.3%) (Zhang et al., 2004). However, the largest double-blind study, carried out by the Veterans Administration multicenter, a placebo-controlled clinical trial (Adler et al., 1999), found vitamin E not to be effective. As a potential prophylactic agent, vitamin E (3200 IU/day) was found not to protect against development of drug-induced parkinsonism (Eranti et al., 1998). Nor was vitamin E treatment able to prevent neuroleptic-induced VCMs in rats (Sachdev et al., 1999). In a small open-label trial combining vitamins E and C, improvement in TD was seen (Michael et al., 2003).

There continue to be reports of TD responding to open-label trials. Gabapentin (Hardoy et al., 1999, 2003), pyridoxine (Lerner et al., 1999), and branched-chain amino acids (Richardson et al., 2003) are such compounds. Levetiracetam was helpful in a small trial (Konitsiotis et al., 2006).

Injections of botulinum toxin into the muscles causing oral dyskinesia have been reported to be effective in reducing the movements (Rapaport et al., 2000). This includes tongue protrusion, which has been successfully treated with injections into the genioglossal portion of the tongue (van Harten and Hovestadt, 2006).

Sporadic reports noted efficacy of electroconvulsive therapy in refractory cases of TD (Price and Levin, 1978), but Yassa and colleagues (1990) reported success in only one of nine patients.

Conclusions on classic tardive dyskinesia

By blocking D2 receptors or depleting dopamine from synaptic terminals, neuroleptics are effective in reducing the abnormal involuntary movements of TD. Depletors do not cause TD and are therefore preferred; their use, while controlling symptoms, allows the brain to heal spontaneously. Avoiding side effects, particularly drug-induced parkinsonism, is a major limiting factor. DRBAs, while controlling symptoms, are the culprits causing TD; the brain does not heal, and TD may continue to worsen in the presence of these agents. If one needs to utilize an antipsychotic, it seems safer to use one that is suspected of having less ability to induce TD, such as clozapine and quetiapine. Olanzapine comes closer to being a typical, rather than an atypical, antipsychotic. When clozapine and quetiapine occasionally reduce dyskinesias, the doses that are used suggest the response is from their D2-blocking activity.

Figures 19.1 and 19.2 are flow charts that provide a useful algorithm for treating TD.

Tardive dystonia

As with classic TD, the most effective medications for tardive dystonia are also antidopaminergic drugs (Kang et al., 1986), but the percentage of patients who improve is smaller. Reserpine and TBZ each produce improvement in about 50% of patients. Some patients who do not respond or have intolerable side effects to one might respond to the other. DRBAs are more effective in suppressing the movements (77%). Symptomatically, those who remained on DRBAs after the onset of tardive dystonia and those who were withdrawn from them do not have a significant difference in their improvement rate. This again is in agreement with the data in classic tardive dyskinesia, in which continued use of DRBAs does not necessarily lead to aggravation of their movements (Casey et al., 1986; Gardos et al., 1988). The atypical antipsychotic clozapine has been helpful in some patients with tardive dystonia (Lieberman et al., 1989, 1991;

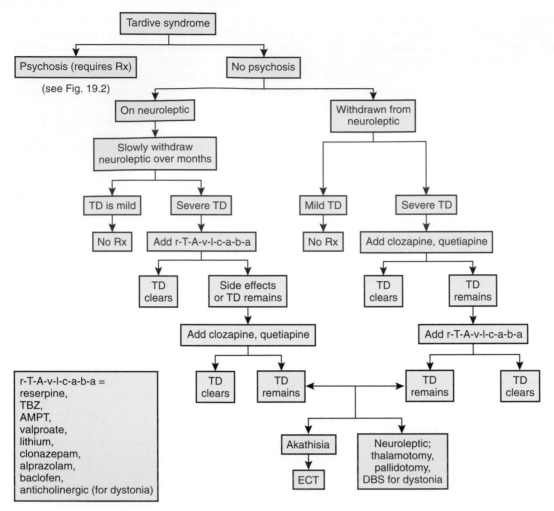

Figure 19.1 Flowchart for treating tardive dyskinesia in the absence of psychosis. AMPT, α-methyl-para-tyrosine; DBS, deep brain stimulation; ECT, electroconvulsive therapy; TBZ, tetrabenazine.

Van Putten et al., 1990; Friedman, 1994; Trugman et al., 1994; Wolf and Mosnaim, 1994; Raja et al., 1996; van Harten et al., 1996a). There are reports of quetiapine's effectiveness as well (Gourzis et al., 2005). It is likely that its treatment of tardive dystonia in some situations is due to its D2 receptor-blocking activity resulting in a masking of the symptoms, because withdrawal would exacerbate the dystonia (Krack et al., 1994). The combination of clozapine and clonazepam has been effective in some patients when either drug alone was much less satisfactory (Shapleske et al., 1996).

In tardive dystonia, antimuscarinics are almost as effective as antidopaminergic drugs. This is different from classic tardive dyskinesia, which may get worse with antimuscarinics (Yassa, 1988). Kang and colleagues (1986) reported a 46% improvement rate on antimuscarinics such as trihexyphenidyl and ethopropazine. CNS side effects of the antimuscarinics include forgetfulness, lethargy, psychosis, dysphoria, and personality changes; elderly patients are more susceptible to these. Peripheral side effects include blurred vision, dry mouth, constipation, urinary retention, and orthostatic dizziness. Those who develop side effects to one anticholinergic drug may tolerate another anticholinergic better. Although there is no evidence that one anticholinergic is

more efficacious than the others, ethopropazine may produce fewer CNS side effects in elderly patients. Although peripheral pharmacokinetics show relatively short half-lives, their central effects have a very slow onset of action and several weeks are often required before benefit is noticed. Therefore, the medications are started at a low dose, 2.5 mg of trihexyphenidyl or 25 mg of ethopropazine, and increased slowly by 2.5 mg of trihexyphenidyl or 25 mg of ethopropazine weekly until sufficient control of dystonia or intolerable side effects are achieved. As in idiopathic dystonia, many patients respond only to a high dose of anticholinergics. Therefore, every attempt must be made to control side effects so that high-dose anticholinergics may be tried. Kang and colleagues (1986) reported use of a maximum of 450 mg ethopropazine or 32 mg of trihexyphenidyl, and higher doses may be tolerated in young patients if judiciously used. Peripheral side effects are often controlled by peripheral cholinergic drugs, such as oral pyridostigmine and pilocarpine eye drops.

The clinical pharmacology of tardive dystonia indicates two subtypes: one group that responds to antidopaminergic drugs like the other tardive syndromes and one that responds to anticholinergics like idiopathic dystonia. Analysis of clinical characteristics of patients who respond to

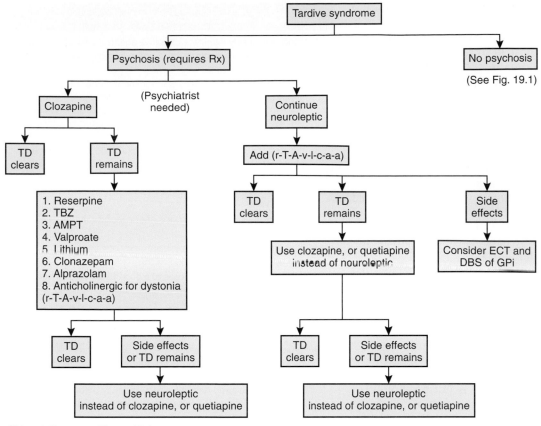

Figure 19.2 Flowchart for treating tardive syndromes in the presence of psychosis.

Flowchart content:

Tardive syndrome
- Psychosis (requires Rx) (Psychiatrist needed)
  - Clozapine
    - TD clears
    - TD remains
      1. Reserpine
      2. TBZ
      3. AMPT
      4. Valproate
      5. Lithium
      6. Clonazepam
      7. Alprazolam
      8. Anticholinergic for dystonia (r-T-A-v-l-c-a-a)
         - TD clears
         - Side effects or TD remains
           - Use neuroleptic instead of clozapine, or quetiapine
  - Continue neuroleptic
    - Add (r-T-A-v-l-c-a-a)
      - TD clears
      - TD remains
        - Use clozapine, or quetiapine instead of neuroleptic
          - TD clears
          - Side effects or TD remains
            - Use neuroleptic instead of clozapine, or quetiapine
      - Side effects
        - Consider ECT and DBS of GPi
- No psychosis (See Fig. 19.1)

Abbreviations, see Figure 19.1

antidopaminergic drugs and those who respond to anticholinergic drugs has not shown any significant difference (Kang et al., 1986). However, the data from Kang and colleagues (1986) are retrospective and the treatment choice between the two classes of drugs was rather arbitrary, partly based on anticipated side effects. For example, patients who were elderly or who had dementia were treated with dopamine-depleting drugs first, because these patients have greater risk for anticholinergic side effects such as memory loss and confusion. Patients with depression might have relapse of their symptoms on dopamine-depleting drugs and were treated preferentially with anticholinergics. This is a reasonable clinical approach, but characterization of subtypes will require a controlled study with random assignment of the treatment. If either a dopamine depletor or antimuscarinic is ineffective by itself, the combination should be tried.

Benzodiazepines are mainly helpful as adjunctive therapy with dopamine-depleting or anticholinergic drugs, and occasionally can be quite beneficial (Yamamoto et al., 2007). Minimal success with propranolol, levodopa, carbamazepine, and baclofen has been noted. Bromocriptine, deanol, clonidine, lisuride, amantadine, and valproate were reported with mixed results. The calcium channel blocker verapamil was reported to be effective in one patient (Abad and Ovsiew, 1993). Opioids do not have lasting value in suppressing tardive dystonia (Berg et al., 2001). But one study found the combination of naltrexone and clonazepam to offer some benefit (Wonodi et al., 2004b).

If any residual dystonia remains that is localized to one or a few parts of the body, injections of botulinum toxin into the affected parts, such as the orbicularis oculi, masseters, or cervical muscles, might be useful (Chatterjee et al., 1997; Tarsy et al., 1997; Kanovsky et al., 1999).

Electroconvulsive therapy (ECT) might be effective in intractable cases (Yoshida et al., 1996), and deep brain stimulation in the globus pallidus interna is often effective (Franzini et al., 2005; Sako et al., 2008; Gruber et al., 2009), as is intrathecal baclofen (Dressler et al., 1997). Surgery is not always effective and it does pose risks of complications (Trottenberg et al., 2001). However, deep brain stimulation in the pallidum can be safe and effective (Capelle et al., 2010; Chang et al., 2010); it is worth considering when medications fail.

A centrally acting muscle relaxant, eperisone, was successful in treating one patient with tardive dystonia (Nisijima et al., 1998). Eperisone is a beta-aminopropiophenone derivative.

Figures 19.1 and 19.2 depict flowcharts for therapy that can be applied to tardive dystonia, as well as to classic TD.

Tardive akathisia

As was noted earlier, variants of akathisia have been the source of confusion in the literature. Most of the papers do not distinguish between acute and tardive akathisia or usually refer to acute akathisia and not tardive akathisia.

Very few studies have focused on the treatment of tardive akathisia.

Tardive akathisia is difficult to treat and does not respond to anticholinergics, which have been reported to help acute akathisia. It and tardive dystonia are the most distressing and disabling features of the tardive symptoms, and their treatment is important. In the study of tardive akathisia by Burke et al. (1989), all of the patients noted that the subjective sensations were distressing. The same study reported that 87% of patients improved on reserpine up to 5 mg/day and 58% on TBZ up to 175 mg/day. In one-third of these patients, the movements were completely suppressed. In this respect the clinical pharmacology is more like that of classic tardive dyskinesia than that of acute akathisia. Opioids were reported to be beneficial (Walters et al., 1986), but the effect has not been persistent (Burke et al., 1989). Electroconvulsive treatment can be effective in those patients whose akathisia has proved to be intractable (Hermesh et al., 1992).

Figures 19.1 and 19.2 depict flowcharts on therapy that can also be applied to tardive akathisia.

Treatment summary

Table 19.14 summarizes a useful approach to treat tardive syndromes in general. The approach to treatment should be earmarked according to whether the patient is psychotic and requires antipsychotic medication, or is not psychotic. For detailed, step-by-step decisions in the treatment of the tardive syndromes, the flowcharts of Figures 19.1 and 19.2 should be helpful.

In summary, since the initial description of tardive dyskinesia as an iatrogenic complication of dopamine receptor antagonists, considerable progress has been made in understanding the risks, epidemiology, and clinical subtypes of the condition. However, pathogenesis and characteristics of distinct subtypes are still poorly understood. Management of tardive syndromes must be based on proper understanding of these aspects of the disorder. The only effective and safe antipsychotic agents that do not produce, or rarely produce, tardive dyskinesia appear to be clozapine and quetiapine. Meanwhile, prevention is possible by avoiding indiscriminate use of DRBAs and limiting their use to disorders for which no other type of medication is available or effective. When prevention and withdrawal of the offending drugs for

eventual remission fail, symptomatic suppression can be achieved in many patients with pharmacologic treatments. New approaches are needed, and prospective controlled clinical trials with particular attention to clinical subtypes are necessary for better management of these conditions.

References available on Expert Consult: www.expertconsult.com

Table 19.14 Treatment for tardive dyskinesia syndromes

1. Taper and slowly eliminate causative agents if clinically possible. Avoid sudden cessation of these drugs, which could exacerbate the tardive syndrome.
2. Avoid drugs, if possible (i.e., wait for spontaneous recovery). This is possible only if the dyskinesia is not severe or there is no accompanying tardive akathisia or tardive dystonia. Akathisia and dystonia are more distressing and disabling than classic tardive dyskinesia (TD).
3. If necessary to treat the symptoms, first use dopame-depleting drugs: tetrabenazine (TBZ), reserpine, α-methylparatyrosine. Attempt to overcome the adverse effects of depression and parkinsonism with antidepressants and antiparkinsonism drugs, respectively.
4. Consider melatonin on the basis of one report (Shamir et al., 2001).
5. Next, consider the true atypical antipsychotic agents, clozapine and quetiapine.
6. If these fail, consider tiny doses of a dopamine receptor agonist to activate only the presynaptic dopamine receptor and reduce the biosynthesis of dopamine.
7. For tardive dystonia, consider antimuscarinics.
8. For intractable tardive akathisia, consider ECT.
9. Typical antipsychotic agents can be used to control the dyskinesias when all previously mentioned approaches fail. Combining this with a dopamine depletor may increase the potency of the antidyskinetic effect, and may theoretically protect against a worsening of the underlying tardive pathology.
10. Thalamotomy, pallidotomy, and deep brain stimulation of the thalamus and pallidum have been performed for tardive dystonia with success. Deep brain stimulation of the pallidum appears to be the preferred surgical procedure if the symptoms remain severe and all medication trials fail.

CHAPTER **20**

Myoclonus
Phenomenology, etiology, physiology, and treatment

Chapter contents

Classification of myoclonus	447	Axial myoclonus	454
Neurophysiologic assessment	448	Multifocal and generalized cortical myoclonus	456
Making the diagnosis	450	Drug treatment of generalized or multifocal myoclonus	462
Focal myoclonus	450		

Literally, myoclonus means "a quick movement of muscle." Sudden, brief jerks may be caused not only by active muscle contractions, positive myoclonus, but also by sudden, brief lapses of muscle contraction in active postural muscles, negative myoclonus or asterixis (Shibasaki, 1995).

The history of myoclonus has been described by Marsden and colleagues (1982), Hallett (1986), and Fahn (2002). Friedreich first defined myoclonus as a discrete entity in a case report published in 1881 of a patient with essential myoclonus. He wanted to separate the involuntary movement that he saw from epileptic clonus, a single jerk in patients with epilepsy, and chorea, which was the only previously described type of involuntary movement. For the next 10–20 years, many other types of involuntary movements, such as tic and myokymia, were also called myoclonus, but in 1903 Lundborg proposed a classification of myoclonus that cleared up much of the confusion. Lundborg classified myoclonus into three groups: symptomatic myoclonus, essential myoclonus, and familial myoclonic epilepsy.

Myoclonus is distinguished from tics because the latter can be controlled by an effort of will, at least temporarily, whereas myoclonus cannot. In addition, many tics are complex movements which are accompanied by a conscious urge to move and by relief of tension after the tic has occurred. Many of the individual movements of chorea may be myoclonic jerks, but in chorea, the movements continue in a constant flow, randomly distributed over the body and randomly distributed in time. Many patients with dystonia have brief muscle spasms, sometimes repetitively (myoclonic dystonia), but these drive the body part into distinctive dystonic postures. Sometimes, myoclonic jerks may be rhythmic, giving a superficial impression of tremor.

Myoclonus is a common movement disorder. Caviness and Maraganore (Caviness et al., 1999) reviewed the record linkage system for Olmsted County at the Mayo Clinic,

Rochester, Minnesota for the years 1976–1990 and found an average annual incidence of myoclonus of 1.3 cases per 100 000, and a prevalence in 1990 of 8.6 cases per 100 000.

Classification of myoclonus

Myoclonus can be classified on the basis of its clinical characteristics, its pathophysiology, or its cause (Table 20.1) (Marsden et al., 1982; Hallett et al., 1987; Fahn, 2002).

Clinical features

The whole body or most of it may be affected in a single jerk (generalized myoclonus). Many different parts of the body may be affected, not necessarily at the same time (multifocal myoclonus); or myoclonus may be confined to one particular region of the body (focal or segmental myoclonus) (Video 20.1). Myoclonic jerks may occur repetitively and rhythmically, or irregularly. They may be evident at rest, on maintaining a posture, or on movement (action myoclonus). Jerks may be triggered by external stimuli (reflex myoclonus), which can be visual, auditory, or somesthetic (touch, pinprick, muscle stretch) (Video 20.2).

Pathophysiology

The clinical features of myoclonus and the results of electrophysiologic investigation allow a relatively precise prediction as to its site of origin in the nervous system (Shibasaki and Hallett, 2005; Hallett and Shibasaki, 2008). On this basis, myoclonus may be shown to arise in the cerebral cortex (cortical myoclonus); in the brainstem (brainstem myoclonus); or in the spinal cord (spinal myoclonus). Rarely,

© 2011 Elsevier Ltd, Inc, BV

DOI: 10.1016/B978-1-4377-2369-4.00020-2

Table 20.1 Classification schemes for myoclonus

Clinical	Pathophysiology	Etiology
Spontaneous	Cortical	Physiological
Action	Focal	Essential
Reflex	Multifocal	Epileptic
Focal	Generalized	Symptomatic
Axial	Epilepsia partialis	Storage diseases
Multifocal	continua	Cerebellar degenerations
Generalized	Thalamic	Basal ganglia
Irregular	Brainstem	degenerations
Repetitive	Reticular	Dementias
Rhythmic	Startle	Viral encephalopathies
	Palatal	Metabolic
	Spinal	encephalopathies
	Segmental	Toxic encephalopathies
	Propriospinal	Hypoxia
	Peripheral	Focal damage
	Ballistic	

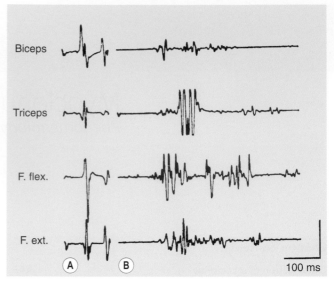

Figure 20.1 EMG patterns underlying two types of myoclonus. **A** is from a patient with post-hypoxic myoclonus, and **B** is from a patient with a type of essential myoclonus (ballistic movement overflow myoclonus). The time scale is the same for both; vertical calibration is 1 mV for **A** and 0.5 mV for **B**. In **A**, the EMG burst is very short and synchronous in antagonist muscles, while in **B**, the EMG bursts are longer and asynchronous. *From Chadwick D, Hallett M, Harris R, et al. Clinical, biochemical, and physiological features distinguishing myoclonus responsive to 5-hydroxytryptophan, tryptophan with a monoamine oxidase inhibitor, and clonazepam. Brain 1977;100(3):455–487, with permission.*

lesions of spinal roots, nerve plexi, or peripheral nerves can cause myoclonus (peripheral myoclonus). Hemifacial spasm might be considered a form of peripheral myoclonus, due most often to neurovascular compression.

Cortical myoclonus, in which the abnormal activity originates in the sensorimotor cortex and is transmitted down the spinal cord in pyramidal pathways, may manifest as focal jerks, sometimes repetitive (epilepsia partialis continua), which can propagate into focal motor seizures; with or without secondary generalization (Hallett et al., 1979; Shibasaki and Hallett, 2005; Hallett and Shibasaki, 2008).

Myoclonus arising in the *brainstem* may take different forms (Hallett, 2002). One employs the pathways responsible for the startle reflex, causing exaggerated startle syndromes and the hyperekplexias. Another is independent of startle mechanisms, but causes generalized muscle jerks (brainstem reticular myoclonus). A third is the palatal myoclonus (tremor) syndrome.

In the *spinal cord*, two forms of myoclonus are now recognized; spinal segmental myoclonus affects a restricted body part, involving a few spinal segments; propriospinal myoclonus produces generalized axial jerks, usually beginning in the abdominal muscles. Rarely, local lesions of peripheral nerves, the plexi, or nerve roots may produce segmental myoclonus.

Finally, one pathophysiologic type of *essential myoclonus* takes the form of spontaneous or action-induced ballistic electromyographic (EMG) bursts in muscles, with inappropriate overflow into other muscles (ballistic movement overflow myoclonus) (Hallett et al., 1977b).

Cause

With regard to etiology, so many neurologic conditions may produce myoclonus that such a classification runs to a textbook of neurology (Table 20.2) (Marsden et al., 1982; Hallett et al., 1987; Fahn, 2002; Hallett and Shibasaki, 2008). It is, however, useful to consider several broad categories.

Physiologic myoclonus refers to muscle jerks occurring in certain circumstances in normal subjects. These include sleep jerks (hypnic jerks) and hiccup. Essential myoclonus consists of multifocal myoclonus in which there is no other neurologic deficit or abnormality on investigation. Epileptic myoclonus refers to conditions in which the major clinical problem is one of epilepsy, but one of the manifestations of the epileptic attacks is myoclonic jerks. Symptomatic generalized myoclonus refers to those many conditions in which generalized or multifocal muscle jerking is a manifestation of an underlying identifiable neurologic disease. Psychogenic myoclonus refers to myoclonus produced as a conversion symptom or as "voluntary" or "simulated" myoclonus (Thompson et al., 1992; Monday and Jankovic, 1993).

In the survey by Caviness et al. (1999), symptomatic myoclonus was most common, followed by epileptic myoclonus and essential myoclonus. Dementing illnesses were the commonest cause of symptomatic myoclonus.

Neurophysiologic assessment

Polymyography (recording the duration, distribution, and stimulus sensitivity of EMG activity in affected muscles) is the first step in assessing a patient with myoclonus (Toro and Hallett, 2004; Shibasaki and Hallett, 2005; Hallett and Shibasaki, 2008). Most myoclonic jerks are due to brief EMG bursts of 10–50 ms. EMG bursts in the 100 ms range are seen in some situations such as essential myoclonus. Longer jerks of more than 100 ms are likely to be dystonic. Agonists and antagonists usually fire synchronously (Fig. 20.1).

Table 20.2 Etiologic classification of myoclonus

I. Physiological myoclonus (normal subjects)

A. Sleep jerks (hypnic jerks)
B. Anxiety-induced
C. Exercise-induced
D. Hiccup (singultus)
E. Benign infantile myoclonus with feeding

II. Essential myoclonus (no known cause other than genetic and no other gross neurologic deficit)

A. Hereditary (autosomal dominant)
B. Sporadic

III. Epileptic myoclonus (seizures dominate and no encephalopathy, at least initially)

A. Fragments of epilepsy
    Isolated epileptic myoclonic jerks
    Photosensitive myoclonus
    Myoclonic absences in petit mal
    Epilepsia partialis continua
B. Childhood myoclonic epilepsies
    Infantile spasms
    Myoclonic astatic epilepsy (Lennox–Gastaut)
    Cryptogenic myoclonus epilepsy (Aicardi)
    Juvenile myoclonus epilepsy of Janz
C. Benign familial myoclonic epilepsy (Rabot)
D. Progressive myoclonus epilepsy (Unverricht–Lundborg)

IV. Symptomatic myoclonus (progressive or static encephalopathy dominates)

A. Storage disease
    Lafora body disease
    Lipidoses, e.g., GM1 and GM2 gangliosidosis, Krabbe
    Ceroid-lipofuscinosis (Batten)
    Sialidosis ("cherry-red spot")
B. Spinocerebellar degeneration
    Unverricht–Lundborg disease
    Ataxia telangiectasia
    Adult-onset cerebellar ataxias
        Autosomal dominant cerebellar ataxia (ADCA) type I
        Sporadic olivopontocerebellar atrophy (OPCA)
    Celiac disease
C. Basal ganglia degenerations
    Wilson disease
    Dystonia
    Pantothenate kinase-associated neurodegeneration
    Progressive supranuclear palsy
    Multiple system atrophy
    Huntington disease
    Corticobasal ganglionic degeneration
    Dentatorubro-pallidoluysian atrophy
    Parkinson disease
D. Dementias
    Creutzfeldt–Jakob disease
    Alzheimer disease
E. Viral encephalopathies
    Subacute sclerosing panencephalitis (SSPE)
    Encephalitis lethargica
    Arbor virus encephalitis
    Herpes simplex encephalitis
    Postinfectious encephalitis
    Opsoclonus–myoclonus syndrome
    Whipple disease
    AIDS
F. Metabolic
    Hepatic failure
    Renal failure
    Dialysis syndrome
    Hyponatremia
    Hypoglycemia
    Infantile myoclonic encephalopathy
    Nonketotic hyperglycemia
    Mitochondrial encephalomyopathy
    Multiple carboxylase deficiency
    Biotin deficiency
G. Toxic encephalopathies
    Bismuth
    Heavy-metal poisons
    Methyl bromide, DDT
    Drugs, including levodopa
    Serotonin syndrome (e.g., SSRIs)
H. Physical encephalopathies
    Post-hypoxic (Lance–Adams)
    Post-traumatic
    Heat stroke
    Electric shock
    Decompression injury
I. Focal CNS damage
    Post-stroke
    Post-thalamotomy
    Tumor
    Trauma
    Dentato-olivary lesions (palatal myoclonus/tremor)

The distribution of muscles involved may suggest that it arises as a result of a lesion of a peripheral nerve, part of a plexus, a spinal root or a restricted number of segments of the spinal cord (*segmental myoclonus*). Myoclonic muscle jerks affecting axial muscles (neck, shoulders, trunk, and hips) may arise in the brainstem as an exaggerated startle response or brainstem reticular myoclonus, or in the spinal cord as propriospinal myoclonus. In *brainstem myoclonus*, there is no preceding cortical discharge. Cranial nerve muscles are usually activated from the XI nucleus up the brainstem; limb and axial muscles are activated in descending order. In *propriospinal myoclonus*, the first muscles activated are usually in the thoracic cord, with slow upward and downward spread. *Cortical myoclonus* is indicated when somatosensory evoked potentials produced by peripheral nerve stimulation are pathologically enlarged, and a cortical correlate can be back-averaged in the ongoing EEG by triggering from the EMG of the muscle jerk (Hallett et al., 1979;

Shibasaki and Hallett, 2005). Stimuli generating giant somatosensory evoked potentials often provoke a subsequent EMG burst of myoclonic activity (the C reflex), at a latency compatible with conduction through fast corticomotoneuron pathways from the motor cortex to muscle. The giant somatosensory evoked potentials usually consist of an enlarged P_{25}/N_{33} component; the first major cortical negative peak (N_{20}), reflecting arrival of the sensory volley in the cortex, usually is of normal size. The motor volleys in cortical myoclonus activate the cranial and limb musculature in descending order via fast conducting corticospinal pathways. Abnormal corticomuscular and intermuscular coupling can also be a sensitive physiologic feature in cortical myoclonus (Grosse et al., 2003). The increased cortical excitability in cortical myoclonus may well be due to loss of inhibitory interneurons (Hanajima et al., 2008). Cortical reflex myoclonus usually consists of positive EMG discharges, but negative cortical reflex myoclonus also occurs (Shibasaki, 1995; Tassinari et al., 1998), where a giant somatosensory cortical potential is time-locked to EMG silence. *Subcortical myoclonus* is suggested when reflex myoclonus triggered by peripheral stimuli occurs after a latency that is too short to involve cortical pathways (Thompson et al., 1994; Cantello et al., 1997).

Psychogenic myoclonus is suggested if stimulus-evoked jerks are of very variable latency and longer than a voluntary reaction time (Thompson et al., 1992; Brown, 2006), and when the Bereitschaftspotential is evident prior to EMG bursts on jerk-locked back-averaging of the EEG, as in voluntary movement (Terada et al., 1995). Monday and Jankovic (1993) reported the clinical features of 18 such patients. There were 13 women and 5 men with an age range of 22–75 years. The myoclonus was present for 1–110 months; and it was segmental in 10, generalized in 7, and focal in 1. Stress precipitated or exacerbated the myoclonic movements in 15 patients; 14 had a definite increase in myoclonic activity during periods of anxiety. The following findings helped to establish the psychogenic nature of the myoclonus: clinical features incongruous with "organic" myoclonus, evidence of underlying psychopathology, an improvement with distraction or placebo, and the presence of incongruous sensory loss or false weakness. Over half of all patients with adequate follow-up improved after gaining insight into the psychogenic mechanisms of their movement disorder.

Making the diagnosis

It is convenient to consider myoclonus according to its clinical distribution, for this is how neurologists first assess the patient. Thus, we will first describe focal myoclonus restricted to one body part, for example, a limb or brainstem-innervated muscles. Then we will describe axial (neck, trunk, and proximal limb muscles) myoclonus, followed by generalized multifocal myoclonus.

Focal myoclonus

Jerking of one body part may arise anywhere from the peripheral nerve to the motor cortex (Table 20.3). With peripheral nerve lesions, the myoclonus may well arise

Table 20.3 Causes of focal myoclonus

Category	Source	Etiology
Peripheral lesions	Peripheral nerve Plexus Nerve roots	Trauma Tumor Electrical injury Surgery Hemifacial spasm
Spinal lesions	(a) Spinal segmental myoclonus	Trauma Inflammation Infection Demyelination Tumor Arteriovenous malformation Ischemic myelopathy Spondylitic myelopathy Spinal anesthesia Idiopathic
	(b) Propriospinal myoclonus	Trauma Tumor Idiopathic
Brainstem lesions	Palatal myoclonus	See Table 20.5
Cortical lesions	Sensorimotor cortex	See Table 20.6
Idiopathic		

because of secondary central nervous system changes (Shin et al., 2007). Another possibility is that there is a peripheral ectopic generator that triggers the myoclonus (Tyvaert et al., 2009). Spontaneous rhythmic focal myoclonus is likely to be *epilepsia partialis continua* or *spinal segmental myoclonus*. Stimulus-sensitive myoclonus, particularly affecting the distal limbs, is most likely to arise in the cerebral cortex. Polymyography, somatosensory evoked potentials, and back-averaging from spontaneous jerks will usually suffice to define the site of origin.

A variety of lesions of the peripheral nerve and spinal cord have been described as causing focal myoclonus (Frenken et al., 1976; Jankovic and Pardo, 1986; Massimi et al., 2009). These include peripheral nerve tumors, trauma or radiation, and spinal cord trauma, tumor, vascular lesions, multiple sclerosis and other inflammatory myelitis. Such spinal segmental myoclonus characteristically is rhythmic (0.5–3 Hz), is confined to muscles innervated by a few spinal segments, and persists during sleep (Fig. 20.2 and Video 20.3). Spinal segmental myoclonus appears to be due to loss of inhibitory interneurons in the posterior horns, which may be demonstrated physiologically (Di Lazzaro et al., 1996). As a result, there is spontaneous bursting of groups of anterior horn cells. Usually it is not stimulus-sensitive, but it can be (Davis et al., 1981). Clonazepam is most likely to help. One case was responsive to topiramate (Siniscalchi et al., 2004). 📹

Palatal myoclonus (alternately referred to as palatal tremor) describes the syndrome of rhythmic palatal movements at about 1.5–3 Hz, sometimes synchronously

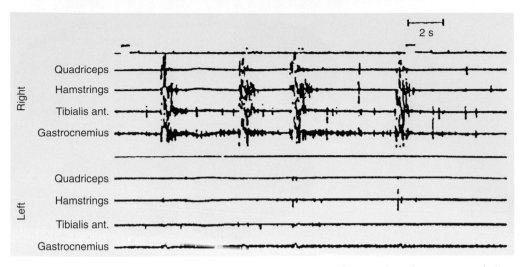

Figure 20.2 Spinal segmental myoclonus. Myoclonic jerking of right leg: surface recording of EMG activity in both legs. This 75 year-old man developed involuntary jerking of the right leg 8 days prior to investigation. He had an abdominal aortic aneurysm, and died 3 months later. Autopsy showed ischemic loss of interneurons in the thoracolumbar cord. *From Davis SM, Murray NM, Diengdoh JV, et al. Stimulus-sensitive spinal myoclonus. J Neurol Neurosurg Psychiatry 1981;44(10):884–888, with permission.*

affecting the eyes, face, tongue and larynx, and even the head, trunk, intercostal muscles and diaphragm (Deuschl et al., 1990, 1994a, 1994b). The movements usually are bilateral and symmetric, occurring between 100 and 150 times per minute, and, in some circumstances, persist during sleep. There are two forms, essential palatal myoclonus and symptomatic palatal myoclonus (Table 20.4 and Video 20.4). The main symptom caused by these movements, seen only in the essential form, is clicking in the ear due to rhythmic contractions of tensor veli palatini which opens the eustachian tube. The tensor veli palatini is innervated by the trigeminal nerve.

In many cases, a focal brainstem lesion can be identified (symptomatic palatal myoclonus/tremor), usually a stroke, encephalitis, multiple sclerosis, tumor, trauma, or degenerative disease (Table 20.5). Often the palatal myoclonus appears some months after the acute lesion. Such patients will have symptoms appropriate to the brainstem damage and to the underlying cause, in addition to the palatal myoclonus. They also may have pendular vertical nystagmus (ocular myoclonus), as well as facial, intercostal, and diaphragmatic jerks in synchrony with the palatal myoclonus. The pathology in symptomatic palatal myoclonus damages the dentato-olivary pathway, often in the brainstem central tegmental tract (Fig. 20.3); the resulting denervation of the inferior olive leads to hypertrophy (Fig. 20.4), which can be seen on brain MRI (Deuschl et al., 1994b). In this situation, the palatal movement is due to contractions of the levator veli palatini (innervated by the nucleus ambiguus). Only rarely can the ear clicking be caused by spontaneous contractions of the levator veli palatini (Jamieson et al., 1996).

In other cases, no cause is evident (essential palatal myoclonus/tremor). The complaint of these patients is the clicking; the eye and other structures are not involved; and there are no other symptoms or signs. These patients tend to be younger and do not appear to develop other diseases. Clonazepam, anticholinergics, or carbamazepine may help some patients with palatal myoclonus (Sakai and Murakami, 1981; Jabbari et al., 1987). Sumatriptan can be

Table 20.4 Differences between essential and symptomatic palatal myoclonus

Essential palatal myoclonus

Ear click

Tensor veli palatini muscle (CN5): elevates the roof of the soft palate and opens eustachian tube

Stops during sleep

Hypertrophy of the inferior olive is NOT found

Symptomatic palatal myoclonus

Levator veli palatini muscle (CN7 or CN9): lifts and pulls back the soft palate

May be accompanied by synchronous activity of adjacent muscles

Continues during sleep

Exerts remote effect on limb muscles

Associated with ipsilateral cerebellar dysfunction

Contralateral hypertrophy of inferior olive

Table 20.5 Causes of palatal myoclonus in 287 patients

Condition	Number
(A) Primary (essential) palatal myoclonus	77
(B) Secondary (symptomatic) palatal myoclonus	210
1. Vascular disease	115
2. Trauma	23
3. Tumor (brainstem)	19
4. Multiple sclerosis	9
5. Degenerations	7
6. Encephalitis	5
7. Other; e.g., arteriovenous malformation, herpes zoster	32

From Deuschl G, Mischke G, Schenck E, Schulte-Monting J, Lucking CH. Symptomatic and essential rhythmic palatal myoclonus. Brain 1990;113(Pt 6): 1645–1672.

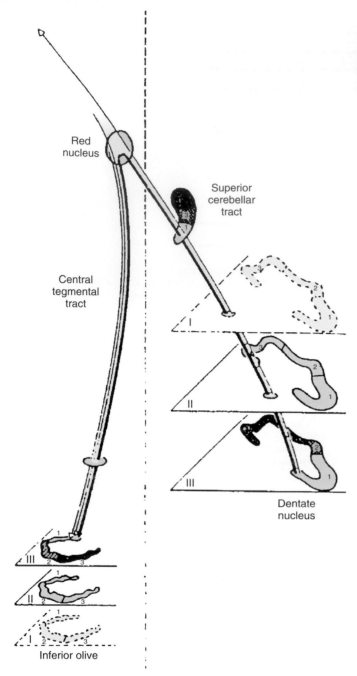

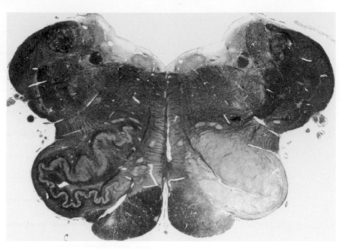

Figure 20.4 Unilateral hypertrophy of the inferior olive in a patient with unilateral symptomatic palatal myoclonus. *From Deuschl G, Toro C, Valls-Solé J, et al. Symptomatic and essential palatal tremor. 1. Clinical, physiological, and MRI analysis. Brain 1994;117:775–88, with permission.*

Figure 20.3 Palatal myoclonus. Dentato-olivary somatotopic relationships in humans are crossed in both horizontal and vertical planes; somatotopic relationships between the dentate nucleus and homolateral superior cerebellar peduncle are direct. The dentato-olivary pathway (continuous dark line) passes from the dentate nucleus through the superior cerebellar peduncle and joins the contralateral central tegmental tract on its way to the inferior olive; in the red nucleus region, this pathway (broken line) passes by the internal and dorsal surfaces of this structure. *Modified from Lapresle J. Palatal myoclonus. Adv Neurol. 1986;43:265–273, with permission.*

effective (Scott et al., 1996), but not in patients with symptomatic palatal myoclonus. Ear clicking can be relieved by injection of botulinum toxin into the appropriate muscles (Deuschl et al., 1991; Jamieson et al., 1996). Ear clicking occasionally may be due to simple partial seizures (Ebner and Noachtar, 1995). Some of these patients may be psychogenic (Pirio Richardson et al., 2006).

Cortical myoclonus produces spontaneous muscle jerks (spontaneous cortical myoclonus), jerks triggered by external stimuli (cortical reflex myoclonus), or jerks on movement (cortical action myoclonus) (Hallett et al., 1979; Obeso et al., 1985). Such patients have neurophysiologic evidence of an abnormal discharge in the sensory motor cortex generating the myoclonic jerks via fast conducting corticomotoneuron pathways (Figs 20.5 and 20.6). Myoclonus arising in the cerebral cortex can be focal affecting one body part, such as a hand or foot, but multiple cortical discharges can cause multifocal jerks, each jerk being due to a discrete discharge in one part of the motor cortex. In addition, cortical discharges can cause generalized muscle jerks, either by intracortical and transcallosal spread to activate both motor cortices (Brown et al., 1991a, 1996; Brown and Marsden, 1996), or by cortico-reticular pathways activating brainstem myoclonic generators. Such multifocal and generalized cortical myoclonus is discussed below. Patients with focal cortical myoclonus also exhibit epilepsia partialis continua (Juul-Jensen and Denny-Brown, 1966), partial motor seizures, and secondary generalization with tonic-clonic grand mal seizures (Cowan et al., 1986) (Fig. 20.7). Focal slow-frequency repetitive transcranial magnetic stimulation has suppressed focal cortical myoclonus in a patient with cortical dysplasia (Rossi et al., 2004).

Epilepsia partialis continua is defined clinically as a syndrome of continuous focal jerking of a body part, usually localized to a distal limb, occurring over hours, days or even years, due to a cerebral cortical abnormality (Cockerell et al., 1996) (Fig. 20.8). The most common etiologies now are Rasmussen encephalitis and cerebrovascular disease. Most, but not all patients, have epileptic or other EEG abnormalities, and over half have identifiable cortical lesions on brain MRI. A similar clinical picture can occur with subcortical lesions, in which case it is suggested that the term "myoclonia continua" be employed (Cockerell et al., 1996). Cortical myoclonus sometimes is so rhythmic as to produce a tremor (Ikeda et al., 1990; Toro and Hallett,

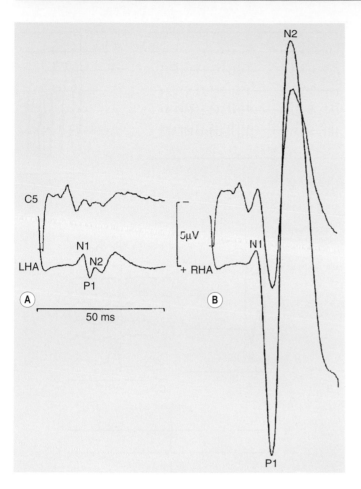

Figure 20.5 Focal cortical myoclonus. Details of short-latency components of somatosensory evoked potentials in cervical (C5; top traces) and cortical hand area of the left and right hand (LHA, RHA; bottom traces) following electrical stimulation of the index finger of the left (**A**) and right (**B**) hand. The patient, a 34-year-old woman, had an undiagnosed left hemisphere lesion. For some 6 years she had experienced rare grand mal seizures but continuous flexor jerking of the right hand and forearm while awake. These jerks occurred spontaneously, on action, or in response to touch of the fingers or a tap with a tendon hammer. On examination, apart from the focal myoclonus of the right hand, there were no other neurologic signs. Brain imaging was normal, as was a carotid arteriogram and CSF examination. Routine EEG showed a focal abnormality over the region of the left sensorimotor area, with spike-sharp-wave discharges. The early cervical potentials, with a peak latency of 13 ms, and the first major cortical response (N1), with a latency of 20 ms, are the same size on both sides. The later components are much enlarged after right hand stimulation (**B**). Traces are the average of 999 sweeps, with the stimulation given at the beginning of the sweep. Electrodes referred to a reference at Fz. The apparent large late responses recorded at the cervical electrode in **B** are due to activity at the Fz reference. *From Rothwell JC, Obeso IA, Marsden CD. Electrophysiology of somatosensory reflex myoclonus. Adv Neurol 1986;43:385–398, with permission*

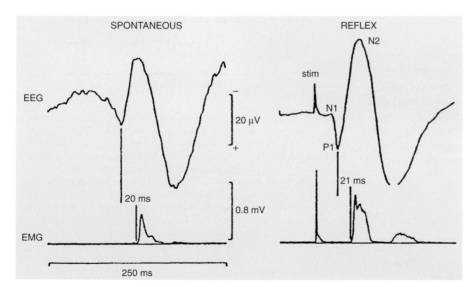

Figure 20.6 Focal cortical myoclonus. Average (of 128) EMG and EEG events associated with spontaneous (left traces) and reflex-evoked (right traces) cortical myoclonus in a patient with a focal dysplastic lesion of the right sensorimotor cortex. The EEG during spontaneous jerks was back-averaged from a trigger point on the rectified EMG record. Reflex jerks were elicited by giving electrical stimuli (stim) to the left forefinger, 50 ms after the start of the recording sweep. The time interval between the large P1 positive wave in the EEG and the start of the myoclonic EMG burst is indicated. EMGs taken from the left first dorsal interosseous; EEG records from the contralateral sensorimotor hand area, referred to a linked mastoid reference. *From Rothwell JC, Obeso JA, Marsden CD. On the significance of giant somatosensory evoked potentials in cortical myoclonus. J Neurol Neurosurg Psychiatry 1984;47(1):33–42, with permission.*

2004) (Video 20.5). A focal cortical lesion produces focal myoclonus in the opposite appropriate body part. Such lesions include those due to vascular disease, tumor, granulomas, and focal encephalitis (Table 20.6) (Thomas et al., 1977; Cockerell et al., 1996). Chronic, prolonged focal myoclonic jerking in children suggests the possibility of Rasmussen encephalitis. 📹

Rasmussen encephalitis is a disorder of childhood and adolescence in which a unilateral focal seizure disorder is accompanied by a progressive hemiplegia due to focal cortical inflammation and destruction (Hart, 2004; Freeman, 2005). The seizures are severe, often with epilepsia partialis continua, partial motor seizures, and secondary generalization. The EEG may show focal epileptiform activity, or

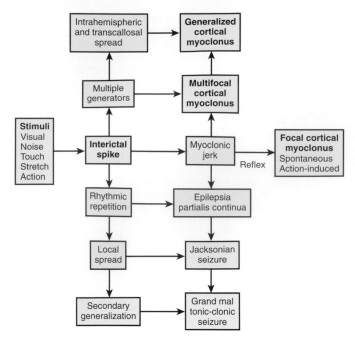

Figure 20.7 Cortical myoclonus. The various manifestations of spike discharges in the motor cortex, and their interrelationships are depicted. The physiologic correlate of the focal cortical myoclonic jerk is a cortical positive wave (an interictal spike) which represents a volley of pyramidal cell discharge in motor cortex. This can occur spontaneously, on voluntary movement, or in response to stimuli. Multiple spikes can cause multifocal myoclonus. The cortical discharge can also spread throughout the motor strip and, via the corpus callosum, to the opposite motor cortex to cause multifocal or generalized cortical myoclonus. If the spike discharge occurs repetitively, the result is epilepsia partialis continua. If it propagates locally it may cause a simple Jacksonian motor seizure, or if it becomes secondarily generalized, a tonic-clonic grand mal seizure occurs.

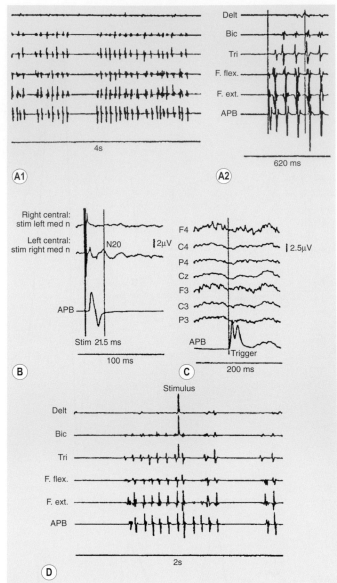

Figure 20.8 Epilepsia partialis continua. **A1** Pattern of spontaneous jerking in the left arm of a case due to cerebral infarction. Hypersynchronous bursts of EMG activity occur at the same time in virtually all muscles of the arm (Delt, deltoid; Bic, biceps: Tri, triceps; F. flex., flexor muscles in the forearm; F. ext., extensor muscles in the forearm; APB, abductor pollicis brevis). The jerks occur in short runs with pauses of 0.5 s or so between each. **A2** Shows the start of a run of activity after one of these pauses. Note that the first jerk of the run occurs only in forearm and hand muscles; the second jerk involves most of the muscles of the left arm (**B**). Lack of enlarged somatosensory evoked potential (SEP) and reflex muscle jerk following stimulation of the left median nerve at the elbow. The top two traces are average (of 256 trials) EEG records from the right central (C4) and left central (C3) electrodes, referenced to linked earlobes. The bottom trace is the EMG from abductor pollicis brevis (APB). The N20 component of the SEP is present and of normal size and latency. **C** Lack of any back-averaged EEG correlate preceding spontaneous jerks of the left APB muscle (rectified EMG record in bottom trace); 350 trials averaged. Linked earlobe reference. **D** Effect of a sub-motor threshold magnetic stimulus over the right motor cortex on an ongoing run of spontaneous jerking. The stimulus occurs at the time of the stimulus artifact. No short-latency muscle response is evident (on this time scale it would merge into the stimulus artifact). A spontaneous jerk of all arm muscles follows the stimulus, but then the upper arm muscles pause for the following two jerks. *From Cockerell OC, Rothwell J, Thompson PD, et al. Clinical and physiological features of epilepsia partialis continua. Cases ascertained in the UK. Brain 1996;119(Pt 2):393–407, with permission.*

periodic lateralized discharges (PLEDs), or both. In addition to the progressive hemiplegia, there often is cognitive decline. The cause appears due to an autoimmune process, specifically to the glutamate receptor (GluR) 3 subunit, with such antibodies acting as a GluR agonist to cause an excitotoxic cascade (Gahring et al., 2001). Immunotherapy (steroids, plasmapheresis, or intravenous human immunoglobulin (IVIg)) may help some, but hemispherectomy may be necessary.

Axial myoclonus

Typically axial myoclonus consists of neck and trunk flexion with abduction of the arms and flexion of the hips.

Axial myoclonic jerks may arise in the spinal cord or brainstem. Propriospinal myoclonus involves long propriospinal fibers in the spinal cord distributed to axial muscles (Brown et al., 1991c) (Fig. 20.9). The most prominent movement of propriospinal myoclonus is truncal flexion, and it can be either spontaneous or stimulus induced (Video 20.6). A review of 60 patients noted a middle-aged male predominance (Roze et al., 2009). The myoclonus tended to be worse when lying down and at wake–sleep transitions. A premonitory sensation might be present before the jerks. The etiology

Table 20.6 Causes of focal cortical myoclonus and epilepsia partialis continua

Etiology	Number	
	Thomas et al. (1977)	Cockerell et al. (1996)
Infarct or cerebral hemorrhage	8	9

Tumor
  Astrocytoma
  Hemangioma
  Lymphoma
  Uncertain
	5	4

Encephalitis (including Rasmussen encephalitis)	5	7
Trauma	2	1
Hepatic encephalopathy	2	–
Subarachnoid hemorrhage	1	–
Unknown	9	9
Total	**32**	**30**
Others		
Subdural hematoma		
Abscess		
Granuloma (TB)		
Multiple sclerosis		
Meningitis		
Nonketotic hyperglycemia		
Focal gliosis		
Spinocerebellar degeneration		
Mitochondrial disease		

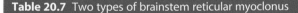

Table 20.7 Two types of brainstem reticular myoclonus

In both types, the myoclonus originates in the caudal brainstem, and muscles are activated up the brainstem and down the spinal cord. The myoclonus is generalized and mainly axial to cause neck flexion, shoulder elevation, and trunk and knee extension.

(1) Exaggerated startle response

Bulbospinal pathways are slow conducting

Evoked by sudden noise or light, or by sensory stimuli to the mantle area

Spontaneous jerks not prominent

(2) Reticular reflex myoclonus

Bulbospinal pathways are fast conducting

Stimulus sensitivity greatest over the limbs

Spontaneous jerks common

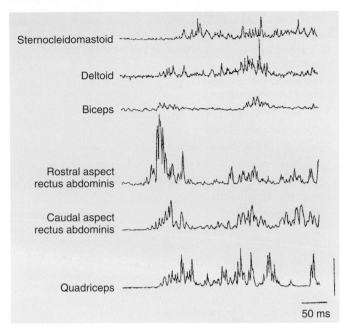

Figure 20.9 Propriospinal myoclonus. EMG record of a single spontaneous jerk in a patient with propriospinal myoclonus. Muscles are sternocleidomastoid, deltoid, biceps, rostral aspect of rectus abdominis, caudal aspect of rectus abdominis, and quadriceps. EMG activity occurred first in rectus abdominis. Contraction of sternocleidomastoid, rectus abdominis, and quadriceps occurred in all jerks, but activity in deltoid and biceps (evident here) was variable. Vertical calibration line = 200 μV and 100 μV for bottom and top three channels, respectively. *From Brown P, Thompson PD, Rothwell JC, et al. Axial myoclonus of propriospinal origin. Brain 1991;114:197–214., with permission.*

of many of these cases is not clear, although injury to the spinal cord from trauma, infection, tumor, and disk herniation has been described (Capelle et al., 2005; Shprecher et al., 2010). Diffusion tensor imaging with fiber tracking of the spinal cord may reveal abnormalities (Roze et al., 2009). The EMG pattern of propriospinal myoclonus can be mimicked voluntarily, indicating that psychogenic myoclonus should be in the differential diagnosis in these cases (Kang and Sohn, 2006), and several such cases have now been reported (Williams et al., 2008; Slawek et al., 2010). In a series of 35 patients referred with axial jerks, 34 of them were considered to be psychogenic (van der Salm et al., 2010). More work is needed in this area to understand this disorder better. The most effective drug for treatment has been clonazepam (Roze et al., 2009).

Brainstem reticular myoclonus (Table 20.7 and Fig. 20.10) may follow cerebral anoxia, and probably is responsible for the generalized muscle jerks that occur in a number of toxic myoclonic syndromes, as for example in uremia and other metabolic disturbances, as well as those precipitated by drugs. It is characterized by a generalized axial myoclonic jerk which starts in muscles innervated by the lower brainstem, then spreading up the brainstem and down the spinal cord (Hallett et al., 1977a). There is no time-locked cortical correlate and sensory evoked potentials are normal. Such brainstem reticular myoclonus may occur after cerebral anoxia, and can be seen in some patients with the stiff-man syndrome (Leigh et al., 1980). Brainstem lesions, such as

Table 20.8 Causes of the startle syndrome

A. Pathologic exaggeration of the normal startle reflex

1. Hereditary hyperekplexia
2. Idiopathic hyperekplexia
3. Symptomatic startle syndromes

Static encephalopathies

    a. Static perinatal encephalopathy with tonic spasms
    b. Post-anoxic encephalopathy
    c. Post-traumatic encephalopathy

Brainstem encephalitis

    a. Sarcoidosis
    b. Viral encephalomyelitis
    c. Encephalomyelitis with rigidity
    d. Multiple sclerosis
    e. Paraneoplastic

Structural

    a. Brainstem hemorrhage/infarct
    b. Cerebral abscess

B. Brainstem reticular reflex myoclonus

Post-anoxic encephalopathy

C. Unknown physiology

1. Hexosaminidase A deficiency
2. Static perinatal encephalopathy with epileptic tonic spasms (startle epilepsy)
3. Gilles de la Tourette syndrome
4. Jumping Frenchmen, Latah, and Myriachit
5. Hysterical jumps

From Brown P, Rothwell JC, Thompson PD, et al. The hyperekplexias and their relationship to the normal startle reflex. Brain 1991;114:1903–1928.

and glycine receptor complex. Additionally, responsible mutations are also found presynaptically in the glycine transporter 2 (Rees et al., 2006). Glycine is an inhibitory neurotransmitter in several spinal interneurons, including Renshaw cells, Ia inhibitory interneurons, and some Ib inhibitory interneurons. Physiologic studies suggest normal recurrent inhibition, but abnormal Ia reciprocal inhibition in hyperekplexia (Floeter et al., 1996). Affected babies are hypertonic and stiff when handled, and have difficulty subsequently with walking. They develop excessive startles, which take two forms; the minor form is a simple brief startle jerk; the major form is a more prolonged tonic startle spasm. In these situations, the normal startle reflex is exaggerated, both in amplitude, and in its failure to rapidly habituate (Brown et al., 1991b; Matsumoto et al., 1992; Matsumoto and Hallett, 1994). The afferent and efferent systems of the startle reflex in hyperekplexia are identical to those of the normal startle response, involving a similar or the same generator in the lower brainstem, probably in the medial bulbopontine reticular formation. However, there may be differences between the minor form and major form of hyperekplexia. First, only the major form appears to be linked to the glycine receptor gene (Tijssen et al., 1995, 2002). Second, the physiologic abnormalities in the minor and major forms appear to differ (Tijssen et al., 1996, 1997). Treatment with clonazepam may be very effective in some patients (Matsumoto and Hallett, 1994). Others have responded to sodium valproate or piracetam.

An exaggerated startle response may be responsible for the motor manifestations of "jumping Frenchmen" and other culturally determined startle syndromes (Andermann and Andermann, 1988; Brown et al., 1991b; Matsumoto and Hallett, 1994). In these syndromes the startle is followed by stereotyped behaviors such as a vocalization or striking out (Video 20.8). Hyperekplexia must be distinguished from startle-evoked epileptic seizures (Matsumoto and Hallett, 1994; Manford et al., 1996).

occur in multiple sclerosis, also may be responsible (Smith and Scheinberg, 1990).

Exaggerated startle syndromes (hyperekplexia) consist of an excessive motor response or jump, to unexpected auditory and, sometimes, somesthetic and visual stimuli (Tables 20.7 and 20.8) (Suhren et al., 1966; Andermann and Andermann, 1988; Brown et al., 1991b; Matsumoto et al., 1992, Matsumoto and Hallett, 1994; Bakker et al., 2006). The jump consists of a blink, contortion of the face, flexion of the neck and trunk, and abduction and flexion of the arm (Fig. 20.11). Such patients jump in response to sound and crash to the ground, injuring themselves. There is no loss of consciousness. An exaggerated startle syndrome may be due to local brainstem pathology (anoxia, inflammatory lesions including sarcoidosis and multiple sclerosis, and hemorrhage), and also occurs as an inherited condition (hereditary hyperekplexia), transmitted as an autosomal dominant trait (Video 20.7). The first abnormal gene found for this disorder was a point mutation in the alpha-1 subunit of the glycine-receptor (Shiang et al., 1993, 1995; Tijssen et al., 1995). This may lead to altered ligand binding or disturbance of the chloride ion-channel part of the receptor. Subsequently other mutations were found in the glycine receptor

Multifocal and generalized cortical myoclonus

Multifocal myoclonus of cortical origin typically affects many parts of the body bilaterally, but not synchronously. Each myoclonic jerk involves only a few adjacent muscles. The movements of the fingers or toes may be small twitches (minipolymyoclonus) (Wilkins et al., 1985); those of more proximal and axial muscles cause bigger movements. Multifocal cortical myoclonus is due to a generalized excitability of the cerebral cortex, particularly of the sensorimotor cortex. The EEG may show multifocal spike discharges, and back-averaging reveals the typical cortical correlate to each focal myoclonic jerk. Somatosensory evoked potentials often are enlarged. The jerks are frequently stimulus-sensitive.

Many patients with multifocal cortical myoclonus also exhibit generalized myoclonic jerks, synchronous in many muscles at the same time. Some of these are of brainstem origin (brainstem reticular myoclonus), perhaps driven by a cortical origin. However, discharge in the sensorimotor cortex may produce a generalized jerk as a result of transcallosal and intracortical spread (Brown et al., 1991a).

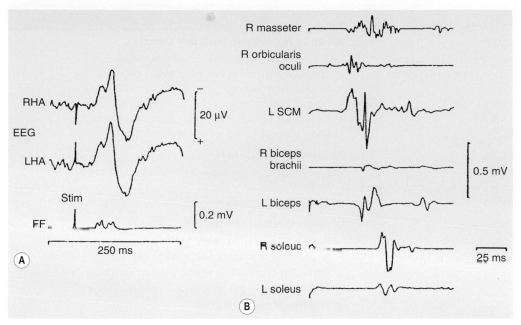

Figure 20.10 Brainstem reticular myoclonus. **A** Average of 128 EEG and EMG responses to electrical stimulation (Stim) of the index finger of the right hand in a patient with reticular reflex myoclonus. EEG recorded monopolarly from over the sensorimotor hand area (RHA, right-hand area; LHA, left-hand area) referred to a linked mastoid reference. Rectified EMG from surface electrodes placed over the flexor carpi radialis (FF). No enlargement of the EEG response is evident preceding the myoclonic muscle jerk. The bilateral late response probably is produced by movement artifact from the generalized muscle jerk. **B** Order of muscle activation on a single generalized myoclonic jerk in the same patient, produced by a light tap with a tendon hammer to the forehead at the start of the sweep. The jerk begins in the sternocleidomastoid (SCM) and travels up the cranial nerves and down the spinal cord.

This 41-year-old man developed increasing generalized muscle stiffness and jerks over a period of about 1 year. Eventually, he became bedridden with severe rigidity but remained alert and, according to his relatives, suitably responsive. On examination, although alert, he was severely dysarthric, and he could not move voluntarily. His limbs were held in flexion and exhibited extreme rigidity. Tendon reflexes were brisk, and the plantar responses were flexor. Any stimulus, including visual menace, load noise, light touch, or a tap with a tendon hammer, evoked massive generalized muscle jerking. All investigations failed to reveal a pathologic diagnosis, although clinically it was suspected that he had a diffuse encephalomyelitis. *From Rothwell JC, Obeso JA, Marsden CD. Electrophysiology of somatosensory reflex myoclonus. Adv Neurol. 1986;43:385–398, with permission.*

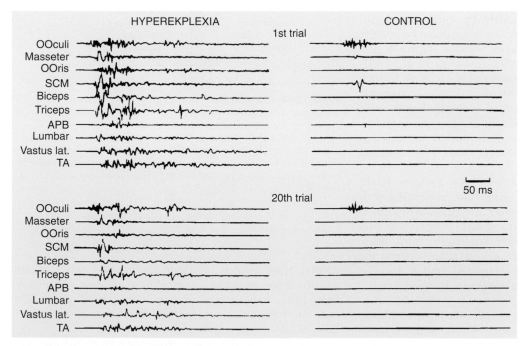

Figure 20.11 EMG in hereditary hyperekplexia. Multichannel surface EMG recordings of startle responses in a 13-year-old girl with hereditary hyperekplexia compared with a normal subject. Top left: An initial 103 dB acoustic stimulus given at the time indicated by the arrow is followed by a generalized EMG startle response. Note the early activation of the orbicularis oculi (OOculi) followed by the sternocleidomastoid (SCM). Bottom left: The twentieth startle response after repetitive acoustic stimuli given at 1-minute intervals shows little habituation. The control subject's recordings on the right show a much more subdued response that reveals marked habituation at the 20th trial. *From Matsumoto J, Hallett M. Startle syndromes. In: Marsden CD, Fahn S (eds) Movement Disorders 3. Oxford: Butterworth-Heinemann; 1994, pp. 418–433, with permission.*

Table 20.9 Characteristics of major primary epileptic myoclonus syndromes

Cryptogenic myoclonic epilepsy

1. Massive myoclonic jerks as the only or major seizure type
2. Bursts of bilateral irregular slow spike/wave at 2.5 Hz or more
3. Onset 6 months to 5 years
4. No signs of brain damage prior to seizures
5. Tonic-clonic seizures, but no tonic seizures
6. Relatively good prognosis

Eyelid myoclonus with absences

1. Photosensitive attacks
2. Marked eyelid jerking, with upward eye deviation, during absences
3. Irregular 3 Hz spike/wave in EEG

Infantile spasms

1. Flexor (extensor) spasms
2. Hypsarrhythmic EEG
3. Onset in first year of life
4. Many causes recognized
5. Learning disability

Juvenile myoclonic epilepsy (Janz)

1. Myoclonus, mainly in arms, especially in the morning
2. Spikes, polyspikes and slow waves in EEG
3. Onset around puberty
4. No signs of brain damage
5. Tonic-clonic seizures, especially at night. Absences in 10%
6. Very good response to sodium valproate

Absences in petit mal

1. Eyelid myoclonus, and more rarely massive myoclonic jerks, with absences
2. 3 Hz spike/wave in EEG

Lennox–Gastaut syndrome

1. Massive myoclonic jerks, tonic spasms and atonic attacks
2. Atypical slow (less than 2.5 Hz) spike/wave in EEG
3. Onset after infantile spasms, and other brain insults, around 2–8 years
4. Tonic-clonic and other seizures
5. Poor prognosis

Many conditions cause multifocal and generalized cortical myoclonus. These include epileptic myoclonus, in which epilepsy dominates and there is no progressive disease of the brain, progressive myoclonus epilepsy and progressive myoclonic ataxia, post-anoxic myoclonus, viral encephalopathies, metabolic disease, and toxic encephalopathies (Table 20.2).

Epileptic myoclonus refers to those epilepsies characterized exclusively, or predominantly by brief myoclonic, atonic, or tonic seizures. Epileptic myoclonus can be positive (with active muscle contractions) or negative (lapses of postural tone) (Guerrini et al., 1993; Tassinari et al., 1995, 1998). Conditions subsumed under this category include infantile spasms, the Lennox–Gastaut syndrome, cryptogenic myoclonic epilepsy, the myoclonus associated with petit mal, and juvenile myoclonic epilepsy of adolescence (Janz). The key features of these various conditions are summarized in Table 20.9 (Aicardi, 1986; Shields, 2004; Nabbout and Dulac, 2008).

Of these conditions, juvenile myoclonic epilepsy (JME) is the most frequent epileptic syndrome presenting with myoclonus, usually in adolescence. The main symptom is myoclonic jerks, usually without loss of consciousness, predominantly in the morning after awakening from sleep. Generalized tonic-clonic seizures also tend to occur in the morning. Linkage studies have identified genetic loci for some patients with JME and other myoclonic epilepsies (Lu and Wang, 2009).

Progressive myoclonus epilepsy refers to a combination of severe myoclonus (spontaneous, action, and stimulus-sensitive), severe generalized tonic-clonic and other seizures, and progressive neurological decline, particularly dementia and ataxia (Berkovic and Andermann, 1986; Berkovic et al., 1986; Marseille Consensus Group, 1990; Ramachandran et al., 2009; Shahwan et al., 2005; Zupanc and Legros, 2004). Progressive myoclonic ataxia (sometimes known as the

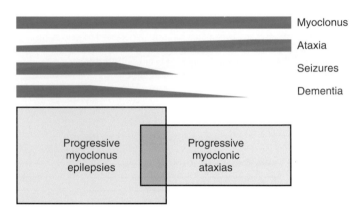

Figure 20.12 Schematic representation of the clinical features and relationship of the syndromes of progressive myoclonic epilepsy (PME) and of progressive myoclonic ataxia (PMA). The bars in the upper part of the figure give a general indication of the prominence of the key clinical signs in the PME and PMA syndromes. Initial recognition of either syndrome then demands an attempt to reach a specific diagnosis. A specific diagnosis can now usually be made in patients with PME, whereas a larger proportion of cases with PMA remain undiagnosed. Previous authors have used the term Ramsay Hunt syndrome to describe different groups of patients within this spectrum. *From Marseille Consensus Group. Classification of progressive myoclonus epilepsies and related disorders. Ann Neurol 1990;28(1):113–116, with permission.*

Ramsay Hunt syndrome) (Marsden et al., 1990) is distinguished from progressive myoclonus epilepsy by seizures being mild or absent, and dementia being mild or nonexistent, but myoclonus and ataxia are the major problems (Fig. 20.12).

The differential diagnosis of progressive myoclonus epilepsy (Table 20.10) and progressive myoclonic ataxia (Table 20.11) is dominated by five main conditions.

Lafora body disease and neuronal ceroid lipofuscinosis generally produce severe neurologic decline with dementia or regression, along with myoclonus and fits (Rapin, 1986).

Table 20.10 Major causes of progressive myoclonus epilepsy

Condition	Age at onset (years)	Diagnostic features		
		Clinical	**Laboratory**	**Diagnostic test**
Unverricht–Lundborg disease	6–15	Severe myoclonus Dementia absent or mild	EEG	Clinical
Lafora body disease	11–18	Occipital seizures Dementia	EEG	Lafora bodies (skin, liver, brain)
Neuronal ceroid lipofuscinosis (Batten) Late-infantile (Jansky–Bielschowsky)	2.5–4 (dead by 6–10)	Severe seizures Rapid regression Macular degeneration	EEG ERG VER	EM of skin, muscle Rectum or brain
Juvenile (Spielmeyer–Vogt)	4–10 (dead by 15–25)	Visual failure Macular degeneration	Dolichols	
Adults (Kufs)	12–50 (long course)	Behavioral change Dementia		
Sialidosis Type I	8–20	Cherry-red spot	Storage in lymphocytes, etc.	Alpha-N-acetyl-neuraminidase
Type II	10–30	Cherry-red spot Dysmorphic	Urinary sialyl-oligosaccharides	
Mitochondrial encephalomyopathy (MERRF)	5–42	Short stature Deafness	Blood and CSF lactate	"Ragged-red" fibers on muscle biopsy DNA tests

EEG, electroencephalogram; ERG, electroretinogram; VER, visual evoked responses; MERRF, myoclonus epilepsy and ragged-red fibers. Genetic testing is now available for many of these disorders.

After Berkovic SF, Andermann F. The progressive myoclonic epilepsies. In: Pedley TA, Meldrum BS, editors. Recent Advances in Epilepsy 3. Edinburgh: Churchill Livingstone; 1986, pp. 157–187.

Lafora body disease (EPM2), inherited as an autosomal recessive trait, is characterized by polyglucosan acid–Schiff (PAS)-positive inclusions in cells of brain, liver, muscle, and skin (eccrine sweat glands). Onset usually is in childhood with behavioral and cognitive change, dementia and seizures, as well as myoclonus; late-onset forms with a more benign onset also occur (Footitt et al., 1997). The gene responsible in about 75% of cases has been localized to chromosome 6q and has now been identified (Minassian et al., 1999) as encoding a protein tyrosine phosphatase (PTP) (Minassian et al., 1998; Serratosa et al., 1999). The protein, called laforin (or EPM2A), localizes at the plasma membrane and the endoplasmic reticulum (Minassian et al., 2001). Laforin presumably metabolizes polyglucosans preventing their aggregation (Chan et al., 2004a) with a mode of action of regulating autophagy (Aguado et al., 2010). A second gene is associated with Lafora body disease, *NHLRC1* (also called *EPM2B*), which encodes malin, a putative E3 ubiquitin ligase with a RING finger domain and six NHL motifs (Chan et al., 2003; Ganesh et al., 2006; Singh and Ganesh, 2009). Laforin is a substrate for malin (Gentry et al., 2005). Both laforin and malin colocalize to the ER, suggesting they operate in a related pathway protecting against polyglucosan accumulation (Delgado-Escueta, 2007; Singh et al., 2008; Moreno et al., 2010). A third locus is predicted on the

Table 20.11 Causes of progressive myoclonic ataxia

Major causes

Unverricht–Lundborg disease
Mitochondrial encephalomyopathy
Sialidosis
Lafora body disease*
Neuronal ceroid lipofuscinosis*
Spinocerebellar degenerations

Rarer causes

Gaucher disease (non-infantile neuronopathic form)
GM$_2$ gangliosidosis*
Biotin-responsive encephalopathy
Neuroaxonal dystrophy (juvenile form)*
Pantothenate kinase-associated neurodegeneration
Atypical inclusion-body disease
Action myoclonus–renal failure syndrome
Dentatorubral–pallidoluysian atrophy
Progressive myoclonic epilepsy and deafness (May–White syndrome)
Progressive myoclonic epilepsy and lipomas
Celiac disease
Whipple disease

*Dementia often prominent, so not typical of progressive myoclonic ataxia.

basis of a family without linkage to the two known sites (Chan et al., 2004b). There is a mouse model of the disorder (Ganesh et al., 2002). Zonisamide has been described as very useful for the myoclonus and epilepsy in these patients (Yoshimura et al., 2001).

Neuronal ceroid lipofuscinosis (Batten disease), inherited as an autosomal recessive condition, also presents with seizures and myoclonus with cognitive impairment and dementia, along with blindness in the late infantile and juvenile forms (Jalanko and Braulke, 2009). The adult form is often dominated by psychiatric and cognitive impairment. Lipopigment accumulates in lysosomes in brain, eccrine glands, skin, muscle, and gut with characteristic inclusions (curvilinear bodies and finger print profiles). Both Lafora body disease and neuronal ceroid lipofuscinosis usually can be diagnosed in axillary skin biopsies with electron microscopy.

Unverricht–Lundborg disease (EPM1) is characterized by stimulus-sensitive myoclonus, tonic-clonic seizures, a characteristic EEG (paroxysmal generalized spike-wave activity, and photosensitivity), and a progressive course with ataxia but only mild intellectual decline (Eldridge et al., 1983; Koskiniemi, 1986; Lehesjoki and Koskiniemi, 1998; Lehesjoki and Koskiniemi, 1999; Kalviainen et al., 2008). In some patients there might be oculomotor apraxia, dystonia, or rapidly progressive dementia (Chew et al., 2008). It is inherited as an autosomal recessive trait, with onset around the age of 6–15 years, and occurs worldwide. Autopsy shows widespread degeneration, with prominent loss of cerebellar Purkinje cells without storage material. The gene for Unverricht–Lundborg disease has now been linked to the long arm of chromosome 21q22.3 in a number of Finnish and Mediterranean families, and the gene involved codes for cystatin B, a small protein that is a member of a superfamily of cysteine protease inhibitors (Lehesjoki and Koskiniemi, 1998, 1999). The most common mutation is an unstable expansion of a dodecamer minisatellite repeat unit in the promoter region of the cystatin B gene. The exact role of cystatin B is not known, but it has been found primarily localized in the nucleus (Riccio et al., 2001). Cystatin B interacts with a variety of proteins and these multiprotein complexes are found in the cerebellum (Di Giaimo et al., 2002). One possible pathophysiologic mechanism is sensitization to oxidative stress (Lehtinen et al., 2009). An animal model has been developed (Shannon et al., 2002). In an Arab family with similar clinical appearance, a cystatin B mutation was ruled out, linkage was identified on chromosome 12, and the disorder named EPM1B (Berkovic et al., 2005).

It is of critical importance in these cases to recognize that phenytoin treatment may be associated with worsening of the condition (Eldridge et al., 1983). Patients can be treated successfully with other anticonvulsants, as described later.

Mitochondrial encephalomyopathy presents in many guises. One phenotype is the myoclonus epilepsy and ragged-red fiber syndrome (MERRF) (Canafoglia et al., 2001; Traff et al., 1995). Symptoms typically commence in the second decade, but onset as late as the age of 40 has been described. Myoclonus and ataxia are typical features, while tonic-clonic seizures and dementia often also occur. Deafness and short stature may be a clue to the diagnosis. Muscle weakness is variable. A raised blood or CSF lactate concentration may suggest the diagnosis. Muscle biopsy reveals the characteristic "ragged-red" fibers. Maternal inheritance can sometimes be evident, and a number of mutations of mitochondrial genes have been identified.

Sialidosis (cherry-red spot myoclonus syndrome) also is inherited as an autosomal recessive condition with onset in childhood or adolescence (Rapin, 1986). The sialidoses are lysosomal storage disorders associated with a deficiency of alpha-N-acetylneuraminidase and, in some, with additional deficiency of alpha-galactosidase.

In adults, another group of conditions, namely spinocerebellar degenerations, may cause myoclonus. For example, one presentation of dentatorubro-pallidoluysian atrophy (DRPLA) is with myoclonus and epilepsy (Becher et al., 1997). Some patients with the autosomal dominant cerebellar ataxias, including type 1, also may have prominent myoclonus. So, too, may patients with multiple system atrophy, where the myoclonus tends to affect the fingers and toes, and is stimulus-sensitive (Rodriguez et al., 1994).

There is an interesting but unexplained association between progressive myoclonic ataxia and celiac disease (Bhatia et al., 1995; Lu et al., 1986). The onset of the neurologic syndrome followed the gastrointestinal and other manifestations of celiac disease while on a gluten-free diet, in the absence of overt features of malabsorption or nutritional deficiency. The neurologic syndrome was dominated by action and stimulus-sensitive myoclonus of cortical origin with mild ataxia and infrequent seizures. The condition progressed despite strict adherence to diet. No treatment is known.

Action myoclonus–renal failure syndrome (AMRF) is a distinctive form of progressive myoclonus epilepsy associated with renal dysfunction. Badhwar et al. (2004) have described 15 individuals who presented with either renal or neurologic features. Segregation analyses suggested autosomal recessive inheritance. Tremor (onset 17–26 years), action myoclonus (onset 14–29 years), infrequent generalized seizures (onset 20.28 years), and cerebellar features were characteristic. Brain autopsy in two patients revealed extraneuronal pigment accumulation. Proteinuria, detected between ages 9 and 30 years in all cases, progressed to renal failure in most patients within 8 years. Renal biopsies showed collapsing glomerulopathy, a severe variant of focal glomerulosclerosis. Dialysis and renal transplantation were effective for the renal but not the neurologic features, which continued to progress even when kidney function was improved.

Other causes of progressive myoclonus epilepsy and progressive myoclonic ataxia are much rarer (Table 20.11). Investigation of patients with these clinical syndromes should include neurophysiology, white cell enzyme assays, and muscle and axillary skin biopsy.

Myoclonus after cerebral anoxia is usually the result of an anesthetic accident, cardiac arrest, or respiratory failure often due to asthma (Lance and Adams, 1963; Werhahn et al., 1997; Frucht, 2002) (Table 20.12). In acute post-hypoxic myoclonus, there is an initial period of coma, sometimes with myoclonic storms. The first three days are crucial to long-term prognosis; generalized myoclonic status epilepticus carries a very poor prognosis (Wijdicks et al., 1994). In those who survive, spontaneous, action-induced and stimulus-sensitive myoclonus may emerge on recovery (Video 20.9). Intellect may be normal, but there may be

Table 20.12 Causes of post-hypoxic myoclonus

Cause	Number of patients
Associated with anesthesia and surgery	32
Myocardial infarct	12
Obstructed airway	11
Drug intoxication	9
Miscellaneous	21
Not stated	3
Total	**88**

From Fahn S. Posthypoxic action myoclonus: literature review update. Adv Neurol 1986;43:157–169.

Table 20.13 The opsoclonus–myoclonus syndrome (dancing eyes and dancing feet)

Opsoclonus: Continuous, arrhythmic, multidirectional, large saccades
Myoclonus: Trunk, limbs, diaphragm, larynx, pharynx and palate
Causes: Viral infections, postinfectious encephalitis, trauma, tumor (metabolic)
50% of children have a neuroblastoma (chest or abdomen)
Only 2% of those with a neuroblastoma have opsoclonus–myoclonus syndrome
20% of adults have an underlying cancer (see Table 20.14)

Table 20.14 "Brainstem encephalitis"

Subacute onset of ataxia, dysarthria, diplopia and ophthalmoplegia, nystagmus, opsoclonus, vertigo, deafness and myoclonus
Viral infection (e.g., herpes simplex), bacterial infection (e.g., *Listeria*), postinfectious, demyelination, vascular disease, tumor, or paraneoplastic syndromes
Paraneoplastic cases have normal imaging, but often have an active CSF with oligoclonal bands. Many have anti-Purkinje cell (e.g., anti-Yo) or anti-Ri antibodies. Common cancers are of ovary and lung

additional cerebellar ataxia as well as the disabling myoclonus. Seizures may persist. Post-anoxic myoclonus may consist of multifocal jerks of cortical origin, or generalized jerks due to intrahemispheric and transcallosal spread, or brainstem reticular myoclonus, or a mixture of all these types (Werhahn et al., 1997; Hallett, 2000). Many patients have prominent negative myoclonus particularly of the legs, causing sudden falls (Video 20.10). An animal model has been developed that should be useful in understanding the pathophysiology of this disorder (Kanthasamy et al., 2000; Nguyen et al., 2000; Truong et al., 2000). 🎥

The clinical syndrome as reported by Lance and Adams noted the precipitating feature of action, and the association with cerebellar ataxia, postural lapses, gait disturbance, and grand mal seizures. Werhahn and colleagues (1997) reported the clinical and neurophysiologic features of 14 patients with chronic post-hypoxic myoclonus. All patients had had a cardiorespiratory arrest, most caused by an acute asthmatic attack. All patients had multifocal action myoclonus, and 11 had additional stimulus-sensitive myoclonus. There was late improvement in the myoclonic syndrome and the level of disability in all but one patient. Cognitive deficits were found in seven patients and were usually mild. Electrophysiologic investigation confirmed cortical action myoclonus in every case, although this could be combined with cortical reflex myoclonus, an exaggerated startle response, or brainstem reticular reflex myoclonus. The site of the responsible lesion in the brain is not certain, but there does appear to be a disorder of serotonin metabolism supported not only by the therapeutic response to 5-hydroxytryptophan, but also by the reduction in CSF levels of 5-HIAA which improves with successful therapy. A study using glucose PET showed a bilateral hypermetabolism in the ventrolateral thalamus and pontine tegmentum relative to controls, but the significance of this is not clear (Frucht et al., 2004).

Multifocal and generalized myoclonus also may occur in a variety of acute encephalitic illnesses or postinfectious disseminated encephalomyelitis (Bhatia et al., 1992). It is characteristic of some of the slow viral encephalopathies such as subacute sclerosing panencephalitis (SSPE) and Creutzfeldt–Jakob disease (Shibasaki et al., 1981; Brown et al., 1986). In SSPE, the myoclonus is often periodic at long intervals (Video 20.11). Carbamazepine might be considered for the myoclonus of SSPE (Yigit and Sarikaya, 2006). In these latter conditions, the myoclonus often has a characteristic hung-up jerk, and periodic EEG discharges are evident in the majority of patients. Myoclonus also is seen in patients with the AIDS–dementia complex (Maher et al., 1997). 🎥

The myoclonic encephalopathy of infants (opsoclonus–myoclonus, or dancing eyes–dancing feet syndrome) appears between the ages of 6 and 18 months and often responds dramatically to steroid or ACTH treatment (Pranzatelli, 1992, 1996; Tate et al., 2005) (Table 20.13). Plasmapheresis may also be effective (Yiu et al., 2001). A recent approach is B cell depletion therapy with rituximab, ACTH, and IVIg (Pranzatelli et al., 2010a, 2010b). About a half of such cases have an underlying neuroblastoma (De Grandis et al., 2009). An autoimmune origin seems likely since it is associated with a distinctive pattern of serum IgM and IgG binding to neural tissues and antigens (Connolly et al., 1997; Blaes et al., 2008; Raffaghello et al., 2008). Reduced levels of the metabolites of serotonin (5-HIAA) and dopamine (HVA) have been found in the CSF (Pranzatelli et al., 1995) and some patients may benefit from treatment with the serotonin precursor 5-hydroxy-L-tryptophan. The incidence of subsequent developmental or neurologic disturbance is high (Rudnick et al., 2001; Krug et al., 2010). A similar syndrome of opsoclonus and myoclonus may occur in adults, whether inflammatory or paraneoplastic (Bataller et al., 2001; Markakis et al., 2008; Sabater et al., 2008) (Table 20.14 and Video 20.12). The "idiopathic" cases have a more benign course than those with cancer. If the cancer is treated, the opsoclonus–myoclonus may resolve. One defined syndrome is breast cancer and anti-Ri antibody (Weizman and Leong, 2004). A patient with large-cell carcinoma of the lung and ANNA-2 antibodies responded well to treatment of the tumor and antibody levels declined (Erlich et al., 2004). Whipple disease also may produce such a clinical picture (Schwartz et al., 1986). A case was seen in a young woman with anti-N-methyl-D-aspartate receptor encephalitis (Kurian et al., 2010). Symptomatic therapy that should be considered includes steroids or ACTH. Plasmapheresis may be effective (Yiu et al., 2001). Trazadone may also be helpful. 🎥

Antibodies to voltage-gated potassium channels (VGKC) may also be found in patients with myoclonus. In a study from the Mayo Clinic where they screened sera from 130 000 patients for markers of paraneoplastic neurologic autoimmunity, 80 patients were identified with VGKC immunoreactivity, and 29% manifested myoclonus (Tan et al., 2008).

Myoclonus and dementia in adults occurs not only in Creutzfeldt–Jakob disease but also in Alzheimer disease (Wilkins et al., 1984). Parkinson disease rarely manifests myoclonus. While the myoclonus appears to be cortical in origin, there is no reflex myoclonus or a giant somatosensory evoked potential (Caviness et al., 1998, 2002). Myoclonus is a well-described feature of dopa-dyskinesias (Luquin et al., 1992), and this would be its most frequent cause in patients with Parkinson disease. Patients with Parkinson disease and unsteadiness when standing may have orthostatic myoclonus (Leu-Semenescu et al., 2007). Myoclonus is more common in multiple system atrophy. Myoclonus can be seen in patients with dystonia, the myoclonus in this situation being a short "burst" of dystonia (Kinugawa et al., 2008) (Video 20.13). It may also be a feature of Huntington disease, and in one case it was shown to be cortical myoclonus (Caviness and Kurth, 1997). Myoclonus is a prominent, characteristic feature of corticobasal degeneration (Kompoliti et al., 1998). The myoclonus is stimulus-sensitive with a short latency that may be helpful in differential diagnosis. Its pathophysiology is still debated as to whether it is cortical or subcortical in origin (Carella et al., 1997; Strafella et al., 1997). 🎥

A wide variety of drugs and toxins may provoke multifocal and generalized myoclonus (Gordon, 2002), as may renal failure (Chadwick and French, 1979). Among drugs, antidepressants (particularly the selective serotonin reuptake inhibitors), anesthetics, anticonvulsants (particularly at toxic levels), withdrawal of benzodiazepines and propranolol, lithium (Caviness and Evidente, 2003), monoamine oxidase inhibitors, and levodopa can all cause myoclonus. Among toxins, bismuth, heavy metals, glue and gasoline sniffing, and toxic cooking oil in Spain can cause prominent myoclonus. Myoclonus is prominent in the "serotonin syndrome," along with confusion, agitation, diarrhea, fever, and sweating. This syndrome has been reported after treatment with tryptophan, monoamine oxidase inhibitors, selective serotonin reuptake inhibitors, and tricyclic antidepressants, alone or in combination (Mason et al., 2000). Myoclonus is also associated with the use of gabapentin, but is generally mild and may not cause any symptomatic problem (Asconape et al., 2000).

Essential myoclonus refers to a syndrome of nonprogressive multifocal myoclonus, without other cognitive or neurologic symptoms or signs, or fits. It may be inherited as an autosomal dominant trait (Fahn and Sjaastad, 1991). Essential myoclonus usually presents in the first or second decade and the course is benign. There are no seizures, dementia or ataxia, and the EEG is normal. In some with essential myoclonus the physiologic abnormality appears to be that of overflow of ballistic movement patterns (Hallett et al., 1977b).

Sporadic cases of essential myoclonus also occur (Bressman and Fahn, 1986). In some families with essential myoclonus, there also are manifestations of dystonia; some individuals have both, others have myoclonus or dystonia. The myoclonus in such families may be very responsive to alcohol – hence the description as alcohol-sensitive myoclonus dystonia (Quinn, 1996). Most families with myoclonus dystonia have an abnormal gene for ε-sarcoglycan (Zimprich et al., 2001). The clinical presentation is relatively homogeneous with this gene defect with myoclonus predominantly of neck and upper limbs and dystonia presenting as cervical dystonia and/or writer's cramp (Asmus et al., 2002; Nardocci et al., 2008; Roze et al., 2008). In one family, however, epilepsy was also seen in affected members so the phenotype may be broad (Foncke et al., 2003). There is clearly genetic heterogeneity (Grimes et al., 2002). See also Chapter 12 for more details on myoclonus–dystonia.

Myoclonus is a frequent presentation of a psychogenic movement disorder, and it is important to keep this in mind in the differential diagnosis (Video 20.14). Psychogenic movement disorders are discussed in Chapter 25, but in the context of discussing myoclonus, it is noteworthy that the clinical neurophysiology is distinctive and can help to resolve the differential diagnosis (Brown, 2006; Esposito et al., 2009; Hallett, 2010). 🎥

Drug treatment of generalized or multifocal myoclonus

Myoclonus, particularly action myoclonus, can be very disabling. It distorts speech, interferes with manual function, and prevents walking. The drugs used to treat myoclonus generally possess anticonvulsant properties (Table 20.15) (Obeso et al., 1989; Brown, 1995; Obeso, 1995; Pranzatelli and Nadi, 1995; Frucht, 2000), usually by enhancing gamma-aminobutyric (GABA) inhibitory activity. In epilepsy, it is currently fashionable to try and manage patients using a single drug rather than polytherapy. However, there are good reasons for the opposite approach in the treatment of myoclonus. Electrophysiologic evidence suggests that antimyoclonic drugs may exert different actions on the sequence of events responsible for myoclonus, at least for those concerned with cortical myoclonus. Some drugs which decrease cortical myoclonus increase the size of the giant sensory evoked potential, while others have the opposite effect. Myoclonus thus often responds best to a combination of drugs (Obeso et al., 1989).

Table 20.16 summarizes the drugs used to treat specific types of myoclonus arising in different parts of the neuraxis.

Epileptic myoclonus and cortical myoclonus respond best to drugs such as sodium valproate and clonazepam, often used in combination in maximum tolerated anticonvulsant doses (Obeso et al., 1989). Sodium valproate is the drug of choice to treat juvenile myoclonic epilepsy (Mantoan and Walker, 2011).

Table 20.15 Appropriate dosages of agents for the treatment of myoclonus

Drug	Dosage (mg/day)
Baclofen	15–100
Benzatropine	4–9
Carbamazepine	800–1600
Clonazepam	Up to 15
Diazepam	5–30
5-hydroxytryptophan	Up to 1500*
Levetiracetam	1000–3000
Phenobarbital	60–180
Phenytoin	100–300
Piracetam	2400–16 800
Primidone	500–750
Tetrabenazine	50–200
Trihexyphenidyl (benzhexol)	Up to 35
Valproic acid (sodium valproate)	1000–1500

*In combination with a peripheral aromatic amino acid decarboxylase inhibitor (such as carbidopa 100–300 mg/day).
Modified from Brown P. Myoclonus: A practical guide to drug therapy. CNS Drugs 1995;3:22–29.

Table 20.16 Drug treatment for specific types of myoclonus

Type of myoclonus	Drug(s) of first choice	Other agents
Cortical myoclonus	Valproic acid (sodium valproate or clonazepam)	Primidone or phenobarbital, levetiracetam, piracetam, 5-HTP*
Brainstem reticular myoclonus	Valproic acid or clonazepam[†]	5-HTP*
Hyperekplexia	Clonazepam	Carbamazepine, phenytoin
Ballistic overflow myoclonus	Benzatropine or trihexyphenidyl (Benzhexol)	Alcohol (ethanol), clonazepam, 5-HTP*
Palatal myoclonus	Phenytoin, carbamazepine, clonazepam, diazepam, trihexyphenidyl or baclofen[†]	5-HTP*, sumatriptan
Propriospinal myoclonus	Clonazepam	
Segmental spinal myoclonus	Clonazepam	Diazepam, carbamazepine, tetrabenazine

*Combined with a peripheral aromatic amino acid decarboxylase inhibitor (such as carbidopa). Usefulness limited by poor tolerability.
[†]Treatment with any agent is often unsuccessful.
5-HTP, 5-hydroxytryptophan.

It is conventional to start with sodium valproate in patients with severe myoclonus, then to add clonazepam. If disability is not adequately improved, piracetam or levetiracetam can then be added. The mechanism of action of piracetam is uncertain, but it undoubtedly possesses antimyoclonic activity (Obeso et al., 1988; Brown et al., 1993; Ikeda et al., 1996; Koskiniemi et al., 1998; Genton et al., 1999; Fedi et al., 2001). Levetiracetam, a molecule related to piracetam that has been approved for the treatment of epilepsy, also is very effective for myoclonus (Genton and Van Vleymen, 2000; Genton and Gelisse, 2000, 2001; Frucht et al., 2001; Krauss et al., 2001; Schauer et al., 2002; Magaudda et al., 2004). There is one report of tizanidine helping two of three patients (Mukand and Giunti, 2004).

Primidone also may be of value as an additional drug in severely affected patients, as may clobazam and acetazolamide (Vaamonde et al., 1992). The potential antimyoclonic activity of newer anticonvulsants, such as vigabatrin, gabapentin, and lamotrigine, remains to be established. However, both vigabatrin and gabapentin may, paradoxically, worsen some types of myoclonus (Asconape et al., 2000). Milacemide, a glycine precursor, has been shown to be ineffective (Brown et al., 1991d; Gordon et al., 1993). One patient with alcohol-responsive post-hypoxic myoclonus responded well to gamma-hydroxybutryic acid (Frucht et al., 2005).

Unfortunately, while spontaneous, action, and reflex positive myoclonus often is helped by drug therapy, negative myoclonus frequently is resistant. As a result, disabling postural lapses in antigravity leg muscles usually persist to cause the typical bouncy unsteady stance and gait, often with falls. Two patients have been described with an excellent response to levetiracetam (Gelisse et al., 2003; Yu et al., 2009). In the setting of childhood partial epilepsy, negative myoclonus can be effectively treated with ethosuximide (Oguni et al., 1998; Capovilla et al., 1999). It is not clear whether this treatment would be useful in other circumstances.

The antioxidant N-acetylcysteine has been claimed to have considerable beneficial effect on the myoclonus in Unverricht–Lundborg disease (Hurd et al., 1996; Ben-Menachem et al., 2000). Alcohol also has been found to be a potent antimyoclonic agent in post-hypoxic myoclonus as well as Unverricht–Lundborg disease (Genton and Guerrini, 1992).

Those with brainstem myoclonus seem to respond best to clonazepam. 5-hydroxytrytophan with a peripheral decarboxylase inhibitor also has been used with some success, although gastrointestinal side effects may be prominent (Chadwick et al., 1977).

Spinal and other segmental myoclonus also responds best to treatment with clonazepam (Obeso, 1995; Devetag Chalaupka and Bernardi, 1999), but tetrabenazine and baclofen occasionally may be helpful. Levetiracetam can be useful (Keswani et al., 2002). One case responded to valproate and serotonergic therapy (Jimenez-Jimenez et al., 1991). If all else fails, botulinum toxin can be used (Lagueny et al., 1999).

Essential myoclonus sometimes improves with alcohol, a beta-blocker such as propranolol, or an anticholinergic agent (Duvoisin, 1984; Chokroverty et al., 1987). In myoclonus–dystonia syndrome, alcohol can be of benefit to the myoclonus, but not to the dystonia with which it may be associated (Quinn, 1996). Myoclonus–dystonia can be improved with bilateral deep brain stimulation of the globus pallidus interna (Cif et al., 2004; Azoulay-Zyss et al., 2011).

References available on Expert Consult: www.expertconsult.com

CHAPTER **21**

Ataxia
Pathophysiology and clinical syndromes

Chapter contents			
Sporadic ataxia	465	Diagnostic plan	474
Genetic ataxia	467	Recovery from cerebellar injury; therapy	474

Ataxia is the type of clumsiness produced by dysfunction of the cerebellum or cerebellar pathways. The pathophysiology of the signs and symptoms has been detailed in the earlier chapter on motor control (Chapter 2). The core symptoms are difficulty with balance and gait, clumsiness of the hands, and dysarthria. The differential diagnosis is very long and includes all types of neurologic pathologic processes. While most patients presenting with ataxia will have a sporadic disorder, recently there has been increased attention on the genetic ataxias because of rapid advances in research.

Sporadic ataxia

Table 21.1 lists the principal categories. A series of 112 patients with sporadic ataxia with the following criteria were studied: (1) progressive ataxia; (2) onset after 20 years; (3) informative and negative family history (no similar disorders in first- and second-degree relatives; parents older than 50 years); and (4) no established symptomatic cause (Abele et al., 2002). Thirty-two patients (29%) met the clinical criteria of possible (7%) or probable (22%) multiple system atrophy (MSA). With genetic testing, Friedreich ataxia was found in five patients (4%), the spinocerebellar ataxia (SCA) 2 mutation in one (1%), the SCA3 mutation in two (2%) and the SCA6 mutation in seven (6%). The disease remained unexplained in 65 patients (58%). Antigliadin antibodies were present in 14 patients, 10 patients with unexplained ataxia (15%) and 4 patients with an established diagnosis (9%); this interesting aspect will be discussed further below.

Degenerative ataxia

MSA is likely the most common disorder, certainly in adults (Bhidayasiri and Ling, 2008; Gilman et al., 2008; Wenning et al., 2008). In addition to ataxia, patients have parkinsonism and autonomic dysfunction (including impotence). The disorder has also been called olivopontocerebellar atrophy

when the emphasis is on ataxia, striatonigral degeneration when the emphasis is on bradykinesia and rigidity, and Shy–Drager syndrome when the emphasis is on autonomic dysfunction. Early falls are a prominent feature. Variable clinical features include pyramidal signs, tremor, dysarthria, dystonia, and mild dementia. There is typically a poor response to levodopa, but clearly at times there is some response, and this can be confusing. Responses are never dramatic and typically unsustained. The pathologic hallmark of the disorder, in addition to neuronal cell loss, is the glial cytoplasmic inclusion (GCI) (Yoshida, 2007). MSA is described in detail in Chapter 9.

Laboratory findings of value are particularly autonomic abnormalities. Studies include the skin sympathetic response, the Valsalva maneuver, and heart rate variation. Rectal sphincter electromyography (EMG) shows denervation, but this test must be done with caution. Women who have been through childbirth may have denervation secondary to their delivery. The specificity of this finding has been called into question. Magnetic resonance imaging (MRI) can show cerebellar and pontine atrophy. The hot-cross bun sign in the pons is due to degeneration of corticocerebellar fibers. Magnetic resonance spectroscopy (MRS) can show decreased N-acetyl aspartate signal in the cerebellum, and positron emission tomography (PET) can show decreased cerebellar metabolism.

Another degenerative cause is progressive myoclonic epilepsy since ataxia is typically a part of this syndrome. Often myoclonus and ataxia become difficult to separate. These syndromes are described in Chapter 20.

Strokes

There are a variety of strokes that produce ataxia. These can be due to lesions of the cerebellum or the cerebellar pathways.

Ataxic hemiparesis is characterized by both weakness and incoordination. Lesions can be in the thalamus and

DOI: 10.1016/B978-1-4377-2369-4.00021-4

Table 21.1 Categories of sporadic ataxia

Degenerative
Stroke
Tumor
Toxic/metabolic
Paraneoplastic
Autoimmune
Infectious/postinfectious
Demyelinating
Other
Ataxia of non-cerebellar origin

Table 21.2 Tumors producing ataxia

Medulloblastoma
Astrocytoma
Ependymoma
Hemangioblastoma
Metastatic tumor
Meningioma
Cerebellopontine angle schwannoma

posterior limb of the internal capsule, upper basis pontis and cerebral peduncle, parietal lobe, and (debated) anterior internal capsule and frontal lobe.

Hemisensory loss and hemiataxia is typically due to a thalamic lesion.

Isolated gait ataxia can be seen with a lesion of the pontomedullary junction.

Ataxia (hemiataxia and/or gait ataxia) with variable cranial nerve involvement can be seen with involvement of several arteries. The superior cerebellar artery affects the upper pontine tegmentum; the anterior inferior cerebellar artery leads to damage of the lateral pontomedullary junction; and the posterior inferior cerebellar artery gives rise to the well-known lateral medullary syndrome.

Tumors

The tumors commonly affecting the cerebellum are listed in Table 21.2.

Toxic/metabolic

Toxic damage to the cerebellum can be caused by alcohol, both acute and chronic. The acute effects of alcohol appear to cause a true ataxia as measured by physiologic studies. In the chronic state, there can be irreversible cerebellar damage, particularly to the cerebellar vermis, leading to particular difficulties with stance and gait. There is also a characteristic prominent anterior-posterior sway when standing.

Hypoxia damages the cerebellum with a particular propensity for the Purkinje cells. These patients may also get myoclonus. Hyperthermia is another cause for Purkinje cell loss.

The childhood hyperammonemias are a cause of intermittent ataxia.

Celiac disease or sprue is an interesting cause of ataxia and possibly myoclonus as well (Hadjivassiliou et al., 1998).

Celiac disease itself is a gluten-sensitive enteropathy with malabsorption. The gastrointestinal disorder can be reversed with a gluten-free diet, but the cerebellar degeneration does not necessarily get better. Curiously, it is now clear that up to 40% of patients with sporadic ataxia have antigliadin antibodies, but no sign of celiac disease (Pellecchia et al., 1999; Burk et al., 2001; Bushara et al., 2001; Hadjivassiliou et al., 2003, 2008c; Lin et al., 2010). This has been disputed, but the power of that study may have been too low (Abele et al., 2003). Antigliadin antibodies have also been seen in a similar percentage of patients with genetic ataxias (Bushara et al., 2001). This has also been disputed (Hadjivassiliou et al., 2003), but the percent abnormal may depend on the numbers of the specific SCA types. It is not clear what this means. In some of these patients, there are abnormalities of the white matter and prominent headache; at least these patients have some symptomatic response to a gluten-free diet (Hadjivassiliou et al., 2001). Antibodies to gangliosides were found in 64% of patients with mixed ataxias, suggesting that the increase in antigliadin antibodies may not be specific (Shill et al., 2003). In gluten-associated ataxia, there can also be antibodies directed to tissue transglutaminase, either type 2 (Hadjivassiliou et al., 2006) or, likely more specifically, type 6 (Hadjivassiliou et al., 2008a). Antigliadin antibodies in patients with ataxia bind to the neural antigen synapsin I (Alaedini et al., 2007). There may well be an increase in autoimmunity in sporadic cerebellar ataxia (Hadjivassiliou et al., 2008b).

There is open-label evidence that a gluten-free diet may benefit patients with antigliadin antibodies (Hadjivassiliou et al., 2008c). Intravenous immunoglobulin (IVIg) has improved the ataxia in three patients with overt celiac disease and ataxia (Souayah et al., 2008). IVIg therapy has appeared to help two patients, as well as two other patients with anti-GAD antibodies (see below for this entity), suggesting a role for immunotherapy (Nanri et al., 2009).

Vitamin deficiencies can cause cerebellar dysfunction including thiamine (vitamin B1), vitamin B12, and vitamin E. Zinc deficiency may also be a culprit.

In the endocrine area, hypothyroidism, hypoparathyroidism, and hypoglycemia (insulinoma) have been associated with ataxia.

Toxic drugs include thallium, bismuth subsalicylate, methyl mercury, methyl bromide, and toluene. Drugs include phenytoin, carbamazepine, barbiturates, lithium, cyclosporine, methotrexate, and 5-fluorouracil. Ataxia can be a component of the serotonin syndrome, from SSRIs (selective serotonin reuptake inhibitors).

Paraneoplastic

The paraneoplastic causes are very important to keep in mind (Anderson et al., 1988; Bolla and Palmer, 1997). The clinical syndrome is often a rapidly progressive one over a relatively short period of time and then a plateau without further change. What appears to be happening is a rapid destruction of Purkinje cells. Even if the cancer is found and successfully treated, the disorder may not improve because the cells are irreversibly damaged. Nevertheless, the best treatment is certainly treatment of the cancer.

In many cases, there will be detectable antibodies in the serum. These antibodies are markers of the cancer and are not specific for cerebellar syndromes. Some cases of paraneo-plastic ataxia have no defined associated antibody.

There are three types of anti-Purkinje cell antibodies. Anti-Yo (PCA-1) is seen with tumors of breast, ovary, and adnexa. Atypical anticytoplasmic antibody (anti-Tr or PCA-Tr) is seen with Hodgkin disease, and tumors of the lung and colon. PCA-2 has been identified mostly with lung tumors; 3 of 10 patients had ataxia (Vernino and Lennon, 2000).

There are three antineuronal antibodies. Anti-Hu (ANNA-1) can be seen in possible conjunction with encephalomy-elitis (Lucchinetti et al., 1998). It is associated with small-cell lung tumor, tumors of breast and prostate, and neuroblast-oma. Anti-Ri (ANNA-2) is found with tumors of breast and ovary. Atypical anti-Hu is seen with tumors of the lung and colon, adenocarcinoma, and lymphoma.

Anti-CV2 (CRMP) antibody is associated with a syndrome of ataxia and optic neuritis (de la Sayette et al., 1998). It has been seen with small-cell lung carcinoma. The CV2 antigen is expressed by oligodendrocytes. Interestingly, this is one syndrome where improvement has been seen with removal of the tumor.

Antibodies directed to a serum protein, Ma1, have been found in patients with testicular and other tumors (Dalmau et al., 1999; Gultekin et al., 2000). The antibodies are anti-Ma and anti-Ta (Ta is Ma2). These patients may also have limbic encephalitis. Ma1 is a phosphoprotein highly limited to brain and testis.

Antibodies directed to amphiphysin are rarely associated with a cerebellar syndrome (Saiz et al., 1999). This is a marker for small-cell lung carcinoma. Antibodies to Zic4 are associated with cerebellar degeneration and small-cell lung cancer (Sabater et al., 2008).

Antibodies against a glutamate receptor can be seen with cancer, and this causes a pure cerebellar syndrome (Sillevis Smitt et al., 2000). Patients with Hodgkin disease can develop paraneoplastic cerebellar ataxia because of the generation of autoantibodies against mGluR1, and this is mediated both by functional and degenerative effects (Coesmans et al., 2003).

Other new antibodies are being identified (Jarius et al., 2010). Tests that are currently commercially available include Hu, Ma, Ta, Yo, Ri, amphiphysin, Zic4 and CV2.

In a series of 50 patients with paraneoplastic cerebellar degeneration out of 137 with any neurologic syndrome, 19 had anti-Yo, 16 anti-Hu, 7 anti-Tr, 6 anti-Ri, and 2 anti-mGluR1 (Shams'ili et al., 2003). While 100% of patients with anti-Yo, anti-Tr, and anti-mGluR1 antibodies had ataxia, 86% of anti-Ri and only 18% of anti-Hu patients had paraneoplastic cerebellar degeneration. In 42 patients (84%), a tumor was detected; the most common were gynecological and breast cancer (anti-Yo and anti-Ri), lung cancer (anti-Hu), and Hodgkin lymphoma (anti-Tr and anti-mGluR1). All patients received antitumor therapy and 7 had some neurologic improvement. The functional outcome was best in the anti-Ri patients, with 3 out of 6 improving neurologi-cally; 5 were able to walk at the time of last follow-up or death. Survival was worse with anti-Yo and anti-Hu com-pared with anti-Tr and anti-Ri.

Autoimmune

Ataxia can be associated with anti-GAD antibodies (Saiz et al., 1997; Abele et al., 1999; Honnorat et al., 2001). There

can be a pure ataxia syndrome and one with an associated peripheral neuropathy. In one series of 14 patients, 13 were women and 11 had late-onset diabetes (Honnorat et al., 2001). Anti-GAD antibodies are better known for association with stiff-person syndrome, but the relationship is not clear. In one case with antibodies in the cerebrospinal fluid, the antibody blocked GABAergic transmission in the rat cerebel-lum (Mitoma et al., 2000). As with stiff-person syndrome, patients can exhibit other forms of autoimmunity. IVIg therapy may be useful (Nanri et al., 2009).

Infectious/postinfectious

Infectious causes include rubella and *Haemophilus influenzae*. Acute postinfectious cerebellitis is generally a childhood condition, most common after varicella. Creutzfeldt–Jakob disease may have an ataxic form.

Demyelinating

Ataxia is common in multiple sclerosis. A patient with leu-koencephalopathy with neuroaxonal spheroids (LENAS), a rare disease of cerebral and cerebellar white matter, had a 14-year course of progressive neurologic decline consistent with a clinical diagnosis of probable MSA, with prominent cerebellar dysfunction and dysautonomia (Moro-De-Casillas et al., 2004).

Other

Other syndromes include Chiari malformation, abscess, hydrocephalus, and superficial central nervous system hemosiderosis.

Ataxia of non-cerebellar origin

What looks like cerebellar ataxia can come from dysfunction outside the cerebellum. Most common causes include neuro-pathies such as the Miller Fisher form of Guillain–Barré syndrome (Lo, 2007) and spinocerebellar tract lesions.

Genetic ataxia

One of the most active areas in movement disorders and genetics is in determining the genes for numerous types of hereditary ataxias. Additionally, we are beginning to under-stand some of the mechanisms of neurodegeneration. On the other hand, specific therapies are still in the future. Many of the genes can be tested commercially. This is helpful, but it is important to remember that genetic testing can have significant consequences, both emotionally and socially – and not only for the individual tested, but also for the family. Hence, testing should be done with care and clear informed consent (Tan and Ashizawa, 2001).

Moseley et al. (1998) determined the incidence of spinoc-erebellar ataxia (SCA) types 1, 2, 3, 6, and 7 and Friedreich ataxia (FA) among a large panel of ataxia families in the United States. They collected DNA samples and clinical data from patients representing 361 families with adult-onset ataxia of unknown etiology. Patients with a clinical diagnosis of FA were specifically excluded. Among the 178 dominant kindreds, they found SCA1 expansion at a frequency of

5.6%, SCA2 expansion at a frequency of 15.2%, SCA3 expansion at a frequency of 20.8%, SCA6 expansion at a frequency of 15.2%, and SCA7 expansion at a frequency of 4.5%. Among patients with apparently recessive or negative family histories of ataxia, 6.8% and 4.4% tested positive for a CAG expansion at one of the dominant loci, and 11.4% and 5.2% of patients with apparently recessive or sporadic forms of ataxia had FA expansions. Among the FA patients, the repeat sizes for one or both FA alleles were relatively small, with sizes for the smaller allele ranging from 90 to 600 GAA repeats. The clinical presentation for these patients was atypical for FA including adult onset of disease, retained tendon reflexes, normal plantar response, and intact or partially intact sensation. The incidence of the SCAs has also been explored in other countries, such as Australia (Storey et al., 2000), Taiwan (Soong et al., 2001), and Thailand (Sura et al., 2009). The pattern does differ somewhat in different countries (Schols et al., 2004). The epidemiologic patterns are updated in the supplementary material in Wardle et al. (2009).

Looking specifically at patients with onset at age 18 or later ("late onset"), a study in the southeast Wales population showed the most frequent defined diagnoses to be SCA6, dentatorubral-pallidoluysian atrophy (DRPLA), and SCA8 (Wardle et al., 2009).

A very detailed compendium of the genetic ataxic disorders can be found at: http://www.neuromuscular.wustl.edu/ataxia/aindex.html.

Here, the principal disorders will be reviewed. There are several good reviews (Di Donato, 1998; Subramony et al., 1999; Evidente et al., 2000; Klockgether, 2000; Stevanin et al., 2000; Devos et al., 2001; Di Donato et al., 2001; Schols et al., 2004; Klockgether, 2008; Manto and Marmolino, 2009; Durr, 2010).

Dominant ataxia

The dominant ataxias were divided into three clinical syndromes by Anita Harding, the autosomal dominant cerebellar ataxias, ADCA I, II, and III. ADCA I is a cerebellar syndrome plus other neurologic degenerations such as pyramidal, extrapyramidal, ophthalmoplegia, and dementia. ADCA II is a cerebellar syndrome with a pigmentary maculopathy. ADCA III is largely a pure cerebellar syndrome, with possible mild pyramidal signs. Subsequently, the genes were identified for these disorders, and they have been called the spinocerebellar ataxias, the SCAs. This terminology is much more common now in clinical use. The identified SCAs are growing rapidly and clearly there are more to be determined.

Table 21.3 gives the identified SCAs and their known genetic disorder. Many of them are due to expanded trinucleotide repeats. SCA3 is identical to Machado–Joseph disease and is often referred to as SCA3/MJD. DRPLA is often included in such lists. It shares the mutation disorder of CAG expansion and may have prominent ataxia as part of its manifestation. Some details about the proteins are known and these are listed in Table 21.4.

Commercial tests are available for SCA1, 2, 3, 5, 6, 7, 8, 10, 12, 13, 14, 17, and DRPLA (and this list is likely to expand).

Generally, the cerebellar syndrome is similar in the different disorders. Patients experience gradual onset of balance and gait difficulty, dysarthria and clumsiness of the hands. There may be visual symptoms such as blurry vision or diplopia. Age of onset is highly variable. Sometimes clinical features can help differentiate the different disorders. SCA12, for example, may be somewhat unique in that it may present with an action tremor that may look like essential tremor (O'Hearn et al., 2001). Other manifestations may help predict the genotype, but virtually any constellation of signs and symptoms can occur with any phenotype. Some guidelines are noted below.

Lining up the ADCAs and the SCAs gives a start (Table 21.5). Subramony has suggested some phenotypic clues (Subramony et al., 1999), and these are updated in Table 21.6.

DRPLA is most common in the Japanese. It is also known as the Haw River syndrome from an African-American family in North Carolina. In addition to ataxia, there may be myoclonus, epilepsy, chorea, athetosis, dystonia, dementia, psychiatric disorders, and parkinsonism.

The pathophysiology of the triplet repeat ataxias has been extensively studied (Koeppen, 2005; Paulson, 2007; Soong and Paulson, 2007; Zoghbi and Orr, 2009). It appears that the mutated protein is toxic to the cell. For example, in a mouse model of SCA1, the gene was made conditional; when the gene was turned off, the animals improved (Zu et al., 2004). Similarly, treatment of a mouse model of SCA1 with RNA interference (RNAi) can improve the disorder. Recombinant adeno-associated virus vectors expressing short hairpin RNAs were injected into the cerebellum with marked benefit (Xia et al., 2004).

There is no treatment for the SCAs. Lithium improved neurologic function and hippocampal dendritic arborization in a mouse model of SCA1 (Watase et al., 2007). Mode of action of lithium in this circumstance is not clear. Human studies have been initiated.

Then there are the autosomal dominant episodic ataxias (Table 21.7) (Evidente et al., 2000; Kullmann et al., 2001; Jen, 2008; Tomlinson et al., 2009).

EA-1 is associated with interictal myokymia. There are brief attacks of ataxia and dysarthria lasting seconds to minutes precipitated by exercise or startle. Onset is in childhood or early adolescence. The myokymia is prominent around the eyes, lips or in the fingers. The myokymia may respond to phenytoin and the ataxia to acetazolamide.

EA-2 has intermittent attacks of ataxia, dysarthria, nausea, vertigo, diplopia, and oscillopsia lasting minutes to days. There may be interictal nystagmus or mild ataxia. Episodes are provoked by stress and exercise, but not startle. About half of the patients also have migraine. The attacks may respond to acetazolamide. The potassium channel blocker 4-aminopyridine can also be effective (Strupp et al., 2004). The gene for EA-2 is the same as the gene for SCA6, but the nature of the mutation differs. A different missense or truncation mutation in this gene causes familial hemiplegic migraine. There can be phenotypic overlaps between all three conditions. Two patients have been described that progressed to a late life dystonia (Spacey et al., 2005). Such patients may also have weakness; a disorder at the neuromuscular junction has been demonstrated with single fiber EMG (Jen et al., 2001; Maselli et al., 2003).

EA-3, called periodic vestibulocerebellar ataxia, is an autosomal dominant disorder characterized by defective smooth

Table 21.3 The SCAs

Name	Chromosome	Mutation	Normal repeat number	Range of repeats in the disorder
SCA1	6p23	CAG expansion	6–44	40–83
SCA2	12q24	CAG expansion	14–31	34–59
SCA3	14q32	CAG expansion	12–38	56–86
SCA4	16q22			
SCA5	11q13	Deletion or point mutation		
SCA6	19p13	CAG expansion	4–20	21–31
SCA7	3p14	CAG expansion	7–17	38–>200
SCA8	13q21	CTG expansion	15–91	100–155
SCA9	Not linked			
SCA10	22q13	ATTCT repeat	10–22	800–3800
SCA11	15q14			
SCA12	5q31	CAG expansion	<29	66–93
SCA13	19q13			
SCA14	19q13.4–qter	Point mutation		
SCA15, 16, 29?	3p26	Deletion or point mutation		
SCA17	6q27	CAG expansion	25–42	45–63
SCA18	7q31			
SCA19, 22	1p21–q21			
SCA20	11			
SCA21	7p21			
SCA23	20p13–12.2			
(SCA24)	Now SCAR4			
SCA25	2p15–p21			
SCA26	19p13			
SCA27	13q34	Point mutation		
SCA28	18p11			
SCA29	3p26			
SCA30	4q34			
SCA31 (SCA4)	16q22	Point mutation		
DRPLA	12p13	CAG expansion	3–36	49–88

pursuit, gaze-evoked nystagmus, ataxia, and vertigo (Damji et al., 1996).

EA-4 is characterized by vestibular ataxia, vertigo, tinnitus, and interictal myokymia; attacks are diminished by acetazolamide (Steckley et al., 2001).

Episodic ataxia with paroxysmal choreoathetosis and spasticity has age of onset of 2–15 years (Auburger et al., 1996). There are attacks of ataxia, with involuntary movements and dystonia of extremities, paresthesias, and headache. Episodes last about 20 minutes and occur twice per day to twice per year. Precipitating factors include alcohol, fatigue, emotional stress, and physical exercise. In some there is spastic paraplegia which may persist between attacks. Treatment is with acetazolamide.

EA-5 has been identified in one family and is due to a mutation in a calcium channel gene (Escayg et al., 2000). In other families with a mutation in this gene, there is epilepsy.

Recessive ataxia

There are a large number of recessive ataxias. The most common of these are discussed here, but even many of these are rare. The ones discussed in this chapter are summarized

Table 21.4 The proteins that are affected in the SCAs

Name	Protein
SCA1	Ataxin-1
SCA2	Ataxin-2
SCA3 (Machado–Joseph disease)	Ataxin-3
SCA4 (with sensory axonal neuropathy)	
SCA5 (Lincoln ataxia)	Beta III spectrin (SPTBN2)
SCA6	α_{1a} component of the voltage-dependent calcium channel: CACNL1A4
SCA7	Ataxin-7
SCA8	(mutation is in noncoding region)
SCA9	
SCA10	Ataxin-10
SCA11	Tau tubulin kinase 2 (TTBK2)
SCA12	Protein phosphatase 2A, regulatory subunit B (PPP2R2B)
SCA13	KCNC3
SCA14	Protein kinase Cγ (PRKCG)
SCA15, 16, 29?	Inositol 1,4,5-triphosphate receptor, type 1 (ITPR1)
SCA17 (also called HDL4)	TATA binding protein (TBP)
SCA18 (with sensorimotor neuropathy)	
SCA19	
SCA20	
SCA21	
SCA22	
SCA23	
(SCA24) Now SCAR4	
SCA25 (with sensory neuropathy)	
SCA26	
SCA27	Fibroblast growth factor 14 (FGF14)
SCA28	ATPase family gene 3-like 2 (AFG3L2)
SCA29 (congenital, non-progressive)	
SCA30	
SCA31 (Japanese form of SCA4)	Pleckstrin homology domain-containing protein, family G, member 4 (PLEKHG4, puratrophin-1)
DRPLA	Atrophin-1 or DRPLA protein

Table 21.5 Relationship between ADCAs and SCAs

ADCA type	SCA type
I (ataxia plus)	1, 2, 3, 4, 8, 9, 12, 17, 27, 28, DRPLA
II (with pigmentary maculopathy)	7
III (pure ataxia)	5, 6, 11, 14, 15, 16, 22, 26, 30, 31
Ataxia and epilepsy	10
Early onset with learning disability	13

Table 21.6 Clues to the SCAs

Age at onset	Young adult: SCA1, 2, 3, 21 Older adult: SCA6 Childhood onset: SCA2, 7, 13, 25, 27, DRPLA
Prominent anticipation	SCA7, DRPLA
Upper motor neuron signs	SCA1, 3, 7,12 Some in SCA6, 8 Rare in SCA2
Slow saccades	Early, prominent: SCA2, 7 Late: SCA1, 3, 28 Rare: SCA6
Extrapyramidal signs	Early chorea: DRPLA Akinetic-rigid, Parkinson: SCA2, 3, 12, 21
Generalized areflexia	SCA2, 4, 19, 21, 22 Late: SCA3 Rare: SCA1
Visual loss	SCA7
Dementia	Prominent: SCA17, DRPLA Early: SCA2, 7 Otherwise: rare
Myoclonus	DRPLA, SCA2, 14, 19
Tremor	SCA2, 8, 12, 15, 16, 19, 27
Seizures	SCA10

in Table 21.8. Others can be found in the genetics table in Chapter 1 (Table 1.5). The full list of designated autosomal recessive ataxias (SCAR) and ataxias with spasticity (SPAX) can be found there. The terminology is rather complex and some disorders have multiple names from appearing in multiple lists. Another abbreviation for autosomal recessive ataxia is ARCA, and below it will be noted that ARCA1 is SCAR8 and ARCA2 is SCAR9.

Friedreich ataxia (FA)

The major autosomal recessive ataxia to consider is FA, the most common cause of hereditary ataxia with a prevalence of about 1 in 50 000 persons (Bradley et al., 2000; Evidente et al., 2000; Pandolfo, 2008; Schulz et al., 2009a). Age of onset is generally before 20 years. The clinical features, in addition to ataxia, are dysarthria, sensory loss, and

Table 21.7 The episodic ataxias

Name	Chromosome	Mutation	Protein
EA type 1 (with myokymia)	12p13	Missense	Potassium channel, KCNA1
EA type 2 (with nystagmus)	19p13	Missense	α_{1a} component of the voltage dependent calcium channel: CACNL1A4
EA type 3 (with vertigo and tinnitus)	1q42		
EA type 4 (PATX)			
EA type 5	2q22		CACNB4β4
EA type 6 (with migraine)	5p13		SLC1A3
EA type 7	19q13		
EA with paroxysmal choreoathetosis and spasticity	1p		

Table 21.8 Some recessive ataxias

Name	Chromosome	Mutation	Protein
Friedreich ataxia (FA)	9q13	Trinucleotide repeat of GAA (some point mutations)	Frataxin
Friedreich ataxia 2 (FA2)	9p23		
Ataxia with isolated vitamin E deficiency (AVED)	8q13	Point mutations and deletions	α-Tocopherol transfer protein (TTP1)
Abetalipoproteinemia	4q22	Point mutation, deletion	Microsomal triglyceride transfer protein (MTP)
Ataxia telangiectasia	11q22	Chromosome breaks	ATM gene that codes for the protein kinase PI-3
(Early onset) ataxia with oculomotor apraxia type 1 (AOA1)	9p13	Insertion, deletion, point mutation	Aprataxin (APTX)
(Early onset) ataxia with oculomotor apraxia type 2 (AOA2) (SCAR1)	9q34	Point mutation, deletion	Senataxin (SETX)
Autosomal recessive spastic ataxia of Charlevoix–Saguenay (ARSACS)	13q12	Deletions, point mutations	SACS gene that codes for sacsin
Cayman ataxia (ATCAY)	19p13	Point mutations	ATCAY gene that codes for caytaxin
Marinesco–Sjögren Syndrome (MSS)	5q31	Various	SIL1
Mitochondrial recessive ataxia syndrome (MIRAS)	15q25	Point mutation	POLG1, a catalytic subunit of the mitochondrial DNA polymerase gamma
Spinocerebellar ataxia with axonal neuropathy (SCAN1)	14q31	Point mutation	Tyrosyl-DNA phosphodiesterase (TDP1)
ARCA1 (SCAR8)	6q25	Point mutation, deletions	Synaptic nuclear envelope protein 1 (SYNE1)
ARCA2 (SCAR9)	1q41	Point mutations	CABC1 (ADCK3)
Familial cerebellar ataxia with muscle coenzyme Q10 deficiency			Some patients have AOA1 or ARCA2

corticospinal tract signs with absent reflexes. There is an axon loss peripheral neuropathy. There may be skeletal abnormalities such as kyphoscoliosis, cardiomyopathy, and diabetes. The cardiomyopathy is hypertrophic with possible associated muscular subaortic stenosis or hypokinetic-dilated left ventricle. Abnormal ECGs are common.

The genetic abnormality is usually an expanded trinucleotide repeat of GAA in a gene on chromosome 9q coding for the protein called frataxin, and a commercial genetic test is available. Normal repeat length is 6–28, and patients have 66–1700. Six percent of the time there is a point mutation. Frataxin is a mitochondrial protein encoded by nuclear

DNA. It is believed that frataxin is involved in iron transport, and in FA there is excessive iron accumulation in mitochondria. Using functional MRI, increased iron has been detected in patients in the dentate nucleus (Waldvogel et al., 1999). The excess iron may lead to toxic free radical damage. There are significant reductions in the activities of complex I, complex II/III, and aconitase in FA heart muscle (Bradley et al., 2000).

For treatment, there has been considerable enthusiasm for idebenone, a molecule structurally related to coenzyme Q10. Early studies showed that it could reduce heart size and improve cardiac function, but without clear effect on the ataxia (Rustin et al., 1999; Lerman-Sagie et al., 2001; Hausse et al., 2002; Rustin et al., 2002; Buyse et al., 2003, Mariotti et al., 2003). There are also negative studies on cardiac function (Schols et al., 2001). Some studies, in children and using higher doses, have begun to show beneficial effects on the ataxia. In an open-label trial of 9 patients, age range 11–19 years, treated with idebenone at 5 mg/kg/day, there was a significant reduction in ataxia scores after 3 months of treatment (Artuch et al., 2002). In a subsequent long-term study with 5–20 mg/kg/day by this same group over a 3–5-year period, 10 children in the age range of 8–18 years showed stable neurologic function (Pineda et al., 2008). Adults of age 18–46 over the same period showed neurologic deterioration.

In another study, 48 FA patients, aged 9–17 years, were enrolled in a 6-month, randomized, double-blind, placebo-controlled study (Di Prospero et al., 2007). The patients received placebo or one of three doses of idebenone (approximately 5 mg/kg, 15 mg/kg, and 45 mg/kg). Whereas an overall analysis did not show a significant neurologic improvement, there were indications of a dose-dependent response. A secondary analysis, excluding patients who required wheelchair assistance, showed a significant improvement in the ICARS (International Cooperative Ataxia Rating Scale). The authors suggested that higher doses may be necessary to have a beneficial effect on neurologic function. Further trials are ongoing (Schulz et al., 2009b), but it is not clear that the drug will really have an impact on quality of life (Brandsema et al., 2010).

There are also some attempts at treatment using coenzyme Q10. Cardiac muscle 31P-MRS has been demonstrated to improve with combination therapy with coenzyme Q10 (CoQ10) and vitamin E (Lodi et al., 2001). Some of these patients were followed for 4 years, and a few of them had suggestive benefit with less progression than predicted (Hart et al., 2005).

There are other approaches being considered in treatment of FA also (Mancuso et al., 2010). Because of the mitochondrial iron accumulation, iron chelation might be useful. A 6-month trial of deferiprone was conducted in nine adolescents (Boddaert et al., 2007). By MRI, there was reduction of iron in the dentate nucleus, and the youngest patients may have had some neurologic improvement. Histone deacetylase (HDAC) inhibitors may increase frataxin expression and this has been tested in a mouse model (Rai et al., 2008).

Now that the gene can be identified, the phenotype has been widened in recent years. (1) Late-onset FA with age of onset more than 25 characterized by a more benign course; (2) FA with retained reflexes (FARR); and (3) the Acadian or Louisiana form with slower progression (Evidente et al., 2000). FA can even present with peripheral neuropathy alone, without ataxia (Panas et al., 2002).

A second gene was identified whose mutation can lead to classic FA. This has been localized to chromosome 9p (Christodoulou et al., 2001).

Ataxia with isolated vitamin E deficiency (AVED)

This is a rare, but important, disorder that has a phenotype similar to FA (Di Donato et al., 2010). Additionally, there can be ophthalmoplegia and retinitis pigmentosa. This disorder is due to a defect in the TTP1 gene coding for α-tocopherol transfer protein. This protein incorporates α-tocopherol into lipoproteins secreted by the liver. As in the conditions when vitamin E is deficient because of malabsorption, this disorder can be treated with vitamin E (Gabsi et al., 2001). It should not be missed!

Abetalipoproteinemia

Abetalipoproteinemia is a rare autosomal recessive deficiency of apoB-containing lipoproteins caused by a microsomal triglyceride transfer protein (MTP) deficiency. Coming on in teenage years or early adulthood, the syndrome is due to vitamin E deficiency. The main characteristics are ataxia and polyneuropathy, as well as acanthocytosis, celiac syndrome, and retinal degeneration (Triantafillidis et al., 1998). It should be treated with high doses of vitamin E.

Ataxia telangectasia (AT)

This disorder is due to a mutation in the ATM gene that codes for a protein kinase that plays an important role in cell cycle control, apoptosis, and DNA double-strand break repair. This abnormality leads to increased incidence of malignancy as well as neurodegeneration. The mutations are scattered over the gene. The disorder begins early in childhood, often age 1–2 years (Woods and Taylor, 1992; Di Donato et al., 2001). There is ataxia, truncal more than appendicular, and dysarthria. Oculomotor apraxia – difficulty in initiating saccades – occurs early. Many other features are associated such as dystonia, masked facies, choreoathetosis, myoclonus, tremor, long tract signs and, eventually, peripheral neuropathy and cognitive decline. There are the well-known oculocutaneous telangectasias as well as immunodeficiencies with reduced immunoglobulins and T-cell deficiencies, recurrent sinopulmonary infections, and malignancies, particularly leukemia or lymphoma. Alpha-fetoprotein levels are elevated and chromosome breaks can be identified.

Early-onset ataxia with ocular motor apraxia and hypoalbuminemia (EAOH or AOA1 and AOA2)

Two disorders recognized in Japan, early-onset ataxia with hypoalbuminemia and ataxia with ocular motor apraxia are now considered the same clinical entity because of the identification of a common mutation in the aprataxin gene (APTX). In six patients from four families, cerebellar ataxia and peripheral neuropathy were noted in all, ocular motor apraxia was observed in five patients, and choreiform movements of the limbs and mental deterioration were observed in five patients (Shimazaki et al., 2002). All patients had hypoalbuminemia and hypercholesterolemia; brain MRI or

CT showed marked cerebellar atrophy. Nerve biopsy revealed depletion of large myelinated fibers in three of the five patients examined. Many other patients have been described (D'Arrigo et al., 2008). This disorder is also common in Portugal, but rare in Germany (Habeck et al., 2004). Genetic testing is available. Ataxia with oculomotor apraxia type 2 (AOA2) has also been identified with a similar clinical picture but with mutations in the senataxin (*SETX*) gene (Criscuolo et al., 2006). In a series of 19 patients, other features noted were a frequent polyneuropathy and elevation of the serum alpha-fetoprotein (Tazir et al., 2009). The *SETX* gene is also mutated in ALS4, a motor neuron disorder with early onset, and some patients may share this phenotype (Schols et al., 2008).

Autosomal recessive spastic ataxia of Charlevoix–Saguenay (ARSACS)

This disorder of ataxia and pyramidal signs with high prevalence in northeastern Quebec is due to a mutation in the gene, *SACS*, that codes for a protein sacsin (Engert et al., 2000). Even in Quebec, the clinical syndrome is genetically heterogeneous (Thiffault et al., 2006).

Although this entity has been thought to be geographically distinct, a family in Tunisia was identified with the disorder (Mrissa et al., 2000), and more cases with variable phenotype are also being recognized (Takiyama, 2007). Commercial genetic testing is available for this disorder.

Cayman ataxia

Cayman ataxia is a recessive congenital ataxia restricted to one area of Grand Cayman Island that appears to be due to one of two mutations (Bomar et al., 2003). The gene *ATCAY* or *Atcay* encodes a neuron-restricted protein called caytaxin. Caytaxin contains a CRAL-TRIO motif common to proteins that bind small lipophilic molecules. Mutations in caytaxin are also responsible for the jittery mouse. Mutations in another protein containing a CRAL-TRIO domain, alpha-tocopherol transfer protein (TTPA), cause a vitamin E-responsive ataxia.

Marinesco–Sjögren syndrome (MSS)

This syndrome is characterized by ataxia, cataracts from infancy, learning disability, myopathy, and short stature. Mutations in the gene for SIL1, a protein in the endoplasmic reticulum, cause the disorder (Senderek et al., 2005). SIL1 appears to function as a nucleotide exchange factor for the heat-shock protein 70 (HSP70) (Anttonen et al., 2005).

Mitochondrial recessive ataxia syndrome (MIRAS)

Most commonly mutations in POLG1, a catalytic subunit of the mitochondrial DNA polymerase gamma, produce progressive weakness of the eye muscles, dysphagia, and some somatic weakness (Cagnoli et al., 2008). Particularly in Finland, mutations can also cause ataxia, perhaps with sensory axonal peripheral neuropathy (Hakonen et al., 2005). An alternate phenotype is SANDO (sensory ataxia, neuropathy, dysarthria, and ophthalmoparesis). A wide spectrum of neurologic disease can be produced by mutations in POLG1 (Milone and Massie, 2010; Tzoulis et al., 2010).

Spinocerebellar ataxia with axonal neuropathy (SCAN1)

This disorder appears due to a mutation in tyrosyl-DNA phosphodiesterase (TDP1), a protein in the DNA repair pathway (Takashima et al., 2002; Hirano et al., 2007).

Autosomal recessive cerebellar ataxia type 1 (ARCA1)

This syndrome is characterized by middle-age onset, slow progression and moderate disability, significant dysarthria, mild oculomotor abnormalities, occasional brisk reflexes in the lower extremities, normal nerve conduction studies, and diffuse cerebellar atrophy on imaging (Dupre et al., 2007). SYNE1 mutations are causative (Gros-Louis et al., 2007).

Autosomal recessive cerebellar ataxia type 2 (ARCA2)

These patients present with progressive ataxia characterized by cerebellar atrophy and seizures, and studies suggestive of coenzyme Q10 deficiency including mildly elevated lactate levels (Lagier-Tourenne et al., 2008; Mollet et al., 2008). Mutations in the same gene were found by two groups, one that called it the *CABC1* gene (Mollet et al., 2008) and the other referring to it as the *ADCK3* gene (Lagier-Tourenne et al., 2008).

Familial cerebellar ataxia with muscle coenzyme Q10 deficiency

Six patients with muscle CoQ10 deficiency (26–35% of normal) presented with cerebellar ataxia, pyramidal signs, and seizures (Musumeci et al., 2001). All six patients responded to CoQ10 supplementation; strength increased, ataxia improved, and seizures became less frequent. In a study of muscle biopsies in 135 patients with undefined cerebellar ataxia, 13 were found to have deficient CoQ10 (Lamperti et al., 2003). The mutation in one family was in the aprataxin gene (Quinzii et al., 2005). This diagnosis is a potentially important cause of familial ataxia because it is at least partially treatable (Artuch et al., 2006). The disorder appears to be recessive, the gene defect is not identified in all cases (Montero et al., 2007), but some of these patients certainly have ARCA2.

Frequency of the autosomal recessive ataxias

In a review of 102 patients with autosomal recessive (or sporadic) ataxia, a diagnosis was made in 57 of them; 36 were affected with FA, seven with AOA2, four with AT, three with AOA1, three with MSS, two with ARSACS, one with AVED, and one with ARCA2 (Anheim et al., 2010). Genetic testing is currently available for FA, AVED, MSS, AOA1, AOA2 and MIRAS.

X-linked ataxia

Fragile X-associated tremor/ataxia syndrome (FXTAS)

Attention has been drawn to the fact that the fragile X premutation has been associated with tremor with appearance

Table 21.9 Evaluation of the ataxic patient

Good history and physical exam including a careful family history
Standard laboratory tests including lipids and thyroid function
MRI (and PET and/or MRS if available)
Autonomic testing, sphincter EMG
Genetic testing
Toxic screen, vitamin levels (especially E)
Paraneoplastic antibodies, antigliadin antibodies

similar to essential tremor (Leehey et al., 2003; Amiri et al., 2008). Ataxia and executive dysfunction are also prominent in this disorder (Hagerman and Hagerman, 2004). Women can be affected as well as men (Hagerman et al., 2004). FXTAS has a similar clinical appearance to MSA, but in a review of 77 patients with an MSA diagnosis, only one person was identified with FXTAS (Biancalana et al., 2005); in another review of 426 patients, only 4 had the premutation (Kamm et al., 2005). Continuing studies show this disorder to be rare (Reis et al., 2008). The neuropathology of this syndrome is characterized by intranuclear inclusions (Greco et al., 2006). An increased signal in the middle cerebellar peduncle can sometimes be seen by MRI.

Diagnostic plan

In the evaluation of a patient with ataxia, Table 21.9 outlines a reasonable approach. After a good history and physical examination, laboratory tests should be done to follow up clinical suspicions. A nice algorithm is presented by Schulz et al., (2009a). A detailed algorithm for recessive or sporadic ataxia is presented by Anheim et al. (2010).

Recovery from cerebellar injury; therapy

Chronic signs and symptoms of cerebellar injury differ from those of the acute phase and signs may disappear entirely, especially when cerebellar damage is sustained early in life or is limited in extent. In general, recovery from lesions limited to regions of the cerebellar cortex, especially of the lateral hemispheres, is potentially greater than lesions that affect the deep nuclei. This may be due to plasticity at other sites within and outside the cerebellum, combined with the fact that cerebral repercussions of cerebellar injury may not be especially apparent on conventional testing.

Weakness, deconditioning, and spasticity are often seen in conjunction with ataxia and contribute substantially to its morbidity. All other factors being equal, stronger, more athletic individuals tend to tolerate moderate ataxia better. Specific physical treatments for ataxia with the application of weights might be helpful. The use of added mass to treat certain tremors has a sound mechanical basis. Because the addition of mass lowers the resonant frequency of a limb, it reduces its response to high-frequency oscillating driving signals. Indeed, Hewer et al. (1972) found better results in patients who had a tremor frequency greater than 7 Hz. In general, the more severe the tremor in terms of amplitude,

the more weight was needed to obtain improvement. With regard to ataxia, up to a point, additional mass also improved ataxia of arm movement and of gait. However, beyond this, increased weight was associated with poorer performance. The optimal weight value varied by individual and was not clearly related to the severity of ataxia. Within the limits of fatigue tolerance, which unfortunately may pose a significant restriction, weight therapy remains a reasonable treatment option for some patients. It is also possible to use devices with incorporated viscous damping (Aisen et al., 1993).

Pharmacologic therapy has been reviewed (Ogawa, 2004), and there has been an evidence-based review (Trujillo-Martin et al., 2009). Unfortunately, there are not any excellent treatments and the evidence itself is generally limited.

Several agents have been reported to show some ataxia-ameliorating effects. Botez et al. (1996) found low levels of the dopamine metabolite homovanillic acid in the cerebrospinal fluid of patients with FA and olivopontocerebellar atrophy. In a double-blind trial, amantadine produced significant improvements in both movement time and reaction time in patients (Botez et al., 1996). Unfortunately, this was not associated with functional improvement. Research conducted largely in Japan has emphasized the potential utility of thyrotropin releasing hormone (TRH) and many analogs in cerebellar ataxia (Sobue et al., 1983), but these results are generally not dramatic and have not been widely reproduced.

The dense and widespread distribution of serotonergic terminals throughout the cerebellum and spinocerebellar tracts suggests that serotonin plays a major role in regulating cerebellar functions. While some studies have shown benefit in ataxic patients from oral administration of L-5-hydroxytryptophan (L-5-HTP) (Trouillas et al., 1995), there have also been a number of negative results (Wessel et al., 1995). Moreover, L-5-HTP has been associated with a somewhat high rate of unpleasant gastrointestinal side effects, chiefly nausea and diarrhea, even when administered with a peripheral decarboxylase blocker. In addition, L-5-HTP has been associated with a syndrome resembling eosinophilia–myalgia although the possible role of contaminants in the preparation has not been fully determined (Michelson et al., 1994). Some attention has shifted toward trials of alternative serotonin agonists. Buspirone is a selective serotonin 1A receptor agonist which has been found by Lou et al. (1995) in an open-label study and Trouillas et al. (1997) in both an open and in a randomized double-blind study to produce some small benefit. There has been a double-blind study at NINDS with negative results (Massaquoi et al., unpublished). Ondansetron, a 5-HT$_3$ antagonist, may help some patients (Mandelcorn et al., 2004).

There have been reports of a small but persistent improvement in ataxia, and possibly arrest of symptom progression in patients treated with physostigmine, either orally or via a transdermal patch (Aschoff et al., 1996), but double-blind studies have failed to demonstrate significant benefit (Wessel et al., 1997). In anecdotal reports (Helveston et al., 1996a, 1996b; Hurd et al., 1996), the antioxidant N-acetylcysteine has been reported to improve ataxia along with a number of other problems in different ataxias, but controlled trials have not been done. There is a double-blind crossover trial of branched-chain amino acid therapy which has suggested some improvement over a 4-week period (Mori et al., 2002).

The proposed explanation of efficacy is that this therapy improved glutamatergic transmission in the cerebellum. A small trial of D-cycloserine was successful (Ogawa et al., 2003), and one patient improved significantly on piracetam (Vural et al., 2003). In an open trial, 10 patients were improved with gabapentin (Gazulla et al., 2004).

Three patients with different types of ataxia have responded favorably to varenicline (Zesiewicz and Sullivan, 2008; Zesiewicz et al., 2009). Varenicline is a highly selective partial agonist at $\alpha_4\beta_2$ nicotinic acetylcholine receptors and a full agonist at α_7 nicotinic receptors. There are acetylcholine receptors in the cerebellum, and stimulation of $\alpha_4\beta_2$ nicotinic acetylcholine receptors can improve alcohol-induced ataxia in an animal model. However, the mechanism of action is not at all certain for any symptomatic effect should this prove useful.

Riluzole has shown some efficacy in a randomized, double-blind, placebo-controlled trial of 40 patients presenting with cerebellar ataxias of different etiologies. Patients were treated with riluzole (100 mg/day) or placebo for 8 weeks. The number of patients with an improvement in ataxia was significantly higher in the riluzole group (Ristori et al., 2010).

Surgical ablation or high-frequency electrical stimulation of the ventral intermediate nucleus of the thalamus (VIM) can be effective in reducing cerebellar tremor (Narabayashi, 1992; Nguyen and Degos, 1993); however, these procedures do not significantly lessen ataxia.

References available on Expert Consult: www.expertconsult.com

CHAPTER **22**

The paroxysmal dyskinesias

Chapter contents

Introduction	476	Paroxysmal exertional dyskinesia (PED)	490
Definitions: transient, paroxysmal, episodic, and periodic	477	Episodic ataxias	491
Historical aspects	477	Molecular genetics of paroxysmal dyskinesias	493
Classification of the paroxysmal dyskinesias	482	Miscellany	494
Paroxysmal kinesigenic dyskinesia (PKD)	483	Summary	495
Paroxysmal nonkinesigenic dyskinesia (PNKD)	487		

Introduction

The overwhelming majority of individuals with hyperkinetic movement disorders have symptoms that are continuous or continual (e.g., chorea, dystonia, tardive dyskinesia), except for relief with sleep, and with some variation in intensity during periods of stress and relaxation, or other factors such as voluntary movements (e.g., action dystonia, intention myoclonus, intention tremor) or maintaining certain postures (e.g., essential tremor). The symptoms and signs of dopa-responsive dystonia sometimes have a diurnal pattern, being absent or slight in the morning hours and becoming more pronounced as the day proceeds (see Chapter 12). Some dyskinesias (Table 22.1) are characterized as occurring intermittently, such as myoclonus (Fahn et al., 1986; Hallett et al., 1987) and startle syndromes (hyperekplexia) (Andermann and Andermann, 1986) that can be triggered by a variety of stimuli. Restless legs syndrome is best described as a diurnal disorder, manifesting itself primarily (1) in the evenings with abnormal crawling sensations that are relieved by the patient moving about and (2) during the night with periodic movements in sleep (Hening et al., 1986; Walters et al., 1991). Sandifer syndrome is a tilting downwards of the head after eating a meal, occurring in boys, and associated with gastroesophageal reflux (Menkes and Ament, 1988). Movements that occur as a result of akathisia relieve the sensation of inner restlessness. These movements occur intermittently and are usually complex (see Chapter 19). Stereotypies are also complex movements, which appear largely in individuals with learning disability, autism, and schizophrenia (Fahn, 1993). They are not always present but occur frequently and almost continually, but in some patients they appear as intermittent bursts (Tan et al., 1997). The explanation as to why these patients make these movements

is not known, but suggestions such as "being in touch with the environment" have been proposed. Perhaps the commonest dyskinesias that occur intermittently are tics, which are suppressible to varying degrees (Koller and Biary, 1989). Although tics and myoclonic jerks, since they commonly occur out of a normal background, could possibly be considered paroxysmal, this term is usually reserved for an entirely different set of hyperkinetic movement disorders, which is the topic of this chapter. The term paroxysmal dyskinesia has been applied to these disorders.

The common neurologic paroxysmal disorders are epilepsy and migraine. Movement disorders that appear "out of the blue" and are transient and recurring are uncommon, and often present to the clinician as confusing diagnostic problems. Not uncommonly, the history that is provided by the patient does not convey the information that the episodes of abnormal movements occur at intermittent intervals, and the clinician might overlook the category of paroxysmal dyskinesias. Therefore, if the examination does not reveal the presence of a movement disorder, the clinician needs to consider the possibility that he or she is dealing with a paroxysmal dyskinesia, and thereby ask the appropriate questions that can lead to the proper diagnosis. To compound the problem, nonfamilial paroxysmal movement disorders are often psychogenic in etiology (Bressman et al., 1988); therefore, the clinician has the problem of determining the etiologic distinction of psychogenic versus organic.

The pathophysiology of paroxysmal dyskinesias is not understood, and "epilepsy of the basal ganglia" has been a serious consideration but difficult to prove. Some paroxysmal dyskinesias are supplementary sensorimotor seizures, including many of the hypnogenic variety (Lüders, 1996). The classification of the paroxysmal dyskinesias is still incomplete and evolving (Demirkiran and Jankovic, 1995),

DOI: 10.1016/B978-1-4377-2369-4.00022-6

Table 22.1 Classic movement disorders that usually appear in bursts or with specific actions, but are not considered paroxysmal dyskinesias

1. Action dystonia
2. Action myoclonus
3. Action and intention tremors
4. Arrhythmic myoclonus
5. Hyperekplexia
6. Periodic movements in sleep
7. Restless legs syndrome
8. Sandifer syndrome
9. Akathitic movements
10. Stereotypies
11. Tics

The movements usually occur so frequently that they are not distinguished with a "paroxysmal" label.

Table 22.2 Transient movement disorders in children (clinic of Fernandez-Alvarez, 1998)

Benign paroxysmal torticollis in infancy
Benign paroxysmal tonic upgaze
Benign myoclonus of the newborn
Benign myoclonus of infancy
Essential palatal myoclonus
Jitteriness
Shuddering
Spasmus nutans
Transient idiopathic dystonia of infancy
Transient tic

and treatment for many of them is often unsuccessful, but treatment for some can be highly successful. A most welcome burst of research on the genetics of the paroxysmal dyskinesias is shedding new light in the classification of these disorders (Nutt and Gancher, 1997), their diagnoses, and their mechanism of action as channelopathies (Griggs and Nutt, 1995) now that the genes that have so far been discovered for these disorders are those that code for some of the ion channels.

Definitions: transient, paroxysmal, episodic, and periodic

Some pediatric neurologists have utilized the term "transient" for a number of movement disorders in children, but the concept of paroxysmal dyskinesias is becoming more widely recognized among pediatric neurologists (Lotze and Jankovic, 2003). Excluding tic disorders, Fernandez-Alvarez (1998) reviewed the 356 movement disorder cases under the age of 18 years that had been seen in his department's clinic and reported that 19% of them were classified as transient dyskinesias (Table 22.2). Sometimes these transient movements can be mistaken for seizures (Donat and Wright, 1990). An accurate diagnosis can be reassuring to the family because these movements are not seizures and are almost always benign. The diagnosis depends on the clinical features; diagnostic tests are normal and unnecessary.

Kotagal and colleagues (2002) evaluated their cases of paroxysmal nonepileptic events. These are reviewed in Chapter 25. These were most common in adolescents and the school-age group. In the preschool group, the most common diagnoses were stereotypies, hypnic jerks, parasomnias, and Sandifer syndrome.

It is not clear how the label "paroxysmal" became the most common terminology applied to the group of dyskinesias of the choreoathetotic and dystonic type and the label "episodic" became commonly used for the ataxic variety. According to *Dorland's Medical Dictionary* a paroxysm is defined as (1) a sudden recurrence or intensification of symptoms and (2) a spasm or seizure. *Webster's Third International Dictionary* gives a similar definition. "Episodic" is not listed in

Dorland's; Webster's defines "episodic" as occurring, appearing, or changing at usually, irregular intervals. This definition is not very different from the definition of paroxysmal, except that the latter includes the word "sudden." Both terms are reasonable and acceptable.

The term "periodic" is defined by both Dorland's and Webster's as recurring at regular intervals of time. Since the paroxysmal dyskinesias do not recur at regular intervals, the term "periodic" would not be appropriate. Despite this, in neurology this term is used for the condition of familial periodic paralysis (Rowland and Gordon, 2005) and familial periodic ataxia (e.g., Vighetto et al., 1988), even though muscle weakness and ataxia, respectively, in these disorders do not occur at regular intervals. Some authors (e.g., Griggs et al., 1978) had used the term paroxysmal ataxia in preference to periodic ataxia, and others use the term episodic ataxia (Zasorin et al., 1983). But the literature today uses "episodic ataxia."

According to dictionary definitions, either "paroxysmal" or "episodic" would be an appropriate term for the dyskinesias that are under discussion here. By common usage, and with few exceptions (e.g., Margolin and Marsden, 1982), "paroxysmal" has been chosen in preference over "episodic" for the choreoathetotic and dystonic types and is used in this chapter. The term "episodic" is also applied here to the ataxias in keeping with the current trend in the literature. The term "paroxysmal" has been utilized to indicate that the symptoms occur suddenly out of a background of normal motor behavior. It does not define the frequency, severity, duration, aggravating factors, or type of dyskinesia of the attack. These features vary and are important in the current nosology and classification of the paroxysmal dyskinesias.

Historical aspects

This is a condensed review of historical highlights of the paroxysmal and episodic dyskinesias. For a more complete discussion, see the review by Fahn (1994). A review of paroxysmal dyskinesias in the Japanese literature is available in English by Hishikawa and colleagues (1973).

Earliest descriptions: reported as epilepsy

Although Gowers (1885) is often credited with the first report of movement-induced seizures, it is possible that his cases actually represented paroxysmal dyskinesia. One of his patients was a boy whose attack lasted 15 seconds, but the boy was said to be unconscious during his initial attack. Later, he remained awake during the attacks. Another patient was a girl whose attacks started at the age of 11 years and occurred when she arose suddenly after prolonged sitting. But at least one of her attacks was said to be associated with a terrified expression, flushed facies, and dilated pupils. Subsequent to Gowers, a number of reports of "movement-induced seizures" appeared in the literature. Many of these reports have been published under the designation of reflex epilepsy and tonic seizures induced by movement. But unlike most motor convulsions, there was no alteration in the state of consciousness. Moreover, some of these reports had more than tonic contraction, namely, they included sustained twisting, athetosis, and chorea. These characteristics are today referred to as paroxysmal dystonia and paroxysmal choreoathetosis, rather than convulsive seizures. Even the presence of choreoathetosis did not lead the earliest interpreters of these brief attacks to conclude they were a movement disorder; instead, they were considered to be a form of epilepsy, the cerebral site of these "seizures" being in the basal ganglia or in the subcortical region.

After the report of Gowers, the next report of movement-induced paroxysmal movements appears to be that of Spiller in 1927. Spiller described two patients with brief tonic spasms that were brought on by voluntary movement of the involved limbs and, in one of them, also by passive manipulation. Spiller called this "subcortical epilepsy." Wilson (1930) described a 5-year-old boy who had brief attacks of unilateral torsion and tonic spasm that lasted up to 3 minutes and were precipitated by fright or excitement. There was no loss of consciousness. The attacks could be preceded by pain. Wilson considered this to be reflex tonic epilepsy and thought it also to be subcortical in origin. In more recent times, the concept that these attacks of tonic, often twisting, contractions without loss of consciousness are uncommon seizure disorders has continued (Whitty et al., 1964; Burger et al., 1972). It would appear that today these movement-induced involuntary movements would be considered paroxysmal choreoathetosis/dystonia rather than convulsive movements of the reflex epilepsy type. Differentiation of the attacks between cortical seizures and paroxysmal dyskinesias is sometimes difficult. Clouding of consciousness, if it occurs, would point to a seizure disorder.

By 1966 and 1967, when papers using the term "paroxysmal choreoathetosis" began regularly to appear (Stevens, 1966; Kertesz, 1967; Mushet and Dreifuss, 1967), particularly those cases induced by movements, there were still occasional papers referring the condition to a seizure disorder. As is discussed below in the section on paroxysmal hypnogenic dyskinesias, nocturnal epilepsy is now considered to be the leading cause.

Reported as a paroxysmal disorder of involuntary movements

In 1940, Mount and Reback (1940) introduced a new concept, that of labeling attacks of tonic spasms plus choreic and athetotic movements as a paroxysmal type of movement disorder. They described a 23-year-old man who had had both large and small "spells" since infancy. Both types were preceded by a sensory aura of tightness in parts of the body or by a feeling of tiredness. The movements involved the arms and legs and were usually a combination of sustained twisted posturing and chorea and athetosis. The small attacks lasted from 5–10 minutes. Longer attacks were considered large and also involved the neck (retrocollis), eyes (upward gaze), face (ipsilateral to the limbs if the limb involvement was unilateral), and speech. These large attacks lasted for as long as 2 hours, and the movements were considered to resemble those seen in Huntington disease. There was never a loss of consciousness or clonic convulsive movements, biting of the tongue, or loss of sphincter control. Drinking alcohol, coffee, tea, or cola would usually bring on an attack. Fatigue, smoking, and concentrating were other precipitating factors. The attacks would clear more rapidly if the patient lay down and would be aborted by sleep. The patient had an average of one large and two small attacks a day. Between attacks, the neurologic examination was normal. Phenytoin and phenobarbital had no effect, and scopolamine was the only drug that was found to reduce the frequency, severity, and duration of the attacks. The family history revealed 27 other members who had similar attacks; the pedigree showed autosomal dominant inheritance with what appears to be complete penetrance. Mount and Reback called this disorder "familial paroxysmal choreoathetosis."

Mount and Reback's paper became the seminal paper in the field of paroxysmal dyskinesias. Following its publication, most of the reports in the literature referenced it over the next five decades. However, the next report of a large family with similar attacks of muscle spasms did not refer to it. In 1961 Forssman (1961) described a family with autosomal dominant inheritance in which there were attacks lasting from 4 minutes to 3 hours.

The next large family was described in 1963 by Lance. Like Forssman (1961), Lance also did not relate this to nor refer to Mount and Reback's report, nor did he mention the report by Forssman. In fact, Lance considered his patients to have a form of epilepsy. Later, Lance (1977) was to write one of the definitive papers in this field, containing a useful classification scheme in which he related his family to those of Mount and Reback (1940), Forssman (1961), and Richards and Barnett (1968).

Although there were reports of patients whose paroxysmal dyskinesias were induced by sudden movement, they were not denoted by any special terminology until 1967, when Kertesz (1967) introduced the label "paroxysmal kinesigenic choreoathetosis" (PKC). This label has developed into a most useful and widely accepted designation, since the kinesigenic feature has proven to be so characteristic. Kinesigenicity has an important place in the classification of the paroxysmal dyskinesias, and Demirkiran and Jankovic (1995) recommended that the term paroxysmal kinesigenic dyskinesia (PKD) be used instead, because the movements can be other than choreoathetotic. That suggestion is followed in this chapter. As is pointed out below, the PKD designation can be applied to some patients who do not have the dyskinesias triggered by sudden movement (or startle).

Kertesz reported 10 new cases of paroxysmal dyskinesia and reviewed the literature. Among the important features of his paper, Kertesz differentiated the kinesigenic variety (induced by sudden movement) from that described by

Mount and Reback, by Forssman, and by Lance, which were aggravated not by movement but by alcohol, caffeine, and fatigue. It should be noted that Kertesz differentiated the kinesigenic type from that reported by Mount and Reback (1940) and by Lance (1963), but he failed to mention the paper by Forssman (1961).

Although phenytoin was recognized earlier as a very useful agent for PKD, carbamazepine was later found to be as useful and was introduced as a treatment by Kato and Araki (1969). This drug currently appears to be the one that is most commonly used for this disorder.

After Lance's paper in 1963, Richards and Barnett (1968) reported the next big family with the same type of paroxysmal dyskinesia as Mount and Reback's case and thought that Lance's family (1963) represented a variant, since there were only tonic spasms and no movements in that family. Richards and Barnett emphasized the nonkinesigenic nature of the attacks and felt that the terms rigidity, tremor, dystonia, torsions spasm, athetosis, chorea, and hemiballism could all be used for such movements, often blending into each other. To emphasize the postural and increased tone, they added "dystonic" to the label. They recommended avoiding the term "epilepsy" until the pathophysiology is better known. Richards and Barnett coined the term "paroxysmal dystonic choreoathetosis" (PDC), which was later adopted by Lance in 1977. The terms "paroxysmal nonkinesigenic choreoathetosis" and "paroxysmal dystonia" are sometimes used instead of PDC (Bressman et al., 1988). We have adopted the term paroxysmal nonkinesigenic dyskinesia (PNKD) proposed by Demirkiran and Jankovic (1995).

The original cases that were reported as PNKD were idiopathic and usually familial. It was not long before symptomatic cases began to be reported in which the attacks of movements were reported as a PNKD: perinatal encephalopathy by (Rosen, 1964), encephalitis (Mushet and Dreifuss, 1967), and head injury (Whitty et al., 1964; Robin, 1977). However, earlier reports of symptomatic PNKD had been described as a manifestation of multiple sclerosis, but considered as a form of epilepsy (Matthews, 1958; Joynt and Green, 1962; Verheul and Tyssen, 1990). Many other etiologies have been reported since the cases in the 1950s and 1960s (see below).

One of the most enlightening papers (Lance, 1977) achieved the following:

1. It discovered Forssman's paper (1961).
2. It placed together as one syndrome the families that Mount and Reback (1940), Forssman (1961), Lance (1963), and Richards and Barnett (1968) had reported, bringing them all in under the term familial paroxysmal dystonic choreoathetosis (PDC), which has a duration of attacks from 5 minutes to 4 hours.
3. It expanded the description of Lance's own previously reported family (1963), which he now classified as having this disorder instead of the seizure disorder that he had originally considered.
4. It added another family with paroxysmal dyskinesia that had attacks induced by continuous exercise rather than sudden movement that affected the legs with a duration between 5 and 30 minutes. (These were the first cases of what is now recognized as paroxysmal exertional dyskinesia.)

5. It classified the paroxysmal dyskinesias into three groups separated primarily by duration of action (prolonged, intermediate, and brief attacks) and secondarily by precipitating factors.
6. It reported the therapeutic response to clonazepam in some patients with the prolonged attacks.
7. It mentioned normal autopsy findings in two individuals with the prolonged attacks.
8. It summarized the literature to that date.
9. It pointed out that the Forssman and Lance families with the prolonged attacks had dystonic postures without choreoathetosis, whereas the Mount and Reback and the Richards and Barnett families had choreoathetosis.
10. It explained that over time, patients with sustained spasms can eventually develop writhing movements thereby linking these phenotypes together.
11. It commented that in all types of paroxysmal dyskinesias, males are more affected than are females.

Instead of Lance's proposed classification (item 5 in the preceding list) based on duration of the attacks, the classification scheme that is adopted here is the one based on precipitating factors suggested by Demirkiran and Jankovic (1995).

The next historical advances were the recognition that (1) idiopathic PNKD can occur sporadically and not just in families (Bressman et al., 1988) and that (2) sporadic PNKD is often psychogenic in origin (Bressman et al., 1988; Fahn and Williams, 1988).

Paroxysmal hypnogenic dyskinesia (PHD)

Horner and Jackson (1969) described two families in which several members of the family had attacks of involuntary movement that occurred during sleep. These appear to be the first cases of paroxysmal hypnogenic dyskinesia (PHD) to be reported. Family W is of particular interest because some affected members had classic PKD, some had hypnogenic, and others had a combination. Case 3 in this family began with the hypnogenic variety at age 8. By age 11, daytime attacks also occurred, sometimes triggered by sudden movement. Gradually, the hypnogenic episodes disappeared, leaving the patient with kinesigenic dyskinesia that responded to anticonvulsants. Lugaresi and his colleagues (Lugaresi and Cirignotta, 1981; Lugaresi et al., 1986) independently rediscovered and eventually popularized the syndrome of paroxysmal hypnogenic dyskinesias.

In addition to these short-duration attacks, Lugaresi and colleagues (1986) reported long-duration hypnogenic attacks. Such long-duration attacks occur in a minority of individuals with paroxysmal hypnogenic dyskinesia. These longer attacks last from 2 to 50 minutes and do not respond to medication, including anticonvulsants, tricyclics, benzodiazepines, and antipsychotics.

There has long been considerable speculation as to whether the short-duration hypnogenic attacks could be a manifestation of epilepsy, since they respond so well to anticonvulsants. The lack of abnormal electroencephalographic (EEG) findings during the attack has been used to argue against this concept. However, there is accumulating evidence that many paroxysmal hypnogenic dyskinesias are indeed due to seizures. Tinuper and colleagues (1990) described three patients with this disorder who had EEG evidence for frontal lobe seizures as a cause of the attacks. Sellal and colleagues (1991) and Meierkord and colleagues (1992) studied a series of patients with hypnogenic dystonia and concluded that these represent seizure disorders, particularly of frontal lobe epilepsy because repeated nocturnal EEG recordings often reveal epileptic patterns of abnormalities. Seizures arising near the mesial posterior frontal supplementary sensorimotor area may be a particular culprit in inducing paroxysmal hypnogenic dyskinesias in children (Bass et al., 1995). These types of seizures tend to be brief, frequent, and with bilateral tonic posturing, gross proximal limb movements, and preserved consciousness. Dystonic and other dyskinetic features may result from spread of epileptic activity from the mesial frontal region to the basal ganglia because there are close anatomic connections between them. It appears that the short-lasting attacks of paroxysmal hypnogenic dyskinesias are most likely due to seizures, but the question remains whether patients without abnormal EEGs and more prolonged hypnogenic attacks could have something more akin to the paroxysmal dyskinesias. In a family with autosomal dominant nocturnal frontal lobe epilepsy, interictal EEGs were normal, but ictal video-EEG studies showed that the attacks were partial seizures with frontal lobe origin (Scheffer et al., 1995). Fish and Marsden (1994) have reviewed epilepsy masquerading as a movement disorder, and they concluded that most cases of hypnogenic dyskinesias are considered to be due to epilepsy, as did Lüders (1996), with cyclic alternating EEG pattern believed to be a provocative factor (Terzano et al., 1997).

The genetics of hypnogenic dyskinesias/seizures is being explored. A large autosomal dominant Australian family (Oldani et al., 1998) and a Norwegian family (Nakken et al., 1999) have been described with mutations in the nicotinic acetylcholine receptor alpha 4 subunit (CHRNA4) gene, located on chromosome 20q13.2–q13.3. A second acetylcholine receptor subunit, CHRNB2, is also associated with autosomal dominant nocturnal frontal lobe epilepsy (Phillips et al., 2001). Another family with autosomal dominant hypnogenic frontal-lobe epilepsy has been mapped to 15q24 (Phillips et al., 1998).

In addition to epilepsy mimicking hypnogenic paroxysmal dyskinesias, there is a syndrome of infantile convulsions and paroxysmal dyskinesias, referred to as the "infantile convulsions with choreoathetosis" (ICCA) syndrome (Lee et al., 1998). The gene for this disorder has been mapped to the pericentromeric region of chromosome 16 (see the discussion in the section on PKD and also the section "Molecular genetics of paroxysmal dyskinesias"). Single photon emission computed tomography (SPECT) studies revealed alterations in local cerebral perfusion in the sensorimotor cortex, the supplementary motor areas, and the pallidum (Thiriaux et al., 2002).

Transient paroxysmal dyskinesias in infancy

Snyder (1969) introduced a new type of paroxysmal dyskinesia that he called "paroxysmal torticollis in infancy." He described 12 cases of intermittent head tilting in young infants. The age at onset was between 2 and 8 months of age, except for three cases, in which the first attacks occurred at 14, 17, and 30 months. The attacks would occur about two to three times a month and last from 10 minutes to 14 days, usually 2–3 days. The head would tilt to either side and often rotate slightly to the opposite side. There is no distress unless a parent attempts to straighten the head, upon which the baby cries. In some cases, the head tilting is associated with vomiting, pallor, and agitation for a short period. The infant is normal between attacks, which disappear after months or years, usually around age 2 or 3 years. Subsequently, a number of similar cases have been described (Gourley, 1971; Sanner and Bergstrom, 1979; Bratt and Menelaus, 1992), including familial cases (Lipson and Robertson, 1978). Sanner and Bergstrom (1979) reported a patient whose father had a similar condition in early infancy, suggesting that this disorder is hereditary.

The clinical picture of paroxysmal torticollis in infancy (Video 22.1) that has evolved is that the trunk can also be involved, with lateral curvature concave to the same side as the head tilting, and the ipsilateral leg can be flexed. Onset can be as early as the first months of life and can recur every couple of weeks until they disappear before the age of 2 years. Each attack can last a couple of hours to a couple of weeks. In between attacks, the child is normal. The main differential diagnosis is a posterior fossa tumor and Sandifer syndrome (Menkes and Ament, 1988).

In 1988, the clinical spectrum expanded with the report by Angelini and colleagues (1988) under the name "transient paroxysmal dystonia in infancy." They described nine patients who had onset of the paroxysmal dyskinesias between 3 and 5 months of age, except for one patient who had an onset at age 1 month. Three had a history of perinatal brain damage, six did not. The attacks consisted of opisthotonus, increased muscle tone with twisting of the limbs, and, in three, neck and trunk twisting, thereby linking this with "paroxysmal torticollis in infancy." The attacks lasted several minutes, with a maximum of 2 hours in one patient. They would occur from several times per day (Video 22.2) to once a month. Remission occurred between the ages of 8 and 22 months, with two not yet having reached a remission.

Dunn (1981) described an infant with head turning and posturing of the right arm lasting from 45 minutes to 18 hours. There were six attacks from age 26 months to age 40 months. The author did not mention the possible diagnosis of paroxysmal torticollis in infancy and made a diagnosis of paroxysmal dystonic choreoathetosis instead. One should consider the possibility that PNKD may occur in infancy and disappear over several months. If so, then the paroxysmal torticollis in infancy of Snyder and the paroxysmal dystonia in infancy of Angelini may represent the lowest age spectrum of PNKD and a benign form of the disorder.

Some patients with benign paroxysmal torticollis of infancy come from kindreds with familial hemiplegic migraine linked to CACNA1A mutation, and after recovering from these episodes as they reach childhood, they might have migraines (Giffin et al., 2002). In fact, a family with individual members of the kindred having one or more of the following: paroxysmal tonic upgaze, benign paroxysmal torticollis of infancy, and episodic ataxia, with familial migraine and a CACNA1A mutation (as in EA-2) has been reported (Roubertie et al., 2008). The clinical picture of benign paroxysmal torticollis of infancy has been summarized to consist of attacks usually lasting less than a week, recurring from every few days to every few months, improving by age 2 years, and ending by age 3; there is very frequently a family history of migraine (Rosman et al., 2009).

Intrauterine cocaine exposure can be associated with multiple transient dyskinesias. Beltran and Coker (1995) described four infants who tested positive for cocaine metabolite at birth with subsequent transient dystonic reactions, beginning at 3 hours to 3 months of age and persisting for several months.

The clinical syndrome of transient paroxysmal dyskinesia of infancy appears distinct from the syndrome referred to as "benign paroxysmal tonic upgaze of childhood" (Ouvrier and Billson, 1988; Deonna et al., 1990; Echenne and Rivier, 1992; Campistol et al., 1993), which is a sustained tonic conjugate upward deviation of the eyes that begins in infancy and eventually disappears in childhood. This appears to be an autosomal dominant disorder (Guerrini et al., 1998). An infant with tonic upgaze was found to have a partial tetrasomy of 15q (Joseph et al., 2005). Ataxia may be present, and there can be clumsiness and delayed walking. The ocular deviations lessen in the morning hours and disappear with sleep. Acetazolamide is not effective; however, Campistol and colleagues (1993) reported levodopa to be effective. Perhaps the tonic upgaze with diurnal fluctuations would be a better term than "paroxysmal." Not all cases of infantile transient tonic upgaze disturbance are benign, although the mean age of offset is 2.5 years (Hayman et al., 1998). Ouvrier and Billson (2005) published a recent review of this disorder. The family reported by Roubertie and colleagues (2008) suggests that tonic upgaze and transient torticollis and EA-2 may be related. A secondary cause of paroxysmal tonic upgaze has been reported: a 1-year-old girl with a hypomyelinating leukoencephalopathy, who presented in the neonatal period with episodes of sustained paroxysmal tonic upward gaze, roving eye movements, pendular nystagmus, and severe hypotonia, with the later appearance of pyramidal and extrapyramidal signs and no development (Blumkin et al., 2007).

Another paroxysmal ocular disorder, known as paroxysmal ocular downward deviation has been described in normal and brain-damaged infants (Yokochi, 1991; Miller and Packard, 1998). The ocular displacement was accompanied by closure of the upper eyelids, and the episode lasted seconds.

The syndrome of "benign myoclonus of infancy" can be mistaken for infantile spasms, but the benign EEG and clinical course allow for a clear distinction. The movements are sudden myoclonic and shuddering episodes of the head and shoulders (Lombroso and Fejerman, 1977; Fejerman, 1984). The jerks often repeat in a series; consciousness remains intact.

Another benign paroxysmal disorder in infants is spasmus nutans. It consists of a slow (2.4 Hz) tremor of the head, usually horizontal, and often an associated pendular nystagmus (Antony et al., 1980). It tends to disappear within 6 months and must be differentiated from congenital nystagmus (Fernandez-Alvarez, 1998).

Episodic (paroxysmal) ataxias and tremor

Intermittent ataxia can be due to metabolic defects such as Hartnup disease (Baron et al., 1956), pyruvate decarboxylase deficiency (Lonsdale et al., 1969; Blass et al., 1970, 1971), and maple syrup urine disease (Dancis et al., 1967). Fever often triggers the attacks of ataxia. In one case with pyruvate decarboxylase deficiency (Blass et al., 1971), choreoathetosis tended to accompany the chorea. Paroxysmal ataxia and dysarthria have also been reported to occur in multiple sclerosis (Andermann et al., 1959; Espir et al., 1966; DeCastro and Campbell, 1967; Miley and Forster, 1974; Gorard and Gibberd, 1989), which as remarked previously, is a disorder that also can cause paroxysmal choreoathetosis/dystonia. The attacks of paroxysmal ataxia due to multiple sclerosis last seconds, and are thus much shorter than the attacks described below. They also can respond to carbamazepine. Paroxysmal ataxia has also been reported in Behçet disease (Akmandemir et al., 1995).

In 1946, Parker described six patients in four families with idiopathic familial paroxysmal ataxia, which he labeled periodic ataxia. The age at onset ranged from 21 to 32 years. The attacks affected gait and speech and lasted from 30 seconds to 30 minutes. There could be several attacks per day, or there could be interval-free periods of several weeks. Vestibular symptoms occurred in some of the patients. Progressive cerebellar ataxia developed in some members.

In 1963, Farmer and Mustian reported a family from rural North Carolina with idiopathic paroxysmal ataxia. The major clinical difference from Parker's cases were the high frequency of accompanying vestibular symptoms of vertigo, diplopia, and oscillopsia and the lack of speech involvement. Farmer and Mustian labeled their family as vestibulo-cerebellar ataxia. The age at onset ranged from 23 to 42 years. The attacks ranged from a few minutes to 2 months in duration. The brief episodes could occur daily, but free intervals could last a year or more. Some affected members also developed progressive ataxia.

A second family from the same region in North Carolina also had ocular motility problems. These were abnormal smooth pursuit with normal saccades, dampened optokinetic nystagmus, inability to suppress the vestibulo-ocular reflex, gaze-evoked nystagmus, and episodic attacks of horizontal diplopia, oscillopsia, ataxia, nausea, vertigo, and tinnitus (Damji et al., 1996). This family's disorder was considered part of the same neurologic disorder that is referred to as periodic vestibulo-cerebellar ataxia, like Farmer and Mustian's family. Of special clinical significance is the lack of dysarthria. Genetic studies showed that the ataxia of this family is distinct from the two types of episodic ataxias (EA-1 and EA-2) that were previously characterized genetically (see below).

Hill and Sherman (1968) described another family, in which onset was in childhood in many of the affected members and there was no development of progressive ataxia. White (1969) described another family that experienced childhood onset and a benign course. All the families showed autosomal dominant inheritance.

An important advance was the discovery by Griggs and colleagues (1978) that acetazolamide can effectively prevent attacks. These authors showed this benefit in one kindred with familial paroxysmal ataxia. The following year, Donat and Auger (1979) had similar results in another kindred. Fahn (1983, 1984) reported a woman who had paroxysmal tremor, both intention and resting, associated with ataxia and postural instability during the attack; acetazolamide eliminated the attacks. Factor and colleagues (1991) reported an infant who had three attacks of coarse tremor and an orofacial dyskinesia that resembled that seen with tardive dyskinesia. Each attack lasted several hours before spontaneously clearing. Tetrahydrobiopterin, the cofactor for the enzymes tyrosine hydroxylase and phenylalanine hydroxylase, was reduced. The child responded to levodopa.

Mayeux and Fahn (1982) reported a patient with PNKD in a background of hereditary ataxia. Onset of PNKD was at age 10; onset of ataxia was at age 19. During an attack, which could last from 10 minutes to 4 hours, there was an accompanying increase of ataxia. Initially there was an 8-month response to acetazolamide. After the drug was no longer effective, the patient's PNKD responded to clonazepam. This patient might be a link between familial PNKD and paroxysmal ataxia.

Several other reports of acetazolamide-responsive familial paroxysmal ataxia have been reported (Aimard et al., 1983; Zasorin et al., 1983; Koller and Bahamon-Dussan, 1987). Although computed tomography (CT) has been normal, magnetic resonance imaging (MRI) studies have revealed selective atrophy in the anterior cerebellar vermis (Vighetto et al., 1988).

Families with a combination of periodic ataxia and persistent, continuous electrical activity in several muscles, reported either as myokymia (Van Dyke et al., 1975; Hanson et al., 1977; Gancher and Nutt, 1986; Brunt and Van Weerden, 1990) or as neuromyotonia (Vaamonde et al., 1991), have been described. Description of the attacks, which are brief and are sometimes preceded by sudden movement, include dyskinetic movements and sustained posturing as well as ataxia, dysarthria, and vertigo. This type of paroxysmal ataxia is now called episodic ataxia 1 (EA-1).

In 1986, Gancher and Nutt (1986) classified the hereditary episodic ataxias into three syndromes. In one group are those cases associated with persistent myokymia or neuromyotonia (now called EA-1). They described the attacks being precipitated by fatigue, excitement, stress, and physical trauma, but the family reported by Vaamonde and colleagues (1991) had attacks triggered by sudden movement, and kinesigenicity is now recognized as a feature. There is no dizziness or vertigo. The attacks last 2 minutes or less. Acetazolamide and anticonvulsants are usually ineffective. The gene for this type of paroxysmal ataxia has been located at chromosome 12p13 (Litt et al., 1994).

The second group (now known as EA-2) is featured by attacks of ataxia (with or without interictal nystagmus and with or without persistent ataxia), responding to acetazolamide or amphetamines. The attacks are precipitated by exercise, fatigue, or stress and occasionally by carbohydrate or alcohol ingestion. In addition to ataxia, the attacks are accompanied by vertigo, headache, nausea, and malaise. The attacks last for several hours or until the patient falls asleep. In recent years, additional families have been reported with these features (Bain et al., 1991; Baloh and Winder, 1991; Hawkes, 1992). The siblings reported by Bain and colleagues (1991) had persistent diplopia due to superior oblique paresis as part of the syndrome. Using [^{31}P] nuclear magnetic resonance spectroscopy, Bain and his colleagues (1992) found the pH levels in the cerebellum to be increased in untreated subjects with acetazolamide-responsive paroxysmal ataxia; the pH dropped to normal with treatment. The gene for this type of paroxysmal ataxia has been mapped to chromosome 19p13 (von Brederlow et al., 1995; Vahedi et al., 1995).

Gancher and Nutt (1986) listed a third group, which is kinesigenic. Typical PKD can occur in some members of the family. The attacks of ataxia last minutes to hours, whereas the PKD lasts seconds. The disorder can resolve with time. Acetazolamide appears to be ineffective, but phenytoin is effective for both the kinesigenic ataxia and the PKD. In their review, Griggs and Nutt (1995) place this third type with associated PKD in the first group of paroxysmal ataxias. Genotyping has now definitively placed this as EA-1 (Nutt and Gancher, 1997).

A case was reported in which a young girl had attacks of ataxia associated with fevers and accompanied by vertical supranuclear ophthalmoplegia (Nightingale and Barton, 1991). The ataxia and eye findings can last days.

Miscellaneous paroxysmal disorders

Keane (1984) reported two patients with post-traumatic periodic, rhythmic movements of the tongue. The attacks occurred about every 20 seconds and each attack lasted 10 seconds. They consisted of three undulations per second. Eventually, the movements diminished. Other cases of episodic lingual dyskinesias were associated with epilepsy (Jabbari and Coker, 1981) and pontine ischemia (Postert et al., 1997).

A few paroxysmal dyskinesias are mentioned here, but are not discussed further. These are Sandifer syndrome (prolonged head tilting in children following eating, due to gastroesophageal reflux) (see the review by Menkes and Ament, 1988); hyperekplexia (excessive startle syndrome with complex movements) (see the review by Andermann and Andermann, 1986 and Chapter 20); stereotypy (Duchowny et al., 1988; Tan et al., 1997), and paroxysmal bursts of myoclonus and tics. Classically, stereotypy, myoclonus, and tics are each recognized as a specific class of movement disorders, and they characteristically present as paroxysmal bursts of their type of movement. As a result, their discussion should be separated from discussion of conditions labeled as "paroxysmal." Shuddering attacks in children (Holmes and Russman, 1986) are brief bursts of rapid shivering-like movements of the head and arms, occurring up to 100 times per day; they can begin in infancy or in older children, and they resolve over time. The attacks lasts several seconds without impairment of consciousness. The frequency of shuddering movements as seen on EMG or EEG was similar to that of essential tremor (Kanazawa, 2000).

Classification of the paroxysmal dyskinesias

Because the various movement phenomena in any of the paroxysmal dyskinesias can vary from chorea/ballism to the sustained contractions of dystonia in any given patient, Demirkiran and Jankovic (1995) suggested that these disorders be labeled with the more generic names paroxysmal kinesigenic dyskinesia (PKD), paroxysmal nonkinesigenic dyskinesia (PNKD) (whether short-lasting or long-lasting), and paroxysmal exertion-induced dyskinesia

(PED) regardless of the duration of the attack. This classification system is used here. But the paroxysmal dyskinesias that last seconds and might not be induced by sudden movement are also included in the PKD category because of their otherwise similar short duration of attacks and response to anticonvulsants.

The highlights of various categories of paroxysmal dyskinesias are presented in outline format in Table 22.3.

Paroxysmal kinesigenic dyskinesia (PKD)

Clinical features

The attacks of PKD consist of any combination of dystonic postures, chorea, athetosis, and ballism. They can be unilateral – always on one side or on either side – or bilateral. Unilateral episodes can be followed by a bilateral episode.

The attacks are brief, usually lasting only seconds, but rarely can last up to 5 minutes. They are precipitated by a sudden movement or a startle, usually after the patient has been sitting quietly for some time (Video 22.3). The attacks can be severe enough to cause a patient to fall down. There can be as many as 100 attacks per day. After an attack, there is usually a short refractory period before another attack can take place. Speech can sometimes be affected, with inability to speak due to dystonia, but there is never any alteration of consciousness. The attacks can sometimes be aborted if the patient stops moving or warms up slowly. Very often, patients report variable sensations at the beginning of the paroxysms. These can consist of paresthesias, a feeling of stiffness, crawling sensations, or a tense feeling. 🎥

Equivalent to PKD are equally brief attacks that are not precipitated by sudden movement or startle. Because the duration and therapeutic response are the same as in PKD, they are listed here under the PKD rubric rather than in an

---

Table 22.3 Categories of paroxysmal dyskinesias

A. Paroxysmal kinesigenic dyskinesia (PKD)

Duration: seconds to 5 minutes

Precipitant: sudden movement, startle, hyperventilation

Treatment: responds well to anticonvulsants

Etiology

Primary – familial, sporadic

Secondary

Genetics

Syndrome of infantile convulsions and PKD (ICCA) (Szepetowski et al., 1997) has been mapped to chromosome 16p11.2–q12.1

The syndrome of PKD without infantile convulsions has been mapped to chromosome 16q13–q22.1 (Valente et al., 2000). There is no overlap

Note: The effectiveness of anticonvulsants correlates with brief duration of the paroxysms rather than their being triggered by sudden movement. New diagnostic criteria for PKD have been proposed (Bruno et al., 2004a)

Variant: A family of paroxysmal kinesigenic atonia has been reported (Fukuda et al., 1999). There was no alteration of consciousness or EEG findings of epilepsy. Anticonvulsants were effective in reducing the attacks

B. Paroxysmal nonkinesigenic dyskinesia (PNKD) (Mount–Reback type)

Duration: 2 minutes to 4 hours

Precipitant: none

Aggravating factors: alcohol, caffeine, and fatigue

Treatment: not sensitive to anticonvulsants

Etiology

Primary – familial, sporadic

Secondary

Alternating hemiplegia of childhood

Psychogenic

Genetics of five familial types

FPD1 (familial paroxysmal dyskinesia type 1) (PNKD1; DYT8) on 2q34; myofibrillogenesis regulator 1 (MR1) gene

CSE (choreoathetosis/spasticity episodica) on 1p (now thought to be the SLC2A1 gene for the glucose transporter, GLUT1)

Familial infantile convulsions on chromosome 16, called infantile convulsions with choreoathetosis (another ICCA) with the gene identified as the sodium/glucose cotransporter

Linkage to chromosome 2q31 (PNKD2; DYT20)

Ca-sensitive potassium channelopathy with epilepsy on chromosome 10q22, KCNMA1 gene

C. Paroxysmal exertional dyskinesia (PED)

Duration: 5–30 minutes

Precipitant: continued exertion

Etiology

Idiopathic – familial, sporadic

Symptomatic

Psychogenic

Genetics

PED and autosomal recessive rolandic epilepsy, chromosome 16p12–p11.2

PED with autosomal epilepsy, due to glucose transporter 1 (GLUT1) deficiency, chromosome 1p35–p31.1, SLC2A1 gene

D. Paroxysmal hypnogenic dyskinesia (PHD)

1. Brief attacks (many are due to supplementary/frontal lobe seizures)

2. Prolonged attacks

Genetics

Chromosome 20q13.2

Chromosome 15q24

Chromosome 1

E. Benign dyskinesias in infancy and childhood

1. Paroxysmal dystonia/torticollis in infancy

2. Paroxysmal tonic upgaze or downgaze

3. Paroxysmal myoclonus of infancy

4. Shuddering attacks

5. Spasmus nutans

6. Sandifer syndrome

7. Stereotypies

Table 22.3 Continued

F. Paroxysmal dyskinesias and epilepsy

1. Hypnogenic paroxysmal dyskinesias as frontal lobe epilepsy (see above)
2. Infantile convulsions and paroxysmal dyskinesias (ICCA) on chromosome 16p12–q12 and 16q13–q22.1

G. Paroxysmal ataxia and tremor

1. EA-1 with myokymia/neuromyotonia

    Attacks: ataxia, dysarthria, or behavioral changes or feeling strange

    Duration: brief; <2 minutes

    Precipitant: sudden movement or startle

    Treatment: sometimes sensitive to acetazolamide and to anticonvulsants

    Interictal: persistent myokymia/neuromyotonia

    Other feature: may be accompanied by PKD

    Genetics: point mutations on chromosome 12p13, involving the ion-gated potassium channel

2. EA-2 with nystagmus

    Attacks: ataxia and dysarthria

    Duration: hours

    Precipitant: exercise, fatigue, stress, alcohol

    Treatment: sensitive to acetazolamide

    Interictal: nystagmus

    Other features: headache, malaise, may develop persistent ataxia

    Genetics: mapped to chromosome 19p

3. EA-3 with tinnitus and headache

    Attacks: ataxia, tinnitus, falling, headache, blurred vision, vertigo, nausea

    Duration: 10–30 minutes

    Precipitant: none

    Treatment: acetazolamide

Other features: myokymia

Genetics: mapped to 1q42

4. EA-4 with ocular motility dysfunction

    Attacks: ataxia, diplopia, oscillopsia, vertigo, nausea, tinnitus

    Duration: minutes to hours

    Precipitant: sudden change in head position, fatigue, and an environment where objects are moving past the patient

    Treatment: lying quietly with eyes closed for 15–30 minutes; no response to acetazolamide

    Other features: the episodes become more frequent and then become constant with progressive ataxia

    Genetics: genetically distinct from other episodic ataxias

5. EA-5 with vertigo and juvenile epilepsy

    Attacks: ataxia, vertigo

    Precipitant: none

    Treatment: acetazolamide

    Other features: juvenile epilepsy; interictal nystagmus

    Genetics: mapped to 2q22–q23, *CACNB4* gene

6. EA-6 episodes of ataxia from birth to 20 years

    Attacks: ataxia, alternating hemiplegia, photophobia, phonophobia

    Precipitant: excitement, exercise

    Treatment: acetazolamide

    Other features: hemiplegic migraine

    Genetics: mapped to 5p13, glutamate transporter, *SLC1A3* gene

7. EA-7 episodes of ataxia in juveniles

    Attacks: ataxia

    Precipitant: excitement, exercise

    Treatment: none

    Other features: attacks accompanied by weakness and dysarthria

    Genetics: mapped to 19p3

entirely new category. Often, these attacks, lasting a few seconds, can be triggered by hyperventilation.

Kinast and colleagues (1980) reported as Case 4 a patient with typical brief dyskinesias occurring many times a day, preceded by paresthesias, and responding to anticonvulsants but not induced by sudden movement. Although this was technically not PKD, because sudden movements did not trigger any attacks, the clinical features otherwise resemble the attacks that are seen in PKD. As was mentioned above, this type of paroxysmal dyskinesia is placed in this category of PKD. Since the attacks of PNKD are usually so prolonged and because they do not ordinarily respond to anticonvulsants, this case does not fit into the PNKD category. See the discussion on the classification of these brief attacks as symptomatic PKD below.

Plant (1983) emphasized the focal and unilateral nature of PKD in many patients (Table 22.4).

In the literature there are many reports of paroxysmal dyskinesia without distinguishing kinesigenic from nonkinesigenic. These episodes have occurred with or without accompanying epilepsy. Without videotapes of the episodes and without a clear clinical description, the placement into PKD or PNKD is done with a degree of uncertainty. This caveat is provided here and applies to the rest of this chapter, including the molecular genetics.

Table 22.4 Laterality of types of paroxysmal kinesigenic dyskinesia (Plant, 1983)

Laterality of attacks	No.
Unilateral – one side only	25
Unilateral – either side	12
Unilateral and bilateral	11
Bilateral only	22
Not stated	3
Total	**73**

Primary paroxysmal kinesigenic dyskinesia

The etiology of most case reports of PKD has been idiopathic and predominantly hereditary, inheritance being autosomal dominant. For some unexplained reason males are more often affected than females, with a ratio of 3.75 : 1 (75 males and 20 females reported in Fahn, 1994). A large series of 150 cases were reported from a questionnaire in Japan. This gender imbalance was supported by the additional 26 cases reported by Houser and colleagues (1999), consisting of 23 men and 3 women, and another 150 case from Japan (Nagamitsu et al., 1999). Adding all these cases together brings the total to 218 men and 53 women or a ratio of 4.1 : 1. Age at onset shows a wide range, usually starting in childhood between the ages of 6 and 16 years, but can range from 6 months to 40 years (Frucht and Fahn, 1999; Li et al., 2005). Excluding the cases by Nagamitsu and colleagues (1999), the mean age at onset is 12 years; the median age is also 12 years. Familial cases might be more common among the Japanese (Kishimoto, 1957; Fukuyama and Okada, 1967; Kato and Araki, 1969) and Chinese (Jung et al., 1973). The survey reported by Nagamitsu and colleagues (1999) found 53 sporadic cases and 97 familial ones.

There is one report of PKD developing in a patient who had essential tremor (Nair et al., 1991). EEGs are generally normal, and CT scans are also normal (Goodenough et al., 1978; Kinast et al., 1980; Suber and Riley, 1980; Bortolotti and Schoenhuber, 1983, Lou, 1989) with a few exceptions, such as the case reported by Watson and Scott (1979) with suggested brainstem atrophy, and the one by Gilroy (1982) with an ill-defined unilateral hemispheric lesion. However, Hirata and colleagues (1991) demonstrated an abnormal EEG with rhythmic 5 Hz discharges over the entire scalp during episodes of PKD, raising the possibility that the PKD might have an epileptogenic basis. A patient was reported who developed PKD shortly after initiation of therapy with methylphenidate for attention-deficit hyperactivity disorder. Attacks persisted long after methylphenidate was discontinued and responded to treatment with carbamazepine (Gay and Ryan, 1994). The authors believe that the patient had a hereditary susceptibility for PKD that was triggered by the drug.

The attacks tend to diminish with age. Fortunately, PKD responds dramatically to anticonvulsants. The early literature indicates that phenytoin was the most popular, followed by phenobarbital and primidone. Carbamazepine appears to be the drug that is most commonly used. Valproate has also been effective (Suber and Riley, 1980), although Hwang and colleagues (1998) report that both carbamazepine and phenytoin were superior to valproate. Other anticonvulsants are effective also, including oxcarbazepine (Gokcay and Gokcay, 2000; Tsao, 2004; Chillag and Deroos, 2009), lamotrigine (Pereira et al., 2000; Uberall and Wenzel, 2000), levetiracetam (Chatterjee et al., 2002), and topiramate (Y.G. Huang et al., 2005). There is one report where high dosage of only phenytoin was effective (Bonakis et al., 2009). There is a report of response to levodopa (Loong and Ong, 1973), but another report of lack of effect with this drug (Garello et al., 1983). Analogously, there is one report of three patients with PKD worsening with haloperidol (Przuntek and Monninger, 1983), but Garello and colleagues (1983) reported no effect from this drug (as well as levodopa) in two brothers. The calcium channel blocker flunarizine, which is also a neuroleptic, was effective in a 7-year-old girl, who did not respond to carbamazepine or methylphenidate (Lou, 1989).

Homan and colleagues (1980) reported that children with PKD need doses of phenytoin that are similar to those used to treat epilepsy, whereas adults can respond to lower doses. These authors also describe a patient who might have had interictal chorea (the patient was described as fidgety) and suggested that this might represent a possible link to benign hereditary chorea. However, the fidgetiness that was described might not have been chorea. Perhaps these movements

might be interictal myoclonus, similar to the two patients with PKD recently reported (Cochen De Cock et al., 2006). Another report of interictal movements was by Bird and colleagues (1978) in which a woman had anxiety-induced dystonia/choreoathetosis and random, adventitious small jerky movements when she was not having an attack (first reported by Perez-Borja and colleagues 1967); her daughter had delayed milestones and persistent choreoathetosis. However, it seems likely that the daughter's choreoathetosis is not idiopathic but secondary, so it seems that paroxysmal dyskinesias and hereditary benign chorea should not be linked on the basis of a couple of these cases.

The pathophysiology of PKD is still unclear, and its relationship with epilepsy remains speculative. Because movement-induced seizures can occur (e.g., the case of Falconer et al., 1963) and because PKD responds dramatically to anticonvulsants, these are not sufficient reasons to consider PKD a form of epilepsy. The retention of consciousness and lack of postictal phenomena, as well as the presence of dystonia and choreoathetosis, should be sufficient to disqualify PKD from the epilepsies. However, Beaumanoir and colleagues (1996) described a boy with PKD and normal EEGs and consciousness, who later had a longer attack with clouding of consciousness and recording of postictal abnormalities on the EEG to support the diagnosis of reflex epilepsy. There is an emerging syndrome of infantile epilepsy, referred to as the ICCA syndrome, followed by childhood paroxysmal dyskinesias, as was mentioned earlier in the chapter (Lee et al., 1998; Thiriaux et al., 2002).

Franssen and colleagues (1983) investigated the contingent negative variation in one patient with PKD. Contingent negative variation is a slow cerebral potential that follows a warning stimulus, which prepares the subject to expect an imperative stimulus requiring a decision or motor response. The slow negative wave component of the contingent negative variation was more pronounced than that in control subjects. It returned to normal after phenytoin treatment. Mir and colleagues (2005) later demonstrated reduced intracortical inhibition, reduced early phase transcallosal inhibition, and reduced first phase of spinal reciprocal inhibition in PKD patients; treatment with carbamazepine normalized the abnormality of transcallosal inhibition.

The differential diagnosis of PKD is focal epilepsy, tetany, hyperekplexia, tics, stereotypies, and hysteria, as was noted in the misdiagnosis of the case reported by Waller (1977). The clinical features are so distinctive, particularly if triggered by sudden movement, that there is little likelihood of not diagnosing the condition correctly once one is aware of its existence. Similarly, the markedly effective response to anticonvulsants sets PKD apart from the other disorders. One case of primary PKD has been observed to be the result of a consistent ictal discharge arising focally from the supplementary sensorimotor cortex, with a concomitant discharge recorded from the ipsilateral caudate nucleus without spread to other neocortical areas (Lombroso, 1995), which suggests that some primary PKDs could be epileptic in origin. The nonkinesigenic, brief attacks of hemidystonia, often precipitated by hyperventilation, and controlled with anticonvulsants, has been considered a sign of epilepsy (Kotagal et al., 1989; Newton et al., 1992). So each case of such suspected nonkinesigenic paroxysmal dyskinesia needs to be evaluated for a convulsive disorder.

In addition to the cases of PKD described in the historical highlights earlier in the chapter, a number of other reports should be cited to make the review complete (Zacchetti et al., 1983; Boel and Casaer, 1984; Lang, 1984). One case of paroxysmal torticollis induced by sudden movement or stimulus appeared 5 years after the onset of classic spasmodic torticollis that had begun at age 20 years (Lagueny et al., 1993). After failing to respond to alcohol, tiapride, haloperidol, carbamazepine, clobazam, and valproate, the patient was treated effectively with injections of botulinum toxin.

There have been reports of two autopsies in PKD. Case 4 of Kertesz (1967) died, apparently by suicide, and a postmortem examination revealed no clear-cut abnormality in brain, just the presence of some melanin pigment in macrophages in the locus coeruleus. Stevens (1966) had earlier reported the postmortem findings of one of his patients, which were also essentially normal, showing only a slight asymmetry of the substantia nigra.

SPECT scans measuring cerebral blood flow were studied in two children with PKD, revealing increased perfusion in the contralateral basal ganglia at the onset of an attack in one (Ko et al., 2001) and in the contralateral thalamus in the other (Shirane et al., 2001). Physiologic studies indicate that there is surround inhibition in PKD (Shin et al., 2010).

Three independent laboratories have mapped autosomal dominant PKD with infantile convulsions (ICCA syndrome) to chromosome 16p11.2–q12.1 (Tomita et al., 1999; Bennett et al., 2000; Swoboda et al., 2000) and labeled EKD1 (episodic kinesigenic dyskinesia 1). A second locus on this chromosome at 16q13–q22.1 has been found in other families, referred to as EKD2 (Valente et al., 2000). This locus does not overlap with those of the other families. This family is distinct from the others by not having infantile convulsions. It has been given the designation of DYT19. Evidence for a third locus, called EKD3, has been suggested because three families did not map to the two known ones on chromosome 16 (Spacey et al., 2002).

A familial atonic form of PKD has been reported (Fukuda et al., 1999).

Secondary paroxysmal kinesigenic dyskinesia

The overwhelming majority of reported cases of PKD are idiopathic or familial. Although not reported as often, symptomatic PKD is probably more common. Table 22.5 lists the most common causes of symptomatic PKD, the most common being associated with multiple sclerosis and head injury. Pseudohypoparathyroidism has recently been added to this list (C.W. Huang et al., 2005). In one family with X-linked mutations in the thyroid hormone transporter gene *MCT8*, paroxysmal dyskinesias accompanied global retardation (Brockmann et al., 2005).

In symptomatic PKD, like primary PKD, attacks that last seconds are sometimes induced not by sudden movement but by hyperventilation. These also usually respond to anticonvulsants, such as carbamazepine, and are also seen in multiple sclerosis (Verheul and Tyssen, 1990; Sethi et al., 1992). Fahn (unpublished) has encountered a patient who had attacks lasting seconds, induced by hyperventilation and without being induced by sudden movement, following a mild cerebral ischemic episode, that also responded to

Table 22.5 Symptomatic paroxysmal kinesigenic dyskinesia
Multiple sclerosis
Head injury
Perinatal hypoxic encephalopathy
Idiopathic hypoparathyroidism
Pseudohypoparathyroidism
Basal ganglia calcifications
Hemiatrophy
Putaminal infarct
Thalamic infarct
Moyamoya disease
Medullary lesion (hemorrhage, subarachnoid cyst)
HIV infection
Hyperglycemia in the presence of a lenticular vascular malformation
Progressive supranuclear palsy
Spinal cord lesion
Huntington disease
Peripheral trauma

carbamazepine. These pharmacologic responses suggest that the briefness of the attack is more important than the sudden movement to distinguish the classification of the paroxysmal dyskinesias. Sethi and colleagues (1992) reported success in treating three patients with paroxysmal dystonia (not induced by movement, but triggered by hyperventilation and lasting many seconds) with acetazolamide with or without a combination of carbamazepine.

Multiple sclerosis

Although few of the paroxysmal dyskinesias that are associated with multiple sclerosis are triggered by sudden movement, an occasional patient with multiple sclerosis will manifest typical PKD (Matthews, 1958). In fact, the presenting symptom of multiple sclerosis can be PKDs as in the case reported by Roos and colleagues (1991); these attacks were associated with a lesion in the caudate nucleus and responded to phenytoin. In three of the eight patients reported by Berger and colleagues (1984) with paroxysmal dyskinesia associated with multiple sclerosis, the attacks were induced by sudden movement; they were relieved by anticonvulsants. The patient with PKD with multiple sclerosis reported by Burguera and colleagues (1991) had a lesion in the left thalamus demonstrated by MRI. The PKD was the presenting symptom, as in other cases of demyelinating disease. Gatto and colleagues (1996) reported medullary lesions in multiple sclerosis and bilateral paroxysmal dystonia.

Head trauma

Case 3 of Whitty and colleagues (1964) was a 13-year-old boy with onset 9 months after mild head trauma. Robin (1977) reported a 33-year-old man with severe head injury who developed PKD 8 months later. In two of the three cases of post-traumatic paroxysmal dyskinesias reported by Drake and colleagues (1986), the movements were induced by sudden movement of the affected body part. Richardson and colleagues (1987) reported another post-traumatic case.

These post-traumatic cases of PKD responded to anticonvulsants, similar to idiopathic PKD. Attacks of dystonia lasting several seconds and induced by tactile stimulation were reported secondary to a head injury; they disappeared within 2 months without treatment (George et al., 1990). Nijssen and Tijssen (1992) reported another case of tactile-induced dyskinesias as a result of a thalamic infarct.

Perinatal hypoxic encephalopathy

Rosen (1964) appears to have been the first to report a case of PKD associated with perinatal hypoxic encephalopathy, with the onset at age 12. This boy's attacks were usually triggered by a combination of startle and body contact. Mushet and Dreifuss (1967) described a 9-year-old boy who developed brief attacks of athetosis and dystonia. They usually occurred when he was startled but also could occur following sudden movement. At age 6 months, he had a febrile illness, which was retrospectively thought to be encephalitis. He had considerable motor regression and was not able to walk, nor did he gain syntactical speech. His dyskinetic attacks were not suppressed by anticonvulsants but did respond to anticholinergics.

Basal ganglia calcifications

PKD has been reported to occur with basal ganglia calcifications with or without hypoparathyroidism (Arden, 1953). Subsequent cases of hypoparathyroidism were reported (Tabaee-Zadeh et al., 1972; Barabas and Tucker, 1988). The clinical syndrome resembles that of primary infantile convulsions and childhood PKD (Hattori and Yorifuji, 2000). Calciferol was effective in controlling these attacks. The case reported by Soffer and colleagues (1977) was not noted to have the attacks induced by sudden movement, but the briefness of the attack resembles that of PKD.

Hemiatrophy

Case 2 of the five cases described by Kinast and colleagues (1980) had attacks of left hemidystonia lasting 1 minute and occurring up to 50 times a day. The major precipitating factor was not sudden movement, but stress and the anticipation of movement (also reported in one patient by Franssen et al., 1983). Technically, like their Case 4 described above, this patient does not fulfill the criterion of attacks induced by sudden movement. This is another example, because of the brief duration, the frequency of the attacks, and their response to phenytoin, that otherwise resembles PKD, and again points out why such nonkinesigenic cases are placed under the PKD rubric in the classification scheme used here. Examination of this revealed left-sided hemiatrophy and hyperreflexia with a normal CT scan. Because the hemiatrophy syndrome can be associated with a delayed-onset movement disorder (Buchman et al., 1988), it seems reasonable to consider it an etiologic factor in this particular case.

Gilroy (1982) reported a 32-year-old man with an abnormal right hemisphere on CT scan who had multiple daily brief attacks of left hemidystonia present since the age of 5 that were typical of PKD. The speculation is that the PKD was secondary to pathology in the involved hemisphere. An arteriogram and cortical biopsy did not shed further light on the pathology.

Cerebral infarcts and hemorrhages

With the advent of magnetic resonance imaging, more cases of PKD have been reported as a result of cerebral infarcts with putaminal infarct (Merchut and Brumlik, 1986), thalamic infarct (Video 22.4) (Camac et al., 1990; Nijssen and Tijssen, 1992; Milandre et al., 1993), an infarct probably in the cortex (Fuh et al., 1991), and medullary hemorrhage (LeDoux, 1997). As was mentioned above, the case of Nijssen and Tijssen (1992) had attacks stimulated by touch of the affected limb. The attacks secondary to infarcts (Merchut and Brumlik, 1986; Fuh et al., 1991) or to multiple sclerosis (Sethi et al., 1992) can be painful tonic spasms. Riley (1996) reported a patient who had paroxysmal attacks of tightening of his throat muscles and elevation of his tongue to the roof of his mouth associated with a remote hemorrhage in the medulla. Moyamoya disease has been reported to cause PKD (and PNKD) (Gonzalez-Alegre et al., 2003).

Other etiologies

PKD has also been reported to occur in a patient with progressive supranuclear palsy (Adam and Orinda, 1986), in hyperglycemia in the presence of a lenticular vascular malformation (Vincent, 1986), in subacute sclerosing panencephalitis (Ondo and Verma, 2002), and in spinal cord lesion (Cosentino et al., 1996). A case of spinal cord glioma was associated with paroxysmal kinesigenic segmental myoclonus (Marrufo et al., 2007). Another case of spinal cord compression was associated with PKD (Yulug et al., 2008). A case of PKD was reported in which it was the first symptom in a patient who developed Huntington disease (Scheidtmann et al., 1997). HIV infection has been reported to be associated with PKD and PKND (Mirsattari et al., 1999). A lesion in the medulla has been associated with PKD (Jabbari et al., 1999). Peripheral trauma to a foot was subsequently followed by paroxysmal hemidystonic episodes (Chiesa et al., 2008). An adult with PKD and cramp-fasciculation syndrome was associated with voltage-gated potassium channel-complex protein antibody encephalitis, with the patient responding to plasma exchange and intravenous immunoglobulin (Aradillas and Schwartzman, 2011).

Paroxysmal nonkinesigenic dyskinesia (PNKD)

Clinical features

As with PKD, the attacks of PNKD consist of any combination of dystonic postures, chorea, athetosis, and ballism. They can be unilateral – always on one side or on either side – or bilateral. Unilateral episodes can be followed by a bilateral one. They can affect a single region of the body or be generalized. Involvement of the neck can be a combination of torticollis and head tremor (Hughes et al., 1991). The major distinctions from PKD are the longer duration of each attack, the smaller frequency of the attacks, and a host of different aggravating factors for the attacks. The attacks last minutes to hours, sometimes longer than a day. Usually, they range from 5 minutes to 4 hours (Video 22.5). They are primed by consuming alcohol, coffee, or tea; by psychological stress or excitement; and by fatigue. There are usually no more than three attacks per day, and attacks may be months apart. The attacks can be severe enough to cause a patient to fall down. Speech is often affected, with inability to speak due to dystonia, but there is never any alteration of consciousness. The attacks can sometimes be aborted if the patient goes to sleep. As with PKD, patients very often report variable sensations at the beginning of the paroxysms. These can consist of paresthesias, a feeling of stiffness, crawling sensations, or a tense feeling. 🎥

A form of PNKD, known as intermediate PDC, and more recently as paroxysmal exertion-induced dyskinesia, is triggered only by prolonged exercise and not the other precipitants. This was first described by Lance (1977) and subsequently reported in another family by Plant and colleagues (1984) and in a sporadic case by Nardocci and colleagues (1989). Under the classification scheme of Demirkiran and Jankovic (1995), this form, which is discussed separately, is called paroxysmal exertional dyskinesia (PED).

Primary paroxysmal nonkinesigenic dyskinesia (Mount–Reback syndrome)

The initial reports of PNKD were familial (Mount and Reback, 1940; Forssman, 1961; Lance, 1963; Weber, 1967; Richards and Barnett, 1968; Lance, 1977; Horner and Jackson, 1969; Tibbles and Barnes, 1980; Walker, 1981; Mayeux and Fahn, 1982; Przuntek and Monninger, 1983; Jacome and Risko, 1984), with hereditary transmission being autosomal dominant. In 1980 Kinast and colleagues (Case 4) and Dunn in 1981 each described a child with PNKD without a positive family history. Bressman and colleagues (1988) later described seven sporadic cases of PNKD, and Nardocci and colleagues (1989) added another one. The familial cases of idiopathic PNKD still greatly outnumber sporadic cases, according to the reports in the literature. However, the sporadic cases are much more difficult to diagnose, and they have the difficulty of the need to be differentiated from a psychogenic etiology (Bressman et al., 1988; Fahn and Williams, 1988). On the basis of the experience of Bressman and her colleagues (1988), the sporadic form may actually be more common than the familial form but is just rarely reported.

For some unexplained reason males are slightly more often affected than females, with a ratio of 1.4:1 (32 males and 23 females reported in the reviewed English language literature) (see Fahn, 1994). Age at onset shows a wide range, usually in childhood between the ages of 6 and 16 years, but can range from 2 months to 30 years. The mean age at onset is 12 years; the median is also 12 years. CT scans are normal (Mayeux and Fahn, 1982; Jacome and Risko, 1984).

The EEGs are generally normal, but the case of Jacome and Risko (1984) may be of interest. The patient had unilateral PNKD and had normal interictal EEGs. Photic stimulation at low frequencies induced paroxysmal lateralized epileptiform discharges from the contralateral hemisphere. From this the authors suggest that the disorder might have some epileptogenic basis.

Sleep aborted the episodes in one family that had myokymia in addition to the PNKD (Byrne et al., 1991). The presence of myokymia links this particular family to several with paroxysmal ataxia, in which myokymia is a feature (Van Dyke et al., 1975; Vaamonde et al., 1991).

A family reported by Kurlan and colleagues (1987) had some atypical features for classic PNKD. The long-duration attacks were painful dystonic spasms that were not precipitated by alcohol, caffeine, or excitement, but could follow exposure to cold or heat or result from exertional cramping. Other members of the family had only exertional cramping without PNKD. The authors suggested that exertional cramping might be a forme fruste of PNKD. It is also possible that the PNKD in this family falls into the category of the intermediate form of paroxysmal dyskinesia that was reported by Lance (1977) and Plant and colleagues (1984). Also unusual was the presence of some fixed dystonia, which had not been reported previously. Bressman and colleagues (1988) also described some sporadic cases of PNKD, in which the patients had some interictal dystonia.

Lance (1977) mentioned that autopsies performed on two patients with PNKD revealed no pathology. His Case II.4 had normal macroscopic findings. His Case IV.2 died of sudden infant death syndrome; macroscopic and microscopic findings were normal.

The attacks can diminish spontaneously with age (Lance, 1977; Kinast et al., 1980; Bressman et al., 1988). Unfortunately, most patients have persistence of their attacks, and they are difficult to treat. As a general rule, PNKD does not respond to the same type of anticonvulsants that so effectively treat PKD. An occasional patient will respond to such agents as carbamazepine, valproate, and gabapentin (Chudnow et al., 1997). Clonazepam, as introduced for PNKD by Lance (1977), appears to be the most successful agent, for both for primary PNKD and symptomatic PNKD. A number of other drugs have been tried, sometimes with success. These include antimuscarinics (Mount and Reback, 1940), chlordiazepoxide (Perez-Borja et al., 1967; Walker, 1981), acetazolamide (Mayeux and Fahn, 1982; Bressman et al., 1988), oxazepam and other benzodiazepines (Kurlan and Shoulson, 1983; Kurlan et al., 1987), sublingual lorazepam (Dooley and Brna, 2004), and L-tryptophan (Kurlan et al., 1987).

Kurlan and Shoulson (1983) treated one patient with familial PNKD on alternate-day oxazepam. He had marked benefit from diazepam but only for 4 weeks. Clonazepam and oxazepam gave relief for 2–3 weeks each. Eventually he was placed on a regimen of 40 mg oxazepam given on alternate days. The concept was that the benzodiazepine receptors became desensitized on daily doses. Alternate-day administration prevented this desensitization.

Przuntek and Monninger (1983) and Coulter and Donofrio (1980) carried out trials of the dopamine receptor antagonist haloperidol and reported benefit. In the obverse, Przuntek and Monninger (1983) found that levodopa worsened one patient.

Levetiracetam was found helpful in one family (Szczałuba et al., 2009).

Chronic stimulation of the ventral intermediate nucleus (VIM) of the thalamus was effective in reducing the frequency, duration, and intensity of attacks in one patient with PNKD (Loher et al., 2001). At least one patient with PNKD has been treated successfully with deep brain stimulation of the globus pallidus interna (Yamada et al., 2006).

In contrast to idiopathic PKD, which is so distinctive, the major difficulty in the diagnosis of sporadic PNKD is to differentiate it from a psychogenic movement disorder. The problem is that the disappearance of the movements with placebo or psychotherapy could be coincidental since the attacks disappear spontaneously. However, if the paroxysms are frequent and the attacks are prolonged, then repeated trials with placebo can be informative. If such trials consistently produce remissions, then one can be convinced that the diagnosis is a psychogenic disorder (see Chapter 25).

Three different genetic mappings have been made for PNKD. The first type, originally described by Mount and Reback (1940), is referred to genetically as familial paroxysmal dyskinesia type 1 (FPD1) and was mapped to 2q33–q35 (Fink et al., 1996; Fouad et al., 1996; Hofele et al., 1997; Matsuo et al., 1999). One of these families (Przuntek and Monninger, 1983; Hofele et al., 1997) shows a fair response to diazepam. The gene for this disorder has been identified as myofibrillogenesis regulator 1 (*MR1*) (Lee et al., 2004). Bruno and colleagues (2007) analyzed 14 families with PNKD and 8 had *MR1* mutations. Patients with PNKD with *MR1* mutations had their attack onset in youth (infancy and early childhood). Typical attacks consisted of a mixture of chorea and dystonia in the limbs, face, and trunk, and typical attack duration lasted from 10 minutes to 1 hour. These attacks resembled the phenotype presented by Mount and Reback (1940). Caffeine, alcohol, and emotional stress were prominent precipitants. Attacks had a favorable response to benzodiazepines, such as clonazepam and diazepam. Attacks in families without *MR1* mutations were more variable in their age at onset, precipitants, clinical features, and response to medications. Several were induced by persistent exercise. A Serbian family with PKND and the *MR1* mutation had similar clinical features, with attacks starting in the first 6 months of life (Stefanova et al., 2006). The frequency and severity of attacks showed an age-dependent incremental decremental pattern with a peak between 13 and 15 years of age. Some of the non-*MR1* affected patients with PNKD are suspected of having paroxysmal exertional dyskinesia (Bruno et al., 2007).

The second type of PNKD has additional clinical features, including perioral paresthesias, double vision, and headache during attacks, and some also have a constant spastic paraparesis; this type was mapped to chromosome 1p (Auburger et al., 1996) and has been called choreoathetosis/spasticity episodica (CSE). The locus is very close to the *SLC2A1* gene, suggesting that the family might be positive for a *GLUT1* mutation. The third type of PNKD has been seen in familial infantile convulsions, in which the gene has been mapped to the pericentromeric region of chromosome 16 (Szepetowski et al., 1997). This has been called infantile convulsions with paroxysmal choreoathetosis (ICCA). The gene has been identified as the sodium/glucose cotransporter (Roll et al., 2002). A fourth type is linked to chromosome 2q31 and has been designated PNKD2 and also listed with the dystonias as DYT20. A fifth type is a family with PNKD and epilepsy, found to be due to a mutation in the Ca-sensitive potassium channel gene on chromosome 10q22 (*KCNMA1* gene) (Du et al., 2005). Further discussion about the genetics of the paroxysmal dyskinesias is in a later section in this chapter.

Secondary paroxysmal nonkinesigenic dyskinesia

The overwhelming majority of reported cases of PNKD are idiopathic or familial in etiology, but a number of cases of

Table 22.6 Symptomatic paroxysmal nonkinesigenic dyskinesia

Multiple sclerosis
Perinatal hypoxic encephalopathy
Psychogenic
Encephalitis
Idiopathic hypoparathyroidism
Pseudohypoparathyroidism
Basal ganglia calcifications
Thyrotoxicosis
Transient ischemic attacks
Infantile hemiplegia
Cystinuria
Succinic semialdehyde dehydrogenase deficiency (Leuzzi et al., 2007)
Head injury
Hypoglycemia
AIDS
Diabetes
Anoxia
Brain tumor
Tardive syndrome?
Alternating hemiplegia of childhood
Antiphospholipid syndrome
Moyamoya disease
Celiac disease
Allan–Herndon–Dudley syndrome (impaired transporter of thyroid hormones)
Streptococcal infection
Sjögren syndrome

symptomatic PNKD have been reported. Table 22.6 lists the most common causes of symptomatic PNKD.

The most common cause of symptomatic PNKD, just like PKD, is multiple sclerosis (Matthews, 1958; Joynt and Green, 1962; Lance, 1963; Berger et al., 1984; Verheul and Tyssen, 1990; Sethi et al., 1992). In multiple sclerosis, the paroxysmal movements may only be ocular, lasting several minutes (MacLean and Sassin, 1973). One patient with paroxysmal hemidystonia associated with multiple sclerosis later developed psychogenic PNKD (Morgan et al., 2005). Another patient had paroxysmal laughter in addition to paroxysmal dyskinesias (Aguirregomozcorta et al., 2008).

The next two most common causes are perinatal encephalopathy (Lance, 1963; Erickson and Chun, 1987; Bressman et al., 1988) and psychogenic (Video 22.6) (Bressman et al., 1988; Fahn and Williams, 1988; Lang, 1995). A longer discourse on psychogenic PNKD is presented in Chapter 25. 📹

Other causes of PNKD are encephalitis (Video 22.7) (Mushet and Dreifuss, 1967; Bressman et al., 1988), cystinuria (Cavanagh et al., 1974), succinic semialdehyde dehydrogenase deficiency (improved with vigabatrin) (Leuzzi et al., 2007), hypoparathyroidism (Soffer et al., 1977; Yamamoto and Kawazawa, 1987; Dragasevic et al., 1997), pseudohypoparathyroidism (Prashantha and Pal, 2009), basal ganglia calcifications without altered serum calcium (Micheli et al., 1986), thyrotoxicosis (Fischbeck and Layzer, 1979), transient ischemic attacks (Margolin and Marsden, 1982; Bennett and Fox, 1989) including basilar ischemia causing episodic tongue and alternating limb movements (Li and Lee, 2009), infantile hemiplegia (Huffstutter and Myers, 1983), head trauma (Perlmutter and Raichle, 1984; Drake et al., 1986), hypoglycemia (Newman and Kinkel, 1984; Winer et al., 1990; Schmidt and Pillay, 1993), AIDS (Nath et al., 1987), diabetes (Haan et al., 1988), anoxia (Bressman et al., 1988), brain tumor (Bressman et al., 1988), hypoglycemia induced by an insulinoma (Shaw et al., 1996; Debruyne et al., 2009), poststreptococcal autoimmune neuropsychiatric disease (PANDAS) (Dale et al., 2002; Senbil et al., 2008), celiac disease (Hall et al., 2007), Sjögren syndrome (Alonso-Navarro et al., 2009), and the Allan–Herndon–Dudley syndrome, which is an X-linked recessive disorder due to a mutation in the monocarboxylate transporter 8 (*MCT8*) gene resulting in decreased transport of thyroid hormone into neurons (Fuchs et al., 2009). The patient with AIDS (Nath et al., 1987) had two attacks of dystonia, but details are lacking in regard to the duration or characteristics of the attacks. Moyamoya disease has been reported to cause PNKD (and PKD) (Gonzalez-Alegre et al., 2003). 🎥

There is a case report of one person who developed paroxysmal hemidystonia after starting fluoxetine, which cleared on discontinuing the drug (Dominguez-Moran et al., 2001). Related to transient ischemic attacks mentioned above is the case of one patient who had paroxysmal hemidystonia precipitated by assuming an upright position after sitting or lying, associated with occlusion of the contralateral internal carotid artery (ICA) and near-total occlusion of the ipsilateral internal carotid artery (Sethi et al., 2002). The authors called this orthostatic paroxysmal dystonia. A SPECT study demonstrated decreased perfusion in the contralateral frontoparietal cortex during the typical dystonic spell. PNKD has now been reported in the antiphospholipid syndrome (Engelen and Tijssen, 2005). A series of 17 cases of secondary paroxysmal dyskinesias was reported by Blakeley and Jankovic (2002), who found that 9 patients had PNKD, 2 patients had PKD, 5 patients had mixed PKD/PNKD, and 1 patient had PHD.

PNKD caused by endocrine disorders responds to appropriate treatment. But in general, treatment of symptomatic PNKD is not often effective.

Micheli and colleagues (1987) reported an interesting case of a youth with learning disability who had received dopamine receptor-blocking drugs since the age of 3. At age 16 he developed paroxysmal dystonia. The attacks could be precipitated by stress but not by movement, caffeine, cold, fatigue, or hyperventilation. The episodes lasted from 30 minutes to 3 hours. They did not respond to anticonvulsants but were abolished with trihexyphenidyl 20 mg/day. It is possible that the PNKD in this youth represented a variant of tardive dystonia (Burke et al., 1982; Kang et al., 1986).

A PET study was performed on one patient with post-traumatic paroxysmal hemidystonia (Perlmutter and Raichle, 1984). Decreased oxygen metabolism, decreased oxygen extraction, increased blood volume, and increased blood flow in the contralateral basal ganglia were found.

The syndrome commonly known as "alternating hemiplegia of childhood" typically contains periods of prolonged dystonic attacks, along with other elements of the syndrome (Bourgeois et al., 1993). The syndrome begins before 18 months of age. In addition to prolonged periods of dystonia,

there are attacks of nystagmus, dyspnea, and autonomic phenomena. Episodes of quadriplegia appear either when a hemiplegia shifts from one side to the other or as an isolated manifestation. The episodes were often followed by developmental deterioration. Eventually, there is cognitive impairment and a choreoathetotic movement disorder. Sleep relieves the weakness and other paroxysmal phenomena, but they can reappear after awakening. The attacks can last from a few minutes to several days. Flunarizine and aripiprazole can be partially effective (Haffejee and Santosh, 2009). Some infants manifest paroxysmal dystonia before the classic features of alternating hemiplegia develop (Andermann et al., 1994). Magnetic resonance spectroscopy was normal in the case reported by Nezu and colleagues (1997). A review of the phenotypic data on 103 patients with this syndrome has been published (Sweney et al., 2009). Paroxysmal eye movements were the most frequent early symptom, manifesting in the first 3 months of life in 83% of patients. Paroxysmal episodes of focal dystonia or flaccid, alternating hemiplegia appeared by 6 months of age in 56% of infants. A European consortium reported that the natural history of alternating hemiplegia is highly variable and unpredictable, and the course is not always steadily progressive and degenerative (Panagiotakaki et al., 2010).

Paroxysmal exertional dyskinesia (PED)

Lance (1977) was the first to describe what he called an intermediate form of PDC (now called PNKD). Today, this family would appear to have PED. The family had attacks that were briefer than those in classic PNKD, lasting from 5 to 30 minutes, and in which the attacks were precipitated by prolonged exercise and not by cold, heat, stress, ethanol, excitement, or anxiety. The spasms affected mainly the legs. Plant and colleagues (1984) reported a second family. In both families, the inheritance pattern was that of autosomal dominant transmission. In neither family did anyone derive any benefit from barbiturates levodopa, or clonazepam. Sporadic cases are also seen (Video 22.8), such as the case reported by Nardocci and colleagues (1989) (Case 3). This patient also had interictal chorea without any family history of a similar condition. This patient was helped by clonazepam. Wali (1992) reported another sporadic case; this was an 18-year-old man in whom attacks of right hemidystonia lasting about 10 minutes were precipitated by prolonged running (about 10 minutes) or by cold. The EEG and the CT scan were normal; anticonvulsants were not helpful. Demirkiran and Jankovic (1995) mentioned seeing five patients, three being females. The largest series of sporadic cases is that by Bhatia and colleagues (1997). Familial cases appear to be autosomal dominant (Kluge et al., 1998). A large family with PED with four affected members had onset at 9–15 years of age and a male : female ratio of 3 : 1 (Munchau et al., 2000). The 26 reported cases consisted of 13 women and 13 men. The age at onset ranged from 2 to 30 years, all but six beginning in childhood. 🎥

Some patients labeled as PKD, e.g., Cases 1 and 3 of Jung and colleagues (1973), and PNKD e.g., the family of Kurlan and colleagues (1987), have attacks that occur after prolonged exercise. It is possible that such patients have a variant of PNKD or a combination of PNKD and one of the other paroxysmal dyskinesias. However, if the attacks last only seconds and respond to anticonvulsants, they fit clinically with these features of PKD.

The family reported by Schloesser and colleagues (1996) supports the notion that PED is a variant of PNKD. The father of the proband was affected by exertional cramping, and two other men in the family had PED. Women in the family had more prolonged attacks, fitting those of PNKD.

Ictal and interictal cerebral perfusion SPECT studies have been conducted (Kluge et al., 1998). During the motor attacks, decreased perfusion of the frontal cortex and increased cerebellar perfusion were observed. The perfusion of the basal ganglia also decreased. No cortical hyperperfusion indicative of an epileptic nature was seen. The authors conclude that PED represents a paroxysmal movement disorder rather than epilepsy. However, an opposite finding in a case of PED has also been reported (Yoon et al., 2007). In this 16-year-old boy, there was increased perfusion in the somatosensory cortex.

In a patient with familial PED, different stimuli and maneuvers in triggering dystonic attacks in the arm were studied. Motor paroxysms could be provoked by muscle vibration, passive movements, transcranial magnetic stimulation, magnetic stimulation of the brachial plexus, and electrical nerve stimulation but not by sham stimulation (Meyer et al., 2001). The authors conclude that dystonic attacks are triggered by proprioceptive afferents.

Guerrini and colleagues (1999) described a family with PED and autosomal recessive rolandic epilepsy, with the gene mapped to chromosome 16p12–11.2. That family's dystonia resembles the ICCA syndrome, and the genetic mapping overlaps with that syndrome. Perniola and colleagues (2001) described another family with autosomal dominant PED and epilepsy; fasting and stress were also precipitating factors.

In a study in which cerebrospinal fluid (CSF) monoamine metabolites were measured before and after the attack, a twofold increase in the concentration of homovanillic acid and 5-hydroxyindoleacetic acid was detected after the attack (Barnett et al., 2002).

A case of PED foot dystonia in an adult was found to be due to the earliest symptom of Parkinson disease, as established by dopamine transporter binding and SPECT, and effectively treated with dopaminergic medication (Katzenschlager et al., 2002). Two other adults (second cousins) who presented with paroxysmal exercise-induced dystonia later developed clinical features of Parkinson disease (Bruno et al., 2004b).

Autosomal dominant PED accompanied by epilepsy was found to be due to glucose transporter 1 (GLUT1) deficiency (Suls et al., 2008; Weber et al., 2008; Zorzi et al., 2008; Leen et al., 2010). The syndrome also includes mild developmental delay, reduced CSF glucose levels, hemolytic anemia with echinocytosis, and altered erythrocyte iron concentrations. The clinical spectrum of GLUT1 deficiency was evaluated by videotape in 57 patients, and a wide range of movement disorders are seen (Pons et al., 2010). These include abnormal gait (ataxic-spastic and ataxic), action limb dystonia (86%), mild chorea (75%), cerebellar tremor (70%), myoclonus (16%), and dyspraxia (21%). Nonepileptic paroxysmal events were encountered in 28% of patients, and included episodes of ataxia, weakness, parkinsonism, and

nonkinesigenic dyskinesias. Alternating hemiplegia has also been reported with GLUT1 deficiency (Rotstein et al., 2009).

PEDs are difficult to treat. Those with GLUT1 deficiency can be treated with a ketogenic diet. Posteroventral pallidotomy has been reported to ameliorate attacks of PED (Bhatia et al., 1998). A pair of homozygous twins with GLUT1 deficiency had PED, migraine, absence seizures and writer's cramp with an excellent response to a ketogenic diet (Urbizu et al., 2010).

Table 22.7 lists the major distinguishing features of nonepileptic PKD, PNKD, and PED.

Episodic ataxias

The paroxysmal ataxias, called episodic ataxias, have been distinguished by their clinical features and by their genotypes. These characteristics are presented and summarized in Table 22.8.

The genes for four of the hereditary episodic ataxias have been determined. In one of them, EA-1, the type associated with myokymia or neuromyotonia, has been found to be due to point mutations in the gene $Kv1.1$ for the voltage-gated potassium channel (KCNA1) (Browne et al., 1994; Comu et al., 1996). The gene is located on chromosome 12p13 (Litt et al., 1994). Different mutations have been found in different families (D'Adamo et al., 1998; Zerr et al., 1998; Eunson et al., 2000). The attacks are brief, lasting seconds to minutes; myokymia is present during and between attacks. The attacks can be triggered by sudden movement (Nutt and Gancher, 1997), and these can respond to anticonvulsants. Some families have episodes of myokymia without ataxia (Eunson et al., 2000). In one family, mutations in the KCNA1 gene can cause severe neuromyotonia resulting in marked skeletal deformities without episodic ataxia, and others in the family had the ataxia (Kinali et al., 2004).

Another episodic ataxia, EA-2, is the type that has a vestibular component and does not have myokymia as an associated feature. The attacks last between 15 minutes and a few days and respond to acetazolamide. The gene was mapped to chromosome 19p13 (Vahedi et al., 1995; von Brederlow et al., 1995) and the syndrome was found to be mutations in the gene for the calcium channel $CACNA1A$ (Spacey et al., 2005). Spontaneous mutations (Yue et al., 1998) as well as familial cases have been described. There is clinical heterogeneity, with attacks varying from pure ataxia to combinations of symptoms that suggest involvement of the cerebellum, brainstem, and cortex. Oculographic findings were localizing to the vestibulocerebellum and posterior vermis. Some affected individuals exhibited a progressive ataxia syndrome that is phenotypically indistinguishable from the dominantly inherited spinocerebellar ataxia (SCA) syndromes. SCA6 has been found to be due to an expanded CAG repeat on the same gene (Zhuchenko et al., 1997). Two patients with childhood onset EA-2 developed adult-onset dystonia (Spacey et al., 2005). About one-half of the affected individuals have migraine headaches and several have episodes that are typical of basilar migraine (Baloh et al., 1997). Both familial hemiplegic migraine and EA2 are caused by mutations in the Ca^{2+} channel gene $CACNL1A4$ and can be

Table 22.7 Clinical features of paroxysmal kinesigenic (PKD), nonkinesigenic (PNKD), and exertional dyskinesia (PED)

Feature	PKD	PNKD	PED
Male:female	4:1	1.4:1	13:13 (N=26)
Inheritance	AD	AD	AD
Genetic mapping	(1) 16p11.2–q12.1 (also designated as DYT10); with infantile convulsions (2) 16q13–q22.1 (gene designated as *EKD2*); PKD without convulsions; (also designated as DYT19)	(1) Mount–Reback syndrome; 2q34 (FPD1) (PNKD1); (also designated as DYT8); myofibrillogenesis regulator 1 (*MR1*) gene (2) With diplopia and spasticity (CSE); chromosome 1p21; (also designated as DYT9); now thought to be due to *GLUT1* mutations (3) With familial infantile convulsions; ICCA; chromosome 16, pericentric; sodium/glucose cotransporter (4) Linkage on chromosome 2q31; (PNKD2); (DYT20) (5) With epilepsy; chromosome 10q22; Ca-sensitive potassium channel (*KCNMA1*)	(1) With autosomal recessive rolandic epilepsy and writer's cramp; 16p12–11.2 (2) Glucose transporter 1; autosomal dominant; developmental delay; hemolytic anemia; echinocytosis; (DYT18); (*SLC2A1*), 1p35–31.1
Age at onset Range: Median: Mean:	<1–40 12 12	<1–30 12 12	2–30 11.5 12
Attacks Duration Frequency	<5 minutes 100/day to 1/month	2 minutes to 4 hours 3/day to 2/year	5 minutes to 2 hours 1/day to 2/month
Trigger	Sudden movement, startle, hyperventilation	Nil	Prolonged exercise; muscle vibration; nerve stimulation; transcranial magnetic stimulation of motor cortex
Precipitant	Stress	Alcohol, stress, caffeine, fatigue	Stress
Movement pattern	Any combination of dystonic postures, chorea, athetosis, and ballism; unilateral or bilateral	Any combination of dystonic postures, chorea, athetosis, and ballism; unilateral or bilateral	Any combination of dystonic postures, chorea, athetosis, and ballism; unilateral or bilateral
Treatment	Anticonvulsants	Clonazepam, benzodiazepines, acetazolamide, antimuscarinics	Acetazolamide, antimuscarinics, benzodiazepines

considered as allelic channelopathies (Ophoff et al., 1996). When progressive ataxia is present, there is cerebellar atrophy on MRI scans, and not all cases have a CAG expansion (Yue et al., 1997). On the other hand, cases with the CAG expansion and cerebellar atrophy can also have EA-2 (Jodice et al., 1997). A family with the phenotype of EA-2 was found not to have a mutation of the *CACNL1A* gene on chromosome 19p13, indicating genetic heterogeneity for this disorder (Hirose et al., 2003).

EA-1 and EA-2 are described above. Not all families with migraine and episodic vertigo could be linked to the EA-2 markers on chromosome 19p, indicating genetic heterogeneity for this type of episodic ataxia (Baloh et al., 1996). EA-3 is an autosomal dominant episodic ataxia manifested by vestibular ataxia, vertigo, tinnitus, and interictal myokymia; attacks are diminished by acetazolamide (Steckley et al., 2001). EA-1 and EA-2 genetics were excluded. The fourth type of paroxysmal ataxia with ocular motility problems can be precipitated by sudden head movement (Damji et al., 1996). The gene for this fourth type of EA has

not yet been mapped, but is genetically distinct from EA-1 and EA-2. The fifth type was seen in a French-Canadian family. The attacks began after age 20 years, but earlier in life there was epilepsy (Escayg et al., 2000). The sixth type ranges from more severe with younger onset with episodes of ataxia, seizures, migraine, and alternating hemiplegia from birth (Jen et al., 2005) to milder forms with attacks accompanied by nausea, vomiting, photophobia, phonophobia, vertigo, diplopia, and dysarthria (de Vries et al., 2009). The seventh type maps to the same region as EA-2, without any interictal symptoms, and without mutations in the potassium channel gene (Kerber et al., 2007).

Another family with episodic ataxia that does not map to the disorders labeled as EA-1 to EA-7 has been described (Damak et al., 2009). This family has not been linked to any chromosomal site yet. It appears to be autosomal dominant, with onset between 48 and 56 years of age; the most severely affected had daily attacks with slowly progressive and disabling permanent cerebellar ataxia and a poor response to acetazolamide. Sporadic cases of episodic ataxias occur. Four

Table 22.8 Clinical and genetic features of episodic ataxias

Type	Age at onset	Clinical	Acetazolamide response	Precipitant	Frequency/ duration	Interictal	Gene
Myokymia, neuromyotonia (EA-1)	2–15	Aura of weightlessness or weakness, then ataxia, dysarthria, tremor, facial twitching	In some kindreds, anticonvulsants may help	Startle, movement, exercise, excitement, fatigue	Up to 15 per day; usually one or fewer per day; seconds to minutes, usually 2–10 minutes	Myokymia, shortened Achilles tendon; PKD	12p13, K^+ channel, different point mutations in KCNA1
Vestibular (EA-2)	0–40, usually 5–15	Ataxia, vertigo, nystagmus, dysarthria, headache, ptosis, ocular palsy, vermis atrophy	Very effective	Stress, alcohol, fatigue, exercise, caffeine	Daily to q 2 months; usually hours; 5 minutes to weeks	Nystagmus, mild ataxia; less common: dysarthria and progressive cerebellar signs	19p13, Ca^{2+} channel, CACNL1A4 familial hemiplegic migraine
Tinnitus (EA-3) (Steckley et al., 2001)	1–41	Ataxia, tinnitus, falling, headache, blurred vision, vertigo, nausea	Effective	None	Daily; 10–30 minutes	Myokymia; some with ataxia	1q42
Ocular (EA-4) (Damji et al., 1996)	20–50	Ataxia, diplopia, vertigo, nausea	No response	Sudden change in head position	Daily to year; minutes to hours	Symptoms gradually become constant	Unknown
Vertigo (EA-5) (Escayg et al., 2000)	20–30	Ataxia, vertigo, juvenile epilepsy	Effective	None	Daily; hours	Nystagmus, mild ataxia, dysarthria	2q22–q23, Ca^{2+} channel, CACNB4
Photophobia (EA-6) (Jen et al., 2005)	Birth to 20	Ataxia, dysarthria, hemiplegic migraine, photophobia	Effective	Fever, emotional stress, fatigue, alcohol, caffeine	Daily; 2–3 hours	Ataxia, nystagmus	5p13, SLC1A3; glutamate transporter EAAT1
Ataxia (EA-7) (Kerber et al., 2007)	<20	Ataxia, weakness, dysarthria	Unknown	Excitement, exercise	Monthly to yearly; hours to days	Normal	19p13

patients with autopsies had ataxia resembling EA-2, but had not responded to acetazolamide, nor did their molecular genetics workup fit EA-2 (Julien et al., 2001).

Molecular genetics of paroxysmal dyskinesias

A number of paroxysmal dyskinesias have been mapped to chromosome 16. PKD with infantile convulsions has been mapped to 16p11.2–q12.1 and called EKD1 and designated as DYT10 (Tomita et al., 1999; Bennett et al., 2000; Swoboda et al., 2000). PKD without convulsions has been mapped to 16q13–q22.1, with the gene referred to as EKD2 and designated as DYT19 (Valente et al., 2000). The ICCA syndrome has been reported without linkage to these two loci (Spacey et al., 2002). A family with infantile convulsions has an associated PNKD, and the abnormal gene has been mapped to chromosome 16 (Szepetowski et al., 1997). The gene in this region that appears to be responsible for ICCA is the sodium/glucose cotransporter gene (KST1) (Roll et al., 2002). It also appears to be responsible for benign familial infantile convulsions. Perhaps this disorder with its genetic

mapping has been referred to by others as PKD with infantile convulsions. Guerrini (2001) proposes that disparate reports of families suggest that the same gene could be responsible for autosomal recessive rolandic epilepsy, PED, writer's cramp (RE-PED-WC), and PNKD, with specific mutations accounting for each of these mendelian disorders. Evidence is for a major gene or a cluster of genes for epilepsy and paroxysmal dyskinesia to the pericentromeric region of chromosome 16. These families need to be tested for the KST1 mutation. Caraballo and colleagues (2001) have diagrammed where the gene loci for these different disorders have been mapped on chromosome 16 (Fig. 22.1).

Six pedigrees with PKD have been found on the Chinese mainland, and they were not linked to the two known loci and so represent another familial form of PKD (Zhou et al., 2008).

An autosomal dominant form of PED with development delay and erythrocyte changes has been found to be due to glucose transporter 1 (GLUT1) deficiency (Weber et al., 2008; Zorzi et al., 2008). There is a cation leak from the erythrocytes that alters the intracellular concentration of sodium, potassium, and calcium. This leads to hemolytic

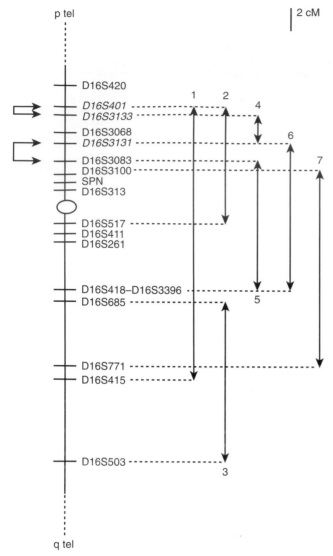

p tel

| 2 cM

D16S420

D16S401
D16S3133

D16S3068

D16S3131

D16S3083
D16S3100
SPN
D16S313

D16S517
D16S411
D16S261

D16S418–D16S3396

D16S685

D16S771

D16S415

D16S503

q tel

Figure 22.1 Schematic representation of the genetic map of human chromosome 16p12–q12. Critical regions are indicated: 1 = benign familial infantile convulsions (BFIC) (7 families, Caraballo et al., 2001); 2 = ICCA (Szepetowski et al., 1997); 3 = PKD (Valente et al., 2000); 4 = reflex epilepsy–PED–writer's cramp (RE-PED-WC) syndrome (Guerrini et al., 1999); 5 = PKD and BFIC (Tomita et al., 1999); 6 = PKD and BFIC (Swoboda et al., 2000); 7 = PKD (Bennett et al., 2000). *From Caraballo R, Pavek S, Lemainque A, et al. Linkage of benign familial infantile convulsions to chromosome 16p12-q12 suggests allelism of the infantile convulsions and choreoathetosis syndrome. Am J Hum Genet 2001;68(3):788–794.*

associated with PNKD in 50 individuals from eight families; they cause changes (Ala to Val) in the N-terminal region of two MR1 isoforms. The MR1L isoform is specifically expressed in the brain and is localized to the cell membrane while the MR1S isoform is ubiquitously expressed and shows diffuse cytoplasmic and nuclear localization. The *MR1* gene is homologous to the hydroxyacylglutathione hydrolase (*HAGH*) gene, which functions in a pathway to detoxify methylglyoxal, a compound that is present in coffee and alcoholic beverages and is produced as a by-product of oxidative stress. The finding of the *MR1* gene locus suggests a mechanism whereby alcohol, coffee, and stress may act as precipitants of attacks in PNKD. However, there is genetic heterogeneity in PNKD, because there is a Canadian family without this mutation, with links to a separate locus at 2q31 instead (Spacey et al., 2006); it has been designated as PNKD2 and also DYT20, while the *MR1* gene disorder is called PNKD1 and DYT8.

Auburger and colleagues (1996) studied a family with PNKD with associated spasticity; their mutated gene was mapped to a potassium channel gene cluster on chromosome 1p. The attacks are said to consist of dystonia of limbs, imbalance, dysarthria, diplopia, and sometimes headache. The attacks last about 20 minutes and can be precipitated by exercise, stress, lack of sleep, and alcohol consumption. Some affected members had persistent spastic paraparesis, which would make this family's condition different from classic Mount–Reback syndrome. This condition has been called choreoathetosis/spasticity episodica (CSE). The locus is very close to the *GLUT1* locus, suggesting that the family might be positive for a *GLUT1* mutation.

A large Australian family with autosomal dominant hypnogenic frontal lobe seizures/dystonia has been found to have a missense mutation in the second transmembrane domain of the nicotinic acetylcholine receptor alpha 4 subunit (CHRNA4) gene, located on chromosome 20q13.2–q13.3 (Oldani et al., 1998). A second locus has been found on chromosome 15q24 (Phillips et al., 1998, 2001) and a third locus has been found on chromosome 1 in a large Italian family (Gambardella et al., 2000).

For a detailed review of the genetics of the paroxysmal dyskinesias, the reader is referred to the article by Weber and Lerche (2009).

Miscellany

There are probably a number of other types of paroxysmal dyskinesias that do not fit well into the classification scheme listed previously (Pourfar et al., 2005). For example, a case of truncal flexion spasms that persist repeatedly in attacks lasting several hours has been described (Brown et al., 1991). These were considered to have a spinal origin, presumably involving the propriospinal pathways. We have seen a patient with multiple brief dystonic spasms, lasting seconds, in a woman following cardiac arrhythmias. These attacks have all the clinical features of symptomatic PKD, except that they were not precipitated by sudden movement or startle. Like PKD, they responded dramatically to low dosages of carbamazepine. Perhaps the major delimiter in classifying the paroxysmal dyskinesias should not be whether they are kinesigenic or not, but the duration of

anemia and echinocytosis as detected by electron microscopy. Many more papers have reported GLUT1 deficiency causing PED (Suls et al., 2008; Schneider et al., 2009; Leen et al., 2010).

Two papers independently reported the mapping of a gene for PNKD to chromosome 2q31–q36 (Fink et al., 1996; Fouad et al., 1996), and the region was narrowed to 2q33–q35 by Fink et al. (1997). Another family was mapped by Raskind and colleagues (1998), who narrowed the region to 2q34. And Jarman and colleagues (1997) mapped the gene to a large British family. Although a cluster of sodium channel genes is near the PNKD locus, the mutated gene has now been found to be the myofibrillogenesis regulator 1 (*MR1*) (Lee et al., 2004). The mutations in this gene were the attacks. Like tics, stereotypies can occur episodically (Video 22.9). 🎥

A syndrome in infant girls is self-stimulatory (previously called masturbatory) behavior that occurs episodically (Fleisher and Morrison, 1990; Mink and Neil, 1995; Nechay et al., 2004; Yang et al., 2005). The episodes appear between 3 and 14 months of age and consist of the child's applying her suprapubic region to a firm edge of furniture, such as the arm of a sofa (Video 22.10). There is often stiffening of the lower extremities. The episodes last less than a minute to hours at a time. Most commonly this behavior is misdiagnosed as epilepsy or paroxysmal dystonia. 🎥

Summary

The paroxysmal dyskinesias are usually divided into kinesigenic dyskinesias (which are induced by sudden movement and are brief in duration, lasting seconds to 5 minutes), the nonkinesigenic dyskinesias (which are not induced by sudden movement), and the exertional dyskinesias. The duration of PNKD is usually prolonged (2 minutes to 4 hours, up to 2 days), and PED is intermediate in duration (5–30 minutes). PNKD is often induced by alcohol, cold, heat, fatigue, caffeine, and stress and is caused by mutations in a gene (*MR1*) that is involved in a stress–response pathway.

The kinesigenic dyskinesias ordinarily respond extremely well to a variety of anticonvulsants, whereas these drugs are usually not beneficial in the other two types. PNKD is sometimes sensitive to clonazepam, benzodiazepines, acetazolamide, anticholinergics, and neuroleptics.

PKD, PNKD, and PED have all been reported also to occur with benign infantile epilepsy (ICCA syndrome); the genes have been mapped to the 16p12 region, and it appears that the involved gene for this syndrome is the sodium/glucose cotransporter gene (*KST1*). PNKD has also been shown to be associated with a mutation to myelofibrillogenesis 1; and PED with mutations of glucose transporter 1.

Variants of these disorders are the paroxysmal dyskinesias that occur during sleep (paroxysmal hypnogenic dyskinesias), for which there is mounting evidence that they are supplementary sensorimotor area seizures, and the transient paroxysmal dystonias (particularly torticollis) in infants.

When the genes have been identified, they involve ion channels. It is likely that all the paroxysmal dyskinesias will be channelopathies.

References available on Expert Consult: www.expertconsult.com

495

CHAPTER **23**

Restless legs and peripheral movement disorders

Chapter contents

Restless legs syndrome and periodic movements of sleep	496
Peripheral movement disorders	500

Restless legs syndrome and periodic movements of sleep

The term "restless legs" has been applied to a number of conditions. Ekbom (1960) originally applied this term to unpleasant crawling sensations in the legs, particularly when sitting and relaxing in the evening, which disappeared on walking. The syndrome was probably first described by Thomas Willis in 1685. "Restlessness" is also a characteristic feature of akathisia, but here the feeling is of inner restlessness not specifically referred to the legs, although this inner feeling can be dissipated by activity. "Inner tension" is also a feature of the urge preceding tics, relieved by the involuntary movement.

The restless legs syndrome (RLS) is characterized by a deep, ill-defined discomfort or dysesthesiae in the legs, which arises during prolonged rest, or when the patient is drowsy and trying to fall asleep, especially at night (Winkelmann et al., 2000; Bassetti et al., 2001, Trenkwalder et al., 2009; Trenkwalder and Paulus, 2010). The disorder is truly diurnal; the symptoms are worse during the night, even when the person tries to stay awake for long periods of time (Hening et al., 1999; Trenkwalder et al., 1999). The discomfort may be difficult to describe – terms such as crawling, creeping, pulling, itching, drawing, or stretching are used, and the feeling usually is felt in the muscles or bones. These intolerable sensations are relieved by movement of the legs or by walking. The feeling usually is bilateral and the arms are rarely involved. Standardized criteria have been put forward by the International Restless Legs Syndrome Study Group (Table 23.1) (Allen et al., 2003). Complaints of restless legs are common, with an estimated prevalence of 3–10% (Phillips et al., 2000; Rothdach et al., 2000; Hening et al., 2004; Bjorvatn et al., 2005). A large population study (over 16 000 adults) showed a prevalence of any restless symptoms to be 7.2%, and moderately or severely distressing symptoms to be 2.7% (Allen et al., 2005). RLS is generally a condition of middle to old age, but at least one-third of

patients experience their first symptoms before the age of 20 years (Kotagal and Silber, 2004). Most patients have mild symptoms to begin with, but these worsen with time, so that they seek aid in middle life. Remission is uncommon, occurring in about 15% (Walters et al., 1996). RLS can even affect a phantom limb (Skidmore et al., 2009; Vetrugno et al., 2010).

The majority of those with RLS also exhibit periodic movements of sleep (Walters, 1995; Trenkwalder et al., 1996) (Table 23.2). These consist of brief (1–2 seconds) jerks of one or both legs, consisting of, at it simplest, dorsiflexion of the big toe and foot. Initially there is a jerk, but subsequently there is sustained tonic spasm. Such events tend to occur in runs every 20 seconds or so for minutes or hours. Sometimes the whole leg or both legs may flex (Fig. 23.1). The movement resembles a flexion reflex (Bara-Jimenez et al., 2000). Such periodic movements often wake the sleeping partner and may cause disturbance of sleep in the affected individual, in which case there may be excessive daytime drowsiness. Generally they appear during periods of arousal during sleep in stage I and II, and decrease during deep sleep during stages III and IV; they are unusual during REM sleep. Sometimes such flexion movements of one or both legs can occur in the waking subject, particularly when drowsy (Hening et al., 1986) (Video 23.1). Note should be made that some patients with RLS have propriospinal myoclonus just before falling asleep (Vetrugno et al., 2005). 📹

While most people with restless legs have periodic movements of sleep (at least in the sleep laboratory), there is a proportion who do not complain of restless legs. The combined syndrome of restless legs and periodic movements of sleep is an age-related condition; its incidence increases in adult and late life. It usually presents after the age of 30, and it is said to affect 5% of those between the ages of 30 and 50 years, and as many as 30% of those over the age of 50. However, in a large proportion of cases, the periodic movements of sleep do not cause complaint and are found incidentally during sleep studies. In many with restless legs the condition is not disabling.

DOI: 10.1016/B978-1-4377-2369-4.00023-8

Table 23.1 Restless legs syndrome

Essential diagnostic criteria for restless legs syndrome

1. An urge to move the legs, usually accompanied or caused by uncomfortable and unpleasant sensations in the legs. (Sometimes the urge to move is present with the uncomfortable sensations and sometimes the arms or other body parts are involved in addition to the legs.)
2. The urge to move or unpleasant sensations begin or worsen during periods of rest or inactivity such as lying or sitting.
3. The urge to move or unpleasant sensations are partially or totally relieved by movement, such as walking or stretching, at least as long as the activity continues.
4. The urge to move or unpleasant sensations are worse in the evening or night than during the day or only occur in the evening or night. (When symptoms are very severe, the worsening at night may not be noticeable but must have been previously present.)

Supportive clinical features of restless legs syndrome

Family history

The prevalence of RLS among first-degree relatives of people with RLS is 3–5 times greater than in people without RLS.

Response to dopaminergic therapy

Nearly all people with RLS show at least an initial response to either levodopa or a dopamine-receptor agonist at doses considered to be very low in relation to the traditional doses of these medications used for the treatment of Parkinson disease. This initial response is not, however, universally maintained.

Periodic limb movements (during wakefulness or sleep)

Periodic limb movements in sleep (PLMS) occur in at least 85% of people with RLS; however, PLMS also commonly occur in other disorders and in elderly people. In children, PLMS are much less common than in adults.

From Allen RP, Picchietti D, Hening WA, et al. Restless legs syndrome: diagnostic criteria, special considerations, and epidemiology. A report from the restless legs syndrome diagnosis and epidemiology workshop at the National Institutes of Health. Sleep Med 2003;4(2):101–19, with permission.

Table 23.2 Periodic movements of sleep

Runs (every 30 seconds or so) of brief (1–2 seconds) jerks in one or both legs

Initial jerk followed by tonic spasm

Dorsiflexion of big toe and foot (or flexion of whole leg)

During arousal (stage I and II sleep)

May occur in awake, drowsy individual

Asymptomatic, may wake sleeping partner or, sometimes, the patient

Prevalence increase with age: rare under 30 years; 5% 30–50 years; 29% over 50 years

There is evidence to suggest that the disorder in many if not most patients is transmitted as an autosomal dominant trait (Walters et al., 1996; Winkelmann et al., 2000; Xiong et al., 2010). For a number of years, family studies have been conducted looking for genes with strong mendelian influence. Linkage on 12q seemed the best defined and has been designated RLS1 (Desautels et al., 2005). Variants in the neuronal nitric oxide synthase gene (NOS1) may be the relevant gene at this locus (Winkelmann et al., 2008). Linkage has been found on 14q for a few families and has been designated RLS2 (Bonati et al., 2003; Levchenko et al., 2004). Linkage on 9p24–22 has been designated RLS3 (Liebetanz et al., 2006; Winkelmann and Ferini-Strambi, 2006). Subsequent linkages have identified on chromosomes 2q, 20p, and 6p and designated RLS4, RLS5, and RLS6 (Kemlink et al., 2008). Specific genes, however, have not been identified.

Association studies in large populations have now identified several common sequence variants (single nucleotide polymorphism, SNP) that convey substantial risk for the disorder (Winkelmann, 2008). These variants explain a considerable amount of the familial incidence, and to some extent explain why the earlier studies were having difficulty, since they did not take these strong genetic effects into account. One SNP was identified by two groups, BTBD9 (Stefansson et al., 2007; Winkelmann et al., 2007). Carriers have a 50% risk of developing RLS. It is possible that this SNP is actually specific for periodic limb movements in sleep (PLMS) rather than RLS (Stefansson et al., 2007). Four other SNPs have been identified, MEIS1, MAP2K5, LBXCOR1, and PTPRD (protein tyrosine phosphatase receptor type delta) (Winkelmann et al., 2007; Schormair et al., 2008). The first three of these SNPs have been confirmed in a large replication study (Kemlink et al., 2009). Their biologic function is not clear.

Some cases have been associated with anemia, pregnancy, chronic myelopathies and peripheral neuropathies, gastric surgery, uremia, and chronic lung disease (Ondo and Jankovic, 1996; Winkelmann et al., 2000). It is not uncommon in Parkinson disease (Ondo et al., 2002) and one epidemiologic study found increased prevalence compared with the general population (Krishnan et al., 2003) while another did not (Tan et al., 2002). A point of confusion in this regard is that wearing-off phenomena may mimic RLS symptoms (Peralta et al., 2009). These symptomatic cases of restless legs should be distinguished from the primary familial form of the condition. Occasionally drugs (neuroleptics and antidepressants, lithium, and anticonvulsants) may precipitate intense restlessness of the legs.

Interestingly, in the idiopathic form of the disorder, Earley and colleagues (2000b) found low CSF ferritin levels and high CSF transferrin levels. There was no difference, however, in serum ferritin and transferrin levels. The findings suggest that there might be low brain iron in these patients. Further investigations by this group have shown that the CSF ferritin is low only in the early-onset RLS patients and that levels are lower at night than during the day (Earley et al., 2005). Neuroimaging studies of iron and a neuropathologic evaluation of seven brains has demonstrated decreased iron and H-ferritin in the substantia nigra (Connor et al., 2003). There was a positive correlation between the serum and CSF ferritin levels in both patients with RLS and normal controls, but the slope of the regression lines for the RLS group was lower. These results indicate low brain iron concentration might be caused by the dysfunction of iron transport from serum to central nervous system (CNS) in patients with idiopathic RLS (Mizuno et al., 2005), and now there is good evidence for this (Connor et al., 2011). Another observation is that the number of mitochondria and the mitochondrial ferritin is increased in the substantia nigra; the authors suggest that the mitochondria might also be partially

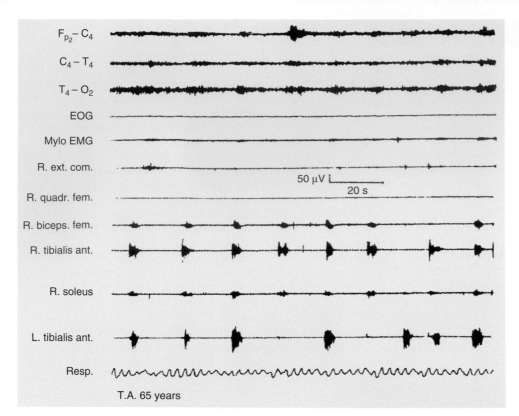

Fp₂– C₄

C₄ – T₄

T₄ – O₂

EOG

Mylo EMG

R. ext. com.

R. quadr. fem.

R. biceps. fem.

R. tibialis ant.

R. soleus

L. tibialis ant.

Resp.

50 µV
20 s

T.A. 65 years

Figure 23.1 Polysomnography recording from a patient with periodic limb movements of sleep. Note the periodic EMG bursts in leg muscles coming about every 20 seconds. *From Lugaresi E, Cirignotta F, Coccagna G, Montagna P. Nocturnal myoclonus and restless legs syndrome. Adv Neurol 1986;43:295–307, with permission.*

responsible for the low cytosolic iron (Snyder et al., 2009). Iron deficiency could well influence dopamine metabolism (Connor, 2008; Connor et al., 2009).

Periodic movements of sleep should be distinguished from hypnic jerks or "sleep starts," which consist of whole-body sudden jerks on falling asleep, and from fragmentary sleep myoclonus. This consists of multifocal myoclonus, which can commonly be observed in the dog asleep on the mat. RLS must be distinguished from the syndrome of painful legs and moving toes, and from painful night cramps.

The pathophysiology of primary restless legs and periodic movements of sleep is unknown (Hening, 2004; Trenkwalder and Paulus, 2004). That dopaminergic mechanisms are involved is strongly suggested by the amelioration of symptoms with dopaminergic therapy. A critical role for the basal ganglia is suggested by the observation that pallidotomy or deep brain stimulation of the pallidum for Parkinson disease ameliorated the sensory symptoms of restless legs (Rye and DeLong, 1999; Okun et al., 2005). (In relation to surgery for Parkinson disease, some patients with deep brain stimulation of the subthalamic nucleus will develop RLS (Kedia et al., 2004). This might be due to the fact that dopaminergic drug therapy is reduced, and this might unmask the disorder.) There is some evidence for D2 receptor binding in the striatum to be low, while presynaptic dopamine function appears normal as indicated by dopamine transporter measurement (Michaud et al., 2002). All studies do not find this D2 receptor abnormality (Eisensehr et al., 2001). Interestingly, there is a strong relationship between iron and dopamine, iron deficiency causing a dopamine deficiency (Allen, 2004).

Voxel-based morphometry (VBM) studies in RLS have produced conflicting results. Etgen et al. (2005) found bilateral increase in gray matter in the pulvinar of the thalamus bilaterally. Unrath et al. (2007) found a decrease in cortical gray matter in the sensorimotor cortex, and the degree of abnormality appeared to correlate with the severity of the disorder. This has some interest since the primary symptom of RLS is sensory. On the other hand, other reports found no apparent relevant abnormality (Hornyak et al., 2008; Celle et al., 2010).

Opioid receptor availability evaluated with positron emission tomography and [¹¹C]diprenorphine, a nonselective opioid receptor radioligand, showed no difference between patients and controls (von Spiczak et al., 2005). However, patients' symptoms were inversely proportional to the binding in the brain medial pain system.

RLS is characterized by abnormal sensations, and sensory testing reveals abnormalities of temperature sensation. Studies suggest that in idiopathic RLS, the abnormality is in the central processing (Schattschneider et al., 2004; Tyvaert et al., 2009).

If the syndrome is distressing, drug treatment may be justified (Satija and Ondo, 2008). A nocturnal dose of a levodopa preparation is beneficial (Tan and Ondo, 2000; Trenkwalder et al., 2003). Dopamine agonists are preferred such as bromocriptine (Earley et al., 1998; Pieta et al., 1998), pergolide (Wetter et al., 1999; Stiasny et al., 2001), pramipexole (Montplaisir et al., 1999; Ferini-Strambi et al., 2008; Inoue et al., 2010), and ropinirole (Adler et al., 2004; Bogan et al., 2006; Hansen et al., 2009). Dopaminergic therapy with the rotigotine patch can be effective (Trenkwalder et al., 2008a). Dopaminergic therapy has efficacy even in patients with complete spinal cord lesions, suggesting some action at the level of the spinal cord (de Mello et al., 1999). Alternatively, a nocturnal dose of an opiate such as codeine phosphate (Becker et al., 1993; Walters et al., 1993; Prinz, 1995), or of a benzodiazepine such as clonazepam may be of help. Carbamazepine also may help (Telstad et al., 1984), as may baclofen (Guilleminault and Flagg, 1984), clonidine (Wagner et al., 1996), gabapentin (Garcia-Borreguero et al., 2002; Albanese and Filippini, 2003), and pregabalin (Allen et al., 2010; Garcia-Borreguero et al., 2010). It may be necessary to change from one drug to another if tolerance develops. Placebo responsiveness in RLS is very high and this must be taken into account when analyzing results from studies (Fulda and Wetter, 2008).

A problem with dopaminergic therapy of RLS is augmentation, an increase in the severity of symptoms, a shift in time for the start of symptoms to earlier in the day, a shorter latency to symptoms when resting, and sometimes spread of symptoms to other body parts (Hogl et al., 2010). The explanation is not completely clear, but one hypothesis is that there is an increase of dopamine concentration in the CNS with dopaminergic overstimulation, particularly of the D1 receptor (Paulus and Trenkwalder, 2006). This suggests that dopaminergic therapeutic levels should be low for optimal therapy (Williams and Garcia-Borreguero, 2009). It is possible to give the dopaminergic therapy earlier in the day to combat this, but this may provoke an even earlier onset of symptoms. Iron supplementation and opiates have also been suggested for therapy.

Pathologic gambling and other compulsive behaviors have been reported in RLS patients on dopamine agonists, similar to that seen in Parkinson disease (Driver-Dunckley et al., 2007; Quickfall and Suchowersky, 2007; Tippmann-Peikert et al., 2007; Pourcher et al., 2010).

Iron also has been recommended for therapy (Ekbom, 1960), and it has been suggested that it may act by virtue of its effect upon dopamine and opiate receptors (Earley et al., 2000a), but one study was negative (Davis et al., 2000). Another open-label study evaluated the effects of a single 1000 mg intravenous infusion of iron dextran (Earley et al., 2004). Therapy significantly improved the mean global RLS symptom severity, total sleep time, hours with RLS symptoms and PLMS, but on an individual basis failed to produce any response in 3 of the 10 subjects who were fully treated. An open-label study of 25 severely refractory patients with iron dextran produced a good response in some, but the effect was highly variable, and two patients had an anaphylactic reaction (Ondo, 2010). A randomized, double-blind, placebo-controlled study of intravenous iron sucrose did not show any efficacy (Earley et al., 2009). Iron should be curative, of course, in those cases associated with iron deficiency. In patients with low ferritin levels, oral ferrous sulfate 325 mg twice daily improved symptoms more than placebo (Wang et al., 2009). Patients with mild to moderate iron deficiency treated with intravenous iron sucrose also improved, but not significantly more than placebo treatment (Grote et al., 2009).

Practice parameters for treatment have been published by the American Academy of Sleep Medicine (Littner et al., 2004). Evidence-based reviews have been published by the European Federation of Neurological Societies (Vignatelli et al., 2006), the Movement Disorder Society (Trenkwalder et al., 2008b), and Cochrane (Scholz, 2011a, 2011b). A review of the dopamine agonists shows their efficacy (Zintzaras et al., 2010). A useful general algorithm has been developed (Fig. 23.2) (Silber et al., 2004).

ALGORITHM FOR MANAGEMENT OF RLS

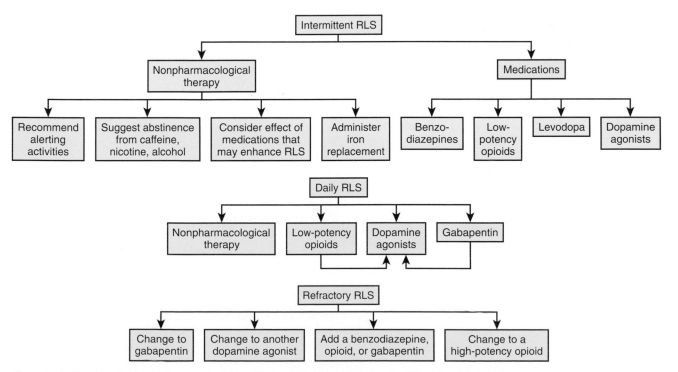

Figure 23.2 Algorithm for therapeutic management of RLS. *From Silber MH, Fhrenberg BL, Allen RP, et al. An algorithm for the management of restless legs syndrome. Mayo Clin Proc 2004;79(7):916–22, with permission.*

Table 23.3 Peripheral movement disorders

Hemifacial spasm
Spinal segmental myoclonus
Root, plexus, nerve lesions
Reflex sympathetic dystrophy
Causalgia–dystonia syndrome
Dystonia triggered by peripheral injury
Jumpy stumps
Belly dancer's dyskinesia
Painful legs and moving toes

Table 23.4 Criteria for a movement disorder to be related to trauma

1. Injury must be severe enough to cause local symptoms persisting for at least 2 weeks or requiring medical evaluation within 2 weeks of the injury
2. The onset of the movement disorder must have occurred within a few days or months (up to 1 year) after the injury
3. The onset of the movement disorder must have been anatomically related to the site of the injury

From Jankovic J. Post-traumatic movement disorders: central and peripheral mechanisms. Neurology 1994;44:2006–14; and Cardoso F, Jankovic J. Peripherally induced tremor and parkinsonism. Arch Neurol 1995;52:263–70.

Peripheral movement disorders

Abnormal involuntary movements (dyskinesias) usually are caused by brain damage or dysfunction. Occasionally, however, lesions of the spinal cord, spinal roots, cervical or lumbar plexus, or even peripheral nerves appear to cause a variety of dyskinesias (Table 23.3). Sometimes the relationship between the trauma and the movement disorder is not definite, and there are no proven rules to relate them. Jankovic and colleagues have proposed some criteria that can be used as guidelines while waiting for more definitive rules (Table 23.4) (Jankovic, 1994; Cardoso and Jankovic, 1995). An example of a definitive peripheral disorder is hemifacial spasm, where compression of the facial nerve by a cerebellopontine angle mass lesion, or by aberrant arteries in the posterior fossa, produces repetitive clonic and tonic contractions of one side of the face. Local pathology in the spinal cord may lead to focal spinal segmental myoclonus. Similar focal myoclonus is sometimes due to damage to spinal roots, the plexus, or peripheral nerves. Such lesions also rarely cause other dyskinesias, such as dystonia and other forms of muscle spasms, sometimes associated with causalgia and reflex sympathetic dystrophy. Finally, a peripheral injury may act as the trigger to the appearance of dyskinesias thought to arise in the brain, as is the case in a significant proportion of patients with primary dystonia. In some way, the peripheral injury alters CNS activity to generate involuntary movements.

Hemifacial spasm

Hemifacial spasm is characterized by synchronous spasms of one side of the face (Table 23.5). Most cases are primary,

Table 23.5 Hemifacial spasm

Unilateral clonic jerks, with tonic spasm of all facial muscles
Starts around eye, spreads to mouth and platysma
Spasms lift eyebrow
Irregular and unpredictable; triggered by facial movement; may occur in flurries
Mild facial weakness develops, with paradoxical synkinesis
Adults. Females more than males (3:2)
95% essential, due to vascular compression of seventh nerve at exit from brainstem
5% symptomatic, due to post-paralytic (Bell palsy), or cerebellopontine angle mass lesions (tumor or arteriovenous malformations), or rarely brainstem lesions (multiple sclerosis: tonic spasms or facial myokymia)
Remissions rare
Treatment:
    Drugs usually do not help
    Botulinum toxin
    Posterior fossa exploration and facial nerve protection

but some are secondary following recovery from facial nerve paresis (Colosimo et al., 2006; Yaltho and Jankovic, 2011). The spasms are usually very brief, but can occur in runs and are occasionally tonic. The disorder typically begins around the eye and this often is the most symptomatic aspect to the disorder (Fig. 23.3 and Video 23.2). The disorder can be bilateral, but then the two sides of the face do not spasm in synchrony. Cases seem to be more common in persons of Asian origin (Poungvarin et al., 1995). Twitching can be brought out by facial muscle contraction. The disorder clearly involves the facial nerve, and the etiology appears to be most frequently (94%) a compression of the nerve by a blood vessel just as the nerve leaves the brainstem (Tan and Chan, 2004; Naraghi et al., 2007). About 4% of cases are due to a tumor compressing the nerve (Han et al., 2010). Biopsy of the compressed nerve shows demyelination. Definitive treatment can be by surgery to decompress the nerve (Samii et al., 2002; Huh et al., 2008; Hyun et al., 2010), although many patients prefer botulinum toxin treatment, which can be highly effective (Poungvarin et al., 1995; Jost and Kohl, 2001; Defazio et al., 2002; Simpson et al., 2008; Bentivoglio et al., 2009; Gill and Kraft, 2010) and can improve quality of life (Tan et al., 2004).

Although the etiology is relatively clear, the pathophysiology is still not certain. There are two main hypotheses and there are good data to support each.

Nerve origin hypothesis

This hypothesis proposes that the abnormal discharges producing the spasms come from the region of demyelinated nerve under the compression (Nielsen, 1984a, 1984b; Nielsen and Jannetta, 1984). It is known that demyelinated nerve can produce spontaneous discharges, called ectopic discharges. In addition, there can be lateral transmission of activity between demyelinated nerve axons, called ephaptic transmission. Ephaptic transmission can be responsible for involvement of much of the face. It is also possible in the transmission all the way to the brainstem and back, rather than just to the site of demyelination (Moller and Jannetta, 1984; Moller, 1987).

Focal myoclonus due to root, plexus, or peripheral nerve lesions

Myoclonic jerking of the paraspinal muscles due to a malignant tumor involving the fifth thoracic root, without long tract signs of spinal cord involvement, has been described (Sotaniemi, 1985). Similar focal myoclonus of the legs has also occurred with lumbosacral radiculopathy, and after lumbar laminectomy for lumbar stenosis and root lesions (Jankovic and Pardo, 1986). Rhythmic myoclonus of the quadriceps muscle has been reported due to a Schwann-cell sarcoma of the femoral nerve (Said and Bathien, 1977).

Focal myoclonus of the right arm due to a brachial plexus lesion has been described following radiotherapy for carcinoma of the breast followed by abduction trauma of the right shoulder (Banks et al., 1985). The latter case exhibited rhythmic muscle jerks at about five per second in the distribution of the axillary and radial nerves, but not in other muscles innervated by the lateral and medial cords of the brachial plexus. Electromyographic analysis of this case indicated that the myoclonus arose from a generator located in a segment of the posterior cord of the brachial plexus, between the departure of the axillary nerve and distal to the emergence of the suprascapular nerve. Another patient developed myoclonus of one arm after an electrical injury to the left brachial plexus (Jankovic and Pardo, 1986). Myoclonus of an arm has even occurred after a thoracic sympathectomy (Jankovic and Pardo, 1986).

The clinical characteristics of myoclonus due to spinal cord, root, plexus, or peripheral nerve diseases are:

1. It is focal, being confined to the muscles innervated by the affected spinal cord segments or peripheral lower motor neurons.
2. It is usually spontaneous and rhythmic, and it often persists in sleep.

These observations suggest that it is the result of repetitive, spontaneous discharge of groups of anterior horn cells.

Swanson et al. (1962) suggested two mechanisms which might be responsible for spinal segmental myoclonus: (1) enhanced neuronal excitability due to direct cellular excitation by inflammation or tumor, or (2) enhanced neuronal excitability due to removal of inhibition. The former seems unlikely, since spinal segmental myoclonus can occur without evidence of damage to anterior horn cells. Loss of inhibition of anterior horn cell pools seems more probable.

Posterior rhizotomy or hemicordectomy leads to abnormal spontaneous discharge of some spinal neurons in the deafferented segments, which tend to fire in bursts at high frequency (Loeser and Ward, 1967). However, these bursting spinal neurons are found in the dorsal, not the ventral horns. Nevertheless, such spontaneous bursting of spinal interneurons following deafferentation might drive anterior horn cells to produce focal myoclonus.

Alternatively, loss of inhibitory spinal interneurons might liberate anterior horn cells to fire spontaneously in a rhythmic burst fashion. In the case described by Davis et al. (1981)

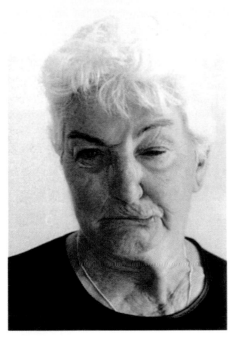

Figure 23.3 Left-sided hemifacial spasm. Note the elevation of the left brow with the spasm due to contraction of the frontalis muscle. Elevation of the brow with closing of the eye is not easily possible voluntarily. The phenomenon was noted by Babinski and has been referred to as the "other Babinski's sign." *From Devoize JL. "The other" Babinski's sign: paradoxical raising of the eyebrow in hemifacial spasm. J Neurol Neurosurg Psychiatry 2001;70(4):516, with permission.*

case of activity in demyelinated axons with ephaptic transmission for trains of activity to be produced following a single action potential. These phenomena could explain many of the clinical features.

Additionally, there are physiological studies that are consistent. If a branch of the seventh nerve is stimulated, in these patients there will be late responses seen in muscles innervated by other branches at latencies consistent with ephaptic transmission at the site of demyelination. This phenomenon is not influenced by botulinum toxin treatment (Geller et al., 1989). Studies of the variability of transmission of this effect, using the technique of jitter, are consistent with only the neuromuscular junction and no intervening synapses (Sanders, 1989).

The final argument in favor of the nerve origin hypothesis is the fact that the disorder very rapidly ameliorates following decompression.

Facial nucleus hypothesis

According to this theory, the peripheral lesion leads to hyperexcitability of the facial nucleus and the discharges arise there. There is a rat model where such a phenomenon has been demonstrated. Perhaps the most persuasive argument for this hypothesis is that there is hyperexcitability of the blink reflex in hemifacial spasm, and this must involve brainstem synaptic circuitry. By this theory, the late responses seen with stimulation of branches of the nerve are enhanced F-waves (Roth et al., 1990; Ishikawa et al., 1994). Lastly, while the calculations deal in differences of only a millisecond or two, conduction times may be more consistent with spinal myoclonus occurred following ischemic damage to the cord, which at autopsy was found to have caused extensive loss of small and medium-sized interneurons, with relative preservation of large anterior horn cells. The loss of inhibitory spinal interneurons could release anterior horn cells to discharge spontaneously, but what then determines their tendency to fire repetitively and rhythmically is less clear (Kiehn, 1991; Kiehn and Eken, 1997). Loss of spinal interneurons also is the pathologic change thought to be responsible for alpha spinal rigidity.

Jumpy stumps

Not only did Weir Mitchell (Mitchell, 1872) describe causalgia after gunshot wounds of peripheral nerves, he also recorded tremor, jerks, and spasms of the remaining stump following amputation, sometimes associated with severe phantom pain. The "painful, jumpy stump" has since been described by others (Russell, 1970; Steiner et al., 1974; Marion et al., 1989; Kulisevsky et al., 1992), and even a phantom dyskinesia induced by metoclopramide has been recorded (Jankovic and Glass, 1985) (Video 23.3).

Jerking of the amputation stump (jactitation), coinciding with lancinating neuralgic stump pains, frequently occurs in the postoperative period but settles over weeks or months (Russell, 1970). The cases referred to above, however, experienced spasms and jerks of the stump for prolonged periods, for example up to 40 years in one of the patients reported by Marion et al. (1989), who also reviewed many similar cases described in the earlier literature. Jerking of the stump frequently was preceded by severe pain in the stump, appearing weeks or months after the surgery. Upper or lower limb stumps could be affected. The stump jerks could be induced by voluntary movement or, sometimes, by cutaneous stimuli.

Steiner et al. (1974) considered involuntary stump movements to be a form of segmental myoclonus, caused by afferent impulses arising from the severed nerves. Marion et al. (1989) concluded that they were due to either "the result of functional changes in spinal (or cortical) circuitry leading to redirection of afferent information through different spinal neurons, or structural reorganization of local neuronal circuitry by axonal sprouting following nerve injury."

Belly dancer's dyskinesia

Belly dancer's dyskinesia, or the moving umbilicus syndrome, is another bizarre condition sometimes related to abdominal trauma. Iliceto et al. (1990) described five patients with odd abnormal movements of the abdomen (Video 23.4). One had diaphragmatic flutter (repetitive contractions at about one per second are seen on diaphragmatic screening), but the remainder did not. The latter exhibited regular rhythmic contractions of the abdominal wall, which had a sinuous, writhing flowing character, often moving the umbilicus from side to side or in a circular rotatory fashion. The intensity of the abnormal movement may vary with respiration. Three of these four patients dated the onset of their abdominal dyskinesia to trauma (cholecystectomy and anal fistula, cystoscopic removal of a renal calculus, and cystectomy), and two had severe pain. Botulinum toxin can be helpful (Lim and Seet, 2009). One patient responded to bilateral deep brain stimulation of the globus pallidus interna (Schrader et al., 2009).

Painful legs and moving toes

There is another condition in which injury to peripheral nerves and roots may cause the combination of pain in the leg and abnormal involuntary movement of the toes (Table 23.6). Spillane et al. (1971) described six patients with severe pain in one or both feet accompanied by characteristic writhing movements of the toes and sometimes of the feet. Three of these patients had a history suggestive of lumbosacral root damage. Subsequently, further patients were described with local peripheral nerve damage, L5 herpes zoster, S1 root compression and cauda equina lesions (Nathan, 1978), generalized peripheral neuropathy (Montagna et al., 1983), as well as minor trauma to the legs (Schott, 1981). It may be associated with the neuropathy of AIDS (Pitagoras de Mattos et al., 1999). A similar condition has been recorded in the upper limb, with a painful arm and moving fingers, one example being due to a brachial plexus lesion associated with a breast carcinoma and radiotherapy (Verhagen et al., 1985).

Dressler et al. (1994) reviewed a series of 18 patients with the syndrome of painful legs and moving toes (Table 23.7).

Table 23.6 Painful legs and moving toes

Adults 30–80 years: males and females

Unilateral or bilateral

Pain in feet first, followed days or years later by movements

Deep ache, burning, throbbing, crushing, tearing

Hyperpathia and allodynia

Sinuous, writhing, athetoid toe movements

Complex 1–2 Hz movement patterns of central origin

Treatments usually fail:

    Nerve blocks, guanethidine infusions, TENS

    Anticonvulsants, antidepressants, adenosine(?)

Table 23.7 Clinical features of patients with painful legs and moving toes

	n = 29*	n = 18[†]
Average age of onset (years)	57.7 (30–80)	60.3 (28–76)
Male/Female	11:18	3:15
Bilateral/unilateral	15:14	10:8
Lesions identified		
Cord	0	0
Cauda equina[‡]	14	8
Peripheral neuropathy	7	3
Peripheral trauma	6	4
Unknown	2	3

*29 cases from various sources (Spillane et al., 1971; Nathan, 1978; Barnett et al., 1981; Schott, 1981; Wulff, 1982; Montagna et al., 1983; Schoenen et al., 1984).
[†]Cases from Dressler et al. (1994).
[‡]Includes disk compression, herpes zoster, sacral cyst, hemangioma, and trauma.

One case followed a bullet injury to the spinal cord and cauda equina; four cases were due to spinal nerve root injury (herpes zoster, two with lumbar disk prolapses, and an L5 hemangioma); four cases were due to peripheral leg trauma; three cases were associated with an axonal peripheral neuropathy; and in six cases no definite cause could be identified (although lumbosacral radiculopathies were suspected in at least four of these patients). Three other patients with identical toe movements but no other pain were also described.

The age of onset usually is in middle or late life. Pain usually is the first symptom, preceding the movements by days to years. The pain has been described as a deep dull ache, burning, throbbing, crushing, searing, surging, or bursting. Sometimes there are associated sensations of pins and needles in the affected limb. The pain is very severe, leading patients to put their feet into refrigerators, wrap them with flannels, or other major measures. The onset may be unilateral, with subsequent spread to the opposite limb, or bilateral. In many patients the pain and the movements appeared to be linked, with increasing pain associated with worsening movements. The pain typically is diffuse, not limited to a peripheral nerve or segmented dermatomal pattern. The characteristics of the pain, and the common coexistence of hyperpathia and allodynia may suggest causalgia (Schott, 1986b).

The moving toes symptom refers to sinuous, athetoid-like dystonic movements of the toes and rarely of the feet. The patient may complain that the toes are working inside the shoe, rubbing to cause blisters. The toe movements consist of complex sequences of flexion, extension, abduction, and adduction, in various combinations at frequencies of 1–2 Hz (Alvarez et al., 2008) (Video 23.5). The electromyographic (EMG) characteristics of such muscle contractions cannot be explained by a peripheral nerve mechanism alone, but point to an origin in the CNS.

The mechanism proposed to explain this condition again is that of peripheral injury to nerves, plexus, or roots, causing an alteration in spinal and/or supraspinal sensory (the pain) and motor (the movements) machinery. However, the nature of the movements (slow, writhing, and sustained, i.e., dystonic) is quite different to the type of movements seen in hemifacial spasm (myoclonic jerks) or, indeed, in spinal myoclonus. Whether the movements in this condition arise in the spinal cord, as suggested by Nathan (1978) and Schott (1981, 1986a), or supraspinally is unknown.

It is the pain that causes the major disability and, unfortunately, this is very difficult to treat. A few patients have responded to sympathetic blockade, but in the majority this is ineffective. A course of guanethidine blocks into the affected limb is worth trying. Transcutaneous electrical nerve stimulation (TENS) applied to the leg or foot may help the pain. Carbamazepine, diphenylhydantoin, amitriptyline, and phenothiazines occasionally help. There is one report of adenosine being useful (Guieu et al., 1994). One patient responded to gabapentin 600 mg three times per day (Villarejo et al., 2004), and another did also at 200 mg three times per day (Aizawa, 2007). Epidural block may be helpful (Okuda et al., 1998), as may epidural spinal cord stimulation (Takahashi et al., 2002). Botulinum toxin injection has been reported useful for both movement and pain in two patients (Eisa et al., 2008).

The syndrome can very rarely involve the upper extremity, in which case it is referred to as painful arm and moving fingers (Supiot et al., 2002) (Video 23.6).

Dystonia induced by peripheral injury

This is a controversial area. There have been a number of case reports of peripheral trauma with or without nerve lesions with subsequent dystonia. There were some early reports of nerve lesions that "appeared to cause" typical arm dystonia (Schott, 1985; Scherokman et al., 1986). Other cases with the association of trauma and the onset of dystonia did not have nerve lesions (Video 23.7). Sheehy and Marsden (1980) described three trauma-induced cases out of a series of 60 patients with torticollis and calculated that 9% of 414 cases of this focal dystonia had suffered preceding injuries. These authors (Sheehy and Marsden, 1982) subsequently reported that writer's cramp could be precipitated by local hand injury, and identified five such cases among 91 patients (Sheehy et al., 1988). Schott (1985) described four patients with axial or arm dystonia after local trauma, and later Schott (1986a) described ten additional patients with movement disorders which appeared to have been precipitated by peripheral trauma; six of these had developed dystonia, including writer's and pianist's cramps, cranial segmental dystonia, axial segmental dystonia, and focal foot dystonia. The interval from injury to development of dystonia ranged from 24 hours to 3 years. Brin and colleagues (1986) briefly reported 23 patients in whom trauma precipitated dystonia in the injured region after an interval of between 1 day and 8 weeks. Jankovic and van der Linden (1988) also described a number of patients with dystonia and tremor induced by peripheral trauma; of 28 cases, 13 had persistent dystonia (four of a hand, five of a foot, one of an arm, one of a leg and two of craniocervical musculature) developing within 1 day to 12 months after a relevant injury. One report focused on post-traumatic cervical dystonia (Tarsy, 1998). In some patients, oromandibular dystonia has appeared after dental treatment (Thompson et al., 1986; Koller et al., 1989; Sankhla et al., 1998; Schrag et al., 1999). Two patients with task-specific musician's cramp have been described following trauma (Frucht et al., 2000). Immobilization has also been described as an antecedent (Okun et al., 2002; Singer and Papapetropoulos, 2005).

Although the dystonia in association with trauma is often similar to that without trauma, there are some differences in many cases (Schrag et al., 2004; Jankovic, 2009). The dystonia tends to be fixed and this may lead to early contractures. Sensory tricks are not common.

There is at least one point of caution in attributing dystonia to a peripheral nerve injury since nerve entrapment may be secondary to dystonia. Thus, for example, some 7% of patients with writer's cramp subsequently develop carpal tunnel compression of the median nerve as a consequence of their dystonia (Sheehy et al., 1988), and secondary entrapment neuropathies are not uncommon in those with any form of dystonia, including athetoid cerebral palsy (Alvarez et al., 1982).

There is no proof that trauma is formally causal for dystonia. Of course, it makes sense only if there is a "reasonable" temporal and spatial relationship. Jankovic and colleagues have proposed a set of arbitrary rules in this regard: (1) the trauma is severe enough to cause local symptoms for at least 2 weeks or requires medical evaluation within 2 weeks after trauma; (2) the initial manifestation of the movement disorder is anatomically related to the site of injury; and (3) the onset of the movement disorder is within days or months (up to 1 year) after the injury (Jankovic, 2009).

There are some controlled epidemiologic studies of this issue, and these are largely negative. A multicenter case-control study was performed using a semi-structured interview in five Italian referral centers (Martino et al., 2007). The presence of a history of head trauma and of post-traumatic sequelae was recorded from 177 patients with primary adult-onset cranial dystonia and from 217 controls with hemifacial spasm. No association was found between vault/maxillofacial trauma and cranial dystonia. Another case-control study was done with 104 consecutive patients with writer's cramp and matched controls (Roze et al., 2009). The risk of writer's cramp increased with the time spent writing and also with head trauma with loss of consciousness, but it was not significantly associated with peripheral trauma.

The matter remains controversial, however, and is often debated (Jankovic, 2001; Weiner, 2001).

Of course, the vast majority of those subjected to local injury do not develop dystonia, so trauma alone is unlikely to be the sole cause. Rather, it seems more probable that trauma acts as a trigger to the appearance of dystonia in those predisposed to develop this illness. One such patient, where this seems to be the case, developed foot dystonia following trauma (Bohlhalter et al., 2007). His brother was already known to have craniocervical dystonia, and both he and the brother had increased cortical excitability with transcranial magnetic stimulation similar to patients with primary focal dystonia. Moreover, on occasion, trauma may trigger a focal dystonia in patients who subsequently progress to develop generalized dystonia.

In blepharospasm, there is often a history of preceding local ocular disease (Grandas et al., 1988; Martino et al., 2005), and in spasmodic dysphonia, there is often a preceding history of sore throat (Schweinfurth et al., 2002). These results do seem to support the idea that local trauma can be a trigger.

Primary torsion dystonia is usually genetic in origin, so trauma may be a significant trigger to onset of the illness in those carrying the abnormal gene. Fletcher et al. (1991b) examined the relationship between trauma and dystonia in 104 patients with primary generalized, multifocal or segmental torsion dystonia. Genetic analysis of this population had indicated that the illness was caused by an autosomal dominant gene with reduced (40%) penetrance in about 85% of cases (Fletcher et al., 1990). Seventeen (16.4%) of these 104 cases reported that their dystonia had been precipitated (14 cases) or exacerbated (5 cases) by local trauma. The dystonia appeared in the injured part of the body within days or up to 12 months after the trauma. Subsequently, the dystonia spread to other body regions. Some patients experienced a new dystonia in a different body part after a subsequent injury to that distant structure. Eight of these 17 patients had affected relatives, so were genetically at risk of developing dystonia before the injury. Brin et al. (1986) and Jankovic and van der Linden (1988) also noted familial cases amongst patients with trauma-induced dystonia (i.e., 9 of 23, and 3 of 13 cases, respectively). All this evidence is consistent with the hypothesis that peripheral injury might precipitate dystonia in those carrying the idiopathic torsion dystonia gene or genes, although trauma amongst those with idiopathic torsion dystonia is no more frequent than in a matched control population (Fletcher et al., 1991a).

The dystonia associated with trauma in these cases was similar in all respects to that occurring spontaneously. Inherited primary dystonia is thought to be due to basal ganglia dysfunction. If this is also the case in those who develop dystonia after injury, then it would seem that trauma may trigger abnormalities of the brain, as well as the spinal cord.

There are possible mechanisms whereby peripheral injury might alter basal ganglia function. A major projection of the spinothalamic tract is to the ventrobasal nucleus of the thalamus, which projects to the somatosensory cortex. This system probably subserves discriminative pain perception, while spinoreticular pathways may be involved in large-scale somatic and autonomic responses to pain. The main projection of the nociceptive component of the spinoreticular tract is to the nucleus gigantocellularis in which (in the rat) nearly all cells respond to noxious stimuli (Benjamin, 1970). Neurons in nucleus gigantocellularis project principally to the centrum medianum and parafascicular thalamic nuclei, which are a major source of projections to the striatum (Guilbaud, 1985). Thus, nociceptive stimuli can gain access to the basal ganglia.

There also is direct experimental evidence that peripheral injury can alter basal ganglia chemistry. De Ceballos et al. (1986) found that a thermal injury to one hind limb in the rat causes early (24 hours) bilateral reduction of leu-enkephalin immunoreactivity in the globus pallidus, and later (1 week) bilateral (but most marked contralaterally) reduction of both met-enkephalin and leu-enkephalin immunoreactivity in globus pallidus, and of met-enkephalin immunoreactivity in caudate and putamen. These late changes in basal ganglia enkephalin content may reflect alterations in basal ganglia function that conceivably may be responsible for peripheral trauma precipitating dystonia in genetically susceptible individuals.

Whether or not the basal ganglia are involved, peripheral injury certainly can lead to CNS plastic changes (Hallett, 1999; Navarro et al., 2007), and some of these might be directly pathologic or interact with other factors to cause dystonia.

Muscle spasms associated with complex regional pain syndrome (CRPS)

This situation is one step more complex than the last topic, in that there is now CRPS in addition to dystonia or other movement disorder. In 1984, five patients were described who developed abnormal involuntary movements of a limb after injury (Marsden et al., 1984). All developed reflex sympathetic dystrophy, which is now preferentially called complex regional pain syndrome, CRPS (Stanton-Hicks et al., 1995) with Sudeck atrophy, and then abnormal muscle spasms or jerks of the affected limb, lasting years. Two exhibited myoclonic jerks of the injured leg; one had both jerks and more prolonged muscle spasms of the injured foot; the remaining two patients developed more complex dystonic spasms of the injured arm. All had severe persistent causalgic pain in the damaged limb, as well as the vasomotor, sudomotor, and trophic changes typical of reflex sympathetic dystrophy. Jankovic and van der Linden (1988), Robberecht et al. (1988) and Schwartzman and Kerrigan (1990) also have drawn attention to a variety of involuntary movements associated with causalgia (CRPS II), where there is nerve injury, and reflex sympathetic dystrophy (CRPS I), where there is not. These include fixed abnormal dystonic postures due to sustained muscle spasms, and tremor. Schwartzman and Kerrigan (1990) collected 43 patients with "dystonia," spasms or tremor from 200 cases of reflex sympathetic dystrophy. Another large series has been published by van Rijn et al. (2007).

Bhatia et al. (1993) reviewed 18 patients with causalgia and dystonia, triggered by injury (usually trivial) in 15, and occurring spontaneously in 3 cases (Table 23.8). Most were young women. All had the typical burning causalgic pain with hyperpathia and allodynia, along with the vasomotor, sudomotor, and trophic changes in skin, subcutaneous tissue and bone, typical of reflex sympathetic dystrophy (Table 23.9). All these patients developed deforming and often

---

Table 23.8 The causalgia–dystonia syndrome

18 cases, aged 12–51 years, 16 women and 2 men

15 followed peripheral injury (often minor); 3 spontaneous

None had a family history of this disorder

All had reflex sympathetic dystrophy (see Table 23.9)

Painful fixed dystonia presented at or following onset of reflex sympathetic dystrophy, initially in the injured limb

Lower limb in 12; upper limb in 6

Contractures developed

Dystonia spread in 10 cases to other limbs, as did causalgia in 7 cases

Brain and spinal cord imaging normal

No response to treatment

Two spontaneous recoveries (4 and 9 years after onset)

From Bhatia KP, Bhatt MH, Marsden CD. The causalgia-dystonia syndrome. Brain 1993;116(Pt 4):843–51, with permission.

Table 23.9 Reflex sympathetic dystrophy

Causalgia (spontaneous burning pain)

Allodynia (hyperpathia or pain on gentle touch)

Trophic changes (edema, cyanosis, hair loss, brittle nails, shiny thin skin)

Sudeck atrophy

Spread of pain

Emotional consequences

Relief by sympathetic block (possibly placebo effect)

Soft tissue injury

Infection

Fractures, sprains, dislocations

Surgery

Immobilization

Myocardial infarction (1%)

Nerve damage (5%)

From Bhatia KP, Bhatt MH, Marsden CD. The causalgia-dystonia syndrome. Brain 1993;116(Pt 4):843–51, with permission.

---

grotesque dystonic postures in the affected limb (the arm in 6, the leg in 12 cases), coincident with or after the causalgia. The dystonic spasms typically were sustained, producing a fixed dystonic posture, in contrast to the mobile spasms characteristic of primary torsion dystonia. Both the dystonia and the causalgia spread to affect other limbs in 7 patients. All investigations were normal and all modes of conventional treatment failed to relieve either the pain or the dystonia, but two patients recovered spontaneously. Thus, there appears to be a relation between causalgia, reflex sympathetic dystrophy, and a variety of involuntary movements, all precipitated by peripheral injury.

The classic clinical features of CRPS have been documented extensively (Schott, 1986b; Schwartzman and McLellan, 1987; Schwartzman, 1993; Maihofner et al., 2010). The mechanisms responsible for CRPS have been the subject of much study and speculation, but are still not certain (Maihofner et al., 2010). One view is that some persisting peripheral abnormality must be responsible, such as a small fiber neuropathy (Oaklander and Fields, 2009). Others believe that this is an inadequate explanation (Schwartzman and McLellan, 1987; Schott, 1995), and that altered central mechanisms, triggered by peripheral trauma, are most important (Lebel et al., 2008).

It is important to note that the whole issue of reflex sympathetic dystrophy is muddled in controversy. Certainly, the notion of a primary sympathetic dysfunction seems unlikely. This whole area has been marked by anecdotal reports and poor science. The view opposing reflex sympathetic dystrophy has been eloquently stated by Ochoa (1995, 1999; Ochoa and Verdugo, 1995). Many patients with this syndrome have significant psychiatric disease and many of the movement disorders appear to be psychogenic. Verdugo and Ochoa (2000) prospectively studied 58 patients with CRPS I or II and a movement disorder. The patients exhibited various combinations of dystonic spasms, coarse postural or action tremor, irregular jerks, and choreiform movements. No case of CRPS II but only cases of CRPS type I displayed abnormal movements. In addition to an absence of evidence of structural nerve, spinal cord, or intracranial damage, all CRPS I patients with abnormal movements typically exhibited pseudoneurologic (nonorganic) signs. In some cases, malingering was documented by secret surveillance. A detailed psychological investigation was carried out in a group of patients with CRPS 1 patients with dystonia. Compared to patients with conversion disorder and affective disorder, the CRPS 1 and dystonia group had elevated scores on somatoform dissociation, traumatic experiences, general psychopathology, but lower scores on some other scales (Reedijk et al., 2008).

Schrag et al. (2004) reported a large series of 103 patients with fixed dystonia. Most patients were female (84%) and had a mean age of onset of 29.7 years. A peripheral injury preceded onset in 63% and spread of dystonia to other body regions occurred in 56%. Pain was present in most patients, was a major complaint in 41%, and 20% had CRPS. No consistent investigational abnormalities were found, and 37% of patients fulfilled classification criteria for documented or clinically established psychogenic dystonia, 29% fulfilled criteria for somatization disorder, and 24% fulfilled both. However, 10% of the prospectively studied and 45% of the retrospectively studied patients did not have any evidence of psychogenic dystonia. Treatment was largely unsuccessful. Some of these patients were followed up after a mean of 7.6 years. About 23% improved and 31% worsened, and there continued to be high rates of neuropsychiatric features (Ibrahim et al., 2009).

Controversies continue. Reports of dystonia in the setting of CRPS appear (Oaklander, 2004; Oaklander and Fields, 2009), and are challenged (Morgan et al., 2005; Reich and Weiner, 2005; Lang and Chen, 2010).

Abnormalities in clinical neurophysiologic testing has been found by one group (van de Beek et al., 2002) but another study reported that changes are not dissimilar to findings that are seen in normal individuals mimicking an abnormal posture (Koelman et al., 1999). In a physiologic analysis of myoclonus in CRPS, EMG burst lengths ranged from 25 to 240 ms, and in two patients there was coherence between the EMG on the two sides of the body (Munts et al., 2008). These elements are consistent with a psychogenic origin (Lang et al., 2009).

The treatment of this disorder is very difficult. There are reports that intrathecal baclofen can be efficacious (van Hilten et al., 2000; van Rijn et al., 2009). Of course, if the disorder is psychogenic, then a psychiatric approach would be appropriate.

The bottom line when there are patients with CRPS and dystonia is to be careful and thoughtful.

References available on Expert Consult: www.expertconsult.com

CHAPTER **24**

Wilson disease

Chapter contents

Wilson disease	507	Hereditary deficiency of ceruloplasmin	512
Treatment of Wilson disease	510		

Wilson disease

Wilson disease is an inborn error of copper metabolism manifest as hepatic cirrhosis and basal ganglia damage (Wilson, 1912). Wilson disease is one of the few curable movement disorders at the present time. It presents in so many guises that any patient with a movement disorder under the age of 50 years should be considered to possibly have Wilson disease. It is sufficiently rare that the diagnosis is often missed. In a review of 307 patients, the average delay to diagnosis was 2 years and misdiagnoses included schizophrenia, juvenile polyarthritis, rheumatic chorea, nephrotic syndrome, metachromatic leukodystrophy, congenital myopathies, subacute sclerosing panencephalitis, and neurodegenerative disease (Prashanth et al., 2004).

Wilson disease is inherited as an autosomal recessive trait. The gene responsible lies on chromosome 13q14.3 (whereas that for ceruloplasmin is located on chromosome 8 (Wang et al., 1988). The Wilson disease gene encodes for a copper-transporting P-type ATPase (ATP7B) (Petrukhin et al., 1993; Tanzi et al., 1993). Over 300 mutations of the gene have been detected, and more are being found regularly (Thomas et al., 1995; Shah et al., 1997; Curtis et al., 1999; Lin et al., 2010). The enzyme binds copper in its large N-terminal domain and aids in intracellular processing in the hepatocyte (Ala et al., 2007).

Intestinal absorption of copper is normal in Wilson disease (normal adults absorb about 1 mg of copper daily), as is subsequent transport into the hepatocyte. Since absorption is about 1 mg per day, and the requirement is for 0.75 mg per day, about 0.25 mg must be excreted from the body each day (Lorincz, 2010). There are two pathways for copper excretion from the hepatocyte aided by ATP7B. One is the attachment to ceruloplasmin in the Golgi apparatus, and subsequent delivery of the copper–ceruloplasmin complex into the serum. A second is promotion of copper excretion into the bile. The mutations lead to failure to excrete copper by both routes, causing build-up of copper in the hepatocyte and eventual spillover of free copper into the circulation. This leads to a substantial positive net copper balance and

systemic copper poisoning (Cuthbert, 1998; Loudianos and Gitlin, 2000). There is increased circulating free copper and excessive urinary excretion of copper, but this is insufficient to prevent copper accumulation (the normal human body contains 80 mg of copper). Excess copper in the liver causes progressive liver damage. Copper also accumulates in brain and other sites (the eye, kidney, bones, and blood tissues being particularly vulnerable to copper toxicity). Some of the toxicity of copper may be due to oxidative mechanisms.

Curiously, monozygotic twins might be discordant for Wilson disease, suggesting that epigenetic or environmental factors must also be important (Czlonkowska et al., 2009).

In most cases, Wilson disease can be diagnosed by measuring the serum concentration of the copper protein ceruloplasmin. Ceruloplasmin (molecular weight 132 000), an alpha-2 globulin glycoprotein, contains six atoms of copper per molecule. Ceruloplasmin contains 0.3% copper in a fixed ratio of metal to protein (330 mg ceruloplasmin carries 1000 µg copper/L). In Wilson disease, there is defective incorporation of copper into ceruloplasmin, and the ceruloplasmin is not normally produced as a consequence. However, it is clear that there is no defect in ceruloplasmin in Wilson disease; indeed, some patients have normal levels, and the gene for the disease lies at a different site for that responsible for ceruloplasmin synthesis.

Drugs that remove copper from the body and/or prevent its absorption can reverse the manifestations of Wilson disease and prevent its appearance in asymptomatic affected siblings. More will be discussed below.

The prevalence of heterozygous carriers, who have inherited only one abnormal gene, is around 1 in 100–200 of the population (Reilly et al., 1993). Heterozygotes do not develop Wilson disease, but may exhibit mild abnormalities of copper metabolism, and prevalence is estimated to be about 17 per million of the population.

The initial manifestations of the illness (Table 24.1) are neurologic in about 40% of patients (usually after the age of 12 years) (Brewer, 2000a; Lorincz, 2010). The remainder present with symptoms of liver disease (about 40%) (usually at an earlier age) (Manolaki et al., 2009) or a psychiatric

DOI: 10.1016/B978-1-4377-2369-4.00024-X

Table 24.1 Presentation of Wilson disease

Liver disease (40%)

95% present under the age of 20 years (usually 7–15)

Acute hepatitis

Fulminant hepatitis

Chronic active hepatitis

Cirrhosis

Neurologic (40%)

30% present over the age of 20 years

Isolated tremor, dysarthria, drooling, clumsiness or gait disturbance (rarely, seizures)

A parkinsonian syndrome

A generalized dystonic syndrome

A "pseudosclerotic" syndrome (postural and intention tremor)

Psychiatric (15%)

Conduct disorder

Cognitive impairment

Dementia

Psychosis

Others (5%)

Ocular: Kayser–Fleischer ring, sunflower cataract

Renal: Aminoaciduria, renal tubular acidosis, calculi

Skeletal: Osteomalacia and rickets (blue nails)

Hematologic: Hemolytic anemia

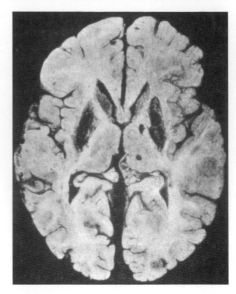

Figure 24.1 Postmortem brain of a patient with Wilson disease showing the cavitary necrosis of the basal ganglia. *From Wilson SAK. Progressive lenticular degeneration: A familial nervous disease associated with cirrhosis of the liver. Brain 1912;34:295–507.*

illness (about 15%). The psychiatric picture may show a change in personality or mood. Psychosis is rare. What determines these individual variations in clinical presentation is not clear. One factor has been determined; patients with ApoE epsilon3/3 genotype have delayed onset of symptoms compared to all other ApoE genotypes (Schiefermeier et al., 2000). Symptoms usually appear between the ages of 11 and 25 years, but can occur as early as 4 and as late as 50+ years (Starosta-Rubinstein et al., 1987; Stremmel et al., 1991; Walshe and Yealland, 1992; Ferenci et al., 2007). Some patients with Wilson disease have autonomic nervous system abnormalities (Bhattacharya et al., 2002; Meenakshi-Sundaram et al., 2002).

The pathologic abnormalities in the brain are primarily in the basal ganglia, with cavitary necrosis of the putamen and caudate, associated with neuronal loss, axonal degeneration and astrocytosis (Fig. 24.1). In addition, there is cortical atrophy. In a recent pathologic study of eight patients, six had neurological manifestations clinically (Meenakshi-Sundaram et al., 2008). Of these six, five had central pontine myelinolysis, five had subcortical white matter cavitations, four had putaminal softening, and six had variable ventricular dilatation. The liver in Wilson disease develops cirrhosis, typically of the nodular type.

A detailed analysis of the psychiatric presentation of 15 patients showed an affective disorder spectrum abnormality in 11 and a schizophreniform illness in 3 (Srinivas et al., 2008). Note was made that while the psychiatric symptoms improved in five patients with de-coppering therapy, seven patients needed symptomatic treatment as well.

Those with neurologic abnormalities usually present in the second or third decade, as (1) an akinetic-rigid syndrome

resembling parkinsonism, (2) a generalized dystonic syndrome (pure chorea is uncommon), or (3) postural and intention tremor with ataxia, titubation and dysarthria (pseudosclerosis) (Table 24.2 and Video 24.1). The tremor may be mild, but is classically a slow, high-amplitude proximal tremor with the appearance of "wing-beating" when the arms are elevated and the hands placed near the nose. Dysarthria and clumsiness of the hands are common presenting features. The speech abnormality may include rapid speech, hypophonia, and slurring. It is most unusual for the illness to present with a gait disorder. No two patients with Wilson disease are ever quite the same. The facile grinning face with drooling saliva is characteristic. Early pseudobulbar features are common. Eye movements can be disordered with slow saccades (Kirkham and Kamin, 1974) and occasionally ophthalmoplegia (Gadoth and Liel, 1980). Vision and sensation are not affected, and paralysis does not occur although pyramidal signs may be evident. Sphincter control is spared. Seizures are infrequent (Smith and Mattson, 1967). Cognitive changes are common, even to the extent of a frank dementia. Changes in school or work performance are often the initial indication of the illness. Impulsiveness or antisocial behavior, and other indices of personality change are common (Dening and Berrios, 1989; Dening, 1991; Akil and Brewer, 1995).

Many of those with neurologic complaints give a history of prior or concurrent liver disease. This may consist of a previous episode of acute hepatitis, chronic active hepatitis, portal hypertension, or asymptomatic hepatosplenomegaly (Scheinberg and Sternlieb, 1984). An unexplained hemolytic anemia, renal disease with hematuria, amino-aciduria, renal tubular defects, and calculi (Wiebers et al., 1979), or skeletal disease with osteoporosis/osteomalacia (Carpenter et al., 1983) are other clues.

Untreated, the condition progresses inexorably to death either from the complications of the liver disease, or from severe neurologic involvement, within a few years.

Table 24.2 Number (percentage) of Wilson disease patients with different initial symptoms and signs

	Juveniles (n = 65)	Adults (n = 71)
Symptoms		
Personality change	21 (32)	23 (32)
Speech defect	63 (41)	42 (30)
Drooling	31 (20)	22 (16)
Dysphagia	14 (9)	7 (5)
Hand tremor	48 (31)	55 (39)
Hand clumsy	32 (21)	20 (14)
Abnormal gait	34 (22)	18 (13)
Fall at work or school	40 (26)	
Signs		
Personality disorder	14 (21)	13 (18)
Dysarthria	34 (52)	19 (27)
Gait abnormal	8 (12)	5 (7)
Eye movement abnormal	4 (6)	4 (6)
Drooling	18 (28)	11 (15)
Parkinsonian facies	15 (23)	5 (7)
Open mouth	10 (15)	0 (0)
Bradykinesia	6 (9)	3 (4)
Tongue abnormal	11 (17)	9 (13)
UL tremor	17 (26)	23 (32)
UL dystonia	14 (21)	13 (18)
UL spontaneous movements	8 (12)	0 (0)
LL tremor	2 (3)	6 (8)
LL dystonia	12 (18)	0 (0)
LL spontaneous movements	1 (1)	1 (1)
Liver disease	19 (29)	8 (11)

UL, upper limb; LL lower limb.
From Walshe JM, Yealland M. Wilson's disease: the problem of delayed diagnosis. J Neurol Neurosurg Psychiatry 1992;55(8):692–696.

Table 24.3 The diagnosis of Wilson disease (WD)

1. Low serum ceruloplasmin (<20 mg/dL)
   False negatives in:
   - 5% of WD patients
   - Pregnancy or birth control pills
   False positives in:
   - Heterozygotes
   - Severe protein loss
   - Severe liver disease
   - Menkes disease
2. Kayser–Fleischer ring
   False negatives in:
   - Liver WD
   - Local eye disease
   False positives in primary biliary cirrhosis
3. Raised 24-hour urinary copper excretion (>100 μg)
   False positives in cholestasis (NB: drugs)
4. Raised liver copper concentration (>250 μg/g dry weight)
   False positives in:
   - Biliary cirrhosis
   - Cholestasis
   - (NB: histology is essential)
5. Genetic linkage studies to chromosome 13

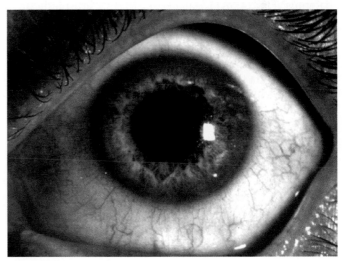

Figure 24.2 Kayser–Fleischer ring in a patient with Wilson disease. The ring is composed of the brown pigment at the outer circumference of the iris.
From Scheinberg IH, Sternlieb I. Wilson's disease. Philadelphia: W.B. Saunders; 1984.

Laboratory testing can make a definitive diagnosis (Mak and Lam, 2008). The diagnosis (Table 24.3) is first tested by looking for reduced serum ceruloplasmin. However, 5% of those with Wilson disease have a normal serum ceruloplasmin. The concentration of this copper protein may be low in heterozygotes, in patients with severe protein loss, and with severe liver disease of other cause. Serum ceruloplasmin may be increased by pregnancy and estrogens. Serum total copper is low in many patients (but nonspecific; Kumar et al., 2007), and urinary copper excretion is nearly always raised. However, anything causing cholestasis (particularly drugs) may raise serum copper and increase urinary copper excretion. When an expert examines the cornea with a slit lamp, virtually all patients with neurologic Wilson disease show Kayser–Fleischer rings in the Descemet membrane (Fig. 24.2) (Wiebers et al., 1977). However, rare patients with neurologic Wilson disease but no Kayser–Fleischer rings have been described (Ross et al., 1985; Demirkiran et al., 1996). A Kayser–Fleischer ring occasionally is only seen in one eye (Madden et al., 1985). The yellow and brown copper deposits are seen at the limbus of the cornea, usually first visible and most dense at the upper and lower poles of the eye. Kayser–Fleischer rings are not present in all patients with the liver manifestations of Wilson disease and other liver disease can produce them (Fleming et al., 1977).

Computed tomography (Harik and Post, 1981; Williams and Walshe, 1981) or magnetic resonance imaging (MRI)

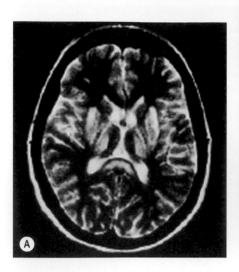 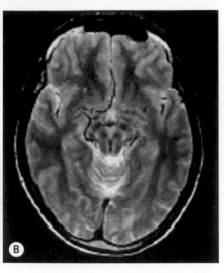

Figure 24.3 MRI scans in Wilson disease.
A T2-weighted image showing hyperintensity of the basal ganglia. **B** T2-weighted image showing the "face of the giant panda sign" due to hyperintensity of the mesencephalon sparing the red nuclei and the lateral part of the substantia nigra. *Modified from Giagheddu M, Tamburini G, Piga M, et al. Comparison of MRI, EEG, EPs and ECD-SPECT in Wilson's disease. Acta Neurol Scand 2001;103(2):71–81.*

(Starosta-Rubinstein et al., 1987; Alanen et al., 1999; Giagheddu et al., 2001) of the brain usually reveals changes in the basal ganglia, which are reversible with treatment. Caudate and putamen show increased T2 signal, and there may be similar changes in the substantia nigra pars compacta, periaqueductal gray, the pontine tegmentum, and the thalamus (Fig. 24.3A) (Saatci et al., 1997). Particularly striking are the putaminal lesions with a pattern of symmetric, bilateral, concentric-laminar T2 hyperintensity. Hyperintensity of the mesencephalon with sparing of the red nuclei and lateral aspect of the substantia nigra gives rise to the "face of the giant panda sign" (Fig. 24.3B) (Giagheddu et al., 2001). A "double panda sign" has also been described (Jacobs et al., 2003; Liebeskind et al., 2003). There can be hyperintensity of the middle cerebellar peduncle (Uchino et al., 2004). Another change has a similar appearance to central pontine myelinolysis, and this will improve with therapy (Sinha et al., 2007b). Diffusion-weighted MRI might also be useful (Favrole et al., 2006). In a study of 100 patients with various extrapyramidal diseases, the MRI features most useful to diagnose Wilson disease were the "face of giant panda" sign (seen in 14.3%), tectal plate hyperintensity (seen in 75%), central pontine myelinolysis-like abnormalities (seen in 62.5%), and concurrent signal changes in basal ganglia, thalamus, and brainstem (seen in 55.3%) (Prashanth et al., 2010).

Positron emission tomography using ^{18}F-fluorodopa shows reduced uptake in the striatum indicating loss of the dopaminergic nigrostriatal pathway (Snow et al., 1991). Transcranial brain parenchyma sonography (TCS) detects lenticular nucleus hyperechogenicity, likely to be caused by copper accumulation, in neurologically symptomatic and asymptomatic Wilson disease patients (Walter et al., 2005). Magnetic resonance spectroscopy is also abnormal (Lucato et al., 2005; Tarnacka et al., 2009).

If there is any doubt about the diagnosis of Wilson disease in a patient presenting with neurologic problems under the age of 50, the first test would be a 24-hour urine copper excretion. In Wilson disease, excretion is typically more than 100 μg/24 hours and less than 50 μg/24 hours would exclude the diagnosis (Brewer and Yuzbasiyan-Gurkan, 1992; Brewer, 2000a). The definitive investigation is a liver biopsy with histologic assessment of tissue, and measurement of copper concentration. Guidelines for diagnosis have been published by the American Association for the Study of Liver Diseases (Roberts and Schilsky, 2008). An algorithm for the diagnosis is presented in Figure 24.4 (Brewer, 2008).

Genetic linkage studies to chromosome 13 may be valuable if other family members are available, and the gene can be closely searched for a mutation (Farrer et al., 1991; Caca et al., 2001; Davies et al., 2008). However, since there are so many possible mutations, such testing is not easily nor currently commercially available. Genotyping microarray is one method for looking for multiple mutations in one test (Gojova et al., 2008). Another technique is high-resolution melting analysis (Lin et al., 2010). Certainly if you know the high-frequency mutations in a population, it is possible to focus on those (Schilsky and Ala, 2010).

All siblings, who have a one in four chance of developing the illness, and cousins of known patients, should be screened for Wilson disease. Clinical signs, the presence of a Kayser–Fleischer ring, and abnormalities of serum and urine copper metabolism indicate the need for prophylactic treatment. If there is doubt, a liver biopsy may be undertaken, although molecular genetic techniques may prove diagnostic. An algorithm for evaluating presymptomatic siblings is presented in Figure 24.5 (Brewer, 2008).

Treatment of Wilson disease

The treatments for Wilson disease have been reviewed (Walshe, 1999; Brewer, 2000b, 2006; Gouider-Khouja, 2009; Lorincz, 2010). Guidelines for treatment have been published by the American Association for the Study of Liver Diseases (Roberts and Schilsky, 2008).

The gold standard of treatment (Table 24.4) is D-penicillamine (Shimizu et al., 1999; Walshe, 1999), building up to around 1 g/day, along with pyridoxine 25 mg/day. D-penicillamine should be introduced gradually because about 20% of patients may develop early side effects. The commonest are fever, a rash, and lymphadenopathy. Gradual reintroduction of D-penicillamine in low dosage under steroid cover may overcome these problems. More serious is

SCREENING AND DIAGNOSIS IN PATIENTS WITH THE NEUROLOGIC/PSYCHIATRIC PRESENTATION

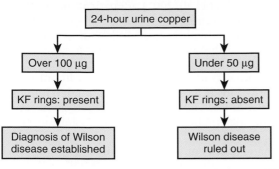

If tests are discordant, i.e. urine copper over 100 µg and KF rings negative, or KF rings positive and urine copper under 50 µg, do liver biopsy and measure hepatic copper

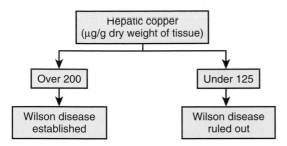

Figure 24.4 An algorithm for screening and definitive diagnosis in patients with suspicion of Wilson disease. KF, Kayser–Fleischer. *From Brewer GJ. Wilson's disease. In: Hallett M, Poewe W (eds), Therapeutics of Parkinson's Disease and Other Movement Disorders. Chichester, UK: Wiley-Blackwell; 2008, pp. 251–261.*

SCREENING AND DIAGNOSIS OF PRESYMPTOMATIC SIBLINGS

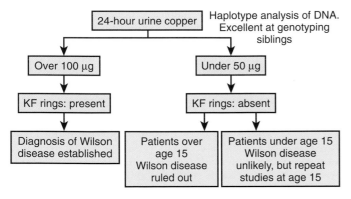

If urine copper between 50 and 100 µg, liver biopsy with measure of copper required

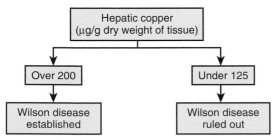

Figure 24.5 An algorithm for screening and diagnosis of presymptomatic siblings. KF, Kayser–Fleischer. *From Brewer GJ. Wilson's disease. In: Hallett M, Poewe W (eds), Therapeutics of Parkinson's Disease and Other Movement Disorders. Chichester, UK: Wiley-Blackwell; 2008, pp. 251–261.*

Table 24.4 Treatment of Wilson disease

1. D-Penicillamine
   Low and slow: 1 g/day (0.5–2.0) before food
   Pyridoxine 25 mg/day
   Avoid copper-rich foods
   Monitor blood count and liver function tests, serum and urinary copper, Kayser–Fleischer ring
   Early side effects: allergy (20%) – fever, rash, glands; marrow depression; neurologic deterioration (20–40%)
   Late problems: nephrotoxicity (proteinuria, nephrotic syndrome); systemic lupus erythematosus; thrombocytopenia; Goodpasture syndrome; dermatopathy; myasthenia
2. Trientine
   1–2 g/daily (250–500 mg four times per day)
   Iron deficiency
3. Zinc (sulfate or acetate)
   50–200 mg three times a day
   Gastrointestinal side effects
4. Tetrathiomolybdate
5. Liver transplant

the development of bone marrow depression. Unfortunately, 20–40% of those with neurologic disability will exhibit deterioration in the initial months of penicillamine treatment (Brewer, 1999). The neurologic deterioration can be severe; in one case the patient developed marked dystonia (status dystonicus) and died (Svetel et al., 2001). However, clinical improvement usually occurs within about 3 months, but it may take 6 months to a year before noticeable change takes place.

Reducing copper intake obviously is wise (Shimizu et al., 1999), but strict diets are rarely followed. Copper-rich foods include liver, nuts, chocolate, coffee, and shellfish.

Successful de-coppering can be monitored by an initial increase in urinary copper excretion, which subsequently falls, a reduction in the concentration of free copper in serum, and the fading of Kayser–Fleischer rings.

Late reactions to penicillamine treatment are usually seen after a year or so of therapy. The commonest is penicillamine dermatopathy, due to damage of collagen and elastin causing weakness of subcutaneous tissue so that slight trauma may cause bleeding, leaving brown papules with excessive wrinkling and thinning of the skin. A minority may develop proteinuria which can progress to a frank nephrotic syndrome. Other problems include the emergence of a form of systemic lupus erythematosus, thrombocytopenia, Goodpasture syndrome, and myasthenia gravis.

An alternative to D-penicillamine is trientine (triethylene tetramine dihydrochloride) (Brewer, 1999; Shimizu et al., 1999), another chelator. Trientine undoubtedly is a valuable alternative in those intolerant to the latter, but it has advantages in that the initial worsening may not occur (Brewer, 1999). It can also be used in children where it can be effective with fewer side effects than with penicillamine (Taylor et al., 2009). Trientine is relatively safe (it can cause a sideroblastic anemia and can reactivate penicillamine-induced lupus), but is expensive and poorly absorbed.

Zinc and tetrathiomolybdate prevent the absorption of copper and are other alternatives. Zinc is an excellent agent for chronic use for mild cases and prevention (Hoogenraad, 2006; Linn et al., 2009), but may not be rapid enough for initiating therapy in someone with severe illness (Brewer, 1999, 2000a). Zinc is also the treatment of choice during pregnancy. Zinc can also be given safely in the pediatric age group (Brewer et al., 2001). Long-term follow-up of neurologically asymptomatic children treated for 10 years shows that zinc is well tolerated; liver disease improves, neurologic disorders do not develop, and growth is normal (Marcellini et al., 2005). Zinc monotherapy may fail and chelators would be needed (Weiss et al., 2011).

Tetrathiomolybdate is not easily available except experimentally (Brewer, 2005, 2009). An open-label study of 55 de novo patients reported treatment with doses of 120–410 mg per day for 8 weeks with follow-up for 3 years (Brewer et al., 2003). Only 2 (4%) showed initial neurologic deterioration, and overall neurologic improvement was excellent. Five patients had bone marrow suppression and 3 had aminotransferase elevation; the authors thought that this may have been precipitated by a too rapid dose escalation. A randomized, double-blind trial of 48 patients compared tetrathiomolybdate with trientine (Brewer et al., 2006). Patients either received 500 mg of trientine hydrochloride two times per day or 20 mg of tetrathiomolybdate three times per day with meals and 20 mg three times per day between meals for 8 weeks. All patients received 50 mg of zinc twice a day. There were more side effects (including neurologic deterioration) with trientine. For those patients that did not deteriorate the improvement was similar, but given the side effects tetrathiomolybdate should be preferred. It has now been demonstrated that free copper levels drop with tetrathiomolybdate therapy, while they might rise with trientine (Brewer et al., 2009). This may explain the early deterioration with trientine.

With therapy, in addition to clinical improvement, there is also radiologic improvement (Sinha et al., 2007a). Magnetic resonance spectroscopy, particularly measuring N-acetylaspartate (NAA), can be helpful in assessment of treatment efficacy (Tarnacka et al., 2008).

In desperate cases, injection of dimercaprol (BAL) still may be life-saving (Scheinberg and Sternlieb, 1995). But because injections are painful, this cannot be used chronically (Walshe, 1999).

The role of these alternative agents in the treatment of Wilson disease is debated, and there is a nice formal debate published in *Movement Disorders* (Brewer, 1999; LeWitt, 1999; Walshe, 1999). Brewer (1999) takes the strong view that D-penicillamine should not be used. He and others favor zinc, or a combination of zinc and trientine, or tetrathiomolybdate, on the grounds that such an approach reduces the chances of initial neurologic deterioration, and causes fewer side effects than D-penicillamine (Czlonkowska et al., 1996; Brewer, 1999, 2000a, 2005; Schilsky, 2001). In a systematic review of the literature, for neurologic Wilson disease, zinc was best tolerated and had good efficacy (Wiggelinkhuizen et al., 2009).

Liver transplantation has also been employed, and cures Wilson disease (Schilsky et al., 1994; Shimizu et al., 1999; Podgaetz and Chan, 2003; Arnon et al., 2011). The neurologic manifestations can be reversed in about 80% of cases, and liver transplantation can be undertaken for the neurologic disorder even with stable liver disease (Stracciari et al.,

2000; Geissler et al., 2003). A series of 21 patients had a mean follow-up of 5.2 years and an actuarial follow-up of 10 years (Schumacher et al., 2001). All patients did well with the neurologic functioning improving over 1–1.5 years. In a series of 24 patients with a mean follow-up period of 92 months, quality of life improved to the same level as controls in the general population (Sutcliffe et al., 2003). In a series of 13 patients, all did well, and those without neurologic manifestations before transplant did not develop them (Pabon et al., 2008). Other series also report good results (Marin et al., 2007; Cheng et al., 2009; Yoshitoshi et al., 2009).

Symptomatic treatment with antiparkinsonian drugs such as levodopa, dopamine agonists, and anticholinergics may be of benefit.

Hereditary deficiency of ceruloplasmin

A rare condition, hereditary deficiency of ceruloplasmin, can cause a movement disorder. In this autosomal recessive disorder due to gene defects in the ceruloplasmin gene (Yazaki et al., 1998), homozygotes develop iron overload (Miyajima et al., 1987; Harris et al., 1995). The disorder is estimated to occur in 0.5 persons per million in Japan (Miyajima et al., 1999). Ceruloplasmin oxidizes ferrous iron to ferric iron (so some call it ceruloplasmin "ferroxidase"), which is stored in ferritin and hemosiderin. Ferric iron can be transported out of cells. Absence of ceruloplasmin leads to a low serum iron with normal total iron binding capacity, and sometimes to anemia. Serum ferritin, and liver and brain iron concentrations are increased. Brain MRI shows increased iron deposition in the striatum, substantia nigra, red nuclei, and dentate nuclei. T2 hypointensities can be marked, including the cerebral cortex (Grisoli et al., 2005). Clinical presentation has been with insulin-dependent diabetes, retinal degeneration, subcortical dementia, and a movement disorder which typically is a facial dyskinesia (blepharospasm and oral dystonia) and torticollis, rigidity, and sometimes ataxia (Miyajima et al., 1987; Kawanami et al., 1996). One patient has presented with parkinsonism (Kohno et al., 2000). A review of 33 patients found the age at diagnosis to be 16 to 71, and there was cognitive impairment in 42%, cranial-facial dyskinesia in 28%, cerebellar ataxia in 46%, and retinal degeneration in 75% of patients (McNeill et al., 2008). Treatment is by iron chelation with desferrioxamine (Miyajima et al., 1997). One patient was successfully treated with repeated infusions of fresh frozen plasma (containing ceruloplasmin) (Yonekawa et al., 1999).

Hypoceruloplasminemia-related movement disorder (HCMD)

There is one report of HCMD without Kayser–Fleischer rings and without the Wilson disease mutation (Lirong et al., 2009). Patients presented with parkinsonism, tremor, dystonia, ataxia, and a tic disorder. It is not clear what these patients have, and whether this is even a homogeneous entity.

References available on Expert Consult: www.expertconsult.com

CHAPTER **25**

Psychogenic movement disorders
Phenomenology, diagnosis, and treatment

Chapter contents

Introduction	513	Psychogenic dystonia	521
Degree of certainty of the diagnosis of a psychogenic movement disorder	516	Psychogenic nondystonic movement disorders	523
Definitions of psychiatric terminology	517	Approaches to the patient suspected of having a psychogenic movement disorder	525
Clues suggesting the presence of a psychogenic movement disorder	518	Results of treatment	526
Diagnostic approach and clinical features	520	Movement disorders caused by psychiatric conditions but not regarded as psychogenic	527

Introduction

An entire international symposium on psychogenic movement disorders was held in late 2004, and the subsequent publication of its proceedings is now available (Hallett et al., 2006). That volume covers all aspects of psychogenic movement disorders, beyond the scope of this chapter, and scholars in the field are encouraged to read it. A second symposium was held in April 2009, and its proceedings will be published soon.

Psychogenic movement disorders are caused by psychological factors rather than by an organic etiology. Other terms such as *functional, nonorganic,* and *medically unexplained symptoms* have been used. Although the term *functional* might be more convenient to convey to patients and their families – because of old stigmas regarding having a psychological disorder – the term *psychogenic* describes the condition best because it refers to the etiology. This is much the same way neurologists label many disorders, such as postencephalitic parkinsonism, vascular parkinsonism, post-traumatic parkinsonism or drug-induced parkinsonism. Why not label parkinsonism due to psychogenic etiology as psychogenic parkinsonism? It places the emphasis on etiology and thereby guides the physician towards appropriate treatment. The term *functional* has been used in the past to denote organic diseases in which a specific cause was not determined, and has been applied to organic illnesses such as chorea, epilepsy, and neuralgias because these were considered physiologic, rather than anatomic, disorders (see historical reviews by Fahn, 2006a; Munts and Koehler, 2010). Today, for most clinicians, the meaning of *functional* is synonymous with *psychogenic,* but this might not be uniformly defined this way, so it would be less ambiguous to use *psychogenic.* The term *organic* is used to mean "not due to a psychogenic etiology," and, thus, the term *nonorganic* refers to psychogenic. More and more the literature in neurology has adopted the term psychogenic, as can be seen by the epilepsy specialty. The terminology debate in epilepsy appears to be not about psychogenic terminology, but about whether the episodes should be called psychogenic nonepileptiform seizures or attacks (Benbadis, 2010; LaFrance, 2010).

Frequency

Movement disorder specialists are seeing increasing numbers of patients with movement disorders whose problems are secondary to psychogenic factors. As one might expect, bradykinetic disorders are less likely than hyperkinetic ones to have a psychogenic etiology unless one were to consider the phenomenon of deliberate slowness to be a bradykinetic disorder. Although deliberate slowness is common in psychogenic disorders, it is not usually the dominant feature, but when it is pure and without accompanying abnormal movements, it is considered in the category of psychogenic parkinsonism. Fixed postures, fairly common in psychogenic dystonia, account for a sizable proportion of psychogenic movement disorders, so a separate section of this chapter is devoted to the psychogenic dystonias.

Psychogenic disorders in neurology have been estimated to occur in 1–9% of all neurologic diagnoses (Marsden, 1986; Lempert et al., 1990). Neurologists usually and appropriately recognize patients with psychogenic movement disorders, but the patients often do not accept this diagnosis and seek other opinions, going from physician to physician, seeking a diagnosis that is more to their liking. Therefore, a strategy is necessary for the best way to inform the patients

DOI: 10.1016/B978-1-4377-2369-4.00025-1

of the diagnosis. This issue is discussed in this chapter. Another common situation is that many physicians do not offer the time-consuming care that is necessary to restore such patients to normality, preferring instead merely to diagnose the condition and have the referring physician deal with the healing.

Like other subspecialties in neurology, psychogenic movement disorders are not uncommon. In one large movement disorder clinic, such patients account for 10% of all non-parkinsonian new patient visits (Portera-Cailliau et al., 2006). Typically, patients are diagnosed by the predominant movement feature, e.g., psychogenic tremor, psychogenic dystonia, psychogenic myoclonus, etc. When evaluated this way, tremor is the most common psychogenic phenomenology, followed by dystonia.

Importance of an accurate diagnosis

The diagnosis of a psychogenic movement disorder is a two-stage process (Lang, 2006). First is to make a positive diagnosis that the movements are psychogenic and not due to an organic illness. Second is to identify a psychiatric disorder or the psychodynamics that could explain the etiology of the abnormal movements and prepare the way to deciding the best course for therapy of the individual patient. Deciding between abnormal movements due to a psychogenic cause and an organic one can be extremely difficult. Never having seen strange movements before and pronouncing them to be psychogenic therefore is not a satisfactory method because not even senior movement disorder specialists have seen the whole gamut of organic abnormal movements. An organic cause of the movements needs to be excluded (Fahn, 1994; Williams et al., 2005). But this alone is insufficient and neurologists in times past and present advise that making a diagnosis of a psychogenic disorder depends on finding positive criteria and not simply failing to finding an organic cause (for historical review, see Fahn 2006a).

An accurate diagnosis of a psychogenic movement disorder, as opposed to diagnosing an organic movement disorder, is often one of the most difficult tasks there is in the movement disorder specialty. It is extremely important to be correct in the diagnosis because only then can the appropriate therapy be initiated. The results of an incorrect diagnosis are detrimental. If a patient has a psychogenic disorder that is misdiagnosed, the patient will be given inappropriate and potentially harmful medication and is also denied the proper treatment to overcome the disabling symptoms. By postponing the appropriate psychiatric treatment, the cycle of disability is perpetuated. Untreated patients with psychogenic movement disorders are at risk for becoming career invalids with chronic disability.

If the obverse occurs – that is, if a patient is given a diagnosis of a psychogenic movement disorder when, in fact, he or she suffers from an organic one – again the wrong treatment is given. In this situation, time-consuming and expensive psychotherapy, psychiatric medications, and possibly electroconvulsive therapy might be initiated instead of more appropriate pharmacotherapeutic agents that could provide relief. Moreover, a diagnosis of a psychogenic disorder can create emotional trauma for the patient and his or her family (Cooper, 1976). It is important to point out that no matter how much experience a clinician has had, encountering a new type of movement disorder for the first time does not automatically make this a psychogenic movement disorder. For example, task-specific jaw tremor (Miles et al., 1997) is rare, and even when it is encountered for the first time, a wise clinician should consider it to be organic (Video 25.1) and not psychogenic (Video 25.2).

Neurologic symptoms and signs are a common result of hysteria, and neurologists have long been fascinated by the brain's ability to be able to produce such clinical expressions on the basis of psychological disturbances. Many great neurologists, such as Charcot and Freud, intensively studied hysterical conversion reactions, using hypnosis as a tool in their investigations and treatment (Goetz, 1987). In their training, neurologists-to-be are taught to differentiate the clinical findings of psychogenic etiology from those of organic disorders (Gowers, 1893; Oppenheim, 1911a; DeJong, 1958a). However, textbooks in the past often considered some dyskinesias, recognized today as organic, such as tics, writer's cramp and other occupational cramps, and some other forms of dystonia, to be examples of hysteria (DeJong, 1958b).

Although there is a modest neurologic literature on psychogenic phenomenology, the literature dealing specifically with psychogenic movement disorders is rather sparse. For example, tremor as the result of a conversion reaction has been long recognized, at least since the days of Gowers (1893), but scientific reports on psychogenic tremor or other movement disorders are rarely described in the literature. Campbell (1979) pointed out that the amplitude of psychogenic tremor is more pronounced when attention is paid to it, and that it lessens and may even disappear when the patient's attention is diverted to another subject or other part of the body. Distraction is a useful part of the examination, and lessening of severity by distraction can be very helpful diagnostically in trying to establish a diagnosis of psychogenic tremor. But in our experience, distraction does not always succeed in making the tremor disappear, so this maneuver is often not successful. Therefore, additional findings on examination are often necessary and can be just as helpful in considering the diagnosis of a psychogenic movement disorder; these are discussed in this chapter.

Although in the great majority of patients with a psychogenic movement disorder, all their clinical features result only from a psychogenic problem, some may have the psychogenic movement disorder on top of an organic movement disorder, as seen in Patient 5 in the series of psychogenic dystonias reported by Fahn and Williams (1988) and the cases of Ranawaya and colleagues (1990). Perhaps 10–15% of patients with a psychogenic movement disorder have an underlying organic movement disorder as well. This overlap is seen in patients with psychogenic seizures ("pseudoseizures"); 10–37% of patients have organic seizures as well (Krumholz and Niedermeyer, 1983; Lesser et al., 1983). Nevertheless, a useful rule of thumb is that if one part of the examination reveals nonorganicity, it is likely that other "abnormalities" on the examination might also be nonorganic.

Perhaps the movement disorders with the highest prevalence rate of a psychogenic origin are the nonfamilial, "idiopathic", paroxysmal nonkinesigenic dyskinesias, as surveyed by Bressman and colleagues (1988). They found that of 18 patients with paroxysmal nonkinesigenic dystonias and with no known symptomatic etiology or positive family history for a paroxysmal dyskinesia, the dystonias were due to psychogenic causes in 11 patients. This represents 61% of such cases. The age at onset in these patients ranged from 11 to 49 years; 8 of the 11 patients were female. Thus, unless accompanied by a clear-cut family history, these paroxysmal dystonias are commonly psychogenic, and their diagnosis is extremely difficult to make for reasons that are explained later in the chapter (Fahn and Williams, 1988).

Kotagal and colleagues (2002) conducted a study of paroxysmal events in children. Over a 6-year period, 883 patients were monitored in their pediatric epilepsy monitoring unit; 134 patients (15.2%) were documented to have paroxysmal nonepileptic events. Children in the preschool group (age: 2 months to 5 years) (n = 26) were eventually diagnosed with stereotypies, hypnic jerks, parasomnias, and Sandifer syndrome. The school-age group (age: 5–12 years) (n = 61) had diagnoses of psychogenic seizures, inattention or daydreaming, stereotypies, hypnic jerks, and paroxysmal dyskinesias. The adolescent group (age: 12–18 years) (n = 48) had a diagnosis of psychogenic seizures in 40 patients (83%). The authors concluded that in patients with paroxysmal nonepileptic events, conversion disorder was seen in children older than 5 years of age, and its frequency increased with age, becoming the most common type of paroxysmal nonepileptic events among adolescents. In adolescents, conversion disorder was more common in females, whereas males predominated in the school-age group. Concomitant epilepsy with nonepileptic events occurred in all three age groups to a varying extent.

Mass hysteria

Today, neurologists encounter individual patients with psychogenic movement disorders. But historically, mass hysteria was common, probably more so than it is today. Mass hysteria still occurs, such as "shell shock" in wartime, as well as during current environmental events such as mass inoculations (Kharabsheh et al., 2001; Khiem et al., 2003). Symptoms can also be generated from mass concerns about medications and breast implants, in part owing to widespread publicity, although legal liability issues may also drive the development of symptoms. Mass hysteria resembling seizures occurred recently in 10 high school girls following the development of organic absence seizures in another student (Roach and Langley, 2004).

It is interesting to note on a historical level that the term *chorea*, meaning dancing in Latin, comes from the dancing mania (a mass hysteria) that was seen in the Middle Ages, and from which the term *St Vitus' dance* was coined; this term subsequently was applied by Sydenham to describe the condition now referred to as *Sydenham chorea* (Hayden, 1981).

For further information, see the 2001 monograph by Halligan and colleagues, which is devoted to the topic of hysteria.

Physiologic basis for psychogenic neurologic dysfunctions – neuroimaging

It is intellectually intriguing that the brain can create neurologic deficits – such as paralysis, sensory loss, blindness, seizures, and movement disorders – from psychological factors. This mysterious ability fascinated pioneers working on hysteria, such as Charcot and Freud. We have not been much enlightened over the ensuing 100-plus years until recently, when newer imaging technologies have shed some light on the mechanism. As stated by Hallett (2010), physiologically, we cannot tell the difference between voluntary and involuntary. The exceptions are electrophysiologic measurements of myoclonus, startle, tremor and blepharospasm. The fast 50–100 ms contractions of organic myoclonus cannot be duplicated by psychogenic myoclonus. Psychogenic startle responses are too delayed and variable to be a physiologic reflex (Thompson et al., 1992). Psychogenic tremor can often be detected by variable width on spiral analysis (Hsu et al., 2009) and by other tests like coactivation sign and tapping (Deuschl et al., 1998, 2006; Zeuner et al., 2003; Criswell et al., 2010). The R2 recovery in the blink reflex is disinhibited in organic blepharospasm and is normal in psychogenic blepharospasm (Schwingenschuh et al., 2011). The Bereitschaftspotential (BP) (readiness potential) is seen with ordinarily voluntary movements, but by itself does not indicate that a movement is voluntary (Hallett, 2010). The electrophysiology of psychogenic dystonia resembles that of organic dystonia (Espay et al., 2006; Quartarone et al., 2009), except for findings of increased plasticity in the latter.

Vuilleumier and colleagues (2001) utilized single photon emission computed tomography (SPECT) to measure regional cerebral blood flow with and without bilateral vibration in seven patients with unilateral psychogenic sensory loss and then again in four subjects after full recovery. These studies revealed a consistent decrease of regional cerebral blood flow in the thalamus and basal ganglia contralateral to the deficit, which reverted to normal when the patients recovered. These results suggest that hysterical conversion deficits might entail a functional disorder in striatothalamocortical circuits controlling sensorimotor function and voluntary motor behavior. The same subcortical premotor circuits are involved in unilateral motor neglect after organic neurologic damage.

In an analogous situation, a patient who was diagnosed with psychogenic reduced visual acuity underwent a SPECT scan that revealed reduced regional cerebral blood flow in the bilateral visual association areas but not in the primary visual areas (Okuyama et al., 2002). The authors concluded that psychogenic visual disturbance is associated with functional suppression of the visual association area. A listing of functional imaging studies carried out in hysteria has been collated by Fink and colleagues (2006). These studies indicate that alterations in regional brain activity may accompany the expression of conversion symptoms. Since then, another study utilizing positron emission tomography (PET) in patients with hysterical anesthesia showed lack of response in the contralateral cortex to sensory stimulation of the affected limb, again indicating the brain physiologically shuts down as a result of the hysterical anesthesia (Ghaffar et al., 2006). Yet when bilateral stimulation is applied, there is bilateral activation of the cortex, indicating that the cortex is indeed intact.

The results in functional imaging studies are complemented by motor physiology studies. When cortical and spinal inhibition was evaluated in psychogenic and organic dystonia, both groups had similar results of reduced inhibition (Espay et al., 2006). Again, this suggests that the central nervous system accommodates its physiology to follow the motor pattern, or the reverse, i.e., that the abnormal psychological problem alters brain physiology, which then produces the abnormal motoric effect.

Degree of certainty of the diagnosis of a psychogenic movement disorder

Fahn and Williams (1988) categorized patients into four levels of certainty as to the likelihood of their having psychogenic dystonia; these categories can be applied to all psychogenic movement disorders. These four degrees of certainty are: (1) documented psychogenic disorder, (2) clinically established psychogenic disorder, (3) probable psychogenic disorder, and (4) possible psychogenic movement disorder. Subsequent authors have used this classification (Koller et al., 1989; Ranawaya et al., 1990; Lang, 1995; Shill and Gerber, 2006). We have incorporated the classification of Fahn and Williams but have expanded the criteria somewhat, taking into account additional observations since the original publication.

Documented psychogenic movement disorder

Just being suspicious that the signs and symptoms are psychogenic is insufficient for the diagnosis of documented psychogenic disorder. For the disorder to be documented as being psychogenic, the symptoms must be completely relieved by psychotherapy, by the clinician utilizing psychological suggestion including physiotherapy, or by administration of placebos (again with suggestion being a part of this approach), or the patient must be witnessed as being free of symptoms when left alone, supposedly unobserved. This last feature would be a major factor in proving psychogenicity in those who are malingering or have a factitious disorder, since such patients would not likely obtain relief of symptoms by manipulation of the examiner. Insurance companies are increasingly using videotaped surveillance to protect themselves against fraud. There is now a published report of a patient with a clinical diagnosis of reflex sympathetic dystrophy who sued for financial compensation despite features of psychogenicity and was videotaped while under surveillance by a private investigator to be completely free of the abnormal movements, allowing the case to be settled for a reduced amount (Kurlan et al., 1997). If the signs and symptoms disappear and do not return, that is fairly good evidence that the underlying psychiatric problem has been relieved. But it is not uncommon for the psychogenic movement disorder to return if the patient does not obtain complete relief of the psychiatric factors that led to the neurologic dysfunction.

A critical issue for using the relief of signs as a criterion for the definition is that most organic movement disorders rarely remit spontaneously and completely except for tics, tardive dyskinesia, infectious (e.g., Sydenham chorea), and drug-induced reactions, and rarely, essential myoclonus (Fahn and Sjaastad, 1991). Other organic disorders, such as Parkinson disease, Huntington disease, and essential tremor, are persistent and even progressive. Idiopathic torsion dystonia, except for torticollis (Jayne et al., 1984; Friedman and

Fahn, 1986; Jahanshahi et al., 1990), rarely totally remits. On occasion, patients with other types of dystonia will show improvement, but this improvement is typically incomplete and temporary (Marsden and Harrison, 1974), although gradual, prolonged, incomplete improvement has been encountered in at least one patient (Eldridge et al., 1984).

The degree of remission that is seen in cases with documented psychogenic movement disorders is usually the dramatic, sudden improvement that occurs within a few days with supportive suggestion or placebo treatment. In a few patients with more chronic symptoms, improvement can be more gradual, occurring over weeks to months of "physiotherapy" used as a means of allowing the patient to relinquish the symptoms in a face-saving manner. Physiotherapy also can have physical benefits for patients who had developed weakness, spasms, or contractures based on chronic disuse and/or abnormal postures for extended periods, even though these were on a psychogenic basis.

Clinically established psychogenic movement disorder

When the movement disorder is inconsistent over time (the features are different when the patient is observed at subsequent examinations) or is incongruent with a classic movement disorder, one becomes suspicious that the movements are psychogenic. If either inconsistency or incongruity is present and, in addition the patient has any of the manifestations listed in Table 25.1, one can feel comfortable in believing that the disorder is psychogenic, and this has been referred to as clinically established psychogenic movement disorder.

It should be noted that item 4 in Table 25.1 by itself is insufficient for a diagnosis of a documented or clinically established psychogenic disorder. This is because some organic movement disorders can be temporarily and voluntarily suppressed (Koller and Biary, 1989). Similarly, akathitic movements and paradoxical dystonia (Fahn, 1989) also tend to disappear with active voluntary movement. The difficulty establishing psychogenic paroxysmal dyskinesias which have a normal interictal pattern is covered below. Fortunately, myoclonus has such a short-duration contraction that it

Table 25.1 Additional manifestations besides inconsistency and incongruity for the diagnosis of clinically established psychogenic movement disorder

1. Other neurologic signs are present that are definitely psychogenic (e.g., false weakness, false sensory findings, and self-inflicted injuries)
2. Multiple somatizations are present
3. An obvious psychiatric disturbance is present
4. The movement disorder disappears with distraction
5. Excessive (appearing deliberate) slowness of movement is present
6. Excessive fatigue that is incompatible with the amount of motor activity.
7. The electrophysiologic analysis of the phenomenology of myoclonus or tremor does not fit with the organic pattern in these phenomenologies

cannot be purposely produced, so electrophysiologic evidence against organic myoclonus could be one of the factors along with inconsistency and incongruity that can lead to a clinically established diagnosis of a psychogenic myoclonus. Psychogenic tremors have features such as a coactivation sign (Deuschl et al., 1998, 2006) or a change in tremor frequency due to entrainment by tapping the contralateral limb (Zeuner et al., 2003). These features would establish the tremor as psychogenic.

Probable psychogenic movement disorder

This definition contains four categories of patients:

1. Patients in whom the movements are inconsistent or are incongruent with any classic movement disorder, and there are no other features to provide further support for such a diagnosis of psychogenicity.
2. Patients in whom the movements are consistent and congruent with an organic disorder, and the movements can be made to disappear with distraction, when ordinarily distraction would not be expected to eliminate the movements if they were organic.
3. Patients in whom the movements are consistent and congruent with an organic disorder, but other neurologic signs are present that are definitely psychogenic (e.g., false weakness, false sensory findings, or self-inflicted injuries).
4. Patients in whom the movements are consistent and congruent with an organic disorder, but multiple somatizations are present.

The last two subdivisions contain psychiatric manifestations that make the clinician highly suspicious that the movements might also be psychogenic, but by themselves they are insufficient to give a higher degree of certainty to the diagnosis of a psychogenic movement disorder.

Possible psychogenic movement disorder

One can be suspicious that the movements are psychogenic if an obvious emotional disturbance is present, but this is not as compelling as the psychiatric features listed above. For the category of a possible psychogenic disorder, the movements would be consistent and congruent with an organic movement disorder.

Summary on the degree of certainty of the diagnosis of a psychogenic paroxysmal movement disorder

Paroxysmal movement disorders present a special and difficult problem. Their natural history characteristically shows prolonged periods of cessation of the abnormal movements, so its disappearance with placebo or by suggestion cannot by itself establish the diagnosis of a psychogenic disorder, since the remission could have been coincidental. However, if the paroxysms are frequent and the attacks are prolonged, then repeated trials with placebo can be informative. If such trials consistently produce remissions, then one can be convinced that the diagnosis is a documented psychogenic disorder.

The criteria for clinically established, probable, and possible psychogenic movement disorders would be the same for paroxysmal movement disorders and continual movement disorders. It is likely when both a paroxysmal movement disorder and a continual movement disorder are present in the same patient that the etiology is psychogenic.

Definitions of psychiatric terminology

Definitions from DSM-IV are used regarding psychogenic movement disorders. Patients with psychogenic movement disorder can be subdivided into three categories: the somatoform disorders, the factitious disorders, and malingering.

Somatoform disorder

A somatoform disorder is one in which the physical symptoms are linked to psychological factors, yet the symptom production is *not under voluntary control* (i.e., *not consciously produced*). The two main types of somatoform disorders that produce psychogenic neurologic problems are *conversion disorder* and *somatization disorder*; the latter is also known as hysteria or as Briquet syndrome. Other somatoform subsets are hypochondriasis, somatoform pain disorder, and body dysmorphic disorder.

In *conversion disorder*, psychological factors may be judged to play a primary etiologic role in a variety of ways. This may be suggested by a temporal relationship between the onset or worsening of the symptoms and the presence of an environmental stimulus that activates a psychological conflict or need. Alternatively, the symptom may be noted to free the patient from a noxious activity or encounter. Finally, the symptom may be noted to enable the patient to get support from the environment that otherwise might not be forthcoming.

A *somatization disorder* involves recurrent and multiple complaints of several years' duration for which medical care has been sought, but that are apparently not due to any physical disorder. The dynamics are presumably the same as those of conversion disorder, and the symptoms may emerge from chronic, recurrent, untreated conversion disorder. There are four separate categories of symptoms that need to be present at some time for the diagnosis of a somatization disorder according to the DSM-IV-TR. They are (1) four sites or functions of pain, (2) two gastrointestinal symptoms, (3) one symptom related to sex or reproduction, and (4) at least one of 13 neurologic complaints, namely problems with coordination, paralysis or weakness, feeling of an object in the throat, aphonia, urinary retention, hallucinations, anesthesia, diplopia, blindness, deafness, seizures, amnesia, and loss of consciousness. It should be noted that various movement disorders, such as tremor and sustained contractions, are not on this list of 13, and they should be included as one of the neurologic complaints. Other requirements are age at onset under 30 years and severe enough symptomatology that the patient has taken medications, consulted a physician, or altered his or her lifestyle because of it.

The abnormal movements of somatoform disorders are involuntary. The knowledge that one is the cause of one's own actions is known as self-agency. Thus, people with abnormal movements due to a somatoform disorder lack self-agency. The right inferior parietal cortex is the brain area believed to play a role in self-agency. Voon and her colleagues (2010) utilized functional magnetic resonance imaging in eight subjects with a conversion disorder (tremor). The right temporoparietal junction was found to be hypoactive compared to those purposefully mimicking the same type of tremor ($P < 0.05$). There was an associated reduced connectivity between this cortical area and the sensorimotor areas and the limbic system.

Factitious disorder

A factitious disorder is one in which the physical symptoms are *intentionally produced* (hence are under voluntary control) owing to psychological need. This group includes Munchausen syndrome. Factitious disorders are due to a mental disorder. They are generally associated with severe dependent, masochistic, or antisocial personality disorders.

Malingering

Malingering refers to *voluntarily produced* physical symptoms in pursuit of a goal such as financial compensation, avoidance of school or work, evasion of criminal prosecution, or acquisition of drugs. Malingering is not considered to be a mental disorder.

When a physician is faced with a patient who has a psychogenic movement disorder, it is often not possible to distinguish with certainty among somatoform, factitious, and malingering disorders. A patient's volitional intent is often impossible to determine with certainty.

Depression

It is worth making some comment about depression. In our experience, many patients with a psychogenic movement disorder also have concurrent depression. Treatment of this depression is essential and is part of the overall strategy in outlining a treatment program for the patient. Often, lifting of the depression is necessary for the patient to obtain relief of the motor symptoms.

Clues suggesting the presence of a psychogenic movement disorder

Often, there are clues from the history and neurologic examination that lead the clinician to suspect a diagnosis of psychogenic dystonia. Fahn and Williams (1988), Koller and colleagues (1989), and Factor and colleagues (1995) have enunciated many of these clues. Tables 25.2 and 25.3 list these clues, as well as some additional ones.

Abrupt onset of the movement disorder is quite common. The presence of more than one type of dyskinesia (item 5 in Table 25.2) is another important clue, often confounding clinicians (Video 25.3). Most of the time, patients with an organic movement disorder present with only a single type. A note of caution is warranted, however. Certain disorders progress to involve more than one type of abnormal movement. For example, Huntington disease can have chorea,

Table 25.2 Clues relating to the movements that suggest a psychogenic movement disorder

1. Abrupt onset
2. Inconsistent movements (changing characteristics over time; pattern, body distribution, rapidly varying severity)
3. Incongruous movements and postures (movements that do not fit with recognized patterns or with normal physiologic patterns)
4. Presence of certain types of abnormal movements that are fairly common among individuals with psychogenic movement disorders, such as:
   rhythmic shaking
   bizarre gait
   deliberate slowness carrying out requested voluntary movement
   bursts of verbal gibberish
   excessive startle (bizarre movements in response to sudden, unexpected noise or threatening movement)
5. Presence of additional types of abnormal movements that are not known to be part of the primary or principal movement pattern that the patient manifests
6. Manifesting exhaustion, excessive fatigue
7. Delayed, often excessive, startle response to a stimulus
8. Spontaneous remissions
9. Decrease or disappearance of movements with distraction
10. Disappearance of tremors when handling treasured objects
11. Entrainment of the tremor to the rate of the requested rapid successive movement the patient is asked to perform
12. Response to placebo, suggestion or psychotherapy
13. Manifestation of a paroxysmal disorder
14. Dystonia beginning as a fixed posture
15. Twisting facial movements that move the mouth to one side or the other (*note*: organic dystonia of the facial muscles usually does not move the mouth sideways)

Table 25.3 Clues relating to other medical observations that suggest a psychogenic movement disorder

1. False (give-way) weakness
2. False sensory complaints
3. Multiple somatizations or undiagnosed conditions
4. Self-inflicted injuries
5. Obvious psychiatric disturbances
6. Employed in the health profession or in health insurance claims
7. Presence of secondary gain, including continuing care by a devoted spouse
8. Litigation or compensation pending

bradykinesia, dystonia, and myoclonus (Penney et al., 1990). Neuroacanthocytosis often is manifested by both chorea and tics (Hardie et al., 1991). Some patients with childhood-onset tics may later develop torsion dystonia (Shale et al., 1986; Stone and Jankovic, 1991). Often, patients with idiopathic torsion dystonia will have dystonic tremor or rapid movements that resemble myoclonus or chorea (Fahn et al., 1987). Patients with tardive dyskinesia may have a combination of rhythmical oral-buccal-lingual movements plus dystonia and akathitic movements (Fahn, 1984). Table 1.17 in Chapter 1 lists the diseases that are composed of multiple types of movement disorders. 📹

The most common types of movements, whether isolated or in the presence of other types of movements, in patients with psychogenic movement disorders are shaking movements (item 4 in Table 25.2) that can resemble organic tremors or peculiar, atypical tremors (Video 25.4). This was the most common type of abnormal movement in the spectrum of psychogenic movement disorders reported by Lang (2006) and by Jankovic et al. (2006b). Another note of caution about unusual tremors is that Wilson disease can also present with unusual tremors (Shale et al., 1987, 1988). Utterances of gibberish can be another useful sign (Videos 25.5 and 25.6). 📹

Item 4 in Table 25.2 also lists bizarre gaits as a feature of psychogenicity. After tremors and dystonia, bizarre gait disorders are the next most common type of unusual movement disorder encountered in patients with mixed features of movements. The psychogenic gait can show posturing, excessive slowness, and hesitation. There could be pseudoataxia or careful walking (like walking on ice). The latter resembles the fear-of-falling syndrome, which is discussed in more detail later. There can be sudden buckling of a leg, as if there is weakness (Vecht et al., 1991), but the failure to produce this dipping movement each time the patient steps on the leg would be evidence of inconsistency. Accompanying this bizarre gait would be a variability of impairment and excessive swaying when tested for the Romberg sign, without actually falling.

Another aspect of item 4 is excessive startle that could mimic hyperekplexia, excessive startle syndrome, the jumping Frenchmen syndrome (Video 25.7), or even reflex myoclonus (Andermann and Andermann, 1986). Thompson and colleagues (1992) determined the physiologic parameters that are typically seen in patients with psychogenic startles. There is a variable latency to the onset of the jerk; the latencies are greater than those seen in reflex myoclonus of cortical or brainstem origin; the latencies are longer than the fastest voluntary reaction time; there are variable patterns of muscle recruitment within each jerk; and there is significant habituation with repeated stimulation. This last point is probably not specific to psychogenic startle, since organic startles may also show habituation. Noise stimuli can induce other abnormal movements besides startle. Walters and Hening (1992) reported a case with psychogenic tremor following sudden, loud noise; the patient had a post-traumatic stress disorder. 📹

Item 11 in Table 25.2 points out that in a patient with psychogenic tremor, when asked to carry out rapid successive movements, such as tapping the index finger on the thumb, the rate of the tremor becomes the same as the rapid successive movements (i.e., the tremor has become entrained). In contrast, an organic tremor is the dominant rate; it will gradually force the voluntary movements to be the same rate as the tremor.

Idiopathic torsion dystonia usually begins with action dystonia (Fahn et al., 1987), but psychogenic dystonia often begins with a fixed posture. Fixed postures are sustained postures that resist passive movement, and the presence of such fixed postures is highly likely to be due to a psychogenic dystonia (Fahn and Williams, 1988; Lang and Fahn, 1990;

Schrag et al., 2004; Schrag, 2006). The posture can manifest so much rigidity that it is extremely difficult to move the limb about a joint (Video 25.8). Often, the psychogenic dystonia resembles reflex sympathetic dystrophy (complex regional pain syndrome, CRPS) because there is accompanying pain, tenderness (allodynia), and skin changes (Lang and Fahn, 1990; Schwartzman and Kerrigan, 1990; Bhatia et al., 1993; Schrag et al., 2004; Schrag, 2006). Nerve injury leading to pain, shiny red skin, and fixed postures was called causalgia by Mitchell et al. (1864). Charcot (1892) considered the disorder hysterical (see Munts and Koehler, 2010). The term "reflex sympathetic dystrophy" was coined by Evans (1946) because the phenotype could occur in the absence of trauma to a major nerve and might be due to sympathetic nerves. "Complex regional pain syndrome" was the recommended term in 1994, with type 1 being reflex sympathetic dystrophy and type 2 being causalgia (Merskey and Bogduk, 1994). 📹

To make matters confusing, in many cases, psychogenic dystonia of a limb follows a minor trauma to that limb, similar to the pattern of reflex sympathetic dystrophy. On the other hand, organic dystonia of a body part can be preceded by an injury to that body part (Schott, 1985, 1986; Scherokman et al., 1986; Gordon et al., 1990; Goldman and Ahlskog, 1993), so it can be difficult to distinguish between organic and psychogenic dystonia. Fixed painful postural torticollis following trauma is not uncommon, and determining whether it is organic or psychogenic is difficult, but analysis indicates that many of these cases appear to be psychogenic in etiology (Sa et al., 2003).

Although a fixed dystonic posture, in which the joint cannot be passively extended or flexed, is often psychogenic, it could also be due to a contracture (which, of course could also be the result of a psychogenic dystonia as well as an organic dystonia). The evaluation of such fixed postures in which the affected joint cannot be passively altered requires the aid of anesthesia to see if contractures are present (Fahn, 2006b). This technique not only aids the diagnosis but also guides the clinician and patient in what to expect during therapy (Video 25.9). The prognosis of fixed dystonia is often poor (Ibrahim et al., 2009), but it depends on recognizing this disorder as likely to be a psychogenic one and then applying treatment according the principles described below. 📹

Debates continue as to whether CRPS is organic or psychogenic. This topic was discussed at the Second Psychogenic Movement Disorder Symposium in 2009. A recent proposal that small fiber neuropathy might be responsible (Oaklander and Fields, 2009) has been countered by the observation that the patient had the phenomenology of a psychogenic dystonia (Lang and Chen, 2010).

In addition to the clues in the history and examination related to the movements themselves presented in Table 25.2, there are often clues in the non-movement history and examination that help the clinician consider a psychogenic disorder. These are presented in Table 25.3.

We have been impressed by the frequency with which patients with psychogenic movement disorders are employed in some capacity working in the health profession (item 6 in Table 25.3). Many are nurses; another large group are employed in the health insurance industry, processing medical claims.

Another point that is worth commenting on is that many of the affected individuals have a devoted spouse who responds readily to their pressing needs (item 7 in Table 25.3). Some spouses carry a pager so that the patient can easily call them while they are at work. Others pamper the patient, who might even be wheelchair bound, especially if the patient has psychogenic dystonia. Such devotion could be a secondary gain from having the movement disorder.

Diagnostic approach and clinical features

Psychogenic movement disorders are usually identified on the basis of (1) unusual motor phenomenology and other clues as listed in Tables 25.2 and 25.3, (2) a discrepancy between the patient's disability and objective signs of motor deficit, and (3) the presence of psychiatric abnormalities. First, the neurologist bases the suspected diagnosis on identifying the different types of abnormal movements that are present in a given patient. The type of movement disorder is assigned the basis of the phenomenology, which can consist of more than one type (item 5, Table 25.2). The neurologist must exclude possible organic causes for the abnormal movements so that both the neurologist and the patient feel comfortable that the diagnosis of a psychogenic movement disorder has been made with confidence. Then the consulting psychiatrist attempts to establish a psychiatric diagnosis. Finally, a suggested strategy for treatment is presented to the patient. In fact, explaining to the patient that the condition has the potential for a more favorable outcome with proper treatment than would an organic movement disorder may help the patient more readily accept the diagnosis of a psychogenic etiology.

Medically unexplained neurologic symptoms are common. About one-third of neurology outpatients receive that diagnosis (Stone et al., 2009). It would appear that neurologists are quite accurate when diagnosing a psychogenic disorder. Of 1144 patients diagnosed as medically unexplained, by 18 months, only 0.4% had acquired an organic disease diagnosis that was unexpected at initial assessment and plausibly the cause of the patients' original symptoms (Stone et al., 2009).

The types of psychogenic movements seen in a review of the publications from eight movement disorders centers are presented in Table 25.4. Tremor was found to be the most common psychogenic phenomenology, followed by dystonia. Tics were the least common.

Williams and colleagues (1995) reviewed the records of 131 patients with psychogenic movement disorders and listed their motor phenomenologies (Table 25.5). In their experience, dystonia, tremor, gait disturbances, paroxysmal dyskinesias, and myoclonus were the major motor types that were encountered. The difference from other centers that found tremor to be more common than dystonia may be because the Columbia group labeled movements on a hierarchical scale, whereby if any dystonia is present, regardless if other movements like tremor are also present, the condition was coded as a dystonic one. Williams and colleagues found that 79% of patients had multiple types of abnormal movements and that only 21% had a single definable type (Table 25.6). Moreover, again in contrast with the vast

Table 25.4 Predominant movement features in psychogenic movement disorders

Predominant movement feature	No.	Percent
Tremor	467	37.5
Dystonia	365	29.3
Myoclonus	146	11.7
Gait disorder	114	9.2
Parkinsonism	60	4.8
Tics	29	2.3
Other	64	5.1
Total	**1245**	**100**

A tabulation of psychogenic movement disorders seen at eight centers; most centers report their patients by a single primary motor feature, but some report multiple features if more than one is present.
Data from Lang AE. General overview of psychogenic movement disorders: epidemiology, diagnosis, and prognosis. In Hallett M, Fahn S, Jankovic J, et al., eds. Psychogenic Movement Disorders – Neurology and Neuropsychiatry. Philadelphia, Lippincott Williams & Wilkins, 2006; pp. 35–41.

Table 25.5 Principal motor phenomenology in 131 patients with psychogenic movement disorders

Movements	No.	Percent of organic cases
Dystonia	82	2.5
Tremor	21	
Gait disorder	14	
Myoclonus	11	
Blepharospasm/facial movements	4	
Parkinsonism	3	<0.1
Tics	2	
Stiff person	1	
Paroxysmal and undifferentiated movements	14	

Total for types of movements = 152, because more than one type was equally prominent.
Data from Williams DT, Ford B, Fahn S. Phenomenology and psychopathology related to psychogenic movement disorders. Adv Neurol 1995;65:231–257.

majority of organic movement disorders, in 55% of the patients the movements were either intermittent or paroxysmal, while only 45% of the patients had only continuous movements. They also reported that the onset was abrupt in 60% of patients, usually with a specific inciting event. In 43% of patients, the movements spread beyond the initial site of involvement.

Factor and colleagues (1995) reviewed their 28 cases of psychogenic movement disorders. These represented 3.3% of all 842 consecutive movement disorder patients seen over a

Table 25.6 Phenomenology of psychogenic movements

Single type	21%
Multiple types	79%
Continuous movements	45%
Intermittent/paroxysmal	55%
15 patients with hand tremor: dominant hand	93%
Abrupt onset (usually inciting event)	60%
Spread from initial site	43%

Data from Williams DT, Ford B, Fahn S. Phenomenology and psychopathology related to psychogenic movement disorders. Adv Neurol 1995;65:231–257.

Table 25.7 Demographics of patients with psychogenic movement disorders

Age at onset
Range: 4–73 years
Mean: 36.9 years

Gender
Males:Females = 22:109
Males = 13%
Females = 87%

Presence of some organic component
13%

Onset to correct diagnosis
Mean: 4.9 years
Trimodal:
    <6 months: 25%
    2 years: 40%
    23 years: 15%

Data from Williams DT, Ford B, Fahn S. Phenomenology and psychopathology related to psychogenic movement disorders. Adv Neurol 1995;65:231–257.

Table 25.8 Clinical features in patients with psychogenic movement disorders

Previously erroneously diagnosed as organic (3 with multiple sclerosis despite negative laboratory tests)	75%
False weakness	37%
False sensory exam	8.7%
Pain & tenderness	17.4%
Startle	29%
Psychogenic seizures	11.6%
Disabled	65%
Head trauma	25%
Peripheral trauma	12.5%

Data from Williams DT, Ford B, Fahn S. Phenomenology and psychopathology related to psychogenic movement disorders. Adv Neurol 1995;65:231–257.

Table 25.9 Psychiatric aspects of psychogenic movement disorders

Conversion disorder	75%
Somatization disorder	12.5%
Factitious disorder	8.3%
Malingering	4.2%
Accompanying depression	71%
anxiety	17%
Hypnotizable highly	36%
mild-moderately	41%

Data from Williams DT, Ford B, Fahn S. Phenomenology and psychopathology related to psychogenic movement disorders. Adv Neurol 1995;65:231–257.

6-year period. Tremor was most common (50%), followed by dystonia, myoclonus, and parkinsonism. Clinical clues included distractibility (86%) and abrupt onset (54%). Distractibility was more important in tremor and least important in dystonia. Other diagnostic clues included entrainment of tremor to the frequency of repetitive movements of another limb, fatigue of tremor, stimulus sensitivity, and a previous history of psychogenic illness.

The demographic pattern of the 131 patients reported by Williams and colleagues (1995) is presented in Table 25.7. Of the 131 patients, 87% were females; the mean age at onset was 37 years, with a range of 4–73 years. An organic component of a movement disorder was present in 13%. The mean duration before a correct diagnosis was made was 5 years.

An organic diagnosis was made originally in 75% of the patients with a psychogenic movement disorder (Table 25.8), including three patients who carried a diagnosis of multiple sclerosis despite the lack of any positive laboratory data detected by the treating neurologist. A number of neurologic findings presented as clues to psychogenicity. The

most common was the presence of give-way weakness (37%). Next most common was a startle reaction that was nonphysiologic (29%). Pain and false sensory findings on examination were also encountered (Table 25.8). Surprisingly, psychogenic seizures were concurrently present in 12% of the patients. The psychogenic movement disorder was disabling in 65% of the patients. A preceding history and inciting event of head trauma and peripheral trauma occurred in 25% and 12.5% of patients, respectively.

Williams and colleagues (1995) found that the most common psychiatric diagnosis was a somatoform disorder, particularly a conversion disorder (Table 25.9). Briquet syndrome (somatization disorder) was diagnosed in 12.5%, and there were even fewer patients with a factitious disorder (8%) or malingering (4%). An accompanying depression or anxiety was found in 71% and 17% of patients, respectively.

Psychogenic dystonia

It is, in some ways, ironic that torsion dystonia can sometimes be due to psychogenic causation. From its earliest beginnings, idiopathic torsion dystonia appeared to have been mistaken as a manifestation of a psychiatric disturbance (Schwalbe, 1908). Soon after Schwalbe's description in 1908 (see English translation by Truong and Fahn, 1988), however, Oppenheim (1911b) and Flatau and Sterling (1911) set matters right by emphasizing the organic nature of this disorder. Although some early publications on dystonia mentioned the "functional" nature of the symptoms (Destarac, 1901) or used the label, *neurosis* (Ziehen, 1911), these terms were employed in those days in a manner different from today. *Functional* referred to a physiologic activation of the abnormal movements with voluntary motor activity, which would otherwise disappear when the patient was quiet at rest. *Neurosis* was a term that was used to indicate a neurologic, rather than a psychiatric, disorder but one without a structural lesion. Today, it is common for the term *functional* to be equivalent to *psychogenic* and for *neurosis* not to be used at all in neurology but to refer to a certain type of psychiatric disorder.

Thus, for many decades, the organic nature of torsion dystonia was emphasized. Yet, possibly beginning in the 1950s, many patients with various forms of focal, segmental, and generalized dystonia began to be misdiagnosed as having a conversion disorder (Table 25.10). Among 44 patients with idiopathic dystonia reviewed by Eldridge and colleagues (1969), 23 patients (52%) had previously been referred for psychiatric treatment (without benefit). Marsden and Harrison (1974) had a similar experience; 43% of their 42 patients were previously diagnosed as suffering from hysteria. Cooper and his colleagues (1976) reviewed their series of 226 patients and found that 56 patients (25%) had a diagnosis of psychogenic etiology at some time during their illness. Lesser and Fahn (1978) reviewed the records of 84 patients with idiopathic dystonia seen at Presbyterian Hospital in New York from 1969 to 1974 and found that 37 patients (44%) had previously been given a diagnosis that their movement abnormalities were due to an emotional disorder. These 37 patients consisted of 11 with generalized dystonia, 14 with segmental dystonia, and 19 with focal dystonia (14 with torticollis, 2 with oromandibular dystonia, and 3 with blepharospasm).

Although some authors (Meares, 1971; Tibbets, 1971) suggested that an underlying psychiatric illness might exist in patients with torticollis, others (Zeman and Dyken, 1968; Cockburn, 1971; Riklan et al., 1976) found no differences between dystonic patients and controls in regard to previous psychiatric history and current life adjustment or on psychiatric testing. Similarly, some authors (Crisp and Moldofsky, 1965; Bindman and Tibbets, 1977) considered hand dystonia (writer's cramp, occupational cramp) to be psychogenic. But Sheehy and Marsden (1982) studied 34 patients with writer's or other occupational cramps affecting the hand or arm. All patients underwent assessment by a psychiatric interview technique; these patients compared favorably with a control group, and the investigators concluded that their disorder was not psychiatric in origin. Another recent study involved psychiatric assessment in 20 subjects with focal hand dystonia and also concluded that none had any serious psychopathology (Grafman et al., 1991). Furthermore, patients with writer's cramp do not have increased anxiety (Harrington et al., 1988).

At the time of the first international symposium on dystonia, held in 1975, Fahn and Eldridge (1976) noted that no case of proven psychological dystonia had been reported. With the realization that patients with dystonia were being misdiagnosed as having a psychiatric disorder, knowledgeable neurologists became sensitive to this problem and, since then, seemed to avoid a diagnosis of hysterical dystonia. However, at the annual meeting of the American Academy of Neurology in 1983, Fahn and colleagues (1983) described ten patients as having documented psychogenic dystonia, five of them identified after the abstract to the meeting was submitted. Batshaw and colleagues (1985) had followed a patient who had been misdiagnosed as having an organic dystonia and who had had a stereotactic thalamotomy based on that diagnosis; these authors eventually recognized that their patient had psychogenic dystonia and reported her as a case of Munchausen syndrome. Fahn and Williams (1988) have described 22 cases of documented or clinically established psychogenic dystonia, including a case of a young girl who underwent a stereotactic thalamotomy. Lang (1995) reported on 18 patients with documented or clinically established psychogenic dystonia, 14 of whom had a known precipitant. Involvement of the legs occurred in 12 patients, despite onset in adulthood. Ten of Lang's patients had paroxysmal worsening of dystonia or other abnormal movements. Pain was a prominent feature in 14 of 16 patients with this complaint.

Psychogenic dystonia is difficult to diagnose, since there are no laboratory tests to establish the diagnosis of organic idiopathic dystonia. A number of cortical and spinal reflex abnormalities have been reported in organic dystonia, all showing lack of inhibition or spread of cortical field (see Chapter 12). These abnormalities could be a useful way to differentiate psychogenic dystonia from organic dystonia. But when these tests were applied to both groups to see their differences, the results were similar in the two groups, that is, both groups showed a reduced inhibition (Espay et al., 2006). This supports the growing findings detected by PET scans in psychogenic neurologic disorders that the central nervous system accommodates its physiology to follow the motor pattern.

Without laboratory analysis, diagnosis depends on clinical skill to differentiate organic and psychogenic dystonia. The clues listed in Tables 25.2 and 25.3 should help to alert the clinician to the possibility of a psychogenic etiology. Clues that often point to an organic diagnosis, such as a sensory trick (*geste antagoniste*) that mitigates dystonia, can be very helpful, but also occasionally can be misleading (Munhoz and Lang, 2004).

In a survey of 22 patients reported by Fahn (1994) on documented and clinically established cases of psychogenic dystonia, he found that 6 patients had paroxysmal dystonia,

Table 25.10 Reports on the misdiagnosis of organic dystonia as being psychogenic

Eldridge et al. (1969)	23/44 (52%)
Marsden and Harrison (1974)	18/42 (43%)
Cooper et al. (1976)	56/226 (25%)
Lesser and Fahn (1978)	37/84 (44%)

and 16 had continual dystonia. Females outnumbered males by a ratio of 20:2. The youngest age at onset was 8 years, and the oldest was 58 years. Those with paroxysmal dystonia were, as a general rule, older than patients with continual dystonia.

Psychogenic nondystonic movement disorders

Psychogenic tremor

As mentioned above, rhythmic movements are the most common abnormal movement in patients with psychogenic movements, often appearing as shaking movements. But what resembles organic tremor is also a common presentation. The tremor tends to be present equally with the affected limb at rest, with posture holding and with action (Video 25.10). This helps differentiate it from organic tremors, which typically dominate in just one of these characteristic features. Also, psychogenic tremor tends to vary in pattern (for example, being vertical in the hands when the arm is at rest, and being horizontal in the hands when the arm is held against gravity in front of the body) (Jankovic et al., 2006b). Distracting the patient with a disappearance of the tremor is a helpful sign that the tremor is psychogenic (Campbell, 1979), but it is not specific enough. Many patients with organic tremor can temporally suppress the tremor, even parkinsonian tremor; furthermore, distractibility is often difficult to observe. Many patients are sophisticated, and it is difficult to eliminate their tremor with distraction. Entrainment of the tremor to a new frequency may sometimes be seen by having the patient touch thumb to the different fingers in a dictated pattern. Of 12 patients with psychogenic tremor compared to 33 with organic essential tremor studied by Kenney and colleagues (2007), psychogenic tremor was significantly more likely to start suddenly and was more likely associated with spontaneous remissions compared to essential tremor; family history of tremor was significantly more common in the essential tremor group, distraction with alternate finger tapping significantly decreased psychogenic tremor, but entrainment did not differentiate the two groups. 🎥

Koller and colleagues (1989) diagnosed 24 patients with psychogenic tremors. They described the tremors as complex; usually they were present at rest, with posture, and with action. The onset was abrupt, and in all but one the tremors lessened or were abolished with distraction. Fahn (1994) described that psychogenic tremors are sometimes paroxysmal and not always continuous. Deuschl and colleagues (1998) reviewed 25 cases of psychogenic tremor. Sudden onset and rare remissions were common. The "coactivation sign" and absent finger tremor were the most consistent criteria to separate them from organic tremors. Whereas most organic tremors show decreasing amplitudes when the extremity is loaded with additional weights, most psychogenic tremors show an increase of tremor amplitude (i.e., coactivation sign). Overall, psychogenic tremor in their series had a poor outcome. Kim and colleagues (1999) reviewed their series of 70 cases of psychogenic tremor. They emphasized the abrupt onset (73%), often with the maximal disability at onset (46%), and then taking static (46%) or fluctuating (17%) courses. Tremor usually started in one limb and spread rapidly to a generalized or mixed distribution. Other features were spontaneous resolution and recurrence, as well as easy distractibility together with entrainment and response to suggestion. McKeon and colleagues (2009) followed up their 62 patients with psychogenic tremor; 33 responded. The outcome was good (mild or no tremor) in 36%, moderate in 24% and severe in 40%. Five patients with the good outcome had spontaneous improvement without psychotherapy.

In addition to tremor in the limbs, psychogenic palatal tremor has been reported (Pirio Richardson et al., 2006). Psychogenic stridor was diagnosed in a boy who developed inspiratory stridor when trying to fall asleep (Vetrugno et al., 2009), but this seems more appropriately to be called anxiety-induced stridor.

Another electrophysiologic approach to aid in distinguishing between psychogenic and organic tremors is with accelerometry. Tremor is measured in one hand while the other hand either rested or tapped to an auditory stimulus at 3 and 4 or 5 Hz. Psychogenic tremors showed larger tremor frequency changes and higher intraindividual variability during tapping (Zeuner et al., 2003). Motor control physiology can be useful to distinguish psychogenic from organic tremor (Deuschl et al., 2006).

About half of the psychogenic tremors are coherent between the two arms, suggesting to the authors that coherent tremors might be voluntary, while noncoherent tremors are involuntary (Raethjen et al., 2004). Voluntary tapping of the contralateral limb usually results in either dissipating the tremor or shifting the tremor frequency to that of the metronome (O'Suilleabhain and Matsumoto, 1998).

A patient who underwent deep brain stimulation for the treatment of essential tremor developed psychogenic tremor following the surgery (McKeon et al., 2008).

Psychogenic gait

An abnormal gait is a common feature in patients with a psychogenic movement disorder. Of 279 patients, 118 (42%) had an abnormal gait (Baik and Lang, 2007). 102 (86%) of these 118 patients had other psychogenic movements, and gait was also abnormal, with slowing of gait (18.6%), dystonic gait (17.8%), bizarre gait (11.9%), astasia–abasia (11.9%), and buckling of the knee (7.6%) as the most common types. Among the pure psychogenic gait disorders, buckling of the knee was the most common feature (31.3%), followed by astasia–abasia (18.8%) (Table 25.11).

Morris and colleagues (2006) described key features of the psychogenic gait. These include exaggerated effort, fatigue with groans and sighs, extreme slowness, appearance of pain with grimaces, knee-buckling, unusual postures, and astasia–abasia. Keane (1989) described 60 cases with psychogenic gait abnormality out of 228 patients with psychogenic neurologic problems. Among these abnormal gaits were 24 patients with "ataxia" (the most common gait abnormality), 9 patients with trembling, 2 patients with "dystonia," 2 patients with truncal "myoclonus," and 1 patient with camptocormia (markedly stooped posture). Among the myriad of associated psychogenic signs were 8 patients with tremor. A knee giving way, with recovery, was seen in 5 patients, and is a feature of a case that presented as an unknown, unusual movement disorder (Vecht et al., 1991). In a video review of

Table 25.11 Types of psychogenic gaits

Clinical feature	Mixed type	Pure type
Number of patients	102	16
Slowing	21	1
Dystonic	20	1
Bizarre	12	2
Astasia–abasia	11	3
Knee-buckling	4	5
Tight-rope walking	7	1
Trembling	4	1
Stiff-legged	5	0
Dragging	4	0
Scissoring	4	1
Truncal myoclonus	4	0
Fatigue	3	0
Waddling	2	1
Ataxic	1	0

Data from Baik JS, Lang AE. Gait abnormalities in psychogenic movement disorders. Mov Disord 2007;22(3):395–399.

psychogenic gaits, Hayes and colleagues (1999) emphasized certain features of the gait: exaggerated effort, extreme slowness, variability throughout the day, unusual or uneconomic postures, collapses, convulsive tremors, and distractibility. On the other hand, it is possible to misdiagnose as psychogenic an abnormal gait that is organic. Such happened to a patient with a gait disorder and episodic weakness that were thought to be psychogenic who was subsequently diagnosed with status cataplecticus due to narcolepsy (Simon et al., 2004).

Fear of falling

According to Keane (1989), Spiller (1933) referred to the syndrome of fear of falling as *staso-basophobia*. Fear of falling is a syndrome in which the patient can walk perfectly well if he or she is holding onto someone, but is unable to walk without leaning against furniture or walls if alone. Sometimes, this could be purely due to a psychiatric problem, such as agoraphobia. Most of the patients we have seen with this problem developed the condition after they had fallen, usually from organic causes (such as loss of postural reflexes or ataxia) and were left with a marked fear of falling when walking without holding on. One of our patients with essential action myoclonus developed this disorder after suffering several falls and continued to have fear of falling even after successful treatment of the myoclonus with clonazepam. The freezing phenomenon (or motor blocks) that is seen in parkinsonism and the gait in action myoclonus patients are the other major conditions in which the gait also normalizes when the patient

holds on to someone. The fear-of-falling syndrome is usually separated from the list of psychogenic movement disorders (see below), and would be characterized as a psychiatric movement disorder. But in many of these patients, the fear of falling is beyond what is rational, so there is a psychogenic component. Women are more affected than men, and often the mistaken diagnosis is Parkinson disease (Kurlan, 2005).

Psychogenic myoclonus

Psychogenic myoclonus should be relatively easy to distinguish from organic myoclonus if access to a motor control physiology laboratory is available (Brown, 2006). PolyEMG is very helpful in distinguishing psychogenic myoclonus from organic myoclonus. The short duration of a myoclonic jerk (usually less than 100 ms) is almost impossible to duplicate voluntarily. The EMG pattern of voluntary jerks exhibits a triphasic pattern of activity between antagonistic muscles, whereas cortical myoclonus consists of short-duration 25–50 ms bursts of cocontracting antagonists muscles (Thompson, 2006). Furthermore, the latency of reflex myoclonus is physiologically short (40–100 ms) whereas abnormal reactive voluntary jerks are much longer (Thompson, 2006).

Monday and Jankovic (1993) reported 18 patients with psychogenic myoclonus (although no EMG observations were reported to indicate that myoclonus was the actual type of abnormal movement), stating that this is the most common form of psychogenic movement disorder encountered in their clinic. The myoclonus was segmental in 10 patients, generalized in 7 patients and focal in 1 patient. Psychogenic myoclonus accounted for 8.5% of the 212 patients with myoclonus in their clinic. Inconsistency with continuously changing pattern anatomically and temporally was common. The movements often increased with stress, anxiety, and exposure to noise or light. A Bereitschaftspotential preceding muscle jerks was found in five of six patients with a diagnosis of psychogenic myoclonus (Terada et al., 1995). The authors suggest that this is a positive sign for the diagnosis of psychogenic myoclonus, but because of the one patient who did not have a Bereitschaftspotential, its absence cannot be used to exclude the diagnosis.

Rhythmical palatal myoclonus has also been reported to be of a psychogenic etiology in rare cases (Williams, 2004; Pirio Richardson et al., 2006). A case of propriospinal myoclonus was presumed be of psychogenic etiology when it disappeared after some minor procedures (Williams et al., 2008).

Psychogenic tics

Psychogenic movements can sometimes resemble tics, but these are one of the least common manifestations of a psychogenic movement disorder (Lang, 2006). It is more complicated when organic tics are also present. Dooley and colleagues (1994) described two children with Tourette syndrome who also had pseudo-tics, in whom the psychogenic movements resolved when the stressful issues in their lives were addressed.

Psychogenic parkinsonism

Psychogenic parkinsonism is relatively uncommon (see Tables 25.4 and 25.5). Lang and colleagues (1995) reported 14 patients with this disorder. Eleven patients had tremor at rest, but the tremor did not disappear with movement of the limb, and the frequency and rhythmicity varied. Rigidity was present in six patients but without cogwheeling. All 14 patients had slowness of movement (bradykinesia) without the typical decrementing feature of organic bradykinesia (Video 25.11). One patient had evidence of some organic parkinsonism as well but required a fluorodopa PET scan to be certain. Other studies also reported the combination of organic and psychogenic parkinsonism and found the dopaminergic SPECT imaging can help in distinguishing this diagnosis from pure psychogenic parkinsonism (Benaderette et al., 2006; Gaig et al., 2006).

Approaches to the patient suspected of having a psychogenic movement disorder

The following treatment plan has been developed over the years for managing patients with psychogenic disorders.

A. Ideally, the patient should be admitted to the hospital, specifically to the neurology unit where the treating neurologist is in control of the treating regimen. Informing the patient of the diagnosis on the initial visit in an outpatient setting often leads to disbelief and distrust by the patient. If this happens, the patient usually never returns and will continue to have symptoms and probably see a number of other physicians, looking for an organic diagnosis. The success rate of outpatient treatment is uncertain, but in this age of managed health care, the difficulty in obtaining permission to admit the patient to a hospital will force many patients to be treated in an outpatient setting.

B. Because of the difficulty in admitting the patient to the hospital, a new strategy has evolved over the last few years that appears to be a reasonable substitute for hospitalization. All necessary and reasonable tests should be performed to ensure that an organic basis for the symptoms has not been overlooked. This includes a sleep study with video recording if the family insists that the movements are present during sleep.

C. When the diagnosis seems certain during an outpatient evaluation, the next step is to inform the patient of the diagnosis. This is usually difficult for the physician and must be done in a tactful manner that will convince the patient and the family without incurring denial by them. It is helpful to ask them if they have any thoughts as to what is the cause of the symptoms. If they mention that it might be due to their "nerves" or to stress, this is an excellent opportunity for the physician to mention that he or she has come to a similar conclusion. If they do not mention stress, the physician needs another approach to inform the patient about the diagnosis. Our approach, in this situation, is to inform the patient that he or she has a movement disorder (specifically naming the disorder – e.g.,

dystonia, tremor, etc.) and that this disorder "can be caused by many different etiologies." Then we proceed to explain that in the patient's situation, all the evidence rules out a structural defect in the brain and that the variety of symptoms indicate they are caused by brain physiology expressing pent-up emotions that need to be expressed and do so by producing these abnormal movements. Explain that the mind controls the body by producing physiologic changes in the brain to allow these symptoms to come out. It is important to mention that because the symptoms are not due to a structural lesion, the chance for reversing the abnormal physiology is great. This provides the positive aspect of the disorder, which is strengthened when the physician points out that if this were due to a structural change in the brain, the chance for full recovery would be almost impossible.

D. At this point, the physician explains the treatment approach, pointing out that it is essential for the neurologist to work with a psychiatrist who can determine what the stress factors are that have allowed the brain physiology to be altered. If the psychiatrist determines there is an underlying depression or anxiety, the psychiatrist has the opportunity to treat those conditions with medications. It is important to explain to the patient that (1) the psychiatrist may want to utilize medications to alter the brain transmitters to hasten a normalization of brain physiology and (2) in addition to working with a psychiatrist, it will be essential to include physiotherapy to teach the muscles (essentially retraining the muscles) to move normally again.

E. Once the diagnosis and the therapeutic strategy has been explained, the physician must determine whether the patient sincerely wishes to improve by an intensive treatment program that entails outpatient psychotherapy and outpatient physiotherapy. It should be explained that it is up to the patient to work on this treatment regimen if improvement is to be achieved. This places pressure on the patient to improve. The patient should be told that unless improvement is seen at each follow-up visit, there is no sense in continuing the program; it would be a waste of time and money.

F. Ideally, the psychiatric consultant should be experienced in and should have had success working with patients with a psychogenic movement disorder. It will be the psychiatrist who will obtain clues about the possible psychodynamics underlying the symptoms; who determines whether the patient has insight that will be important for estimating the prognosis; who utilizes hypnosis or conducts an amobarbital interview in order to obtain more psychodynamic information; who discusses possible pharmacotherapeutic approaches; and who establishes the rapport with the patient that will be necessary for psychotherapy. A psychiatrist who has an interest in treating psychogenic movement disorders is critical to successful therapy.

G. It is important to recognize that a psychiatrist cannot make the diagnosis of a psychogenic movement disorder. This diagnosis can be made only by the neurologist.

H. The severity of the underlying psychiatric illness should not be underestimated by the neurologist. These patients are prone to committing suicide.

I. The presence of joint contractures does not exclude the diagnosis of a psychogenic movement disorder (Fahn and Williams, 1988; Ziegler et al., 2008). This feature would require examination under deep anesthesia to determine whether there is an actual contracture (Fahn, 2006b). Knowing this information allows one to calculate the maximum amount of motor improvement that can be expected. Arrangements are made with an anesthesiologist to carry out the evaluation.

J. There is controversy about using placebos in the diagnosis or treatment of patients with psychogenic movement disorders (Jankovic et al., 2006a). Although their use can be an easy approach to make the correct diagnosis, their use also often angers patients, stating that they have been "tricked." If used to help make the diagnosis, disclosure is necessary afterwards, explaining the rationale and that the physician wants to be certain with the diagnosis so that proper treatment can be initiated. Patients will not have further trust in the treating physician if the patients discover placebos on their own. Placebos can also be used to exacerbate the abnormal movements as well as to relieve them (Levy and Jankovic, 1983). Using placebos to treat the symptoms can lead to mistrust also; this approach is no substitute for important psychotherapy to get to the root cause and cure of the problem. If placebos were used to treat the condition, and the patient improves, it can be difficult to then explain to the patient what was done. Patients can have a serious clinical reversal when they learn what has happened. If placebos were used to treat the symptoms, it would, therefore, be important to inform the patient as soon as possible keep the patient's confidence that you were working with the patient to help them to a speedy recovery. For many reasons, then, it is better to avoid the use of placebos and strive to obtain successful results without them (Ford et al., 1995). Nonetheless, if really in doubt about the diagnosis, judicious use of a placebo can aid in making the correct diagnosis (Tan, 2004) and thereby lead to proper treatment.

K. If the patient is admitted to hospital before receiving the diagnosis of a psychogenic movement disorder, the patient should not be allowed to leave the hospital without being informed of the diagnosis. The diagnosis should be discussed with the patient in the presence of the psychiatric consultant, if necessary. It is usually incorrect to anticipate that the referring physician is in a better position to discuss the diagnosis and manage treatment. When outpatient treatment is the only available choice, the patient needs to be informed of the diagnosis before being referred to the psychiatrist. As mentioned above, psychiatrists cannot make the diagnosis of a psychogenic movement disorder; their role is to establish the psychodynamics and provide psychiatric treatment.

L. It is important to be consistently positive and absolute with the patient once the diagnosis is certain. If any uncertainty is conveyed, the patient will continue to doubt the diagnosis and fail to respond to therapy.

Positive reinforcement should be given to assure the patient that the symptoms will progressively improve with time as the muscles "are being retrained to move more appropriately." However, if there is uncertainty about the diagnosis, another opinion should be sought.

M. As was mentioned previously, treatment should be initiated in the hospital if at all possible. But if hospitalization is not feasible, treatment may be given in the outpatient setting. Any combination of psychotherapy, positive reinforcement, physiotherapy, relaxation techniques, and *desensitization therapy* may be used. Desensitization therapy is a mechanism of treatment for patients who are stimulus-sensitive, such as having excessive startle, shakes, or myoclonus after exposure to a sensory stimulus. Introducing the stimulus in a mild, subclinical form that fails to induce the abnormal response is the starting point. Then the intensity of the stimulus should be increased over time until the patient is desensitized. Patients who are depressed will usually benefit from psychotherapy or antidepressant medication. For long-term care, often the patient has a need to belong to a group and will join the local chapter of the lay organization that deals with this disorder.

N. Factitious disorders and malingering are usually not benefited. Symptoms will disappear only when the patient is ready to give them up.

O. Somatoform disorders can usually be treated. In some patients, the symptom may return despite the patient being aware that it is due to an emotional problem.

Results of treatment

Psychotherapy is the major treatment approach that is best suited for permanent benefit. Somatoform disorders have the best results from treatment. Factitious disorders and malingering yield poor results, and the patient improves only when he or she is ready to relinquish the symptoms. Williams and colleagues (1995) utilized psychotherapy in all patients, along with the following supplemental approaches: family sessions, 58%; hypnosis, 42%; physical therapy, 42%; and placebo therapy, 13% (Table 25.12).

Table 25.12 Treatment of psychogenic movement disorders

Accepted diagnosis and treatment	70%
Refused diagnosis and treatment	30%
Psychiatrically treated patients	
Family sessions	58%
Hypnosis	88%
Physiotherapy	42%
Placebo	13%
Antidepressants	71%
ECT	8%

Data from Williams DT, Ford B, Fahn S. Phenomenology and psychopathology related to psychogenic movement disorders. Adv Neurol 1995;65:231–257.

Table 25.13 Results of treatment of psychogenic movement disorders

Permanent, complete relief	25%
Permanent, considerable relief	21%
Permanent, moderate relief	8%
Relapse	4%
Partial relapse	17%
No improvement	12%
Previously employed	
Now working full-time	25%
Now working part-time	10%
Functioning at home	15%
Now disabled	30%

Data from Williams DT, Ford B, Fahn S. Phenomenology and psychopathology related to psychogenic movement disorders. Adv Neurol 1995;65:231–257.

Table 25.14 Movement disorders that are symptoms of psychiatric conditions and not classified as psychogenic movement disorders

Psychiatric condition	Psychiatric movement disorder
Schizophrenia, depression	Catatonia
Depression	Psychomotor slowness
Obsessive-compulsive disorder	Obsessional slowness, stereotypies
Agoraphobia, anxiety	Fear of falling
Schizophrenia, autism	Stereotypies

Psychotropic medication (antidepressants) was utilized in 71%. Two patients with treatment-resistant major depression received ECT; one responded completely, and the other responded only partially. One-quarter of the patients required more extensive psychiatric hospitalization because of suicidal ideation or because there was a poor response in reversing the psychodynamic pathology while on the neurology service.

Treatment by Williams and colleagues (1995) resulted in a permanent, meaningful benefit in 52% of patients, with complete relief, considerable relief, and moderate relief in 25%, 21%, and 8% of patients, respectively (Table 25.13). Some relapse occurred in 21% of patients, and no improvement was seen in 12%. Of those who had been previously employed, 25% were able to resume full-time work, and 10% were able to work part-time, with 15% functioning at home (see Table 25.13).

In the series of 28 cases of psychogenic movement disorders reported by Factor and colleagues (1995), 35% resolved, and this subgroup had a shorter duration of disease than those who did not resolve. Of 56 patients with any type of psychogenic neurologic disorder other than pseudoseizures, Couprie and colleagues (1995) found that the long-term outcome was good in 96% of those who improved during a hospital stay and in only 30% of others, and that rapid improvement was related to recent onset of symptoms. In a longitudinal study of 228 patients evaluated in the Baylor College of Medicine Movement Disorders Clinic, after a mean duration of follow up of 3.4 ± 2.8 years, improvement of symptoms was noted in 56.6% patients, 22.1% were worse, and 21.3% remained the same at the time of follow-up. Positive social life perceptions, strong suggestion by the physician of effective treatment, elimination of stressors, and treatment with antidepressant medications contributed to a favorable outcome. Using a "blinded" review of videos, psychiatric rating scales, and psychogenic movement disorder scale, Hinson and colleagues (2006) demonstrated the efficacy of psychotherapy and medications in the treatment of patients with psychogenic movement disorders.

We can compare treatment of psychogenic movement disorders with that of psychogenic nonepileptiform seizures. In a double-blind study, cognitive-behavioral therapy was more effective than standard medical care in reducing seizure frequency in these patients (Goldstein et al., 2010). This contrasts with limited or no special treatment. About one-third became seizure free, one-sixth worsened, and the others were unchanged (McKenzie et al., 2010).

Movement disorders caused by psychiatric conditions but not regarded as psychogenic

A number of movement disorders are due to diseases that are classified as mental or psychiatric disturbances, in which the abnormal hypokinesia or hyperkinesia is not listed as a psychogenic movement disorder. Table 25.14 lists these, as well as the common underlying causes.

Table 25.14 shows that, basically, none of the aforementioned psychiatric conditions is either a somatoform disorder, a factitious disorder, or a malingering state. Thus, we can distinguish the psychogenic movement disorders from the conditions listed in Table 25.14 on the basis of the underlying psychiatric state. It should be noted that even if a somatoform disorder, a factitious disorder, or a malingering state is only suspected and not officially diagnosed, the diagnosis of a psychogenic movement disorder can still be made. Also, even if a psychiatric consultant cannot detect one of these disorders, a neurologist may still make the diagnosis on the grounds listed in Tables 25.2 and 25.3.

References available on Expert Consult: www.expertconsult.com

Index

Page numbers followed by "f" indicate figures, "t" indicate tables.

A

A8 neurons, 82
AAV-GAD gene therapy, 181–182
Abdominal dyskinesias, 25, 502
Abetalipoproteinemia, 472
Abnormal involuntary movements (AIMs), 1
  see also Dyskinesias
Abulia, 20, 54, 78, 189–190
Acamprosate, 297
Acanthocytosis see Neuroacanthocytosis
Aceruloplasminemia, 275t–276t, 276, 276f
Acetylcholine (ACh), 58–59
  interneurons and, 61
  in Parkinson disease, 98, 98t
  see also Cholinergic system
Acetylcholinesterase inhibitors see
    Cholinesterase inhibitors
Acquired parkinsonism see Parkinsonism,
    secondary
ACR16 (pridopidine), 331–332
Acrobatic gait, 248
  see also Gait, psychogenic
Action dystonia, 27, 263
Action myoclonus, 29
Action myoclonus–renal failure syndrome
    (AMRF), 460
Action tremors, 389, 390t, 394–412
Adaptation learning, 52
Adenosine, 60
  in progressive supranuclear palsy, 206
Adenosine A[2A], 121, 125
Adiadochokinesia see Dysdiadochokinesia
α-Adrenergic agonists
  in acute akathisia, 428
  in ADHD, 376–377
β-Adrenergic blockers
  in acute akathisia, 428
  in essential tremor, 405
Afferent pathways, 36–37, 37f
Aging, essential tremor and, 403–404
Akathisia, 25, 185, 387, 416, 426–428
  tardive, 25, 416, 426, 440, 445–446
Akinesia, 18–21
  acute, 85
  pathophysiology of, 39–41
  in progressive supranuclear palsy, 199
  pure, 22, 199
  see also Freezing phenomenon
Akinetic mutism, 54
Alcohol
  causing ataxia, 466
  in essential tremor, 404–405, 410–411
  in myoclonus, 463–464
Alien hand phenomenon, 54, 218–219

Alien limb phenomenon, 21, 218–219
Alper syndrome, 239–240
Alpha motoneurons, 36–38, 37f
Alternating hemiplegia of childhood, 490
Alternative therapies, 298
Alzheimer disease (AD)
  corticobasal degeneration and, 220
  dementia with Lewy bodies and, 223–224
  neurodiagnostic studies, 230
  neuropathology of, 230–231
  Parkinson disease and, 192–193, 222–223
  progressive supranuclear palsy and,
      204–206, 228
Amantadine
  antiglutamatergic actions, 125
  in cerebellar ataxia, 474
  dopaminergic actions, 124, 137
  in Huntington disease, 333
  in levodopa-associated dyskinesias, 153
Amisulpride, 423
Amputated limbs, 28, 502
Amyloid-β (Aβ) precursor protein (APP),
    223
Amyotrophic lateral sclerosis (ALS), 232–233
Anarthria
  in anterior opercular syndrome, 239
  syndrome of slowly progressive, 220
Anesthesia
  hysterical, 515
  peripheral deafferentiation with, 297, 407
Animal models
  of acute dystonia, 426
  of classic tardive dyskinesia, 435–437
  of dystonias, 280, 292
  of Huntington disease, 320–322, 324,
      326–328
  of multiple system atrophy, 216
  of Parkinson disease, 81, 118
  of progressive supranuclear palsy, 206–207
  of Rett syndrome, 386
  of tau pathology, 229
  of tremors, 408–409
Animals, stereotypies in, 364, 366, 380–381
Anoxia, post-hypoxic myoclonus, 460–461,
    461t
Anterior cervical rhizotomy, 308–309
Anterior horn cells, 36
Anterior opercular syndrome, 239
Anti-amphiphysin antibodies, 254
Antibodies
  in autoimmune ataxia, 467
  botulinum toxin and, 300–301, 301t
  in celiac disease, 466
  chorea and, 344–345
  neuromyotonia and, 256
  in paraneoplastic ataxia, 466–467
  stiff-person syndrome and, 254
  Tourette syndrome and, 363–364

Anticholinergics see Antimuscarinics/
    anticholinergics
Anticonvulsants
  in dystonia, 295, 297
  in essential tremor, 405–406
  in kinetic tremor, 407–408
  in myoclonus, 462–463
  in paroxysmal dyskinesias, 485–486, 488
  in rest tremors, 393
  in restless legs syndrome, 498–499
  in Tourette syndrome, 373–374, 374f
Antidepressants
  in ADHD, 376
  in Parkinson disease, 122, 126, 153, 190
  in rest tremors, 393
Antidopaminergic drugs see Dopamine
    receptor-blocking agents
Antiglutamatergics
  in Huntington disease, 327–328, 333
  in Parkinson disease, 121, 125, 131, 153
Antihistaminics
  in dystonia, 296
  in Parkinson disease, 121, 125
Antihypertensives, 109–110
Antimuscarinics/anticholinergics
  in acute akathisia, 428
  in drug-induced parkinsonism, 429
  in dystonia, 295–296, 426, 444–445
  in Parkinson disease, 121, 125, 134,
      137–138
  progressive supranuclear palsy and, 207
  in rest tremors, 393
  in tardive akathisia, 446
Antioxidant vitamins
  ataxia with isolated vitamin E deficiency,
      472
  in classic tardive dyskinesia, 443
  in Parkinson disease, 121, 125, 127–131,
      128t
Antiphospholipid syndrome, 344–345
Antipsychotics
  in dystonia, 295–296
  in Huntington disease, 329
  in Parkinson disease, 126, 153, 195
  in parkinsonism-dementia syndromes,
      232
  in rest tremors, 393
  side effects, 423–424
    acute akathisia, 427
    acute dystonia, 285, 425–426
    neuroleptic malignant syndrome, 24,
        429–430
    parkinsonism, 236, 415, 428–429
    tardive see Antipsychotics, tardive
        syndromes and
    withdrawal dyskinesia, 435
  tardive syndromes and, 415–416, 418–424,
      430–440

classic tardive dyskinesia, 387, 430–439, 441–443
tardive akathisia, 416, 426, 440, 445–446
tardive dystonia, 285, 416, 425, 439–440, 443–445, 490
tardive tremor, 392–393
terminology, 417
treatment, 440–446
in tics, 371–373
Anxiety
Parkinson disease and, 75–77, 190–191
drugs for, 122, 126, 191
Apathy
in Parkinson disease, 75–78, 189–190
drugs for, 122, 126
in progressive supranuclear palsy, 201–202
Aphasia, in corticobasal degeneration, 219–220
Apnea, in Parkinson disease, 187
ApoE ε4 allele, 224
Apomorphine
in dystonia, 295
in Huntington disease, 331–332
in Parkinson disease, 124
levodopa complications and, 148, 151
as test for Parkinson disease, 85
Apoptosis
in Huntington disease, 323–326
in Parkinson disease, 99–100, 99f, 108f, 133
in Tourette syndrome, 362
Applause sign, 201–202
Apraxia, 21
in corticobasal degeneration, 218–219
equilibrium, 248
of eyelid opening, 19, 23, 288
ignition, 248
mixed gait, 248
types of, 21, 54t
Argyrophilic grain disease (AGD), 205–206
Aripiprazole, 372, 423
Arm
freezing phenomenon of, 23
manifestation of bradykinesia in, 19
myoclonus in, 501
painful, 28, 502–503
Ascorbate, 125, 131
Asperger syndrome, 368–369, 383–384
Astasia–abasia, 248
see also Gait, psychogenic
Asterixis, 28–29
Asthenia, 45–46
Astrocytic plaques, 221
Asymmetry of symptoms
in corticobasal degeneration, 218
in Parkinson disease, 67
see also Hemiballism; Hemidystonia; Hemifacial spasm; Hemiparkinsonism–hemiatrophy syndrome
Asynergia, 47–48
see also Ataxia
Ataxia, 26, 465–475
abetalipoproteinemia, 472
autoimmune, 467
autosomal dominant cerebellar, 468, 470t
see also Ataxia, spinocerebellar

autosomal dominant episodic see Ataxia, episodic
autosomal recessive, 6t–17t, 50, 343, 467–473, 471t
Cayman, 473
celiac disease and, 460, 466
degenerative, 217–218, 465
demyelinating, 467
diagnostic plan, 474, 474t
early-onset with ocular motor apraxia and hypoalbuminemia, 472–473
episodic, 30, 468–469, 471t, 481–482, 483t–484t, 491–493, 493t
familial cerebellar with muscle coenzyme Q10 deficiency, 473
Fragile X-associated tremor/ataxia syndrome, 412–413, 473–474
Friedreich, 50, 467–468, 470–472
gait, 26, 51–52, 246, 411, 466
genetic, 5t–18t, 210, 467–474
infectious, 467
with isolated vitamin E deficiency, 472
Marinesco Sjögren syndrome, 473
mitochondrial recessive ataxia syndrome, 473
multijoint movements, 47–48, 50–51
of non-cerebellar origin, 467
paraneoplastic, 466–467
pathophysiology of, 44–53
prevalence of, 5t
progressive myoclonic, 29, 458, 458f, 459t, 460
spinocerebellar, 6t–17t, 210, 337–338, 467–468, 469t–470t
spinocerebellar with axonal neuropathy, 473
sporadic, 465–467
stroke causing, 465–466
therapy for, 474–475
toxins causing, 466
tumors causing, 466, 466t
Ataxia with isolated vitamin E deficiency (AVED), 472
Ataxia telangiectasia (AT), 343, 472
Athetosis, 6t–17t, 26, 178–179, 347–348
ATN1 (DRPLA) gene, 336
Atomoxetine, 376–377
ATP1A3 gene, 284
Attention deficit disorder (ADD), 358
Attention deficit hyperactivity disorder (ADHD)
dopamine reward pathway, 363
management of, 375–377
stereotypies and, 382
Tourette syndrome and, 354–358, 356f, 357t
pathogenesis of, 360, 364–365
Atypical antipsychotics, 420–424
in dystonia, 295–296
in Huntington disease, 329
in Parkinson disease, 126, 195
levodopa-associated dyskinesias in, 153
in parkinsonism-dementia syndromes, 232
in rest tremors, 393
side effects, 423–425
acute akathisia, 427
acute dystonia, 285, 425

neuroleptic malignant syndrome, 429–430
parkinsonism, 428–429
tardive syndromes and, 387, 416, 418–424, 434, 442–444
in tics, 371–373
Autistic spectrum disorders, 368–369, 380, 383–386
Autoimmune ataxia, 467
Autoimmune choreas, 336t, 343–346
Autoimmunity
parkinsonism and, 239
Tourette syndrome and, 363–365
Automatic movements, 1–2, 351
Autonomic dysfunction
in multiple system atrophy, 74, 209, 211–212, 216–217
in Parkinson disease, 74–75, 113–114, 185–187
drugs for, 122t, 126
treatment-related, 141–143, 141t, 186–187
Autophagy, Parkinson disease and, 100, 108, 108f, 115, 116f
Autosomal recessive cerebellar ataxia type 1 (ARCA1), 473
Autosomal recessive cerebellar ataxia type 2 (ARCA2), 473
Autosomal recessive spastic ataxia of Charlevoix–Saguenay (ARSACS), 473

B

Baclofen
in dystonia, 296–297
in Huntington disease, 333
in tics, 373
Balance, 241–242
assessment, 20, 85–87, 241–242
in ataxia, 50–51
in Parkinson disease, 20, 71–72, 156, 174
in progressive supranuclear palsy, 199
sway, 50–51, 241–242, 242f
Ballism, 26, 346–347
Barany pointing test, 47
Basal ganglia
calcification of, 239, 487
functional neuroanatomy of, 55–65, 157–159
circuitry of, 38, 38f–39f, 62–64, 158f, 159
components of, 60–62
neurotransmitters, 55–60
oscillatory activity, 159
physiology of, 64–65
see also Basal ganglia, in physiology of movement
in movement disorders, 2, 38, 44
athetoid cerebral palsy, 26
ballism, 26
bradykinesia in PD, 82
dystonia, 158f, 159, 290, 292, 504
hypothetical models, 158f
Parkinson disease, 92, 94–99, 158f
psychogenic, 515
restless legs syndrome, 498
stereotypies, 380–381

Tourette syndrome, 158f, 359, 360f, 361–364, 366
tremor-at-rest, 41–42, 82
Wilson disease, 509–510, 510f
in physiology of movement, 38, 38f–39f, 65
center-surround mechanism, 38, 39f
loop anatomy, 38, 38f
see also Globus pallidus; Pedunculopontine nucleus; Striatum; Substantia nigra; Subthalamic nucleus
Basal ganglia calcification
familial, 239
paroxysmal dyskinesias and, 487
Base of support (BOS), 241
Batten disease (neuronal ceroid lipofuscinoses), 6t–17t, 459t, 460
Behavioral therapy, 370–371
see also Cognitive-behavioral therapy
Belly dancer's dyskinesia, 25, 502
see also Abdominal dyskinesias
Benserazide, 121–123
Benserazide/levodopa, 122–123, 139
Bent spine, 70–71
Benzodiazepines
in classic tardive dyskinesia, 442–443
in dystonia, 296
in essential tremor, 405–406
in myoclonus, 462–463
in Parkinson disease, 125–126, 193
in paroxysmal nonkinesigenic dyskinesia, 488
in restless legs syndrome, 498–499
in stiff-person syndrome, 254
in tardive dystonia, 445
in tics, 373
Bereitschaftspotential (readiness potential), 1–2, 515, 524
Beta-blockers
in acute akathisia, 428
in essential tremor, 405
Biballism, 26
Bilateral striopallidodentate calcinosis, 239
Bilirubin encephalopathy, 347
Binswanger disease, 237–238
Bipolar disorder, 179
Bladder function
in multiple system atrophy, 208, 217
in Parkinson disease, 75, 126, 185–186
in progressive supranuclear palsy, 204
Blepharospasm, 27, 272t, 273
botulinum toxin for, 302–303
diffusion tensor imaging in, 292
hemifacial spasm contrasted with, 27–28, 273
medical treatment of, 298t, 302–303
pathoanatomy of, 289
pathophysiology of, 43, 288
peripheral trauma and, 504
prevalence of, 5t
in progressive supranuclear palsy, 200–201
surgical treatment of, 309
Blink reflex see Eye blink reflex
Blocking (holding) tics, 21, 351–352
Bobble-head doll syndrome, 414
Botulinum toxin (BTX), 298–306
in blepharospasm, 302–303
in cervical dystonia, 301, 301t, 303–305

in classic tardive dyskinesia, 443
in essential tremor, 406–407
indications for, 305–306, 306t
in limb dystonias, 305
in rest tremors, 393
in spasticity, 252
in tics, 374–375
Bouncing gait, 247
Bovine spongiform encephalopathy (BSE), 234–235
Boxer's parkinsonism, 238
Braak staging system, 92, 110–114, 183–184, 192–193
Braces, in dystonia, 294
Brachial plexus lesions, focal myoclonus due to, 501
Bradykinesia, 18–21, 78
deep brain stimulation surgery in, 168–169
in Huntington disease, 312–313
Parkinson disease and, 82–83, 98–99, 162
pathophysiology of, 39–41, 69, 82
psychogenic, 513
rigidity and, 24
Bradyphrenia
in obsessive-compulsive disorder, 357–358
in Parkinson disease, 20, 40, 191–192
Brain grafting
in Huntington disease, 333–334
in Parkinson disease, 179–182
Lewy body pathology, 116–117
Brain-derived neurotrophic factor (BDNF), 150, 323–324
Brainstem
basal ganglia circuitry, 63
dystonia and, 289–290
freezing phenomenon and, 72–73
myoclonus arising in, 448–451, 454–456, 455t, 457f
Parkinson disease and, 110–114
startle syndromes and, 456
tremor generation in, 409
see also Locus coeruleus; Raphe nuclei; Substantia nigra
Breast cancer
myoclonus and, 461–462
stiff-person syndrome and, 254
Briquet syndrome see Somatization disorder
Bromocriptine, 121t, 124, 135–137
Burning sensation in Parkinson disease, 184

C

Cabergoline, 121t, 124, 135, 151
Caffeine consumption, Parkinson disease and, 107
CAG repeats
in episodic ataxias, 491–492
in Huntington disease, 312, 316, 319–322, 319f, 328–329
in Huntington disease-like disorders, 336–339
Calcium influx
in Huntington disease, 325
in Parkinson disease, 108–110, 134
Calcium spike bursts, in tremor generation, 409

Calcium-channel blockers
in essential tremor, 405–406
Huntington disease and, 317
mechanisms of action, 418–419
Parkinson disease and, 109–110, 134
in postural tremors, 405–406
Camptocormia, 70–71, 246
Cancer
ataxia and, 466–467
chorea and, 345
myoclonus and, 461–462
Parkinson disease and, 75, 123
stiff-person syndrome and, 254
Cannabinoids, in tics, 373–374
Carbamazepine
in dystonia, 295
in kinetic tremor, 407–408
Carbidopa, 121–123
Carbidopa/levodopa (Sinemet), 122–123, 139–140
in levodopa-associated dyskinesias, 153–154
in levodopa-associated motor fluctuations, 150–152, 154
in levodopa-associated yo-yo-ing, 154
Carbidopa/levodopa/entacapone (LCE), 123–124, 140
Carbon monoxide parkinsonism, 236
Cardiac MIBG uptake, 91–92, 113, 186
Cardiac surgery, post-pump chorea, 345
Cardiac valvulopathy, 135
Caspase inhibitors, 326–327, 329
Caspases, 323–324, 326
Cataplexy, 21–22
Catatonia, 22, 386
malignant see Neuroleptic malignant syndrome
Catechol-O-methyltransferase (COMT), 56–58, 59f
Catechol-O-methyltransferase (COMT) inhibitors, 121, 123–124, 140, 150
Caudate, 55, 57f, 60–61, 64, 82, 98t, 157–159
dystonia and, 289–291
Huntington disease and, 315–317
Tourette syndrome and, 361, 363, 366
Causalgia-dystonia syndrome, 286, 504–505, 505t, 519
Cautious gait, 23, 248
Cayman ataxia, 473
Celiac disease, 460, 466
Center of mass (COM), 241
Center of pressure (COP), 241, 242f
Center-surround mechanism, 38, 39f
Cerebellum, 2, 38, 44, 45f
ataxia and, 26, 44–53, 246, 465–475
dystonia and, 289–291
tremors and, 50, 52–53, 407, 410–412
Cerebral cortex
apraxia and, 21
basal ganglia circuitry and, 38, 38f–39f, 62–64
corticobasal degeneration and, 21, 218–222
deep brain stimulation surgery and, 166–167
dystonia and, 42–43, 288–290
frontal gait disorders and, 23
frontotemporal dementias and, 225–227

in Huntington disease, 315–317, 324–326
myoclonus and, 29, 411–412, 448–450, 452–453, 453f–454f, 455t, 456, 458, 462
Parkinson disease and
Braak staging system, 110–113
dementia, 224
extradural stimulation, 179
paroxysmal dyskinesias and, 487
physiology of movement, 53, 53f
abnormal plasticity in dystonia, 43–44
in center-surround mechanism of motor control, 39f
control of alpha motoneurons by, 37–38
cortico-cerebellar-cortical loop, 44, 45f
corticobasal ganglia network, 38, 38f
loss of inhibition in dystonia, 42–43, 288
reaction time in Parkinson disease, 40
progressive supranuclear palsy and, 201–202
reflex myoclonus, 29, 411–412, 449–450, 452
in restless legs syndrome, 498
self-agency, 517–518
spasticity and, 250–251
in Tourette syndrome, 358–363, 366
tremor generation in, 411–412
Cerebral hemorrhages/infarcts, paroxysmal dyskinesias and, 487
Cerebral palsy, athetoid, 26, 178–179, 347–348
Cerebrospinal fluid (CSF)
in classic tardive dyskinesia, 437
in normal pressure hydrocephalus, 238–239
in progressive supranuclear palsy, 201–202
Ceruloplasmin
hereditary deficiency of, 512
hypoceruloplasminemia-related movement disorder, 512
in Wilson disease, 507, 509
Cervical dystonia (spasmodic torticollis), 27, 262–263, 272–273
diffusion tensor imaging in, 292
genetics of, 272, 272t
interstitial nucleus of Cajal and, 288
non-dystonic, 277
pain in, 264
pathoanatomy of, 289
platelet mitochondria in, 292
secondary causes, 285–286
sensory tricks, 264, 272–273
treatment of, 298t
botulinum toxin, 301, 301t, 303–305
physical therapy, 294–295
surgical, 308–309
tremor and, 265
CHAP syndrome, 345
Chaperone proteins, 324
Chaperone-mediated autophagy (CMA), 100, 108, 108f, 115, 116f
Cheese effect, 125, 130–131
Cherry-red spot myoclonus syndrome (sialidosis), 459t, 460
Chin tremor, hereditary, 414
Choice reaction time, 40, 69
in Huntington disease, 312

Cholinergic system, 58–59
interneurons and, 61
Parkinson disease and, 72, 98, 113
progressive supranuclear palsy and, 206
Cholinesterase inhibitors
in parkinsonism-dementia syndromes, 126, 193, 232
in tics, 373
Chorea, 26, 335
athetosis and, 6t–17t, 178–179, 347–348
autoimmune, 336t, 343–346
ballism and, 346
diagnostic evaluation of, 338f
differential diagnosis, 336t–337t
drug-induced, 152–153, 345
essential (senile), 343
familial dyskinesia and facial myokymia, 343
gait, 247
hereditary, 6t–18t, 336t–337t
ataxia telangiectasia, 343
benign (BHC), 342–343
Huntington disease, 26, 178–179, 311–313, 335
Huntington disease-like disorders, 335–339, 336t
infantile bilateral striatal necrosis, 343
neuroacanthocytosis, 27, 339–341
neurodegeneration with brain iron accumulation, 341
infectious, 336t, 343
mass hysteria and, 515
metabolic, 345
Morvan's fibrillary, 256
myclonus contrasted with, 26, 447
"negative" (motor impersistence), 26
neuroferritinopathy and, 345–346
paraneoplastic, 345
postinfectious, 336t, 344–345
in pregnancy, 344–345
prevalence of, 5t
Sydenham disease, 26, 343–344, 363–365
tics contrasted with, 26, 31, 344
treatment of, 346
vascular, 336t, 345–346
voluntariness of, 54
withdrawal emergent syndrome, 26, 416
Chorea–acanthocytosis see Chorea, hereditary, neuroacanthocytosis
Choreoathetosis, 6t–17t, 178–179, 347–348
Choreoathetosis/spasticity episodica (CSE), 494
Ciliary neurotrophic factor, 333–334
Cinnarizine, 419
Classic tardive dyskinesia see Tardive syndromes, classic tardive dyskinesia
Clinical rating scales see Rating scales
Clonidine
in acute akathisia, 428
in ADHD, 376
Clozapine, 416, 419–421
in dystonia, 295–296
in Huntington disease, 329
in Parkinson disease, 126, 153, 156, 195
in parkinsonism-dementia syndromes, 232
in rest tremors, 393

side effects, 421, 423–424
in tardive syndromes, 416, 442–444
in tics, 372
Coenzyme Q10 (CoQ10), 132, 207–208
familial cerebellar ataxia with deficiency of, 473
in Huntington disease, 327–328
Coffee consumption, 107
Cognitive function
in essential tremor, 399
in frontotemporal dementias, 225, 232
in Huntington disease, 313–314
in obsessive-compulsive disorder, 357–358
in Parkinson disease, 74–79, 191–192
after deep brain stimulation surgery, 174–175
after pallidotomy, 162–163
bradyphrenia, 20, 40, 78
driving and, 87, 124
drugs for, 122t, 126, 192
loss of postural reflexes and, 71–72
in progressive supranuclear palsy, 201–202
in Tourette syndrome, 356–358
in Wilson disease, 508
see also Dementia
Cognitive-behavioral therapy, 377
Cogwheel rigidity, 23–24, 70
Cold hands/feet sign, 211
Color vision, 81
Complementary therapies, 298
Complex regional pain syndrome (CRPS), 504–506, 519
Comprehensive Behavioral Intervention for Tic Disorders (CIBT), 370–371
Compulsive behaviors, 31
in Parkinson disease, 78–79, 193–194
in restless legs syndrome, 499
tics, 31, 352
see also Obsessive-compulsive disorder
Conceptual apraxia, 54t
Conduction apraxia, 54t
Constipation
in multiple system atrophy, 217
in Parkinson disease, 75, 113, 126–127, 187
"rancho recipe", 187
Continuous muscle fiber activity (neuromyotonia), 24, 255–258, 255t
Conversion disorder, 54, 514–515, 517–518, 521
Copper metabolism
in dystonia, 292
Wilson disease, 5t–17t, 32, 507–512
Coprolalia, 352–353, 355–356
Copropraxia, 32, 352, 355–356
Cortical reflex myoclonus, 29, 411–412, 449–450, 452
Corticobasal degeneration (CBD), 218–222, 225
clinical features of, 21, 218–220, 462
genetics of, 228
neurodiagnostic studies, 220–221
neuropathology of, 219, 221–222, 227
progressive supranuclear palsy and, 204–206, 221–222, 228
treatment of, 222

Corticobasal ganglionic degeneration (CBGD), 218
see also Corticobasal degeneration
Corticofugal syndrome, 250–252
Corticoreticulospinal tract, 37–38, 250–251
Corticospinal tract, spasticity and, 250–251
Cramps
  musician's see Musician's dystonia
  painful, 153–154, 184
  writer's see Hand dystonia
Creatine
  in Huntington disease, 326–327
  in Parkinson disease, 133
Creutzfeldt–Jakob disease (CJD), 234–236
Cryptogenic myoclonic epilepsy, 458t
CTG/CAG trinucleotide repeats, 337–338
Cyclic adenosine monophosphate (cAMP), 58, 60
Cytokines, in Huntington disease, 318
Cytosine-adenine-guanine (CAG) trinucleotide repeats see CAG repeats

D

Dancing (choreic) gait, 247
Dancing eyes (opsoclonus), 29, 461–462
Dancing eyes, dancing feet syndrome, 29, 461–462
DAT imaging, 89–92, 399–400
DCTN1 gene, 104, 105t–106t
Deafness, in essential tremor, 399
Decarboxylase inhibitors, 121–123
  see also Carbidopa
Deep brain stimulation (DBS) surgery
  advantages of, 164t
  assessing response to, 164–165
  complications of, 174–176, 189
  disadvantages of, 164t
  in dyskinesias, 177–179
  in dystonia, 177–178, 306–308
  in dystonia–choreoathetosis in CP, 178–179, 348
  emerging indications for, 178–179, 179t
  hardware for, 164
  in Huntington disease, 178–179, 333
  mechanisms of, 165–166, 166t
  MRI scans and, 166–167, 176
  in Parkinson disease, 164–176, 246–247, 393–394
    sleep and, 189
    subthalamotomy compared with, 163–164
    thalamotomy compared with, 160, 167–168
  in paroxysmal nonkinesigenic dyskinesia, 488
  patient selection for, 173, 173t
  programming the parameters for, 168
  safety of, 174–176
  targets for, 164, 164t
  in Tourette syndrome, 178, 378–379
  in tremors, 167–168, 170, 179, 393–394, 407–408
Delayed-onset dystonia, 275
Dementia
  Huntington disease and, 313–314
  myoclonus and, 462

parkinsonian disorders and, 20, 74–77, 191–193, 222–224
  clinical features, 222–224
  drugs for, 122, 126
  neurodiagnostic studies, 230
  parkinsonism–dementia–amyotrophic lateral sclerosis complex of Guam, 232–233
  tauopathies, 201–202, 219, 224–232
  see also Alzheimer disease
Dementia with Lewy bodies (DLB)
  Lewy body pathology, 230
  neurodiagnostic studies, 230
  Parkinson disease and, 192–193, 222–224
    Braak staging system, 113, 192–193
  treatment, 232
Dementia pugilistica, 238
Demyelinating ataxia, 467
Dentatorubral-pallidoluysian atrophy (DRPLA), 335–337, 337t, 460, 468
Deprenyl see Selegiline
Depression
  deep brain stimulation surgery and, 175, 179
  Huntington disease and, 313, 331
  Parkinson disease and, 20, 75–78, 190
    drugs for, 122, 126, 190
    mental health therapy, 121
  psychogenic movement disorders and, 518, 526–527
  psychomotor, 22
  SSRI safety, 377–378
  TBZ treatment and, 331
Desensitization therapy, 526
Dextroamphetamine, 375–376
Diabetes mellitus, 253–254
Diffuse Lewy body disease see Dementia with Lewy bodies
Diffusion tensor imaging
  in dystonia, 292
  in Tourette syndrome, 361
Diffusion weighted imaging (DWI)
  in Creutzfeldt–Jakob disease, 235
  in multiple system atrophy, 212–213
  in Parkinson disease, 89
Dihydroxyphenyl-acetaldehyde (DOPAL), 107
3,4 dihydroxyphenylacetic acid (DOPAC), 56–58
Dimercaprol, 512
Dissociation (verbal-motor) apraxia, 54t
DJ-1 gene, 102, 105t–106t, 116
Domperidone, 124–127, 151
  acute dystonic reactions to, 285
Dopamine agonist withdrawal syndrome (DAWS), 136
Dopamine agonists, 121t
  in classic tardive dyskinesia, 442
  complications of, 124, 135–136
    compulsive behaviors, 124, 193–194, 499
    dopamine agonist withdrawal syndrome, 136
    drugs for, 126
    dyskinesias, 136
    edema, 136
    orthostatic hypotension, 136
    psychosis, 195
    punding, 194

respiratory distress, 187
  in restless legs syndrome, 499
  St Anthony's fire, 184
  sleep attacks, 124, 135–136, 189
  valvulopathy, 135
  in dystonia, 295
  in Huntington disease, 331–332
  in levodopa-induced complications
    dyskinesias, 153–154
    motor fluctuations, 151, 154
    yo-yo-ing, 154
  in Parkinson disease, 124
    complications of see Dopamine agonists, complications of
    in the early stage, 133–134
    with levodopa, 124, 133–134, 151
    levodopa compared, 124, 133–135, 139, 148
    in the mild stage, 134–137
    therapeutic principles, 120
  in progressive supranuclear palsy, 207
  in restless legs syndrome, 498–499
  in tics, 373
Dopamine (DA) and dopaminergic system, 55–58
  in Alzheimer disease, 230
  basal ganglia circuitry, 62–63, 63f
  in corticobasal degeneration, 222
  in dystonia, 282, 283f, 291, 295
  in Huntington disease, 317–318, 331–332
  metabolism of, 56–58, 59f, 107, 107f
  in multiple system atrophy, 215
  in Parkinson disease, 41, 66, 95–99, 98t
    animal models, 118
    autopsy findings, 92
    biomarkers, 90–91
    bradykinesia, 69, 98–99
    brain grafting, 116–117, 179–182
    circadian factors, 79–80
    etiology/pathogenesis, 99–100, 104–110
    exercise and, 120
    fetal dopaminergic neurons, 116–117, 180–181
    freezing phenomenon, 72–73
    hedonistic homeostatic dysregulation and, 79
    infantile dystonia-parkinsonism disorder, 104
    levodopa complications, 144–145, 147–150
    multiple hit hypothesis, 117, 117f
    neuroimaging, 89–92
    obsessive-compulsive disorder and, 78–79
    premorbid parkinsonian personality and, 78
  in parkinsonism–dementia–amyotrophic lateral sclerosis complex of Guam, 233
  in progressive supranuclear palsy, 206
  projection systems, 55, 58f, 60–62
  in restless legs syndrome, 498
  in stereotypies, 381
  tardive syndromes and, 419–421, 435–438
    see also Dopamine receptor-blocking agents (DRBAs), tardive syndromes
  in Tourette syndrome, 361–363, 366
Dopamine precursor agents see Levodopa

Dopamine receptor-blocking agents (DRBAs), 121, 124–127, 151, 415, 418–420
  adverse effects, 417t, 424–430
    acute dystonia, 285, 425–426
    akathisia, 25, 416, 426–428
    neuroleptic malignant syndrome, 24, 429–430
    oculogyric crises, 27, 425
    parkinsonism, 236, 415, 428–429
    tardive syndromes see Dopamine receptor-blocking agents (DRBAs), tardive syndromes
  in ballism, 347
  in chorea, 346
  in dystonia, 295–296
  in Huntington disease, 329–331
  in Parkinson disease, 126, 195
    levodopa-associated dyskinesias in, 153
  in parkinsonism-dementia syndromes, 232
  in rest tremors, 393
  tardive syndromes, 415, 417t, 418–420, 430–440
    atypical antipsychotics, 420–424
    classic tardive dyskinesia, 387, 415–416, 430–439, 441–443
    tardive akathisia, 416, 426, 440, 445–446
    tardive dystonia, 285, 416, 425, 439–440, 443–445, 490
    terminology, 416–418
    treatment of, 440–446
    withdrawal dyskinesia, 435
  in tics, 371–374
  to treat tardive dystonia, 443–444
Dopamine releasers, 121, 124, 137
Dopamine transporter (DAT) imaging, 89–92, 399–400
Dopaminergic agents, 121t
  catechol-O-methyltransferase inhibitors see Entacapone; Tolcapone
  decarboxylase inhibitors see Benserazide; Carbidopa
  dopamine agonists see Dopamine agonists
  dopamine precursor see Levodopa
  dopamine receptor blockers see Dopamine receptor-blocking agents
  dopamine releasers see Amantadine
  dopamine synthesizers see Zonisamide
  long-term effects, 122, 122t
  monoamine oxidase inhibitors see Monoamine oxidase (MAO) inhibitors
Dopa-responsive dystonia (DRD; DYT5), 261, 264, 270, 280–283, 295
DRD3 gene, 402–403
Driving, Parkinson disease and, 87, 124, 189
Drooling, in Parkinson disease, 75, 126–127, 187
Drop attacks, 21–22
Droxidopa, 217
DRPLA (ATN1) gene, 336
Drug-induced disorders
  akathisia, 25, 416, 426–428, 440, 445–446
  chorea, 152–153, 345
    see also Dyskinesias, (hyperkinesias, abnormal involuntary movements), levodopa-induced

parkinsonism, 27, 155–156, 236, 415, 428–429
  stereotypies (punding), 387
  tremors, 414
  see also Tardive syndromes
DuoDopa levodopa infusion, 154–155
Dysarthria
  after deep brain stimulation, 175
  cerebellar, 51
  Parkinson disease-related, 73
Dysautonomia see Autonomic dysfunction
Dysdiadochokinesia, 26, 48–49, 52–53
Dyskinesias (hyperkinesias, abnormal involuntary movements), 1
  abdominal, 25, 502
  ataxia see Ataxia
  athetosis, 26, 347–348
  ballism, 26, 346–347
  chorea see Chorea
  differential diagnosis of, 25–34, 33t–35t
  dopamine agonists causing, 136
  dystonia see Dystonia
  evaluation of, 24–25, 32–34
  genetics of, 6t–18t
  historical perspective on, 3t–4t
  Huntington disease see Huntington disease
  levodopa-induced, 139, 141–142, 141t
    chorea, 152–153, 345
    clinicopathologic correlation of, 143
    deep brain stimulation surgery in, 168–171
    diphasic, 142, 153
    end-of-day, 142
    fluctuations and (yo-yo-ing), 154–155
    in multiple system atrophy, 217–218
    myoclonus, 142, 155
    "off" dystonia, 142, 153–154, 184
    "off" painful cramps, 153–154, 184
    pallidotomy for, 161–163
    pathogenesis of, 149–150
    peak-dose, 142–143, 149–150, 152–153
    risk factors for, 143, 149–150
    simultaneous dyskinesia and parkinsonism, 142, 155
    somatotopically-specific, 155
    treatment, 152–155, 161–162, 168–171
  list of, 2t
  myoclonus see Myoclonus
  paroxysmal see Paroxysmal dyskinesias
  pathology of, 42–53
  peripheral see Peripheral movement disorders
  prevalence of, 5t
  restless legs syndrome see Restless legs syndrome
  stereotypies see Stereotypies
  tardive see Tardive syndromes
  Tourette syndrome see Tourette syndrome
  tremors see Tremors
  use of term, 1
Dysmetria, 26, 46–48, 50, 52–53
  see also Ataxia
Dysphagia
  in Parkinson disease, 75, 187
  in progressive supranuclear palsy, 200
Dysphonia, 272t
  spasmodic (laryngeal dystonia), 298t, 303
Dyspnea, in Parkinson disease, 187

Dysrhythmia, 48–49
Dyssynergia, 47–48
  see also Ataxia
Dystonia, 26–27, 259–292
  action, 27, 263
  acute, 285, 425–426
  age at onset, 266
  in alternating hemiplegia of childhood, 490
  athetosis and, 178–179, 347
  basal ganglia models in, 158f, 159
  causalgia-dystonia syndrome, 286, 504–505, 505t, 519
  cervical see Cervical dystonia
  chorea contrasted with, 26
  classification of, 260t, 266–277, 267t
  complex regional pain syndrome and, 504–506, 519
  in conditions unlabelled as DYT, 262t
  delayed onset, 273
  distribution of, 265–268, 267t
  dopa-responsive, 261, 264, 270, 280–283, 295
  dystonic storm, 265, 298
  early-onset dystonia–parkinsonism, 261, 272
  epidemiology of, 5t, 265–266, 267t
  essential tremor and, 396–397, 400
  etiologic classification of, 268–277
    dystonia in other neurologic diseases, 268, 276–277, 277t
    dystonia-plus syndromes, 268, 269t–271t, 273–274
    heredodegenerative diseases, 268, 269t–271t, 274–276
    primary dystonias, 268–273, 269t–271t
    secondary dystonias, 268, 269t–271t, 274–275
  focal, 27, 42, 262–263, 266–268, 268t, 272–273, 272t
    medical treatment of, 297, 298t, 301–305, 301t
    physical therapy for, 294–295
    surgical treatment of, 308–309
    see also Blepharospasm; Cervical dystonia; Hand dystonia; Oromandibular dystonia
  gait, 247
  generalized, 27, 262–263, 266, 298t
  genetics of, 6t–17t, 260–262, 269, 269t–271t, 278
    see also specific dystonias
  geste antagoniste for, 27, 264, 272–273
  hemidystonia, 27, 265–266
  historical background, 259–260
  hypnogenic paroxysmal, 28
  laryngeal (spasmodic dysphonia), 298t, 303
  levodopa-associated, 141, 152–154
  Lubag, 233, 261, 271, 286–287
  medical treatment of, 294t
    acamprosate, 297
    alternative therapies, 298
    anesthetics, 297
    anticholinergic, 296, 426
    anticonvulsants, 295, 297
    antidopaminergic, 295–296
    baclofen, 296–297

benzodiazepines, 296–297
botulinum toxin, 298–306
complementary therapies, 298
dopaminergic, 295
gamma-hydroxybutyrate, 297
intrathecal baclofen, 296–297
morphine sulfate, 297
muscle-necrotizing drugs, 297
novel therapies, 309
phenol injections, 297
therapeutic guidelines, 309–310
multifocal, 27, 266
in multiple system atrophy, 210–211
myoclonus–dystonia syndrome, 261–262,
269t–271t, 284–285, 297, 464
"off", 141, 153–154, 184
Oppenheim, 261, 269t–271t, 277–280,
284, 291
oromandibular, 273, 298t, 303, 439
orthostatic hemidystonia, 265
pain in, 264
paradoxical, 27, 264
with parkinsonism see
Dystonia–parkinsonisms
peripheral injury causing, 503–505, 519
phenomenology of, 262–265
physical therapy for, 294–295
postural changes in, 26–27, 263–264
primary
biochemistry of, 291–292
etiologic classification of, 268–273,
269t–271t
genetics of, 261, 269–272, 269t–271t
neuroimaging of, 291–292
pathoanatomy of, 289–291
pathophysiology of, 42–44, 287–289
prevalence, 265–266
progression of, 263–264, 263t
see also Dystonia, Oppenheim
in progressive supranuclear palsy, 200–201
pseudodystonia, 277, 277t
psychogenic, 264, 274, 286, 286t, 515–516,
519, 521–523
psychopathology in, 265, 284
rapid-onset dystonia–parkinsonism, 261,
283–284
secondary, 285–286
etiologic classification of, 268, 269t–
271t, 274–275
see also Dystonia, psychogenic; Dystonia,
tardive
segmental, 27, 262–263, 266, 268t, 298t
status dystonicus, 265, 298
sudden onset, limited duration see
Paroxysmal dyskinesias
surgical treatment of, 306–309
deep brain stimulation, 177–178,
306–308
pallidotomy, 163, 306–308
peripheral denervation procedures,
308–309
thalamotomy, 306
therapeutic guidelines, 309–310
tardive, 285, 416, 425, 439–440, 443–445,
490
task-specific, 263, 273, 288, 298t, 305, 503
tics in, 265, 276–277
see also Dystonic tics

torsion, 259–260, 266–277
trauma causing, 275, 285–286, 503–504,
519
treatment choices in, 293–294, 309f
see also Dystonia, medical treatment of;
Dystonia, physical therapy for;
Dystonia, surgical treatment of
treatment evaluation in, 293
treatment guidelines for, 309–310
tremors and, 30, 264–265, 268–269,
396–397, 400, 402
X-linked dystonia–parkinsonism (Lubag),
233, 261, 271, 286–287
Dystonia–parkinsonisms, 104, 231
early-onset (DYT16), 261, 272
Lubag (X-linked), 233, 261, 271,
286–287
rapid-onset, 261, 283–284
truncal deformities in, 71
Dystonic myorhythmia, 30
Dystonic storm, 265, 298
Dystonic tics, 32, 351–352
Dystonic tremors, 30, 264–265, 268–269,
396–397, 402

E

Early-onset ataxia with ocular motor apraxia
and hypoalbuminemia (EAOH,
AOA1), 472–473
Early-onset dystonia–parkinsonism (DYT16),
261, 272
Early-onset Parkinson disease (EOPD) see
Young-onset Parkinson disease
Eating, compulsive, 194
Echolalia, 352–353, 355–356
Echopraxia, 352, 355–356
Edema, with dopamine agonists, 136
EIF4G1 gene, 103, 105t–106t
Electroconvulsive therapy (ECT), 190
Electromyograph-guided (EMG) BTX
injections, 303–305
Electromyograph-guided (EMG) phenol
injections, 297
Electronic instruments, disease severity
assessment, 18
Embouchure dystonia, 263, 273
Encephalitis
dystonia and, 286
myoclonus and, 461
parkinsonism and, 233–234
paroxysmal nonkinesigenic dyskinesia and,
489–490
Encephalitis lethargica, 234
Encephalomyelitis with rigidity, 24, 254–255
Entacapone, 123–124, 140, 150
Environmental enrichment, 326–327
Environmental factors
in dystonias, 274, 285
in multiple system atrophy, 216
in Parkinson disease, 104–107
in parkinsonism–dementia–amyotrophic
lateral sclerosis complex of Guam,
232–233
in Tourette syndrome, 368
toxin-induced parkinsonism, 236–237
trauma-induced parkinsonism, 238
Ephatic transmissions, 500–501

Epilepsia partialis continua, 452–453, 454f,
455t
Epilepsy
and paroxysmal dyskinesias, 477–478, 480,
483t–484t, 485, 491, 493
psychogenic, 513, 515
see also Seizures
Epileptic myoclonus, 448, 458–460, 458f,
458t–459t, 462
Episodic ataxias (EAs), 30, 468–469, 471t,
481–482, 483t–484t, 491–493, 493t
Erectile dysfunction, 186
Essential chorea, 343
Essential myoclonus, 448, 449t, 462
Essential palatal myoclonus (EPM), 392,
450–452
Essential tremor (ET), 394
assessment of, 391
classification of, 389, 390t, 395t
diagnosis of, 395–402
epidemiology of, 394–395
genetics of, 402–404
pathophysiology of, 410–412
rest tremor and, 392
therapeutic algorithm, 404f
treatment of, 404–407
Ethyl-eicosapentaenoate (ethyl-EPA), 329
Etilevodopa, 151
Excessive movements see Dyskinesias
Excitotoxicity
in classic tardive dyskinesia, 438
in Huntington disease, 324–326
in Parkinson disease, 99–100
Executive loop, basal ganglia circuitry, 64,
64f
Exercise therapy, 120
Exertional paroxysmal dyskinesias (PED), 30,
479, 482–483, 483t–484t, 488,
490–491, 492t, 493–494
Extrapyramidal disorders, use of term, 55
Extrapyramidal syndrome (EPS) see Drug-
induced disorders, parkinsonism
Eye blink conditioning, 52
Eye blink reflex
dystonia and, 43
hemifacial spasm, 501
Parkinson disease, 19, 73
Eye of the tiger sign, 203, 220–221, 275–276
Eyebrow spasm
dystonic see Blepharospasm
hemifacial, 27–28, 273, 501f
Eyelid freezing, 19, 23, 200–201, 273, 288
Eyelid myoclonus with absences, 458t
Eyelid spasms, dystonic see Blepharospasm
Eyes
focal dystonia, 27
in Huntington disease, 312
Kayser–Fleischer rings, 509, 509f
myoclonus, 28–29
myorhythmia, 30
oculogyric crises, 27, 32, 425
opsoclonus (dancing eyes), 29, 461–462
in parkinsonian disorders, 19, 23, 40, 81
corticobasal degeneration, 219
progressive supranuclear palsy,
199–200
paroxysmal ocular downward deviation,
481

paroxysmal tonic upgaze of childhood, 481
saccades *see* Saccades
supranuclear ophthalmoparesis (gaze palsy), 199–200
tics, 31–32
see also Eyebrow spasm; Eyelid freezing
Eyes-closed instability, 50–51, 242

F

Face of the giant panda sign, 509–510, 510f
Facial dystonia *see* Blepharospasm
Facial effects of progressive supranuclear palsy, 200–201, 201f
Facial myoclonus, repetitive, 27–28
Facial myokymia, 29
Facial myorhythmia, 30
Facial nucleus hypothesis, 501
Facial spasm, hemifacial, 5t, 27–28, 273, 500–501, 500t, 501f
Facial synkinesis, 29
Factitious disorder, 518, 521, 526–527
FAHN, 275t, 276
Fahr disease, 239
Falling
  fear of, 23, 248, 524
  in Parkinson disease, 71–73, 156, 196
Familial dyskinesia and facial myokymia (FDFM), 343
Fasciculations, 29
Fatal familial insomnia (FFI), 234–236
Fatigue
  in cerebellar ataxia, 46, 50
  in Parkinson disease, 78, 189
    drugs for, 122, 126, 189
FBX07 gene, 103, 105t–106t, 231
Fear of falling, 23, 248, 524
Festination, 245
  in parkinsonism, 20, 72, 156
Fetal tissue grafting
  in Huntington disease, 333–334
  in Parkinson disease, 116–117, 179–182
Fingers
  minipolymyoclonus, 456
  painful arm and moving, 28, 502–503
  pseudoathetosis, 26
Flexed posture, parkinsonism, 20, 70–71
Flexor reflex afferents (FRAs), 36, 37f
Fluctuations ("offs"), levodopa-related, 141–142, 141t
  clinicopathologic correlation of, 143
  delayed "on", 151–152
  dyskinesias and (yo-yo-ing), 154–155
  episodic response failures, 151
  freezing, 152
  meal-related, 152
  on-off (sudden "off") phenomenon, 141–145, 147–148, 151, 154–155
  pathogenesis of, 143–149
  random, 151
  "super offs", 152
  treatment, 150–152
  weak end-of-day response, 152
  wearing-off phenomenon (end-of-dose failure), 141, 143–151, 154–155, 196
Flunarizine, 419
Foix–Chavany–Marie syndrome, 239

Food
  cheese effect, 125, 130–131
  meal-related responses to levodopa, 152
  parkinsonism–dementia–amyotrophic lateral sclerosis complex of Guam and, 232–233
Foot
  cold feet sign, 211
  dancing eyes, dancing feet syndrome, 29, 461–462
  dystonia, 305, 504
  edema with dopamine agonists, 136
  freezing phenomenon, 20, 22–23
  gait ataxia, 51
  painful legs and moving toes syndrome, 28, 502–503
  striatal toe deformity, 70
Force-rate deficit, 46–47
Fracture risk, in Parkinson disease, 196
Fragile X-associated/ataxia syndrome (FXTAS), 412–413, 473–474
Freezing phenomenon, 20, 22–23, 72–73, 245
  deep brain stimulation surgery in, 174, 246–247
  levodopa-associated, 152
  "on" and "off" types, 152
  primary freezing gait (gait ignition failure), 22–23, 199, 247–248
  primary progressive freezing gait, 248
  selegiline and, 128
  treatment, 246–247
Friedreich ataxia (FA), 50, 467–468, 470–472
FRM1 gene, 412
Frontal gait disorders, 23, 247–248
Frontotemporal dementias (FTDs), 225–232
  clinical features of, 225–226
  genetics of, 225–231
  neuropathology of, 222f, 230–231
  prevalence of, 225
  treatment, 232
FTL1 gene, 345–346
Functional movement disorders, 513
  see also Psychogenic movement disorders

G

GABA agonists
  in classic tardive dyskinesia, 442–443
  in essential tremor, 407
Gait, 241–244
  ataxic, 26, 51–52, 246, 411, 466
  bouncing, 247
  cautious, 23, 248
  choreic, 247
  classification of disorders of, 245–248
  dystonic, 247
  epidemiology of disorders of, 244–245, 244t
  evaluation of, 245
  freezing, 245
    see also Gait, parkinsonian, freezing phenomenon
  frontal disequilibrium of, 23, 247–248
  frontal gait disorders, 23, 247–248
  hemiparetic, 246
  hesitant (uncertain), 23
  ignition failure, 22–23, 199, 247–248

initiation, 243–244
  in normal pressure hydrocephalus, 248
  paraparetic, 246
  parkinsonian, 246–247
    deep brain stimulation surgery in, 174, 189, 246–247
    freezing phenomenon, 20, 22–23, 72–73, 128, 152, 174, 246–247
    levodopa-associated tachykinesis, 156
    loss of postural reflexes and, 72
    prevalence of, 5t
    in progressive supranuclear palsy, 199
    ten steps test, 68–69
  psychogenic, 248, 519, 523–524
  running, 156
  senile gait disorder, 23
  stiff-legged, 246
  subcortical disequilibrium of, 23, 247
  terms used to describe, 243
  therapeutic considerations, 249
Gait cycle, 243, 243f–244f
GALOP syndrome, 245
Gambling, pathologic, 78–79, 175, 193–194
Gamma knife (GF) surgery, 161
Gamma-aminobutyric acid (GABA), 60
  basal ganglia circuitry, 62–63, 63f
  Huntington disease and, 318, 324
  interneurons and, 61
  in loss of inhibition in dystonia, 42–43
  in presynaptic inhibition, 36–37
  stiff-person syndrome, 253–254
Gamma-hydroxybutyrate, 296–297
Gastric emptying, in Parkinson disease, 151, 187
Gastrointestinal dysfunction
  in multiple system atrophy, 217
  in Parkinson disease, 75, 113, 187
    dopaminergic agents for, 122–127, 151
    nondopaminergic agents for, 122t, 126–127, 187
Gaucher disease, 103
Gaze palsy (supranuclear ophthalmoparesis), 199–200
GBA gene, 103, 105t–106t
GCH gene, dopa-responsive dystonia, 280–283
Gegenhalten, 23–24
Geldanamycin, 328
Gene therapy, 181–182
Genetics of movement disorders, 2–18, 6t–18t
  see also specific disorders
Geniospasm, hereditary, 414
Gerstmann–Sträussler–Scheinker (GSS) disease, 234–236
Geste antagoniste (sensory tricks), 27, 264, 272–273
Gestures, 31, 380
  obscene (copropraxia), 32, 352, 355–356
Gilles de la Tourette syndrome *see* Tourette syndrome
Glabellar tap reflex, 19, 73
Glial cell line-derived neurotrophic factor (GDNF), 131, 181–182
Glial cytoplasmic inclusions (GCI), 208, 214–216
Glioma, facial myokymia in pontine, 29

Globus pallidus (GP; paleostriatum), 55, 61–62, 157–159
  basal ganglia circuitry, 62–65, 63f, 159
  bradykinesia and, 69
  cellular activity in, 65
  in classic tardive dyskinesia, 436–437
  deep brain stimulation surgery
    in dyskinesias, 177–179
    in dystonia, 307–308, 307f
    in Parkinson disease, 164t, 168–175
    in paroxysmal nonkinesigenic dyskinesia, 488
    in Tourette syndrome, 378–379
  in dystonia, 291
    pallidotomy for, 163, 306–308
  in Huntington disease, 318
    pallidotomy for, 333
  in Parkinson disease
    biochemical pathology, 98t
    clinical–pathological correlations, 82
    deep brain stimulation surgery in, 164t, 168–175
    pallidotomy for, 159–164, 173, 394
  in progressive supranuclear palsy, 204
  in Tourette syndrome, 361–362, 378–379
  tremor generation in, 408–410
Glucose transporter 1 (GLUT1) deficiency, 491, 493–494
Glutamate (Glu), 59–60
  basal ganglia circuitry, 62–63, 63f
  Huntington disease and, 324–325
  medium spiny neurons and, 60–61
  Parkinson disease and
    antiglutamatergics, 121, 125, 131
    biochemical pathology, 98t
    excitotoxicity, 100
Glutamic acid decarboxylase (GAD)
  in classic tardive dyskinesia, 436–437
  stiff-person syndrome and, 254
Glutathione (GSH), 99
Glutethimide, 407–408
Glycogen synthase kinase (GSK-3β; tau protein kinase I), 207, 227
GPI-1046 (neuroimmunophilin), 131–132
Group A β-hemolytic streptococcus (GABHS) infection, 343–344, 363–365
Guadeloupean tauopathy, 232–233
Guam dementia, 232–233
Guanfacine, 376–377

H

H reflexes, 251–253
Habenula, 62–63
Habit-reversal training (HRT), 370–371
Hallervorden–Spatz disease see Neurodegenerations with brain iron accumulation (NBIA)
Hallucinations
  in dementia with Lewy bodies, 223–224, 232
  in Parkinson disease, 77–78, 194–196
Hand
  alien hand phenomenon, 54, 218–219
  behavior in corticobasal degeneration, 21
  cold hands sign, 211

focal dystonia of see Hand dystonia
painful arm and moving fingers syndrome, 28, 502–503
  striatal deformity of, 70, 71f
Hand dystonia (writer's cramp), 27, 272t, 273
  botulinum toxin treatment, 305
  loss of inhibition, 42–43, 288
  neuroimaging of, 292
  pathoanatomy of, 289–290
  peripheral injury causing, 503–504
  physical therapy for, 294–295
  sensory dysfunction, 44, 288
  task-specific tremor and, 402
Harmaline-induced tremors, 408–409
HARP syndrome, 341
Haw River syndrome see Dentatorubral-pallidoluysian atrophy (DRPLA)
HDC gene, 366–367
Head drop, 70–71
Head trauma
  causing dystonia, 275, 285–286, 504
  paroxysmal dyskinesias and, 486–487
Headaches, Tourette syndrome and, 359
Head-shaking nystagmus, 393
Health-related quality of life (HRQoL), 78, 87, 134, 171–172, 196
Hearing loss, in essential tremor, 399
Hedonistic homeostatic dysregulation, 79
Helicobacter pylori, 123
Hemiatrophy, paroxysmal dyskinesias and, 487
Hemiballism, 26, 346
  model of basal ganglia dysfunction in, 158f
  prevalence of, 5t
Hemidystonia, 27, 265–266
  paroxysmal, 490
Hemifacial spasm, 5t, 27–28, 273, 500–501, 500t, 501f
Hemiparesis, ataxic, 465–466
Hemiparetic gait, 246
Hemiparkinsonism–hemiatrophy syndrome, 5t, 67, 238
Hemiplegia, alternating of childhood, 490
Hemorrhages, cerebral, 487
Heredodegenerative dystonias, 268, 269t–271t, 274–276
Heredodegenerative parkinsonism, 86t, 198t, 233
Hesitant (uncertain) gaits, 23
  cautious, 23, 248
  frontal disequilibrium, 23
  frontal gait disorders, 23, 247–248
  gait ignition failure, 22–23, 199, 247–248
  senile gait disorder, 23
  subcortical disequilibrium, 23, 247
Hiccups, 25
Histone deacetylase inhibitors, 322–323, 328
Holding (blocking) tics, 21, 351–352
Holmes tremor see Midbrain tremor
Homocysteine, levodopa therapy and, 123
Hot cross bun sign, 212–213, 214f
HS1-BP3 gene, 402–403
5-HT see Serotonin
Htt-associated protein (HAP1), 326
Hufschmidt phenomenon, 47

Hummingbird sign, 202–203, 203f
Huntingtin (Htt), 317–318
  genetics of Huntington disease, 318–322
  pathogenesis of Huntington disease, 322–326
Huntingtin (Htt; IT15) gene, 318–319, 325
  CAG repeats, 312, 316, 319–322, 319f, 328–329
  RNA interference, 334
Huntington disease (HD), 311–334
  chorea in, 26, 178–179, 311–313, 335
  clinical aspects of, 311–314
  genetics of, 6t–18t, 318–322
  HD-like phenotypes see Huntington disease-like (HDL) disorders
  historical background, 311
  juvenile, 314
  natural course of, 314–315, 320
  neurochemistry of, 316–318
  neuroimaging of, 315–316
  neuropathology of, 44, 316–318
  pathogenesis of, 322–326
  prevalence of, 5t, 311
  progressive supranuclear palsy contrasted, 201–202
  treatment of, 326–333, 332f, 334t
    deep brain stimulation surgery, 178–179, 333
    experimental therapeutics, 333–334
  voluntariness of movement in, 54
Huntington disease-like (HDL) disorders, 335, 336t, 337–339
  dentatorubral-pallidoluysian atrophy, 335–337, 460
  HDL1, 337
  HDL2, 337–338
  HDL3, 338
Hydrocephalus-associated parkinsonism, 238–239, 248
5-hydroxytryptamine see Serotonin
Hyperekplexia ("startle disease"), 6t–17t, 24, 28, 456, 456t, 457f, 519
Hyperhidrosis, 74–75, 187
Hyperkinesias, use of term, 1
  see also Dyskinesias
Hypermetria, 46–47
Hypersexuality, pathologic, 194
Hypertension, Parkinson disease and, 109–110
Hypertonia, spastic, 250–252
Hypnic jerks (sleep starts), 498
Hypnogenic dyskinesias
  paroxysmal (PHD), 28, 479–480, 483t–484t
  periodic movements in sleep, 28, 496–499
Hypnotics, in Parkinson disease, 125–126, 193
Hypoceruloplasminemia-related movement disorder (HCMD), 512
Hypohidrosis, 74–75
Hypokinesias, 1
  definitions of, 1
  differential diagnosis of, 18–24
  genetics of, 6t–17t
  historical perspective on, 3t–4t
  list of, 2t
  prevalence of, 5t

quantitative assessments of, 18
stiffness syndromes, 250–258
see also Akinesia; Apraxia; Bradykinesia; Parkinsonism
Hypometria, 46
Hypophonia, 175
Hyposmia, 80–81, 113–114, 185, 398
Hypotension, orthostatic *see* Orthostatic hypotension
Hypothyroid slowness, 23
Hypotonia, 45–46, 250
Hypoxia
causing ataxia, 466
perinatal hypoxic encephalopathy, 487, 489
post-hypoxic myoclonus, 460–461, 461t
Hysteria, 514–515
see also Somatization disorder

I

Ideational apraxia, 21, 54t, 218–219
Ideomotor apraxia, 21, 53, 54t, 218–219
Idiopathic dystonia *see* Dystonia, primary
Idiopathic parkinsonism *see* Juvenile parkinsonism; Parkinson disease
Immobilization therapy, in dystonia, 294
Immunologic mechanisms
in Huntington disease, 318
in Tourette syndrome, 363–365
Impaired check sign, 47
Impotence, 186
Impulse control, 358–359, 362
Impulse control disorders (ICD), 193–194, 366–367
Infantile bilateral striatal necrosis (IBSN), 343
Infantile convulsions with choreoathetosis (ICCA) syndrome, 480, 485–486, 495
Infantile dystonia-parkinsonism disorder, 104
Infantile neuroaxonal dystrophy (INAD) *see* PLA2G6-associated neurodegeneration
Infantile spasms, 458t
Infections
ataxia and, 467
infectious chorea, 336t, 343
myoclonus and, 461
PANDAS and PITANDS, 364–365
Parkinson disease and, 104–107
parkinsonism with, 233–234
postinfectious chorea, 336t, 344–345, 365
Tourette syndrome and, 363–365
Infectious protein hypothesis, 116–117, 180–181
Inflammation, in Parkinson disease, 99–100, 99f, 133
Inhibition
alpha motoneuron and, 36–37, 37f
in basal ganglia circuitry, 38, 38f–39f, 44, 62–63
long intracortical, 42–43
loss of in dyskinesias, 43–44, 288
presynaptic, 36–37
reciprocal, 36–37, 301
recurrent, 36–37
short intracortical, 42–43
surround, 43–44, 288
in Tourette syndrome, 358–360, 362, 366

Intention tremors *see* Kinetic tremors
Intermanual conflict, 21
Interneurons, 61, 64–65
Inter-onset latency (IOL), 40
Intraduodenal pumps, 154–155
Intrathecal baclofen (ITB), 296–297
Involuntary movements, 1–2, 36–54, 351
Iron, 231, 342f
hereditary deficiency of ceruloplasmin, 512
restless legs syndrome and, 497–499
see also Neurodegenerations with brain iron accumulation
Isaacs syndrome *see* Neuromyotonia
Isometric tremors, 389
Istradefylline, 121, 125
IT15 gene, 337–338

J

Jaw tremor, task-specific, 514
Jerks
hypnic (sleep starts), 498
myoclonic *see* Myoclonus
JPH3 gene, 337–338
Jumping disorders, 28, 369, 456, 519
Jumpy stumps, 28, 502
Juvenile myoclonic epilepsy (JME), 458
Juvenile parkinsonism, 20, 96, 240
dopa-responsive dystonia and, 281–282, 282t

K

Karak syndrome, 231
Kayser–Fleischer rings, 509, 509f
Kernicterus, 347
Kinesigenic paroxysmal dyskinesia *see* Paroxysmal dyskinesias, kinesigenic
Kinesthesia, 39
Kinetic tremors, 389, 407–408, 412
Kufor–Rakeb syndrome (PARK9), 103, 105t–106t, 231, 275t
Kuru, 234

L

L-dopa *see* Levodopa
Lactate accumulation, 325
Lafora body disease, 458–460, 459t
Lamotrigine, 333
Lance–Adams syndrome, 29
Language problems
in corticobasal degeneration, 219–220
in frontotemporal dementias, 225
Laryngeal dystonia (spasmodic dysphonia), 298t, 303
Lateral habenula, 62–63
Latrepirdine, 329
LAX-101 (ethyl-eicosapentaenoate), 329
Lazabemide, 125
Lead-pipe rigidity, 23–24
Learning
cognitive decline in Parkinson disease and, 76
motor, 52, 65, 65f
Leg
complex regional pain syndrome, 504–506
edema with dopamine agonists, 136

manifestation of bradykinesia in, 19
myoclonus in, 29, 501
painful, 28, 502–503
periodic movements in sleep, 28, 496–499
restless syndrome *see* Restless legs syndrome
Lennox–Gastaut syndrome, 458t
Lenticular nucleus, 55
Levine–Critchley syndrome choreoacanthocytosis *see* Neuroacanthocytosis
Levodopa
in metabolism of dopamine, 56–58, 59f
Parkinson disease and, 107, 107f, 110
therapeutic use of *see* Levodopa treatment
Levodopa treatment
in athetosis, 348
dopa-responsive dystonia, 261, 264, 270, 280–283, 295
in drug-induced parkinsonism, 429
in Parkinson disease, 119, 122–123
in the advanced stage, 141–156
age at onset predicting response to, 84
compliance, 196
complications of *see* Levodopa treatment complications
with COMT inhibitors, 123–124, 140
with decarboxylase inhibitors, 122–123
see also Carbidopa/levodopa (Sinemet); Carbidopa/levodopa/entacapone (LCE)
diagnostic use of, 85, 88–89, 140
with dopamine agonists, 124, 133–134, 151
dopamine agonists compared, 133–135, 139
during surgery, 140, 156
Helicobacter pylori and, 123
life expectancy and, 85
malignant melanoma and, 123
with MAO inhibitors, 128–131, 134, 190
in the mild stage, 134–135, 138–139
in the moderate stage, 139–141
therapeutic principles, 120, 120t
in Parkinsonism-plus syndromes
corticobasal degeneration, 222
multiple system atrophy, 216–218
progressive supranuclear palsy, 207
in tyrosine hydroxylase deficiency, 283
Levodopa treatment complications, 120t, 123, 138–139, 141–156
autonomic "offs", 141–143, 141t, 186–187
behavioral "offs", 141–143, 141t, 191
in dementia, 192
dyskinesias, 141–142, 141t
chorea, 152–153, 345
clinicopathologic correlation of, 143
deep brain stimulation surgery in, 168–172
diphasic, 142, 153
end-of-day, 142
fluctuations and (yo-yo-ing), 154–155
in multiple system atrophy, 217–218
myoclonus, 142, 155
"off" dystonia, 142, 153–154, 184
"off" painful cramps, 153–154, 184
pallidotomy for, 161–163
pathogenesis of, 149–150

537

peak-dose, 142–143, 149–150, 152–153
risk factors for, 143, 149–150
simultaneous dyskinesia and
    parkinsonism, 142, 155
somatotopically-specific, 155
treatment, 152–155, 161–162, 168–172
efficacy over time, 155
falling, 156
fluctuations ("offs"), 141–142, 141t
    clinicopathologic correlation of, 143
    delayed "on", 151–152
    dyskinesias and (yo-yo-ing), 154–155
    episodic response failures, 151
    freezing, 152
    meal-related, 152
    on-off (sudden "off") phenomenon,
        141–145, 147–148, 151, 154–155
    pathogenesis of, 143–149
    random, 151
    "super offs", 152
    treatment, 150–152
    weak end-of-day response, 152
    wearing-off phenomenon (end-of-dose
        failure), 141, 143–151, 154–155, 196
increased parkinsonism, 155–156
in multiple system atrophy, 217–218
psychosis, 195
punding, 194
sensory "offs", 141–143, 141t, 184–185,
    191
sleep, 188–189
tachyphemia, 156
treatment of, 126, 143, 150–156, 161–162,
    168–174
Lewy bodies (LBs)
dementia with see Dementia with Lewy
    bodies (DLB)
essential tremor and, 411
neuropathology, 230
Parkinson disease and
    anatomical pathology of, 94–97, 95f,
        97f, 97t
    autopsy findings, 92, 114
    Braak staging system, 110–114, 192–193
    clinical features of, 74–75, 77
    dementia, 192–193
    fetal dopaminergic neurons, 116–117,
        180–181
    infectious protein hypothesis, 116–117,
        180–181
    pathogenic mechanisms, 99–103, 101f,
        108, 108f, 110–117, 180–181, 230
    α-synuclein, 100–102, 101f, 108, 108f,
        110–117, 180–181
Lewy body variant of Alzheimer disease see
    Dementia with Lewy bodies
Lewy neurites, 110–115
Lidocaine
    in dystonia, 297
    in essential tremor, 407
Limb amputations, 28, 502
Limb behavior
    in ataxia, 26
    in ballism, 26
    in complex regional pain syndrome,
        504–506
    in corticobasal degeneration, 21, 218–219
Limb kinetic apraxia, 21, 54t, 218–219

Limbic loop, basal ganglia circuitry, 64, 64f
Limbic system
    stereotypies and, 380–382
    Tourette syndrome and, 362–363, 366
LINGO1 gene, 403
Lingual dyskinesias, 417, 432–433
Lingual dystonia, 273
Lingual feeding dystonia, 27, 339
Lisdexamfetamine dimesylate (LDX),
    375–376
Lisuride, 121t, 124
Lithium, 329
Liver damage, in Wilson disease, 507–508,
    508t, 512
Liver transplantation, 512
Local field potentials (LFPs), 65
Locus coeruleus (LC), 62–63
    in pathology of Parkinson disease
        anatomical, 95–97
        autopsy findings, 92
        biochemical, 97
        Braak staging system, 110, 113
Long intracortical inhibition (LICI), 42–43
Lower body parkinsonism, 237–238,
    247–248
LRRK2 gene, 73–74, 80–81, 90–91, 96,
    102–103, 105t–106t, 113, 116
Lubag dystonia (X-linked dystonia–
    parkinsonism, XDP), 233, 261, 271,
    286–287
Lytico-bodig, 232

M

Magnetic resonance imaging see MRI
Magnetic resonance spectroscopy (MRS), 213
Malignant catatonia see Neuroleptic
    malignant syndrome
Malignant melanoma, 75, 123
Malingering, 518, 521, 526–527
Manganese parkinsonism, 236–237, 237f
Mania, deep brain stimulation surgery and,
    175, 179
Mannerisms, 31, 380, 382
MAO inhibitors see Monoamine oxidase
    (MAO) inhibitors
MAPT gene, 225–227
Marché à petit pas, 245
Mariana dementia, 232
Marinesco–Sjögren syndrome, 473
Mass estimation impairments, 49
Mass hysteria, 515
Masticatory muscle myorhythmia, 30
Maternal imprinting, 284–285
Meal-related levodopa responses, 152
Mechanical instruments, disease severity
    assessment, 18
MECP2 gene, 385–386
Median raphe nucleus (MRN), 62–63
Medium spiny neurons (MSN), 60–61, 61f,
    64–65
Melanoma, 75, 123
Melatonin, 418–419
Memantine, 333
Menkes protein, 292
Mental slowness see Bradyphrenia
[123]I-metaiodobenzylguanidine (MIBG) uptake,
    91–92, 113, 186

Methazolamide, 405–406
1-methyl-4-phenyl-1,2,3,6-tetrahydropyridine
    see MPTP
Methylene blue, 207–208
Methylphenidate, 375–376
Metoclopramide, 424–426
Mexiletine, 297
Meyerson sign, 19, 73
MIBG uptake, 91–92, 113, 186
Midbrain tremor, 32, 82, 392
Migraine headaches, 359
Milk-maid grip, 26
Milodrine, 216–217
Mini-Mental State Examination (MMSE), 76
Minipolymyoclonus, 29, 456
Minocycline, 327–329
Mitochondrial disorders, parkinsonism and,
    239–240
Mitochondrial dysfunction
    in classic tardive dyskinesia, 437
    in Huntington disease, 321–322, 324–325
    in Parkinson disease, 99–100, 99f, 115,
        132–133
    in progressive supranuclear palsy, 206–208
Mitochondrial encephalomyopathy, 459t, 460
Mitochondrial enhancers, 121, 132–133
Mitochondrial recessive ataxia syndrome
    (MIRAS), 473
Modafinil
    in ADHD, 377
    in Parkinson disease, 126
Monoamine oxidase (MAO), metabolism of
    dopamine by, 56–58, 59f, 107
Monoamine oxidase (MAO) inhibitors, 121,
    125
    in ADHD, 376–377
    in depression in Parkinson disease, 190
    type A, 125–126, 129–131, 134
    type B, 125–131, 150
Montreal Cognitive Assessment (MoCA), 76,
    191
Mood, after deep brain stimulation surgery,
    175, 179
    see also Depression
Morning glory sign, 202–203
Morphine sulfate, 297
Morvan syndrome (Morvan's fibrillary
    chorea), 256
Motion prediction, 49
Motivation, loss of see Apathy
Motor blocks see Freezing phenomenon
Motor control, 36–54
    alpha motoneurons' role in, 36–38
    in apraxias, 53, 54t
    basal ganglia circuitry for, 38, 44, 65
    cerebellar, 38, 44–53, 45f
    cerebral cortical, 37–38, 38f–39f, 42–44,
        45f, 53, 53f
    in dyskinesias, 44
        ataxia, 44–53
        dystonia, 42–44
    in Parkinson disease, 38–42
    of voluntary movement, 36, 46–47, 54
Motor impersistence ("negative chorea"), 26
Motor learning, 65, 65f
    impaired, 52
Motor loop, basal ganglia circuitry, 64, 64f
Motor neuron disease, 232

Motor neuron disease-inclusion body dementia (MIND-ID), 220
Motor tics, 30–32
    with phonic see Tourette syndrome
Mount–Reback syndrome, 488–489
Movement amplitude scaling deficits, 46–47
Movement Disorders, 1
Movement disorders
    clinical overview of, 1–35
    definitions of, 1
    differential diagnosis of dyskinesias, 25–34
    differential diagnosis of hypokinesias, 18–24
    epidemiology of, 2, 5t
    evaluation of dyskinesias, 24–25
    genetics of, 2–18, 6t–18t
    historical perspective on, 2, 3t–4t
    origins of, 2
    physiology of movement in, 38–53
    quantifying severity of, 18
    see also specific disorders
Movement Order Society, MDS-UPDRS, 85–87
Movement time (MT), 39, 69
    in Huntington disease, 312
Movement variability, ataxic, 50
Movements
    categories of, 1–2, 351
    physiology of see Motor control
Moving toes syndrome, 28, 502–503
Moving umbilicus syndrome (belly dancer's dyskinesia), 25, 502
Moyamoya, 237–238
MPTP (1-methyl-4-phenyl-1,2,3,6-tetrahydropyridine), 99–100, 104, 118, 236
MR1 gene, 494
MRI (magnetic resonance imaging)
    in classic tardive dyskinesia, 438
    in corticobasal degeneration, 220–221
    Creutzfeldt–Jakob disease, 235
    deep brain stimulation surgery and, 166–167, 176
    in dystonia, 292
    eye of the tiger sign, 203, 220–221, 275–276
    hot cross bun sign, 212–213, 214f
    hummingbird sign, 202–203, 203f
    in Huntington disease, 315
    morning glory sign, 202–203
    in multiple system atrophy, 212–213, 214f
    neurodegenerations with brain iron accumulation, 275–276, 276f, 276t
    panda signs, 509–510, 510f
    in Parkinson disease, 89–92
    in progressive supranuclear palsy, 202–203, 203f
    in Tourette syndrome, 361
    in Wilson disease, 509–510, 510f
Multi-infarct progressive supranuclear palsy, 202–203
Multiple sclerosis
    facial myokymia in, 29
    paroxysmal dyskinesias and, 486–487, 489
Multiple system atrophy (MSA), 208–218
    clinical features of, 208–212
    epidemiology of, 212
    genetics of, 216

natural history of, 211–212
    neurodiagnostic studies of, 212–214
    neuropathology of, 214–216
    prevalence of, 5t
    treatment for, 216–218
Multisystem degenerations see Parkinsonism-plus syndromes
Multitasking, in Parkinson disease, 73
Muscarinic acetylcholine receptors (mACHR), 59
Muscle relaxants
    in dystonia, 296
    in Parkinson disease, 121, 125
Musician's dystonia (musician's cramps), 263, 273, 288, 503
    physical therapy for, 294
Mutism, akinetic, 54
Myerson sign, 19, 73
Myoclonus, 28–29, 447–464
    action, 29
    axial, 454–456
    bouncing gait in, 247
    brainstem, 448–451, 454–456, 455t, 457f
    chorea contrasted with, 26, 447
    clinical classification of, 447, 448t
    cortical, 448–450, 452–453, 453f–454f, 455t, 456, 458, 462
    cortical reflex, 29, 411–412, 449–450, 452
    in corticobasal degeneration, 219, 462
    drugs provoking, 462
        levodopa, 142, 155
    dystonia and see Myoclonus–dystonia
    epileptic, 448, 458–460, 458f, 458t–459t, 462
    essential, 448, 449t, 462
    essential tremor and, 400
    etiologic classification of, 448, 448t–449t
    focal, 450–454, 501–502
    generalized, 456–464
    genetics of, 6t–17t
    historical background, 447
    in juvenile Huntington disease, 314
    multifocal, 456–464
    in multiple system atrophy, 210–211
    negative, 28–29
    neurophysiologic assessment of, 448–450
    nocturnal, 28
        see also Periodic movements in sleep
    ocular, 28–29
    orthostatic, 248
    palatal, 28–30, 392, 450–452, 452f, 524
    pathophysiologic classification of, 447–448, 448t
    physiologic, 448, 449t
    post-hypoxic, 460–461, 461t
    prevalence of, 5t
    progressive myoclonic ataxia (Ramsay Hunt syndrome), 29, 458, 458f, 459t, 460
    progressive myoclonus epilepsy, 458–460, 458f, 459t
    propriospinal, 29, 449–450, 454–455, 455f, 524
    psychogenic, 448, 450, 462, 515, 524
    reflex, 29, 219
    respiratory, 29
    rhythmic, 29
    segmental, 449–450
    segmental abdominal, 25

segmental palatal, 28–30, 392
    spinal, 29, 454–455, 463
    spinal segmental, 450, 451f, 501–502
    subcortical, 449–450
    symptomatic, 448, 449t
    tics contrasted with, 31, 447
    treatment of, 462–464
    with viral encephalopathies, 461
    voluntariness of, 54
Myoclonus epilepsy and ragged-red fiber syndrome (MERRF), 459t, 460
Myoclonus of infancy, benign, 481
Myoclonus–dystonia, 261–262, 269t–271t, 284–285, 297, 464
Myoglobinuria, 298
Myokymia, 29
    in episodic ataxias, 468, 482, 491
    familial dyskinesia and facial, 343
    with impaired muscle relaxation see Neuromyotonia
Myorhythmia, 30, 392

N

Neostriatum see Striatum
Nerve growth factor, 333–334
Nerve origin hypothesis, 500–501
Neuroacanthocytosis, 27, 339–341, 339t, 386
Neurodegenerations with brain iron accumulation (NBIA), 275–276, 275t, 341
    deep brain stimulation surgery in, 178–179
    PARK9 (Kufor–Rakeb), 103, 105t–106t, 231, 275t
    type 1 (NBIA1, PKAN), 231, 275–276, 276f, 276t, 341
    type 2 (NBIA2, PARK14, PLAN, INAD), 103, 105t–106t, 231, 275t–276t, 276, 276f, 341
    type 3 (neuroferritinopathy), 275t–276t, 276, 276f, 345–346
    type 4 (aceruloplasminemia), 262t, 275t–276t, 276f
Neuroferritinopathy, 275t–276t, 276, 276f, 345–346
Neurofibrillary tangles (NFTs)
    in parkinsonism–dementia–amyotrophic lateral sclerosis complex of Guam, 233
    in progressive supranuclear palsy, 204–205, 207, 228
    tau gene and, 228–231
Neuroimmunophilin, 131–132
Neuroleptic malignant syndrome (NMS), 429–430
    rigidity in, 24
Neuroleptics see Antipsychotics
Neuromelanin, 62, 94–96, 107–108
Neuromuscular disorders, involuntary movements, 36, 37t
Neuromyotonia, 24, 255–258, 255t
Neuronal ceroid lipofuscinoses (Batten disease), 6t–17t, 459t, 460
Neuronal intermediate filaments inclusion disease, 227
Neuronal intranuclear inclusion disease, 240

Neuronal intranuclear inclusions
  in DRPLA, 336–337
  in Huntington disease, 317, 321, 323–324, 326
Neuropathic tremors, 413
Neuropeptides, stereotypies and, 381–382
Neuroprotection
  deep brain stimulation surgery in, 173
  in Huntington disease, 317, 321–323, 326
  use of term, 127, 127f
Neuroprotective agents
  in Huntington disease, 326–329
  in Parkinson disease, 127–134
Neurotransmitters, 55–60, 157–159
  Huntington disease and, 317–318, 318t, 321–322, 324–325
  Parkinson disease pathology, 97–99
  progressive supranuclear palsy pathology, 206
  see also specific neurotransmitters
Neurotransplantation see Brain grafting
Neurotrophins
  in Huntington disease, 323–324, 333–334
  in Parkinson disease, 121, 131–132, 181–182
Neurturin
  in Huntington disease, 334
  in Parkinson disease, 181–182
New variant Creutzfeldt–Jakob disease (nvCJD), 234–235
Nicotine, in tics, 373–374
Nicotinic acetylcholine receptors (nACHR), 59
3-Nitropropionic acid (3-NP), 325
N-methyl-D-aspartate (NMDA)
  in classic tardive dyskinesia, 436
  in Huntington disease, 324–325
N-methyl-D-aspartate (NMDA) antagonists, in Huntington disease, 333
NMSQuest, 87
Nocturnal dyskinesias, 28
  paroxysmal hypnogenic, 28, 479–480, 483t–484t
  periodic movements in sleep, 28, 496–499
  RBD see REM sleep behavior disorder
Nonkinesigenic paroxysmal dyskinesia see Paroxysmal dyskinesias, nonkinesigenic (PNKD)
Noradrenergic system
  freezing phenomenon and, 72–73
  pathogenesis of PD and, 99, 113
Norepinephrine (NE), 60, 97, 98t
  dystonia and, 291
Normal pressure hydrocephalus (NPH), 238–239, 248
Nottingham Health Profile, 87
Numbness in Parkinson disease, 184
Nurr1 protein, 92

O

Obsessive-compulsive disorder (OCD)
  compulsions, 31
  deep brain stimulation surgery and, 175, 179, 378–379
  obsessional slowness, 22
  Parkinson disease and, 78–79
  postinfectious, 365

stereotypies and, 382, 386–387
Tourette syndrome and, 354–359, 356f
  genetics of, 367–368
  pathogenesis of, 360, 363–365
  treatment, 377–378
Occupational hazards
  dystonia, 263, 273, 288
  parkinsonism and, 104, 236–237
  see also Musician's dystonia
Occupational therapy, 326–327
Ocular features of movement disorders see Eyes
Oculofaciomasticatory myorhythmia, 30
Oculogyric crises, 27, 32, 425
Olanzapine, 416, 419–421
  in classic tardive dyskinesia, 442
  in Parkinson disease, 126, 153, 195
  in parkinsonism-dementia syndromes, 232
  side effects, 422–424
Olfactory apparatus, in Parkinson disease, 110, 114
Olfactory loss, in Parkinson disease, 80–81, 113–114, 185, 398
Olivopontocerebellar atrophy (OPCA), 208–218
Ondansetron, 195–196
Ophthalmoparesis, supranuclear, 199–200
Oppenheim dystonia (DYT1), 261, 269t–271t, 277–280, 284, 291
Oppenheim, Hermann, 259
Opsoclonus (dancing eyes), 29, 461–462
Opsoclonus-myoclonus syndrome, 29, 461–462
Oral dyskinesias
  differential diagnosis, 431, 431t
  oral-buccal-lingual, 417, 432–433
  spontaneous, 432–433
Oromandibular dystonia (OMD), 273, 298t, 303, 439
Orthostatic hemidystonia, 265
Orthostatic hypotension (OH)
  in multiple system atrophy, 209, 216–217
  in Parkinson disease, 74, 186
    dopamine agonists causing, 136
    drugs for, 122, 126, 186
Orthostatic myoclonus, 248
Orthostatic paroxysmal dystonia, 490
Orthostatic tremor, 400–401, 406
Osler, Sir William, 1
OSU6162, 331–332
Overflow phenomena, 26–27, 263–264
Oxidative stress
  in classic tardive dyskinesia, 438
  in Huntington disease, 324–326
  Parkinson disease and, 99–100, 99f, 107–108, 109f, 110, 131
  paroxysmal nonkinesigenic dyskinesia and, 494

P

Pain
  in dystonia, 264
  as part of Parkinson disease, 153–154, 184
  thresholds of in Parkinson disease, 81
Pain syndrome, complex regional, 504–506, 519
Painful arm and moving fingers, 28, 502–503

Painful legs and moving toes syndrome, 28, 502–503
Paired associative stimulation (PAS), 43
Palatal myoclonus, 28–30, 392, 450–452, 452f, 524
Paleostriatum see Globus pallidus
Palilalia, parkinsonian, 23
Pallido-pyramidal (Parkinsonism-pyramidal) syndrome, 103, 231
Pallidonigroluysial atrophy (PNLA), 204–205
Pallidotomy
  in dystonia, 163, 306–308
  in Huntington disease, 333
  in Parkinson disease, 159–164, 173, 394
Palmomental reflex, 73
Panda signs, 509–510, 510f
PANDAS, 364–365
Panic, Parkinson disease and, 190–191
PANK2 gene, 231, 275–276, 341
Pantothenate kinase-associated neurodegeneration (PKAN) see Neurodegenerations with brain iron accumulation (NBIA), type 1
Paraballism, 346
Paradoxical dystonia, 27, 264
Parakinesia, 26
Paraneoplastic disorders, 239, 345, 466–467
Paranoia, in Parkinson disease, 194–196
Paraparetic gait, 246
Paresthesia in Parkinson disease, 184
Parietal lobe, motor functions of, 53, 53f
PARK1 (SNCA), 101–102, 105t–106t, 114–115
PARK2 see Parkin (PARK2) gene
PARK3, 101–102, 105t–106t
PARK4, 102, 105t–106t, 114–115
PARK5, 102, 105t–106t, 115
PARK6, 102, 105t–106t, 116
PARK7, 102, 105t–106t, 116
PARK8, 102, 105t–106t, 116
PARK9, 103, 105t–106t, 231, 275t
PARK10, 103, 105t–106t
PARK11, 103, 105t–106t
PARK12, 103, 105t–106t
PARK13, 103, 105t–106t
PARK14, 103, 105t–106t, 231, 275t–276t, 276
PARK15, 103, 105t–106t
PARK16, 103, 105t–106t
Parkin (PARK2) gene, 73–74, 80–82, 99–102, 105t–106t, 115
Parkinson, James, 66, 93
Parkinson disease (PD)
  age at onset, 20, 67, 93–94
    disease progression and, 82–84
  asymmetry of symptoms in, 67
    see also Hemiparkinsonism–hemiatrophy syndrome
  clinical rating scales for, 18, 76, 85–87, 183
  diagnosis of
    at autopsy, 88–89, 92
    biomarkers, 90–92
    criteria for, 88–89, 88t, 96–97
    neuroimaging for, 90–92, 230, 399–400
    nonmotor symptoms, 183–185
    presymptomatic, 90–92, 90f, 185
  differential diagnosis, 85, 90–91, 140
  early-onset see Parkinson disease (PD), young-onset

epidemiology of, 88–89, 93–94
  prevalence, 5t, 20–21, 93–94
essential tremor and, 396–400, 397f
etiology/pathogenesis of, 99f
  animal models, 118
  apoptosis, 99–100, 108f
  Braak's staging system, 110–114
  clues from monogenic PD, 114–116
  endogenous factors, 104, 107–110
  environmental factors, 104–107
  excitotoxicity, 99–100
  genetics, 99–104, 114–117
  infectious protein hypothesis, 116–117,
    180–181
  inflammation, 99–100
  interconnection of mechanisms, 96f,
    99–100, 117
  mitochondrial dysfunction, 99–100, 115
  multiple hit hypothesis, 117
  oxidative stress, 99–100, 99f, 107–108,
    109f, 110
  timeline, 114f
  toxic protein accumulation, 99–100, 101f
exercise therapy for, 120
eye movement in, 19, 40
genetics of, 6t–17t
  anatomical pathology and, 96
  animal models, 118
  clinical features and, 73–74, 80–82, 85
  dementia and, 223
  etiology/pathogenesis and, 99–104,
    114–117
  levodopa-induced dyskinesia, 150
historical background of, 66, 93
juvenile parkinsonism, 20
laboratory tests for, 89–90
medical treatment of, 119–156
  in the advanced stage, 141–156
  available medications, 121–127
  compliance with, 196
  during surgery, 140, 156
  individualized, 120–121
  in the mild stage, 134–139
  in the moderate stage, 139–141
  neuroprotection in the early stage,
    127–134
  postoperatively, 156
  see also specific agents
mental health therapy for, 119
mirror movements in, 66–67
mortality, 20–21, 85, 94
motor symptoms, 19, 66–69, 73–74, 86t
  akinesia, 19, 39–41, 85
  Braak staging system and, 113–114, 183
  bradykinesia, 19–20, 39–41, 69
  disease progression, 82–85
  dual task impairment, 73
  flexed posture, 20, 70–71
  freezing, 20, 23, 72–73, 246–247
  genetic background and, 73–74
  loss of postural reflexes, 20, 71–72,
    156
  pathologic correlations with, 81–82,
    88–89
  primitive reflexes, 73
  rating scales see Parkinson disease (PD),
    clinical rating scales for
  rest tremors see Tremor-at-rest

rigidity, 20, 70–71
  speech, 73
  see also Gait, parkinsonian
myoclonus and, 462
natural history of, 67, 68f, 82–85, 119,
    120f
nonmotor symptoms, 67–68, 74, 86t,
    183–196
  animal models, 81
  anxiety, 75–77, 190–191
  apathy, 75–78, 189–190
  assessment of, 87
  autonomic, 74–75, 113, 185–187
  Braak staging system and, 113–114,
    183–184, 192–193
  cognitive, 20, 40, 74–79, 87, 191–192
  comorbid medical conditions, 75
  compulsive behaviors, 78–79, 193–194
  dementia, 20, 74–77, 192–193, 222–224
  depression, 75–78, 190
  fatigue, 78, 189
  frequency of, 183–184, 184t
  personality change, 189–191
  psychosis, 77–78, 194–196
  respiratory distress, 187
  sensory, 80–81, 113–114, 184–185, 191
  sleep, 79–80, 187–189
  weight loss, 81
obsessional slowness contrasted with, 22
pathology of, 38–42, 65
  anatomical, 94–97, 158f
  autopsy findings, 81–82, 88–89, 92
  basal ganglia in, 92, 94–99, 158f
  biochemical, 97–99
  Braak's staging system, 110–114
  bradykinesia and, 69, 82, 99
  circadian factors, 79–80
  clinical correlations with, 81–82, 88–89
  historical background, 66, 93
  olfactory impairment and, 80–81,
    113–114
  premorbid parkinsonian personality and,
    78–79
  see also Parkinson disease (PD), etiology/
    pathogenesis of
quality of life with, 78, 87, 134, 171–172,
    196
sex ratio of, 20–21, 89, 93–94, 94f
subtypes of, 68–69, 68f, 73–74, 81–85, 392
surgical treatment of, 157–182
  brain grafting, 116–117, 179–182
  deep brain stimulation, 164–176, 189,
    246–247, 393–394
  evidentiary standards, 157
  functional anatomy of the basal ganglia,
    157–159
  historical background, 157, 158t
  pallidotomy, 159–164, 173, 394
  stereotactic techniques, 159–160
  thalamotomy, 160–161, 167–168,
    393–394
  vagus nerve stimulation, 179
therapeutic choices for, 121
  see also Parkinson disease (PD), medical
    treatment of; Parkinson disease
    (PD), surgical treatment of
therapeutic principles, 119–121
young-onset, 20, 79, 82, 84

Parkinson disease dementia (PDD), 192–193,
    222–224
Parkinsonian palilalia, 23
Parkinsonism, 66–92
  acquired see Parkinsonism, secondary
  atypical, 197–240
    neuroimaging of, 89–90
    prognosis of, 68–69
    see also Parkinsonism,
      heredodegenerative; Parkinsonism,
      secondary; Parkinsonism-plus
      syndromes
  catatonia contrasted with, 22
  classification of, 19t, 85, 86t, 197, 198t,
    199f
  clinical features of, 18–21, 19t
  clinical rating scales for, 18, 76, 85–87
  diagnostic criteria, 67t
  differential diagnosis, 85, 90–91, 140
  drug-induced, 27, 155–156, 236, 415,
    428–429
  epidemiology of, 5t, 88–89
  essential tremor and, 396–397
  freezing phenomenon, 20, 22–23, 72–73,
    128, 152
  genetics of, 6t–17t, 73–74, 80–82, 85, 96,
    99–104, 105t–106t
  heredodegenerative, 86t, 198t, 233
  historical background of, 66
  in Huntington disease, 312–313
  idiopathic see Juvenile parkinsonism;
    Parkinson disease
  juvenile, 20, 96, 240
    dopa-responsive dystonia and, 281–282,
      282t
  laboratory tests in, 89–90
  levodopa-induced, 155–156
  multiple system degenerations see
    Parkinsonism-plus syndromes
  obsessional slowness contrasted with,
    22
  pathologic findings in, 92
  primary see Juvenile parkinsonism;
    Parkinson disease
  psychogenic, 513, 525
  psychomotor depression contrasted with,
    22
  secondary, 27, 86t, 198t, 233–240
  tardive, 428–429
Parkinsonism–dementia syndromes,
    222–232
  see also Dementia, parkinsonian disorders
    and
Parkinsonism–dementia–amyotrophic lateral
    sclerosis complex of Guam
    (PDACG), 232–233
Parkinsonism-plus syndromes, 19, 86t,
    197, 198t
  anatomical pathology of, 95–96
  corticobasal degeneration, 218–222
  frontotemporal dementias,
    225–232
  genetics of, 6t–17t, 103, 198,
    206–207, 216, 225–230
  levodopa response in, 140
  multiple system atrophy, 208–218
  Parkinsonism–dementia syndromes,
    222–232

Parkinsonism–dementia–amyotrophic lateral sclerosis complex of Guam, 232–233
progressive supranuclear palsy, 197–208
taupathies, 225–232
Parkinsonism-pyramidal (pallido-pyramidal) syndrome, 103, 231
Paroxetine, 326–328
Paroxysmal dyskinesias, 27, 30, 476–495
  ataxia and, 30
  benign in infancy and childhood, 480–481, 483t–484t, 493, 495
  classification of, 482–483, 483t–484t, 494–495
  definitions, 477
  and epilepsy, 477–478, 483t–484t, 485, 491, 493
  episodic ataxias, 477, 481–482, 483t–484t, 491–493, 493t
  exertional (PED), 30, 479, 482–483, 483t–484t, 488, 490–491, 492t, 493–494
  genetics of, 6t–17t, 483t–484t, 486, 489, 491–494, 492t
  historical aspects, 477–482
  hypnogenic, 28, 479–480, 483t–484t
  kinesigenic (PKD), 30, 478, 482–483, 483t–484t
    clinical features of, 483–484, 492t
    genetics of, 6t–17t, 483t–484t, 486, 493
    primary, 484–486
    secondary, 486–487
    truncal flexion spasms and, 494–495
  nonkinesigenic (PNKD), 30, 479, 482–483, 483t–484t
    clinical features of, 487–488, 492t
    genetics of, 6t–17t, 483t–484t, 489, 493–494
    primary (Mount–Reback syndrome), 488–489
    secondary, 489–490
  periodic, 477
  prevalence of, 5t
  psychogenic, 488–489, 514–517
  self-stimulatory behavior, 495
  transient, 477, 477t, 480–481
  treatment, 298t
  tremor and, 30
Paroxysmal ocular downward deviation, 481
Paroxysmal tonic upgaze, 27, 481
Past-pointing sign, 47
Pathologic gambling, 78–79, 175, 193–194
Paucity of movements see Hypokinesias
Pediatric autoimmune neuropsychiatric disorders associated with streptococcal infections (PANDAS), 364–365
Pediatric infection-triggered autoimmune neuropsychiatric disorders (PITANDS), 364
Pedunculopontine nucleus (PPN), 55, 58f, 62–63, 64f
  deep brain stimulation surgery on, 173–174, 189
  gait and, 242–243
Pemoline, 375–376
D-Penicillamine, 510–512

Pergolide, 121t, 124, 133, 135–137
  in levodopa-associated fluctuations, 151
  in tics, 373
Perinatal hypoxic encephalopathy, 487, 489
Periodic movements in sleep, 28, 496–499
Periodic paroxysmal dyskinesias, 477
Periodic vestibulocerebellar ataxia (EA-3), 468–469
Peripheral deafferentiation with anesthesia
  in dystonia, 297
  in essential tremor, 407
Peripheral movement disorders, 500–506
  belly dancer's dyskinesia, 25, 502
  causalgia-dystonia, 286, 504–505, 519
  complex regional pain syndrome, 504–506, 519
  dystonia induced by peripheral injury, 503–505
  focal myoclonus due to nerve lesions, 501–502
  hemifacial spasm, 5t, 27–28, 273, 500–501, 500t, 501f
  jumpy stumps, 28, 502
  painful legs and moving toes syndrome, 28, 502–503
  spinal segmental myoclonus, 450, 451f, 501–502
Peripheral nervous system, 2
  denervation procedures, 308–309
  myoclonus arising from, 450, 501–502
Perry syndrome, 104, 239–240
Personality
  in frontotemporal dementias, 225–226
  in Parkinson disease, 189–191
  premorbid parkinsonian, 78
Pervasive developmental (autistic spectrum) disorders, 368–369, 380, 383–386
Pesticides, parkinsonism and, 104, 118
PET scans
  in classic tardive dyskinesia, 437
  in dystonia, 291–292
  in Huntington disease, 315–316
  in multiple system atrophy, 212–214
  in Parkinson disease, 89–92
    biochemical pathology of, 97–99, 98f
    Braak hypothesis and, 113
  in psychogenic movement disorders, 515
  in tauopathies
    corticobasal degeneration, 220–221
    progressive supranuclear palsy, 203–204
  in Tourette syndrome, 361–363
  in Wilson disease, 510
Petit mal, 458t
PGC-1a gene, 321–322
PGRN gene, 229–230
Phenol injections, 297
Phenylalanine-loading test, 283
Phenylbutyrate, 329
Phonations, involuntary, 25, 32
  in progressive supranuclear palsy, 200
  see also Phonic tics; Tourette syndrome (TS), motor and phonic tics in
Phonic tics, 31–32
  combined with motor see Tourette syndrome
Physical therapy
  in dystonia, 294–295
  in Parkinson disease, 120

Physiologic myoclonus, 448, 449t
Physiologic tremors, 394, 409
Pick disease, 225
  corticobasal degeneration and, 221–222
  tau pathology, 227
Pick-like bodies, 221
Pimozide, 371–373
PINK1 gene, 73–74, 82, 96, 99–100, 102, 105t–106t, 115–116
Piribedil, 124
Pisa syndrome, 71, 210–211
PITANDS, 364
PKAN see Neurodegenerations with brain iron accumulation (NBIA), type 1
PLA2G6 gene, 103, 105t–106t, 231, 341
PLA2G6-associated neurodegeneration (PLAN), 103, 105t–106t, 231, 275t–276t, 276, 341
Placebos, 526
Plasticity, abnormal, 43–44
Polymyoclonia see Opsoclonus-myoclonus syndrome
Porcine fetal mesencephalic transplants, 181
Positron emission tomography see PET scans
Posterior ramisectomy, in cervical dystonia, 308–309
Posteroventral pallidotomy (PVP), 159, 161–162, 394
Post-hypoxic myoclonus, 460–461, 461t
Poststreptococcal acute disseminated encephalomyelitis (PSADEM), 234, 344–345, 363–364
Postural changes
  in catatonia, 22
  cerebellar tremors and, 50
  in depression, 22
  in dystonia, 26–27, 263–264
  in obsessional slowness, 22
  in parkinsonian disorders, 20, 70–72, 156
    corticobasal degeneration, 21
    deep brain stimulation surgery in, 174
    multiple system atrophy, 210–211
Postural hypotension see Orthostatic hypotension
Postural instability and gait difficulty (PIGD), 68–69, 82–83, 192, 392
Postural reactions, exaggerated, 47
Postural sway, 50–51, 241–242, 242f
Postural tremors, 389, 390t, 394–407, 410–412
Posturography, 241–242, 242f
Pramipexole, 121t, 124, 133–137, 137t, 139
  in levodopa-associated fluctuations, 151
Prediction deficits, motion, 49
Pregnancy, chorea in, 344–345
Presynaptic inhibition, 36–37
Pridopidine (ACR16), 331–332
Primary parkinsonism see Juvenile parkinsonism; Parkinson disease
Primary progressive aphasia (PPA), 219–220, 225
Primidone
  in essential tremor, 405
  in myoclonus, 463
Primrose syndrome, 386
Prion diseases, 234–236, 337
Prion-like mechanism, in Parkinson disease, 116–117, 180–181

Prism glasses, 52
PRNP gene, 235–236, 337
Procerus signs, 200
Progressive myoclonic ataxia (Ramsay Hunt syndrome), 29, 458, 458f, 459t, 460
Progressive myoclonus epilepsy (PME), 458–460, 458f, 459t
Progressive supranuclear palsy (PSP), 197–208, 225
  clinical features of, 197–202, 204
  dementia and, 201–202, 224
  epidemiology of, 5t, 202
  genetics of, 198, 206–207, 227–229
  Guadeloupean tauopathy and, 232–233
  natural history of, 202
  neurodiagnostic studies in, 202–204
  neuropathology of, 204–207
    corticobasal degeneration and, 204–206, 221–222, 222f
    tau abnormalities, 204–207, 227–229
  treatment for, 207–208
Propanolol
  in acute akathisia, 428
  in essential tremor, 405
Propriospinal myoclonus, 29, 449–450, 454–455, 455f, 524
Protein accumulation
  in Huntington disease, 317, 323–326
  in Parkinson disease, 99–100, 99f, 101f, 115, 116f–117f
Pseudoathetosis, 26
Pseudodystonias, 277, 277t
Pseudomyotonia and myokymia *see* Neuromyotonia
Psychiatric movement disorders, 527t
  catatonia, 22, 386
  fear of falling, 23, 248
  obsessional slowness, 22
  psychomotor depression, 22
  see also Stereotypies
Psychiatric symptoms
  in dystonia, 265, 284
  in Huntington disease, 313–315, 329, 331, 333
  Parkinson disease and, 20, 75–78, 122, 126, 190
  psychogenic movement disorders and, 527
  in Sydenham disease, 344
  in Wilson disease, 508
  see also Autistic spectrum disorder; Depression; Obsessive-compulsive disorder; Schizophrenia
Psychogenic movement disorders, 513–527
  categorization of patients with, 516–517
  clinical features of, 520–521
  clinically established category of, 516–517
  conversion, 54, 514–515, 517–518, 521
  depression and, 518, 526–527
  diagnosis of, 520–521
    certainty in, 516–517
    importance of, 514–515
    informing the patient of, 525–526
    suggestive clues, 518–520
    use of placebos in, 526
  documented category of, 516
  DSM-IV definitions, 517–518
  dystonia, 264, 274, 286, 286t, 515–516, 519, 521–523

excessive startle, 515, 519
factitious, 518, 521, 526–527
fear of falling, 524
gait, 248, 519, 523–524
malingering, 518, 521, 526–527
mass hysteria, 515
myoclonus, 448, 450, 462, 515, 524
neuroimaging, 515–518
parkinsonism, 513, 525
paroxysmal dyskinesias, 488–489, 514–517
possible category of, 517
prevalence of, 5t, 513–514
probable category of, 517
psychiatric conditions and, 527
self-agency, 517–518
somatization, 517, 521
somatoform, 517–518, 521, 526–527
terminology, 513, 517–518
tics, 524
treatment of, 525–527
tremors, 413–414, 514–515, 517–519, 523
Psychomotor depression, 22
Psychosis
  in Huntington disease, 329
  Parkinson disease-associated, 77–78, 122, 126, 194–196, 194t, 232
Psychotherapy
  in Parkinson disease, 119
  in psychogenic movement disorders, 525–527
Pull test, 20, 85–87, 242
Punding, 78–79, 194, 387
Pure akinesia, 22, 199
Purkinje cells, 215, 385–386, 411, 466
Push and release test, 85–87
Putamen, 55, 57f, 60–61, 64, 82, 97, 98t, 157–159
  dystonia and, 282, 283f, 289–291
  Huntington disease and, 315–316, 324
  infarcts, paroxysmal dyskinesias and, 487
  in Wilson disease, 509–510
Pyruvate dehydrogenase deficiency, 275

Q

Quality of life
  Huntington disease and, 314–315
  Parkinson disease and, 78, 87, 134, 171–172, 196
Quetiapine, 416, 419–421
  in Parkinson disease, 126, 195
  in parkinsonism-dementia syndromes, 232
  side effects, 421, 423–424
  in tardive syndromes, 416, 442–444
  in tics, 372

R

Radicicol, 328
Ramsay Hunt syndrome *see* Progressive myoclonic ataxia
"Rancho recipe", 187
Random "off" phenomenon, 151
Rapamycin, 323–324, 329
Raphe nuclei, 62–63, 95
Rapid-onset dystonia–parkinsonism (RDP; DYT12), 261, 283–284
Rasagiline, 125, 129–130, 130f, 133, 150

Rasmussen encephalitis, 453–454
Rating scales, 18
  for essential tremor, 391
  for Huntington disease, 311–312
  for multiple system atrophy, 208
  for Parkinson disease, 18, 76–77, 85–87, 191
  for progressive supranuclear palsy, 199
  in surgery response assessment, 164–165, 171–172
Reaction time (RT)
  in Huntington disease, 312
  in Parkinson disease, 39–41, 69
Rebound, 47
Reciprocal inhibition, 36–37, 301
Reemergent tremor, 389, 398
Reflex connections onto alpha motoneurons, 36–37, 37f
Reflex myoclonus, 29, 219, 411–412, 449 450, 452
Reflex sympathetic dystrophy *see* Complex regional pain syndrome
Reflexes
  long-latency, 41
  loss of postural in PD, 20, 71–72, 156, 174
  reemergence of primitive in PD, 73
REM sleep, PD-associated psychosis and, 77–78
REM sleep behavior disorder (RBD), 28
  dementia with Lewy bodies and, 223–224
  Parkinson disease and, 79, 188
    Braak staging system, 113
    drugs for, 122, 126, 188
Remacemide, 327–328
Renshaw cells, 36–37, 37f
Repetitive behavior, 194
Reserpine, 415
  acute dystonia and, 425
  in animal models of Parkinson disease, 118
  in classic tardive dyskinesia, 441
  in Huntington disease, 329–330
  in tardive akathisia, 446
  in tardive dystonia, 443–444
Respiratory distress
  in multiple system atrophy, 211, 217–218
  in Parkinson disease, 187
Rest tremors *see* Tremor-at-rest
Restless legs syndrome (RLS), 28, 30, 496–499
  akathisia and, 185
  genetics of, 6t–17t, 497
  Parkinson disease and, 79, 126, 185, 497
    drugs for, 122, 126, 185
  periodic movements in sleep and, 28, 496
  prevalence of, 5t, 496
  therapeutic management, 498–499, 499f
  Tourette syndrome and, 360
Reticular formation, 37–38
Rett syndrome, 384–386
Rhes protein, 326
Rheumatic chorea, 343–344, 365
Rhinorrhea, 187
Richardson syndrome, 200
Rigidity, 23–24
  cogwheel, 23–24, 70
  with encephalomyelitis, 24, 254–255
  lead-pipe, 23–24
  in neuroleptic malignant syndrome, 24

in parkinsonism, 20, 70–71
  interconnected pathogenic mechanisms of PD, 99
  pathophysiology of, 41
  spinal alpha, 255
Riluzole
  in cerebellar ataxia, 475
  in Huntington disease, 327–328
  in Parkinson disease, 131
Rippling muscle disease, 256
Risperidone, 371–372, 416, 419–424
RNA interference (RNAi), 334
Romberg quotient, 50
Romberg test, 242
Ropinirole, 121t, 124, 133, 135–137, 137t
  in levodopa-associated fluctuations, 151
  in tics, 373
Rotenone, 118
Rotigotine, 124, 135–136, 137t
Rubral tremor see Midbrain tremor
Running gait, 156

S

Saccades
  in corticobasal degeneration, 219
  in Huntington disease, 312
  in progressive supranuclear palsy, 199–200
  in Tourette syndrome, 356
St Anthony's fire, 135, 184
St Vitus dance, 515
  see also Sydenham disease
Saliva drooling, 75, 126–127, 187
Sandifer syndrome, 476
Satoyoshi syndrome, 258
Savant syndrome, 383
Scales for Outcomes in Parkinson's Disease (SCOPA), 85–87
  cognition (SCOPA-COG), 76
SCGE gene, 284–285
Schizophrenia, 386, 432–433
Schwartz–Jampel syndrome, 256–258
Scoliosis, 71, 71f
Seborrhea, 187
Secondary parkinsonism see Parkinsonism, secondary
Second-generation antipsychotics see Atypical antipsychotics
Segmental dysfunction, disorders arising from, 37t
Segmental dystonia, 27, 262–263, 266, 268t, 298t
Segmental inputs onto alpha motoneurons, 36–37, 37f
Segmental myoclonus, 449–450
  abdominal, 25
  palatal, 28–30, 392
Seizures
  in progressive supranuclear palsy, 202
  see also Epilepsy
Selective serotonin reuptake inhibitors (SSRIs)
  in Huntington disease, 326–328, 333
  in OCD, 377–378
  in Parkinson disease, 126, 153, 190
  parkinsonism induced by, 428
  paroxysmal hemidystonia with, 490

Selegiline (deprenyl), 125, 127–131, 133, 150, 376–377
Self-agency, 517–518
Self-injurious behavior (SIB)
  in stereotypies, 380–382, 384
  in Tourette syndrome, 359
Semantic dementia (SD), 225–226
  see also Primary progressive aphasia
Semivoluntary (unvoluntary) movements, 1–2, 351
  tics as, 32
Senile chorea (essential chorea), 343
Senile dementia of Lewy body type see Dementia with Lewy bodies
Senile gait disorder, 23
Sensory dysfunction
  in cerebellar ataxia, 49
  in dystonia, 44, 288
  in essential tremor, 398–399
  in Parkinson disease, 80–81, 113–114, 184–185, 398
    treatment-related, 141–143, 141t, 184–185, 191
  psychogenic, 515
  in restless legs syndrome, 498
Sensory feedback therapy, 294
Sensory tricks (geste antagoniste), 27, 264, 272–273
Serotonergic agents
  in acute akathisia, 428
  acute akathisia with, 427
  acute dystonia with, 285
  in cerebellar ataxia, 474
  see also Selective serotonin reuptake inhibitors
Serotonergic system
  atypical antipsychotics and, 420–421
  dopamine agonists and, 135
  levodopa-associated dyskinesias and, 153
  pathogenesis of PD and, 99, 113
Serotonin (5-hydroxytryptamine, 5HT), 60
  biochemical pathology of Parkinson disease, 97, 98t
  tremor in PD and, 82
  see also Serotonergic system
Sex hormones, Tourette syndrome and, 366, 373
Sexual dysfunction, 75, 186
  drugs causing, 194
  drugs for, 122, 126
Shopping, compulsive, 194
Short intracortical inhibition (SICI), 42–43
Short Parkinson's Evaluation Scale (SPES), 85–87
Shy–Drager syndrome (SDS), 208, 215–216
  see also Multiple system atrophy
Sialidosis (cherry-red spot myoclonus syndrome), 459t, 460
Sialorrhea, 75, 126–127, 187
Silent period (SP), 42
Single photon emission computed tomography see SPECT imaging
SLC6A3 gene, 104, 105t–106t
Sleep
  in dementia with Lewy bodies, 223
  in multiple system atrophy, 212
  oculofaciomasticatory myorhythmia in, 30

painful legs and moving toes syndrome in, 28
palatal myoclonus in, 28, 392
in Parkinson disease, 79–80, 187–189
  drugs for, 122t, 126, 188–189
  psychosis and, 77–78
paroxysmal hypnogenic dyskinesia in, 28, 479–480
periodic movements in, 28, 496–499
in progressive supranuclear palsy, 202
RBD see REM sleep behavior disorder
RLS see Restless legs syndrome
in Tourette syndrome, 360
Sleep attacks, 189
  dopamine agonists causing, 124, 135–136, 189
Sleep starts (hypnic jerks), 498
SLITRK1 gene, 366–367
Small ubiquitin-like modifier (SUMO)-1, 328
Smell, decreased sense of see Hyposmia
Smoking, Parkinson disease and, 107
SNCA gene
  multiple system atrophy and, 216
  Parkinson disease and, 101–102, 105t–106t, 114–115, 223
Somatization disorder, 517, 521
Somatoform disorder, 517–518, 521, 526–527
Sonography see Ultrasonography
Spasmodic dysphonia (laryngeal dystonia), 298t, 303
Spasmus nutans, 393, 481
Spasticity, 250–252
  with paroxysmal nonkinesigenic dyskinesia, 494
SPECT imaging
  in classic tardive dyskinesia, 437
  in corticobasal degeneration, 220–221
  in essential tremor, 399–400
  in multiple system atrophy, 212–213
  in Parkinson disease, 89–92, 98–99, 399–400
  in psychogenic movement disorders, 515
  in Tourette syndrome, 362–363
Speech
  in anterior opercular syndrome, 239
  in corticobasal degeneration, 219–220
  dysarthric, 51
    after deep brain stimulation surgery, 175
  in Parkinson disease, 73
  freezing phenomenon in, 23
  in jumping disorders, 28
  levodopa-associated tachyphemia, 156
  primary progressive aphasia, 219
  in progressive supranuclear palsy, 200
Spinal alpha rigidity, 255
Spinal cord, 2
  myoclonus arising in, 448, 450, 501
  paroxysmal dyskinesias and, 487
  spasticity and, 250–251
  stiff-person syndrome and, 253
Spinal interneuronitis see Encephalomyelitis with rigidity
Spinal myoclonus, 29, 454–455, 463
Spinal segmental myoclonus, 450, 451f, 501–502
Spine, bent, 70–71

Spinocerebellar ataxia with axonal neuropathy (SCAN1), 473
Spinocerebellar ataxias (SCAs), 6t–17t, 210, 337–338, 467–468, 469t–470t
Splints, in dystonia, 294
Spongiform encephalopathies, transmissible, 234–236
Stance, 241
Startle responses, psychogenic, 515, 519
Startle syndromes
    hyperekplexia, 6t–17t, 24, 28, 456, 456t, 457f, 519
    jumping disorders, 28, 369, 456
Staso-basophobia, 524
    see also Fear of falling
Statins, Parkinson disease and, 134
Status dystonicus, 265, 298
Stem cell technology, 181
Stereotactic surgery techniques, 159–160
Stereotypies, 30–31, 380–388
    akathisia and, 387
    in animals, 364, 366, 380–381
    classification of, 380, 381t
    in developmental disorders, 382–386
        autism, 380, 383–384
        Rett syndrome, 384–386
        Williams syndrome, 386
    genetics of, 6t–17t
    obsessive-compulsive disorder and, 382, 386–387
    pathophysiology, 380–382
    physiologic, 382
    prevalence of, 5t
    punding, 387
    schizophrenia and, 386
    tardive see Tardive syndromes, classic tardive dyskinesia
    tics and, 30–31, 380, 386–387
        see also Tourette syndrome
    treatment of, 388
Stiff-legged gait, 246
Stiffness syndromes, 24, 250–258
    causes of, 251t
    continuous muscle fiber activity (neuromyotonia), 24, 255–258, 255t
    spasticity, 250–252
    stiff-baby, 24
    stiff-person, 5t, 24, 250, 252–255, 252t, 253f
        encephalomyelitis with rigidity, 24, 254–255
        spinal alpha rigidity, 255
        stiff leg syndrome variant, 255
Stimulation therapies, 294–295
Streptococcal infections
    choreas after, 344–345
    PANDAS and PITANDS, 364–365
    Tourette syndrome and, 363–365
Stress
    Parkinson disease and, 122, 126
    psychogenic movement disorders and, 525
Stretch reflexes, long-latency, 41
Striatal hand deformity, 70, 71f
Striatal toe deformity, 70
Striatonigral degeneration (SND), 208, 215–216
    see also Multiple system atrophy

Striatum, 55, 60–61, 64–65, 157–159
    in classic tardive dyskinesia, 435–436
    in Huntington disease, 315–318, 323–326, 333–334
    in Parkinson disease
        autopsy findings, 92
        biochemical pathology of, 97–99
        clinical–pathologic correlations, 82
        infectious protein hypothesis, 116–117
        interconnected pathogenic mechanisms, 99
        neuroimaging of, 89–91
    in progressive supranuclear palsy, 206
    in psychogenic movement disorders, 515
    in Tourette syndrome, 361–363, 366
Stridor, in multiple system atrophy, 211, 217–218
Striosomes, 61, 61f
Stroke
    ataxia and, 465–466
    hemiballism and, 346
    tremors and, 413
Subacute sclerosing panencephalitis (SSPE), 461
Subcortical disequilibrium, 23, 247
Subcortical myoclonus, 449–450
Substantia nigra (SN), 55, 57f, 62, 157–159
    basal ganglia circuitry, 62–63, 63f
    effects of stimulation of, 179
    essential tremor and, 399–400
    grafting fetal nigral tissue in Parkinson disease, 116–117, 179–182
    neuroimaging in Parkinson disease, 89–92
    paraneoplastic degeneration of, 239
    in pathology of Parkinson disease
        anatomical, 94–97
        animal models, 118
        autopsy findings, 92
        biochemical, 97
        Braak staging system, 110
        calcium influx, 108–110, 134
        clinical correlations with, 82
        pathogenic mechanisms, 99–100, 101f, 107–110, 109f
    as source of dopamine, 55, 58f
        see also Substantia nigra (SN), in pathology of Parkinson disease
Substantia nigra pars compacta (SNc), 55, 62
    basal ganglia circuitry, 62–63, 63f
    in pathology of Parkinson disease
        anatomical, 95–97
        animal models, 118
        autopsy findings, 92
        biochemical, 97, 98t
        calcium influx, 108–110, 134
        pathogenic mechanisms, 99–100, 101f, 107–110, 109f
Substantia nigra pars reticulata (SNr), 62
Subthalamic nucleus (STN), 55, 57f, 61, 157–159
    AAV-GAD gene therapy for PD, 181–182
    basal ganglia circuitry, 62–63, 63f, 65, 159
    cellular activity in, 65
    deep brain stimulation surgery on, 159, 164t, 166, 168–176, 179, 378–379, 394

    origins of movement disorders in, 159
        ballism, 26
        bradykinesia, 69
        tremors, 408–409
    subthalamotomy in Parkinson disease, 163–164
    in Tourette syndrome, 361, 378–379
Subthalamotomy, 163–164
Sudden "off" phenomenon, 141–145, 147–148, 151, 154–155
Suicidal behavior
    after deep brain stimulation surgery, 175
    Huntington disease and, 313
"Super off" phenomenon, 152
Supranuclear ophthalmoparesis (gaze palsy), 199–200
Surround inhibition, 43–44, 288
Swallowing difficulty
    in Parkinson disease, 75, 187
    in progressive supranuclear palsy, 200
Sway, 50–51, 241–242, 242f
Sweating dysfunction, 74–75, 187
Sydenham disease (Sydenham chorea), 26, 343–344, 363–365
Symptomatic palatal myoclonus (SPM), 392, 450–451, 452f
Symptomatic parkinsonism see Parkinsonism, secondary
Synesthesia, 219
Synkinesis, facial, 29
α-Synuclein
    multiple system atrophy and, 208, 215–216
    Parkinson disease and
        accumulation of toxic proteins, 100
        altered degradation in, 115, 116f
        animal models, 118
        Braak staging system, 110–114
        calcium influx, 110
        dementia, 223
        genetic etiology of, 101–102, 101f, 114–115
        infectious protein hypothesis, 116–117, 180–181
        interaction with dopamine, 108, 110, 116–117, 180–181
        multiple hit hypothesis, 117
        pathway to fibrillogenesis, 108, 108f
    tau and, 229
Systemic lupus erythematosus (SLE), 344–345

T

Tachykinesia, 156
Tachyphemia, 156
Tardive syndromes, 415–446
    classic tardive dyskinesia, 31, 387, 415–417, 430–439
        abnormal movements in schizophrenia and, 432–433
        anatomical pathology of, 435–436
        biochemical pathology of, 437–439
        clinical features of, 431–432
        dopamine deficiency states, 438
        epidemiology of, 433–435
        excitotoxicity, 438
        genetics of, 437

imaging studies, 437–438
natural history of, 433–435
oxidative stress, 438
risk factors for, 433–435
with tardive akathisia, 25
treatment of, 440–443
definitions, 416–418
epidemiology of, 5t, 418, 433–435
nature of the drugs producing, 418–424
phenomenology of, 415–416
tardive akathisia, 25, 416, 426, 440,
445–446
tardive dystonia, 285, 416, 425, 439–440,
443–445, 490
tardive parkinsonism, 428–429
tardive stereotypy see Tardive syndromes,
classic tardive dyskinesia
tardive tremor, 392–393, 430
treatment of, 440–446, 444f–445f, 446t
withdrawal emergent syndrome, 26, 416,
430
Task-specific dystonia, 263, 273, 288, 298t,
305, 503
Task-specific tremors, 389, 390t, 402, 514
Tau gene, 225–229, 232–233
Tau pathology, 227–228, 230–231
in corticobasal degeneration, 219, 221,
227
in frontotemporal dementias, 225–227
in progressive supranuclear palsy, 204–207,
227–229
Tauopathies, 225–232
classification of, 225t
clinical features of frontotemporal
dementias, 225–226
genetics of, 225–231
geographically specific, 232–233
neuropathology of, 222f, 230–231
see also Tau pathology
treatment of, 232
see also Corticobasal degeneration; Pick
disease; Primary progressive aphasia;
Progressive supranuclear palsy
TBP gene, 337–338
TDP-43, 229–230, 239–240
Ten steps test, 68–69
Testosterone treatment, in Parkinson disease,
77
Tetrabenazine (TBZ)
acute dystonia with, 425
in ballism, 347
in chorea, 346
in classic tardive dyskinesia, 441–442
in dystonia, 295–296
in Huntington disease, 329–331
in tardive akathisia, 446
in tardive dystonia, 443–444
in tics, 372, 372f
Tetrathiomolybdate, 512
Thalamotomy, 160–161, 167–168
in dystonia, 306
in kinetic tremors, 408
in rest tremors, 393–394
Thalamus
ablative procedures see Thalamotomy
anatomy, 57f, 157–159
astasia (subcortical disequilibrium), 23,
247

basal ganglia circuitry, 39f, 62–64, 63f,
159
cellular activity in, 65
in classic tardive dyskinesia, 436–437
deep brain stimulation surgery on
in kinetic tremors, 408
in Parkinson disease, 164t, 167–168,
178
in rest tremors, 393–394
in Tourette syndrome, 178, 378–379
in dystonia, 291, 306
infarcts, paroxysmal dyskinesias and,
487
in kinetic tremors, 408
in progressive supranuclear palsy, 204,
206
in psychogenic movement disorders, 515
in Tourette syndrome, 361–363, 366,
378–379
tremor generation in, 41–42, 408–411
THAP1 gene, 261, 269–272
Thyroid disorders, 23
Tic status, 31
Tics, 31–32
blocking (holding), 21, 351–352
chorea contrasted with, 26, 31, 344
classification of, 353, 353t
clonic, 351–352
compulsions and, 31, 352
deep brain stimulation surgery in, 178
with dystonia, 265, 276–277, 351–352
dystonic, 32, 351–352
etiology of (secondary tourettism),
368–369
genetics of, 6t–17t
management of, 371–375
mannerisms and, 31
motor, 30–32
with phonic see Tourette syndrome
myoclonus distinguished from, 31, 447
phenomenology of, 351–353
phonic, 31–32
with motor see Tourette syndrome
psychogenic, 524
stereotypies and, 30–31, 380, 386–387
voluntariness of, 54
Timing errors
in cerebellar ataxia, 48–49
in freezing phenomenon, 72–73
Tip of the tongue phenomenon, 191–192
TITF1 gene, 342–343
Titubation, 50–51, 407
Tocopherol (Vitamin E)
ataxia with isolated vitamin E deficiency,
472
in classic tardive dyskinesia, 443
in Parkinson disease, 125, 127, 128t, 129,
131
Toe
minipolymyoclonus, 456
painful legs and moving, 28, 502–503
pseudoathetosis, 26
striatal deformity of, 70
Tolcapone, 123, 150
Tongue
dystonia, 273
feeding dystonia, 27, 339
O-B-L dyskinesia, 417, 432–433

Tonic tics see Tics, dystonic
Tonic upgaze, paroxysmal, 27, 481
Tonically active neurons (TANs), 61,
64–65
Topiramate
in essential tremor, 406
in Tourette syndrome, 373–374, 374f
TorsinA, 278–280, 279t
inhibiting expression of, 309
Torsion dystonia see Dystonia
Torticollis
paroxysmal in infancy, 480–481
spasmodic see Cervical dystonia
Tourette syndrome (TS), 350–379
autistic spectrum disorders and, 368–369,
383–384
behavioral symptoms in, 356–359,
370–371, 375–378
comorbidities of, 354–359, 356f, 365,
382
historical background of, 350
impulse control in, 358–359, 362
malignant, 355, 355t, 359
motor and phonic tics in, 31, 178, 344,
350, 353–356
adult-onset, 355
childhood-onset, 354–355
classification of, 353, 353t
deep brain stimulation surgery in,
378–379
diagnostic criteria, 353–354
epidemiology of, 5t, 369
etiology of secondary tourettism,
368–369
genetics of, 6t–17t, 366–368
impulse control and, 358
management of, 370–375
pathogenesis of see Tourette syndrome
(TS), pathogenesis of
phenomenology of, 351–353
natural course of, 354–355, 356f
pathogenesis of
basal ganglia involvement, 158f, 359,
360f, 361–364, 366
etiology of secondary tourettism and,
368
immunology, 363–365
neurochemistry, 362–363
neuroimaging, 361–362
neurophysiology, 359–360
stereotypies in animals and, 364,
366
premonitory sensations in, 352
self-injurious behavior in, 359
stereotypies and, 364, 366, 382
Sydenham disease and, 344, 363–365
treatment of, 369–379
behavioral symptoms, 370–371,
375–378
motor symptoms, 370–375
surgical, 178, 378–379
Toxins and toxicity
ataxia and, 466
botulinum see Botulinum toxin
delayed-onset dystonia and, 275
Guadeloupean tauopathy and,
232–233
Huntington disease and, 317, 321–326

multiple system atrophy and, 216
Parkinson disease and, 99–100, 99f, 101f, 104–107, 110, 114–115, 116f, 117
parkinsonism with, 236–237
Tracking impairments, 49
Transcranial magnetic stimulation (TMS)
in dystonia, 294–295
in Parkinson disease, 179
in tics, 375
in Tourette syndrome, 360
Transcranial sonography (TCS)
in multiple system atrophy, 213–214
in Parkinson disease, 90–92
in Wilson disease, 510
Transcutaneous electrical stimulation, 295
Tranylcypromine, 131, 134
Trauma
causing dystonia, 275, 285–286, 503–504, 519
causing parkinsonism, 238
causing tremors, 413
paroxysmal dyskinesias and, 486–487
peripheral movement disorders and, 500–506
Trehalose, 328
Tremor-at-rest (rest tremors), 32
classification of, 389, 390t
diagnosis of, 391–393
in Parkinson disease, 19, 41–42, 66–67, 69–70, 81–82
deep brain stimulation surgery in, 160, 167–168, 170, 393–394
diagnosis of, 391–392
disease progression and, 82–84
drugs for, 125–126, 156
pallidotomy for, 161, 394
pathophysiology of, 410
thalamotomy for, 160–161, 167–168, 393–394
pathophysiologic mechanisms, 408–412
treatment of, 393–394
see also under Tremor-at-rest (rest tremors), in Parkinson disease
Tremors, 32, 389–414
action, 389, 390t, 394–412
assessment of, 391
in ataxia, 50–51, 246
cerebellar, 50, 52–53, 407, 410–412
classification of, 390t
by anatomic distribution, 389–391
by phenomenology, 389
deep brain stimulation surgery in, 167–168, 170, 179, 393–394, 407–408
differential diagnosis, 390t
drug-related, 414
dystonic, 30, 264–265, 268–269, 396–397, 402
episodic, 30
essential, 389, 391, 394–407, 410–412
Fragile X–associated/ataxia syndrome, 412–413, 473–474
genetics of, 6t–17t, 402–404
intention see Tremors, kinetic
isometric, 389
kinetic, 389, 407–408, 412
midbrain ("rubral"), 32, 82, 392
myoclonus contrasted with, 29

neuropathic, 413
orthostatic, 400–401, 406
pathophysiology of, 408–412
physiologic, 394, 409
position-specific, 389, 390t
postural, 389, 390t, 394–407, 410–412
prevalence of, 5t
psychogenic, 413–414, 514–515, 517–519, 523
reemergent, 389, 398
rest see Tremor-at-rest
rhythmic myoclonus contrasted, 29
stroke causing, 413
tardive, 392–393, 430
task-specific, 389, 390t, 402, 514
trauma causing, 413
treatment of, 393–394, 404–408
in Wilson disease, 32, 508
Tricyclic antidepressants, 190
Trientine, 511–512
Trimethobenzamide, 151
Trinucleotide repeats, 2–18, 18t
see also CAG repeats
Trunk
camptocormia, 70–71, 246
deformities in Parkinson disease, 70–71
focal dystonia in, 273
manifestation of bradykinesia in, 19
myoclonus in, 454–455
paroxysmal kinesigenic dyskinesia in, 494–495
Pisa syndrome, 71, 210–211
Tryptophan, in Tourette syndrome, 362
Tyramine, 125, 130–131
Tyrosine hydroxylase (TH) deficiency, 282–283

U

Ubiquinone see Coenzyme Q10
Ubiquitin-proteasomal system, 100, 102, 115, 116f–117f
Huntington disease and, 323–324
in tauopathies, 206
UCHL1 gene, 102, 105t–106t, 115
Ultrasonography
in multiple system atrophy, 213–214
in Parkinson disease, 90–92
in Wilson disease, 510
Uncertain gaits see Hesitant (uncertain) gaits
Unified Parkinson's Disease Rating Scale (UPDRS), 18, 85–87, 183
Unnatural movements see Dyskinesias
Unverricht–Lundborg disease, 29, 459t, 460
Unvoluntary (semivoluntary) movements, 1–2, 351
tics as, 32
Upgaze, paroxysmal tonic, 27, 481
Uric acid, Parkinson disease and, 99, 107
Urinary symptoms
in multiple system atrophy, 208–209, 217
in Parkinson disease, 75, 185–186

V

Vagus nerve stimulation, 179
Varenicline, 475

Variant Creutzfeldt–Jakob disease (vCJD), 234–235
Vascular ballism, 346
Vascular chorea, 336t, 345–346
Vascular parkinsonism, 237–238
Vascular paroxysmal dyskinesias and, 487
Vascular progressive supranuclear palsy, 202–203
Ventral intermediate (VIM) nucleus of the thalamus
deep brain stimulation surgery in, 167–168, 393–394
thalamotomy, 160, 393–394, 408
tremor generation by, 41–42
Ventral striatum, 60–61, 64
Tourette syndrome and, 362–363, 366
Ventral tegmental area (VTA), 108–109
Visual impairment
in Parkinson disease, 81
in progressive supranuclear palsy, 199–200
psychogenic, 515
Visual-motor tasks, in assessing learning, 52
Vitamins
ataxia and, 466, 472
in classic tardive dyskinesia, 443
in Parkinson disease, 121, 125, 127–131
Vocal cords
dystonia of, 273
in multiple system atrophy, 211, 217–218
Vocalizations see Phonations, involuntary; Phonic tics; Speech
Voluntary movements, 1–2, 351
physiology of, 36, 46–47, 54
VPS13A gene, 339–340

W

Walking see Gait
Wartenberg sign, 20
Weakness, in cerebellar ataxia, 45–46
Wearing-off phenomenon, 141, 143–151, 154–155, 196
Weight determination ability, 49
Weight gain, after DBS surgery, 175
Weight loss
in Huntington disease, 314
in Parkinson disease, 81, 194
West Nile encephalitis, 234
Whipple disease
myorhythmia in, 30
repetitive facial myoclonus in, 27–28
Williams syndrome, 386
Wilson disease, 507–512
diagnosis of, 509–510, 509t, 511f
genetics of, 6t–17t, 507, 510
natural course of, 508
pathology of, 508, 508f
presentation of, 507–508, 508t–509t
prevalence of, 5t
treatments for, 510–512
tremor in, 32, 508
Wilson protein, dystonia and, 292
Withdrawal dyskinesia, 435
Withdrawal emergent syndrome, 26, 416, 430
Woodhouse–Sakati syndrome, 275
Worster–Drought syndrome, 239

Writer's cramp *see* Hand dystonia
Writing tremor, 402

X

X-linked conditions
    dystonia-parkinsonism (Lubag, DYT3), 233,
        261, 271, 286–287
    Fragile X-associated/ataxia syndrome,
        412–413, 473–474

neuroacanthocytosis (McLeod syndrome),
    339–340, 386
Rett syndrome, 384–386

Y

Young-onset Parkinson disease (YOPD), 20,
    79, 82
    disease progression in, 84
Yo-yo-ing phenomenon, 154–155

Z

Zinc, in Wilson disease, 511–512
Ziprasidone, 420t, 422–423
    in tics, 371–372
Zolpidem, 126
Zona incerta (ZI), 62–63, 165f
    deep brain stimulation surgery on,
        173–174
Zonisamide, 151, 406